FOURTH EDITION

# COMMUNITY HEALTH NURSING
## A CANADIAN PERSPECTIVE

### LYNNETTE LEESEBERG **STAMLER**

University of Nebraska Medical Center

### LUCIA **YIU**

University of Windsor

### ALIYAH **DOSANI**

Mount Royal University

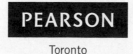

**PEARSON**

Toronto

Editorial Director: Claudine O'Donnell
Acquisitions Editor: Kimberley Veevers
Marketing Manager: Michelle Bish
Program Manager: John Polanszky
Project Manager: Susan Johnson
Developmental Editor: Paul Donnelly
Media Editor: Paul Donnelly
Media Developer: Olga Avdyeyeva
Production Services: Mohinder Singh, iEnergizer Aptara®, Inc.
Permissions Project Manager: Sarah Ellen Horsfall
Photo Permissions Research: Lokesh Bisht, iEnergizer Aptara®, Inc.
Text Permissions Research: Phyllis Padula, iEnergizer Aptara®, Inc.
Interior Designer: iEnergizer Aptara®, Inc.
Cover Designer: Anthony Leung
Cover Image: (clockwise from top left): StockLite/Shutterstock, itsmejust/Shutterstock, Ocskay Bence/
    Shutterstock, WavebreakmediaMicro/Fotolia

Vice-President, Cross Media and Publishing Services: Gary Bennett

Credits and acknowledgments for material borrowed from other sources and reproduced, with permission, in this textbook appear on the appropriate page within the text.

If you purchased this book outside the United States or Canada, you should be aware that it has been imported without the approval of the publisher or the author.

4 16

Library and Archives Canada Cataloguing in Publication

Community health nursing (2015)
    Community health nursing: a Canadian perspective/
[edited by] Lynnette Leeseberg Stamler, Lucia Yiu, Aliyah
Dosani. —Fourth edition.

Includes bibliographical references and index.
ISBN 978-0-13-315625-6 (paperback)

    1. Community health nursing—Canada—Textbooks.    I. Stamler,
Lynnette Leeseberg, 1952-editor    II. Yiu, Lucia, 1951-editor
    III. Dosani, Aliyah, 1977-editor    IV. Title.

RT98.C644 2015        610.73'430971        C2015-906525-9

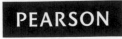

ISBN 978-0-13-315625-6

# Brief Contents

# Contents

# List of Canadian Research Boxes

1.1 McBain, L. (2012). Pulling up their sleeves and getting on with it: Providing health care in a northern remote region. *Canadian Bulletin of Medical History*, *29*(2), 308–328.

1.2 Boschma, G. (2012). Community mental health nursing in Alberta, Canada: An oral history. *Nursing History Review, 20,* 103–135.

2.1 Cohen, D., Huynh, T., Sebold, A., Harvey, J., Neudorf, C., & Brown, A. (2014). The population health approach: A qualitative study on conceptual and operational definitions for leaders in Canadian health care. *SAGE Open Medicine, 2*(Jan–Dec), 1–11. Reproduced by permission of SAGE Publications Ltd.

2.2 Pinto, A., Manson, H., Pauly, B. Thanos, J., Parks, A., & Cox, A. (2012). Equity in public health standards: A qualitative document analysis of policies from two Canadian provinces. *International Journal of Equity in Health, 11*(28), 1–10.

3.1 Hoffart, C., Kuster-Orban, C., Spooner, C., & Neudorf, K. (2014). Intra-professional practice education using a community partnership model. *Journal of Nursing Education, 52*(2), 104–107. Published by Slack, Inc., © 2014.

3.2 Doran, D. M., Reid-Haughian, C., Chilcote, A., Bia, Y. Q. (2013). A formative evaluation of nurses' use of electronic devices in a home care setting. *Canadian Journal of Nursing Research, 45*(1), 54–73.

4.1 Kim, E., Hoetmer, S. E., Li, Y., & Vandenber, J. E. (2013). Relationship between intention to supplement with infant formula and breastfeeding duration. *Canadian Journal of Public Health, 104*(5), e388–e393.

4.2 Stooke, V. D. (2013). Sharing the air: The legal and ethical considerations of extending tobacco legislation to include multi-unit dwellings in Alberta. *Public Health Nursing, 31*(1), 6068. doi:10.1111/phn/12068.

5.1 Markle-Reid, M., Browne, G., & Gafni, A. (2013). Nurse-led health promotion interventions improve quality of life in frail older home care clients: Lessons learned from three randomized trials in Ontario, Canada. *Journal of Evaluation in Clinical Practice, 19*(1), 118–131. doi: 10.1111/j.1365-2753.2011.01782.x.

5.2 Gifford, W., Davies, B., Graham, I., Tourangeau, A., Woodend, A. K., & Lefebre, N. (2013). Developing leadership capacity for guideline use: A pilot cluster randomized control trial. *World Views on Evidence-Based Nursing, 10,* 51–65. doi: 10.1111/j.1741-6787.2012.00254.x. Copyright © by Wiley Publishing, Inc. Used by permission of Wiley Publishing, Inc.

6.1 Nielsen, L. S., Angus, J. E., Gastaldo, D., Howell, D., & Husain, A. (2013). Maintaining distance from a necessary intrusion: A postcolonial perspective on dying at home for Chinese immigrants in Toronto Canada. *European Journal of Oncology Nursing, 17*(5), 649–656. doi:http://dx.doi.org/10.1016/j.ejon.2013.06.006.

6.2 Browne, A. J., Varcoe, C. M., Wong, S. T., Smye, V. L., Lavoie, J., Littlejohn, D., . . . Lennox, S. (2012). Closing the health equity gap: Evidence-based strategies for primary health care organizations. *International Journal for Equity in Health, 11*(59), 1–15.

7.1 Falk-Rafael, A., & Betker, C. (2012a). Witnessing social injustice downstream and advocating for health equity upstream: "The trombone slide" of nursing. *Advances in Nursing Science, 35*(2), 98–112.

Falk-Rafael, A., & Betker, C. (2012b). The primacy of relationships: A study of public health nursing practice from a critical caring perspective. *Advances in Nursing Science, 35*(4), 315–332.

7.2 Funk, L. & Stajduhar, K. (2013). Analysis and proposed model of family caregivers' relationships with home health providers and perceptions of the quality of formal services. *Journal of Applied Gerontology, 32*(2), 188–206.

8.1 Markle-Reid, M., Browne, G., & Gafni, A. (2013). Nurse-led health promotion interventions improve quality of life in frail, older home care clients: Lessons learned from three randomized trials in Ontario, Canada. *Journal of Evaluation in Clinical Practice, 19*(1), 118–131.

8.2 Haines, R. J., Bottorff, J. L., McKeown, S. B., Ptolemy, E., Carey, J., & Sullivan, K. (2010). Breast cancer messaging for younger women: Gender, femininity and risk. *Qualitative Health Research, 20*(6), 731–742.

Perth District Health Unit. Retrieved from http://www.pdhu.on.ca/wp-content/uploads/2015/04/Teen-Esteem-Evaluation-Report-2014.pdf

18.1 Parke, B. I., Hunter, K. F., Bostrom, A. M., Chambers, T., & Manraj, C. (2014). Identifying modifiable factors to improve quality for older adults in hospital: A scoping review. *International Journal of Older People Nursing, 9*(1), 8–24. doi:10.1111/opn.12007

18.2 Macdonald, M., & Lang, A. (2014). Applying risk society theory to findings of a scoping review on caregiver safety. *Health & Social Care in Community, 22*(2), 124–133. Retrieved from http://onlinelibrary.wiley.com/doi/10.1111/hsc.12056/pdf

19.1 Knight, R., Shoveller, J. A., Oliffe, J. L., Gilbert, M., & Goldenberg, S. (2012). Heteronormativity hurts everyone: Experiences of young men and clinicians with STI testing. *Journal of Men's Health, 7*(5), 441–459. doi:10.1177/1363459312464071.

19.2 Creighton, G., Oliffe, J. L., Butterwick, S., & Saewyc, E. (2013). After the death of a friend: Young men's grief and masculine identities. *Social Science & Medicine*, 84, 35–43. http://dx.doi.org/10.1016/j.socscimed.2013.02.022.

20.1 Bauer G. R., Scheim A. I., Deutsch M. B., & Cassarella C. (2014). Reported emergency department avoidance, use, and experiences of transgender persons in Ontario, Canada: Results from a respondent-driven sampling survey. *Annals of Emergency Medicine, 63*(6), 713–720. http://dx.doi.org/10.1016/j.annemergmed.2013.09.027.

20.2 Saewyc, E., Konishi, C., Rose, H., & Homma, Y. (2014). School-based strategies to reduce suicidal ideation and attempts among lesbian, gay, and bisexual, as well as heterosexual adolescents in western Canada. *International Journal of Child, Youth and Family Studies, 5*(1), 89–112.

21.1 Ross, P., Humble, A., & Blum, I. (2013). Sexuality and HIV/AIDS: An exploration of older heterosexual women's knowledge level. *Journal of Women & Aging, 25*, 165–182. doi:0.1080/08952841.2013.760366. Reproduced by permission of Taylor & Francis LLC (http://www.tandfonline.com).

21.2 Ducharme, F., Kergoat, M. J., Antoine, P., Pasquier, F., & Coulombe, R. (2013). The unique experience of spouses in early onset dementia. *American Journal of Alzheimer's Disease and Other Dementias, 28*(6), 634–641. doi:10.1177/1533317513494443.

22.1 Gates, M., Hanning, R. M., Martin, I. D., Gates, A., & Tsuji, L. J. S. (2013). Body mass index of First Nations youth in Ontario, Canada: Influence of sleep and screen time. *Rural and Remote Health, 13*, 2498.

22.2 Charania, N. A., & Tsuji L. J. S. (2013). Assessing the effectiveness of implementing mitigation measures for an influenza pandemic in remote and isolated First Nations communities: A qualitative community-based participatory research approach. *Rural and Remote Health, 13*, 2566. Retrieved from http://www.rrh.org.au

23.1 Perreault, M., Provencher, H., Roberts, S., & Milton, D. (2012). Predictors of caregiver satisfaction with mental health services. *Journal of Community Mental Health, 48*, 232–237.

23.2 Bender, A., Guruge, S., Hyman, I., & Janjua, M. (2012). Tuberculosis and common mental disorders: International lessons for Canadian immigrant health. *Canadian Journal of Nursing Research, 44*(4), 56–57.

24.1 Kulig, J., Edge, D., & Smolenski, S. (2014). Wildfire disasters: Implications for rural nurses. *Australasian Emergency Nursing Journal. 17*(3), 126–134. Copyright © 2014 by Elsevier Ltd. Used by permission of Elsevier Ltd. doi: 10.1016:j.aenj.2014.04.003.

24.2 O'Connell, M. E., Crossley, M., Cammer, A., Morgan, D., Allingham, W., Cheavins, B., . . . Morgan, E. (2013). Development and evaluation of a telehealth videoconferenced support group for rural spouses of individuals diagnosed with atypical early-onset dementias. *Dementia: The International Journal of Social Research and Practice, 13*(3). Reproduced by permission of SAGE Publications Ltd., London, Los Angeles, New Delhi, Singapore and Washington DC. Copyright © SAGE Publications Ltd., 2013. doi:10.1177/1471301212474143.

25.1 Baillot, A., Pelletier, C., Dunbar, P., Geiss, L., Johnson, J., Leiter, L., & Langlois, M. (2014). Profile of adults with type 2 diabetes and uptake of clinical care best practices: Results from the 2011 survey on living with chronic diseases in Canada – diabetes component. *Diabetes Research and Clinical Practice, 103*, 11–19. doi:10.1016/j.diabres.2013.11.22

25.2 Williams, A., Wang, L., & Kitchen, P. (2014). Differential impacts of caregiving across three caregiver groups in Canada: end-of-life care, long-term care, and short-term care. *Health and Social Care in the Community, 22*(2), 187–196. Used by permission of John Wiley & Sons, Ltd. doi:10.1111/hsc.12075.

26.1 Usher, A. M., & Stewart, L. A. (2014). Effectiveness of correctional programs with ethnically diverse offenders: a meta-analytic study. *International Journal of Offender Therapy and Comparative Criminology, 58*(2), 209–230. Reprinted by permission of SAGE Publications, Inc. doi:10.1177/03066 24X12469507.

# Preface

We would like to begin by thanking both students and faculty who welcomed the first three editions and provided excellent and insightful feedback for this fourth edition. This book has been useful not only at multiple levels within a basic or post-RN curriculum, but also in preparation for the Canadian Nurses Association certification examination in community health. To know that each of our previous editions was informative and easy to read yet encouraged learners' thinking made developing this new edition even more meaningful.

In the preface to the first edition we posed the question, "Why should we choose to write a community health nursing book from a Canadian perspective?" The response to the first and subsequent editions has solidified our beliefs. We believe that there are historical, political, legislative, cultural, and social influences that are unique to Canadians. They have shaped the evolution of Canada as a society, our definitions of health, and our expectations relative to healthcare delivery. Community health nurses are both a product of those influences and an influence themselves. Community health nursing has evolved differently in Canada than in other countries. We believe that as practitioners in community health nursing we must understand these influences to better prepare ourselves to help shape community health nursing in Canada.

## OUR APPROACH

Over time there has been much discourse on the terms "community health nursing" versus "public health nursing." The Community Health Nurses of Canada has discriminated these terms based on factors such as who is the client, what is the setting, and who is the employer. Historically, "community health nursing" was used to describe all nursing outside the hospital setting. In this book, community health nursing is defined as a specialty in nursing that encompasses a number of sub-specialties, such as public health nursing and home health nursing.

The community client may be an individual, group, community, system, or population, but care is rendered with an eye to the health of the population. The setting may be a home, institution, community, or agency serving the population. The common academic preparation is the basic baccalaureate education leading to the designation, Registered Nurse. The employer may be an individual, family, community, government, nongovernmental, or not-for-profit agency. When our chapter authors address a specific health issue or a particular population or aggregate in this book, each is speaking through the lens of her or his perspective about a segment within the larger whole of community health nursing.

We believe that community health nursing functions within a multiplicity of theories and understandings. Some theories are common to all facets of the nursing profession, such as ethical treatment of clients, family assessment, or the meaning of health. In some cases, nursing drove the development of the theory; in others, we have used the work of theorists in other disciplines. This text reflects that multiplicity, and the authors have described how the theories relate to community health nursing.

*Community Health Nursing: A Canadian Perspective*, Fourth Edition, has been written with the undergraduate student in mind. The work on this edition is in response to the needs expressed by faculty and students for a broad, comprehensive, and yet concise textbook providing an overview of community health nursing. Each topic is written on with the understanding that this will be the student's first foray into the community health nursing arena. We have chosen to incorporate the individual, family, community, system, and population as client perspectives throughout the text.

## NEW TO THE FOURTH EDITION

The new edition brings many changes. The first and most important change is the wonderful addition of Aliyah Dosani, PhD, RN, as an editor. Her expertise brings fresh ideas to this book.

As is appropriate to the pace of change in community health and community health nursing, we have made extensive updates to various chapters, with new content, statistics, and Canadian research. We continue to focus on the health of the aggregate or population, rather than on the specific clients. We made further emphasis on the importance of application of theory to practice; we addressed the growing needs of our community clients, and we further clarified the distinct specialty practices of public health and home health nursing. We therefore have added four new chapters to this edition:

- Chapter 4: Public Health Nursing
- Chapter 5: Home Health Nursing in Canada
- Chapter 8: Health Promotion
- Chapter 25: Chronic Care, Long-Term Care, and Palliative Care

With this edition we sought to focus more on prevention—primary, secondary, and tertiary—as it relates to the various topics of the chapters. Canadian Research Boxes and Case Studies throughout the text have been thoroughly updated.

We also have new contributors, who offer a fresh perspective and insights to various chapters.

## ABOUT THE CONTRIBUTORS

This fourth edition brings new and former authors to the book. As before, some hold academic positions, some are in management or policy positions, and others are front-line practitioners. All came with a commitment to share their work with the readers as they contribute to this Canadian community health nursing text, and this further demonstrates the cyclical nature of theory and practice. Each brings expertise and knowledge to a particular chapter and topic. Each has presented the various historical, geographical, social, political, and theoretical perspectives that assist in explaining and describing community nursing practice. You will find a list of the contributors, their affiliations, and the chapters they authored following the preface. To provide context regarding the varied experience and expertise of our contributors, we have also provided a short biographical sketch of each contributor immediately following the chapter(s) they wrote.

## CHAPTER ORGANIZATION

The chapters in *Community Health Nursing: A Canadian Perspective* are organized into five parts:

Part I: The Context of Community Health Nursing in Canada

Part II: Foundations and Tools for Community Health Nursing Practice

Part III: Nursing Care of Selected Populations

Part IV: Selected Community Problems

Part V: Looking Ahead

**Part I: The Context of Community Health Nursing in Canada** introduces students to the general topic area. **Chapter 1: The History of Community Health Nursing in Canada** presents an historical perspective on Canadian community health nursing so that students may be enlightened by lessons from the past. In this edition, a timeline is the organizing frame for the chapter. **Chapter 2: Financing, Policy, and Politics of Healthcare Delivery** presents the administration of community health from legislative, cultural, and political perspectives. The importance of strong leadership to assist in meeting healthcare delivery challenges has been highlighted. This chapter is followed by an Appendix, which outlines healthcare delivery to Aboriginal populations. **Chapter 3: Nursing Roles, Functions, and Practice Settings** introduces the students to the Community Health Nursing Practice Model and the Standards of Practice. In response to reader and teacher requests, **Chapter 4: Public Health Nursing** and **Chapter 5: Home Health Nursing in Canada** are new additions to this book and this section. Part 1 ends with **Chapter 6: Advocacy, Ethical, and Legal Considerations**, the authors

of which have used the Canadian Community Health Nursing Standards of Practice (found in Appendix A) to frame a discussion on legal and ethical issues for CHNs. The chapters in Part I form the underpinning for the subsequent sections.

**Part II: Foundations and Tools for Community Health Nursing Practice** builds the base upon which the subspecialties rest. **Chapter 7: Theoretical Foundations of Community Health Nursing** outlines several current theories that students can use to guide their CHN practice. The earlier versions of Chapters 5, 6, and 7, have been subsumed into a new chapter, **Chapter 8: Health Promotion**, which incorporates the concepts previously found in those three chapters. **Chapter 9: Cultural Care** adds current critiques of transcultural nursing and includes the Community Health Nurses Association of Canada's Public Health Nursing category of Diversity and Inclusiveness, and provides explicit discussion of cultural safety, cultural competencies, intersections, and diversity. Guided information on finding, appraising, and using community health nursing research is the focus of **Chapter 10: Research**. **Chapter 11: Epidemiology** describes the science of epidemiology and how it can inform community health nurses' practice. New to this edition is a section on screening and surveillance. **Chapter 12: Communicable Diseases** describes concepts related to communicable disease and includes the updated Public Health Agency of Canada Guidelines for Infection Prevention and Control. **Chapter 13: Community Nursing Process** provides an overview of the community health nursing process, including community assessment, selected community health practice models, population health promotion, community development, and community participatory tools. In **Chapter 14: Community Health Planning, Monitoring, and Evaluation**, the authors examine specifics around planning, monitoring, and evaluating community health programs, with additional information on the logic model and Gantt charts. This portion of the textbook concludes with **Chapter 15: Information Technology**. Here you will find a discussion of information technology and how it contributes to community nursing practice. In this edition additional discussion of social media has been included, as well as the most recent ICT competencies. We believe the topics in Parts I and II are essential for an understanding of community health nursing.

Parts III and IV, composed of focus chapters, examine groups and issues that make the picture of community health nursing more complete. In **Part III**, the spotlight is on **Nursing Care of Selected Populations**, which has been deliberately focused on health rather than challenges. **Chapter 16: Maternal, Infant, and Child Health** examines population health promotion approaches with socio-environmental perspectives on enhancing maternal and child health. **Chapter 17: School Health** draws attention to the common health concerns in school settings. In this edition additional theoretical frameworks have been expanded, and the CNHC standard around capacity building is highlighted. **Chapter 18: Family Health** provides an overview of the social and cultural context of the family in family care. **Chapter 19: Gender and Community Health** focuses on applying a gender lens to community health nursing practice, in such diverse topics as gender expression and cardiovascular health. **Chapter 20: Lesbian, Gay, Bisexual, Transgender, and Queer Clients** gives further explanation about the genetic and social influences on sexual orientation and gender identity development. **Chapter 21: Older Adult Health** highlights the aging population in Canada and expands on factors related to the assessment, maintenance, and promotion of the health of older adults. **Chapter 22: Aboriginal Health** examines the historical and current influences on the health of Aboriginal populations in Canada. First Nations healthcare, including cultural issues for CHNs in Aboriginal communities, are discussed. **Chapter 23: Mental Health** discusses challenges facing persons with mental illness, available services, and strategies to promote mental health within Canadian society. It now has more emphasis on mental health among refugees and immigrants. **Chapter 24: Rural Health** looks at the large portion of Canada's population that lives in rural settings. One of the highlights of this edition is the section of "a day in the life" of a rural nurse. **Chapter 25: Chronic Care, Long-Term Care, and Palliative Care** is a new chapter that examines issues for those community clients who receive extended or end-of-life care in the community. **Chapter 26: Correctional Health** looks at nursing within a controlled environment. Highlighted in this edition are working with youth, looking at alternative measures and restorative justice, the management of substance abuse within a correctional facility, and the containment of contagious diseases such as novovirus. **Chapter 27: Environmental and Occupational Health** includes discussion of the environmental burden of disease, as well as the nurse's role in assessment and prevention.

In contrast, **Part IV** focuses on **Selected Community Problems** that may apply to a variety of populations. Each chapter focuses on one of five specific issues. In this edition, **Chapter 28: Violence in Societies** highlights the links between violence in societies and the social determinants of health. In **Chapter 29: Poverty, Homelessness, and Food Security** sections on food insecurity and childhood poverty have been added, and research on healthcare utilization of homeless individuals is examined. Retitled **Chapter 30: Substance Use, Abuse, and Addictions** looks at licit as well as illicit drug use in Canada. In this edition, information about energy drinks and alcohol and gambling as an addiction are presented. The debate around harm reduction is enhanced. **Chapter 31: Sexually Transmitted Infections and Blood-Borne Pathogens** presents the variety of infections, as well as how public policy in Canada has been developed around these illnesses. Social marketing as a prevention strategy is highlighted. **Chapter 32: Emergency Preparedness and Disaster Nursing** provides an overview of the role of CHNs in community emergency preparedness planning and in disaster situations. Competencies for emergency preparedness for public health nursing are highlighted.

The final section, **Part V: Looking Ahead**, contains **Chapter 33: Global Health**. In this edition, new foci of globalization, global heath and economics, culture, and politics alert the learner to the wider picture. The text concludes with a brief look at where the field of community health nursing is headed and the coming opportunities and challenges in **Chapter 34: Challenges and Future Directions**.

Through the book, you will notice that some concepts and items are mentioned in several of the chapters. This is because they are often seminal documents or definitions that may be viewed through the lenses of the various topics and authors. For instance, many of the chapters will talk about the Lalonde Report, the Epp Report, or the Declaration of Alma-Ata. You will note that each author views the reports differently, depending on the chapter topic. For example, cross-cultural nursing is mentioned in the family health, mental health, and the cultural care chapters but may also be mentioned in the Aboriginal health chapter and the violence in society chapter. We anticipate that students and teachers will see this not as redundancy, but rather as an example of multiple perspectives and how and why a multiplicity of theory and practice exists in community health nursing.

## A Note on Appendices

As in the previous edition, the core competencies for public health can be found in MyNursingLab. These were developed with broad national consultation that led to the creation of the discipline specific competencies that are included in the text. As in previous editions, we have included the Canadian Community Health Nursing Standards of Practice, as shown in Appendix A (revised March 2011). This document explicitly reflects the current practice standards for Canadian community health nurses. In several chapters, contributors have made reference to the standards to enhance the discussion.

Appendices B and C are the discipline specific competencies. Appendix B is the Public Health Nursing Discipline Specific Competencies published by the Community Health Nurses of Canada in 2009. They were developed using several source documents and a Delphi process to arrive at consensus. Appendix C includes the Home Health Nursing Competencies. They were developed by the Community Health Nurses of Canada (CHNC) in partnership with the CHNC Certification, Standards and Competencies Committee and Advisory Group.

## Chapter Features

A special effort has been made with this book to incorporate features that will facilitate learning and enhance an understanding of community health nursing in Canada.

- **Learning Outcomes** outline what will be learned within each chapter.
- **Canadian Research Boxes** present specific studies from the literature or the authors' knowledge to illustrate or augment the material covered in the chapter. Either the researchers themselves are nurses, or we have chosen

Canadian health research that community health nurses can use in their practice. Each Research Box is followed by a few Discussion Questions to assist students in using the results.

---

**CANADIAN RESEARCH BOX 2.1**

**What does "population health approach" mean?**

Cohen, D., Huynh, T., Sebold, A., Harvey, J., Neudorf, C., & Brown, A. (2014). The population health approach: A qualitative study on conceptual and operational definitions for leaders in Canadian health care. *SAGE Open Medicine, 2*(Jan–Dec), 1–11. Reproduced by permission of SAGE Publications Ltd.

"Population health approach" is a broad term used to describe strategies and actions that are developed in recognition of the multitude of factors that affect the health of a population. These factors and forces are both within and outside of the scope of the healthcare system. Canada has b̶e̶e̶n̶ ̶r̶e̶c̶o̶gnized as a leader in the dev̶e̶l̶o̶p̶m̶e̶n̶t̶ ̶a̶n̶d̶ ̶c̶r̶

---

- **Case Studies** illustrate a practice application of the information presented in the chapter, followed by Discussion Questions.

---

**CASE STUDY**

**Public Health Chief Nursing Officer Working Group Report**
(Ontario Ministry of Health and Long-Term Care, 2011b)

Over the last two decades, discussions regarding the need for and establishment of designated nursing leadership roles in Ontario public health units have abounded. In February 2000, the then chief medical officer of health and provincial chief nursing officer endorsed the implementation of a chief nursing officer (CNO) position in each public health unit as a preferred model within the public health system and recognized it as a best practice (Peroff-Johnson, & Tober, 2012).

I̶t̶s̶ May 2006 f̶i̶n̶a̶l̶ report, the p̶u̶b̶l̶i̶c̶ ̶h̶e̶a̶l̶t̶h̶ ̶C̶N̶O̶

---

- **Key Terms** are boldfaced where they are introduced and defined in the body of the text. For convenience, the key terms are listed alphabetically at the end of each chapter.

---

**KEY TERMS**

accessible, p. 18
Canada Health Act, p. 18
Canadian Nurses Association (CNA), p. 18
comprehensive, p. 18
determinants of health, p. 20
health promotion, p. 19
home care, p. 24
interprofessional relationships, p. 27
leadership, p. 17
medicare, p. 18

---

- **Study Questions** test students' knowledge of the facts and concepts in the chapter. Answers to the study questions are included in the eText.

---

**STUDY QUESTIONS**

1. Identify the origins of medicare in Canada and summarize the laws that created the present Canadian healthcare system. What is considered to be phase 2 of the implementation of medicare?

2. Discuss the events that led up to and necessitated passage of the Canada Health Act.

3. What role did organized nursing play in the passage of t̶h̶e̶ Canada Health Act?

---

- **Individual** and **Group Critical-Thinking Exercises** challenge students to reflect on the content of the chapter and apply it in different situations.

---

**INDIVIDUAL CRITICAL-THINKING EXERCISES**

1. List your core values for healthcare in Canada. How do your values compare with the values reflected in the five key funding criteria described in the Canada Health Act (1984)?

2. How would your life be different if healthcare in this country were provided based on ability to pay rather than need?

3. This chapter has shown that health p̶o̶l̶i̶c̶y̶ ̶decisions l̶e̶d̶

---

- **References** cited in the chapter are presented in APA format.
- **Additional Resources** direct students to further information on the chapter topic. These include references to books, or journal articles. Students will also find references to specific government and nongovernmental agencies relevant to the chapter topics. These are included in the eText only.

## TEACHING SUPPORT

These Instructor's Resource Manual, Computerized Test Bank, PowerPoint® Presentations, and Image Library are all available for download from a password-protected section of Pearson Canada's online catalogue (www.pearsoncanada.ca/highered). Navigate to your book's catalogue page to view a list of those supplements that are available. See your local Pearson Canada sales representative for details and access.

- **Instructor's Resource Manual.** Each chapter begins with an overview, a list of learning objectives from the text, and an outline. This is followed by suggestions for classroom activities and discussion points for the Individual and Group Critical-Thinking Exercises found at the end of each chapter, as well as the discussion questions found in the Case Studies and Canadian Research Boxes throughout the text. The lecture suggestions, classroom activities, and out-of-class assignments tied to each of the five parts in the text have been updated to reflect changes made to the fourth edition.

- **Computerized Test Bank.** Pearson's computerized test banks allow instructors to filter and select questions to create quizzes, tests, or homework. Instructors can revise questions or add their own, and may choose print or online options. These questions are also available in Microsoft Word format.
- **PowerPoint® Presentations.** A variety of PowerPoint® slides accompany each chapter of the textbook.
- **Image Library.** The Image Library provides access to many of the images, figures, and tables in the textbook.
- **Learning Solutions Managers.** Pearson's Learning Solutions managers work with faculty and campus course designers to ensure that Pearson technology products, assessment tools, and online course materials are tailored to meet your specific needs. This highly qualified team is dedicated to helping schools take full advantage of a wide range of educational resources by assisting in the integration of a variety of instructional materials and media formats. Your local Pearson Canada sales representative can provide you with more details on this service program.

# MyNursingLab

Each MyNursingLab course matches the organization of the accompanying textbook. Preloaded content for every chapter of the accompanying textbook allows instructors to use MyNursingLab as is or to customize MyNursingLab with their own materials.

## FEATURES FOR STUDENTS

- **Pearson eText.** Pearson eText gives students access to the text whenever and wherever they have access to the Internet. eText pages look exactly like the printed text, offering powerful new functionality for students and instructors. Users can create notes, highlight text in different colours, create bookmarks, zoom, click hyperlinked words and phrases to view definitions, and view in single-page or two-page view. Pearson eText allows for quick navigation to key parts of the eText using a table of contents, and provides full-text search. The eText may also offer links to associated media files, enabling users to access videos, animations, or other activities as they read the text.
- **Study Plan.** Every chapter includes a two-part study plan with Practice questions to help students identify the areas and topics where more study is required and a Quiz to ensure that they've mastered the chapter content. Students can take advantage of the following Chapter Resources to make the most of their learning experience and succeed in their course:
  - eText
  - Clinical Guidelines
  - Videos and Real-Life Stories
  - Weblinks
  - Glossary Flashcards
  - Assessment Tools including
    - Test Your Terminology
    - Review Questions
  - Case Studies

## ACKNOWLEDGMENTS

In the creation of a book such as this, there are so many people to thank. First, we need to thank students and colleagues for encouraging us to start the project and then move on to a fourth edition. As this edition began to take shape, we were thankful for the many authors who once again agreed to contribute to the book or suggested others who had the expertise we required. Many of our authors took time from other projects to add their knowledge to the book, making this book a priority.

We are grateful to the talented team at Pearson Canada. Ms. Lisa Rahn and Mr. Paul Donnelly guided us through the whole process of development of this edition. Ms. Susan Johnson provided expertise, ideas, and support, which were invaluable in moving through production. The reviewers, who were nameless to us at the time, contributed significant time and effort in assisting us to make this text strong and representative of Canadian community health nursing. Their names are listed below. Each of us had particular friends and family members who were supportive as we moved through the process of completing a major text. We are grateful to all of you. We would like to extend our thanks to Corinne Hart and Pina Newman for their feedback on Chapter 20, Lesbian, Gay, Bisexual, Transgender, and Queer Clients. Finally, as teachers, we thank our students, who were guiding forces in considering the project at all.

Many nurses across the country have contributed countless hours to portray community health nursing with passion and pride. We are very excited with this new edition. We hope teachers and learners will also be excited as they continue to learn, explore, and discuss community health nursing as a distinct specialty in Canadian nursing.

Lynnette Leeseberg Stamler, Lucia Yiu, and Aliyah Dosani

## REVIEWERS

Marilyn Evans, University of Western Ontario
Donna Malyon Ginther, Kwantlen Polytechnic University
Corinne Hart, Ryerson University
Michelle Hogan, University of Ontario Institute of Technology
Anne Kearney, Memorial University

Jo-Ann MacDonald, University of Prince Edward Island
Ann MacLeod, Trent University
Helena Myllykoski, Mount Royal University
Cathy O'Brien-Larivee, UNB Saint John

Sheila Profit, Cape Breton University
Edward Venzon Cruz, Centennial College
Cindy Versteeg, Algonquin College
Jane Williamson, Cambrian College

*This edition is dedicated to my parents, Martin and Irma Leeseberg, who had high expectations of what we could accomplish. It is also dedicated to my husband Allan, for his unwavering support, and to all past and present community health nurses who inspired the book. Lastly, it is dedicated to the students and teachers who use this book, that they may experience the joy of nursing and contribute further to the profession.*
—L.L.S.

*This book is dedicated to my daughters, Tamara, Camillia, and Tiffany who love to learn; to the community health nurses who devote themselves to teaching and promoting the health of their communities; and to our students whose love for learning will help shape the future directions for community health nursing.*
—L.Y.

*This book is dedicated to my parents, Abdulrasul and Almas Mawji, who taught me that nothing is impossible to achieve. To my husband, Naushad Dosani, who gave me many encouraging smiles when I needed to write and edit chapters during evenings and weekends. Lastly, to our students, instructors, and community health nurses across Canada—the energy and passion with which you learn and teach, and the exceptional work that you do, ignites a flame in my soul that will never be extinguished!*
—A.D.

# Contributors

**Mary Ellen Andrews, RN(NP), PhD**
Acting Associate Dean North and North-Western
Saskatchewan Campus Rural and Remote Engagement &
Director Nurse Practitioner Program, College of Nursing,
University of Saskatchewan
Chapter 24—Rural Health

**Claire Betker, RN, BN, MN, PhD(c), CCHN(C)**
Senior Knowledge Translation Specialist, National
Collaborating Centre for Determinants of Health
Chapter 2—Financing, Policy, and Politics of Healthcare
Delivery
Chapter 7—Theoretical Foundations of Community Health
Nursing

**Diane Bewick, RN, BScN, MScN, DPA, CCHN(C)**
Director, Family Services and Chief Nursing Officer,
Middlesex-London Health Unit, Ontario
Chapter 2—Financing, Policy, and Politics of Healthcare
Delivery

**Kathleen Carlin, RN, MSc, PhD**
Assistant Professor, Department of Philosophy, Ryerson
University
Chapter 6—Advocacy, Ethical, and Legal Considerations

**Catherine Carter-Snell, RN, BScN, MN, PhD, ENC-C, SANE-A**
Nurse Education Scholar, School of Nursing and Midwifery,
Faculty of Health, Community and Education
Mount Royal University, Calgary Alberta
Chapter 28—Violence in Societies

**Glen Chenard, RN , BHSc, CDE , CCHN(C), CHPCN(C), CVAA(C)**
Advanced Practice Consultant – Chronic Disease Management,
Saint Elizabeth Health Care
Chapter 5—Home Health Nursing in Canada

**Donna Ciliska, RN, PhD**
Professor, School of Nursing, McMaster University
Chapter 10—Research

**Genevieve Currie, RN, BN, MN**
Associate Professor, School of Nursing and Midwifery, Faculty of
Health, Community and Education, Mount Royal University;
Board member of Community Health Nurses of Canada
Chapter 3—Nursing Roles, Functions, and Practice Settings

**Aliyah Dosani, RN, BN, MPH, PhD**
Associate Professor, School of Nursing and Midwifery, Faculty
of Health, Community and Education, Mount Royal
University
Chapter 4—Public Health Nursing
Chapter 16—Maternal, Infant, and Child Health
Chapter 19—Gender and Community Health
Chapter 33—Global Health
Chapter 34—Challenges and Future Directions

**Susan M. Duncan, RN, PhD**
Associate Professor, Nursing, Thompson Rivers University
Chapter 1—The History of Community Health Nursing in
Canada

**Suzanne Dupuis-Blanchard, RN, PhD**
Associate Professor, École de science infirmière/School of
Nursing
Chapter 21— Older Adult Health

**Kathryn Edmunds, RN, BN, MSN, PhD(c)**
Doctoral Candidate, Aurthur Labatt Family School of Nursing,
Western University, Adjunct Assistant Professor, Sessional
Instructor, Faculty of Nursing, University of Windsor
Chapter 9—Cultural Care

**Nancy Edwards, RN, PhD**
Scientific Director Institute of Population and Public Health
Canadian Institutes of Health Research Professor, School of
Nursing, and the Department of Epidemiology and
Community Medicine, University of Ottawa
Chapter 14—Community Health Planning, Monitoring, and
Evaluation

**Josephine Etowa, RN, PhD**
Loyer DaSilva Chair in Public Health Nursing Associate Professor,
School of Nursing, Faculty of Health Sciences, University of Ottawa
Chapter 14—Community Health Planning, Monitoring, and
Evaluation

**Linda Ferguson, RN, PhD**
Professor, College of Nursing, University of Saskatchewan
Chapter 15—Information Technology

**Aaron Gabriel, RN, BA, BSN, MSN**
Clinical Instructor, College of Nursing, University of
Saskatchewan
Chapter 29—Poverty, Homelessness, and Food Security

**Rebecca Ganann, RN, MSc**
Assistant Clinical Professor & Research Assistant, School of Nursing, McMaster University
Chapter 10—Research

**Judith Gleeson, RN, PhD**
Associate Professor, School of Nursing and Midwifery, Faculty of Health, Community and Education, Mount Royal University
Chapter 33—Global Health

**Mary E. Hill, RN, BScN, PhD(c), MEd**
Graduate Student, School of Nursing, University of Victoria
Chapter 7—Theoretical Foundations of Community Health Nursing

**Lorraine Holtslander, RN, PhD, CHPCN(C)**
Associate Professor, College of Nursing, University of Saskatchewan
Chapter 25—Chronic Care, Long-Term Care, and Palliative Care

**Megan Kirk, RN, PhD(c), MSc, BScN**
Graduate Student, School of Nursing, University of Victoria
Chapter 7—Theoretical Foundations of Community Health Nursing

**Kelley Kilpatrick, RN, PhD**
Assistant Professor, Faculty of Nursing, Université de Montréal
Chapter 24—Rural Health

**Judith Kulig, RN, PhD**
Professor and University Scholar, Faculty of Health Sciences, University of Lethbridge
Chapter 24—Rural Health

**Yvette Laforêt-Fliesser, RN, BScN, MScN, CCHN(C)**
Consultant, Community and Public Health Vice-President
Chapter 17—School Health

**Nancy Lefebre, RN, BScN, MScN**
Chief Clinical Executive and Senior Vice-President, Saint Elizabeth Health Care
Chapter 5—Home Health Nursing in Canada

**Melanie Lind-Kosten, RN, BSN, MEd**
Nursing Practice Instructor, Faculty of Nursing, University of Calgary
Chapter 8—Health Promotion

**Candace Lind, RN, BN, MN, PhD**
Assistant Professor, Faculty of Nursing, University of Calgary
Chapter 8—Health Promotion

**Sylvia Loewen, RN, BN, MN**
Senior Instructor, University of Calgary, Faculty of Nursing
Chapter 8—Health Promotion

**Wendi Lokanc-Diluzio, RN, BN, MN, PhD**
Sexual & Reproductive Health Services, Calgary Health Region/Alberta Health Services, Calgary, Alberta
Chapter 31—Sexually Transmitted Infections and Blood-Borne Pathogens

**Marjorie MacDonald, RN, PhD**
Professor and CIHR/PHAC Applied Public Health Chair in Public Health Education and Population Intervention Research
Chapter 7—Theoretical Foundations of Community Health Nursing

**Carol MacDougall, RN, BScN, MA**
Public Health Manager
Chapter 17—School Health

**Cheryl MacLeod, RN, BScN, MEd, CCHN(C)**
Area Manager for the East Calgary Health Centre and Sheldon M Chumir Health Centre.
Chapter 17—School Health

**Martha L. P. MacLeod, RN, PhD**
Professor, Schools of Nursing and Health Sciences, University of Northern British Columbia
Chapter 24—Rural Health

**Deborah Mansell, RN, MN**
Assistant Professor, School of Nursing and Midwifery, Faculty of Health, Community and Education, Mount Royal University
Chapter 16—Maternal, Infant, and Child Health
Chapter 19—Gender and Community Health

**Kim Miller, RN, BScN, MScN**
Lead, Educational program, Saint Elizabeth Health Care
Chapter 5—Home Health Nursing in Canada

**Elaine Mordoch, RN, PhD**
Associate Professor, Faculty of Nursing University of Manitoba
Chapter 23—Mental Health

**Janet Morrison, RN, PhD, M.Ad.Ed., COHN(C)**
Program head, Occupational Health Nursing Specialty Program, The B.C. Institute of Technology
Chapter 27—Environmental and Occupational Health

**Marianna Ofner-Agostini, RN, BScN, MHSc, PhD**
Senior Advisor Centre for Chronic Disease Prevention Public Health Agency of Canada Adjunct Professor, Epidemiology Dhalla Lana School of Public Health, University of Toronto
Chapter 12—Communicable Diseases

**Shelley Peacock, RN, BSc, PhD**
Assistant Professor, College of Nursing, University of Saskatchewan
Chapter 25—Chronic Care, Long-Term Care, and Palliative Care

**Elizabeth Peter, RN, BScN, BA, MScN, PhD**
Associate Professor Lawrence S. Bloomberg Faculty of Nursing
Chair, Health Sciences Research Ethics Board Member, Joint
Centre for Bioethics University of Toronto
Chapter 6—Advocacy, Ethical, and Legal Considerations

**Cindy Peternalj-Taylor, RN, BScN, MScN, DE-IAFN**
Professor, College of Nursing, University of Saskatchewan
Chapter 26—Correctional Health

**Wendy Peterson, RN, PhD**
Associate Professor, School of Nursing, Faculty of Health
Sciences, University of Ottawa
Chapter 14—Community Health Planning, Monitoring, and
Evaluation

**Caroline J. Porr, RN, BScN, MN, PhD**
Assistant Professor, School of Nursing, Health Sciences Centre,
Memorial University of Newfoundland
Chapter 4—Public Health Nursing

**Karen L. Ray, RN, BScN, MSc**
Manager, Knowledge Translation Saint Elizabeth Health Care
Chapter 5—Home Health Nursing in Canada

**Tracie Risling, RN, PhD**
Assistant Professor, College of Nursing, University of
Saskatchewan.
Chapter 15—Information Technology

**Rose A. Roberts, RN, PhD**
Member of the Lac La Ronge Indian Band, Saskatchewan
Chapter 22—Aboriginal Health

**Candace Martin Ryan, RN, BSc, BScN, MSc**
Faculty Advisor, University of Windsor; NICU Nurse,
Windsor Regional Hospital
Chapter 18—Family Health

**Elizabeth M. Saewyc, RN, PhD, PHN(Minn.), FSAHM,
FCAHS**
CIHR/PHAC Chair in Applied Public Health Research
Professor, School of Nursing & Division of Adolescent Health
and Medicine Director, Stigma and Resilience Among
Vulnerable Youth Centre and Research Director, McCreary
Centre Society
Chapter 20—Lesbian, Gay, Bisexual, Transgender, and Queer
Clients

**Betty Schepens, RN, BScN, DPA**
Program Manager, Infectious Disease and Emergency
Preparedness Programs, Chatham-Kent Public Health Unit |
Municipality of Chatham-Kent
Chapter 32—Emergency Preparedness and Disaster
Nursing

**Ruth Schofield, RN, BScN, MSc(T)**
Assistant Professor, McMaster School of Nursing, Past
President of Community Health Nurses of Canada, Board
member of Community Health Nurses of Canada
Chapter 3—Nursing Roles, Functions, and Practice Settings

**Shirlee Sharkey, RN, BScN, MHSc**
President and CEO, Saint Elizabeth Health Care
Chapter 5—Home Health Nursing in Canada

**Lynnette Leeseberg Stamler, RN, PhD, FAAN**
Professor and Associate Dean for Academic Programs, College
of Nursing, University of Nebraska Medical Center
Chapter 11—Epidemiology
Chapter 29—Poverty, Homelessness, and Food Security

**Norma J. Stewart, RN, PhD**
Professor, College of Nursing, University of Saskatchewan.
Chapter 24—Rural Health

**Marilyn A. Sutton, RN, BScN, MA**
Faculty Advisor, Faculty of Nursing, University of Windsor
Chapter 18—Family Health

**Louise R. Sweatman, RN, BScN, LLB, MSc**
Director, Regulatory Policy, Canadian Nurses Association,
Ottawa
Chapter 6—Advocacy, Ethical, and Legal Considerations

**Tammy Troute-Wood, RN, BScN, MN**
Sexual & Reproductive Health Services, Calgary Health
Region/Alberta Health Services, Calgary, Alberta
Chapter 31—Sexually Transmitted Infections and Blood-Borne
Pathogens

**Erin Wilson, RN(NP[F]), MSN, PhD(c)**
Assistant Professor, School of Nursing, University of Northern
British Columbia
Chapter 24—Rural Health

**Hélène Philbin Wilkinson, RN, BScN, MN**
Director, Mental Health and the Law Division North Bay
Regional Health Centre
Chapter 30—Substance Use, Abuse, and Addictions

**Phil Woods, RPN, PhD**
Professor, Associate Dean Research, Innovation and Global
Initiatives, College of Nursing, University of Saskatchewan
Chapter 26—Correctional Health

**Lucia Yiu, RN, BScN, BA, BSc, MScN**
Associate Professor, Faculty of Nursing, University of Windsor
Chapter 13—Community Nursing Process
Chapter 18—Family Health
Chapter 32—Emergency Preparedness and Disaster Nursing
Chapter 34—Challenges and Future Directions

# The History of Community Health Nursing in Canada

*Susan Duncan*

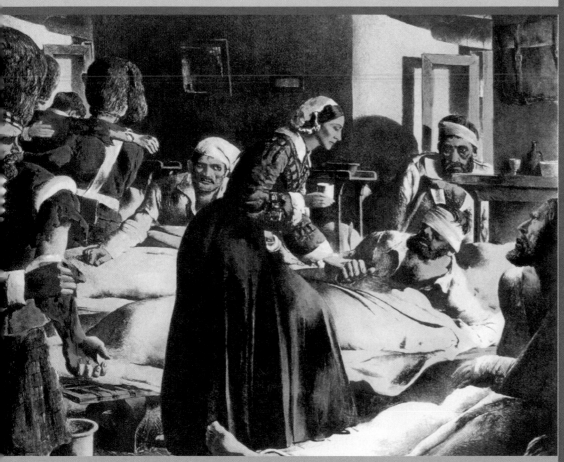

*Source: Everett Historical/Shutterstock*

LEARNING OUTCOMES

**After studying this chapter, you should be able to:**

1. Identify the social, political, and economic contexts of the development of community health nursing in Canada.

2. Appraise how early community health nursing practice relates to current models and standards of community health nursing practice.

3. Identify the contributions and attributes of community health nurses that shaped the evolution of nursing practice.

4. Explain how public health nursing influenced the development of nursing education.

5. Identify the milestones of community health nursing's contribution to primary health care.

6. Envision a future for community health nursing.

## INTRODUCTION

Community health nursing has evolved within dynamic sociopolitical and economic contexts in Canada over the past five centuries. As a practice discipline and profession, nursing history inspires reflection on the questions and issues that persist through time. Nurse historian Patricia D'Antonio (2006) describes how research into nursing's past sheds light on challenges and opportunities in nursing's achievement of its social mission. Community health nurses (CHNs) advocate for the provision of primary health care and provide sociopolitical leadership for the development of the health system and global health in their practice (Armstrong-Reid, 2014; Falk-Rafael, 2005). Community health nursing has been challenged to fulfill its mission in meeting the health needs of diverse communities over time.

The purpose of this chapter is to describe community health nursing practice in a historical context as a foundation for understanding subsequent chapters in this text. This

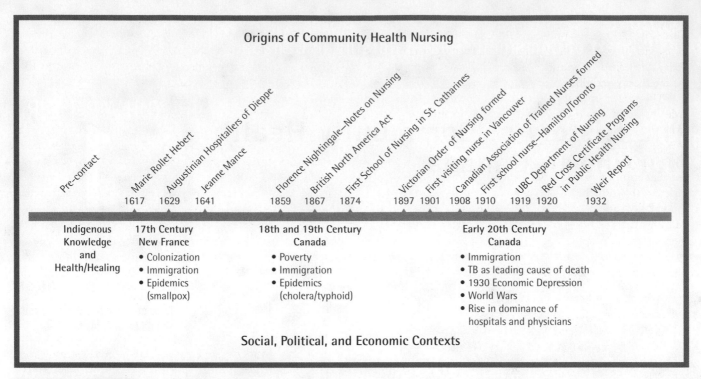

**FIGURE  1.1**  Origins of Community Health Nursing

chapter will examine the evolution and milestones of community health nursing in Canada (see Figure 1.1) and the challenges that confronted CHNs as they advanced their role in their profession. The chapter will also illustrate how CHNs develop relationships with individuals, families, and communities; provide leadership for health services; and promote the health of their clients. Their contributions to health and public policy through political advocacy will be examined.

## ORIGINS OF COMMUNITY HEALTH NURSING

The earliest forms of healthcare in Canada were the practices of Aboriginal peoples involving indigenous medicine and healing practices that met the health needs of communities (Aboriginal Nurses Association of Canada, 2007; Bourque Bearskin, 2011). Later, Aboriginal women provided essential healthcare, including curative midwifery services to European settlers in the western and northern regions of pre-Confederation Canada (Burnett, 2008). These practices have yet to be acknowledged within the history and modern practices of nursing and healthcare despite a growing awareness of their enduring value (Bourque Bearskin, 2014; Kelm, 1998). Epidemics of infectious diseases introduced by European settlers, wars, and the denigration of Aboriginal culture and identity during colonization of Canada by European immigrants have led to social, health, and economic disparities among Aboriginal peoples that persist today. The history of the relationship between colonization and Aboriginal people must be understood in the present-day context of Aboriginal health. (See Chapter 22.)

Community health nursing was known as the earliest form of nursing practised in Canada and has a long and proud history. Canadian nurse historian Margaret Allemang (2000) traces the introduction of community-oriented nursing to 17th century New France and the Duchesse d'Aiguillon sisters, who established "essential health care and carried out work in homes, hospitals and communities" (p. 6). This early work of the sisters is emulated by the CHN practice of today with a focus on the determinants of health, community outreach, and advocacy. Therefore, it is important for nurses to understand the significance of these origins of community health nursing and how they relate to current trends in nursing, healthcare, and health equity.

Historians generally refer to the earliest forms of community health nursing as those practices in 17th century New France and the notable work and contributions of women and sisterhoods (Allemang, 2000). Gibbon and Mathewson (1947) chronicled the lasting and significant influence of the French on providing the earliest forms of organized community health nursing as practised by sisterhoods, including a small group of Augustinian Hospitallers of Dieppe, who worked to establish a hospital and provide care in villages and homes. Allemang (2000) further refers to "the Grey Nuns, established in 1738 by Marguerite d'Youville as Canada's first community nursing order" (p. 6). Also significant were the contributions of a laywoman, Marie Rollet Hebert, who worked alongside her surgeon husband in the early 17th century. Early accounts of Hebert's work include relationships with the Aboriginal people and how she learned about health and healing, including the "value of evergreen trees as a source of vitamin C during the long winter months" (Paul & Ross-Kerr, 2011, p. 20).

Although there is not complete agreement among historians, Canada's first nurse is most often identified as Jeanne Mance (1606–1673). After receiving practical training in nursing in France, Mance came to Canada and confronted the political, social, and economic forces to establish a range of community health services that included the founding of the Hotel-Dieu Hospital of Montreal, and she is also described as the co-founder of Montreal (Allemang, 2000; Gibbon & Mathewson, 1947). This early nursing leader provided direct nursing care, advocated for essential services, and was the administrator of the hospital. Today, the Canadian Nurses Association (CNA) grants its highest and most prestigious award in her name.

The Grey Nuns were Canada's first community nursing order who made significant contributions to providing access to health services, food, shelter, and education for the most vulnerable, including those immigrating and settling the western regions of the province. Hardill (2006) refers to the order as the first form of "street outreach nursing to be found in the early 1700s when the Grey Nuns began public health visits to the sick poor in what is now Quebec" (p. 91). Nurse historian Pauline Paul has undertaken extensive historical research on the contributions of the Grey Nuns and other religious nursing orders to the development of health services, nursing education, and hospital administration across the country:

> Nursing sisters were the first to provide health care in remote and frontier areas, and, when these areas became more settled, they were also among the first to establish and operate modern and urban hospitals. . . . Religious nursing orders have also been significant contributors to Canadian nursing education, operating schools of nursing within hospitals (such as the School of Nursing run by the hospital at the Edmonton General Hospital) and establishing university level nursing programs. (Paul, 2005, p. 137).

The origins of community health nursing encompassed a broad focus on the social determinants of health and concerns for vulnerable populations' access to housing, food, and the essentials of life. Healthcare delivery was not clearly demarcated as separate entities of institutional and community-based care. Rather, the establishments of sick bays and hospitals were considered part of a continuum of health services that also included education, home visiting, clinics, and other avenues of access in the provision of services and advocacy for the essentials of life and health, including immunizations.

## NATION BUILDING AND THE NIGHTINGALE ERA (MID- TO LATE 19TH CENTURY)

This period was marked by the political context of Canada's development as a nation, immigration extending within western Canada, ongoing challenges of providing basic health services to settlers, and Aboriginal peoples experiencing a wave of epidemics introduced by immigrants. The 1867 British North America Act (BNA Act) made only limited provisions for the establishment and maintenance of a healthcare system. The Act specified that the federal government was responsible for taxes, laws, quarantine, and the establishment of marine hospitals. All other responsibilities for the organization of healthcare, including public health services, devolved to the provinces. Healthcare responsibilities were not specified within the Act, nor did the provinces, in the early years after Confederation, make much effort to undertake them. Such organized healthcare as did exist was provided at the local (municipal) level through public welfare or, more frequently, charitable organizations.

Many provinces passed legislation in the late 19th century to allow for the establishment of local and provincial departments of health. Poverty, poor health and self-care, and social unrest created by industrial capitalism, immigration, and urbanization shaped the organization and financing of the public health system and the nature of community health nursing.

The second half of the century was characterized by the development of the nursing profession, predominantly influenced by Florence Nightingale and the commitment of women's groups. There was also a rise in the dominance of medicine and hospitals as the centre of healthcare delivery. All played a role in the development of community health nursing as it exists today.

The Nightingale era in Canada is marked by the establishment of the first school of nursing in St. Catharines, Ontario, in 1874. The introduction of the Nightingale model of training nurses was a significant milestone in the development of the profession, as it offered formal training to nurses to acquire the needed skills and knowledge for practice. During this period, nursing also confronted the dominance of medicine and hospitals, as well as issues of class and gender, which remain today (Larsen & Baumgart, 1992; McPherson, 1996). Health promotion was present in the earliest forms of community health nursing practice, including Florence Nightingale's conceptualization of nursing. She was a visionary epidemiologist, who wisely collected and used statistics to identify population health concerns among soldiers during the Crimean war. An environmentalist, she identified "the five essential points in securing the health of houses as pure air, pure water, efficient drainage, cleanliness and light" (Nightingale, 1859/1946, p. 14).

Women's groups and individual women played a vital role in the development of community health services for the rural and poor communities and immigrant women in Canada in the late 19th and early 20th centuries. One such individual was Lady Aberdeen, wife of the Governor General of Canada, who led the development of the Victorian Order of Nurses. The Victorian Order of Nurses for Canada (VON) was founded in 1897 "to supply nurses, thoroughly trained in Hospital and District Nursing, and subject to one Central Authority, for the nursing of the sick who are otherwise unable to obtain trained nursing in their own homes, both in town and country districts" (Lady Aberdeen, cited in Gibbon, 1947, p. 8). The National Council of Women of Canada advocated for the development of the nursing profession through training and education. However, significant points of conflict emerged between Lady Aberdeen's view of how to best meet the needs of prairie women and that of the National Council of Women. Her view that skilled, practical "home helpers" trained in midwifery and basic care could best reach rural women was opposed by physicians, nurses, and the National Council of Women. This opposition resulted in the creation of the VON. This was followed by the evolution of district and home nursing care in the country and resulted in the extinction of lay midwifery and the medicalization of obstetrics (Boutillier, 1994).

The VON's capacity to respond to local needs stemmed from its organizational structure that included local branches with volunteers in various communities to sustain the organization. The VON encouraged local branches to seize opportunities to extend their work and to demonstrate their capacity to deliver the wide range of community health nursing services. Visiting nursing services became the backbone of these local branches and offered bedside nursing care to families who could not afford to hire private-duty nurses. The difference between the actual cost of the service and what was paid in fees by families was underwritten by charitable donations, fundraising, and, in some cases, grants from city or provincial governments. By doing so, the local branches fulfilled a dual mandate: charitable work among the poor and the provision of affordable nursing care to the working and middle classes. The history of the VON has been documented in two monographs, one written on the occasion of its 50th anniversary (Gibbon, 1947) and one to celebrate its 100th year of service in Canada (Penney, 1996).

## EARLY 20TH CENTURY EVOLUTION OF COMMUNITY HEALTH NURSING

By the late 19th and early 20th century the nursing profession was seen as three distinct sectors: hospital nurses, private-duty nurses, and public health and home-visiting nurses (McPherson, 1996). Community health nursing emerged as a distinct specialty and the majority of nurses were self-employed as private-duty nurses. Public health and home-visiting nurses were considered among the profession's elite. Employment in this specialty practice required additional clinical skills such as midwifery training and, particularly after World War I, post-diploma training at a university (Baldwin, 1997; Green, 1974; McPherson, 1996; Miller, 2000; Penney, 1996). Both public health and home-visiting nurses were different from nurses employed in other sectors of the healthcare system in several ways. They tended to remain in their community practices longer than those employed in hospitals and private-duty nursing. They also enjoyed greater financial stability and higher salaries (McPherson, 1996). Their sense of adventure, independence, courage, and humanitarianism led pioneering Canadian community health nurses (CHNs) to offer their services to those living in Canada's poorest urban districts and most isolated rural communities.

Pioneer CHNs worked to meet the immediate needs of communities for direct care and midwifery while also providing health education and prevention to individuals and families. Therefore, the early practice of community health nursing was characterized by considerable overlap between what we now identify as distinct public health nursing roles and district or home-visiting nursing roles. Over time, there was increased differentiation among the community health nursing roles as district and home healthcare and public health evolved within government-run health organizations. There was a growing distinction between direct care of individuals and families in the community and the focus on the health of the community as a whole as both district or home-visiting nursing and public nursing became specialized as forms of community health nursing that exist today (McKay, 2005). Less well documented but also significant was the emergence of other community health nursing roles, including occupational health nursing, outpost nursing, midwifery, Aboriginal nursing, and, later in the century, community mental health nursing (Benoit & Carroll, 2005; Boschma, 2012; Dodd, Elliot, & Rousseau, 2005; Keddy & Dodd, 2005).

The role of women's volunteerism and leadership in communities continued to be an integral part in the development of community health nursing. At the local level, rural women's groups such as the Women's Institute and the United Farm Women made community development and the development of healthcare services a priority. These women lobbied local officials, served tea at child welfare clinics, sewed layettes for destitute families, provided transportation, made referrals, raised funds, and in untold other ways tried to enable CHNs to fulfill their professional obligations to the fullest extent possible (Miller, 2000; Riddell, 1991; Stuart, 1987).

## Public Health Nursing as a Nursing Specialty

The term **public health nurse** (PHN) was first coined by American nurse Lillian Wald, who, with her nursing colleague Mary Brewster, founded the Henry Street Visiting Nurse Service in the late 19th century. Their conception of practice was broad as they attended to the issues of poverty, culture, and living conditions of the poor (Fee & Bu, 2010). In Canada, PHNs were civil servants employed by the local, provincial, or federal government. Public health nursing emerged in Canada in the early 20th century when civic departments of health established health education and preventive programs to combat communicable diseases, infant mortality, and morbidity in school-age children. Nurses were perceived as the ideal professionals to deliver these programs because of their medical knowledge and their ability to interact with women and children in private homes and in the public school setting (Sears, 1995).

In the early 20th century, community health nursing evolved from the specialties of tuberculosis (TB) nursing and school nursing to programs focused on reducing infant mortality. Despite all efforts to improve urban sanitation and to regulate food and milk supplies, infant mortality rates in Canadian cities continued to climb until well into the second decade of the 20th century. Public health officials identified health education as another strategy to combat unnecessary disease and death. TB was the leading cause of death at the turn of the century, and it was at this point that nurses were first employed as civil servants in local health departments. Although the exact chronology varies from one city to another, the first PHNs were responsible for TB control, child hygiene programs, and school inspection programs.

Zilm and Warbinek (2002) refer to TB nursing and school nursing as the first two public health nursing specialties. The breadth and depth of these nursing specialties are revealed in the earliest issues of the *Canadian Nurse Journal* beginning in 1910, with the appointment of the first school nurses in Hamilton and Toronto. The first PHNs participated in initiatives to preserve and promote the health of school-age children. As working-class children were removed from economic production and placed in the public school system, their significant health problems became fully visible (Peikoff & Brickey, 1991). Programs for the medical inspection of school children were established in major cities across Canada, and nurses were hired by boards of education. In many cities, such as Montreal, Toronto, Winnipeg, and Vancouver, school health programs were initially established by the board of education. They were subsequently taken over by the health department as part of the process of consolidating all public health programs under one jurisdiction (City of Winnipeg Health Department, 1910; MacDougall, 1990).

Early accounts of school nursing indicate a broad focus on the health of children and families related to conditions of living, including poverty. Early school-based initiatives often included medical inspections of children augmented by home visits to educate the parents and to ensure that all recommendations were followed (Sutherland, 1981). One school nurse described how home visiting in connection with school nursing was an important part of community work:

> The child, having been examined by the School Medical Officer and being found to have any physical abnormality such as defective nasal breathing, defective vision or hearing, bad teeth or enlarged tonsils, etc., a notice is sent home to that effect and a visit is made to the parents of the child by the school nurse as soon as possible. She notes the home conditions and family circumstances, enquires as to the child's sleeping apartment, and often gives a few simple instructions in hygiene. When necessary she advises the mother to have treatment for the child, and although a great many of the parents are unable to afford even the simplest of treatments, we are able to a certain extent to overcome this difficulty through the kindness of the different specialists in the city. . . . Often the nurse finds great poverty in the home, and sometimes the children have no boots or suitable clothing in which to come to school, or no sufficient food. (Ewart, 1916, p. 308)

The earliest maternal child health programs were the well-baby clinics, established by the Red Cross Peace Program, and they remain a signature program of public health nursing today. As in the present, these early clinics were run by nurses who assessed the growth and development of children and provided mothers and caregivers with health teaching for the care and promotion of child health. Early accounts of these clinics indicate the involvement of physicians who at times challenged the autonomy of nurses in the delivery of this primary care program. Local physicians sometimes did not support public health programs because they feared that the PHNs would provide primary care and thus compete with them for both patients and income. It took considerable effort on the part of the nurses to lessen these concerns. Stuart (1987) found that PHNs often avoided giving advice to families about the prevention of communicable diseases, even when they knew more about immunization programs than did the local physicians. One of the strategies employed to silence the protests of local physicians was to refer all individuals found to have "abnormal" conditions to the attending physician for further follow-up, even in cases where the nurses could have provided this care themselves (Riddell, 1991). (See Photos 1.1 and 1.2.)

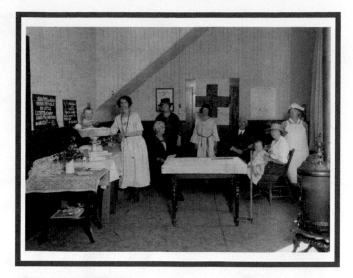

PHOTO 1.1 Article in the *Kamloops Daily News* (Saturday, October 19, 1991): In the early 1920s, Christine Thom became the first Red Cross public health nurse to offer a well-baby clinic, at an annual salary of $166.72.

*Source: Kamloops Museum and Archives photograph collection #1724.*

Public health officials and maternal feminists also turned their attention to the care that infants received from their mothers (Meigs, 1916). They concluded that many parents, particularly the mothers, were "ignorant" and barely capable of providing a safe and healthy environment for the nation's future citizens. Because removing children from their parents was no longer a viable option, educating mothers about infant feeding and hygiene became the intervention of choice (Peikoff & Brickey, 1991). Infant and child welfare and hygiene programs were carried out at milk depots, at well-baby clinics, and in private homes (Locke, 1918; MacNutt, 1913). Visiting nurses (VNs) staffed the clinics and visited the homes of newborn infants in the early postnatal period. They assessed the health of the infant and mother, the family's child-care practices, and the hygienic conditions in the home. A major focus was to promote breastfeeding of newborn infants.

Women volunteers played essential roles in developing the social, cultural, and healthcare services in smaller communities. As written by Yarmie (2013), the Red Cross established the first well-baby clinic with nurse Christina Thom in 1922, and "at the initial clinic over a dozen mothers had their babies' weight and height recorded . . ." (p. 114). Similar well-baby clinics developed across Canada, contributing to the health and wellness of Canada's infants and children and reducing mortality.

The establishment of public health nursing programs had limited success in rural and isolated areas. Many communities wanted the visiting nurses to provide bedside nursing care, rather than the PHNs, who focused on health education and prevention of illness (Matthews, 1920; Stuart, 1987). By the beginning of World War II, the essential elements of community health nursing services were in place across the country. Provincial health departments had been organized, and local health departments operated in the majority of Canadian cities.

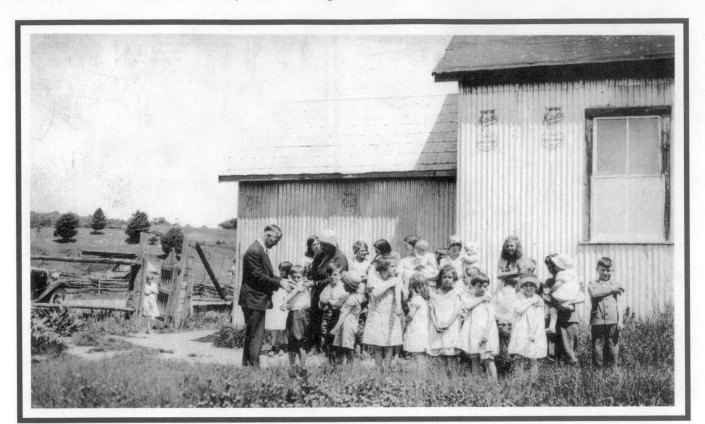

**PHOTO 1.2** Immunization of school-age children was an important part of a rural PHN's work. Small schools and long distances made this a challenging task. In 1932, public health nurse Ina Grenville and an unidentified physician were photographed immunizing a group of school children at Algoma School in northern Ontario.

*Source:* Archives of Ontario. Reference code: RG 10-30-2, 2.15.3/Children lined up to receive their needles at an immunization clinic, Algoma District, Ontario, 1932/Copyright Crown.

The scope of work in health education and prevention of illness had grown to include programs such as mental health, control of venereal diseases, preschool health, and prenatal education. The VON continued to flourish by providing bedside nursing care in the home as a springboard to also providing public health programs in communities. Although the VON had been envisioned by its founders as a nursing service for those living in rural and isolated "country districts," it had attained its greatest success and stability in Canada's urban centres.

In the interwar years, the development of public health services was uneven and often unsuccessful. The time available for individual and family health education or preventive services was limited, and the nurses' ability to provide long-term follow-up in complex situations was significantly constrained. The need for home care and midwifery in rural and isolated areas also limited the successful establishment of public health nursing programs.

## District and Visiting Nursing

Early programs of district or visiting nursing, the foundation of home health nursing as it exists today, were organized and operated by laywomen and charitable organizations, such as the Margaret Scott Nursing Mission in Winnipeg, to provide care to poor and destitute families (McKay, 2008). Working-class and lower-middle-class families also were recipients of visiting nursing services. These families could not afford to hire full-time private-duty nurses, and their homes were not large enough to provide accommodation for a nurse during the term of her employment. **District or visiting nursing** therefore provided a comprehensive array of services from bedside nursing to preventive health teaching across geographic and cultural boundaries and complexities. Pioneer nursing services such as Alberta's district nursing service provided essential emergency and obstetrical care and midwifery (Richardson, 1998). This was an early form of **primary health care**, as it encompassed access to essential curative, preventive, and health promotion services for people in their most immediate community setting—the home (World Health Organization, 1978) (see Chapter 8).

Rural community health nurses faced formidable challenges created by distance and climate. Although their urban counterparts, particularly in the early years, often walked many miles to visit homes at considerable distances from streetcar routes, urban nursing districts were measured in mere city blocks. Rural districts were enormous. One nurse stated, "I have a car for my school inspection. . . . It is the only way of covering 925 miles twice a year and paying home visits" (Matthews, 1920, p. 16). The first-hand accounts of early rural CHNs contain vivid descriptions of the various modes of transportation

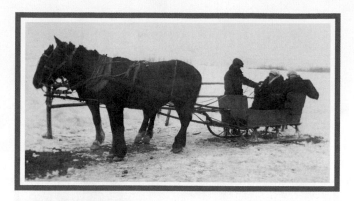

**PHOTO 1.3** Travelling by Sleigh, 1919

*Source: Glenbow Archives NA-3956-1*

used in the course of their work and the dangerous road and weather conditions in which they travelled (Colley, 1970; Giovannini, 1988; Miller, 2000; Nevitt, 1978) (see Photo 1.3).

Publicly funded healthcare programs also changed the organization and work of visiting nursing associations in several ways (McKay, 2012). In the decade immediately following World War II, most programs were unable to sustain either their funding or the quality of their nursing programs (Richardson, 1997). Although the VON continued to grow during the postwar years, it was also forced to respond to the changing face of healthcare in Canada. Expanded local and provincial departments of health took over public health programs that previously had been provided by the VON (Penney, 1996). Hospital admission became the norm for most Canadians requiring obstetrical, medical, or surgical care. This development shifted the VON visiting nursing caseloads to the care of convalescent and chronically ill individuals. Further, the erosion of charitable donations, which had at least partially offset the cost of caring for the poor in the past, meant that visiting nurses were more likely to be providing care to those who could afford to pay for these services either directly or through third-party insurance arrangements.

## Military Nursing

During the influenza epidemics, military nurses often were called upon to help care for the sick in hospitals, medical units, refugee camps, and so on. Canadian nurse Elizabeth Smellie (1884–1968), who provided leadership for the war effort, was "the first woman in the world to become a full colonel and her later career included leadership in public health, VON, and the CNA" (Toman, 2005, p. 171). **Military nursing,** in the past and today, requires the nurse to demonstrate the attributes and competencies of community health nursing: a broad vision; population health approaches; ability to adapt practice in diverse settings across the spectra of primary, secondary, and tertiary prevention; and the ethical comportment to address complex conflicts that involve violence and human justice and rights. Today, emergency preparedness and disaster nursing are essential competencies for military nurses (see Chapter 32).

## Outpost Nursing

**Outpost nursing** refers to nurses providing services in the most remote geographic locations, serving settlers and Aboriginal communities (Drees & McBain, 2001). As with district and visiting nurses, outpost nurses worked in nursing stations that often lacked the backup of physicians or emergency care services. Nonetheless, they rose to the challenge of providing essential services, including emergency care. In situations where acute medical needs took precedence, the time and resources these nurses had to deliver preventive and health promotion services were more limited (Daigle, 2008).

The relationships of these outpost nurses with the people and the communities were complex. Historians describe how these nurses were committed to learn from and integrate their nursing practice with the values and cultures of the people within the political context of the time (Drees & McBain, 2001; Rutherdale, 2008). They actively sought opportunities that combined challenging work with travel and adventure, while fulfilling their desire to use their knowledge and skills in a meaningful way (Banfill, 1967; Colley, 1970; Giovannini, 1988; Miller, 2000). (See Canadian Research Box 1.1).

### CANADIAN RESEARCH BOX 1.1

**What challenges did outpost nurses face in delivering essential health services in the rural and remote regions of Canada?**

McBain, L. (2012). Pulling up their sleeves and getting on with it: Providing health care in a northern remote region. *Canadian Bulletin of Medical History, 29*(2), 308–328.

This research on the practice and working conditions of northern Saskatchewan outpost nurses is based on an analysis of correspondence between nurses in the nursing stations and their supervisors. In the period following World War II, governments extended health services to northern and remote regions of Canada with the mission to "modernize" the people, including Aboriginal peoples and their health practices. This was to be accomplished by situating nurses in remote nursing stations. Nurses' letters to their supervisors indicate how they worked in different ways with diverse communities and how they varied in their relationships with the cultures and values of those they served. There are numerous examples of how the nurses advocated for improved conditions of their practice and resources to support their ability to provide safe care. The findings point to the challenges and hardships endured by the nurses, despite which they rose to the challenge of providing essential care and advocating for the social determinants of health for poor communities in the areas of water, sanitation, and housing. The socioeconomic welfare of the communities and of the nurses was in conflict with government resource allocation priorities and points to the importance of a professional nursing voice and power in addressing nursing practice standards and advocating for resources for underserved communities.

### Discussion Questions

1. To what extent are community health nursing services, including health promotion, accessible to people in rural, remote, and Aboriginal communities?

2. To what extent do you think that today's health education and health promotion programs contain cultural, racial, and gender biases that limit their effectiveness and create barriers between CHNs and the populations that they serve?

3. How has the nursing profession made progress in expressing its voice and power with regard to the conditions of practice and advocacy for underserved and poor communities?

## NURSING EDUCATION

The first formal nurse training program was established at the General and Marine Hospital in St. Catharines, Ontario, in 1874. Early in the development of the nursing education program, hospital-based education had a limited breadth and a limited focus on public health nursing practice. Recognizing a need, the Red Cross played a pivotal role in advancing the education of PHNs by providing funding for certificate courses in public health at five Canadian universities as early as 1919 (see Photo 1.4). Nurses, including Ethel Johns, who was the first director of the Department of Nursing at the University of British Columbia (UBC), and other Canadian nurse leaders, such as Edith Kathleen Russell, had a remarkable vision for the breadth and depth of education needed to prepare nurses and contributed to significant educational reforms needed to prepare CHNs (Carpenter, 1982; Kirkwood & Bouchard, 1992; Street, 1974; Zilm & Warbinek, 1994). In the same year, the first baccalaureate program in nursing was approved to begin at UBC; it was a five-year program in which, during the fifth and final year, students could elect a focus on public health nursing. The box (at right) shows the original outline of the short course in public health nursing, as cited in the UBC calendar. This historical record of academic and field work, similar to some of the realities of community health nursing today, required PHNs to possess the knowledge and scope of practice with a focus on maternal child programs, communicable diseases, school health, and social welfare issues.

As a specialist in education, Weir (1932) was commissioned to undertake a review of nursing education across the country and make recommendations. The report describes the types of community nursing roles, activities, salaries, and numbers of nurses who were practising public health nursing at the time. Included in the classification were "visiting nurse, school nurse, industrial nurse, Red Cross, VON, director, staff nurse and supervisor" (Weir, 1932, p. 118). One of Weir's many recommendations is that "in the immediate health interests of Canadians, as well as in their future economic interests, the number of public health nurses in Canada should at least be doubled within the next five or ten

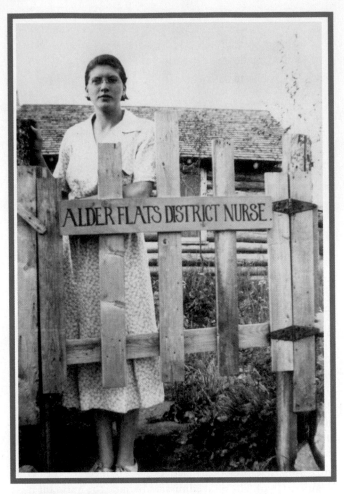

**PHOTO    1.4    Nursing student at Alder Flats, Alberta, 1937**

*Source:* Glenbow Archives NA-3952-5

### OUTLINE OF THE SHORT COURSE IN PUBLIC HEALTH NURSING, NOVEMBER 1920–MARCH 1921

*Academic Work:*

1. **Twelve lectures on each of the following:**
   a. Public Health Nursing
   b. School Hygiene
   c. Communicable Diseases
   d. Modern Social Problems
2. **Six lectures on each of the following:**
   e. Teaching Principles
   f. History of Nursing Education
   g. Social Service Problems
   h. Personal Hygiene
   i. Medical Aspects of Infant and Maternal Welfare
   j. Tuberculosis
   k. Mental Hygiene
   l. Sanitation

3. Occasional lectures on provincial legislation, municipal health departments, voluntary organizations, delinquent and deserted children, etc.

4. Excursions to special health features in and around Vancouver.

*Field Work:* For field work, the class was divided into sections of appropriate size, each of which received from one to two weeks' instruction and experience under trained workers in the actual operation of each of the following branches:

1. Urban School Nursing
2. Tuberculosis Problems
3. District Nursing
4. Health Centres and Rural School Nursing
5. Child Welfare
6. Medical, Social Service, and Relief Organizations

*Source:* UBC Calendar, 7th session, p. 36. Cited by G. Zilm & E. Warbinek. (1994). *Legacy: History of nursing education at the University of British Columbia, 1919–1994* (p. 186). Vancouver, BC: UBC Press. Copyright © 1994 by University of British Columbia. Used by permission of University of British Columbia.

years" (p. 143). The report also contains recommendations for university standards of education and support of public health nursing as a nursing specialty (Duncan, Leipert, & Mill, 1999).

Initially, diploma programs in public health nursing were also established in several Canadian universities to prepare nurses to meet the demands of the specialized practice. These programs prepared nurses without baccalaureate degrees to practice public health nursing. In the later part of the 20th century, the diploma programs in public health nursing were phased out and the baccalaureate degree became an established requirement of entry-level public health nursing.

Questions about the unique nature of public health nursing practice and competencies remain a critical nursing education issue in the 21st century. In 2014, the Canadian Association of Schools of Nursing (CASN) convened an expert task force of educators and practitioners to identify the following entry-level competencies in public health nursing practice for undergraduate nursing students:

■ public health sciences in nursing practice;
■ population and community health assessment and analysis;
■ population health planning, implementation and evaluation;
■ partnerships, collaboration and advocacy; and
■ communication in public health nursing (CASN, 2014).

Each competency domain encompasses the knowledge, skill, and attitudes essential for nursing practice (Tardif, 2006). Specific indicators contained within each domain further define the competency domains. These competencies emphasize the importance of developing and applying knowledge to address the determinants of health, building relationships with communities, and understanding the critical relationships among individual, family, and population health. It is significant to ponder how the competencies required of today's graduating students compare with those of early CHNs. Today's nursing education programs are challenged to balance opportunities for practice education in institutional settings and illness care with that of community health nursing and health promotion. Although these competencies relate specifically to the discipline of public health nursing, it is recognized that all nursing graduates have this preparation. In the face of these educational goals and challenges, one is reminded of the central role of community health nursing practice as the impetus for the ongoing evolution and advancement of baccalaureate nursing education.

## MID-20TH CENTURY: EVOLUTION OF COMMUNITY HEALTH NURSING

Increased government responsibility for the healthcare of Canadians also had a significant impact on public health nursing. Between 1940 and 1970, health departments focused on the expansion of existing programs. However, this process also included a general shift of emphasis from traditional programs such as child health, immunization, and communicable disease control to programs focusing on the reduction of morbidity and mortality from chronic illnesses and injuries. The early postpartum discharge home-visiting program placed significant demands on the time and resources of PHNs. In some instances, staffing patterns in health units and community health centres were modified to provide seven-day-a-week early postpartum services to mothers and neonates.

In the early 1970s, rising hospital costs created both an opportunity and a crisis for the VON. Patients were discharged from the hospital earlier and required longer and more complex follow-up care in the community. However, these individuals were often unable to obtain bedside nursing care in their homes during their convalescence. No publicly insured programs for home care services existed until 1974, when the first such program was established in Manitoba (Shapiro, 1997). The VON realized that participation in publicly insured home care programs provided an opportunity to both consolidate and strengthen its organization. It commissioned a national report, which recommended that Canada's oldest and most experienced visiting nursing organization be given the mandate to deliver publicly insured home care programs (Pickering, 1976). However, individual provincial governments made a variety of decisions about the organization and funding of home care programs, and these decisions did not always include the VON. Today, as it did in the past, the VON continues to function by offering a mix of services shaped by local circumstances, with a particular focus on creating programs to respond to unmet needs among specific segments of the population (Penney, 1996).

During this time, community mental health nursing emerged in the 1960s and 1970s in response to the deinstitutionalization of patients with mental illnesses. Community mental health nurses practising through this transition pioneered their new roles in the complex interface between psychiatry and nursing and between community and institutional care (Boschma, 2012).

Significant pressures on healthcare systems arising from the economic recession of the 1980s caused widespread loss of nursing positions in all sectors of healthcare, which was most evident in the downsizing of hospitals. Particularly problematic was the trend to replace nurses who provided clinical leadership with managers who lacked this capacity, a trend that continues to impact the development of nursing today. The mantra of governments was, and continues to be, replacement of hospital-based care with community health services and home care, although this trend has yet to be fully realized. Publicly funded home care programs had resulted in some growth in the number of nurses working in community settings. However, the role of home health nurses, who provide nursing care and health education to the sick and convalescent in the home, is similar to that fulfilled by the visiting nurses of the late 19th and early 20th centuries. The number of PHNs, however, had not increased. Their mandate has continued to emphasize health promotion, communicable disease control, healthy child development, prevention of chronic illness, and identification of other factors that cause morbidity and mortality in the population.

The reduction in government spending during the 1980s and 1990s affected CHNs in all programs, both directly and indirectly. Static or reduced nursing staff numbers decreased the levels of service for many programs. Infrastructure for communicable disease control was particularly hard hit. The loss of capacity to monitor, identify, and follow up on communicable diseases has been identified as one of the major reasons for the resurgence of TB and the recent emergence of new diseases such as acquired immune deficiency syndrome (AIDS), severe acute respiratory syndrome (SARS), and H1N1 influenza (Garrett, 1994, 2000). Deinstitutionalization of patients from acute care and psychiatric institutions has resulted in the need for innovative and comprehensive community-based healthcare programs and systems. Nursing leadership for the development of essential programs to meet client needs has become more important than ever. (See Canadian Research Box 1.2.)

### CANADIAN RESEARCH BOX 1.2

**How did nurses provide leadership for the development of community mental health nursing services within the policy context of deinstitutionalization?**

Boschma, G. (2012). Community mental health nursing in Alberta, Canada: An oral history. *Nursing History Review, 20,* 103–135.

This nursing history case study chronicles the role transition of nurses within the institutional setting of the large psychiatric hospital to their leadership in establishing community mental health services in the 1960s and 1970s. The policy context of deinstitutionalization of patients with chronic psychiatric illnesses included the poor conditions in large psychiatric institutions and the advent of psychotropic drugs. During this period of transformative and social change in psychiatry and mental healthcare, nursing leadership played a key role in establishing community-based services and a continuum of mental health services. As there are today, there were issues of inadequate funding of community-based services despite the needs of a vulnerable population living with mental health challenges and psychiatric illnesses. The author concluded that communities and institutions were closely connected, although in new and different forms.

#### Discussion Questions

1. How would one characterize the relationship between institutional or hospital-based care and community health services in today's context of community mental health or home care?

2. How do nurses provide essential leadership for the establishment of community-based services, and what inspiration can be taken from nurses who have accomplished this in the past?

## LATE 20TH CENTURY: THE NEW PUBLIC HEALTH—PRIMARY HEALTH CARE AND HEALTH PROMOTION

The WHO adopted the Declaration of Alma-Ata at the 1978 International Conference on Primary Health Care and declared primary health care as the guiding vision for achieving health for all people. Since then, the WHO has consistently recognized nursing as the essential global workforce for achieving primary health care goals (WHO, 1978; 1989). Harnessing the skills and knowledge of community health nurses is essential to achieving health equity, building on the historic foundation of how nurses have contributed to building essential services for people in their communities and advancing health systems.

CHNs have provided leadership for advancing the understanding and integration of primary health care principles in our Canadian healthcare system (see Chapter 2). The CNA (1980) submitted an influential brief titled "Putting Health into Health Care" to the federal government to review its health system. This was CNA's nationwide lobbying effort to endorse primary health care and health promotion.

Canada has provided leadership in the evolution of health promotion. Its landmark documents, the Lalonde Report (1974) and the Ottawa Charter for Health Promotion (WHO, 1986), sparked a public health movement that focused the understanding of health and its determinants as value-based processes and identified broad health promotion strategies that remain foundational to community health nursing practice and to nursing education (see Chapter 3).

In 1987, the formation of the **Community Health Nurses Association of Canada (CHNAC)**, an official interest group of the CNA, marked a significant period of progress. Since that time, the CHNAC has evolved to become the Community Health Nurses of Canada (CHNC), with a vision for developing strategic organizational partnerships, advancing the practice of community health nursing, and refining the role and the standards of practice. The CHNC (2011, revised) has a mandate to advance the practice of community health nursing through role definition, the development of standards and theory development, and research. It has also developed a professional practice model for Canadian community health nursing, specifying seven standards as "benchmarks of excellence that define the practice of a registered nurse in the specialty area of community health nursing" (CHNC, 2011, revised, p. 7) (Appendix A). These current standards and competencies relate to the practice of public health nurses and home health nurses with a minimum of two years' experience (Appendices B and C). In the standards there is continuity with the early practice of nurses working in the community to promote health, prevent illness, advocate for services, partner with community organizations and women's groups, and provide courageous leadership for the establishment of essential services for vulnerable populations. Canadian CHNs build on the legacy of the early nurses as they advance their practice to achieve the present-day goal of global health equity (Reutter & Kushner, 2010).

## 21ST CENTURY PROSPECTIVE: CONTINUITY WITH THEMES OF THE PAST

Events in the first decade of the 21st century continue to shape community health nursing. The Romanow Commission's report titled "Building on Values: The Future of Health Care in Canada" continues to be recognized as a visionary document with recommendations for shifting resources and policy in the direction of primary health care, home healthcare, and health promotion, with nurses as the key players in the transformation of systems and services (Romanow, 2002). However, many of these recommendations have been slow to take shape. Another pivotal event was the formation of the Public Health Agency of Canada (PHAC) in 2004 after the SARS crisis. It was created "in response to growing concerns about the capacity of Canada's public health system to anticipate and respond effectively to public health threats" (PHAC, 2014, para. 1). In its first decade, the PHAC has drawn attention to the need to develop a sustainable public health workforce, including nursing, while emphasizing a vision of intersectoral policy development and interprofessional collaboration.

As in the past, CHNs of today must assume a strong policy advocacy role to ensure that essential nursing care and services are accessible to communities. PHNs must increasingly focus their practice on the social determinants of health and examine the evidence pointing to the causes of poor health that are rooted in societal inequities and how marginalized populations experience homelessness, addiction, poverty, and injustice (Reutter & Kushner, 2010). This mandate is often difficult to

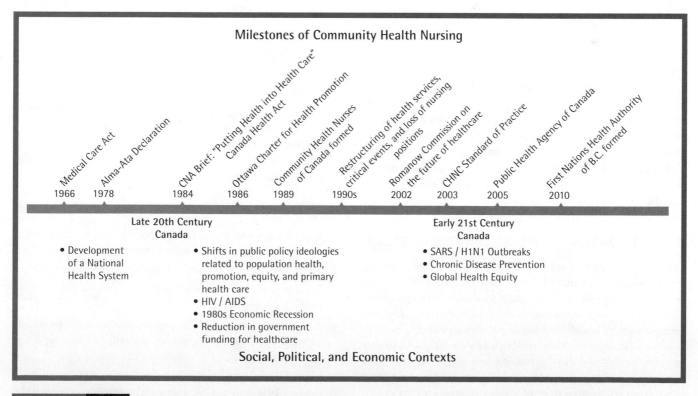

**FIGURE 1.2** Critical Events Influencing the Milestones of Community Health Nursing, Mid-1960s to Present

achieve in hierarchical organizational structures, where there may be barriers to nurses voicing concerns and taking political action for change (Falk-Rafael & Betker, 2012).

Hardill (2006) pointed out that, besides PHNs and the VON from the early days, CHNs can be inspired by the earliest forms of "street nursing" practised by the Grey Nuns who cared for the "sick poor, in 18th century Quebec" (p. 91). Modern street nursing has been traced to Vancouver in 1946, when nurses began to provide antibiotic treatment and contact tracing for venereal diseases. Today, there is a strong legacy of CHNs' outreach, care, and advocacy to address the social and living conditions of those most vulnerable members of society. CHNs can therefore be inspired by their roots of activism, advocacy, and outreach while finding ways to meet their standard of "facilitating access and equity and ensuring that resources are distributed equitably throughout the population and reach the people who need them the most" (CHNC, 2011, revised, p. 20).

In its earliest form, school nursing encompassed issues of the nurses' relationships with children, families, and the community as a whole. In fact, general public health nursing programs emerged from school nursing, whereas today PHNs are working to redefine their roles in schools, which became narrow and diminished in scope during the latter part of the 20th century. A renewed vision of comprehensive school health is revitalizing and extending the work of PHNs in schools; nurses can refer with pride to their legacy of contributions to school health over the past century (see Chapter 18).

It is significant that the early practice of community health nursing was generalist in nature, consisting of a comprehensive range of services, including home healthcare and health promotion. Nursing roles became differentiated and specialized over time in response to social, economic, and political forces, including the expanding knowledge of society.

Today, the competencies and role descriptions for public health, home health, community mental health, and occupational health are distinct forms of community health nursing in Canada (see Chapters 3–5, 23, and 27). Home health nursing is also undergoing specialization in the key areas of palliative care, chronic illness prevention and care, and long-term care. CHNs must also be equipped with knowledge about Aboriginal health, emergency disaster preparedness, and global health (see Chapters 22, 32, and 33). In all areas, there is significant advancement in theory and research to support best practices and the development of the nursing profession into the 21st century. (See Figure 1.2.)

## CONCLUSION

CHN practice has evolved to address the impact that political, economic, and other macrosystems have on individual, family, aggregate, and population health. Knowledge development in health promotion, advocacy, healthy public policy, and the determinants of health enabled nurses to shape their practices in ways that sought to engage both healthcare professionals and community members in finding new and innovative ways to achieve health for all. More about these ideas and their application to the practices of CHNs is presented in subsequent chapters of this text.

As one reflects on the legacy of CHNs over the past three centuries, it is easy to recognize how the early practice of nurses was focused on promoting the health of individuals, families, populations, and communities, and included the prevention of infectious diseases. These nurses worked in partnership with women's groups and the communities they served to develop essential services, address what is now referred to as the social determinants of health, and advocate for marginalized and vulnerable people. The education for CHNs was developed by courageous leaders who had the vision for the difference that these nurses can make. It is this legacy that positioned CHNs to continue and expand to meet the health goals for the 21st century.

Many factors that influenced the early development of community health nursing exist even today. The need to address health and social inequities among First Nations communities, immigrant and refugee health, and communicable and non-communicable disease prevention remain priorities today as in the past. A source of inspiration is found in the history of how nurses worked in partnership with, and gained strength from, dominant social movements and women's groups, and how they influenced policy in the development of health programs and organizations. Advocacy to increase the numbers of CHNs in all roles must remain a priority.

Finally, while the past inspires a vision for community health nursing in the 21st century, one must also acknowledge the vision and contributions of present-day leaders, including students who will move community health nursing forward to new heights. In their final editorial after editing the journal *Public Health Nursing* for a decade, editors Abrams and Hays (2013) leave us with the vision that can apply to all forms of community health nursing today: "On the shoulders of younger giants, public health nursing moves forward" (p. 475).

## KEY TERMS

Community Health Nurses Association of Canada (CHNAC), p. 11
district or visiting nursing, p. 6
military nursing, p. 7
outpost nursing, p. 7
primary health care, p. 6
public health nurse, p. 4

## STUDY QUESTIONS

1. Describe the two forms of community health nursing that evolved in Canada in the early 20th century.

2. Summarize the early forms of community health nursing.

3. Which populations were the focus of early community nursing programs?

4. Briefly describe three of the earliest public health programs in which nurses were involved and the reasons for their implementation.

5. How did the British North America Act (1867) and 19th century beliefs about the role of government influence the development of community health services?

6. Discuss how community health nursing contributed to the advancement of nursing education.

7. Describe the role that non-governmental organizations, such as the VON, the Red Cross, and local philanthropic agencies, played in the development of community health nursing programs.

After working through these questions, go to the MyNursingLab at www.pearsoned.ca/mynursinglab to check your answers.

## INDIVIDUAL CRITICAL-THINKING EXERCISES

The sources listed at the end of some of these questions are cited in full in the references section. Each source will provide additional insights into the controversies and debates surrounding the history of public health and visiting nursing.

1. Meryn Stuart (1987), in her analysis of the development of rural public health nursing in northern Ontario, states, "The Board's focus on health education, however delivered by the nurses, would not erase the effects of poverty. . . . Health education was a facile solution to the serious problem of the lack of permanent human and material resources" (p. 111). Analyze the apparent lack of congruency between the needs of the populations that public health programs served and the typical services that these programs offered. (*Sources:* Piva, 1979; Stuart, 1987)

2. Physicians and nurses assumed different roles in early community health organizations. What role did gender play in the assignment of these roles? (*Sources:* McPherson, 1996, Chapter 1; Stuart, 1992)

3. Community health nursing has frequently been described as more autonomous than nursing practice in institutional settings. However, Eunice Dyke, Toronto's first supervisor of public health nursing, once stated that "public health nursing has in the medical profession its greatest friend and not infrequently its greatest stumbling block." How autonomous was the practice of early community health nurses? (*Sources:* Comacchio, 1993; Stuart, 1992)

4. What role did middle-class ideas about class, ethnicity, and gender play in the development of public health programs to protect the health of infants and children? (*Sources:* Comacchio, 1993; Gleason, 2002; Chapter 3)

5. Reflecting on community health nursing education in your nursing program, what issues do you see that are continuous with the past as described in this chapter?

6. Examine the community health nursing programs available in your community. Taken as a whole, do all of these programs cover the practice of community health nursing as discussed in this text? Is the breadth of competencies of public health and home health nursing roles expressed?

## GROUP CRITICAL-THINKING EXERCISES

1. Social historians such as Alan Hunt (1999) argue that charity, philanthropy, and welfare programs are essentially efforts by the elite and middle classes to impose their behaviour, values, and culture upon others. Hunt describes these programs of moral or social regulation as being inspired by ". . . the passionate conviction that there is something inherently wrong or immoral about the conduct of others" (p. ix). Locate an issue of an early public health or nursing journal such as *The Public Health Journal* (now the *Canadian Journal of Public Health*) or *The Canadian Nurse* (particularly the section on public health). Conduct a brief content analysis of the issue, paying close attention to how the recipients of public health interventions are described. What conclusions can be drawn about the attitudes of healthcare professionals? What anxieties seem to underlie the interventions they describe and recommend to other healthcare practitioners?

2. Nurses were the intermediaries between the clients they served and the social and political elite who employed them to work in the community. However, their perspective on the objectives and effectiveness of community health programs is often absent from published histories of public health. To fill this gap in the historical record, do one of the following: (1) locate a biographical account written by an early visiting or public health nurse, (2) locate an oral history of an early visiting or public health nurse in an archive, or (3) interview a retired visiting or public health nurse. How do their accounts resemble or differ from the history of community health nursing presented in this chapter? How would you account for any differences you identify?

3. Based on what you have learned about the history of community health nursing in Canada, what do you believe are the greatest challenges facing nurses in this practice setting today and in the future?

## REFERENCES

Aboriginal Nurses Association of Canada. (2007). *Twice as good: A history of Aboriginal nurses.* Ottawa, ON: Author.

Abrams, S. E., & Hays, J. C. (2013). On the shoulders of younger giants public health nursing moves forward. *Public Health Nursing, 30*(6), 475–476. Published by John Wiley & Sons, Inc, © 2013.

Allemang, M. (2000). Development of community health nursing in Canada. In M. J. Stewart (Ed.), *Community nursing: Promoting Canada's health* (2nd ed., pp. 4–32). Toronto, ON: W. B. Saunders.

Armstrong-Reid, S. (2014). *Lyle Creelman: The frontiers of global nursing.* Toronto, ON: University of Toronto Press.

Baldwin, D. O. (1997). *She answered every call: The life of public health nurse Mona Gordon Wilson (1894–1981).* Charlottetown, PE: Indigo Press.

Banfill, B. J. (1967). *Pioneer nurse.* Toronto, ON: Ryerson Press.

Benoit, C., & Carroll, D. (2005). Canadian midwifery: Blending traditional and modern practices. In C. Bates, D. Dodd, & N. Rousseau (Eds.), *On all frontiers: Four centuries of*

*Canadian nursing* (pp. 27–41). Ottawa, ON: University of Ottawa Press.

Boschma, G. (2012). Community mental health nursing in Alberta, Canada: An oral history. *Nursing History Review, 20,* 103–135. doi:10.1891/1062-8061.20.103. Copyright © 2012 by University of British Columbia. Used by permission of University of British Columbia.

Bourque Bearskin, R. L. (2011). A critical lens on culture in nursing practice. *Nursing Ethics,* 1–12. doi:10.1177/0969733011480048

Bourque Bearskin, R. L. (2014). *Mâmawoh kamâtowin: Coming together to help each other: Honouring indigenous nursing knowledge.* (Unpublished doctoral dissertation). University of Alberta Faculty of Nursing, Edmonton, Alberta.

Boutillier, B. (1994). Helpers or heroines? The National Council of Women, Nursing and "Women's Work" in late Victorian Canada. In D. Dodd & D. Gorham (Eds.), *Caring and curing: Historical perspectives on women and healing in Canada* (pp. 17–48). Ottawa, ON: University of Ottawa Press.

Burnett, K. (2008). The healing work of Aboriginal women in indigenous and newcomer communities. In J. Elliot, M. Stuart, & C. Toman. (Eds.), *Place and practice in Canadian nursing history* (pp. 40–52). Vancouver, BC: UBC Press.

Canadian Association of Schools of Nursing. (2014). *Entry-to-practice public health nursing competencies for undergraduate nursing education.* Ottawa, ON: Author.

Canadian Nurses Association. (1980). *Putting health into health care: Submission to the Health Services Review.* Ottawa, ON: Author.

Carpenter, H. (1982). *A divine discontent: Edith Kathleen Russell, reforming educator.* Toronto, ON: University of Toronto Faculty of Nursing.

City of Winnipeg Health Department. (1910). *Annual report for the year ending December 1909.* Winnipeg, MB: City of Winnipeg.

Colley, K. B. (1970). *While rivers flow: Stories of early Alberta.* Saskatoon, SK: Prairie Books.

Comacchio, C. (1993). *Nations are built of babies: Saving Ontario's mothers and children 1900–1940.* Montreal, QC: McGill-Queen's University Press.

Community Health Nurses of Canada. (2011, revised). *Canadian community health nursing professional practice model and standards of practice.* St. John's, NL: Author.

Daigle, J. (2008). The call of the North: Settlement nurses in the remote areas of Quebec. In J. Elliot, M. Stuart, & C. Toman (Eds.), *Place and practice in Canadian nursing history* (pp. 111–135). Vancouver, BC: UBC Press.

D'Antonio, P. (2006). History for a practice profession. *Nursing Inquiry, 13*(4), 242–248.

Dodd, D., Elliot, J., & Rousseau, N. (2005). Outpost nursing in Canada. In C. Bates, D. Dodd, & N. Rousseau (Eds.), *On all frontiers: Four centuries of Canadian nursing* (pp. 139–152). Ottawa, ON: University of Ottawa Press.

Drees, L. M., & McBain, L. (2001). Nursing and native peoples in northern Saskatchewan, 1930s–1950s. *Canadian Bulletin of Medical History, 18,* 43–65.

Duncan, S. M., Leipert, B. D., & Mill, J. E. (1999). Nurses as health evangelists? The evolution of public health nursing in Canada, 1918–1939. *Advances in Nursing Science, 22*(1), 40–51.

Ewart, M. (1916). Home visiting in connection with school nursing. *The Canadian Nurse, XII*(6), 307–309.

Falk-Rafael, A. (2005). Speaking truth to power: Nursing's legacy and moral imperative. *Advances in Nursing Science, 28*(2), 222.

Falk-Rafael, A., & Betker, C. (2012). The primacy of relationships: A study of public health nursing from a critical caring perspective. *Advances in Nursing Science, 35*(4), 315–332. doi:10.1097/ANS.ObO13e318271d127

Fee, E., & Bu, L. (2010). The origins of public health nursing: The Henry Street Visiting Service. *American Journal of Public Health, 100*(7), 1206–1207.

Garrett, L. (1994). *The coming plague: Newly emerging diseases in a world out of balance.* New York, NY: Penguin Books.

Garrett, L. (2000). *Betrayal of trust: The collapse of global public health.* New York, NY: Hyperion Press.

Gibbon, J. M. (1947). *The Victorian Order of Nurses for Canada: 50th anniversary, 1897–1947.* Montreal, QC: Southam Press.

Gibbon, J. M., & Mathewson, M. (1947). *Three centuries of Canadian nursing.* Toronto, ON: Macmillan Co. of Canada.

Giovannini, M. (1988). *Outpost nurse.* St. John's, NL: Memorial University Faculty of Medicine.

Gleason, M. (2002). Race, class and health: School medical inspection and "healthy" children in British Columbia, 1890–1930. *Canadian Bulletin of Medical History/Bulletin Canadien d'histoire de la médicine, 19*(1), 85–112.

Green, H. G. (1974). *Don't have your baby in the dory! A biography of Myra Bennett.* Montreal, QC: Harvest House.

Hardill, K. (2006). From the Grey Nuns to the streets: A critical history of outreach nursing in Canada. *Public Health Nursing, 24*(1), 91–97.

Hunt, A. (1999). *Governing morals: A social history of moral regulation.* Cambridge, UK: Cambridge University Press.

Keddy, B., & Dodd, D. (2005). The trained nurse: Private duty and VON home nursing (Late 1800s to 1940s). In C. Bates, D. Dodd, & N. Rousseau (Eds.), *On all frontiers: Four centuries of Canadian nursing* (pp. 43–56). Ottawa, ON: University of Ottawa Press.

Kelm, M. E. (1998). *Colonizing bodies: Aboriginal health and healing in British Columbia 1900–50.* Vancouver, BC: UBC Press.

Kirkwood, R., & Bouchard, J. (1992). *"Take counsel with one another": A beginning history of the Canadian Association of University Schools of Nursing 1942–1992.* Ottawa, ON: Canadian Association of University Schools of Nursing.

Lalonde, M. (1974). *A new perspective on the health of Canadians.* Ottawa, ON: Government of Canada.

Larsen, J., & Baumgart, A. J. (1992). Introduction to nursing in Canada. In A. Baumgart & J. Larsen (Eds.), *Canadian nursing faces the future* (pp. 3–22). St. Louis, MO: Mosby.

Locke, H. L. F. (1918). The problem of our infant population with special reference to the opportunity of the welfare nurse. *American Journal of Nursing, 18*(7), 523–526.

MacDougall, H. (1990). *Activists and advocates: Toronto's Health Department, 1883–1983.* Toronto, ON: Dundurn Press.

MacNutt, J. S. (1913). The Board of Health nurse: What she can do for the public welfare in a small city. *American Journal of Public Health, 3*(4), 344–350.

Matthews, O. (1920). Child welfare. *The Canadian Nurse, 16*(1), 15–16.

McKay, M. (2005). Public health nursing. In C. Bates, D. Dodd, & N. Rousseau (Eds.), *On all frontiers: Four centuries of Canadian nursing* (pp. 107–123). Ottawa, ON: University of Ottawa Press.

McKay, M. (2008). Region, faith and health: The development of Winnipeg's visiting nursing agencies. In J. Elliot, M. Stuart, & C. Toman (Eds.), *Place and practice in Canadian nursing history* (pp. 70–90). Vancouver, BC: UBC Press.

McKay, M. (2012). The history of community health nursing in Canada. In L. L. Stamler & L. Yiu (Eds.), *Community health nursing: A Canadian perspective* (3rd ed., pp. 1–20). Toronto, ON: Pearson Canada.

McPherson, K. (1996). *Bedside matters: The transformation of Canadian nursing, 1900–1990.* Toronto, ON: Oxford University Press.

Meigs, G. L. (1916, August). Other factors in infant mortality than the milk supply and their control. *American Journal of Public Health, 6,* 847–853.

Miller, G. L. (2000). *Mustard plasters and handcars: Through the eyes of a Red Cross outpost nurse.* Toronto, ON: Natural Heritage/Natural History.

Nevitt, J. (1978). *White caps and black bands: Nursing in Newfoundland to 1934.* St. John's, NL: Jefferson Press.

Nightingale, F. (1859/1946). *Notes on nursing.* London, UK: Harrison & Sons; Philadelphia, PA: Lippincott.

Paul, P. (2005). Religious nursing orders of Canada: A presence on all western frontiers. In C. Bates, D. Dodd, & N. Rousseau (Eds.), *On all frontiers: Four centuries of Canadian nursing* (pp. 125–138). Ottawa, ON: University of Ottawa Press.

Paul, P., & Ross-Kerr, J. C. (2011). Nursing in Canada, 1600 to the present: A brief account. In J. C. Ross-Kerr & M. J. Wood (Eds.), *Canadian nursing issues and perspectives* (5th ed., pp. 18–41). Toronto, ON: Elsevier.

Peikoff, T., & Brickey, S. (1991). Creating precious children and glorified mothers: A theoretical assessment of the transformation of childhood. In R. Smandych, G. Dodds, & A. Esau (Eds.), *Dimensions of childhood: Essays on the history of children and youth in Canada* (pp. 29–61). Winnipeg, MB: Legal Research Institute of the University of Manitoba.

Penney, S. (1996). *A century of caring: The history of the Victorian Order of Nurses for Canada.* Ottawa, ON: Victorian Order of Nurses for Canada.

Pickering, E. A. (1976). *A case for the VON in home care.* Ottawa, ON: Victorian Order of Nurses for Canada.

Piva, M. J. (1979). *The condition of the working class in Toronto, 1900–1921.* Ottawa, ON: University of Ottawa Press.

Public Health Agency of Canada. (2014). *History.* ©All rights reserved. Public Health Agency of Canada. Reproduced with permission from the Minister of Health, 2015. Retrieved from http://www.phac-aspc.gc.ca/about_apropos/history-eng.php

Reutter, L., & Kushner, L. (2010). Health equity through action on the social determinants of health: Taking up the challenge in nursing. *Nursing Inquiry, 17,* 269–280.

Richardson, S. (1997). Women's enterprise: Establishing the Lethbridge Nursing Mission, 1909–1919. *Nursing History Review, 5,* 105–130.

Richardson, S. (1998). Political women, professional nurses, and the creation of Alberta's district nursing service, 1919–1925. *Nursing History Review, 6,* 25–50.

Riddell, S. E. (1991). *Curing society's ills: Public health nurses and public health nursing in rural British Columbia, 1916–1946.* Unpublished master's thesis, Simon Fraser University, Vancouver, BC.

Romanow, R. (2002). *Building on values: The future of health care in Canada.* Ottawa, ON: Government of Canada.

Rutherdale, M. (2008). Cleansers, cautious caregivers, and optimistic adventurers: A proposed typology of Arctic Canadian nurses 1945–70. In J. Elliot, M. Stuart, & C. Toman (Eds.), *Place and practice in Canadian nursing history* (pp. 53–69). Vancouver, BC: UBC Press.

Sears, A. (1995). Before the welfare state: Public health and social policy. *Canadian Review of Sociology and Anthropology/Revue canadienne de sociologie et d'anthropologie, 32*(2), 169–188.

Shapiro, E. (1997). *The cost of privatization: A case study of home care in Manitoba.* Ottawa, ON: Canadian Centre for Policy Alternatives.

Street. M. (1974). *Watch-fires on the mountains.* Toronto, ON: University of Toronto Press.

Stuart, M. E. (1987). *"Let not the people perish for lack of knowledge": Public health nursing and the Ontario rural child welfare project, 1916–1930.* (Unpublished doctoral dissertation). University of Pennsylvania, Philadelphia.

Stuart, M. (1992). "Half a loaf is better than no bread": Public health nurses and physicians in Ontario, 1920–1925. *Nursing Research, 41*(1), 21–27.

Sutherland, N. (1981). "To create a strong and healthy race": School children in the public health movement, 1880–1914. In S. E. D. Short (Ed.), *Medicine in Canadian society: Historical perspectives* (pp. 361–393). Montreal, QC: McGill–Queen's University Press.

Tardif, J. (2006). *L'évaluation des compétences: Documenter le parcours de développement.* Montréal, QC: Chenelier Education.

Toman, C. (2005). "Ready, Aye, Ready": Canadian military nurses as an expandable and expendable workforce (1920–2000). In C. Bates, D. Dodd, & N. Rousseau (Eds.). *On all frontiers: Four centuries of Canadian nursing* (pp. 169–182). Ottawa, ON: University of Ottawa Press.

Weir, G. M. (1932). *Survey of nursing education in Canada.* Toronto, ON: University of Toronto Press.

World Health Organization. (1978, September). *Primary health care: Report on the international conference on primary health care, Alma Ata, USSR, 6–12 September.* Geneva, Switzerland: Author.

World Health Organization. (1986, November). *The Ottawa charter for health promotion.* First International Conference on Health Promotion, Ottawa, ON. Retrieved from http://www.who.int/healthpromotion/conferences/previous/ottawa/en/index1.html

World Health Organization. (1989). *The role of nursing and mid-wifery personnel in the strategy of health for all.* Geneva, Switzerland: Author.

Yarmie, A. (2013). *Women caring for Kamloops 1890–1975.* Kamloops, BC: Textual Studies in Canada and the Kamloops Museum and Archives.

Zilm, G., & Warbinek, E. (1994). *Legacy: History of nursing education at the University of British Columbia, 1919–1994.* Vancouver, BC: UBC Press.

Zilm, G., & Warbinek, E. (2002). Profile of a leader: Elizabeth Breeze. *Canadian Journal of Nursing Leadership, 15*(3), 28–29.

**ABOUT THE AUTHOR**

**Susan Duncan**, RN, PhD, holds baccalaureate, master's, and doctoral degrees in nursing. She began her career as a public health nurse on the east side of Vancouver. She teaches and conducts research in the areas of population health, health ethics and policy, and community health nursing education. She is a Professor in the School of Nursing at Thompson Rivers University in Kamloops, British Columbia, where she has for many years shared her passion for public health nursing practice, history, and research. She contributes to the development of public health nursing nationally as a member of the Canadian Association of Schools of Nursing Task Force on Public Health Nursing Education.

## ACKNOWLEDGEMENT

The author acknowledges nurse historian Dr. Marion McKay, the author of the previous version of this chapter, whose work continues to provide a foundation for this presentation of the history of community health nursing in Canada.

# Financing, Policy, and Politics of Healthcare Delivery

*Claire Betker and Diane Bewick*

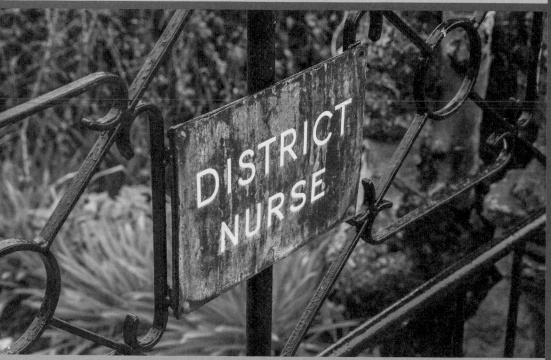

*Source: Mr Doomits/Shutterstock*

LEARNING OUTCOMES

**After studying this chapter, you should be able to:**

1. Summarize milestones in the development of the Canadian healthcare system with a focus on community health.

2. Identify federal, provincial or territorial, regional, and municipal responsibilities for healthcare in Canada.

3. Identify models for the delivery of community healthcare that are used in Canada.

4. Examine delivery models and funding mechanisms for healthcare in Canada, specifically those that apply to community healthcare.

5. Discuss the leadership role that community health nurses (CHNs) play in promoting the health of people, communities, and populations.

6. Discuss the leadership role that organizations and associations play in supporting community health nursing practice that promotes the health of people, communities, and populations.

## INTRODUCTION

A community health nurse's professional practice can occur in a wide range of settings. In their professional practice, CHNs are "accountable to a variety of authorities and stakeholders—the public, the regulatory body, and the employer—and are governed by legislative and policy mandates from multiple sources both internal and external to their employment situation" (Meagher-Stewart et al., 2004, p. 3). The structure, process, and leadership within the organizations and agencies in which CHNs work affect their practice, enabling and constraining it through funding, governance, values, policies, goals, and standards (Ganann et al., 2010; Meagher-Stewart et al., 2004; Molina-Mula & De Pedro-Gómez, 2012; Underwood et al., 2009). **Leadership** is about influence at all levels of an organization.

Almost every day, reports in the media suggest that healthcare in Canada is in crisis, that spending is out of control, that wait times are unreasonable, and that substantive changes are needed to ensure sustainability of the healthcare system. At the same time, there has been a repetitive chorus regarding the significance of health promotion and prevention as well as the critical role of public and community health in addressing the determinants of health and advancing health equity (Canadian Nurses Association, 2012b; Mahony & Jones, 2013; Reutter & Kushner, 2010; World Health Organization, 2008). It is important for CHNs to understand how Canada's healthcare system evolved and what factors influence how it is governed today. The impact of leadership at all levels has been identified as a particularly significant factor in the evolution of the healthcare system and in supporting community health nursing practice (Bekemeier, Grembowski, Yang, & Herting, 2012; Cummings et al., 2010). Throughout this evolution, CHN practice has changed. The last section of the chapter will discuss key issues in Canada for CHNs at this time in history.

## HISTORICAL MILESTONES IN CANADIAN HEALTHCARE

Between the 16th and 18th centuries, tens of thousands of people immigrated to Canada, "the new world," in search of a better future. With them came significant communicable diseases and social issues. In 1832, the first quarantine station, known as Grosse Isle, was established in an attempt to assess all newcomers and isolate those arriving with communicable diseases such as cholera and typhus. This island, located in the St. Lawrence River near Quebec City, remained in operation until 1932 and is now a national historic park. The realization that individuals and communities could do something to stop the spread of disease and benefit from early detection was known as the "sanitary" idea.

Following Confederation in Canada, additional community health strategies were introduced, such as public education; gathering and analyzing statistics; sewage and drinking water management; and maternal, infant, and child health care. In 1882, Ontario became the first provincial government to establish a full-time provincial board of health (with a $4000 budget). The Hudson's Bay Company took on the role and functions of the public health board in western Canada.

Although the 1867 Constitution Act (also known as the British North America Act) did not explicitly assign responsibility for health policy to either the federal government or the provincial governments, both levels of government have been involved in ensuring the availability of and funding for health services. The Act does contain an equalization clause requiring provinces to provide "reasonably comparable levels of public service for reasonably comparable levels of taxation" (Sullivan & Baranek, 2002, p. 21).

Canada currently has a national, universal health insurance program, with the first policy implemented at the provincial level in Saskatchewan, where, in 1947, Tommy Douglas and the Cooperative Commonwealth Federation (CCF) party introduced legislation to institute **medicare**, or publicly funded healthcare, in that province. This is why Tommy Douglas is referred to as the "father of medicare." It was not until 10 years later, in 1957, that similar legislation, the Hospital Insurance and Diagnostic Services Act (HIDS), was passed by the Government of Canada (Rachlis & Kushner, 1994). This legislation provided for the federal government's payment of half the costs of insurance plans if key criteria were met.

Because provincial and territorial wealth varies considerably, the federal government's involvement has been necessary to equalize services across provinces and territories. Since 1957, the federal government has done that in two ways: first, by contributing money (in effect, transferring money from wealthier to poorer provinces and territories) and, second, by stipulating specific conditions that the provinces and territories must meet in order to receive that money. On December 12, 1983, Monique Bégin, the then Federal Minister of Health and Welfare, introduced Bill C-3, or the Canada Health Act, to Parliament. This piece of legislation was to be current for 30 years (to April 16, 2014), and it provided direction for the cash contributions to be made by the federal government. The purpose of the Act was to "establish criteria and conditions in respect of insured health services and extended healthcare services provided under provincial law that must be met before a full cash contribution may be made" (Canada, House of Commons, 1984, p. 5). Bégin faced tough opposition to the Act from lobby groups, opposition parties, and even from members of the Liberal cabinet (Bégin, 2002). Intense lobbying and support by the Canadian Nurses Association was instrumental in the bill being passed. In the words of Begin, "Nursing became a big player during the Canada Health Act. They made the difference; it's as simple as that" (Rafael, 1997). The **Canadian Nurses Association (CNA)** is the national professional voice of registered nurses in Canada. The invaluable support provided by Canadian nurses was acknowledged by the Honourable Monique Bégin at the Canadian Public Health Association (CPHA) conference in Toronto in June 2010. She noted that not only were nurses instrumental in passing the Canada Health Act into law, but they were also successful in having it amended. As it was introduced to Parliament in 1983, Bill C-3 identified only physicians as providers of insurable services. The CNA amendment changed the language to include other healthcare workers as potential providers of insurable services (Mussallem, 1992).

Under the Canada Health Act, federal funding for essential medical services would continue so long as the provinces' health insurance plans met the following five criteria: (1) **publicly administered** (accountable to the public), (2) **comprehensive** (must cover necessary in-hospital, medical, and surgical–dental services), (3) **universal** (available to all), (4) **portable** (available after a maximum of three months of residency, and no extra charge for care out of province), and (5) **accessible** (no user fees, and healthcare providers must be reimbursed adequately). The **Canada Health Act** has ensured that Canadians have access to healthcare regardless of their ability to pay or where they live. It is held up as a symbol of the values that represent Canada. It articulates a social contract that defines healthcare as a basic right and reflects the values of social justice, equity, and community (Auditor General of Canada, 2002).

However, the Canada Health Act identified only essential medical and hospital services as qualifying for federal cost sharing. Health promotion, prevention of disease and injury, health protection, and home health were not emphasized. Tommy Douglas had envisioned a second, more ambitious phase to medicare—one with a focus on keeping people well, as he understood that illness prevention and improved health were essential to controlling healthcare costs (Campbell & Marchildon, 2007). To realize this vision, a shift in the focus from individual conditions and behaviours to the social and economic determinants of health, such as education, poverty, hunger, and inadequate housing, is required (McBane, 2004).

In October 2006, the CNA again spoke up, with the then president, Dr. Marlene Smadu, presenting to the House of Commons Standing Committee on Finance. This CNA presentation outlined the position of nurses in Canada, stating that health promotion, funding to address the determinants of health, and support for control of drug costs were considerations as important as wait times and fears about financial sustainability (CNA, 2006).

In assessing the degree to which the Canada Health Act has been successful in ensuring that all Canadians have access to the healthcare they need, we need to look at the purpose of the Act and the extent to which other aspects of healthcare addressed by the Act have been implemented. In addition to its stated purpose, the Canada Health Act implicitly and explicitly suggests a broader purpose. For example, Section 3 of the Act endorses **health promotion**, stating that the "primary objective of Canadian healthcare policy" is twofold: to facilitate reasonable access to health services and "to protect, promote, and restore the physical and mental well-being of the residents of Canada" (Canada, House of Commons, 1984, Section 3, p. 5). Despite this, the focus on adequate funding of community health services has been limited. Because the Canada Health Act establishes that only medically necessary physician services and hospital services are publicly funded, services such as home care fall outside the legislation. Provision of the funding for these services lies within the jurisdiction of each province and territory.

Because protective, preventive, and health promotion services were not required to meet the five criteria of medicare, they were not subject to the conditions of the Act. As a result, these services were left unprotected by federal legislation and are provided largely by provincial and territorial public health systems, even though it is well recognized that these services add a critical balance to the treatment-focused insured service delivery addressed by the Canada Health Act. Each province, territory, and region determines what services are covered and to what extent. The result has been varied and fragmented community health service across the country (Tsasis, 2009). Today, **public health systems** in Canada continue to be confronted by ideologies that favour efficiency, effectiveness, and short-term outcomes, which tend to overshadow health promotion and prevention values, strategies, and activities (Kirk, Tomm-Bonde, & Schreiber, 2014). Demonstrating measurable indicators of relationship building with marginalized populations and capacity building within neighbourhoods and communities is difficult, especially in the short term.

Canada's life expectancy at birth, for women and men combined, ranks among the highest in the world at 82 years (World Health Organization, 2011). However, while the Canadian infant mortality rates have dropped since 1970, the 2013 rate of 4.78 deaths per 1000 live births is still higher than the rate in a number of other developed countries (Henry J. Kaiser Family Foundation, 2014). There is room for improvement.

In 2011, the United States spent more per capita on healthcare than any of the other 29 countries compared by the Organisation for Economic Cooperation and Development (OECD) (OECD, 2013). Data analyses suggest that Canada's universal health coverage is less costly and more effective than the privatized U.S. healthcare system (Evans, 2008; Rachlis, 2008; Rachlis, Evans, Lewis, & Barer, 2001; Starfield, 2010). Health expenditures in the United States also represented the highest percentage of gross domestic product (GDP) (OECD, 2013). Yet American health outcomes compare poorly with those of other countries. Japan, for example, spends less than one-half as much per capita on healthcare as the United States and yet it ranks very high on all three measures of health outcomes (male life expectancy, female life expectancy, and infant mortality).

The World Health Organization (WHO) reported that the total expenditure on health in 2011 in Canada was $4520 per capita (WHO, 2011), representing about 11.2% of the GDP. Canada's per capita spending in 2011 was about 54% of that of the United States and less than 17.7% of the U.S. GDP (OECD, 2013). Even though the spending was lower, Canada fared substantially better than the United States on all three health outcomes. This is perhaps related to the fact that the American healthcare industry relies to a larger extent on private funding (53.5%) than any of the other countries. When comparing healthcare outcomes to expenditures, one message is very clear—increased spending on healthcare does not result in better health.

When we first started debating medicare 40 years ago, "medically necessary" healthcare could be summed up in two words: *hospitals* and *doctors*. Today, hospital and physician services account for less than one-half of the total cost of the healthcare system. More money is spent on drugs than on physicians. There are more specialists and more care is delivered in homes, in communities, and through a wide array of healthcare providers. In short, the practice of healthcare has evolved. "And despite efforts to keep pace, medicare has not" (Romanow, 2002, p. 2). Effective chronic disease prevention and management will require broad policy options, including amending the Canada Health Act; promoting interdisciplinary teamwork; and supporting further integration of public health, home care, and other sectors of the healthcare system (Tsasis, 2009). Palliative care and community mental health services are areas that need to be strengthened within the Canada Health Act (Marchildon, 2005). The review of the Act will require the involvement of professionals, citizens, and communities to provide insight and direction for the delivery and funding of healthcare.

# A PARADIGM SHIFT TO PREVENTION, PROMOTION, AND THE SOCIAL DETERMINANTS OF HEALTH

When the legislative pillars of Canadian medicare were enacted in 1957, 1966, and 1984, the biomedical model dominated public and political thinking about health. The clinical definition of health was "the absence of disease," and the term "health promotion" was often used interchangeably with "disease prevention." Labelling the illness-oriented, treatment-focused physician and hospital services that were insured under the Act as "healthcare" contributed to this confusion. As challenges to the idea that health was related exclusively to the country's illness emerged, the federal government responded and provided leadership for the development of health promotion policies and resources.

An important acknowledgement of the limitations of the primacy of the funded medical/treatment system in Canada was the Lalonde Report of 1974 (Lalonde, 1974). This bold report presented a vision for health promotion services as a critical component of Canada's healthcare system. The forward-thinking framework identified four determinants of health: environment, lifestyle, human biology, and the healthcare system. This was the first acknowledgement that health was influenced by the social, economic, and environmental conditions in which people lived, worked, and played. The Lalonde Report was considered revolutionary by the global community and led to a reconceptualization of health promotion.

Four years later, in 1978, Canada and other countries around the world met at the International Conference on Primary Health Care in Alma-Ata, USSR. Governments were urged to take action to "protect and promote the health" of the people of the world, and the Declaration of Alma-Ata (WHO, 1978) was issued. Canada was a signatory. The goal of primary health care is the attainment of better health services for all, which will be discussed in Chapter 7. The CNA continues to advocate for primary health care policy and practice that is consistent with the principles outlined in the WHO declaration (CNA, 2012a).

In the years following Alma-Ata, federal leadership in forming a health promotion policy continued. In 1986, the federal Minister of Health, the Honourable Jake Epp, published the document "Achieving Health for All: A Framework for Health Promotion" (Epp, 1986), also known as the "Epp Framework." The Epp Framework expanded Lalonde's definition of health promotion; incorporated some of the tenets of primary health care; and emphasized the role of broad social, environmental, and political **determinants of health** (conditions that contribute to disease and disability). The document concluded with a denouncement of strategies that focus on individual responsibility for health, or "blaming the victim," while ignoring the social and economic determinants.

The Epp Framework formed the basis for the Ottawa Charter for Health Promotion that emerged from the First International Conference on Health Promotion, hosted by the federal government in Ottawa in November 1986 (Epp, 1986). The **Ottawa Charter** (WHO, 1986), authored jointly by Health Canada, the CPHA, and the WHO, identified prerequisites for health, strategies for promoting health, and outcomes of those strategies (Kirk, Tomm-Bonde, & Schreiber, 2014). The release of the Ottawa Charter marked a dramatic shift in health promotion. Peace, education, shelter, income, and food were among the determinants identified, and this broader view of health shifted the focus from providing illness care and identifying risk factors to an inclusive approach that also focused on socio-environmental factors.

The Ottawa Charter acknowledged that caring for one's self and others is conducive to health, and it identified caring, holism, and ecology as essential concepts in health promotion (WHO, 1986). Federal government support for health promotion through policy making and development of resources has continued. Many of the resources that have been developed, such as the Population Health Template (Health Canada, 2001) and the Population Health Promotion Model (Hamilton & Bhatti, 1996), have been used to guide policy development as well as the practice and education of CHNs. More than 30 years after the Declaration of Alma-Ata, the eighth Global Conference on Health Promotion was held in Helsinki in June 2013. At this international conference, participants affirmed that "Health for All is a major societal goal of governments and the cornerstone of sustainable development" (WHO, 2013, p. 1). (See Canadian Research Box 2.1). They called for a "Health in All Policies" approach and a commitment to equity in health. Governments have a responsibility for the health of their people, and equity in health is an expression of social justice (WHO, 2013). Research Box 2.1. This raises important questions: How is this "call to action" put into practice? What are the system and organizational requirements? How is Canada's healthcare system organized, and can it meet the call?

---

### CANADIAN RESEARCH BOX 2.1

#### What does "population health approach" mean?

Cohen, D., Huynh, T., Sebold, A., Harvey, J., Neudorf, C., & Brown, A. (2014). The population health approach: A qualitative study on conceptual and operational definitions for leaders in Canadian health care. *SAGE Open Medicine, 2*(Jan–Dec), 1–11. Reproduced by permission of SAGE Publications Ltd.

"Population health approach" is a broad term used to describe strategies and actions that are developed in recognition of the multitude of factors that affect the health of a population. These factors and forces are both within and outside of the scope of the healthcare system. Canada has been recognized as a leader in the development and operationalization of the population health approach. It has been used in community and public health for decades, but recently it has been used throughout the whole healthcare system. With this more widespread consideration and use comes the need for clarity about what is meant by the term itself. With that in mind, this study set out to "examine the conceptual and operational definitions of a population health approach among senior leaders in Canada to determine a future foundation for common language and understanding" (p. 2).

The study used a qualitative, descriptive method with thematic analysis of the data. The research team identified "lead users" as those study participants who were at the leading edge of the use of this approach. Semi-structured interviews were conducted with senior leaders (n = 21) from across Canada and included the question, "What does a population health approach look like from your perspective?"

Following thematic analysis, themes were identified and subsequently validated at two pan-Canadian workshops with a broad range of health system actors. Six core themes emerged:

1. Focusing on health and wellness and prevention rather than on illness.
2. Taking a population rather than an individual orientation.
3. Understanding needs and solutions through community outreach.
4. Addressing equity, health disparities, and health in vulnerable groups.
5. Addressing the social and multiple determinants of health.
6. Embracing intersectoral action and partnerships (p. 4).

Many of the senior leaders interviewed pointed out that the population health approach was grounded in their personal and organizational values, an approach that represented an active shift toward a "way of thinking rooted in social justice" (p. 6) and supported them in carrying out their "moral responsibility to stay focused on the health of populations in the face of continued pressure to focus on clinical care" (p. 6). Knowledge sharing and networking opportunities were identified as strategies to facilitate other leaders in addressing the unique challenges they face in operationalizing the population health approach.

### Discussion Questions

1. What is the population health approach? What evidence would you look for to ascertain if the population health approach is being used?
2. Are any of the six core themes identified in this study evident in your practice setting? Describe them, and consider what supports them from an organizational and CHN perspective.
3. What strategies could leaders at all levels in an organization use to support the population health approach?

## ORGANIZATION OF COMMUNITY HEALTHCARE

### Public Health Agency of Canada

Over the past several decades, a number of health emergencies have illuminated the problems in and the limitations of the community health system in Canada, and these have been highlighted in several national reports. The report of the Expert Panel on SARS and Infectious Disease Control (Walker, 2004), the National Advisory Committee on SARS and Public Health (Naylor, 2003), and the two interim SARS Commission Reports (Campbell, 2004, 2005) highlighted the central importance of public health in preventing the spread of diseases. These reports posed questions about the funding, governance, and management of public health in Canada. They monitored a series of communicable disease outbreaks, and their focus was on the health system's ability to respond adequately given the impact of the outbreaks on the communities,

the healthcare system, and the economy. In response to the concerns raised, the Public Health Agency of Canada (PHAC) was established in September 2004 to strengthen public health in Canada. Confirmed as a legal entity in December 2006 through the Public Health Agency of Canada Act, it reports to the Parliament of Canada through the Minister of Health. By 2014, more than 2400 PHAC staff members were working in the national headquarters in Ottawa and in six regions distributed across Canada.

The PHAC is led by the Chief Public Health Officer (CPHO), who is the lead federal public health professional tasked with communicating directly with Canadians and government on important public health matters. The mission of the PHAC is to promote and protect the health of Canadians, and it brings together scientists, researchers, policy makers, and public health professionals, including physicians, nurses, and epidemiologists, to do so. The PHAC is committed to the well-being of specific communities and the Canadian population as a whole. The development of a public health agency has strengthened public health leadership in Canada, which is required to address factors that contribute to illness and injury in times of crisis and emergency as well as in other times. The PHAC concentrates, within one agency, the required resources to focus efforts to advance public health nationally and internationally.

While the PHAC was a federal response, each province and territory also responded to the above-mentioned outbreaks and took steps to review and strengthen the public health component of the health system within its jurisdiction. In Ontario, for example, the provincial government launched Operation Health Protection in 2003 (Ontario Ministry of Health and Long-Term Care, 2004), a three-year plan to rebuild public health. The intent was to address the concerns of infectious disease control as well as concerns related to disease prevention and health promotion. Related activities included the establishment of two provincial committees to move public health renewal forward. The first committee, the Capacity Review Committee, was to assess and make recommendations as to the capacity and organizational framework for public health, and the second was to provide recommendations and a plan to establish a provincial arm's-length agency that would focus on research and practice excellence in public health. Public Health Ontario (PHO) provides provincial leadership on funding, policy, standards setting, and accountability in public health programs. All these directly impact the practice of community health nursing in Ontario.

### Community Health Services

"A strong community health system has the potential to effectively and efficiently address disease and injury issues upstream to prevent them from occurring, delay their onset, or care for those affected closer to home to restore health" (Community Health Nurses of Canada, 2011a, p. 17). In a submission to the CNA National Expert Commission (CNA, 2012b), the Community Health Nurses of Canada (CHNC) (CHNC, 2011b) stated that any health reform would require proactive planning in anticipation of population trends and need.

Further, the CHNC identified community-based health organizations as a driving force for the type of innovation (health and social) to create a just, prosperous, and caring society.

Many factors have influenced how community health services are organized and delivered across Canada. Most Canadian provinces and territories have moved to regional health authority structures for all health service delivery. This approach strives to integrate most or all health services (including CHN services) into a single organization. The timing, organization, and, in many cases, repeated reorganization of the regional health authorities and health regions have been unique to each province or territory. While community health services are organized and delivered differently across Canada, each province and territory provides primary health care, primary care, public health, and home care services. These will be briefly discussed in the next section.

# 1. Primary Health Care and Primary Care

In the Declaration of Alma-Ata, **primary health care** is defined as accessible, acceptable, affordable healthcare (WHO, 1978). Other tenets of primary health care include a basis in research; a continuum of services from promotive to rehabilitative; the identification of health education, proper nutrition, disease prevention and control, and maternal and child healthcare as minimum services; the recognition that intersectoral and interdisciplinary approaches are necessary for success; and an emphasis on community participation and empowerment. Primary health care encompasses the determinants of health and their influence on health and well-being (WHO, 1978). The practice of a CHN encompasses these tenets, and CHNs have participated in primary health care and are well prepared to play a leadership role.

**Primary care**, on the other hand, refers to services commonly accessed at the first point of contact with the health system. Primary care, a core component of primary health care, is more narrowly focused. In many developed countries, primary care services focus on acute care and treatment of diseases. While the largest group of primary care providers in Canada is composed of physicians, other primary care providers include nurses, nurse practitioners, dentists, chiropractors, pharmacists, dietitians, midwives, optometrists, and public health nurses. Current funding mechanisms favour physicians, and as a result, most Canadians access primary care in the community physicians' office, commonly through a family or general practitioner, who is reimbursed on a fee-for-service basis.

Physicians' fees account for 15% of overall healthcare spending, and in the 2011–2012 period these costs increased by 9% (Canadian Institute for Health Information, 2013). The most expensive form of remuneration for physicians' services is fee for service; the overwhelming majority of physicians earn almost all their income in this way. Hutchinson, Abelson, and Lavis (2001) noted that "for the 89% of Canadian family physicians or general practitioners who receive some fee-for-service income, fee-for-service payments account for an average of 88%

of their total income" (p. 117). Increasing criticism of this traditional and costly reimbursement model of primary care has led to some innovations over the past quarter century. However, these are often local in nature and have not resulted in a comprehensive nationwide model.

Primary care reform began at a national level and sought to move toward an integrated systems approach, which would more broadly provide the full spectrum of health services in communities or neighbourhoods. It was envisioned that health promotion and disease and injury prevention services would be enhanced as the focus shifted "upstream" with the implementation of primary health care.

In the early 1970s, community health centres (CHCs) were recognized for more "fully reflecting the objectives, priorities, and relationships which society wishes to establish for healthcare in the future" (Canadian Council on Social Development, Research and Development Branch, 1972, p. ii). An inquiry was commissioned to examine the place of CHCs as part of a plan aimed at restructuring healthcare delivery and funding mechanisms. Quebec introduced one of the first primary care reforms in the form of a model based on Centres Locaux de Services Communautaires (CLSCs). Philosophically, CLSCs are based on the ideal of a global, integrated system of care, delivering a broader, less-costly range of services (Hutchinson et al., 2001) to neighbourhoods across the province. In addition to providing primary care treatment, these local community service centres emphasized health promotion, disease prevention, and the provision of expanded services, including social services and mental health services (Shah, 2003).

In Ontario, CHCs focus on the determinants of health and provide interdisciplinary primary health care services, including health promotion, illness prevention, health protection, chronic disease management, and individual and community capacity building. There are 101 CHCs in Ontario, a number of them with satellite offices, each serving an average of 5 to 500 individuals. "Each centre is an incorporated, nonprofit agency governed by a volunteer board of directors" (Ontario Ministry of Health and Long-Term Care, 2013).

The most recent primary care reform initiative of the Ontario government has been to establish family health teams (FHTs). Family health teams are composed of physicians, nurse practitioners, nurses, social workers, dietitians, and other professionals who work together to provide healthcare to a community. Each team is set up on the basis of local health and community needs, and focuses on chronic disease management, disease prevention, and health promotion, as well as on working with other organizations such as public health, home care, and hospitals. Since April 2005, 184 teams have been created across the province, and this is expected to result in improved healthcare for over three million Ontarians. In 2011, the "Ontario Public Health Organizational Standards" was published, mandating that a chief nursing officer position be created in each Ontario health unit by 2013. Nurse practitioners (NPs) have contributed significantly to primary care reform and frequently practice in CHCs, FHTs, and primary health care centres. NPs are registered nurses with advanced education, and they provide a full range of services, including assessing, diagnosing, and treating illnesses (CNA, 2009).

NPs also focus on many health promotion and illness-prevention efforts. The Canada Health Act allows the provinces to establish reimbursement mechanisms for healthcare professionals other than physicians and dentists. Although all provinces and territories have enacted legislation that defines an extended scope of practice for NPs, only some provinces have established associated funding mechanisms for their reimbursement (Canada, House of Commons, 1984). New roles for NPs are emerging across Canada in response to specific needs and populations (CNA, 2009).

## 2. Public Health

Whereas hospital and physicians' services have been governed by federal legislation for the last half of the 20th century, public health was decentralized at the outset. Thus, across Canada, the responsibility for public health services rests with the provinces or territories and, in some cases, municipalities. The principles of comprehensiveness, universality, portability, public administration, and accessibility have been hallmarks of Canadian public health services. **Public health** augments medicare by ensuring that health promotion, illness and injury prevention, and health protection services are among the affordable, acceptable, essential health services that are "universally accessible to individuals and families in the community" (WHO, 1978). Together, Canada's public health services and national healthcare system are providing health services that are consistent with the tenets of primary health care. There is limited evidence on the relationships among public health organization, funding, performance, and health outcomes (Hyde & Shortell, 2012). (See Canadian Research Box 2.1).

However, the public health infrastructure in Canada has been severely eroded over the past several decades, and in 1996, the CPHA warned of the erosion by noting that in some jurisdictions, "public health units and specific categories of workers (e.g., public health nurses) are disappearing" (Canadian Public Health Association, 1996, pp. 1–12). In 2001, the CPHA identified "increasing complexity and decreased funding" as challenges facing public health (CPHA, 1996, p. 7). Sullivan (2002) reported on the key findings of the report of the Federal, Provincial, and Territorial Advisory Committee on Population Health that identified severe problems in public health in Canada, such as disparities among provinces and regions, severely inadequate and decreasing funding, critical human resource issues, and the development of public health policies without consideration of relevant data. There was consensus that the water contamination in Walkerton, Ontario, in 2000 was a "wake-up call" for Canadian public health and had occurred because "institutions vital to the infrastructure of public health were neglected" (Schabas, 2002, p. 1282). Funding of public health services depends, in large part, on provincial governance and delivery structures. Funds are distributed to regions and municipalities through various funding formulas.

The CPHA (2010a) proposed the development of a National Public Health Infrastructure Fund as a "transfer payment scheme dedicated to public health that demands a certain percentage of matching dollars from the provinces and

### CANADIAN RESEARCH BOX 2.2

**Is equity in public health the same across the country?**

Pinto, A., Manson, H., Pauly, B. Thanos, J., Parks, A., & Cox, A. (2012). Equity in public health standards: A qualitative document analysis of policies from two Canadian provinces. *International Journal of Equity in Health, 11*(28), 1–10.

Under the Constitution Act, the provincial and territorial governments in Canada have responsibility for healthcare. Within that responsibility, these governments set the direction for public health programs and determine the funding levels. Recently, there have been calls for the renewal of public health systems in Canada to meet emerging issues, threats, and needs. A coordinated and collaborative approach among jurisdictions (municipal, provincial or territorial, and federal governments) has been identified as desirable. Standards have long been seen as a way to improve accountability and facilitate collaboration and co-operation. However, standards for public health are inconsistently developed across Canada. The development of standards has been influenced by many factors, including legislation, mandates, leadership, and history. Standards review and development has been used as a strategy for systems renewal.

This article reports on one part of a larger study that looked at the renewal of public health systems in Canada. Using document analysis, the researchers' purpose was to gain insight into how and to what extent an equity lens is incorporated into public health standards and to specifically answer the question, "How is equity conceptualized and integrated into key public health documents in British Columbia and Ontario?" The research team of academic researchers and public health knowledge-user partners conducted an inductive content analysis of two sets of key standards documents from the two provinces. The method included the use of constant comparative analysis. A set of questions guided coding and analysis.

Despite several limitations to this study, it does provide insight into two provincial perspectives on health equity. There were similarities between the two sets of documents in the overall goals, how the issues were framed, and the need to look beyond public health and work intersectorally to address inequities. Differences were present in how an equity lens was used, the use of language and terms such as "vulnerable" or "marginalized," and the legislation (or lack thereof) that supported the standards. An interesting finding was that both sets of documents did not include an analysis of the systemic factors that are contributing to the inequities.

### Discussion Questions

1. Access the public health program or organizational standards in your health jurisdiction. Is health equity defined? If so, how is health equity described?

2. Do the standards provide guidance in terms of how equity is addressed in areas such as access to services, intersectoral collaboration, and the social determinants of health?

3. How do standards enhance accountability of organizations to their funders? Are they an effective strategy to increase accountability in the diverse world of today?

territories in order to ensure a stable level of funding for the public health system across the country" (CPHA, 2010a, p. 9). This funding model is in the context of accumulating evidence on the widening gap in health between populations and a recognition of the importance of addressing the determinants of health and advancing health equity for the health of all (Hosseinpoor, Stewart Williams, Itani, & Chatterji, 2012; National Collaborating Centre for Determinants of Health, 2014; National Collaborating Centre for Public Health, 2012; WHO, 2008). Public health organizations and workers are expected to provide leadership in health equity endeavours. See Chapter 4 for additional information on public health.

## 3. Home Health

Health Canada defines **home care** as "a wide range of health services delivered at home and throughout the community to recovering, disabled, chronically, or terminally ill persons in need of medical, nursing, social, or therapeutic treatment and/or assistance with the essential activities of daily living" (Health Canada, 2010). "Home health nurses are committed to the provision of accessible, responsive, and timely care which allows people to stay in their homes with safety and dignity" (CHNC, 2010c, p. 4). The use of home care services has been steadily growing in Canada over the past 35 years; government spending on home care reached $3.4 billion in 2003–2004 (Canadian Institute of Health Information, 2007), and it is estimated that it was close to $4 billion in 2010 (Canadian Alliance for Sustainable Health Care, 2012).

These economic calculations are made difficult in Canada by a general lack of publicly available data that concisely report on public and private contributions made to deliver home care services. The most current data source for public spending on home health services and home support services across the country is 2003–2004 data from the 2007 report produced by the Canadian Institute for Health Information (CIHI) called "Public-Sector Expenditures and Utilization of Home Care Services in Canada: Exploring the Data." These data will become more readily available as more provinces join the home care reporting system, which is part of the CIHI.

With home care broadly accepted as a vital component of the healthcare system, every jurisdiction in Canada provides publicly funded home care to its constituents (CNA, 2013). The vast majority of recipients of home care services in Canada are seniors, and as the population ages, the numbers are predicted to increase. Following an extensive process, the CNA recommended that governments shift their funding and policy emphasis to new community-based, integrated models of healthcare that enable Canadians to remain at home (CNA, 2013). These models must support integration with primary care and provide state-of-the-art home care.

The increase in use of and funding for home care has been attributed to several factors, most significantly the belief that services provided in the home are both less costly and a more desirable means of delivering necessary care. These claims, however, have yet to be proven. Another issue is that as the services shift to the home and community they shift beyond the boundaries of public insurance (Deber, 2003). All of the provinces offer a package of basic services, but there are significant provincial variations in the degree to which services are publicly funded versus privately financed. This results in significant inequity in accessing publicly funded home care across different regions of the country. Although the actual figure is difficult to verify, the CASHC calculated that private payment (a combination of out-of-pocket payment and private insurance coverage) for home care services in Canada was close to $2 million and represented approximately 23% of total home care expenditures in 2010 (Canadian Alliance for Sustainable Health Care, 2012). Thus, savings associated with the provision of services in the home versus in an acute care setting may not reflect an actual decrease in cost so much as a transfer of costs to patients and their families (Shah, 2003).

Nursing care, pharmaceuticals, and physiotherapy and occupational therapy services are some of the services that are being debated (Deber, 2003). Some provinces have legislation to address the financing and provision of home care services at provincial and regional levels (Public Health Agency of Canada, 2006). However, in the absence of national standards, legitimate concerns exist in relation to access to type, amount, and quality of home care services (Sullivan & Baranek, 2002). Adding to the concerns, home care is an expanding area of health spending in Canada. The share of home care spending in provincial and territorial government health expenditures in Canada rose from 3.1% in 1994–1995 to 4.2% in 2003–2004 (CIHI, 2007) and 4.54% in 2010. Even with this growth, spending on home care remains less than 5% of healthcare expenditure.

In all 13 provinces and territories, the ministries or departments of health and social or community services maintain control over home care budgets and funding levels. As part of regionalization, most provinces and territories have delegated the responsibility for service delivery decisions to the regional or local health authorities while maintaining control over policy guidelines, standards for regional service delivery, reporting requirements, and monitoring outcomes. For example, in British Columbia, Alberta, Saskatchewan, Manitoba, Newfoundland and Labrador, Nunavut, and the Northwest Territories, the delivery of home care services is devolved to local or regional health authorities. In Quebec, the services are provided through the local community service centres (CLSCs) or health and social services centres (CSSSs). In New Brunswick, the Extra-Mural Program (EMP), known by many as the "hospital without walls," provides home health services through the regional health authorities. In Nova Scotia, home care service is offered through the continuing care offices in each District Health Authority. In the Yukon, the Continuing Care Division under the Department of Health and Social Services administers home care.

In Ontario, home care is provided through Community Care Access Centres (CCACs), which manage healthcare services for those at home, at work, or in school. In April 2014, the Ontario Ministry of Health and Long-Term Care committed to ensuring a "reliable, robust and accessible home and community care sector," acknowledging the growing demand for this type of service and the need for the services to provide better care for better value (Ontario Ministry of Health and Long-Term Care, 2014). In Ontario, funding for many components of the health system was transferred to the Local Health Integration Networks (LHINs), including funding for home care and the CCACs. Each is staffed by professionals, including nurses, who assess individual health needs, determine requirements for care, answer questions, and develop a customized health plan with the client. The range of professional services provided include nursing, physiotherapy, social work, dietetics, occupational therapy, speech therapy, personal support, and case management. Denton, Zeytinoglu, Davies, and Lian (2002) found that while there is increased demand for home care, there is a paucity of research on the impact of restructuring. The impact of the changing governance and organizational structures on the quality of care and on the workers (including nurses) requires investigation. Across Canada, home care services are delivered using several funding frameworks. While each of the models provides some element of streamlining (intake, assessment, referral, case management), the approaches to delivery of care, most significantly in the degree to which services are contracted out to private agencies (both for-profit and not-for-profit), vary. Within its healthcare budget, each region must decide how much is allocated to home care versus acute care services versus public health and health promotion services. Public funding for home care is allocated to home care organizations, which then coordinate and deliver home care services. While major budgetary decisions are made at the regional level, case managers are then required to make decisions at the individual or family level. Service providers, a mix of for-profit and not-for-profit agencies, compete for contracts to provide the required in-home services. This process allows private, for-profit agencies to profit from public funding earmarked for the delivery of health services. This new situation, sometimes referred to as "passive privatization," has sparked significant debate and concern. A number of papers have challenged the competitive bidding process. While the expectation is that the competitive process will lead to efficiencies, it can result in downward pressure on wages, skill mix, and working conditions (Deber, 2003). The process by which service providers are obtained will have a significant impact on the quality of care individuals will receive. See Chapter 5 for additional information on home care.

## CURRENT AND FUTURE CHALLENGES FOR COMMUNITY HEALTH NURSES

Over the past decade, there has been significant growth in research and literature that describes the current situation for CHNs across Canada. The literature points to the strengths CHNs bring to positively influencing the health of individuals, families, communities, and society as a whole. It also paints a picture of numerous challenges, including health system challenges, lack of role clarity, need for strong leadership, and issues in interprofessional relationships.

## Health System Challenges

Community health nursing practice occurs in a sociopolitical environment. Nurses' ability to shape this environment, thus taking an active role in evolving healthcare so that it positively impacts the health of communities, is often met with multiple challenges and barriers. Despite numerous calls for strengthening primary health care (Romanow, 2002) and shifting toward community health and preventive care, an emphasis on illness care provided in institutions remains the current paradigm (Mahony & Jones, 2013). Inadequate funding and resources for disease prevention and health promotion remains an issue, and what exists is under constant and real threat. The lack of stable, long-term funding is cited as a major barrier to effective practice and service delivery (Dingley & Yoder, 2013; Underwood et al., 2009). CHNs themselves identify as priority items the need for advocacy and collective action to shape system change (CHNC, 2010a; CHNC, 2011a; Schofield et al., 2011).

**Role Clarity** Despite its long and rich history, community health nursing is in a vulnerable position today. The CHNC, the national voice to promote community health nursing in Canada, conducted a survey in 2008 to establish a vision for community health nursing in the year 2020 in Canada (CHNC, 2009a; Schofield et al., 2011). This visioning initiative included a national survey and several focus groups that included CHNs in different regions across Canada. The resulting document, "Community Health Nursing Vision 2020: Shaping the Future" (CHNC, 2009a), contains the following expressions of how community nurses experience their roles:

> I think public health nurses are undervalued by the community, by the consumer, by the nursing profession, by colleagues in different areas of nursing . . . people view it (community health nursing) as not really nursing, while it is really and truly the highest level of nursing that you're going to do. (p. 9)

This undervaluing mirrors the diminished funding and resources of previous decades. Others have identified the relative invisibility of CHNs. Two such examples can be found in post-SARS national and provincial reports. Campbell's report spoke generally of the public health system as "broken and need[ing] to be fixed . . . [T]he overall system is woefully inadequate . . . unprepared, fragmented, poorly led, uncoordinated, inadequately resourced, professionally impoverished and generally incapable of discharging its mandate" (Campbell, 2005, p. 24). Naylor (2003), in his report "Learning from SARS: Renewal of Public Health in Canada," stated that "the essential role of public health nurses throughout and following SARS received little attention" (p. 131).

Role clarity includes components such as shared common language to describe the role, working to the full scope of practice within the role, and an understanding of the role by others within the health system and the public. The ability to describe with confidence the CHN's role can contribute to a greater valuing of it by other professionals, the community, and the policy makers. The need for greater role clarity for CHNs is consistently noted in the literature

(Brookes, Davidson, Daly, & Hancock, 2004; Kennedy et al., 2008; Kulbok, Thatcher, Park, & Meszaros, 2012), and this provides the basis for articulating the value of community health nursing.

Across Canada, there are differences in how CHNs are identified on official registration forms and in organizational structures, and therefore enumeration of CHNs is difficult. It remains unknown how many nurses actually work in the various sectors of community health and any associated demographics. A 2010 synthesis paper reviewed eight recent community health nursing reports, examining the common issues associated with community health nursing (CHNC, 2010b). Of the eight reports reviewed, seven specifically identified role clarity as an issue. As clear professional roles are foundational to both a strong healthcare system and the ability to work effectively on interprofessional teams, CHNs, the organizations within which they work, and the professional associations that support them must continue to address this challenge.

In response to this issue, the CPHA and CHNC released an updated role document for public health nursing in Canada (CPHA, 2010b) to provide a common vision for the role and activities of community and public health nursing in Canada. The PHAC supported the development of discipline-specific competencies for public health nursing (CHNC, 2009b) and home health nursing (CHNC, 2010c) to support efforts toward role clarity.

**Leadership** A second challenge is the decline in visible community health nursing leadership. In 2005, Falk-Rafael et al. surveyed the changing roles of public health nurses in Ontario. Thirty-nine percent of public health nurses (PHNs) who responded to the survey did not know if their health unit had a designated chief nursing officer or a designated senior nurse leader. A further 25% answered "no" when asked if such a role existed in their agency. These results followed a directive from the provincial medical officer of health directing each health unit to appoint a senior nurse to a chief nursing officer role (see Case Study). In this same study, PHNs ranked themselves ninth on a list of 10 possible groups that could influence nursing practice in their organization. In 2005 a survey of all public health employees was conducted in Ontario as part of a review to assess the capacity of public health in Ontario (Capacity Review Committee, 2006). Keeping in mind that nurses comprise over 55% of the workforce, the following key issues were identified:

- need for stronger discipline-specific communities of practice and more opportunities to meet with peers to discuss and solve professional issues,
- substantial level of concern regarding leadership within health units and management skills at the senior management level, and
- lack of career paths and opportunities for advancement.

The areas most cited as needing attention were organizational culture, a sense of being valued and appreciated, the quality of leadership, the quality of supervision and management, and access to ongoing education and training (Capacity Review Committee, 2005, p. 34).

A national study of community health nursing using an appreciative inquiry process found three important organizational attributes that support community and public health nursing practice (Meagher-Stewart et al., 2009; Underwood et al., 2009):

- management practice;
- local organizational culture, which includes values and leadership characteristics; and
- government policy, including system attributes.

The results of surveys such as the ones identified above spur dialogue about options for action on the issues. One proposal is the development of a national centre of excellence for public health nursing with an initial mandate to "research and understand the best mix of staff, services, programs, and settings to achieve optimal outcomes for persons, families, communities and the health system" (CHNC, 2011a, p. 18–19). Development and support of strong and effective leadership for community health nursing is another important recommendation. Short residency programs for leadership development and the creation of a community of practice for leadership development are strategies that could be undertaken by a centre of excellence (CHNC & the National Collaborating Centre for the Determinants of Health, 2013).

---

### CASE STUDY

**Public Health Chief Nursing Officer Working Group Report** (Ontario Ministry of Health and Long-Term Care, 2011b)

Over the last two decades, discussions regarding the need for and establishment of designated nursing leadership roles in Ontario public health units have abounded. In February 2000, the then chief medical officer of health and provincial chief nursing officer endorsed the implementation of a chief nursing officer (CNO) position in each public health unit as a preferred model within the public health system and recognized it as a best practice (Peroff-Johnson & Tober, 2012).

In its May 2006 final report, the public health Capacity Review Committee recommended that the Ministry of Health and Long-Term Care "enforce the 2000 directive regarding the appointment of a senior nurse leader role in each health unit" (p. 19). In February 2011 the ministry issued the Ontario Public Health Organizational Standards (Ontario Ministry of Health and Long-Term Care, 2011a), which established management and governance requirements for all boards of health. These standards required that all 36 boards of health designate a CNO "to be responsible for nursing quality assurance and nursing practice leadership" (p. 21), and within a year, all health units reported the appointment of a nurse in this role in their agencies.

The CNO mandate in the Ontario Public Health Organizational Standards (Ontario Ministry of Health and Long-Term Care, 2011a), with funding support, is aimed at enabling consistency in the designation, accountability, role, and functions of CNOs. Through this position, health outcomes of the community at individual, group, and population levels will be enhanced through CNO contributions to organizational strategic planning and decision making; facilitating recruitment and retention of qualified, competent public health nursing staff; and enabling quality public health nursing practice. The CNO models, articulates, and leads the way toward a vision of excellence in public health nursing practice.

The first provincial meeting of all 36 CNOs, held in Toronto, resulted in the establishment of a Chief Nursing Officers Provincial Association for Ontario, with an executive that is elected and regionally representative, and the development of key strategic directions for the association. Activities are currently under way in each health unit to move forward nursing practice and leadership initiatives.

### Discussion Questions

1. What factors would contribute to the provincial decision to establish CNO positions in each public health unit?

2. Within the first three years of initiating these positions, what key goals and activities will establish the effectiveness of this nursing leadership role?

3. As a new initiative, working within a province with over 2800 nurses (over 50% of all public health front-line staff), how might the CNO role impact the practice of nursing and improve the health of the province? What outcomes would indicate that the goals of this initiative were successfully met?

**Interprofessional Relationships** The relationships nurses have with each other and with other professionals that enable them to achieve a common vision to deliver care and to strengthen the health system and those who are impacted by it are referred to as **interprofessional relationships**. Developing and strengthening these relationships, including intersectoral partnerships, is critical to achieving effective community health outcomes. The future success of CHNs and nursing in leading the health system—from individual client and family care to broad population health interventions—requires a focus on the significance of professional, client, and community collaboration and partnership.

Nurses regard interprofessional and intersectoral partnerships as important, and foundational to effective partnerships is an understanding of the roles of healthcare partners and the contribution each can make. Contributions include the ability to make or influence care and service decisions, implement organizational change, empower policy and administrative decisions, and develop educational curricula. Establishing positive and effective partnerships and processes for working together requires time, leadership, and mutual understanding.

# ROLE OF LEADERSHIP IN RESPONDING TO CHALLENGES FOR CHNS

As described in the preceding sections, community health nursing in the current healthcare system faces significant challenges, but it also has many opportunities to make a significant difference. Leadership at all levels is required to realize the opportunities and address the challenges. Leadership is about influence that moves individuals, groups, communities, and systems toward achieving goals that will result in better health. While senior leaders occupy formal leadership positions, all CHNs have the opportunity within their practice to be leaders and have influence. Leadership is proposed as a strategy for all CHNs to embrace and develop.

While the key attributes of leaders have been articulated (Ganann et al., 2010), awareness of oneself is of key importance. Developing insight into one's beliefs, strengths, weaknesses, and style of relating is fundamental to effective leadership. Leadership occurs within relationships, so understanding the impact of one's behaviour on others and being able to moderate and modify that behaviour or style are essential to effectively steering people and organizations toward a vision (Willcocks, 2012). Creating and articulating a clear purpose and vision is critical, and to do that effectively, CHNs must be able to see the long view, incorporating multiple aspects of the communities, the political environment, and the larger health and social systems. Conceptualizing oneself such that leadership is seen as a dimension of practice for all nurses is important to building leadership capacity in community health nursing (Scott & Miles, 2013).

Strategic thinking and action as well as hearing the perspectives or voices of others, including staff, other sectors, and members of the community, must be evident in the vision. Multiple perspectives must be taken into account. The ability to lead others involves the ability to engage their hearts, minds, and feet through expertise in building, sustaining, and sometimes mending relationships. Strong problem solving, conflict management, and interpersonal skills promote emotional engagement and foster motivation. Leaders understand their role in developing a team or organizational culture and do so in a deliberate, intentional fashion, grounded in clear, strong values and principles that encompass respect, trust, honesty, and integrity.

An effective leader not only copes with change but also understands change and the change process (Cummings et al., 2008). Effective leaders bring energy, enthusiasm, action, and humour to the process and to the tasks at hand while keeping a focus on the desired results (Brody, Barnes, Ruble, & Sakowski, 2012; Cummings et al., 2010). The literature does not identify people from any single discipline as having superior leadership skills; rather, each brings a unique set of perspectives, experiences, knowledge, skills, and attitudes that can be used to develop effective and collaborative leadership.

The outcomes of leadership have been described extensively. One such document is the Registered Nurses' Association of Ontario's (RNAO's) "Best Practice Guideline: Developing and Sustaining Nursing Leadership" (RNAO, 2013), which discusses the significant impact of leadership in the workplace and community. For example, professionals working in health service organizations with strong leadership demonstrate increased organizational commitment, higher levels of organizational effectiveness, greater sense of affiliation with organizational goals, and increased ability to lead a diverse workforce.

Personal resources for nurse leaders in a community health setting that contribute to effective leadership practice include the personal characteristics one brings to a leadership role as well as personal supports, learned behaviours, and expertise (knowledge and skills) that have been honed over time. Personal growth is dependent on individual self-awareness and understanding of how your behaviour influences those around you as well as events in an organization and in the broader community. As community health work is so interconnected with organizations and political bodies, self-awareness and self-concept are critical to effectively influence or lead within these systems (Cummings et al., 2010).

Research completed through the development of the best practice guideline on nursing leadership (RNAO, 2013) found that the following attributes of nurse leaders contribute to effectiveness:

- communication and listening skills;
- resilience, persistence, and hardiness;
- comfort with ambiguity, uncertainty, and complexity;
- willingness to take risks;
- working from a foundational moral framework;
- confidence in own values and beliefs;
- self-confidence, self-awareness, social awareness;
- knowledge; and
- cultivation of professional and personal supports.

A conceptual model (see Figure 2.1) identifies contextual and personal factors that impact a nurse's approach to transformational leadership (Weberg, 2010). The model outlines individual and system components that contribute to effective nursing leadership (RNAO, 2013). For example, a nurse leader who strongly values professional nursing supports will approach relationship building in a way that is more likely to result in healthy and effective outcomes than a nurse leader who values individual successes and works alone in a chaotic environment where budgets are unstable. Leadership growth builds on organizational supports, personal resources, and past outcome experiences.

## Organizational Supports

An organizational assessment tool is contained in Table 2.1. This tool can be used to assess organizational supports for leadership and invite reflection and dialogue on local and larger systems. It builds on the leadership conceptual model, particularly the components of organizational support, and provides a series of activities that leaders may champion as essential to ensuring effective and healthy work environments. These strategies (left column) support a focus on developing personal resources as well as on assisting managers and leaders (right column) to develop system-wide infrastructure. The individual strategies focus on the community health nurse as an individual who is growing within his or her discipline. The strategies highlight formalized communication networks, broader community partnerships, and meaningful involvement of staff in organization and agency decision making. As leaders of organizations, it is important to continually assess the current strategies to ensure

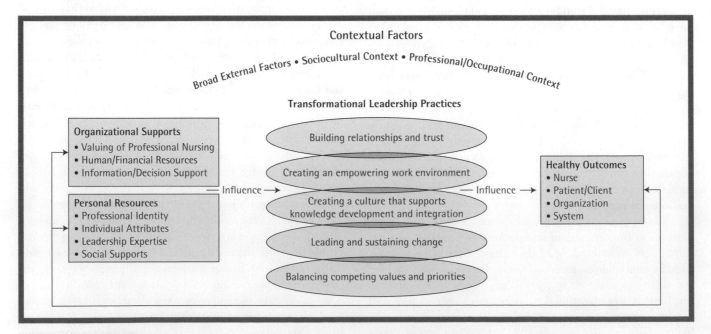

**FIGURE 2.1** Conceptual Model for Developing and Sustaining Leadership

*Source:* Registered Nurses' Association of Ontario. *Best practice guideline: Developing and sustaining nursing leadership* (2nd ed., p. 16). Toronto, ON: Author. Used by permission of Registered Nurses' Association of Ontario.

| Table 2.1 | Organizational Supports | | | | | | |
|---|---|---|---|---|---|---|---|
| A. Employee Development/Enrichment | | Yes | No | B. Community Health Organization | | Yes | No |
| 1. Employee retention plan | | —— | —— | 1. Clear connection between agency vision, mission, mandate, and service delivery | | —— | —— |
| 2. Recruitment and succession plan | | —— | —— | 2. Articulated cultural vision and implementation plan to support workplace environment | | —— | —— |
| 3. Orientation and mentoring program for all new and transferring staff | | —— | —— | 3. Committee/planning structures, which include all levels of staff in a meaningful way | | —— | —— |
| 4. Regular performance feedback mechanisms that include a variety of inputs (e.g., manager, peer, client, colleague, community partner) | | —— | | 4. Stable and predictable funding resources dedicated to a systematic organizational review (e.g., accreditation) | | —— | —— |
| 5. Personal learning plans/professional development plans | | —— | —— | 5. Clear boundaries/program mandates with flexibility to address realities of individual community | | —— | —— |
| 6. Employee satisfaction feedback systems and a process for addressing outcomes | | —— | —— | 6. Opportunities to nurture discussions on relevant research and practice changes | | —— | —— |
| 7. Continuing supportive education policies | | —— | —— | 7. Encouragement to engage with communities and form joint ventures and partnerships | | —— | —— |
| 8. Staff education and training opportunities that include development of affective domain (i.e., values, assumptions, feelings) | | —— | —— | 8. Opportunities for disciplines to work together based on collaborative practice principles | | —— | —— |
| 9. Formalized career development opportunities | | —— | —— | 9. Formalized student preceptor programs | | —— | —— |
| 10. Leadership development plan | | —— | —— | 10. Formalized agreements with the academic community, which include cross-appointments, joint research, and student clinical experiences | | —— | —— |
| 11. Opportunities for communities of practice to meeting together regularly | | —— | —— | 11. Infrastructure support—technical, informational, health and safety, media, communication | | —— | —— |
| 12. Appreciation/acknowledgement events where achievements are recognized (department, team, individual) | | —— | —— | 12. Mechanisms for regular meetings with unions and other associations | | —— | —— |
| 13. Development and role modelling aimed at mid-career nurses and late-career nurses | | —— | —— | 13. Quality practice council(s) | | —— | —— |
| | | | | 14. Formalized communication mechanisms (e.g., all-staff meetings, newsletter, bulletin board, department updates) to engage staff | | —— | —— |
| | | | | 15. Well-established networks within the organization and with key community organizations | | —— | —— |

that effective individual and organizational systems are in place to achieve excellence in practice and outcomes.

Within the context of community health nursing practice, important organizational supports that positively influence practice include a work culture that

■ values the unique and combined contribution of staff,
■ deliberately establishes leadership and mentoring plans,
■ has a clear vision engendering commitment, and

■ has stable funding and access to necessary resources to accomplish work.

Collaborative leadership at a national level will be strengthened by developing intersectoral relationships, promoting community health solutions across sectors, and addressing the wider determinants of health (PHAC, 2006). Mentoring is consistently identified as contributing to leadership development (Cooper & Wheeler, 2010).

## CONCLUSION

To varying degrees, the federal, provincial, territorial, regional, and municipal levels of government are involved in Canadian healthcare. Medicare is one of the great achievements of Canada, and it is more than a public insurance program (Campbell & Marchildon, 2007). A universally accessible, publicly funded, not-for-profit healthcare system is steeped in Canadian values and embraced by the Canadian public. Efforts to enshrine those values in federal legislation began as early as 1919. The present legislation, the Canada Health Act, is limited in that its principles of public administration, portability, accessibility, universality, and public administration apply only to essential medical and hospital services. Nevertheless, the publicly funded and largely privately delivered healthcare system has served Canadians well with respect to both health outcomes and cost-effectiveness (Starfield, 2010).

Pressures to reform medicare have come about not only because of its narrow focus on hospital and medical services but also because some favour augmenting the public system with services provided by the for-profit sector. Numerous reports at the provincial or territorial and federal levels have recommended reforms to the healthcare system. The most comprehensive of those, the Romanow Commission Report, made 47 recommendations for both the immediate future and the next 20 years (Romanow, 2002).

The federal government has played a leadership role, not only in Canada but also in the world, in health promotion policy. However, a coordinated approach to implementing health promotion policy at the community and population levels has been hampered by the lack of a national public health plan. Prior to the SARS outbreak in 2004, there had been a steadily declining emphasis on the role of community health in the Canadian health system, in large part due to the exclusion of community health from the Canada Health Act. Restructuring of provincial health systems to regional models that include community health has played a role as community health issues compete with more pressing acute care concerns. There is, however, a growing awareness of the need to address the upstream issues or root causes of illness if the current healthcare system is to be sustainable. Demands on limited home health and primary health care nursing services have challenged the community health system. Serious erosions to the public health system in Canada have led to the withdrawal and reduction of many public health nursing services and CHN presence in key settings such as schools, community places, and workplaces.

Community health nurses practice at the intersection of public policy and private lives and are thus in a position to include political advocacy and efforts to influence healthy public policy in their practice (Falk-Rafael, 2005). The call for a revitalized public health and community health system is being made. Strong leadership and action at all levels is required to answer this call. CHNs are well positioned and, in fact, morally obligated to act and provide leadership (Falk-Rafael, 2005).

## KEY TERMS

accessible, p. 18
Canada Health Act, p. 18
Canadian Nurses Association (CNA), p. 18
comprehensive, p. 18
determinants of health, p. 20
health promotion, p. 19
home care, p. 24
interprofessional relationships, p. 27
leadership, p. 17
medicare, p. 18
Ottawa Charter, p. 20
portable, p. 18
primary care, p. 22
primary health care, p. 22
public health, p. 23
public health systems, p. 19
publicly administered, p. 18
universal, p. 18

## STUDY QUESTIONS

1. Identify the origins of medicare in Canada and summarize the laws that created the present Canadian healthcare system. What is considered to be phase 2 of the implementation of medicare?

2. Discuss the events that led up to and necessitated passage of the Canada Health Act.

3. What role did organized nursing play in the passage of the Canada Health Act?

4. Discuss the federal and provincial responsibilities for health according to the Canadian Constitution Act.

5. Contrast the funding mechanisms for public health and home health nursing services with the rest of the system.

6. Describe how the Canada Health Act was or was not successful in achieving the intended goals. Are there issues with it?

> After working through these questions, go to the MyNursingLab at www.pearsoned.ca/mynursinglab to check your answers.

## INDIVIDUAL CRITICAL-THINKING EXERCISES

1. List your core values for healthcare in Canada. How do your values compare with the values reflected in the five key funding criteria described in the Canada Health Act (1984)?

2. How would your life be different if healthcare in this country were provided based on ability to pay rather than need?

3. This chapter has shown that health policy decisions leave a legacy for generations. Describe briefly one policy revision you would make in the areas of primary care/primary health care, public health, and home care.

4. What examples can you describe of nurses' work to bring about healthcare systems change?

5. What opportunities have you encountered to promote the second phase of medicare development?

6. Leadership development is an ongoing process. What ideas do you have to develop your leadership skills and knowledge?

## GROUP CRITICAL-THINKING EXERCISES

1. What are the values on which the healthcare system is founded? How do your own values fit with the societal values that are reflected in the five funding criteria described in the Canada Health Act (1984)?

2. What are some of the solutions that you and your group can generate to address the real issues in Canada's healthcare system? What role can community health nurses play?

3. In an ideal world, create a healthcare system designed to provide the best care, to the most people, in the most cost-effective manner. Describe the mechanisms for financing, allocation, and delivery. Compare and contrast this system with the current Canadian system.

## REFERENCES

Auditor General of Canada. (2002). *1999 report of the Auditor General of Canada to the House of Commons* (Chapter 29). Retrieved from http://www.oag-bvg.gc.ca/internet/English/parl_oag_199911_29_e_10158.html

Peroff-Johnson, N., & Tober, J. (2012). *The public health chief nursing officer initiative: Building capacity in the public health nursing workforce in Ontario.* The Ontario Public Health Conference. Retrieved from http://neltoolkit.rnao.ca/sites/neltoolkit/files/Presentation_The%20Public%20Health%20Chief%20Nursing%20Initiative_Building%20Capacity%20in%20the%20Public%20Health%20Nursing.pdf

Begin, M. (2002). *Revisiting the Canada Health Act (1984): What are the impediments to change?* Address to the Institute for Research on Public Policy, 30th Anniversary Conference, Ottawa, ON. Retrieved from http://moniquebegin.telfer.uottawa.ca/files/032.pdf

Bekemeier, B., Grembowski, D., Yang, Y., & Herting, J. R. (2012). Leadership matters: Local health department clinician leaders and their relationship to decreasing health disparities. *Journal of Public Health Management and Practice, 18,* E1–E10.

Brody, A. A., Barnes, K., Ruble, C., & Sakowski, J. (2012). Evidence-based practice council's potential path to staff nurse empowerment and leadership growth. *Journal of Nursing Administration, 42*(1), 28–33.

Brookes, K., Davidson, P., Daly, J., & Hancock, K. (2004). Community health nursing in Australia: A critical literature review and implications for professional nursing. *Contemporary Nursing, 16*(3), 195–207.

Campbell, A. (2004). *SARS Commission Interim report: SARS and public health in Ontario.* Toronto, ON: Ministry of Health and Long-Term Care. Retrieved from http://www.health.gov.on.ca/en/common/ministry/publications/reports/campbell04/campbell04_2.aspx

Campbell, A. (2005). *SARS Commission second interim report: SARS and public health legislation.* Toronto, ON: Ministry of Health and Long-Term Care. Retrieved from http://www.health.gov.on.ca/en/common/ministry/publications/reports/campbell05/campbell05.aspx

Campbell, B., & Marchildon, G. (2007). *Completing Tommy's vision.* Canadian Centre for Policy Alternatives. Retrieved from http://www.policyalternatives.ca/publications/commentary/completing-tommys-vision

Canada, House of Commons. (1984). *An act relating to cash contributions by Canada in respect of insured health services provided under provincial health care insurance plans and amounts payable by Canada in respect of extended health care services and to amend and repeal certain acts in consequence thereof (the Canada Health Act).* Ottawa, ON: Government of Canada. Retrieved from http://laws-lois.justice.gc.ca/PDF/C-6.pdf

Canadian Alliance for Sustainable Health Care. (2012). *Home and community care in Canada: An economic footprint.* Ottawa, Ontario: Conference Board of Canada.

Canadian Council on Social Development, Research and Development Branch. (1972). *Case studies in social planning: Planning under voluntary councils and public auspices.* Ottawa, ON: Author.

Canadian Institute for Health Information. (2007). *Government home care spending reaches $3.4 billion in 2003–2004.* Retrieved from http://www.newswire.ca/en/story/106227/government-home-care-spending-reaches-3-4-billion-in-2003-2004-cihi-study-is-the-first-of-its-kind-to-look-at-government-spending-on-home-care

Canadian Institute for Health Information. (2013). *Number of doctors in Canada rising, as are payments for their services.* Retrieved from http://www.cihi.ca/cihi-ext-portal/internet/en/document/spending+and+health+workforce/workforce/physicians/release_26sep13

Canadian Nurses Association. (2006). Report of Dr. Marlene Smadu (President, Canadian Nurses Association) at the Finance Committee. Retrieved from https://openparliament.ca/committees/finance/39-1/30/dr-marlene-smadu-1/only

Canadian Nurses Association. (2009). *Position statement: The nurse practitioner.* Ottawa, ON: Author. Retrieved from http://cna-aiic.ca/~/media/cna/page-content/pdf-en/ps_nurse_practitioner_e.pdf

Canadian Nurses Association. (2012a). *Primary health care: A position statement.* Retrieved from http://www.cna-aiic.ca/~/media/cna/page-content/pdf-en/ps123_primary_health_care_2013_e.pdf?la=en

Canadian Nurses Association. (2012b). Expert Commission (June, 2012). *A nursing call to action: The health of our nation, the future of our health system.* Retrieved from https://www.cna-aiic.ca/~/media/cna/files/en/nec_report_e.pdf

Canadian Nurses Association. (2013). *Optimizing the role of nursing in home health.* Retrieved from https://cna-aiic.ca/~/media/cna/page-content/pdf-en/optimizing_the_role_of_nursing_in_home_health_e.pdf?la=en

Canadian Public Health Association. (1996). *Focus on health: Public health in health services restructuring.* Ottawa, ON: Author.

Canadian Public Health Association. (2010a). *Enhancing the public health human resource infrastructure in Canada.* A presentation by CPHA to the House of Commons Standing Committee on Health. Ottawa, ON: Author. Retrieved from http://www.cpha.ca/uploads/policy/enhance_ph_e.pdf

Canadian Public Health Association. (2010b). *Public health, community health nursing practice in Canada: Roles and activities* (4th ed.). Ottawa: ON. Author. Retrieved from http://www.cpha.ca/uploads/pubs/3-1bk04214.pdf

Capacity Review Committee. (2005). *Interim report: Revitalizing Ontario's public health capacity: A discussion of issues and options.* Toronto, ON: Author. Retrieved from http://www.health.gov.on.ca/en/common/ministry/publications/reports/capacity_review05/capacity_review05.pdf

Capacity Review Committee. (2006). *Final report: Revitalizing Ontario's public health capacity.* Toronto, ON: Author. Retrieved from http://www.health.gov.on.ca/en/common/ministry/publications/reports/capacity_review06/capacity_review06.pdf

Community Health Nurses of Canada. (2009a). *Vision statement and definition of community health nursing practice in Canada.* Toronto, ON: Author. Retrieved from http://www.chnig.org/documents/Definition_vision_Final.pdf

Community Health Nurses of Canada. (2009b). *Public health nursing discipline specific competencies: Version 1.0.* Toronto, ON: Author. Retrieved from https://www.chnc.ca/documents/CHNC-PublicHealthNursingDisciplineSpecificCompentencies/index.html

Community Health Nurses of Canada. (2010a). *Community health nurses speak out! Key findings from an environmental scan about the future of community health nursing in Canada.* Retrieved from http://www.chnc.ca/documents/Environmentalscan-CHNsspeakout.pdf

Community Health Nurses of Canada. (2010b). *A synthesis of Canadian community health nursing reports.* Retrieved from http://www.chnc.ca/documents/CommunityHealthNursing-keyreportssynthesis2010.doc

Community Health Nurses of Canada. (2010c). *Home health nursing competencies: Version 1.0.* Toronto, ON: Author. Retrieved from http://chnc.ca/documents/HomeHealthNursingCompetenciesVersion1.0March2010.pdf

Community Health Nurses of Canada. (2011a). *A blueprint for action for community health nursing in Canada: Release 1.1.* Retrieved from http://chnc.ca/documents/Blueprint-FinalWordwRevisedGraphic2014-Final2014January6.pdf

Community Health Nurses of Canada. (2011b). *Creating a system for (community) health.* Submission to the Canadian Nurses Association's National Expert Commission. Retrieved from http://www.chnc.ca/documents/CHNC_CNAExpert-Commission_FINAL_CHNCdistribution_000.pdf

Community Health Nurses of Canada & the National Collaborating Centre for the Determinants of Health. (2013). *Public health nursing leadership development.* Toronto, ON: Author. Retrieved from https://www.chnc.ca/documents/PHNLeadershipDevelopmentinCanadaFinalReportwlogo-andacknowledgements2014Fub27.pdf

Cooper, M., & Wheeler, M. M. (2010). Building successful mentoring relationships. *Canadian Nurse, 106*(7), 34–35.

Cummings, G., Lee, H., MacGregor, T., Davey, M., Wong, C., Paul, L., & Stafford, E. (2008). Factors contributing to nursing leadership: A systematic review. *Journal of Health Service Research and Policy, 13,* 240–248.

Cummings, G., MacGregor, T., Davey, M., Lee, H., Wong, C., Lo, E., & Stafford, E. (2010). Leadership styles and outcome patterns for the nursing workforce and work environment: A systematic review. *International Journal of Nursing Studies, 4,* 363–385.

Deber, R. (2003). Health care reform: Lessons from Canada. *American Journal of Public Health, 93*(1), 20–24.

Denton, M., Zeytinoglu, I. U., Davies, S., & Lian, J. (2002). Job stress and job dissatisfaction of home care workers in the context of health care restructuring. *International Journal of Health Services, 32*(2), 327–357.

Dingley, J., & Yoder, L. (2013). The public health nursing work environment: Review of the research literature. *Journal of Public Health Management Practice, 19,* 308–321.

Epp, J. (1986). *Achieving health for all: A framework for health promotion.* Ottawa, ON: Health and Welfare Canada.

Evans, R. (2008). Reform, re-form, and reaction in the Canadian health care system. *Health Law Journal, Special Edition,* 265–286.

Falk-Rafael, A. (2005). Speaking truth to power: Nursing's legacy and moral imperative. *Advances in Nursing Science, 28*(3), 212–223.

Falk-Rafael, A., Fox, J., & Bewick, D. (2005). Report of a 1999 survey of public health nurses: Is public health restructuring in Ontario Canada moving toward primary health care? *Primary Health Care Research & Development, 6*(2), 172–183.

Ganann, R., Underwood, J., Matthews, S., Goodyear, R., Stamler, L. L., Meagher-Stewart, D., & Munroe, V. (2010). Leadership attributes: A key to optimal utilization of the community health nursing workforce. *Canadian Journal of Nursing Leadership, 23*(2), 60–71.

Hamilton, N., & Bhatti, T. (1996). *Population health promotion.* Ottawa, ON: Health Canada, Health Promotion and Development Division. Retrieved from http://www.phac-aspc.gc.ca/ph-sp/php-psp/index-eng.php

Health Canada. (2001). *The population health template: Key elements and actions that define a population health approach.* Retrieved from http://www.phac-aspc.gc.ca/ph-sp/pdf/discussion-eng.pdf

Health Canada. (2010). *Home and continuing care.* © All rights reserved. Health Canada, 2010. Adapted and reproduced with permission from the Minister of Health, 2015. Retrieved from http://www.hc-sc.gc.ca/hcs-sss/home-domicile/index-eng.php

Henry J. Kaiser Family Foundation. (2014). *Global health facts—infant mortality rate.* Retrieved from http://kff.org/global-indicator/infant-mortality-rate

Hosseinpoor, A. R., Stewart Williams, J. A., Itani, L., & Chatterji, S. (2012). Socioeconomic inequality in domains of health: Results from the World Health Surveys. *BMC Public Health, 12,* 198.

Hutchinson, B., Abelson, J., & Lavis, J. (2001). Primary care in Canada: So much innovation, so little change. *Health Affairs, 20*(3), 116–131. Published by Project Hope: The People-to-People Health Foundation, Inc.

Hyde, J. K., & Shortell, S. M. (2012). The structure and organization of local and state public health agencies in the U.S.: A systematic review. *American Journal of Preventive Medicine, 42,* S29–S41.

Kennedy, C., Christie, J., Harbison, J., Maxton, F., Rutherford, I., & Moss, D. (2008). Establishing the contribution of nursing in the community to the health of the people of Scotland: Integrative literature review. *Journal of Advanced Nursing, 64*(50), 416–439.

Kirk, M., Tomm-Bonde, L., & Schreiber, R. (2014). Public health reform and health promotion in Canada. *Global Health Promotion, 21*(2), 15–22.

Kulbok, P. A., Thatcher, E., Park, E., & Meszaros, P. (2012). Evolving public health nursing roles: Focus on community participatory health promotion and prevention. *Online Journal of Issues in Nursing, 17*, 1.

Lalonde, M. (1974). *A new perspective on the health of Canadians: A working paper.* Ottawa, ON: Health and Welfare Canada.

Mahony, D., & Jones, E. J. (2013). Social determinants of health in nursing education, research, and health policy. *Nursing Science Quarterly, 26*, 280–284.

Marchildon, G. (2005). *Health systems in transition: Canada.* Toronto, ON: University of Toronto Press.

McBane, M. (2004). December 2004: Medicare still on life-support. *Canadian Centre for Policy Alternatives.* Retrieved from http://www.policyalternatives.ca

Meagher-Stewart, D., Aston, M., Edwards, N., Smith, D., Young, L., & Woodford, E. (2004). *Fostering citizen participation and collaborative practice: Tapping the wisdom and voices of public health nurses in Nova Scotia. The study of public health nurses primary health care practice.* Dalhousie University, Halifax, NS: Author.

Meagher-Stewart, D., Underwood, J., Schoenfeld, B., Lavoie-Tremblay, M., Blythe, J., MacDonald, M., . . . Munroe, V. (2009). *Building Canadian public health nursing capacity: Implications for action.* Hamilton, ON: McMaster University, Nursing Health Services Research Unit (Health human resources series No. 15).

Molina-Mula, J., & De Pedro-Gómez, J. (2012). Impact of the politics of austerity in the quality of healthcare: Ethical advice. *Nursing Philosophy, 14*(1), 53–60.

Mussallem, H. K. (1992). Professional nurses' associations. In A. J. Baumgart & J. Larsen (Eds.), *Canadian nursing faces the future* (2nd ed., pp. 495–518). Toronto, ON: Mosby.

National Collaborating Centre for Determinants of Health. (2014). *About the social determinants of health.* Retrieved from http://nccdh.ca/resources/about-social-determinants-of-health

National Collaborating Centre for Public Health. (2012). *What are the social determinants of health?* Retrieved from http://www.nccph.ca/docs/NCCPHSDOHFactsheet_EN_May2012.pdf

Naylor, D. (2003). *Learning from SARS: Renewal of public health in Canada: A report of the National Advisory Committee on SARS and Public Health.* Ottawa, ON: Health Canada.

Ontario Ministry of Health and Long-Term Care. (2004). *Operation health protection: An action plan to prevent threats to our health and to promote a healthy Ontario.* Retrieved from http://health.gov.on.ca/en/common/ministry/publications/reports/consumer_04/oper_healthprotection.aspx

Ontario Ministry of Health and Long-Term Care. (2011a). *Ontario public health organizational standards.* Retrieved from http://www.health.gov.on.ca/en/pro/programs/publichealth/orgstandards/docs/org_stds.pdf

Ontario Ministry of Health and Long-Term Care. (2011b). *Public health chief nursing officer working group report.* Retrieved from http://www.health.gov.on.ca/en/pro/programs/publichealth/performance/docs/rep_cno.pdf

Ontario Ministry of Health and Long-Term Care. (2013). *Community health centres.* Retrieved from http://www.health.gov.on.ca/en/common/system/services/chc/default.aspx

Ontario Ministry of Health and Long-Term Care. (2014). *A vision for home and community care in Ontario.* Retrieved from http://www.health.gov.on.ca/en/public/programs/ccac/ccac_vision.pdf

Organisation for Economic Cooperation and Development. (2013). *OECD Health Statistics 2013: Frequently requested data.* Retrieved from http://www.scribd.com/doc/151954800/OECD-Health-Data-2013-Frequently-Requested-Data#scribd

Public Health Agency of Canada. (2006). *Health is everyone's business.* Retrieved from http://www.phac-aspc.gc.ca/ph-sp/collab/index-eng.php

Rachlis, M. (2008). *Operationalizing health equity: How Ontario's health services can contribute to reducing health disparities.* Wellesley Institute. Retrieved from http://www.wellesleyinstitute.com/wp-content/uploads/2011/11/Operationalizing-HealthEquity.pdf

Rachlis, M., Evans, R. G., Lewis, P., & Barer, M. L. (2001). *Revitalizing medicare: Shared problems, public solutions.* Tommy Douglas Research Institute. Retrieved from https://www.leg.bc.ca/cmt/39thparl/session-4/health/submissions/Rachlis_Revitalizing_Medicare_2001.pdf

Rachlis, M., & Kushner, C. (1994). *Strong medicine: How to save Canada's health care system.* Toronto, ON: Harper Perennial.

Rafael, A. (1997). *Every day has different music: An oral history of public health nursing in Southern Ontario, 1980–1996.* (Unpublished doctoral dissertation). University of Colorado, Denver, CO.

Registered Nurses' Association of Ontario. (2013). *Best practice guideline: Developing and sustaining nursing leadership* (2nd ed.). Toronto, ON: Author. Retrieved from http://rnao.ca/sites/rnao-ca/files/LeadershipBPG_Booklet_Web_1.pdf

Reutter, L., & Kushner, K. E. (2010). Health equity through action on the social determinants of health: Taking up the challenge in nursing. *Nursing Inquiry, 17*(3), 269–280.

Romanow, R. (2002). *Shape the future of health care: Interim report.* Retrieved from http://dsp-psd.pwgsc.gc.ca/Collection/CP32-76-2002E.pdf

Schabas, R. (2002). Public health: What is to be done? *Canadian Medical Association Journal, 166*(10), 1282–1283.

Schofield, R., Ganann, R., Brooks, S., McGugan, J., Dalla Bona, K., Betker, C., . . . Watson, C. (2011). Community health nursing vision for 2020: Shaping the future. *Western Journal of Nursing Research, 33*(8), 1047–1068.

Scott, E. S., & Miles, J. (2013). Advancing leadership capacity in nursing. *Nursing Administration Quarterly, 37*, 77–82.

Shah, C. P. (2003). *Public health and preventive medicine in Canada* (5th ed.). Toronto, ON: Saunders Canada.

Starfield, B. (2010). Reinventing primary care: Lessons from Canada for the United States. *Health Affairs, 29*(5), 1030–1036.

Sullivan, P. (2002). Canada's public health system beset by problems: Report. *Canadian Medical Association Journal, 166*(10), 1319.

Sullivan, T., & Baranek, P. (2002). *First do no harm: Making sense of Canadian health reform.* Toronto, ON: Malcolm Lester & Associates.

Tsasis, P. (2009). Chronic disease management and the home-care alternative in Ontario, Canada. *Health Services Management Research, 22*, 136–139.

Underwood, J. M., Mowat, D. L., Meagher-Stewart, D. M., Deber, R. B., Baumann, A. O., MacDonald, M. B., . . . Munroe, V. J. (2009). Building community and public health nursing capacity: A synthesis report of the National Community Health Nursing Study. *Canadian Journal of Public Health, 100*(5), I-1–I-13.

Walker, D. (2004). *For the public's health: A plan for action. Final report of the Ontario Expert Panel on SARS and Infectious Disease Control.* Toronto, ON: Ministry of Health and Long-Term Care. Retrieved from http://www.health.gov.on.ca/en/common/ministry/publications/reports/walker04/walker04_mn.aspx

Weberg, D. (2010). Transformational leadership and staff retention: An evidence review with implications for healthcare systems. *Nursing Administration Quarterly, 34*(3), 246–258.

Willcocks, S. G. (2012). Exploring leadership effectiveness: Nurses as clinical leaders in the NHS. *Leadership in Health Services, 25*(1), 8–19.

World Health Organization. (1978). *Declaration of Alma-Ata.* Retrieved from http://www.who.int/publications/almaata_declaration_en.pdf

World Health Organization. (1986). *Ottawa charter for health promotion.* Ottawa, ON: Author. Retrieved from http://www.who.int/healthpromotion/conferences/previous/ottawa/en

World Health Organization. (2008). *Closing the gap in a generation: Health equity through action on the social determinants of health.* Commission on the Social Determinants of Health, Geneva, Switzerland: Author.

World Health Organization. (2011). Country profile: Canada. Retrieved from http://www.who.int/countries/can/en

World Health Organization. (2013). *The Helsinki statement on health in all policies.* The 8th international conference on health promotion, Helsinki, Finland. Reprinted with permission from World Health Organization. Retrieved from http://www.healthpromotion2013.org/images/8GCHP_Helsinki_Statement.pdf

## ABOUT THE AUTHORS

**Claire Betker**, RN, BN, MN, PhD(c), CCHN(C), has worked in community health for more than 30 years at the local, regional, provincial, and national levels in mental health, home health, primary health care, and public health. Most recently she was the senior knowledge translation specialist with the National Collaborating Centre for Determinants of Health. Claire has been very involved with the Community Health Nurses of Canada in Manitoba and nationally, participating in several standing committees and serving as president. Claire served on the board of directors of the Canadian Nurses Association as the representative for the Canadian Network of Nursing Specialties. In 2010, Claire was awarded the Canadian Public Health Association and the Public Health Agency of Canada's Human Resources Individual Award for her contribution to public health workforce development in Canada. She is currently a PhD student at the University of Saskatchewan, where her interest is in theory and its contribution to public health nursing practice and leadership development.

**Diane Bewick**, RN, BScN, MScN, DPA, CCHN(C), has extensive experience working in community health. She is currently the director of family health services and the chief nursing officer with the Middlesex-London Health Unit in Ontario. Diane has been an active member of numerous boards and commissions such as the Registered Nurses' Association of Ontario (RNAO) expert panel developing the Leadership Best Practice Guideline, the Canadian Nurse Practitioner Initiative Advisory Panel, and the Ontario Public Health Association (OPHA). Diane is an assistant professor in the Faculty of Health Sciences at the University of Western Ontario and is the recipient of the Sigma Theta Tau Leadership Award (Nursing Honor Society). She is currently working with others to strengthen community health nursing leadership nationally, including developing a centre for public health nursing excellence.

# Appendix 2A
## Funding for Health Services for First Nations and Inuit in Canada  *Rose Alene Roberts*

First Nations and Inuit Health Branch (FNIHB), a branch within Health Canada (HC), is responsible for the delivery of health services in First Nations and Inuit communities. Services are federally funded and regionally managed. FNIHB is divided into seven regions (Atlantic, Quebec, Ontario, Manitoba, Saskatchewan, Alberta, and British Columbia) that roughly correspond to the provincial boundaries. The Atlantic region includes all four Atlantic provinces. The Yukon, Northwest Territories, and Nunavut are overseen by the northern secretariat.

FNIHB regions are separate, parallel structures to the HC regional offices that exist in each region. Authority is decentralized, and each region has a unique organizational structure and relationship to its First Nations (FN) constituents. The majority of the First Nations and Inuit (FN/I) communities manage their own healthcare services in whole or in part. In the remainder, the non-transferred, community-based health services are managed by the regional office.

First Nations people are Canadian citizens and as such, have access to provincially and territorially funded health services that fall under the Canada Health Act, 1984. Aboriginal people, who include the Métis and Inuit, are included in the per capita allocations of federal funding that are transferred to the provinces for "medically necessary" health services. However, FN communities (legally known as "reserves") below the 60th parallel are on federal, or Crown, land. For this reason, the federal government has historically funded public health and primary health care services on reserves. "North of 60" Aboriginal people comprise most of the population of the Canadian territories, reserves are largely absent, and health services for Aboriginal people are completely integrated into the health and social services systems.

## Indian Health Policy, 1979

The Federal Indian Health policy is one of the cornerstones of current policy regarding FN people and the Canadian government. The Indian Health Policy of 1979 stated that it was based on the special relationship of the FN people to the federal government and to the Crown (First Nations and Inuit Health, 2005). This relationship is committed to addressing access issues and health disparities that exist for this specific population.

Policy (including health policy) for federal programs for FN people flows from constitutional and statutory provisions, treaties, and customary practice. It also flows from the commitment of FN people to preserve and enhance their culture and traditions. It recognizes the intolerable conditions of poverty and community decline, which affect many communities, and seeks a framework in which communities can remedy these conditions.

The federal government recognizes its legal and traditional responsibilities to Aboriginal populations and seeks to promote the ability of Aboriginal communities to pursue their aspirations within the framework of Canadian institutions (First Nations and Inuit Health, 2005).

Many First Nations communities exhibit conditions that are comparable with the level of poverty and community decline present in many rural and remote parts of Canada. Combined with this economic disadvantage are cultural isolation and the effects of a colonial past. For this reason, addressing the determinants of health is a key feature of federal policy for FN communities. Thus, the Indian Health Policy of 1979 noted that improving the level of health in FN communities is founded on three pillars

- community development (socioeconomic, cultural, and spiritual) to remove the conditions of poverty and powerlessness that prevent the members of the community from achieving a state of physical, mental, and social well-being;
- the traditional relationship of the FN people to the federal government, in which the federal government promotes the capacity of FN communities to manage their own local health services; and
- the Canadian health system, consisting of specialized and interrelated services funded by federal, provincial, or municipal governments, FN bands, or the private sector.

The federal government role lies in public health activities on reserves, health promotion, and the detection and mitigation of hazards to health in the environment. The most significant provincial and private roles are in the diagnosis and treatment of acute and chronic diseases and rehabilitation services (First Nations and Inuit Health, 2005). In 1989, the "Treasury Board approved authorities and resources to support the transfer of Indian health services from Medical Services, Health and Welfare Canada (now Health Canada) to First Nations and Inuit wishing to assume responsibility" (First Nations and Inuit Health, 2005). This "transfer process" (also called the "transfer initiative")

- permits health program control to be assumed at a pace determined by the community—that is, the community can assume control gradually over a number of years through a phased transfer;
- enables communities to design health programs to meet their needs;
- requires that certain mandatory public health and treatment programs be provided; and
- strengthens the accountability of Chiefs and Councils to community members.

Further, the transfer process

- gives communities the financial flexibility to allocate funds according to community health priorities and to retain unspent balances,
- gives communities the responsibility for eliminating deficits and for annual financial audits and evaluations at specific intervals,
- permits multi-year (three- to five-year) agreements,
- does not prejudice treaty or Aboriginal rights,
- operates within current legislation, and
- is optional and open to all FN communities south of the 60th parallel (First Nations and Inuit Health, 2005).

## Community Types

In order to better allocate resources, communities have been classified according to their degree of access to provincial or territorial health services. For example, a remote, isolated community may require professional nursing services on a 24-hour-a-day, seven-day-per-week basis. However, funding for these services also depends on community size:

- Type 1: Remote-Isolated: No scheduled flights, minimal telephone or radio services, and no road access.
- Type 2: Isolated: Scheduled flights, good telephone services, and no year-round road access.
- Type 3: Semi-Isolated: Road access greater than 90 km to physician services.
- Type 4: Non-Isolated: Road access less than 90 km to physician services.

Remote, isolated communities of fewer than 200 people may have only a lay community health representative (CHR) on site, who consults with a community health nurse in a neighbouring community nursing station. Alternatively, a nurse may visit for one or more days a month. Larger centres may have a nursing station with two or more nurses. Nurses in these settings function in an expanded role and provide essential public health, primary care, and physician and pharmacist replacement services on a 24-hour-a-day, seven-day-per-week basis. Larger, less-isolated communities have community health centres that provide more typical public health and primary care services during standard business hours. A physician may visit on a regular basis or clients may be referred out for doctor visits. Rarely, a community health centre may provide expanded role nursing services after hours. In both cases, FNIHB's Non-Insured Health Benefits (NIHB) program provides funding for medical transportation for the community member to visit a doctor or a hospital, when required.

## Other Federally Funded Programs

Health Canada currently funds 52 National Native Alcohol and Drug Abuse Program (NNADAP) treatment centres with approximately 700 beds (First Nations and Inuit Health, 2013b) and 10 National Youth Solvent Abuse Programs (NYSAP) with an additional 120 beds (First Nations and Inuit Health, 2005). NNADAP provides over 550 programs, including prevention, intervention, and aftercare activities. Over 700 workers, the majority of whom are First Nations and Inuit, are employed by NNADAP (First Nations and Inuit Health, 2013). Health Canada provides funding under its category of family health for early childhood development through its Head Start Programs, both on and off reserve, a children's oral health program, and fetal alcohol spectrum disorder (FASD) programs. There are also targeted programs for diabetes, HIV/AIDS, influenza, tuberculosis (TB), and West Nile virus (First Nations and Inuit Health, 2013a). Many of these programs are allocated to the communities on a per capita basis, which can result in very small sums for tiny communities.

Other government departments and branches provide funding to FN/I communities, which contributes to addressing determinants of health. FNIHB and Aboriginal Affairs and Northern Development Canada (AANDC) jointly resource on-reserve water quality; FNIHB is accountable for monitoring and testing, and AANDC is responsible for infrastructure. For the years 2007–2013, an amount of $234 million was allocated to support infrastructure, such as roads and bridges, energy systems, planning and skills development projects, and solid waste management (Aboriginal Affairs and Northern Development Canada, 2013). AANDC is responsible for housing and community-based education. The office of the Solicitor General funds community policing or support from the Royal Canadian Mounted Police. Human Resources Development Canada has an Aboriginal division that works with FN/I communities on strategies to improve access to trades.

In these ways, the federal government attempts to address the determinants of health, while FNIHB ensures access to community-based health services and supports community development.

## REFERENCES

Aboriginal Affairs and Northern Development Canada. (2013, November 5). *First Nation Infrastructure Fund. Aboriginal Affairs and Northern Development Canada Community Infrastructure.* Retrieved from http://www.aadnc-aandc.gc.ca/eng/1100100010656/1100100010657

First Nations and Inuit Health. (2005, April 8). *National Youth Solvent Abuse Program. First Nations and Inuit Health.* Retrieved from http://www.hc-sc.gc.ca/fniah-spnia/substan/ads/nysap-pnlasj-eng.php

First Nations and Inuit Health. (2013a, October 1). *First Nations and Inuit Health.* Retrieved from http://www.hc-sc.gc.ca/fniah-spnia/index-eng.php

First Nations and Inuit Health. (2013b, January 4). *National Native Drug and Alcohol Program. First Nations and Inuit Health.* Retrieved from http://www.hc-sc.gc.ca/fniah-spnia/substan/ads/nnadap-pnlaada-eng

# Nursing Roles, Functions, and Practice Settings

*Genevieve Currie and Ruth Schofield*

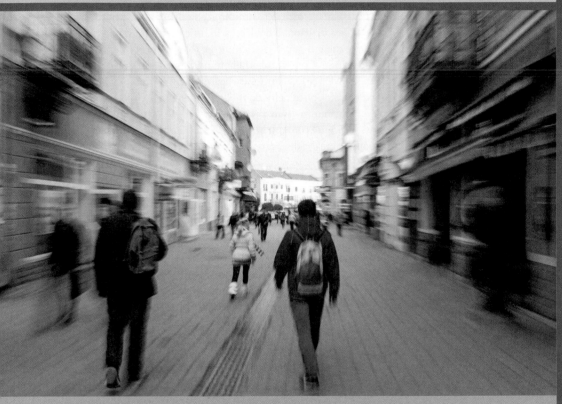

*Source: Vbaleha/Fotolia*

## INTRODUCTION

Community health nursing practice describes the work of registered nurses who work in a variety of settings within the community. **A community health nurse (CHN)** works with people where they live, work, learn, worship, and play to promote health (Community Health Nurses of Canada, 2009). CHNs partner with individuals, families, groups, communities, systems, and populations in various settings such as homes, schools, workplaces, streets, shelters, churches, field hospitals, community health centres, and outpost nursing stations and work with community members to determine and address their priorities. These nurses view health as a dynamic process of physical, mental, spiritual, and social well-being and as a resource for everyday life that is influenced by circumstances, beliefs, and determinants of health (CHNC, 2011a). The title CHN most often refers to nurses working in northern, rural, and remote areas of Canada and it is a generalist role. Other nurses within Canada might have the title of **public health nurse** or **home health nurse**.

As indicated in Chapter 8, Health Promotion, nurses work to promote health at various levels, sometimes implementing multiple interventions at different levels at the same time. This complex interplay of individual, group, community, and population-level interventions in promoting, protecting, or restoring health and preventing illness makes community health nursing unique and challenging. CHNs may undertake many roles and implement a range of interventions within the broad goal of promoting health.

This chapter describes the community health nursing professional practice model, standards of practice, national framework and action plan, and competencies. Examples of a broad range of community nursing roles, functions, and practice settings are also discussed. The range of roles includes primary care or primary health care nurse, PHC nurse practitioner, occupational health nurse, and rural or northern nurse, as well as some of the other community nursing roles. Also included in this chapter are trends affecting community health nursing practice.

# BLUEPRINT FOR ACTION FOR COMMUNITY HEALTH NURSING IN CANADA

The **Blueprint for Action for Community Health Nursing in Canada** was released by CHNC in 2011 (CHNC, 2011a). The Blueprint for Action provides a framework and a point of reference for ongoing dialogue on the development of community health nursing practice in Canada. With extensive collaboration, the voices of educators, policy makers, leaders in health services administration, researchers, and CHNs were heard. To provide further understanding of the context and challenges facing community health nursing practice, a literature review was completed and eight CHNC reports were synthesized and incorporated. The intent of the framework is to inform decisions about community health nursing practice and, ultimately, to promote and protect the health of Canadians. The Blueprint for Action identifies six arenas of action (CHNC, 2011a):

1. CHNs need to work at full scope and with greater clarity for the role in all domains of practice, such as common scope of practice, practice roles, and nomenclature, across provinces and territories;

2. support nursing leadership development and positions to advance community health nursing practice and to provide a voice for the profession;

3. build on successful collaboration within nursing and strengthen partnerships with other professionals and sectors;

4. transform the healthcare system into a system for (community) health;

5. support strong educational preparation in community health nursing; and

6. improve access to a range of professional development resources to advance community health nursing capacity.

# COMMUNITY HEALTH NURSING PRACTICE MODEL AND STANDARDS OF PRACTICE

Community health nursing is one of 20 nursing practice specialties recognized in Canada (Canadian Nurses Association, 2014a). Before World War II, about 60% of all nurses practised in private homes and community-based settings, but by 1989, with technological changes and medicare, about 85% of nurses were employed by hospitals (Bartfay, 2010). The trend toward hospital-based practice is slowly changing once again as a result of changes in PHC in Canada. The CNA predicts that by 2020, 60% of nurses will be working outside the acute care setting (2008). According to the Canadian Institute of Health Information, in 2013, 15.2% of registered nurses (RNs) were employed in the community health sector (2014). This includes community health, public health, home health, occupational health, and telehealth nursing. CHNs embrace their nursing practice within a diversity of roles and practice settings. Combining their foundational nursing education with knowledge of community health nursing concepts, including a variety of service delivery models, nursing care spans the complete continuum from primary prevention (true prevention of illness or injury through health promotion activities and protective actions before the disease or injury) to secondary prevention (screening and early detection and treatment) and tertiary prevention (maintaining and/or restoring health of clients with a chronic illness or condition) in their practice (Public Health Agency of Canada, 2013; Vollman, Anderson, & McFarlane, 2012).

The **Community Health Nurses of Canada (CHNC)** is an associate member of the CNA and a leader in community health nursing practice in Canada. The mission of CHNC, as a national nursing organization for community health RNs, is to advance practice and to improve the health of Canadians. CHNC members view their values as ideals or beliefs that help to define and guide the organization. The values include health that is defined as a human right for all Canadians and a healthcare system that requires a balance of health promotion and illness care; leadership that is a requirement for system change and fundamental to supporting community health nursing practice; engagement of the voice of all populations so that they are full partners in determining approaches to health and wellness; and **social justice** that is foundational to health equity and central to community health nursing practice.

The CHNC represents the voices of community health nurses. The members of CHNC promote practice excellence and create opportunities for partnerships across sectors and networks through national conferences, webinars, local workshops, and online resources. The CHNC provides opportunities for strengthening community health nursing leadership by implementing leadership preferences at their national conferences for community health nursing. They advocate for healthy public policy to address **social and environmental determinants of health** and promote a publicly funded, not-for-profit system for (community) health (CHNC, 2012). Through substantial funding from the Public Health Agency of Canada, many structures and tools, such as standards, competencies, and a Blueprint for Action, have been developed with the intent of strengthening the community health nursing workforce.

In 2011 the CHNC released the components of the Canadian community health nursing professional practice model. Later in 2013, the model was completed with a visual presentation (see Figure 3.1). The CHNC (2011b, revised) outlines a professional practice model that includes a structure, process, and values supporting nurses' control over nursing care delivery and the environment in which care is delivered. The community health nursing professional model of practice describes thirteen components organized in four main categories: the client, CHNs and nursing practice, community organizations, and the system. The core of practice is the client, which includes individuals, families, groups, communities, systems, and populations. Informing the work of CHNs and nursing practice with clients is a code of ethics (CNA, 2008a), theoretical foundations, values and principles, professional regulatory standards, and community health nursing standards of practice and discipline-specific competencies. In the context

of community organizations, community health nursing practice is influenced by management practices, delivery structures and process, and professional relationships and partnerships. The last category is the system that includes government support and determinants of health. The definition of each component is found in Figure 3.1. During the development of the professional practice model, nurses reported that the model would provide them with a common framework for practice and would enable them to speak in a unified manner.

In 2003 the CHNC developed **standards of practice** through a national consultation process with community health nurses (CHNC, 2011b, revised). In 2008 the standards were reformatted, and then in 2011 the standards were revised and updated based on information from a literature review, focus groups, and a national Delphi consensus process with 443 CHNs from all domains of practice. The Delphi technique involves collecting information from selected experts

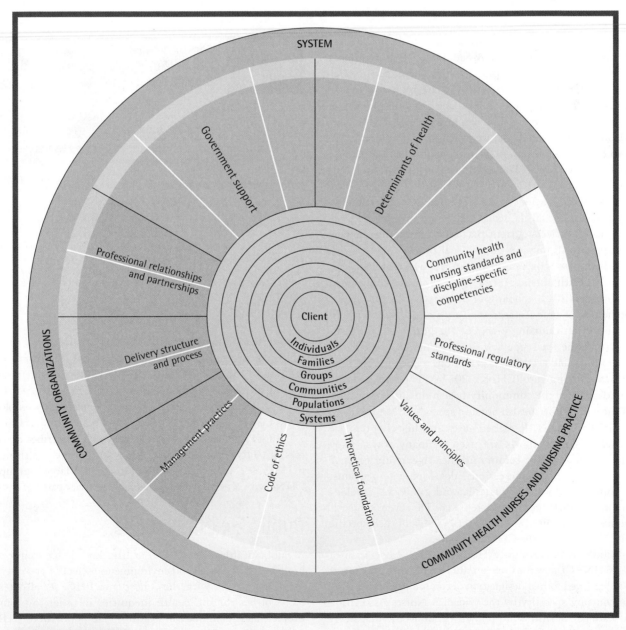

**FIGURE   3.1** Canadian Community Health Nursing Professional Practice Model

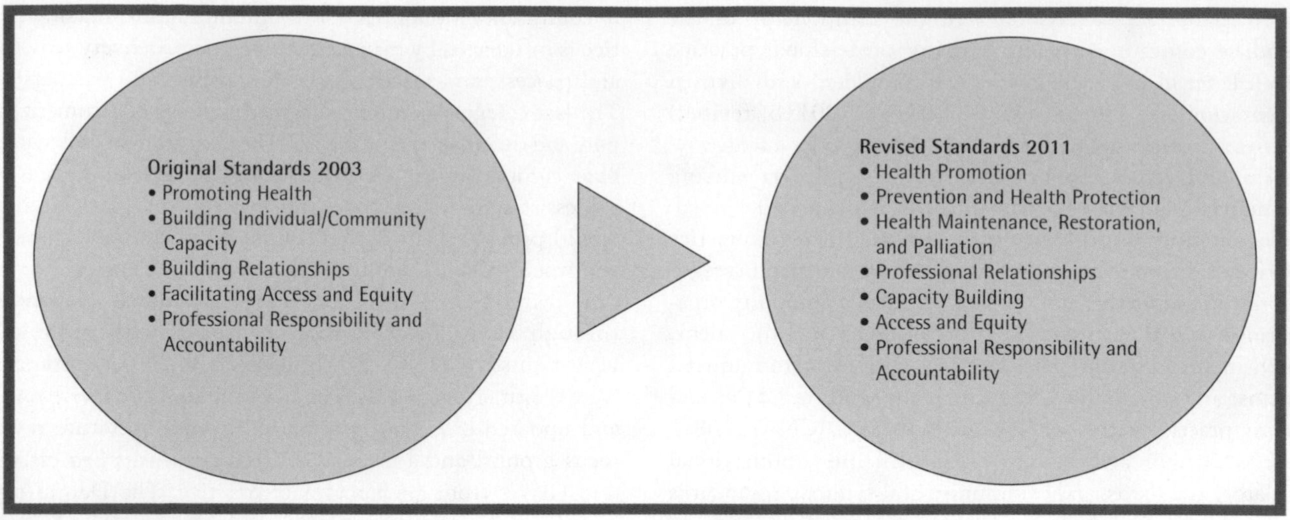

Original Standards 2003
• Promoting Health
• Building Individual/Community Capacity
• Building Relationships
• Facilitating Access and Equity
• Professional Responsibility and Accountability

Revised Standards 2011
• Health Promotion
• Prevention and Health Protection
• Health Maintenance, Restoration, and Palliation
• Professional Relationships
• Capacity Building
• Access and Equity
• Professional Responsibility and Accountability

**FIGURE 3.2** Comparison of 2003 and 2011 Canadian Community Health Nursing Standards of Practice

using a cycle of questionnaires until an agreement on the topic of investigation is reached (Hsu & Sandford, 2007). **Domains of practice** include clinical practice, education, administration, and research. The rationale for the revisions to the standards is noteworthy and reflects the growing practice of community health nursing. By changing the number of standards from five to seven, equal weighting and importance was given to health promotion, prevention and health protection, and health maintenance. The re-ordering of the original standards two and three reflects that professional relationships are an essential initial step in capacity building. A greater emphasis on social justice and the social and environmental determinants of health reflects current practice. Combining the new community health nursing professional practice model with the standards was a necessary step in the overall scheme for community health nursing. (See Figure 3.2 for the comparison of the 2003 and 2011 standards of practice.)

Standards of practice represent a vision for excellence in community health nursing practice. The purpose of the standards is to define the scope and depth of nursing practice in the community and establish expectations for acceptable, safe, and ethical nursing care (CHNC, 2011a). The standards are the foundation for the community health nursing competencies in the community health nursing specialty CNA certification exam, which is described later in this chapter (see Table 3.1). The standards are used in many ways. They measure performance of community health nursing practice by employers, support professional development programs, inform nursing education curricula, and guide the development of new knowledge through research. The seven standards of practice are presented in Table 3.1. Details of each specific standard are found on the CHNC website.

In 2005 the Community Health Nurses Association of Canada (CHNAC), now the Community Health Nurses of Canada (CHNC), received formal designation of community health nursing as a nursing specialty by the Canadian Nurses Association (CNA) national certification program. In 2006 the first CNA community health nursing certification examination was offered. Community health nursing is now one of 20 recognized specialty

| Table 3.1 | Canadian Nurses Association Community Health Nursing Competencies for the Certification Exam |
|---|---|

1. Health promotion
2. Prevention and health protection
3. Health maintenance, restoration, and palliation
4. Building capacity
5. Professional relationship
6. Access and equity
7. Professional responsibility and accountability

Source: Canadian Nurses Association. (2014). *Introduction – Blueprint for the Community Health Nursing Certification Exam*. Ottawa, ON: Author. Published by Canadian Nurses Association, © 2011. Retrieved from http://www.nurseone.ca/en/certification/what-is-certification/competencies-per-specialty-area/community-health-nursing

nursing areas in Canada (CNA, 2014b). The number of certified CHNs has increased steadily over the past five years, from 338 in 2008 to 907 in 2014 (CNA, 2014b). It is a voluntary national nursing credential based on national standards released by CNA in 2003 but it is now often required or preferred by employers across Canada. National certification is valid for five years.

In its standards of practice the CHNC describes two sectors of CHNs: public health nurses and home health nurses (CHNC, 2011c). These two sectors are the largest groups of CHNs with a new, growing sector in primary care.

## Public Health Nursing

A public health nurse (PHN) utilizes knowledge from public health, nursing, social and environmental sciences, and research, integrating these with the concepts of PHC, social determinants of health, and health inequities in order to promote, protect, and maintain the health of the population (CHNC, 2011b, revised). The *goal of public health nursing*, as with public health, is to increase the health of the public (i.e., reduce mortality and morbidity rates) by preventing disease and promoting healthy behaviours and environments. PHNs work under the mandate of provincial public health legislation within official public health agencies (i.e., a health unit or health department of municipal, regional, or provincial governments). Their clients include individuals, families, groups, communities, systems, and populations.

PHNs work with clients of all ages throughout the lifespan and provide a range of health promotion activities, such as prenatal care, postpartum home visiting, routine immunization, school and workplace healthcare, infectious disease control, healthy lifestyle promotion, substance abuse prevention, injury prevention (including infant and child injury and fall prevention with seniors), and environmental health (CHNC, 2011b, revised).

PHNs work with interdisciplinary team members who may include public health professionals, such as public health inspectors, dietitians, epidemiologists, environmental health practitioners, health promoters, dentists, and physicians. They also work closely with other sectors, such as education, industry, housing, and social services to address determinants of health impacting populations or communities at a local, provincial, or national level. Community members and community agency representatives are also an integral part of the team. In smaller agencies and rural or remote communities, PHNs often assume a generalist role, providing a variety of services to a geographic area as opposed to the specialist roles found in larger agencies and settings. Over the years, various initiatives have undertaken to define the areas of practice for community health nursing. Standards define the scope of practice or professional expectations (CHNC, 2011c), while competencies encompass the knowledge, skills, and attitudes required for practice (Public Health Agency of Canada, 2007). Refer to Chapter 4 for the public health nursing discipline-specific competencies, as well as for more information on public health nursing.

## Home Health Nursing

**Home health nursing** is a specialized area of community health nursing practice in which the nurse, employed by a home health agency, provides clinical care in the client's home, school, or workplace. Home health nurses (HHNs) provide the resources to promote their clients' optimal level of well-being and functioning, and empower their clients and caregivers or families to take charge of their own care. Home health nursing activities include chronic disease management and curative practices, health promotion and health education, palliative care, rehabilitation, support and maintenance, social support, and support for the family so that the client can continue to live in the community (Canadian Home Care Association, 2014).

The broad spectrum of services provided by HHNs aims at "providing accessible, responsive, and timely care which allows people to stay in their homes with safety and dignity" (CHNC, 2010, p. 7). Home health nursing "encompasses disease prevention, rehabilitation, restoration of health, health protection, and health promotion with the goal of managing existing problems and preventing potential problems" (p. 7). The aim is to help individuals experiencing any number of health problems to remain in their home environment and familiar surroundings. Such home care services may help to prevent a hospital visit or shorten a hospital stay, thus saving the healthcare system money in the longer term.

Although the role of the HHN is commonly categorized as generalist in nature, the trend toward care from nurses specializing in relevant clinical areas has given rise to numerous specialty roles for HHNs. These include chronic disease specialist, wound ostomy resource nurse, psychogeriatric nurse, continence adviser, diabetes nurse educator, palliative care nurse consultant, hospice nurse, respiratory nurse specialist, and many others. These specialty HHNs provide expert client assessment and care, and plan guidance that contributes to client care excellence while augmenting the generalist nurse's knowledge base and competencies.

Unlike public health, which is government funded, home healthcare is delivered by not-for-profit and for-profit agencies. Some programs receive funding from government(s); however, the remaining funding is delivered through private insurance coverage and fundraising initiatives. The Victorian Order of Nurses (VON) is an example of a not-for-profit organization that has been providing community healthcare services across Canada for well over 100 years (VON, 2009). Paramed (2011) is the largest for-profit home care agency in Canada, offering services in Alberta and Ontario.

The various home healthcare agencies generally have similar philosophies that include the delivery of holistic, evidenced-based healthcare to individuals, families, and groups in community settings. Programs and services vary across agencies and geographical sites as these reflect identified community needs and agency resources. A set of home health nursing competencies was developed in 2010 by CHNC. These competency domains are clinical decision making; care planning and coordination; health maintenance, restoration, and palliation; teaching and education; communication and relationships; access and building capacity; health promotion; illness prevention; and health protection. Refer to Chapter 5 for a complete description of these competencies. More details on the role of the home healthcare nurse can also be found in Chapter 5.

Regardless of specialty areas within community health nursing, key characteristics of CHNs are reflected in the standards and include a high level of independence, autonomy, resourcefulness, collaboration with the client and his or her family and community, strong community and individual health assessment skills, critical thinking and problem solving, and an understanding of the community and its resources, as well as of the overall healthcare system. All CHNs work within an array of provincial or territorial legislations and regulatory professional standards, but the concepts of health promotion and PHC are the foundation of their practice. These will be defined next.

The most commonly used definition of health promotion is that used in a global context by the World Health Organization (WHO) (WHO, 1984): "the process of enabling people to increase control over and to improve their health" (n.p.). It is a broad definition and includes the complete spectrum of health promotion activity, including health enhancement, health protection, disease prevention, health restoration or recovery, and care and support. **Primary health care (PHC)**, on the other hand, was defined at the 1978 Alma-Ata conference as healthcare that is scientifically sound, socially acceptable, universally accessible to individuals and families through their full participation, and at a cost the community and country can afford within the spirit of self-reliance and self-determination (WHO, 1978). This definition has evolved to include all broad social health determinants and the services that can influence health, such as income, housing, education, and social and physical environments (National Collaborating Centre for the Determinants of Health, 2014; Raphael, 2012). A more in-depth discussion of health promotion is found in Chapter 8. All CHNs have a mandate to integrate the principles of PHC into their care of individuals, groups, communities, and populations. The CHNC (2011a) describes the following roles of a CHN in one of the components of the Canadian CHN Professional Practice Model:

■ promote, protect, and preserve the health of individuals, families, groups, communities, and populations in the settings where they live, work, learn, worship, and play in an ongoing and/or episodic process;

■ consider and address the impact of the determinants of health within the political, cultural, and environmental context on health;

■ support capacity building approaches focused on client strengths and client participation;

■ protect and enhance human dignity, respecting social, cultural, and personal belief and circumstances of their clients;

■ advocate and engage in political action and healthy public policy options to facilitate healthy living;

■ incorporate the concepts of inclusiveness, equity, and social justice as well as the principles of community development;

■ participate in knowledge generation and knowledge translation, and integrate knowledge and multiple ways of knowing;

■ engage in evidence-informed decision making;

■ work at a high level of autonomy; and

■ practice with an emphasis on teamwork, collaboration, consultation, and professional relationships (p. 4).

There are differences in the roles and functions of the CHNs among the provinces and territories. For example, in Quebec, there is a blended community health nursing model where a nurse may function within both hospital and community health domains. Figure 3.3 depicts the various types of community nursing and Table 3.2 describes the various characteristics in the practice areas.

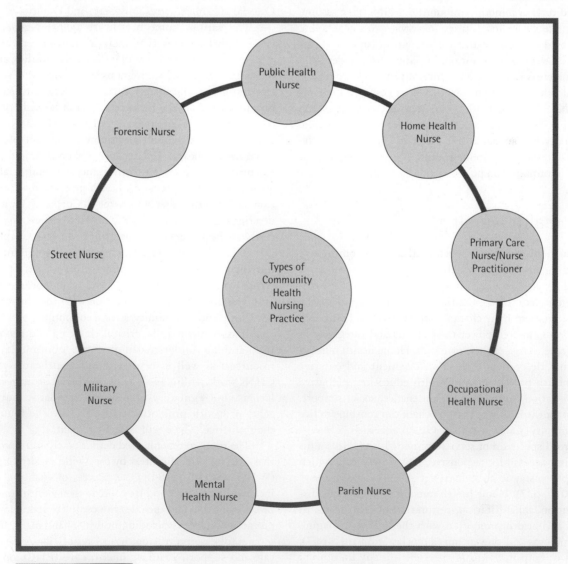

**FIGURE  3.3**  Types of Community Health Nursing Practice

**Table 3.2** Characteristics of Selected Community Health Nurses in Varied Practice Settings

| CHNs | Work Setting | Aims | Roles/Function | Client Focus | Funding |
|---|---|---|---|---|---|
| Public Health Nurse | Client homes, schools, workplaces, shelters, streets, clinics | PHNs focus on promoting, protecting, and preserving the health of the populations. The PHN links the health and illness experiences of individuals, families, and communities to population health promotion (CPHA, 2010). | Performs a variety of roles: <br>– Health promotion (e.g., supports healthy public policy to modify physical and social environments) <br>– Disease and illness prevention (e.g., encourages healthy lifestyle choices) <br>– Health protection (e.g., controls infectious diseases) <br>– Health surveillance (e.g., collects and reports health data for tracking and forecasting health events) <br>– Population health assessment (e.g., collects information about the population to initiate or evaluate services) <br>– Emergency preparedness and response (e.g., plans for and evaluates the public health's response to disasters) | Individual, family, group, community, or larger population | Municipal and/or provincial government funding |
| Home Health Nurse | Client homes, schools, workplaces, clinics, streets | HHNs focus on health promotion, prevention, health restoration and maintenance, or palliation and end-of-life care. | Performs a variety of roles: <br>– Manages chronic and terminal illness across the lifespan (e.g., management of intravenous infusion therapy, complex dialysis regimes) <br>– Health teaching (e.g., new diabetics) <br>– Rehabilitation (e.g., wound care clinics) <br>– Palliation and end-of-life care <br>– Support for individuals and caregivers | Individuals and families | Not-for-profit and for-profit agencies |
| Outpost Nurse / Community Health Nurse | Client homes, schools, clinics, streets, hospitals, or any location in the community | Outpost/CHNs in the North focus on the roles of a PHN; in rural and remote communities, they also focus on the roles of an HHN and acute care nurse. | See the roles identified under PHNs and HHNs <br>– Direct primary health clinical care | Individual, family, group, or larger population | Federal government |

*(continued)*

| Table 3.2 | Continued | | | | |
|---|---|---|---|---|---|
| **Characteristics** | | | | | |
| **CHNs** | **Work Setting** | **Aims** | **Roles/Function** | **Client Focus** | **Funding** |
| Occupational Health Nurse | Workplace | Occupational health nurses focus on health promotion, maintenance and restoration, and injury and disease prevention in the workplace. | – Needs assessments (e.g., health and safety risk assessments of workplace)<br><br>– Injury prevention (e.g., establish policies and procedures)<br><br>– Health promotion (e.g., healthy lifestyles programs)<br><br>– Coordination (e.g., occupational health services) | Individual workers and worker populations | Employer |
| Mental Health Nurse | Client homes, community health centres, various community locations | Mental health nurses focus on mental healthcare of people with serious mental illness living in the community, in collaboration with caregivers and the mental healthcare team. | Therapeutic relationship (e.g., long-term involvement)<br><br>– Diagnoses and monitoring (e.g., risk assessment for alteration in mental health status)<br><br>– Education (e.g., medication in partnership with healthcare team)<br><br>– Teacher/coach (e.g., plan and support choices to maximize mental health)<br><br>– System navigation (e.g., advocate and support access to community resources)<br><br>– Treatment (e.g., administering medication) | Individual, family, group, or population | Provincial government, through facilities such as CHC and the regional health authority |
| Primary Health Care Nurse Practitioner (PHCNP) | Family health teams, NP-led clinics, public health units/departments, regional health authorities, post-secondary medical clinics, outposts | Primary health care nurse practitioners (PHCNPs) are RNs with advanced university nursing education. | PHCNPs focus on health promotion, injury and disease prevention, as well as supportive, curative, rehabilitative, and palliative care. Advanced practice functions include the following:<br><br>– Health screening (e.g., performing Pap smears)<br><br>– Diagnoses (e.g., order and interpret diagnostic tests for ear and bladder infections)<br><br>– Disease management (e.g., prescribe medications) | Individuals, families | Provincial government<br><br>Federal government |

| Table 3.2 | Continued | | | | |
|---|---|---|---|---|---|
| **Characteristics** | | | | | |
| **CHNs** | **Work Setting** | **Aims** | **Roles/Function** | **Client Focus** | **Funding** |
| | | | – Family practice nurses (FPN NPs) are RNs. FPN NPs focus on health promotion, injury and disease prevention, and management. | | |
| | | | – Case management (e.g., helping clients navigate the healthcare system) | | |
| | | | – Health education | | |
| | | | – Triage and referral | | |
| | | | – Treatment (e.g., dressing changes, injections) | | |
| | | | – Counselling (works collaboratively with physician and healthcare team.) | | |
| Forensic Nurse | Prisons, hospital emergency rooms, police departments, coroner's office, lawyers | Forensic nurses focus on the nursing care and forensic sciences in the judicial system. | – Assessment (e.g., collect DNA evidence from victims of accidents or from crime scenes) | Individuals, families | Correctional facility or privately funded |
| | | | – Preservation (e.g., DNA evidence for court) | | |
| | | | – Assist with autopsies | | |
| | | | – Trial expert/consultant (e.g., attend court as witness) | | |
| Nurse Entrepreneur | Any setting where hired to provide services | Nurse entrepreneurs are self-employed professionals who organize, manage, and assume the risks of a business enterprise. They work independently and are self-directed and goal focused. | – Direct patient care | | Private funding |
| | | | – Research | | |
| | | | – Education | | |
| | | | – Administration | | |
| | | | – Consultation | | |
| Military Nurse/ Nursing Officer | Military bases, operational units, outpatient or tertiary care facilities, overseas | Nursing officer is the title for a military nurse who is a commissioned member of the Canadian Forces Medical Service (CFMS). | – Focus on sick and injured patients, not only in static facilities such as a garrison, base, or wing in a healthcare centre, but also in operational facilities such as a field hospital | Military personnel and civilians | Federal government |
| | | | – Direct patient care | | |
| | | | – Policy development | | |
| | | | – Training and education | | |

(*continued*)

**Table 3.2** Continued

| CHNs | Work Setting | Aims | Roles/Function | Client Focus | Funding |
|---|---|---|---|---|---|
| Parish Nurse | Faith communities | Parish nurses are called to minister and are affirmed by a faith to promote health, healing, and wholeness. | Health advocacy<br>– Health education<br>– Health counselling<br>– Referrals to community resources | Individuals and families within a parish community | Private funding |
| Telehealth | A variety of healthcare services offered through information communication technologies | Telehealth nurses focus on support services across a spectrum of healthcare services, including diagnosis, treatment, and prevention of diseases using information communication technologies. They facilitate increased access to healthcare services and enhance coordination of services across the continuum of care. | – Health assessment<br>– Triage<br>– Health education<br>– Monitor client status<br>– Health counselling | The public and professionals | Provincial government<br>Federal government<br>Private funding through physician offices |
| Outreach/Street Nurse | Streets, parks, homeless shelters, drop-in centres | Street nurses focus on mostly secondary and tertiary healthcare services with people who are homeless. | – Prevention (e.g., harm reduction through needle exchange)<br>– Outreach<br>– Counselling<br>– System advocacy (facilitate access to services)<br>– Legal support<br>– Education | All ages of homeless population | Federal and provincial governments |

Characteristics

Depending on the settings they work in, CHNs engage in the following activities: advocacy; building capacity; building coalition and networks; care and counselling; case management; communication; community development; consultation; facilitation; health education; health threat response; leadership; social marketing and outreach; policy development and implementation; referral and follow-up; research; resource management; program planning, coordination, and evaluation; screening; surveillance; and team building and collaboration.

---

**CANADIAN RESEARCH BOX 3.1**

**What are "intra-professional practice education opportunities using a community partnership model"?**

Hoffart, C., Kuster-Orban, C., Spooner, C., & Neudorf, K. (2014). Intra-professional practice education using a community partnership model. *Journal of Nursing Education, 52*(2), 104–107. Published by Slack, Inc., © 2014.

This pilot project reports on an intra-professional practice education model, including acute and community placement experiences. It involved faculty and students from three designations—LPNs, RNs, and RPNs—in the context of a rural First Nations community. The pilot project was conducted in Saskatchewan. The project used the partnership model of community health nursing education (PMCHNE). Three students from each of the three programs participated over an eight-week period, with weekly four-hour conferences with faculty. Triad debriefing meetings with students, faculty, and community advisers were held. Common competencies were identified among the three programs, as well as common learning pathways. The learning pathways were holistic health, professional and ethical practice, cultural safety, therapeutic relationship, critical thinking, and clinical judgment. The results indicated that students and faculty felt welcomed in the First Nations community. Students expressed a greater understanding of primary health care, determinants of health, cultural diversity, holism, the continuum of care and rural nursing, and various roles as well as the value of interdependence of the roles in improving the health of clients, families, and the community. Please read the article to enhance your understanding of the findings.

### Discussion Questions

1. What community health nursing concepts did these students identify in the community placement experience?

2. What Canadian community health nursing standards of practice apply for the registered nurse?

3. What intra-professional competencies might be common between the three nursing designations? Which are distinct for the registered nurse?

---

**CASE STUDY**

You are a nursing student in your final year of study and will soon obtain your baccalaureate degree in nursing. You are determining your final focus for the nursing practicum. You have decided you would like to focus on the broader influences of health and work in the domain of social justice and overcoming health inequities. You are aware of the diversity in practice settings in the community, and the concept of working collaboratively, which seems to be a consistent feature among them, really appeals to you. You want to make your choice for the clinical practicum a good match for your clinical interests, skills, and the roles of the CHN within the specialty.

### Discussion Questions

1. From reading all the descriptions of roles of CHNs in this chapter, assess which one appeals to you in terms of the kind of nursing roles and functions described.

2. What nursing knowledge, skills, and attitudes are required from you if you were working in the various specialties?

3. How would you prepare for practising in the community health nursing role you have chosen? What skill sets and theoretical knowledge would you review?

## EXPANDING COMMUNITY HEALTH NURSING PRACTICE

Five nursing specialty areas were chosen to illustrate the expansion of community health nursing practice in Canada. The historical and practice perspectives, including roles and challenges, are described for primary care nursing, rural or outpost nursing, occupational health nursing, parish nursing, forensic nursing, and military nursing.

## Primary Care Nursing

*Historical Perspectives:* Demand for primary care services has increased in developed countries such as Canada over the last 15 years due to an aging population, rising patient expectations, and a shift in focus from hospital to community care. Due to the high degree of specialization required for care of individuals, families, and communities, **primary care nursing** has also become specialized with regard to nursing knowledge, roles, and functions. Some of the titles for RNs in primary care settings in Canada are family practice nurses, primary care nurses, or **primary health care nurses**. The title for advanced practice nurses can be **primary health care nurse practitioners (PHCNP)**, an area which will be described later in this chapter. Areas of expertise within primary care nursing include chronic disease management nurses, telehealth nurses, and outreach/street nurses. These are described in this section.

*Practice Perspective:* Primary care nurses provide the first contact with healthcare. This first contact often occurs within primary care settings, such as primary care networks, ambulatory care centres, long-term care facilities, physician offices, family health clinics, community health centres, and community clinics in urban, rural, and remote communities (Primary Care Initiative, 2013). Primary care nurses might also focus on vulnerable groups, such as the Aboriginal and Inuit communities, with specific evidence-based interventions that are designed for work with them (Health Canada, 2014). Primary care nursing focuses on health promotion, disease and injury prevention, cure, rehabilitation, and support. These CHNs work with other healthcare providers within a multidisciplinary and multi-sectoral clinic, or they might work independently for a community agency or within a vulnerable population.

**Chronic Disease Nurses** One specialized title within primary care nursing is that of **chronic disease management nurse**. These nurses manage the care of individuals with chronic diseases that require them to be closely followed by a healthcare provider. The nurses often work in collaboration with the individual, family, and healthcare team, including a physician, to closely monitor and manage the disease with the individual and family members. This often occurs in the client's home setting within the community. Diseases that have been identified for nurses to manage can include diabetes; cardiovascular disease, including hypertension and chronic obstructive pulmonary disease; renal disease; mental illness; obesity; and others. The nurse supports patients in learning new behaviours and provides them with the knowledge, tools, and skills to manage their disease. The home care nurse also coordinates referrals to appropriate services, such as nutritionists, the chronic pain clinic, smoking cessation programs, cholesterol educators, exercise specialists, and social workers, and also provides case or disease management according to clinical practice guidelines, focusing on overall health and well-being. An example of a chronic disease program that nurses are involved in is Alberta's Better Choices, Better Health program, which is based on work done at Stanford University using a model of self-management of chronic illness (Stanford University, 2015). Better Choices, Better Health includes supervised exercise and disease-specific education in the areas of problem solving, dealing with difficult emotions, coping with pain and fatigue, symptom management, and making informed treatment decisions for people with ongoing health problems (Alberta Health Services, 2014a).

Use of the **5 A's of behaviour change** approach found in the Registered Nurses' Association of Ontario (RNAO) best practice guideline on self-management of chronic conditions is another common evidence-informed approach applied by CHNs in some provinces (RNAO, 2010). The 5 A's stand for assess, advise, agree, assist, and arrange. CHNs working in home health and primary care settings will be guided by this self-management approach to chronic disease management when working with clients with a chronic illness and their families to assist in improved health outcomes.

Targeted interventions exist within some jurisdictions in Canada for certain populations dealing with high incidences of chronic illnesses as well as facing financial, social, and cultural access barriers in managing these diseases. Some such groups are Aboriginal populations, homeless populations, adolescents, and certain cultural groups, such as the Hutterites, Indo-Asians, and Chinese populations (Alberta Health Services,

2014b). Nurses provide support in accessible community-based sites, utilizing numerous culturally sensitive and credible educational tools that have been developed. Some of the nurses provide services in the patient's native language, such as Punjabi and Spanish, and are called **diversity nurses**. The content of the educational materials is developed in accordance with clinical practice guidelines.

**Telehealth Nurses** Another specialized area of practice in primary care nursing is **telehealth**. **Telehealth nursing** arose out of the need to provide timely access to health information, counselling, health assessment, health promotion, and coordination of services to the appropriate healthcare providers. Telehealth nursing supports the principles of PHC, particularly accessibility of health services, health promotion, and use of appropriate technology, along with telephone-based nurse triage. Eight provinces and two territories use a telecare service, providing nursing support 24 hours a day, 7 days a week (Scott, 2009). Nurses practising within telehealth use strong communication, assessment, and critical-thinking skills while they determine the healthcare needs of individuals over the phone, computer, audio and video conferencing, and the Internet (CNA, 2014c). Nurses provide health illness risk assessments; chronic disease management; support for early postpartum care; acute illness and emergency assessments; wellness promotion; communicable disease control; employee health and monitoring; home clinical monitoring of people with chronic illnesses, such as with the use of ECGs, BP, swallow assessments, and SPO2; and employee health (Scott, 2009). A goal of telehealth nursing is self-care management and support for individuals and families living within the community and being monitored at home. Challenges for telehealth nursing have included lack of standardized accredited and approved clinical practice guidelines in some regions of Canada. This has improved greatly over the last 10 years with the use of algorithms and care maps for managing the assessment, triage, and referral of complex medical issues (CNA, 2014c).

**Outreach/Street Nurses** Another specialized primary care nursing practice area is **outreach/street nursing**. Outreach/street nursing can included RNs or nurse practitioners (NPs), home health nurses, or PHNs. They work in many large city centres across Canada with disenfranchised individuals and the greater populations of homeless individuals within shelters, needle exchange sites, harm reduction clinics, community agencies, jails and remand centres, medical clinics, and rehabilitation clinics. (See Photo 3.1.)

*Historical Perspectives:* This area of practice arose after World War II in an effort to meet the needs of marginalized individuals, and it grew in the 1970s and 80s to address the high rates of sexually transmitted infections (STIs) and the emerging HIV problem within inner city populations, such as in Vancouver and Toronto (BC Centre for Disease Control, 2012a). Nurses were required to provide nursing care using health promotion, disease prevention, and harm reduction strategies specific to vulnerable population groups with accessibility issues and general mistrust of healthcare providers. Thus, CHNs saw the need for development of the specific role of the street nurse (Hardill, 2007).

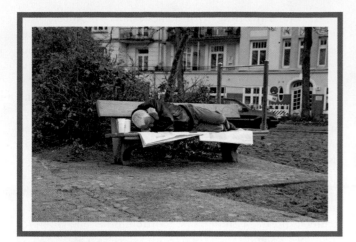

**PHOTO 3.1** Street nursing with people who are homeless

*Source: Britta60/Fotolia*

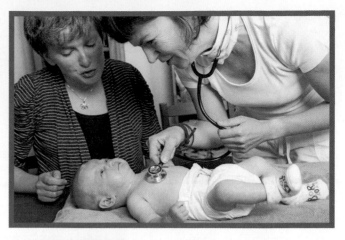

**PHOTO 3.2** Primary health care nurse doing a well-baby check

*Source: Edler von Rabenstein/Fotolia*

*Practice Perspective:* Outreach/street nursing involves care focused on building relationships while maintaining the dignity of and respect for the clients, and creating an environment of cultural safety and empowerment. This relationship-building work often takes place between people who are homeless and community and government agencies. Street nurses rely on partnerships, community collaboration, and a client-centred approach in order to be successful and create change. They work closely with government sectors and community services to provide access to primary care, mental health services, job skills and retraining, housing, communicable disease support for those with HIV and tuberculosis, STI follow-up and care, birth control and prenatal and postnatal supports, and drug and alcohol rehabilitation. Through the lens of health promotion and harm reduction, street nurses use creative and innovative prevention strategies with individuals living on the streets and in shelters in Canada to provide clinical care, such as wound and diabetic care. They also work with larger systems, such as the federal government, to advocate for reform and provide access to the basic necessities of life, such as the affordable housing framework for Canada 2011–2014 (Canadian Mortgage and Housing Corporation, 2011). As an example, nurses from across Canada, including professional partnerships with the CNA, the Registered Nurses' Association of Ontario, the Association of Registered Nurses of British Columbia, and the B.C. Nurses Union, acted as advocates in support of Insite, a harm reduction clinic within Vancouver's Downtown Eastside neighbourhood, and lobbied the Supreme Court of Canada. Outreach and street nurses across Canada supported the subsequent decision by the Supreme Court which ruled in favour of Insite remaining open (Canadian Drug Policy Coalition, 2012). Outreach and street nurses also have a role in mentoring and educating the public, healthcare providers, and higher levels of government on the larger influences of health on individuals and populations (BC Centre for Disease Control, 2012b).

**Primary Health Care Nurse Practitioners** Advanced practice nurses who are nurse practitioners are also called primary health care nurse practitioners (PHCNPs). This NP role is specific to working within the community and often remote areas. (See Photo 3.2.)

*Historical Perspective:* The work of NPs evolved from decades of nurses working in isolated and remote areas in Canada, often as outpost nurses. In the 1970s, interest and expansion in rural and remote nursing grew. In 1971 the Boudreau Report made the implementation of the expanded role of the RN a high priority in Canada's healthcare system. Many education programs began graduating NPs, but in the absence of supporting regulatory legislation, these nurses functioned as RNs working under medical directives (Nurse Practitioners' Association of Ontario, 2011). In the 1990s, the need for additional education for nurses working in specialty areas was recognized and educational institutions began to offer certificate and graduate programs for advanced practice nursing as NPs (CNA, 2011). In an attempt to streamline practice expectations, optimize the contribution of PHCNPs and all NPs, and develop some consistency in advanced nursing practice across the country, in 2006, through federal funding, the CNA established the Canadian Nurse Practitioner Initiative (CNPI) (CNPI, n.d.). The goal of this initiative was to ensure sustained integration of the NP role in the health system. The original recommendations have been updated and revised into four action areas: legislation and regulation, education, communication, and health human resources (CNA, 2011). Major outcomes of the CNPI project evolved around a legislative and regulatory framework that allows for a Canada-wide, consistent, principle-based approach in regulating NP practice, which at the same time gives each provincial and territorial jurisdiction some flexibility in implementation. It also provides a basis for facilitating mobility between jurisdictions and provides clarity for admitting internationally educated NPs (CNA, 2011).

The Canadian Nurse Practitioner Core Competency Framework (CNA, 2011) establishes core competencies as the basis for NP educational programs and a national NP exam, as well as a competency assessment framework for ongoing quality assurance of NP practice. It also recommends title protection for the NP so that only nurses with the defined qualifications are able to use the title NP. Therefore, Canadian

PHCNPs, as NPs, have a framework of consistent practice expectations and must demonstrate specific competencies in the expanded scope of their practice.

*Practice Perspective:* An NP is an RN with additional education, often at the graduate level, and strong clinical experience. It is a different RN class, known as "the extended class" by their regulatory body. They demonstrate the following competencies: autonomously diagnose, order, and interpret certain diagnostic tests, prescribe most pharmaceuticals but not controlled substances, and perform specific procedures within the legislated scope of practice (CNA, 2009). All NPs, including the class of PHCNPs, work both autonomously and in collaboration with an interdisciplinary healthcare team to ensure optimal client care. The PHCNP as an NP is not a second-level physician or a physician's assistant but works within the scope of practice for advanced practice nursing. NPs complement the roles of other health professionals with their advanced level of clinical skills, in-depth knowledge of nursing theory, and regulatory autonomy (CNA, 2011). PHCNPs have the additional role of providing health promotion, illness and injury prevention, and rehabilitation support to the individuals, families, communities, and systems they are collaborating with (NPAO, 2014).

According to the Canadian Institute of Health Information, in 2013, 32% of NPs worked in the community (Canadian Institute of Health Information, 2014). In 2010, only 17.2% of NPs in Canada worked in areas of community health nursing, such as community health centres, home care, public health, telehealth, ambulatory care, and long-term care. Other areas of work include family practice settings, mental health clinics, rural nursing stations, home visiting organizations, public health units, remote and northern communities, and interprofessional family practice settings, such as family health teams and primary care networks (CNA, 2012a).

The focus of PHCNP care in these settings varies considerably. Some provide care to individuals of all ages and stages of life while others work in settings with a specific health focus, such as sexual health, lactation support services, primary health care in secondary schools, or palliative care. Opportunities for PHCNPs in the community continue to expand. For example, in Ontario there are 27 nurse practitioner–led clinics. Consistent with other primary care delivery models, NP-led clinics provide family healthcare services such as annual physicals, episodic illness care, falls-prevention programs for older persons, immunizations, smoking cessation, injury prevention, and monitoring and management of chronic diseases such as diabetes, arthritis, asthma, heart disease, and mental health conditions (NPAO, 2014). This innovative and progressive interprofessional model for the delivery of comprehensive primary health care is designed to improve access to care for the thousands of individuals and families who do not currently have a primary health care provider. Another example of a practice setting for the PHCNP is the Community Health Bus provided by The Alex, a not-for-profit community health centre in Calgary, Alberta. This bus delivers a mobile health program with a team of healthcare providers, including NPs, to provide direct services, education, and advocacy for populations living in poverty and struggling with homelessness in Calgary. Care includes full physical and mental health assessments, pregnancy and prenatal care, lab testing and ECG monitoring, screening for infectious diseases, and referral to specialists and community resources (The Alex, 2015).

PHCNPs are well-suited to working with individuals and families with significant health and social needs and have been an essential part of healthcare delivery in underserviced and rural and remote areas. NP care will become more and more an essential part of primary health care in Canada as barriers to practice are addressed and numbers of NPs increase. Regulatory legislation and standards may vary depending upon the province or territory. As a minimum, PHCNPs can diagnose a common disease, disorder, or condition; order and interpret prescribed diagnostic and screening tests, such as X-rays or ultrasounds; and prescribe specific medication. The authority to perform these advanced acts is subject to limits and conditions outlined by the regulatory body and the NP's expertise. The PHCNP will consult with a physician when the diagnosis or treatment plan is unclear or beyond the scope of the PHCNP to determine (CNA 2012b). In Ontario, Bill 179 (the Regulated Health Professions Statute Law Amendment Act, 2009) introduced significant changes to nursing practice for NPs (College of Nurses of Ontario, 2014). Since 2011, as a result of this legislative change NP practice includes admitting persons to hospital; broadly prescribing drugs; dispensing, compounding, and selling drugs; setting or casting bone fractures or joint dislocations; ordering any laboratory tests; ordering diagnostics and treatments for hospital in-patients and discharge patients from hospital; and ordering services for which patients are insured (CNO, 2014).

## Rural/Outpost Nursing

*Historical Perspective:* In Canada, nurses have been providing healthcare to remote and isolated communities such as the Northwest Territories and Newfoundland and Labrador as well as to northern communities within the Canadian provinces since the 1890s (Higgins 2008). Visiting nurses often covered large geographic areas, travelling by horseback and eventually railway to provide healthcare to physically and socially isolated populations. In the early 1900s, programs became established in small towns or were set up temporarily on railway cars to handle disease outbreaks and teach families and communities about communicable diseases, proper nutrition, child development, school assessments, handling of drinking water, and proper disposal of sewage. Milk and food programs for vulnerable children were also set up (Abrams, 2008).

*Practice Perspective:* Nurses working in rural and northern Canada often call themselves CHNs. Provision of nursing care in these parts of Canada continues to be a challenge due to health disparities and subsequent health inequities that continue to the present day. The majority of Canada's land mass continues to be rural and isolated. CHNs work within large geographic areas containing small numbers of inhabitants. A large portion of these populations are disenfranchised and have poor access to employment, transportation, healthcare services, clean water, and fresh food sources. Populations within the Territories, such as First Nations, Inuit, and Metis, and populations within the Atlantic Canada region are largely rural. The rural locations present challenges for the provision of adequate healthcare services, including midwifery and urgent care. According to Statistics Canada (2013), between 2007 and 2010, First Nations, Inuit, and Métis people living off-reserve reported a high incidence of chronic illnesses. About 56% of First Nations and 55% of Métis were diagnosed with one or more chronic conditions, compared with 48% of non-Aboriginal people. Preterm labour, stillbirths, and infant mortality rates are much higher in rural and isolated locations as compared with the rest of Canada. Infant mortality rates are 2.66 times higher in Inuit inhabited areas than in the rest of Canada (Luo et al., 2010). Life expectancy for First Nations peoples has improved over the last decade but continues to be 6 to 7 years less than for non-Aboriginals living in urban parts of Canada (Health Canada, 2014).

The role of the **rural/outpost nurse** is centred around primary care, chronic disease prevention and management, substance abuse prevention and management, suicide prevention, public health programs, personal practices and coping skills, low income supports, access to housing, and management of environmental constraints (Canadian Association of Rural and Remote Nurses, 2014). Their role is complex and requires strong clinical skills, critical-thinking skills, and the ability to work with established communities with community development initiatives. Health promotion and disease prevention are underdeveloped in rural and isolated locations due to other healthcare priorities within these communities. Access to physician care is scarce and CHNs must work to their full scope of practice with the limited resources that they have to provide care (CNA, 2014c). Partnerships between nursling education and rural communities have been developed and studied to prepare LPN, RN, and RPN students in rural nursing (see Canadian research box 3.1).

According to the nursing database kept by the Canadian Institute for Health Information (CIHI) (CIHI, 2012), 10.5% of the RN workforce (including NPs) and 15% of the registered psychiatric nurse workforce were employed in a rural or remote area in 2012, which corresponds to 34 302 regulated nurses working in rural areas and small towns in Canada. Nurses may experience difficulty with the high levels of responsibility, constraints, and isolation of a small-town lifestyle and experience burn-out due to the complex social and economic issues they are working with (Martin-Misener et al., 2008). They have also expressed frustration with the lack of attention, awareness, and research that exists for this specialty within community health nursing (MacLeod et al., 2008). The emergence of telehealth technology has reduced travel for clients in rural and northern regions by enabling medical and nursing specialists to provide assessment, diagnosis, and treatment protocols via technology. This has aided in delivering some primary care nursing to remote areas in Canada.

**Nursing Programs and Regulation** In order to legitimize the expanded role of nurses working in isolated areas, provincial nursing programs across Canada developed specific nursing programs for providing health services in remote areas of northern Canada, and developed other programs that focused on expanding the role of nurses in primary care within community settings (Kaasalainen et al., 2010). In 1967, Dalhousie University in Nova Scotia established the first certification in midwifery and outpost nursing. Other universities followed suit in the early 1970s with nursing programs available in universities in Alberta, Manitoba, western Ontario, Toronto, Montreal, and Sherbrooke (Kaasalainen et al., 2010). Little has been documented about the role of nurses working in rural and northern parts of Canada, and the role for CHNs in these regions has been largely undefined right up to the present day (MacLeod et al., 2008). Much debate has occurred over a definition of rural and remote nursing practice in Canada. In 2003 a group of nurses achieved associate group status as the Canadian Association for Rural and Remote Nursing (CARRN) under the auspices of the Canadian Nursing Association (CARRN, 2014). CARRN also developed and disseminated standards of practice regarding the roles and functions of the rural or remote nurse in Canada due to the complex and unique nature of this role and in order to increase awareness of it within community health nursing practice.

## Occupational Health Nursing

*Historical Perspective:* A significant milestone in the history of **occupational health nurses** was the formation of a national association in Canada that began over 30 years ago. In this period of time there have been three national associations: the Canadian Council for Occupational Health Nurses (CCOHN), the National Association of Occupational Health Nurses (NAOHN), and the Canadian Occupational Health Nurses Association/Association Canadienne des Infirmières et Infirmiers en Santé du Travail (COHNA/ACIIST). The CCOHN was responsible for certification until 1992. In 1994 the NAOHN was renamed as the Canadian Occupational Health Nurses Association (COHNA) (COHNA, 2014). This association is a voice for influencing health and safety policy for Canadian workers and for advancing occupational health nursing practice excellence through conferences, national standards of practice, certification, and resources like the Disability Management Practice Standard Book. Please refer to Chapter 27, Environmental and Occupational Health, for more details.

*Practice Perspective:*

■ *Conceptual Framework*
Occupational health nurses base their practice on a nursing conceptual framework. This conceptual framework expresses their values and beliefs in four interrelated components: the individual, health, occupational health nursing, and the environment (COHNA, 2014). The individual is viewed holistically, with rights to confidentiality and a healthy and safe workplace. The WHO's definition of health has been adopted wherein health is viewed as a resource for everyday life. Occupational health nursing is defined as a specialty area of nursing practice that focuses on the worker or worker group by promoting health, preventing illness or injury, protecting workers from risks, and recommending a safe and healthy work environment (see Photo 3.3). Environment

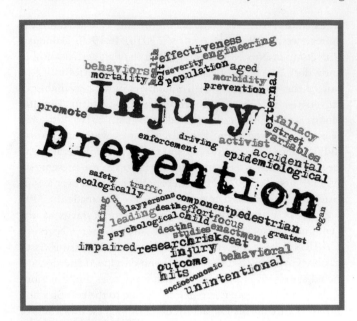

is described as a dynamic interaction between workers and their workplace, recognizing the interplay of social, physical, cultural, economic, and political factors. Health hazards are a particular focus (COHNA, 2014).

■ *Certification*

Occupational health nurses established certification in Canada in 1984 and received international recognition. As was previously noted, the CCOHN was accountable for certification and transferred this accountability to the CNA in 1992. The first national exam was written in 1982 (COHNA, 2014). There were 716 certified occupational health nurses as of July 2014 (CNA, 2014b).

■ *Standards*

In 2003, occupational health nurses released their standards of practice (COHNA, 2014). The standards of practice described two overarching standards: professional responsibility and accountability, and clinical decision making. The organizing framework of the indicators for each standard uses the categories of structure, process, and outcomes.

## Parish Nursing

*Historical Perspective:* **Parish nursing** began in Europe and moved to United States in the mid-1980s. More recently, in 1992 this aspect of community health nursing arrived in Canada (Canadian Association for Parish Nursing Ministry, 2014a). Reverend Granger Westberg is considered the founder of parish nursing (Solari-Twadell & McDermott, 1999). Westberg found that the professional knowledge and skills of RNs made a significant contribution to the health of people within faith communities. The term "faith community" refers to a community of people who share similar history, values, and beliefs around their relationship with a higher power and

with others in the world. They often gather for purposes of worship and to support one another. "Ministry" refers to someone who represents the mission and purposes of a particular faith community, carries out his or her role in accordance with established standards, and is accountable to the public served rather than working in isolation or carrying out a personal agenda. Parish nurses in Canada began annual national conventions in 1998. In 2001 they became incorporated as the Canadian Association for Parish Nursing Ministry (CAPNM). In 2004, parish nurses established core learning competencies and standards of practice. In 2007 they became an associate member of the Canadian Nurses Association.

*Practice Perspective:* A parish nurse is an RN who is hired or recognized by a faith community and integrates faith and health into nursing practice. Parish nurses often have additional training, such as parish nursing courses. The CAPNM (2014a) defines a parish nurse as a registered nurse with specialized knowledge to promote health, healing, and wholeness. The CAPNM (2014b) outlines 11 core competencies for basic parish nursing education programs and five standards of practice. The core competencies for preparation to be a parish nurse include the following: (a) baccalaureate of science in nursing (BScN), (b) orientation to parish nursing, (c) spiritual maturity and theological reflection, (d) personal and interpersonal skills, (e) teaching and facilitation, (f) worship, (g) faith community context, (h) collaboration, (i) management, (j) practicum, and (k) continuing education. The standards of practice for a parish nurse are very similar to the community health nursing standards of practice. In addition to health promotion and professional accountability, they are expected to practise facilitation of spiritual care, collaboration, and advocacy.

## Forensic Nursing

*Historical Perspective:* **Forensic nursing** has its own distinct body of knowledge with a specific scope of practice and nursing standards, which have been developing since the 1970s (Zalon, Constantino, & Crane, 2013). To formalize this specialization, the Forensic Nursing Society of Canada (FNSC) was formed in 2006. This society facilitates networking information for forensic nurses across Canada and internationally to provide educational resources and collaborate on research topics related to forensic nursing practice. FNSC is an associated member of the CNA (FNSC, 2015). For further information on the role of forensic nurses and sexual assault nurse examiners (SANES) see Chapter 28, Violence in Societies.

*Practice Perspective:* "Forensic" refers to the application of medical and nursing scientific knowledge to the care of both the patients and their offenders, whose health issues have intersected with the law. The goals of forensic nurses are to provide for healthcare needs and to collect evidence for police and the legal system in a way that respects clients' dignity, right to choice, and self-determination. As well, within this nursing specialty, forensic nurses address the consequences of violence and trauma within society and work to prevent the reoccurrence of further liability incidents through advocacy and promotion of individuals' knowledge and coping skills. Forensic nurses also engage in the following activities: (a) community education regarding risk factors for violence, (b) social activism to prevent violence at the community and population levels, and (c) influencing healthy public policy to overcome challenges within social, economic, and cultural systems associated with violence (Speck & Faugno, 2013). Forensic nurses are part of a larger professional team and foster coalitions and networks with healthcare, law enforcement, social services, and community and government agencies. Finally, forensic nurses work with survivors of crime and their families in settings such as the emergency room, intensive care, pediatrics, general medical and surgical care, long-term care, schools, prisons, and outreach community settings (Zalon et al., 2013).

Within the specialty of forensic nursing are **sexual assault nurse examiners (SANEs)**. SANEs respond specifically to calls relating to sexual assault or domestic violence in the emergency room and community settings. They provide comprehensive care to patients, collect evidence, and provide expert testimony during court cases that are brought forward in the legal system. Members of SANE teams are on call around the clock on a daily basis, and they respond quickly to calls from the emergency room and urgent care centres for survivors who are triaged as clinically stable but needing assessment, treatment, and possible referral for matters relating to sexual assault or domestic

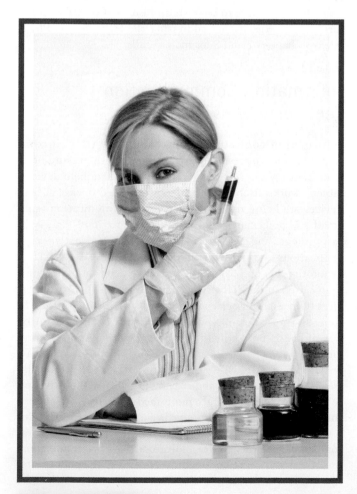

**PHOTO 3.4** Forensic nurse

*Source: Leah-Anne Thompson/Fotolia*

violence. SANEs aim to return control to survivors very early in the assessment phase of the interaction and strive to maintain a client-led approach throughout the intervention (Speck & Faugno, 2013; Zalon et al., 2013). SANEs possess knowledge of community resources and act as an initial liaison between survivors and community personnel and their agencies. SANEs must be non-judgmental and able to explain to the survivors the implications of reporting their violent event; this often is the concern of the survivors. Candid discussion of the possible consequences of reporting or not reporting incidents can assist the survivor in making informed decisions. SANEs must also possess confidence; knowledge; expert communication, assessment, and treatment skills; and knowledge of legal procedures. Care is taken to protect evidence, and documentation of assessment findings must be relevant, clear, objective, and for the physical assessment, detailed (Speck & Faugno, 2013). (See Photo 3.4.)

## Military Nursing

*Historical Perspective:* **Military nursing** has its formalized roots in one of the founders of nursing practice, Florence Nightingale, who practised during the Crimean War in the 1850s. Nightingale published her *Notes on Nursing,* which paved the way for major reforms in providing care for those injured or dying in field hospitals, and which also provided basic principles of epidemiology applied to nursing practice and considered the larger environmental factors influencing health (Nightingale, 1859). The first recorded instance of military nursing in Canada was at the Northwest Rebellion in 1885 with the Métis uprising led by Louis Riel against the Canadian government, where nurses organized themselves to help the wounded. Nurses served as military nurses during World War I within the Royal Canadian Army. Nurses paid their own way to travel overseas when serving in organizations such as the Red Cross, Victorian Order of Nurses, and St. John's Ambulance (Canadian Military History Gateway, 2011). Nurses have since served as military nurses in areas of conflict where Canadians are represented.

*Practice Perspective:* Military nurses are nursing officers who are commissioned members of the Canadian Forces Medical Service. They are expected to possess leadership skills and, like civilian nurses, their primary duty is to care for sick and injured patients, and in this case, the population of Canadian Armed Forces members and insurgents either within Canada or on operations abroad. Nursing officers may work within military hospitals and outpatient health clinics or in moveable facilities, such as field hospitals, while caring for their colleagues in the forces. Nursing officers work in several domains of nursing practice, including direct patient care within perioperative nursing, intensive care, mental health, air evacuation, and community health. Nursing officers are also involved in policy development, administrative duties, health education, and research. They provide preventive, occupational, and environmental healthcare services while working collaboratively with a larger healthcare team including physicians and medical technicians. Other career options for military nurses include humanitarian work and advocacy for the populations in which they serve. Military nursing goes beyond providing healthcare. A nurse working in the Canadian Forces needs to be physically fit, clinically adaptable to many different work environments with limited equipment and varied responsibilities, socially adaptable, and able to be deployed at short notice. Military nursing is challenging and provides nurses with the opportunity to use critical thinking and leadership skills in a variety of healthcare settings that nurses working with civilians are unlikely to experience (National Defence and the Canadian Forces, 2015).

# TRENDS IN COMMUNITY HEALTH NURSING

Established and emerging trends in healthcare and nursing will continue to challenge CHNs to evolve their practice in order to continue to play a central role in the health system and provide effective and relevant care to their clients. Several such trends are described next.

## Focus on Health Equity and Social Justice

Community health nurses historically have addressed **health inequities** and are aware of the need to change the living and working conditions for their clients and populations. Nurses such as Florence Nightingale, Lillian Wald, the Henry Street nurses and, more recently, the Toronto street nurse advocate Cathy Crowe were leaders in nursing and advocating for **community justice** and **social action** (Abrams, 2008; Crowe, 2007; Fee & Bu, 2010 ). Within healthcare's reorganizational trends toward breaking down the nurse's role into a group of skills, tasks, or specialties, such as postpartum care and immunization, this focus on social action has changed. However, one of the mandates of community health nursing is to work with individuals, families, communities, systems, and populations to change underlying conditions that are contributing to health disparities (CHNC, 2011a). It is part of the practice standards for community health nurses to be politically competent, and to use **political and social advocacy** to not just accept the conditions that contribute to marginalization and inequities but to change them (CHNC, 2011a). When differences in health status are experienced by various groups or populations and result from social conditions that are modifiable and seen to be unjust or unfair, this is termed a health inequity. Health equity implies that everyone, regardless of socially determined circumstances, has an equal opportunity to attain their full health potential without being disadvantaged. This requires an understanding of, and ability to analyze and advocate for, policies that increase access to health, as well as the ability to develop policies that address health disparities (Reutter & Kushner, 2010).

Nurses can become socialized to accept marginalization and oppression as part of their day-to-day practice, but instead, when working with population groups such as the homeless, the impoverished, immigrants, and the vulnerable, nurses need to take up CNA's call to action (CNA 2012c). The National Expert Commission was set up in 2011 by the CNA to meet with Canadians and strategize how our healthcare system can better meet the needs of Canadians. As a result, an action plan was developed for nurses and other interdisciplinary professionals to work collectively and collaboratively with other Canadians to focus on health and the factors that influence health. National health goals, a blueprint of best practices, and targeted health outcomes were developed and disseminated within this call to action, as Canada approaches its 150-year birthday in 2017. The report discusses the top five important health outcomes for RNs to tackle: recognizing health inequities and determinants of health within many of our population groups and working to address access to primary care services, transition to community-based care, manage chronic disease care more effectively within community settings, champion primary and preventive-based care, and strengthen the nurse's role as an advocate for vulnerable Canadians, such as First Nations populations and those with chronic disease. All nurses need to be aware of the issues that impact health beyond traditional healthcare if they are to make a meaningful difference in people's lives. This requires an understanding of equity and social justice issues and how the populations that nurses are working with are impacted by the larger influences on health. This should be occurring wherever nurses encounter clients and families. Nurses need to consider how they can work with others to change the conditions that contribute to poor health instead of contributing to further inequities by not addressing the larger issues. Please refer to Chapters 7 and 8 for more details.

## Information Communication Technology Advances

**Information communication technology** (ICT) innovation continues to expand in community health nursing practice. CHNs work with technology such as handheld devices, tablets, workstations, and Bluetooth-enabled devices. These devices are being used for electronic communication (e.g., email and voicemail), multimedia presentations (e.g., podcasts, blogs, and YouTube videos), and social networking applications (e.g., Twitter and Facebook). ICT assists CHNs in information and knowledge management and with communication in the delivery of community health nursing services (Canadian Association of Schools of Nursing, 2012). In some settings, nurses update the client's health record by way of laptop or handheld electronic devices. As stated previously, for nurses working in the far North or rural outposts, it is now possible to send test results electronically and receive a diagnosis and treatment order without having to transport a client to a remote medical centre. Telemonitoring applications are providing new opportunities for remote assessments of wound healing, cardiac and respiratory status, or other health indicators, thus making optimal use of scarce nursing and medical resources. Telephone nursing services are now available in many regions of Canada. CHNs are identifying and developing telehealth nursing competencies that continue to support a therapeutic nurse–client relationship.

Social networking is the expansion of contacts by making connections through individuals and has been going on for centuries. Yet its full potential as a result of the Internet is just starting to be fully recognized. Social networking has become a very popular method of reaching out to a wide variety of audiences. Different sites tend to attract differing age groups. Knowledge of, comfort with, and use of this technology by nurses is expected of CHNs in order to identify, generate, manage, and process relevant data to support nursing practice (CHNC, 2011a). The challenge will be in keeping up with the trends and having organizational policies that both support and protect staff and the public. Please refer to Chapter 15 (Information Technology) for more details.

## Increase in Acuity of Clients in the Community

Caring for individuals and families within their homes and other community settings is an increasing trend within Canada (Schofield et al., 2011). Clients are being discharged from the hospital earlier with shorter hospital stays—early discharge in the postpartum period is an example (PHAC, 2009)—or being cared for at home or within outpatient settings as long as possible to prevent admission to in-patient settings. In addition, Canada has a growing population of older Canadians with a longer life expectancy who are trying to manage chronic conditions. Furthermore, children have chronic and debilitating health conditions and this has contributed to the continued shift of healthcare to the community and home setting. With the advances of technology, more and more can be done to monitor and treat clients using complicated procedures (e.g., central lines) within the community setting. This has led to the specialty of pediatric home healthcare, chronic disease management specialists, as well as telehealth nurses within many jurisdictions within Canada. (See Canadian Research Box 3.2.)

## Emphasis on Evidence-Informed Practice

Community health nursing practice is grounded in a number of community health theories and conceptual frameworks, like the Ottawa Charter, Jakarta Declaration, Bangkok Charter of Health Promotion, Population Health Promotion Model, Pender's Health Belief Model, Behaviour Change Theory, and Systems Theory (CHNC, 2011a). Please refer to Chapter 7 for details on community health nursing theory. With the growing expectation of examining and practising evidence-informed decision making, CHNs access a number of reliable sources. Accordingly, best practice guidelines, systematic reviews, Cochrane reviews, and the website www.healthevidence.org are key resources to inform nursing practice. An excellent example of nursing-led development of best practice guidelines is that of the Registered Nurses' Association of Ontario (RNAO). There are a number of guidelines that apply to community health nursing practice, such as "Supporting and Strengthening Families through Expected and Unexpected Life Events." For a list of guidelines, go to www.rnao.org. The use of current evidence

is expected in the community health nursing standards of practice and also is recognized as part of the community health nursing professional practice model (CHNC, 2011a).

In 2010, the Canadian Nurses Association released a position paper stating, "evidence-informed decision making is an important element of quality care in all domains of nursing practice and is integral to effect changes across the health-care system" (CNA, 2010, p. 1). To enable CHNs to integrate evidence in their practice, various tools are available; for example, engaging citizens for decision making (National Collaborating Centre for Methods and Tools, 2015).

## The Changing Profile of Undergraduate Nursing Education

The preparation for community health nursing practice in undergraduate nursing programs is more important than ever with the shift to community health nursing practice. Several factors are influencing the community health nursing education. In a scan of the integration of community health nursing education within undergraduate nursing programs in Canada, enablers and barriers were identified. Valaitis et al. (2008) found strong community–academic partnerships, supportive curriculum structures and processes, and faculty champions that were enablers, while challenges identified were the devaluing of community health versus acute care, lack of community health placements, lack of qualified faculty, and weak community health education leadership in academia. Further challenges were identified in a Canadian qualitative, descriptive national study of community health nursing leaders regarding practice, education, and research. The findings indicated a devaluing of community health nursing education in the curriculum contributing to insufficient time in theoretical and clinical placements, something that is necessary to developing competencies in health promotion and disease prevention of individuals, families, and communities (Schofield et al., 2011). CHNs in this study boldly recommended a reorientation of basic baccalaureate content to strengthen community health nursing.

On a promising note, the Public Health Agency of Canada (PHAC) recognizes and funds mechanisms to strengthen community health nursing education. With the rising rates of chronic preventable diseases such as diabetes, obesity, heart disease, tobacco-related illness, and the prevalence of new strains of infectious diseases, the PHAC developed long-term plans for public health human resource planning (PHAC, 2005). The top building block in their plan identifies accreditation standards. To this end, PHAC funds organizations like the CASN. One example of strengthening nursing curriculum in the preparation of nurses is the Guidelines for Quality Community Health Nursing Clinical Placements, which is available to schools of nursing to ensure quality community clinical placements for nursing students (CASN, 2010). Another example is the competencies for entry to the practice of public health nursing, to be released in 2015. CASN likewise recognizes the relevance of and need for the preparation of nursing students in population health competencies based on the experience outlined in the SARS and other epidemiology reports (CASN, 2010).

**CANADIAN RESEARCH BOX 3.2**

### How satisfied are nurses in the use of electronic devices in a home care setting?

Doran, D. M., Reid-Haughian, C., Chilcote, A., Bia, Y. Q. (2013). A formative evaluation of nurses' use of electronic devices in a home care setting. *Canadian Journal of Nursing Research, 45*(1), 54–73.

This study evaluated the implementation of a clinical information system (CIS) in a community setting using a mixed method research design. Through interviews, focus groups, and surveys, 118 nurses evaluated the use of information technology for documentation of client assessment, discharge, and reassessment information, as well as for administrative information such as scheduling and accessing best practice evidence-based resources. The findings indicate that nurses were satisfied with the access to structural and electronic resources and with the formal interactions or social capital. Younger nurses researched the resources more. Less satisfaction was associated with research use for evaluation and feedback. The evaluation recognized the importance of educational support, user-centred designs, and responsiveness to the implementation of devices.

#### Discussion Questions

1. What were the four uses of information technology for CHNs?

2. Give an example from the Canadian community health nursing standards of practice indicating the relevance to community health nursing practice.

3. Why is research related to information technology important?

## CONCLUSION

This chapter has described a range of the roles and practice settings of Canada's CHNs, recognizing public health and home health nursing, and further profiling five community health nursing roles in different settings: primary care nursing, rural/outpost nursing, occupational health nursing, parish nursing, and forensic nursing and military nursing. In addition, the future direction of community health nursing is outlined in the Blueprint for Action for Community Health Nursing in Canada (CHNC, 2011a) and the revised Canadian community health nursing standards of practice (CHNC, 2011c). Trends in community health nursing describe the focus on health equity and social justice, increased acute care in the community, information communication technology advances, use of evidence-informed decision making, and the changing profile of undergraduate nursing education.

## KEY TERMS

## STUDY QUESTIONS

1. Identify 10 types of practice settings for nurses working in community health nursing.

2. List five broad roles nurses working in community health nursing may perform in the various practice areas discussed in this chapter, and explain why each is important.

3. Apply practice examples from any of the community health nursing practice areas discussed in this chapter to the five community health nursing standards.

After working through these questions, go to the MyNursingLab at www.pearsoned.ca/mynursinglab to check your answers.

## INDIVIDUAL CRITICAL-THINKING EXERCISES

1. Which area of community health nursing interests you most and why?

2. Identify five key roles or functions or competencies of community health nursing that work toward achieving a healthier community.

3. Describe some examples from your own community where public health has empowered groups to achieve a healthier community.

4. What personal characteristics would draw nurses toward community health nursing rather than hospital-based nursing?

5. What questions would you ask of a community health nursing organization before accepting employment in that setting? How would you prepare for an interview?

## GROUP CRITICAL-THINKING EXERCISES

1. Create a concept map that interconnects the multiple roles and functions of nurses working in a variety of community health settings in their work with individuals, families, groups, communities, and populations to promote health.

2. Identify strategies to promote an understanding of community health nursing roles among nurses in other sectors.

3. Debate the merits of legislation similar to the Canada Health Act that would provide standardized community healthcare services across Canada.

## REFERENCES

Abrams, S. E. (2008). The best of public health nursing, circa 1941. *Public Health Nursing, 25*(3), 285–291.

Alberta Health Services. (2014a). *Better choices, Better health.* Alberta: Author. Retrieved from http://www.albertahealthservices.ca/services.asp?pid=service&rid=1054851

Alberta Health Services. (2014b). *Chronic disease management.* Alberta: Author. Retrieved from http://www.albertahealthservices.ca/7736.asp

The Alex. (2015). *Mobile health program.* Calgary, AB: Author. Retrieved from http://www.thealex.ca/programs-services/health/health-bus-program/

BC Centre for Disease Control. (2012a). *Outreach street nurse program: History.* Vancouver, BC: Author. Retrieved from http://www.bccdc.ca/SexualHealth/Programs/StreetOutreachNurseProgram/SNHistory.htm

BC Centre for Disease Control. (2012b). *Outreach street nurse program.* Vancouver, BC: Author. Retrieved from http://www.bccdc.ca/SexualHealth/Programs/StreetOutreachNurseProgram/default.htm

Bartfay, W. J. (2010). A brief history of community health nursing in Canada. In J. E. Hitchcock, P. E. Schubert, S. A. Thomas, & W. J. Bartfay (Eds.), *Community health nursing: Caring in action* (1st Canadian ed.). Toronto, ON: Nelson Education Ltd.

Canadian Association of Rural and Remote Nurses. (2014). *Rural and remote nursing practice parameters.* Retrieved from http://www.carrn.com/files/NursingPracticeParameters-January08.pdf

Canadian Association for Parish Nursing Ministry. (2014a). Historical Overview. Retrieved from http://www.capnm.ca/historical_overview.htm

Canadian Association for Parish Nursing Ministry. (2014b). Core Competencies. Retrieved from http://www.capnm.ca/historical_overview.htm

Canadian Association Schools of Nursing. (2010). *Guidelines for quality community health nursing clinical placements for baccalaureate nursing students.* Ottawa, ON: Author. Retrieved

from http://casn.ca/wp-content/uploads/2014/12/CPGuidelinesFinalMarch.pdf

Canadian Association of Schools of Nursing. (2012). *Nursing informatics entry-to-practice competencies for registered nurses.* Ottawa, ON: Author. Retrieved from http://casn.ca/wp-content/uploads/2014/12/NursingInformaticsEntryToPracticeCompetenciesFINALENG.pdf

Canadian Drug Policy Coalition. (2012). *Canadian nurses lead the way in harm reduction.* Vancouver, BC: Author. Retrieved from http://drugpolicy.ca/2012/06/nurses-lead-the-way-in-harm-reduction/

Canadian Home Care Association. (2014). *Community home care association on the issues: Access to care.* Retrieved from http://www.cdnhomecare.ca/content.php?doc=180

Canadian Institute for Health Information. (2012). *Regulated nurses 2012—Summary report.* Ottawa, ON: Author. Retrieved from https://secure.cihi.ca/free_products/RegulatedNurses2012Summary_EN.pdf

Canadian Institute of Health Information. (2014). RN workforce, by place of work and jurisdiction, Canada, 2009 to 2013. Retrieved from https://secure.cihi.ca/estore/productFamily.htm?pf=PFC2646&lang=en&media=0

Canadian Mortgage and Housing Corporation. (2011). *Federal, provincial, territorial ministers responsible for housing announce a new framework for affordable housing.* Ottawa, ON: Author. Retrieved from http://www.cmhc-schl.gc.ca/en/corp/nero/nere/2011/2011-07-04-0930.cfm

Canadian Military History Gateway. (2011). *Nurses: Canadian military.* Ottawa, ON: Author. Retrieved from http://www.cmhg.gc.ca/flash/gl-ga/index-eng.asp?letter=N&page=2

Canadian Nurses Association. (2008). *CNA's preferred future: Health for all.* Ottawa, ON: Author. Retrieved from http://cna-aiic.ca/~/media/cna/page-content/pdf-en/preferred_future_webcast_e.pdf

Canadian Nurses Association. (2009). *The nurse practitioner: A position statement.* Ottawa, ON: Author. Retrieved from http://cna-aiic.ca/~/media/cna/page-content/pdf-fr/ps_nurse_practitioner_e.pdf

Canadian Nurses Association. (2010). *Position statement: Evidence-informed decision-making and nursing practice.* Ottawa, ON: Author. Retrieved from http://www.nanb.nb.ca/PDF/CNA-Evidence_Informed_Decision_Making_and_Nursing_Practice_E.pdf

Canadian Nurses Association. (2011). *Collaborative integration plan for the role of nurse practitioners in Canada.* Ottawa, ON: Author. Retrieved from http://www.npnow.ca/docs/Integration_Plan_for_the_Nurse_Practitioner_Role-En.pdf

Canadian Nurses Association. (2012a). *Certification bulletin.* Ottawa, ON: Author. Retrieved from http://nurseone.ca/en/certification

Canadian Nurses Association. (2012b). *Workplace profile 2010 of nurse practitioners in Canada.* Ottawa, ON: Author. Retrieved from http://www.cna-aiic.ca/en/download-buy/nursing-statistics

Canadian Nurses Association. (2012c). *A nursing call to action.* Ottawa, ON: Author. Retrieved from www.cna-aiic.ca/~/media/cna/files/en/nec_report_e.pdf

Canadian Nurses Association. (2014a). *CNA certification.* Ottawa, ON: Author. Retrieved from http://nurseone.ca/en/certification/what-is-certification/statistics

Canadian Nurses Association. (2014b). *Certification statistics.* Ottawa, ON: Author. Retrieved from http://nurseone.ca/~/

media/nurseone/page-content/pdf-en/certification_stats_july_2014_e.pdf?la=en

Canadian Nurses Association. (2014c). *Nurse One: Rural and remote nursing.* Ottawa, ON: Author. Retrieved from http://www.nurseone.ca/en/knowledge-features/rural-and-remote-nursing

Canadian Nurse Practitioner Initiative. (n.d.). *Technical report: Nurse practitioners: The time is now.* Retrieved from http://www.npnow.ca/docs/tech-report/section5/01_Education.pdf

Canadian Occupational Health Nurses Association. (2014). *The scope.* Red Deer, AB: Author. Retrieved from http://www.cohna-aciist.ca/our-scope/

College of Nurses of Ontario. (2014). *Frequently asked questions: (FAQ): Bill 179.* Toronto, ON: Author. Retrieved from http://www.cno.org/what-is-cno/regulation-and-legislation/legislation-governing-nursing/faq-bill-179/

Community Health Nurses of Canada. (2009). *Vision and definition of community health nursing in Canada.* St. John's, NL: Author.

Community Health Nurses of Canada. (2010). *Home health nursing competencies.* St. John's, NL: Author. Used by permission of Community Health Nurses Association of Canada.

Community Health Nurses of Canada. (2011a). *Blueprint for action for community health nursing in Canada.* St. John's, NL: Author. Retrieved from http://www.chnc.ca/documents/2011March03Blueprint_Final.pdf

Community Health Nurses of Canada. (2011b, revised). *Canadian community health nursing: Professional practice model and standards of practice.* St. John's, NL: Author. Retrieved from http://www.chnc.ca/documents/chnc-standards-eng-book.pdf

Community Health Nurses of Canada. (2011c). *Standards of practice in community health nursing: A literature review undertaken to inform revision to the Canadian community health nursing standards of practice.* St. John's, NL: Author. Retrieved from http://www.chnc.ca/documents/ALitReviewUndertakentoInformRevisionstotheCdnCHNStdrsofPracticeMarch03.pdf

Community Health Nurses of Canada. (2012). *Community health nurses of Canada strategic plan 2012–2015.* St. John's, NL: Author. Retrieved from www.chnc.ca.

Crowe, C. (2007). *Dying for a home: Homeless activists speak out.* Toronto, ON: Between the Lines.

Fee, E. & Bu, L. (2010). The origins of public health nursing: The Henry Street visiting nurse service. *The American Journal of Public Health, 100*(7), 1206–1207.

Forensic Nursing Society of Canada. (2015). *About the forensic nursing society of Canada.* Retrieved from http://Porensicnurse .ca/about/

Hardill, K. (2007). From the Grey Nuns to the streets: A critical history of outreach nursing in Canada. *Public Health Nursing. 24*(1), 91–97.

Health Canada. (2014). *First Nations and Inuit Health: Clinical practice guidelines for nurses in primary care.* Ottawa, ON: Author. Retrieved from http://www.hc-sc.gc.ca/fniah-spnia/index-eng.php

Higgins, J. (2008). *Grenfell Mission: Newfoundland and Labrador heritage.* Retrieved from http://www.heritage.nf.ca/society/grenfellmission.html

Hsu, C. C., & Sanford, B. A. (2007). The Delphi technique: Making sense of consensus. *Practical Assessment, Research and Evaluation, 12*(10), 1–8.

Kaasalainen, S., Martin-Misener, R., Kilpatrick, K., Harbman, P., Bryant-Lukosius, D., Donald, F., Carter, N., & DiCenso, A. (2010). An historical overview of the development of advanced practice nursing roles in Canada. *Nursing Leadership, 23*, 25–60.

Luo, Z. C., Senécal, S., Simonet, F., Guimond, E., Penney, C., & Wilkins, R. (2010). Birth outcomes in the Inuit inhabited areas of Canada. *CMAJ: Canadian Medical Association Journal 23*(3), 235–242.

MacLeod, M. L. P., Martin-Misener, R., Banks, C., Morton, M., Vogt, C., & Bentham, D. (2008). "I'm a different kind of nurse": Advice from nurses in rural and remote Canada. *Canadian Journal of Nursing Leadership, 21*(3), 40–53.

Martin-Misener, R., MacLeod, M., Banks, C., Morton, M., Vogt, C., & Bentham, D. (2008). There's rural and then there's rural. *Nursing Leadership, 21*(3), 54–63.

National Collaborating Centre for the Determinants of Health. (2014). *About the social determinants of health.* Antigonish, N.S.: Author. Retrieved from http://nccdh.ca/resources/about-social-determinants-of-health

National Collaborating Centre for Methods and Tools. (2015). *Engaging citizens for decision making.* Hamilton, ON: McMaster University. Author. (Updated 13 April, 2011). Retrieved from http://www.nccmt.ca/registry/view/eng/86.html

National Defence and the Canadian Forces. (2015). *Nursing officer.* Ottawa, ON: Author. Retrieved from http://www.forces.ca/en/job/nursingofficer-53?s=68&t=21#info-1

Nightingale, F. (1859). *Notes on nursing: What it is and what it is not.* Glasgow & London: Blackie and Sons Ltd.

Nurse Practitioners' Association of Ontario. (2011). *Nurse practitioner history in Ontario.* Toronto, ON: Author. Retrieved from http://npao.org/nurse-practitioners/history/#.VUvZJ2d0x9A

Nurse Practitioners' Association of Ontario. (2014). *Nurse practitioner led clinics.* Toronto, ON: Author. Retrieved from http://npao.org/nurse-practitioners/clinics/#.UnElhb7D-cw

Paramed. (2011). *Paramed get better.* Retrieved from http://www.paramed.ca/homecare/about

Primary Care Initiative. (2013). *What is a primary care initiative?* Retrieved from https://www.scpcn.ca/primary-care-initiative

Public Health Agency of Canada. (2005). *Building the public health workforce for the 21st Century.* Ottawa, ON: Author. Retrieved from http://publications.gc.ca/collections/collection_2008/phac-aspc/HP5-12-2005E.pdf

Public Health Agency of Canada. (2007). *Building the public health workforce: Core competencies and skills enhancement programs for public health.* Ottawa, ON: Author. Retrieved from http://www.phac-aspc.gc.ca/php-psp/ccph-cesp/index-eng.php

Public Health Agency of Canada. (2009). *What mothers say: The Canadian maternity experiences survey.* Retrieved from http://www.phac-aspc.gc.ca/rhs-ssg/survey-enquete/concl-eng.php

Public Health Agency of Canada. (2013). *Implementing the population health approach.* Retrieved from http://www.phac-aspc.gc.ca/ph-sp/implement/index-eng.php

Raphael, D. (2012). Educating the Canadian public about the social determinants of health: The time for local public health action is now! *Global Health Promotion, 19*(3), 54–59.

Registered Nurses' Association of Ontario. (2010). *Strategies to support self-management in chronic conditions: Collaboration with clients.* Toronto, ON: Author. Retrieved from http://rnao.ca/sites/rnao-ca/files/Strategies_to_ Support_Self-Management_in_Chronic_Conditions_-_ Collaboration_with_Clients.pdf

Ruetter, L., & Kushner, K. E. (2010). Health equity through action on the social determinants of health: Taking up the challenge in nursing. *Nursing Inquiry, 17*(3), 269–280.

Schofield, R., Ganann, R., Brooks, S., McGugan, J., Dalla Bona, K., Betker, C., . . . Watson, C. (2011). Community health nursing vision 2020: Shaping the future. *Western Journal of Nursing Research., 33*(8), 1047–1068. doi:0.1177/ 0193945910375819

Scott, L. (2009). *Telenursing in Canada: History and emerging roles.* Retrieved from http://www.medetel.lu/down-load/2009/parallel_sessions/presentation/day2/telehealth_ evolution_canada.pdf

Solari-Twadell, P. A., & McDermott, M. A. (1999). *Parish nursing: Promoting whole-person health within faith communities.* Thousand Oaks, CA: Sage.

Speck, P., & Faugno, D. (2013). Intimate partner, child, and elder violence and the three levels of prevention. In R. Constantino et al. (Eds.), *Forensic nursing: Evidence based principles and practice* (1st ed., pp. 117–139). Philadelphia: F. A. Davis.

Statistics Canada. (2013). *Select health indicators of First Nations people living off the reserve, Metis and Inuit 2007 to 2010.* Ottawa, ON: Author. Retrieved from http://www.statcan .gc.ca/daily-quotidien/130129/dq130129b-eng.htm

Stanford University. (2015). *Chronic disease self-management program.* Retrieved from http://patienteducation.stanford.edu/ programs/cdsmp.html

Valaitis, R., Rajsic, C. J., Cohen, B., Leeseberg Stamler, L., Meagher-Stewart, D., & Froude, S. A. (2008). Preparing the community health nursing workforce: Internal and external enablers and challenges influencing undergraduate nursing programs in Canada. *International Journal of Nursing Education Scholarship, 5*(1), 1–23.

Vollman, A., Anderson, E., & McFarlane, J. (2012). *Canadian community as partner: Theory and multidisciplinary practice.* Philadelphia: Wolters Kluwer Health.

Victorian Order of Nurses. (2009). *About VON.* Retrieved from http://www.von.ca

World Health Organization. (1978). *Declaration of Alma-Ata: International conference on primary health care, Alma-Ata, USSR, 6-12.* Geneva, Switzerland: Author. Retrieved from http://www.who.int/topics/primary_health_care/en

World Health Organization. (1984). *Health promotion: A discussion document on the concepts and principles.* Copenhagen, Denmark: WHO Regional Office for Europe.

Zalon, M., Constantino, R., & Crane, P. (2013). Fundamentals of contemporary forensic nursing practice, education and research. In R. Constantino et al. (Eds.), *Forensic nursing: Evidence based principles and practice* (1st ed., pp. 2–26). Philadelphia: F.A. Davis.

## ABOUT THE AUTHORS

**Genevieve Currie**, RN, BN, MN, is an Associate Professor in the School of Nursing and Midwifery, Faculty of Health, Community and Education at Mount Royal University in Calgary, Alberta. She is presently on the Board of Community Health Nurses of Canada and is vice-president, provincial, of Community Health Nurses of Alberta. She has over 30 years in nursing practice as a public health nurse, nurse manager, and educator. Her scholarship and research focus areas are community health nursing, family-newborn nursing, and nursing education.

**Ruth Schofield**, RN, BScN, MSc(T), is an Assistant Professor at McMaster University and clinical instructor at Western University. For the past 14 years she has developed, implemented, and evaluated innovative undergraduate curriculum in community health nursing education. She was president of Community Health Nurses of Canada from 2011 to 2013 and has over 23 years of public health nursing practice experience in various programs and positions from front line to management. Her research focuses on community health nursing, mental health and housing, and nursing education.

# Public Health Nursing

*Caroline J. Porr and Aliyah Dosani*

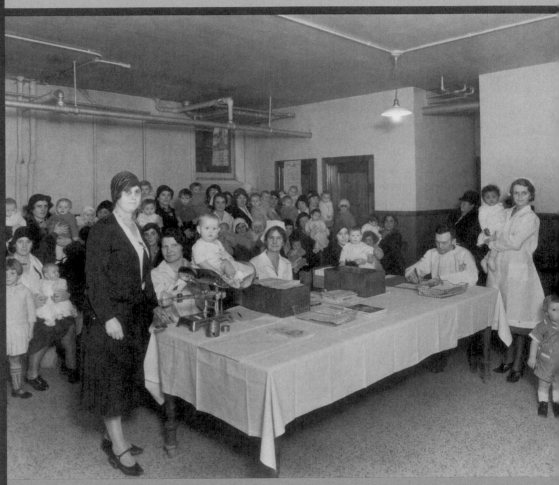

*Source: Archives of Ontario. Reference code: RG 10-30-2, 1.14.5/Well Baby Clinic, Hamilton, Ontario, 1930.*

## INTRODUCTION

**Public health** is most commonly defined as the organized efforts of society to keep people healthy and prevent injury, illness, and premature death. It is a combination of programs, services, and policies that protect and promote the health of all Canadians (Last, 2001). In September 2004, the Public Health Agency of Canada was established with the mission to "promote and protect the health of Canadians through leadership, partnership, innovation, and action in public health" (Government of Canada, 2006; Public Health Agency of Canada, 2015). In 2006, the Public Health Agency of Canada Act confirmed the agency as a legal entity and appointed a chief public health officer (CPHO). This legislation requires that the CPHO report annually on the state of public health in Canada. Under the leadership of the CPHO, various public health

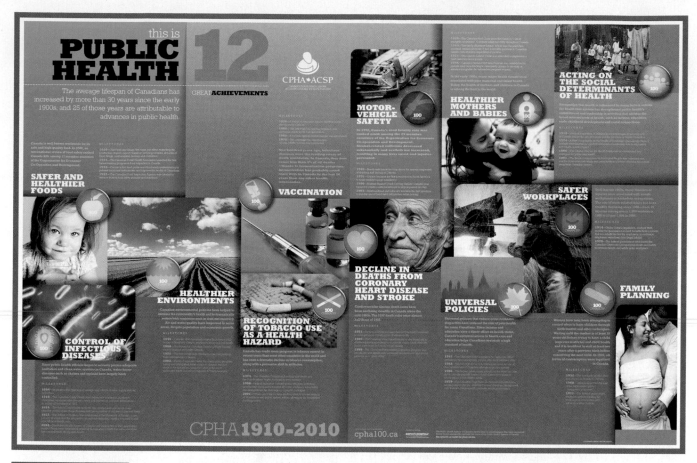

**FIGURE 4.1** The 12 Great Achievements of Public Health

*Source:* Canadian Public Health Association. (n.d.). *This is public health: A Canadian history.* Ottawa, ON: Canadian Public Health Association. Retrieved from http://www.cpha.ca/uploads/history/cpha100-poster_e.pdf

professionals focus on the health of the entire population in Canada to do the following:

- promote health;
- prevent and control chronic diseases and injuries;
- prevent and control infectious diseases;
- prepare for and respond to public health emergencies;
- serve as a central point for sharing Canada's expertise with the rest of the world;
- apply international research and development to Canada's public health programs; and
- strengthen intergovernmental collaboration on public health and facilitate national approaches to public health policy and planning (Public Health Agency of Canada, 2015).

Canada has a remarkable record of public health achievements. The Canadian Public Health Association (Canadian Public Health Association, n.d.) lists the 12 great achievements of public health in Canada (see Figure 4.1). It is significant to note that the average lifespan of Canadians has increased by more than 30 years since the early 1900s, and 25 of those years are attributable to advances in public health and the work of public health professionals (CPHA, n.d.). One type of public health professional is the **public health nurse** (PHN). As discussed in Chapter 3, the PHN is one type of community health nurse. The PHN

applies public health science, the **principles of primary health care**, nursing science, and the social sciences to promote, protect, and preserve the health of populations (CPHA, 2010).

Having briefly introduced you to public health, we will now explore the roles and responsibilities of the PHN, beginning with the historical evolution of public health nursing in Canada. Concepts, principles, and values fundamental to public health nursing practice are interwoven throughout the chapter. At the end of the chapter are real-life exemplars from jurisdictions across Canada to illustrate the nature, diversity, and significant contributions of public health nursing practice. These exemplars will be discussed in terms of primary, secondary, and tertiary prevention.

## HISTORICAL EVOLUTION OF PUBLIC HEALTH NURSING

The earliest documented references to public health occurred before Canada became a nation. In 1831, the Colonial Office in England corresponded with the executive government in Quebec concerning the possible arrival of immigrants to Upper Canada with Asiatic sporadic cholera. In response, a sanitary commission and Canada's first board of health were immediately established and directives were issued for the "preservation

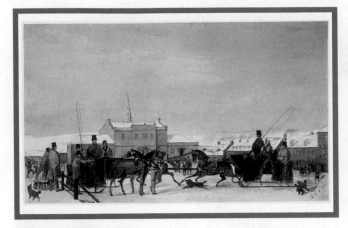

PHOTO 4.1 A Canadian scene in the 19th century

*Source: Library and Archives Canada, Acc. No. R9266-45, Peter Winkworth Collection of Canadiana*

of health" (Bryce, 1910, p. 288). During this period there was little understanding of the nature, origin, and transmission of disease. Infectious diseases, particularly the cholera epidemic, accounted for the deaths of countless indigenous peoples and early settlers. By the 1880s (see Photo 4.1), with scientific discoveries in the growing field of bacteriology, it became evident that personal hygiene and community sanitation were key to preventing malignant, contagious, and infectious diseases. Influenced by England's sanitary movement, Canadian sanitary reformers worked diligently to clean up water supplies and manage sewage removal, and in so doing, championed public health development in Canada. Public health initiatives that followed included legislation with detailed regulations for personal and environmental cleanliness (Allemang, 1995).

## First Provincial Public Health Act

After Canadian Confederation in 1867, health and social welfare matters were the delegated responsibility of the provinces. In 1882, Dr. Peter Henderson Bryce (Photo 4.2) was appointed the first secretary of the Provincial Board of Health of Ontario. He prepared the first Public Health Act, which was passed in Ontario in 1884. This Public Health Act became the model for legislation in other provinces across Canada (Bryce, 1910).

Other provinces in Canada soon established health acts and local boards of health. Local boards of health hired medical officers of health to protect Canadian citizens by responding to communicable disease outbreaks. Public health inspections and regulatory frameworks (e.g., environmental policies addressing contaminated water and sewage disposal systems) were soon added to the mandate of local boards of health. Local public health units were to oversee proper pasteurization of milk, tuberculin testing of cows, tuberculosis isolation and quarantine practices, and the tracking of sexually transmitted infections. World War I made it necessary for preventive medicine to be integrated with clinical medicine to control the spread of disease. A national Department of Health was founded by the Government of Canada at this time to

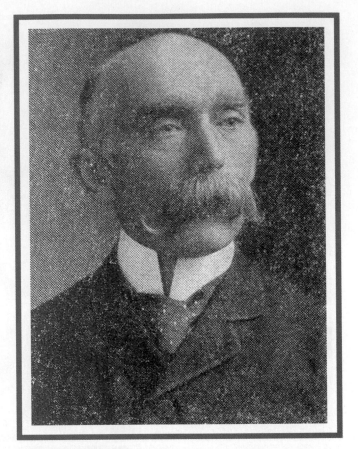

PHOTO 4.2 Dr. Peter Henderson Bryce

*Source: Canadian Public Health Association*

enact legislation concerning disease surveillance and control measures as well as to safeguard public administration of food and drugs (Her Majesty the Queen in Right of Canada, represented by the Minister of Health, 2008).

## The First Public Health Nurses in Canada

Lillian Wald coined the term "public health nurse." Wald was an American nurse and founder of the Henry Street Settlement in New York City. In 1893, Wald described nurses who worked with low-income communities as PHNs, setting them apart from nurses who cared for sick individuals in hospitals or in high-income homes (McKay, 2009). In Canada, public health nursing grew out of the religious persuasion and social conscience of the social gospel movement and maternal feminism. PHNs focused primarily on improving physical environmental conditions to reduce maternal and child morbidity and mortality. In the late 19th century, one out of every five infants died and the rate of maternal deaths was high as well. In addition, at this time, women were not recognized as people under the British North American Act (Ontario Ministry of Government Services, n.d.). Maternal feminists "were seeking sweeping social reform, particularly to protect the interests of women, children and families" (Harrison, 2011, p. 23).

**Charitable Organizations** While little is known about Canada's first PHNs, it is certain that they worked for charitable or religious organizations in several regions of the country. They were known as visiting nurses or district nurses. In 1885, there was a diet dispensary in Montreal that employed a district nurse. The district nurse would have carried out nutrition counselling and assisted with volunteer distribution of nutritious meals to disadvantaged pregnant women and their families. Located in Toronto in 1889, the Nursing-at-Home Mission hired district nurses to visit disadvantaged families who lived close to the Children's Hospital. The Victorian Order of Nurses was founded in 1897 in Ottawa and served as a national district nursing association. It was not uncommon for PHNs to volunteer their expertise at Winnipeg's Margaret Scott Nursing Mission (constructed in 1905) or at the Lethbridge Nursing Mission (built in 1909), for example. Volunteer PHNs were also members of the St. Elizabeth Visiting Nurses' Association that was established in 1910 (McKay, 2009).

**Civic Health Departments** Increasingly, the delivery of public health programs to address complex issues of the more vulnerable populations (e.g., immigrants, urban poor, infants and children, and rural isolated families) was becoming too great a financial burden for charitable organizations. Many organizations sought government funding to maintain their programs. In 1910, Winnipeg's civic health department, through yearly grants, financed the local district nursing association and the milk depot to support their public health programs for children. The district nurse or PHN would have made visits to families armed with milk supplies, health messages, and parenting instruction. The PHNs assisted mothers with childbirth, infant feeding, and childcare, including bathing children (Ontario Ministry of Government Services, n.d.). Universal public schooling in Canada began in the late 19th century. Local school boards began sponsoring school health programs and hired PHNs to conduct physical inspections of children and to provide health education in the classroom. Children who were at risk were identified at schools, and PHNs often used this information to engage in home visits with vulnerable families. PHNs were instrumental in reducing high mortality rates among school-aged children by combatting tuberculosis and controlling other communicable diseases. Civic health departments across Canada eventually took over voluntary public health programs, and before World War I, PHNs were hired to work in specific departments like Winnipeg's Child Hygiene Department. Nurse leader Eunice Henrietta Dyke (see Photo 4.3) spearheaded the opening of the Department of Public Health in the City of Toronto (McKay, 2009).

Families in rural regions of Canada received few PHN services because of a lack of municipal finances. Women's groups (e.g., Women's Institute or the United Farm Women) are cited as organizations that interceded and hired PHNs or physicians to hold child health clinics or to conduct school inspections. Public health programs and public health nursing services were solely the responsibility of the provinces. In 1916, Manitoba became the first province in Canada to establish a provincially funded public health nursing service. In 1919, Alberta provided its citizens with district nursing services and British

Columbia, in the same year, set up health centres for several communities that were staffed with PHNs (Allemang, 1995).

**Vaccination Campaigns** PHNs continued to battle diseases including cholera, smallpox, typhoid fever, and several other bacteria and viruses that have since been eradicated. By the mid-1920s, following the discovery of diphtheria, pertussis, tetanus, and polio toxoids, PHNs were responsible for delivering substantial childhood immunization and vaccination programs. Polio, poliomyelitis, or infantile paralysis all refer to a disease that was terrifying for parents and children alike prior to the vaccine. This is because within a few hours of becoming ill a child could die or be permanently paralyzed (Harrison, 2011). In addition to delivering immunizations, PHNs were working in well-baby clinics, delivering prenatal classes, and conducting postnatal home visits where they discussed issues in parenting and the importance of childhood nutrition (PHAC, n.d.).

## Comprehensive System of Child and Family Health and Welfare Services

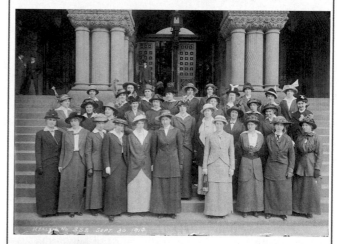

**PHOTO  4.3**  Eunice Henrietta Dyke (front row, 6th from the left)

*Source: City of Toronto Archives, Fonds 200, Series 372, Subseries 32, Item 353*

Eunice Henrietta Dyke was a Toronto-born Canadian who, in 1905, attended nursing school in the United States (Johns Hopkins School for Nurses in Baltimore, Maryland). In 1911, Nurse Dyke began her employment with the Department of Public Health of the City of Toronto. She pioneered the idea of positioning child welfare services as the nucleus of the department's child health centres. The child's family became the focus of public health nursing services, and PHNs were responsible for families on a district basis. Decentralization of public health nursing services was truly innovative and was soon recognized around the world. Nurse Dyke also championed the coordination of public health and community welfare and social services.

*Source. Canadian Public Health Association. (n.d.). Profiles in public health. Retrieved from http://resources.cpha.ca/CPHA/ThisIsPublicHealth/profiles/pages.php?l=E*

## Travelling Public Health Nurse Served Manitoba for 41 Years

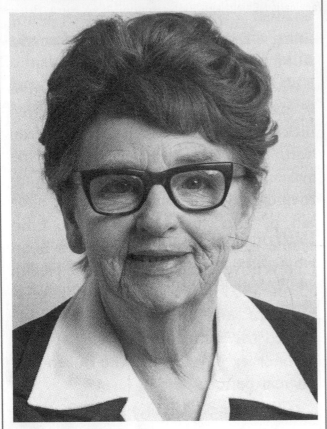

PHOTO 4.4 Lynn Blair

*Source: Canadian Public Health Association*

Lynn Blair grew up in Alexander, Manitoba. She received her nursing training from the Children's Hospital in Winnipeg, graduating in 1928. Nurse Blair obtained a diploma in public health nursing from the University of Minnesota 20 years later. Her nursing career included working at the San Haven State Sanatorium in North Dakota in 1928 and then at the new Department of Health and Welfare in Manitoba in 1929. As a PHN, she travelled extensively throughout Manitoba and assumed diverse responsibilities, including delivering veterinarian services, and she performed some services that were usually carried out by physicians at that time. She met health needs of handicapped children and, as a nursing consultant in venereal disease, worked to prevent the spread of sexually transmitted infections. In 1940, Nurse Blair travelled 1000 miles a week seeking family placement for children evacuated from war-torn Britain. Nurse Blair was awarded the Canadian Public Health Association's Honorary Life Membership in 1975.

*Source: Canadian Public Health Association. (n.d.). Profiles in public health. Retrieved from http://resources.cpha.ca/CPHA/ ThisIsPublicHealth/profiles/pages.php?l=E*

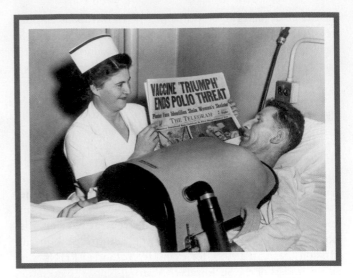

PHOTO 4.5 A patient in an iron lung: The "iron lung" was an artificial respirator used with patients suffering from paralytic polio. Patients with paralytic polio experienced paralysis of the diaphragm and intracostal muscles, which are essential for respiration.

*Source: March of Dimes Canada*

was both exciting and exhausting (see Photos 4.4 and 4.5; see Figure 4.2). It was not uncommon for PHNs to walk several miles in snow storms or travel by dog sled or horseback to

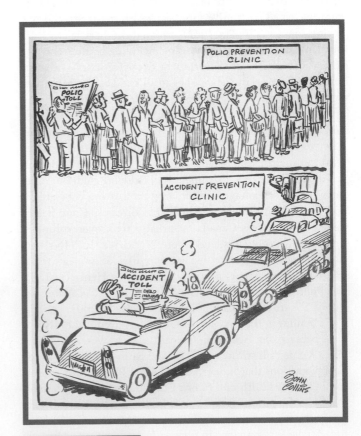

FIGURE 4.2 Polio Vaccination Campaign

*Source: Collins, J. (circa 1959). Too bad we can't have shots for this, too. M965.199.6054 © McCord Museum, Montreal.*

Public health nursing practice required advanced education, and the early PHNs were respected as "elite members of the nursing profession" (McKay, 2009, p. 250). Their work

carry out their diverse roles and responsibilities. Gwen Thomas was a district nurse in Newfoundland after World War II. Her account is a captivating portrayal of a PHN:

> When I went to La Scie, it was 1949, and there was a lot of tuberculosis in Newfoundland. In quite a few families, one person or another was in bed with TB and eventually died. . . . The only way to get into La Scie was either by plane or in the winter by dog team, in the spring and summer by boat, or else across the woods road. I remember one time going to Shoe Cove, which was about four and a half miles, and we had to walk because there were no roads. When I arrived the patient was in labour. She had twins, which I delivered. (Marsh, Walsh, & Beaton, 2008, p. 183)

## PRIMARY HEALTH CARE AND PUBLIC HEALTH NURSING

The motivation behind the World Health Organization's (WHO) Health for All movement was the disturbing reality of health inequalities worldwide. In 1977, the World Assembly announced that the "main social target of governments and of the WHO should be attainment by all people of the world by the year 2000 a level of health that permits them to live socially and economically productive lives" (Little, 1992, p. 198). Assembly members, including Canada, endorsed the primary health care principles of public participation, intersectoral and interdisciplinary collaboration, health promotion, appropriate technology, and accessibility as key to achieving their goal. Former health minister Jake Epp's (1986) "Achieving Health for All" document and the release of the WHO, Health & Welfare Canada, and the Canadian Public Health Association (1986) document, "Ottawa Charter for Health Promotion," were the impetus for Canadian health reform and the foundation of the "new" public health movement.

PHNs were to reduce and challenge health inequalities by enabling citizens to take action to improve their health (see Photo 4.6). PHNs were called on to make a concerted effort to enact the principles of primary health care, to think upstream (i.e., to think about the many risk factors contributing to sickness and disease in an effort to prevent illness or injury) by addressing barriers to health (Butterfield, 2002; Raphael, 2011). Mahler (1985), then director general of the WHO, was confident PHNs could make a difference: "If millions of nurses in a thousand different places articulate the same ideas and convictions about Primary Health Care, and come together as one force, then they could act as a powerhouse for change" (p. 10).

As Canadian provinces began preparing for major healthcare reform, nursing associations actively endorsed primary health care principles by submitting recommendations to provincial advisory committees, task forces, and commissions. "Health for all Canadians: A Call for Health Care Reform" by the Canadian Nurses Association (CNA) (1988) led to position statements and projects pushing for nursing roles reflective of primary health care. Community nurses' resource centres, for example, were created in Manitoba.

### Promoting Public Health Nursing and Primary Prevention

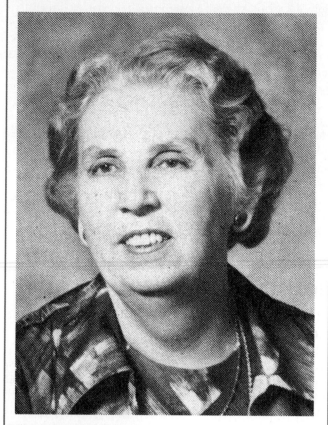

**PHOTO 4.6** Eleanore Louise Miner

*Source: Canadian Public Health Association*

Eleanore Louise Miner of Regina, Saskatchewan, was a public health nursing leader. Her career spanned 35 years and within that time she advanced primary prevention efforts and expanded the staff of public health professionals by including dental hygienists, nutritionists, speech therapists, psychologists, and physiotherapists. She focused on meeting the public health needs of vulnerable groups. From 1959 to 1961, she was president of provincial and national nursing associations. Nurse Miner published a series of articles on public financing of PHNs in the *Canadian Journal of Public Health*, documenting the important contributions of PHNs.

*Source: Canadian Public Health Association. (n.d.). Profiles in public health. Retrieved from http://resources.cpha.ca/CPHA/ ThisIsPublicHealth/profiles/pages.php?l=E*

Alberta took steps to implement plans for the "Increased Direct Access to Nursing Services" project and reallocated $110 million from acute care to community health services. Between 1985 and 1995, the Canadian nursing profession lobbied for the shift from the medical model to a primary health care model.

Healthcare reform and healthcare restructuring in Canada since the mid-1990s have moved healthcare services from institutions to communities and have led to a greater emphasis on health promotion, disease prevention, and public participation (Reutter & Ford, 1998). Public participation is a primary health care principle that is integral to PHNs' achieving sustained change. The PHN's role is not just to educate, consult, or "do for" by providing services, but to collaborate with individual citizens, families, and communities as active partners, addressing problems to promote, maintain, and restore health (Underwood, 2010). The principle of public participation is based on the premise that citizens, collectively, have the knowledge and capacity to identify barriers to health and to determine options to overcome those barriers. PHNs assume a strengths-based orientation by seeking information about capabilities of individual citizens, families, and communities, and by assisting them in mobilize resources. Capitalizing on strengths fosters a sense of optimism and hope, and citizens are apt to take charge and forge a healthier future for themselves (Gottlieb, 2013).

# PUBLIC HEALTH NURSING DISCIPLINE-SPECIFIC COMPETENCIES

PHNs practise in community health centres, homes, schools, workplaces, street clinics, youth centres, outpost settings, and as part of community groups. Disease prevention, particularly infectious diseases, including preventing the introduction and spread of pandemic infections such as SARS and influenza A virus subtype H1N1, remains the responsibility of PHNs. Non-communicable chronic diseases (e.g., coronary heart disease and diabetes), injuries, and lifestyle risks to health due to tobacco, alcohol, and drug consumption require considerable time, effort, and expertise. PHNs continue to promote and to advocate for the health and quality of life of mothers and children, in particular younger mothers and mothers of low socio-economic status. The health of the environment is also a priority focus, especially with the threats brought on by global climate change, deterioration of ecosystem services, and land-use change. Such threats are interacting to create grave risks to community and population health, including exposure to infectious disease, water scarcity, food scarcity, natural disasters, and population displacement (Myers & Patz, 2009). In addition, food safety, sanitation, and occupational hazards remain part of the PHN's responsibilities. Finally, PHNs focus on the prerequisites for health because they seek social justice for individual citizens, families, communities, and populations. PHNs are committed to working collaboratively to help balance the benefits of health throughout society (McKay, 2009).

Today, PHNs are the largest group of public health employees. PHNs function under the laws and regulations of various government bodies that oversee public health. Historically, public health programs have been delivered according to provincial mandates, and variance among programs and across jurisdictions continues. Sometimes PHNs must challenge current laws, regulations, or policies within their jurisdiction to better support the health of individual citizens, families, communities, and population groups. For this reason, the PHN needs to be knowledgeable about how federal, provincial, and territorial governments operate. Additionally, the PHN must have a working knowledge of the local operations of municipalities and Aboriginal organizations (CPHA, 2010). Politics and public health administration are just some of the necessary elements of the PHN's knowledge base.

The PHN is expected to possess a comprehensive knowledge base in order to intervene effectively to contribute to the health of the population as a whole. For example, while the hospital nurse will require human pathophysiology to promote patient healing, the PHN requires the science of epidemiology to assess the magnitude of population-level health threats of specific diseases in society. Being population oriented also means that the PHN is focused on the community origins of health problems, such as those related to nutrition, employment, or the environment. PHNs look for risk factors that could be altered to prevent or delay illness or premature death. Similar to the systematic health assessment of a patient by the acute care nurse, the community is assessed systematically by the PHN. Using a population oriented approach also equips PHNs for effective intersectoral collaboration, which means partnering with representatives from several sectors of society in addition to health (e.g., education, government, industry, recreation, nongovernmental agencies) to deal with, oftentimes, a vast array of factors (PHAC, n.d.).

The **public health nursing discipline-specific competencies** were established in 2009. This work was funded by the Public Health Agency of Canada and led by members of the Community Health Nurses of Canada. The discipline-specific competencies include the following:

1. knowledge derived from public health and nursing science;

2. skills related to assessment and analysis;

3. conducting policy and program planning, implementation, and evaluation;

4. achieving partnerships, collaboration, and advocacy;

5. promoting diversity and inclusiveness;

6. effective communication exchange;

7. leadership capabilities; and

8. professional responsibility and accountability.

All of the eight discipline-specific competencies require that PHNs possess certain knowledge, skills, and attitudes, as outlined in Table 4.1. The PHN may have to rely on several competencies on a day-to-day basis to promote, protect, and preserve the health of the population. The attitudes are critical to the role, as are the broad knowledge base and diverse skills. A PHN would likely draw on all of the knowledge, skills, and attitudes presented in Table 4.1 while completing work that falls under one or more of the public health nursing discipline-specific competencies. Each PHN discerns which knowledge, skills, and attitudes are essential as he or she carries out responsibilities reflecting the competencies. Accordingly, a PHN may place more emphasis on certain knowledge, skills, and attitudes to inform his or her nursing practice.

| Table 4.1 | Public Health Nursing Discipline-Specific Competencies and Corresponding Knowledge, Skills, and Attitudes | | |
|---|---|---|---|
| **Competencies** | **Knowledge** | **Skills** | **Attitudes** |
| 1. Public health and nursing science | *The public health nurse has knowledge of* | *The public health nurse is equipped with skills to* | *The public health nurse considers* |
| 2. Assessment and analysis | • behavioural and social sciences | • apply knowledge, critically appraise knowledge, and research new sources of knowledge | • health as multi-dimensional |
| 3. Policy and program planning, implementation, and evaluation | • biostatistics | | • the influence of physical, sociocultural, political, and economic environments on health |
| | • epidemiology | | |
| | • environmental public health | • collect, assess, analyze, and apply data, facts, concepts, and theories to determine individual, family, group, and community health concerns | |
| 4. Partnerships, collaboration, and advocacy | • demography | | • support needs of individuals, families, groups, and communities to help them improve conditions conducive to health |
| 5. Diversity and inclusiveness | • workplace health | | |
| 6. Communication | • prevention of chronic diseases | | |
| 7. Leadership | • infectious diseases | | |
| 8. Professional responsibility and accountability | • psychosocial problems and injuries | • assess individual, family, group, and community levels of capacity to address health concerns | • opportunities to address health inequities and promote social justice |
| | • nursing theory | | • accommodating diverse sociocultural, economic, and educational backgrounds |
| | • change theory | | |
| | • economics | • identify and recommend appropriate interventions, including health promotion, health protection, and disease and injury prevention | |
| | • politics | | |
| | • public health administration | | |
| | • community assessment | • lead policy and program planning, implementation, and evaluation | |
| | • management theory | | |
| | • program planning and evaluation | | |
| | • population health principles | • collaborate effectively with diverse individuals, families, groups, and communities | |
| | • primary health care | | |
| | • determinants of health | | |
| | • community development theory | • promote positive team functioning | |
| | • social justice | • initiate interdisciplinary and intersectoral partnerships and networks | |
| | • history of public health | | |
| | | • work to achieve interagency and intergovernmental co-operation | |
| | | • act as spokesperson as needed on public health issues | |
| | | • respond to public health emergencies | |

## PUBLIC HEALTH NURSING AND LEADERSHIP

As indicated in the previous section, leadership is one of the core competencies of public health nurses (Community Health Nurses of Canada, 2009). A leader in public health has the aptitude to influence, motivate, and enable others to achieve goals. Nurses work at the "intersection where societal attitudes, government policies, and people's lives meet . . . [and this] creates a moral imperative to not only attend to the health needs of the public but also, like Nightingale, to work to change the societal conditions contributing to poor health" (Falk-Raphael, 2005, p. 219). Public health nurse leaders have "courage, vision, strategic agility, passion, and a moral core. They have substantial networks, keen understanding of issues and are solution focused while seeking root causes of problems" (Community Health Nurses of Canada, 2013, p. 23). It seems fitting, then, that PHNs use their relationships with their diverse range of clients to work at various levels (individual, family, community, and system/sector) on the determinants of health to ultimately impact the health of society (Cohen & Reutter, 2007; Falk-Raphael and Betker, 2012). Community Health Nurses of Canada (2015) recently released the Leadership Competencies for Public Health Practice in Canada. There are five domains of leadership competency:

1. systems transformation,
2. achieve results,
3. lead self,
4. engage others, and
5. develop coalition.

More information regarding these leadership competencies can be found at http://chnc.ca/documents/LCPHPC-EN. The following section provides an overview of how PHNs function to create change in population health status through the six essential functions of public health systems in Canada.

## PUBLIC HEALTH NURSING ROLES

PHNs combine the knowledge, skills, and attitudes of the above discipline-specific competencies to promote, protect, and preserve the health of all Canadians. PHNs perform the roles and responsibilities as outlined in the **six essential functions of public health** (CPHA, 2010):

1. **health protection,**
2. **health surveillance,**
3. **population health assessment,**
4. **disease and injury prevention,**
5. **health promotion, and**
6. **emergency preparation and response.**

PHNs concentrate their efforts on the population and the several prerequisites or determinants of health. Through ongoing surveillance and by examining vital statistics and other population data, the PHN decides when and where to intervene. PHNs carry out the essential public health functions listed above by assuming various roles and employing an array of strategies, as illustrated in Table 4.2.

## LEVELS OF PREVENTION

It is important to note that PHNs intervene at three levels of prevention: primary, secondary, and tertiary. At the level of **primary prevention**, risks of illness, disease, and injury are eliminated. Sometimes the resistance to illness, disease, and injury may be enhanced (Vollman, Anderson, & McFarlane, 2012). Examples of the primary prevention work of PHNs may include the following:

- Breastfeeding campaigns during which PHNs publicly advocate breastfeeding for up to two years and beyond. Breast milk provides infants with "optimal nutritional, immunological, and emotional benefits for growth and development" (CPHA, n.d.). Nutrition gained from breast milk enhances childhood resistance to illness and disease (see Canadian Research Box 4.2).
- The Government of New Brunswick has adopted the "Baby-Friendly Initiative" as a strategy to support breastfeeding. Breastfeeding support services are offered by New Brunswick's Miramichi Region in the form of breastfeeding clinic drop-ins where breastfeeding mothers can meet with PHNs who are lactation consultants.
- PHNs working at public health district offices across Canada prevent children from acquiring communicable diseases by implementing effective vaccination programs.
- PHNs providing education sessions to a group of middle-aged men about how low-salt, low-fat, and low-sugar nutrient-rich foods combined with smoking cessation and exercise will eliminate risk factors for arthrosclerosis.
- PHNs working broadly with the determinants of health advocate for communities to have access to iodized salt, perhaps in the form of enriched flour, to prevent iodine-deficiency goiter.
- Home visiting by PHNs allows for risk assessment and observation related to home safety and environmental hazards. For example, PHNs often work with families to identify factors in the home that may put aging and elderly family members at risk for falls. As another example, PHNs may identify drawstrings on blinds as a choking hazard for small children. PHNs will problem solve with family members to mitigate such risks.

In **secondary prevention**, the disease process is suspended before symptoms occur. Causal factors are not eliminated, but permanent sequelae (a pathological condition) is prevented through early detection for treatment or by public health programs to control the disease (Vollman et al., 2012). Examples of secondary prevention work of PHNs may include the following:

- screening for lead levels in blood samples of employees exposed to environmental contaminants in their workplace;
- screening for cholesterol and blood pressure levels of employees in the workplace (Shah, 2003); and
- working in early detection programs, including mammography to detect breast cancer and papanicolaou smears to detect cervical cancer (McKeown & Messias, 2008).

| Table 4.2 | Public Health Nursing Roles | | |
|---|---|---|---|
| **Public Health Essential Functions** | **Description** | **Public Health Programming** | **Public Health Nursing Roles** |
| Health protection | Health protection is a chief function of public health. Canada's water supply and food are protected from contamination. Regulatory frameworks protect the population from infectious diseases and from environmental threats. | • Water purification and monitoring<br>• Air quality monitoring/enforcement (Environmental Protection Act)<br>• Restaurant inspections<br>• Childcare facility inspections<br>• Smoking cessation through public health policies, tobacco taxes, anti-smoking advertising campaigns, and product labelling | *Collaborator:*<br>• Partners with health inspectors, government officials, and agency representatives to ensure all citizens have safe drinking water and food, and live, work, and play in safe environments<br>• Establishes coalitions and networks as needed to enact or enforce public health legislation<br><br>*Leader:*<br>• Initiates action<br>• Encourages citizens, the community, and those with power to initiate action<br><br>*Policy Formulator:*<br>• Identifies health protection issues in need of policy development<br>• Participates in implementing and evaluating policy |
| Health surveillance | Public health professionals use health surveillance techniques to collect population data on an ongoing basis to detect early signs of illness and disease trends or outbreaks. Surveillance data provide the information needed to intervene in an effective manner to mitigate disease impact. | • Periodic health surveys<br>• Cancer and other disease registries<br>• Communicable disease reporting<br>• Ongoing analysis of data to identify trends or emerging problems (e.g., recognition of increasing syphilis cases)<br>• Reporting health threats to practitioners, what they need to look for, and intervention required | *Epidemiologist:*<br>• Seeks health surveillance data<br>• Coordinates systematic and routine collection and reporting of health data<br>• Analyzes surveillance data for risk and forecasting of threatening events<br>• Conducts surveillance of broad determinants of health<br>• Disseminates surveillance findings and health implications to citizens, communities, and decision makers |
| Population health assessment | Public health professionals are well versed in what facilitates and what hinders the health of the Canadian population. Population health assessment is a tool to ensure public health programs, services, and policies are adequately meeting goals and objectives. | • Population or community health needs assessment<br>• Health status report; system report card | *Epidemiologist:*<br>• Applies health surveillance data to public health nursing practice<br>• Conducts population health assessments and community health assessments<br>• Justifies new initiatives or revisions to current programs or services with needs assessment |

*(continued)*

| Table 4.2 | Continued | | |
|---|---|---|---|
| **Public Health Essential Functions** | **Description** | **Public Health Programming** | **Public Health Nursing Roles** |
| | | | *Outreach Worker:* <br>• Actively seeks information about the health of populations, communities, or aggregates <br>• Uses health assessment findings to target issues (actual or potential) and to plan steps to address issues <br>• Willing to reach out to high-risk communities (e.g., harm reduction strategies) if information indicates public health nursing interventions are warranted |
| Disease and injury prevention | Public health professionals contribute to the longevity and quality of life of Canadians through disease and injury prevention. | • Immunizations <br>• Investigation and outbreak control <br>• Screening for nutritional (e.g., scurvy), occupational (e.g., cancer of scrotum), and environmental (e.g., lead poisoning) diseases <br>• Encouraging healthy behaviours (e.g., smoking cessation during pregnancy, healthy eating, breastfeeding, physical activity, bicycle helmet use) | *Service Provider:* <br>• Manages and controls communicable diseases using prevention techniques, infection control, behaviour change counselling, outbreak management, and immunization <br>• Conducts screening for disease <br>• Informs individuals about screening procedures, rationale, and results <br>• Monitors, documents, and evaluates screening activities <br>• Uses effective strategies to reduce risk factors that may contribute to chronic disease, injury, and disability <br><br>*Health Educator:* <br>• Offers formal presentations, educational programs, and informal teaching sessions about healthy lifestyle behaviours <br>• Applies teaching/learning principles to address health education needs and to ensure readiness of learner to change at-risk behaviours <br>• Evaluates effectiveness of health education interventions <br>• Uses marketing techniques to promote both community health programs and healthy living |
| Health promotion | Public health professionals improve the health of Canadians through healthy public policy, public participation, and community-based interventions. | • Intersectoral community partnerships (e.g., Heart & Stroke Foundation) to address factors affecting health <br>• Advocacy for healthy public policies | *Capacity Builder:* <br>• Involves communities, aggregates, and individual citizens in planning and priority setting of health promotion programs and services <br>• Shares information about community resources <br>• Fosters skill development of community members to mobilize resources, establish social networks, and navigate political processes |

| Table 4.2 | Continued | | |
|---|---|---|---|
| **Public Health Essential Functions** | **Description** | **Public Health Programming** | **Public Health Nursing Roles** |
| | | • Catalyzing the creation of physical and social environments to support health (e.g., bike paths, promoting access to social networks for institutionalized seniors) | **Community Developer:**<br>• Uses community development strategies to engage community members in identifying and addressing social, economic, cultural, and physical environment issues<br>• Uses a strengths-based approach that supports community empowerment and decision making<br><br>**Facilitator:**<br>• Fosters interagency links and working relationships<br>• Uses mediation skills to facilitate interagency and intergovernmental co-operation |
| Emergency preparedness and disaster response | Public health professionals are aware of the immediate and secondary threats to population health incited by natural disasters. Emergency preparedness and disaster response safeguard water supplies or food sources from contamination. | • Disaster planning to prepare communities to respond to floods, earthquakes, and fires<br>• Leading institutions in emergency preparedness to respond to explosives or biological threats | **Consultant:**<br>• Uses knowledge and expertise in emergency preparedness and disaster response planning to inform individual citizens, non-profit agencies, organizations, institutions, the public, and all levels of government of measures required to reduce the impact of public health emergencies<br>• Acts as a resource person to communities, aggregates, and individual citizens<br>• Plans for, is part of, and evaluates the response to both natural disasters (e.g., floods, earthquakes, fires, or infectious disease outbreaks) and man-made disasters (e.g., those involving explosives, chemicals, radioactive substances, or biological threats) to minimize serious illness, death, and social disruption<br>• Uses effective risk-communication techniques to inform individual citizens and the public |

Source: Based on Public Health Agency of Canada (n.d.) and the Canadian Public Health Association (2010). *Public Health – Community Health Nursing Practice in Canada: Roles and Activities* (4th ed.). Copyright © 2010 by Canadian Public Health Association. Used by permission of Canadian Public Health Association. Retrieved from https://www.chnc.ca/documents/PublicHealthCommunityHealthNursinginCanadaRolesandActivities2010.pdf

In **tertiary prevention,** the impairment or disability from the disease process is halted (Vollman et al., 2012). Examples of tertiary prevention work of PHNs may include the following:

■ implementing a control strategy with individuals who are diagnosed with active tuberculosis and who live in communities with a high incidence of tuberculosis;

■ providing treatment, education, self-management, and support to adults and children diagnosed with various infectious diseases, including human immunodeficiency virus (HIV) or hepatitis; and

■ designing, planning, and implementing social marketing campaigns to de-normalize tobacco use (CPHA, 2011) (see Canadian Research Box 4.2).

### CANADIAN RESEARCH BOX 4.1

**What is the relationship between a mother's intention to supplement with infant formula and breastfeeding duration?**

Kim, E., Hoetmer, S. E., Li, Y., & Vandenber, J. E. (2013). Relationship between intention to supplement with infant formula and breastfeeding duration. *Canadian Journal of Public Health, 104*(5), e388–e393.

Health Canada and the Canadian Paediatric Society recommend infants be exclusively breastfed for the first six months with continued breastfeeding for two years and beyond. In this study, Kim, Hoetmer, Li, and Vandenber examined the relationship between a mother's intention to supplement with infant formula and the risk of discontinuing breastfeeding during the first 12 months of the postpartum period. The researchers surveyed 345 mothers at six weeks, six months and 12 months postpartum as part of York Region's Infant Feeding Survey. The relationship between a mother's, prenatal intention to supplement with infant formula and breastfeeding duration was examined using Cox proportional hazards regression. Various factors were controlled for including mother's age, prenatal education, immigration status, parity, household income, mother's ethnicity, and education. Nearly one-third of mothers intended to supplement with infant formula. Of those mothers, 69% actually supplemented their breastfeeding with infant formula within 12 months postpartum. Intention to supplement was found to be associated with shorter breastfeeding duration (hazard ratio = 2.64, 95% CI 1.83-3.81). First-time mothers experienced shorter breastfeeding durations compared to experienced mothers (hazard ratio = 2.13, 95% CI 1.39-3.27). The authors concluded that a mother's prenatal intent to supplement may be associated with shorter breastfeeding duration.

#### Discussion Questions

1. What level of prevention are measures to promote breastfeeding?

2. What types of strategies could PHNs implement to ensure mothers breastfeed exclusively for the first six months postpartum?

3. Hospital policies exist that allow infant formula products to be made readily available to new mothers. What role(s) should the PHN assume in order to promote breastfeeding?

### CANADIAN RESEARCH BOX 4.2

**What are the legal and ethical considerations of extending tobacco legislation to include multi-unit dwellings in Alberta, and what does this mean for public health nursing practice?**

Stooke, V. D. (2013). Sharing the air: The legal and ethical considerations of extending tobacco legislation to include multi-unit dwellings in Alberta. *Public Health Nursing, 31*(1), 6068. doi:10.1111/phn/12068

Stooke explores the legal and ethical considerations of extending tobacco legislation to include multi-unit dwellings (MUDs) in Alberta, and the implications for public health nursing practice. The tobacco legislation in Canada currently protects individuals in public places but not in private dwellings. In Alberta, there are over one million individuals living in MUDs who are exposed to environmental tobacco smoke. Children are particularly vulnerable to the negative health effects of tobacco smoke. As well, many apartment fires in Alberta are related to smoking, which makes expanding tobacco legislation to include MUDs an important public health issue. There are many potential barriers to the adoption of this tobacco legislation, including legal, ethical, and civil rights concerns, and the bureaucracy of the political process. Stooke articulates the position that it is both legal and ethical to expand provincial tobacco legislation to include MUDs after considering individual civil rights. This approach is also aligned with the Canadian Nurses Association code of ethics for registered nurses (2008) that is used to guide nursing practice. PHNs must advocate for change in the current legislation by becoming politically active and building community capacity to promote social justice.

#### Discussion Questions

1. What level of prevention is tobacco legislation?

2. Does social justice include restricting citizens from smoking when living in MUDs?

3. When reading the primary values outlined in the CNA code of ethics one might suggest that stipulating individual lifestyle choices means that PHNs are violating the code. Explain why you agree or do not agree.

### CASE STUDY

Molly Styles is a 20-year-old single mother. She has one child who is two months old. Her home is a dilapidated one-bedroom basement apartment in downtown Toronto. Ms. Styles relies on public assistance, but monthly cheques barely cover the costs of rent, food, and transportation. By the end of the month she has to take a trip to the local food bank. Ms. Styles quit high school when she found out she was pregnant. Her boyfriend, whom she was living with, left before the baby was born. She has been estranged from her parents for several years. Isolated and caring for her child, her life is bittersweet, because on the one hand becoming a mother has given her a reason for living, and on the other hand life is very different now with the demands of raising her child alone. During the baby's two-month immunization appointment, the PHN noticed that Ms. Styles seemed downcast. The PHN was also concerned about the baby's poor weight gain and wondered if Ms. Styles was still breastfeeding.

## Discussion Questions

1. Do you think that you are witnessing health inequalities or social inequities, or both, in this case study?

2. Which public health essential functions and public health nursing roles are most relevant to this case study? Which of the discipline-specific competencies do you think you would need as a PHN to work with Ms. Styles and why?

## CONCLUSION

PHNs have played and continue to play instrumental roles in the health and well-being of Canadians. Earliest documented accounts attest to the dedication, commitment, and visionary leadership of Canada's public health nursing pioneers. Today's PHNs face complex health-related issues locally, nationally, and globally. Safeguarding the health of the Canadian population entails assuming several roles and PHNs must be equipped with diverse competencies. The career of the PHN will continue to be both challenging and exciting as PHNs work to fulfill the essential functions of health protection, health surveillance, population health assessment, disease and injury prevention, health promotion, and emergency preparation and response for the betterment of all Canadians.

## KEY TERMS

disease and injury prevention    p. 68

emergency preparedness and disaster response    p. 68

health promotion    p. 68

health protection    p. 68

health surveillance    p. 68

population health assessment    p. 68

primary prevention    p. 68

principles of primary health care    p. 61

public health    p. 60

public health nurse (PHN)    p. 61

public health nursing discipline-specific competencies    p. 66

secondary prevention    p. 68

six essential functions of public health    p. 68

tertiary prevention    p. 71

## STUDY QUESTIONS

1. What is the definition of public health?

2. When was the Public Health Agency of Canada established and why?

3. What is the role of the Public Health Agency of Canada?

4. What are the six functions of public health in Canada?

5. What are the public health nursing disciplinary-specific competencies?

6. Discuss what you think are two of the important contributions early PHNs have made and why.

After working through these questions, go to the MyNursingLab at www.pearsoned.ca/mynursinglab to check your answers.

## INDIVIDUAL CRITICAL-THINKING EXERCISES

1. Consider the definition of public health presented in this chapter. Is there another component you think is critical to include in this definition?

2. Although the Public Health Agency was established relatively recently, are there other organizations you know of (or may find) that also contributed to public health around the turn of the previous century?

3. How do you think PHNs may contribute to the work of the Public Health Agency of Canada?

4. Discuss the importance of the six functions of public health.

5. Why do you think it is important to have public health nursing disciplinary-specific competencies?

## GROUP CRITICAL-THINKING EXERCISES

1. Discuss what course concepts you have learned in class that relate to the public health nursing discipline-specific competencies (version 1.0).

2. What public health activities are you able to identify in the communities in which you live?

3. Discuss the differences in the definition of the role of community health nurses in general and PHNs.

## REFERENCES

Allemang, M. (1995). Development of community health nursing in Canada. In M. J. Stewart (Ed.), *Community nursing: Promoting Canadians' health* (pp. 2–36). Toronto, ON: W. B. Saunders.

Bryce, P. (1910). History of public health in Canada. *The Canadian Therapeutist and Sanitary Engineer, 1*, 287–291. Retrieved from http://www.cpha.ca/uploads/history/book/History-book-print_chapter1_e.pdf

Butterfield, P. G. (2002). Upstream reflections on environmental health: An abbreviated history and framework for action. *Advances in Nursing Science, 25*(1), 32–49.

Canadian Nurses Association. (1988). *Health for all Canadians: A call for health-care reform.* Ottawa, ON: Author.

Canadian Nurses Association. (2008). *Code of ethics for registered nurses (2008 centennial edition).* Ottawa, ON: Author. Retrieved from http://www.cna-aiic.ca/~/media/cna/files/en/codeofethics.pdf

Canadian Public Health Association. (n.d.). 12 great achievements. Ottawa, ON: Author. Retrieved from http://www.cpha.ca/en/programs/history/achievements.aspp

Canadian Public Health Association. (2010). *Public health/Community health nursing practice in Canada: Roles and activities* (4th ed.). Ottawa, ON: Author. Retrieved from http://www.cpha.ca/uploads/pubs/3-1bk04214.pdf

Canadian Public Health Association. (2011). The winnable battle: Ending tobacco use in Canada. Ottawa, ON: Author. Retrieved from http://www.cpha.ca/uploads/positions/position-paper-tobacco_e.pdf

Cohen, B., & Reutter, L. (2007). Development of the role of public health nurses in addressing child and family poverty: A framework for action. *Journal of Advanced Nursing, 60*(1), 96–107. doi: http://dx.doi.org/10.1111/j.1365-2648.2006.04154.x

Community Health Nurses of Canada. (2009). *The public health nursing discipline specific competencies,* version 1.0. St. John's, NL: Author. Retrieved from http://www.chnc.ca/documents/competencies_june_2009_english.pdf

Community Health Nurses of Canada. (2013). *Public health nursing leadership in Canada: Report to the National Collaborating Center on the Determinants of Health.* St. John's, NL: Author. Retrieved from https://www.chnc.ca/documents/PHNLeadershipDevelopmentinCanadaFinalReportwlogoandacknowledgements2014Fub27.pdf

Community Health Nurses of Canada. (2015). Leadership competencies for public health practice in Canada. Version 1.0. St. John's, NL: Author. Retrieved from http://chnc.ca/documents/LCPHPC-EN/

Epp, J. (1986). *Achieving health for all: A framework for health promotion in Canada.* Toronto, ON: Health and Welfare Canada.

Falk-Raphael, A. (2005). Speaking truth to power: Nursing's legacy and moral imperative. *Advances in Nursing Science, 28*(3), 212–223.

Falk-Raphael, A., & Betker, C. (2012). Witnessing social injustice downstream and advocating for health equity upstream: The trombone slide of nursing. *Advances in Nursing Science, 35*(2), 89–112. doi:10.1097/ANS.0b013e31824fe70f

Gottlieb, L. (2013). *Strengths-based nursing care: Health and healing for person and family.* New York, NY: Springer.

Government of Canada: *Public Health Agency of Canada Act,* S.C., c. 5, 2006, c. Article 12. Retrieved from http://laws-lois.justice.gc.ca/eng/annualstatutes/2006_5/page-1.html

Harrison, C. (2011). *A passion for prevention: Public health nursing in Skeena health unit, 1937–1997.* Victoria, BC: First Choice Books.

Her Majesty the Queen in Right of Canada, represented by the Minister of Health. (2008). *The chief public health officer's report on the state of public health in Canada 2008. Addressing health inequalities.* Ottawa, ON: Author. Retrieved from http://www.phac-aspc.gc.ca/cphorsphc-respcacsp/2008/fr-rc/index-eng.php

Last, J. M. (2001). *A Dictionary of epidemiology* (4th ed.). New York, NY: Oxford University Press.

Little, C. (1992). Health for all by the year 2000: Where is it now? *Nursing and Health Care, 13*(4), 198–201.

Mahler, H. (1985). "Nurses lead the way." *New Zealand Nursing Journal, 78*(10), 10–11.

Marsh, M., Walsh, J., & Beaton, M. (2008). *A life of caring: Sixteen Newfoundland nurses tell their stories.* St. John's, NL: Breakwater Books.

McKay, M. (2009). Public health nursing in early 20th century in Canada. *Canadian Journal of Public Health, 100*(4), 249–250. Retrieved from http://journal.cpha.ca/index.php/cjph/issue/view/267

McKeown, R. E., & Messias, D. K. H. (2008). *Epidemiology.* In M. Stanhope & J. Lancaster (Eds.), *Public health nursing: Population-centered health care in the community* (7th ed., pp. 241–277). St. Louis, MI: Mosby.

Myers, S. S., & Patz, J. A. (2009). Emerging threats to human health from global environmental change. *Annual Review of Environment and Resources, 34,* 223–252. doi:10.1146/annurev.environ.033108.102650

Ontario Ministry of Government Services. (n.d.). *Public health nurses: Bringing health home.* Retrieved from http://www.archives.gov.on.ca/en/explore/online/health_promotion/health_home.aspx

Public Health Agency of Canada. (n.d.). Chapter 3: The role and organization of public health [archived]. Ottawa, ON: Author. Retrieved from http://www.phac-aspc.gc.ca/publicat/sars-sras/naylor/3-eng.php#s3a

Public Health Agency of Canada. (2015). *About the agency.* Ottawa, ON: Author. © All rights reserved. Public Health Agency of Canada, 2015. Reproduced with permission from the Minister of Health, 2015. Retrieved from http://www.phac-aspc.gc.ca/about_apropos/index-eng.php

Raphael, D. (2011). *Poverty in Canada: Implications for health and quality of life* (2nd ed.). Toronto, ON: Canadian Scholars' Press.

Reutter, L., & Ford, J. S. (1998). Perceptions of changes in public health nursing practice: A Canadian perspective. *International Journal of Nursing Studies, 35*(1–2), 85–94. doi:10.1016/S0020-7489(97)00036-9

Shah, C. P. (2003). *Public health and preventive medicine in Canada* (5th ed.). Toronto, ON: Elsevier Canada.

Underwood, J. (2010). *Maximizing community health nursing capacity in Canada: A research summary for decision makers.* [Report of the national community health nursing study.] Ottawa, ON: Canadian Health Services Research Foundation. Retrieved from http://www.cfhi-fcass.ca/Migrated/PDF/ResearchReports/11510_Reiss_report_en_FINAL.pdf http://site.ebrary.com/lib/memorial/Doc?id=10374331&ppg=10

Vollman, A. R., Anderson, E. T., & McFarlane, J. M. (2012). *Canadian community as partner: Theory and multidisciplinary practice* (2nd ed.). Philadelphia, PA: Lippincott Williams & Wilkins.

World Health Organization, Health & Welfare Canada, & Canadian Public Health Association. (1986). *Ottawa charter for health promotion.* Ottawa, ON: Canadian Public Health Association.

## ABOUT THE AUTHORS

**Caroline J. Porr**, RN, BScN, MN, PhD, is an Assistant Professor in the School of Nursing at Memorial University in Newfoundland and Labrador. During her PhD research at the University of Alberta, she formulated a theoretical model of relationship building to inform public health nurses of how to establish therapeutic rapport when working with vulnerable and potentially stigmatized clients. One of her research pursuits has been to disseminate and test the model for its utility for front-line public health nursing practice. Dr. Porr has since facilitated several relational skills training workshops focused on helping public health nurses develop therapeutic relationships with lower-income lone-parent mothers.

**Aliyah Dosani**, RN, BN, MPH, PhD, is an Associate Professor in the School of Nursing and Midwifery, Faculty of Health, Community and Education at Mount Royal University in Calgary, Alberta. She holds a PhD from the University of Calgary with a specialization in population/public health. Her nursing practice includes instructing students in the Bachelor of Nursing program, population/public health, community health nursing, and legal issues in nursing. Her work focuses on maternal, newborn, and child health. Her research interests include working with vulnerable populations through community-based programs and interventions. She also shares a passion for global health issues.

# Home Health Nursing in Canada

*Shirlee Sharkey, Nancy Lefebre, Karen L. Ray, Kim Miller, and Glen Chenard*

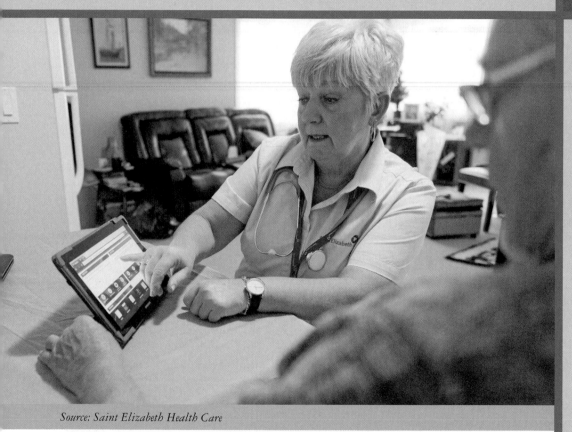

Source: Saint Elizabeth Health Care

## LEARNING OUTCOMES

**After studying this chapter, you should be able to:**

1. Summarize the evolution of home care and home health nursing in Canada.

2. Describe the role and unique characteristics of home health nursing.

3. Outline the key competencies of home health nurses and the application of these in the community.

4. Explain some of the key areas of practice and desired outcomes.

5. Outline the individual, local, and organizational infrastructures and supports that are required for home health nurses to deliver high quality care.

6. Articulate the opportunities and future for home health nursing.

## INTRODUCTION

To understand the role of the **home health nurse** (HHN) in the current healthcare system, it is important to appreciate how home care evolved in Canada and the different ways home care has been implemented across the country. Today, Canada's publicly funded healthcare system is based on values of fairness and equity and established through federal legislation, the **Canada Health Act**, passed in 1984. The Canada Health Act sets the requirements that must be met by provinces and territories in order to ensure "reasonable access to medically necessary hospital and doctors' services" anywhere in Canada. Through five core principles—portability, accessibility, universality, comprehensiveness, and public administration—the intent is to provide Canadians with healthcare "according to need and irrespective of their ability to pay" (Canadian Museum of Civilization, 1966). **Home care** is recognized as an "extended health service," and as such, is not an insured health service to which the principles of the Act apply. This foundational fact has influenced the development of home care services in Canada.

1970 Ontario
1972 Quebec
1974 Manitoba
1975 Newfoundland and Labrador
1978 British Columbia, Alberta, Saskatchewan, Northwest Territories
1979 New Brunswick
1981 Veterans Affairs Canada
1986 Prince Edward Island
1988 Nova Scotia, Yukon
1999 Nunavut (newly formed Territory), First Nations and Inuit Health Branch, Health Canada, Royal Canadian Mounted Police
2005 Canadian Forces

**FIGURE 5.1** Year of Initiation of Publicly Funded Home Care Programs in Canada

As described in Chapter 1, home care was first evident in Canada in the early 17th century when nuns from religious orders arrived in Quebec to provide both direct care and disease prevention services (Community Health Nurses' Initiatives Group, 2000). By 1988, the federal government and all provinces and territories had launched home care programs for their constituents either through legislation or policy (Canadian Home Care Association, 2008). (See Figure 5.1.)

Since its inception, home care has evolved in response to a policy shift toward providing healthcare services "closer to home" (see below box), with consumer preference and research demonstrating improved clinical outcomes and quality of life for people who receive home care. This commitment was achieved after several key initiatives highlighted the need for home care as integral to the healthcare system in Canada. For instance:

- In 2002, the Honourable Michael J. L. Kirby, Chair of the Standing Committee on Social Affairs, Science and Technology, tabled the committee's final report, "The Health of Canadians: The Federal Role." The **Kirby**

## UPDATING THE DEFINITION OF HOME CARE AND HOME HEALTH NURSING

As identified in Chapter 1, home care services help with prevention, health restoration, and health maintenance for clients who require acute or palliative care. But today, with the aging population, home care is more focused on chronic and rehabilitative healthcare needs in order for people to live independently in their communities, and on coordinating and managing admission to facility care when living in the community is not a viable alternative (Canadian Home Care Association, 2008).

**Report** (2002) recognized the need for home care, proposing federal, provincial, and territorial collaboration to develop national home care standards, financing models to support home care, and incentives for home care consumers and informal caregivers. The report also recommended a national palliative care home care program.

- In the same year, the **Romanow Commission** released a report entitled "Building on Values: The Future of Health Care in Canada – Final Report (2002)." Home care was described as the next essential service and one of the fastest growing components of the healthcare system.
- In 2003, all these initiatives culminated with a significant milestone in the creation of the **First Ministers Accord on Health Care Renewal** (Health Canada, 2003). This agreement established a commitment to provide first dollar coverage for "a basket of services for acute and end-of-life care." The following year, a "10-year plan to strengthen health care," known as the 2004 Accord, was established between the federal, provincial, and territorial governments (Health Canada, 2004). The Accord specified public funding for two weeks of short-term acute home care after discharge from hospital, two weeks of short-term acute community mental health home care, and end-of-life care at home.

Between 2003 and 2013, home care saw a number of major changes:

- technological advances that allowed for remote monitoring and better communication with staff in the community;
- a philosophic shift to home-based care as the preferred setting of care resulting in programs to enable faster discharge of people, even those with complex needs, and home-based interventions to prevent premature facility placement; and
- the adoption of quality processes for monitoring and benchmarking performance, clinical outcomes, and system performance. For example, accreditation by an external third party became the expectation in Alberta and Ontario, making it mandatory for all providers of publicly funded home care.

As identified in Chapter 2, jurisdictions in Canada subscribed to a common definition of home care but continued to have variations in mandate, principles, and services (Canadian Home Care Association, 2013). As an extended service, home care policy and funding were a reflection of jurisdictional priorities, available resources, and context. There were no expectations across the country regarding the model of program delivery; all jurisdictions administered home care programs publicly. Provinces either delivered care (see Chapter 2 for full description) through regional health authority employees or, in the case of Ontario, contracted service provider organizations (see the box titled "Definition of Service Provider Organizations").

## DEFINITION OF SERVICE PROVIDER ORGANIZATIONS

Service provider organizations (SPOs) are usually incorporated entities and can be a non-profit organization, private corporation, municipal government, or Aboriginal organization. SPOs are responsible for providing nursing care, home support services, personal care, physiotherapy, occupational therapy, social work, dietetics, speech language therapy, and medical equipment and supplies in the home to individuals of all ages.

*Source:* www.health.gov.on.ca/en/public/programs/ltc/5_glossary.aspx

## HOME HEALTH NURSING

Home health nursing is a specialized area of nursing practice that is delivered in the client's home, school, workplace, or other community setting and requires nurses to travel from place to place to care for individuals. Home health nursing focuses on the provision of care to acute, chronically ill, and well clients of all ages. The care provided integrates community health nursing principles that focus on health promotion as well as environmental, psychosocial, economic, cultural, and personal health factors affecting an individual and family's health status (Humphrey & Milone-Nuzzo, 1996). Further, these nurses work with an interprofessional team and other members of the community, such as police services or community workers, to meet client needs.

According to the Ontario Home Care Association (2011), the unique contribution of home health nurses (HHNs) is their ability to combine knowledge from primary health care, such as the determinants of health (Chapter 1 and others), nursing science, and social science to focus on prevention of health deterioration or disease and on health restoration, maintenance of health, or palliation. HHNs incorporate teaching and counselling into their clinical care, and initiate, manage, and evaluate the resources needed for each client to reach optimal well-being and function. Health conditions today are changing from management of acute conditions to those more common in older adults, such as chronic diseases or dementia. Although HHNs focus their interventions on the client, they do so within the context of family and with other designated caregivers.

## Who Are Home Health Nurses?

**Registered Nurses** HHNs are one of seven groups who use the title "community nurse" (Underwood et al., 2009). In 2010, 77.9% of registered nurses (RNs) were employed as staff nurses and community health nurses and 7362 RNs, representing 2.8% of the total nursing workforce, were employed in home care (Canadian Institute for Health Information, 2010) (see Table 5.1). The average age for an HHN was 47.4 years (Canadian Institute for Health Information, 2010), with older nurses working in home care.

Having both RNs and licensed practical nurses (LPNs) and registered practical nurses (RPNs) provide care in the

| Table 5.1 | Regulated Nurses: Canadian Trends, 2006 to 2010 |
|---|---|

**Registered Nurses**

In 2010 a total of 7362 RNs were employed in home care, a decrease of 0.2%.

Percentage of RNs in community health[1] in 2010

| BC | AB | SK | MB | ON | QC | NB | NS | PE | NL |
|---|---|---|---|---|---|---|---|---|---|
| 12.5% | 14% | 18.1% | 17.7% | 16.3% | 10.4% | 11.6% | 10.2% | 3.1% | 12.6% |

Percentage of RNs in other place of work[2] in 2010

| 8.6% | 13.5% | 12.9% | 11.1% | 10.1% | 20.7% | 11.2% | 12.1% | 24% | 11.1% |
|---|---|---|---|---|---|---|---|---|---|

**Licensed Practical Nurses/Registered Practical Nurses**

In 2010 a total of 1710 LPNs were employed in home care, a growth of 5.4%.

Percentage of LPN/RPNs in community health[1] in 2010

| BC | AB | SK | MB | ON | QC | NB | NS | PE | NL |
|---|---|---|---|---|---|---|---|---|---|
| 5.7% | 25.9% | 9.2% | 10.4% | 11.5% | 1.9% | 4.0% | 14.5% | | 3.4% |

Percentage of RNs in other places of work[2] in 2010

| 6.6% | 9.2% | 2.8% | 6.0% | 6.2% | 11.8% | 3.0% | 2.6% | | 1.6% |
|---|---|---|---|---|---|---|---|---|---|

[1] Community health includes data from community health centre, home care agency, nursing station (outpost or clinic), and public health department/unit.

[2] Other place of work includes data from business/industry/occupational health office, private nursing agency/private duty, self-employed, physician's office/family practice unit, educational institution, association/government, and other.

Source: Canadian Institute for Health Information. (2010). *Regulated Nurses: Canadian Trends, 2006 to 2010.* Ottawa, ON: Canadian Institute for Health Information.

home allows both groups of nurses to fully utilize their skills, provide high quality and safe care to clients, assume supervisory responsibility for unregulated staff, and experience more job satisfaction (Canadian Nurses Association, 2012). For example, care for some home care clients may require advanced assessment and critical decision making skills consistent with RN practice. When the outcomes of care are predictable, such as in chronic disease management, self-care, and wound care, other clients benefit from the knowledge, skills, and expertise of LPN/RPNs.

## Features of Home Health Nursing

HHNs are an important part of the healthcare system and assist in keeping people at home where they want to be. Today, Canada is a very diverse and multicultural nation (Li, 2000), and although awareness of diversity is important in all healthcare settings, the unique aspect for HHNs is working one-on-one with clients and families as "guests" in their homes in both urban and rural settings. In particular, HHNs must strive to be aware of all types of cultural diversity and collaborate with minorities to avoid any type of discrimination, whether clients are of a different sexual orientation (see Chapter 20) or are Canadians of colour, First Nations peoples, immigrants, older adults, those with physical or mental challenges, or other vulnerable populations. HHNs must be aware of different cultural norms and traditions (see Chapter 9) and of differing values and beliefs about health, illness, and treatment that influence their clients' views about healthcare (Registered Nurses' Association of Ontario, 2007), and the need for this is heightened when the nurse is in the client's home.

To provide effective care, HHNs work on the client and family's terms (see Chapter 17). The family plays an integral role in promoting and maintaining the health of family members, as well as providing physical and emotional support. Focusing on the family is an integral component of home health nursing practice, as entire families are affected when members experience health issues (Registered Nurses' Association of Ontario, 2002). Restructuring of healthcare systems and budget cuts to healthcare organizations have resulted in the fundamental expectation that home care only supplements the caregiving of families even when a family member is hospitalized (Canadian Hospice Palliative Care Association, 2013). As well, an important role of the HHN is facilitating the development of partnerships with the family, the healthcare team, and other community resources. This is often referred to as **case management**, and in this the nurse works directly with the client and his or her family to identify healthcare needs, goals, and the resources necessary to meet their goals.

Achieving good health outcomes also requires that HHNs work collaboratively with other members of the interprofessional team, which might include rehabilitation experts, personal support workers, and multiple physicians, from primary care to specialists. This allows for care to be integrated, person-centred, and delivered by the right professional at the right time. Such an approach involves good communication and puts the client at the centre of decision making and care planning. Some HHNs are supported in this work by the organizations that employ them, not only assisting clients but also integrating processes and organize care in a different way (see Chapter 2).

Like all professions, home health nursing has both rewards and challenges, yet for most HHNs, the therapeutic relationship they are able to develop with the client and his or her family in the home keeps them working in the community rather than in institutional care. Most HHNs love the autonomous nature of the role, and when possible, enjoy working to their full scope of practice. However, some nurses find the extended hours of home health difficult, along with the fact that they often work alone and must provide care in all kinds of weather.

Recruiting and retaining new nursing graduates into home health nursing has also been difficult. In the past, new graduates were not hired directly out of college or university programs but were required to gain two years of hospital experience before they would be considered for home healthcare positions. Yet today, with the ability to support, validate, and provide feedback (Sneltvedt, Odlang, & Sorlie, 2010; Wagensteen, Johansson, & Nordstrom, 2008) for nurses through orientation, preceptorship programs, and technology, such as eLearning modules, smartphones, and mobile applications, new graduates can make the transition from dependent to independent practice much more easily (Patterson, Hart, Bishop, & Purdy, 2013).

## What Do Home Health Nurses Do?

To better understand the employment status of community health nurses, Underwood et al. (2010) used a broad definition to encompass all nurses who worked outside hospitals and long-term care institutions, such as in community health, public health, home care, ambulatory care, or occupational health. What they found was that job titles and how community nurses described their workplaces varied. However, they did identify that most RNs work in community health centres or home care while licensed or registered practical nurses typically work in home care and physicians' offices. They also found that most nurse practitioners work in community health centres, nursing stations, or physicians' offices.

The researchers also found that there are skills, knowledge, and attitudes common to all community nurses, including HHNs (Community Health Nurses Canada, 2011). A critical part of community nursing practice is to mobilize resources to support health by coordinating care and planning services, programs, and policies with individuals, caregivers, families, other disciplines, organizations, communities, and government(s) (Community Health Nurses Canada, 2011). However, Mildon and Underwood (2010) did find that the uniqueness of the home health nursing practice could partially be attributed to the range of ages as well as diversity of diagnosis and conditions among home care clients. Although there are variations across Canada, Table 5.2 may assist in more clearly defining the roles of community health nurses, especially those in home health.

| Table 5.2 | Clarifying Community Health Nursing Roles | | | | | |
|---|---|---|---|---|---|---|
| Title | Setting for Care | Primary Area of Focus | Defined Competencies | Funding | Target Population | RN/LPN |
| Public Health Nurse | Community venues such as schools, churches, community health centres, and homes | Disease and injury prevention, health promotion, and community development; program planning and policy development | Yes | Public health agency<br><br>In Ontario this is provincial and municipal funding.<br><br>Rare federal funding for programs such as Canada Prenatal Nutrition Program (CPNP) | Individuals (babies, those with communicable diseases); population-based groups and the larger community | RN, some RPNs |
| Home Health Nurse | Home, school, clinic, and other residential settings, including shelters and on the street | Treatment of diseases or conditions that require surgical or medical interventions; care coordination | Yes | Differs by province; some are employed by regional health authorities, while others are employed by not-for-profit and for-profit home care provider organizations | Individuals and their families or supports | RN<br><br>LPN |
| Community Health Nurse | Community health centres (CHC) | Varies by CHC; could be disease prevention, treatment, health promotion, or community development; program planning | No | Provincial health budget | Individuals, families, and members of the local community, which quite often includes vulnerable groups | RN<br><br>LPN |
| Ambulatory Care Nurse | Outpatient departments and free-standing physician offices or clinics | Varies by AC centre; usually disease prevention or treatment | No | If connected with a hospital, may receive provincial funding; if a private clinic, through physician billing | Individuals; may be disease based | RN<br><br>LPN |
| Occupational Health Nurse | All businesses where worker health and safety is a concern | Disease and injury prevention/ protection or treatment; may include program planning for health and wellness and policy development for occupational health and safety | No | Paid by employing organization | Individuals within organization | RN<br><br>LPN |
| Nurse Practitioner | Primary care clinics | Disease prevention and treatment, health promotion | Yes | Government funded | Individuals and their families | NP |

# HOME HEALTH COMPETENCY

In 2010 the **Community Health Nurses of Canada (CHNC)** developed discipline-specific competencies for HHN (see Appendix C). These arose out of the public health competencies developed earlier by the Public Health Agency of Canada (2007). The **Competencies for Home Health Nursing** place a strong emphasis on the highly independent and autonomous, flexible, and adaptive nature of home health nursing in the context of being a "guest in the home."

The Home Health Nursing Competencies consist of three overarching categories: elements of home health nursing, foundations of home health nursing, and quality and professional responsibility. Within these categories there are 78 home health nursing discipline-specific competencies divided into 12 specific domains.

The first competency category, **Elements of Home Health Nursing**, consists of eight competency domains and 53 individual competencies. These competencies "focus on the nursing activities, functions, goals and outcomes that are central to home health nursing practice" (Community Health Nurses of Canada, 2010, p. 9). Competencies within this category emphasize the HHN's assessment, monitoring, and clinical decision-making abilities, with a focus on autonomous practice in the context of the environment and social supports of clients and their families. Specific competencies include the following:

■ the HHN establishes and maintains a therapeutic nurse–client relationship, working effectively and non-judgmentally in a wide range of environments;

■ the HHN has a focus on health maintenance, restoration, and palliation, often requiring a complex mix of strategies to address health needs and an ability to perform and adapt complex procedures in the home setting; and

■ the HHN provides individualized health teaching and education to promote independence, enhance self-efficacy, and engage clients and families as active participants in self-care and management.

The second category of competencies, **Foundations of Home Health Nursing**, "focuses on the core knowledge and primary health care philosophy that is central to home health nursing practice" (CHNC, 2010, p. 12). This includes the domains of health promotion, illness prevention, and health protection. Education and strategies to support clients in addressing gaps in the social determinants of health occurs as the nurse interacts with clients and families in their home. Advanced critical-thinking skills are needed by the HHN to apply these interventions with the client and family, while recognizing the personal, social, environmental, and cultural impacts of the client's home and community.

The third and final category of competencies, **Quality and Professional Responsibilities**, "focuses on practice activities and/or strategies by which the HHN promotes quality of care and demonstrates professional responsibility" (CHNC, 2010, p. 13). The HHN is pivotal in the identification and mitigation of client risks at home, such as falls or medication errors (Canadian Patient Safety Institute, 2013).

Quality improvement designed to measure effectiveness of services, cost implications, and processes in home care requires creativity and participation from the HHN. For example, some outcome indicators may be measured virtually using technology. The HHN understands the concept of quality monitoring and its relationship to client education, care provision, evaluation, and improvement strategies. Recognition and management of areas of learning opportunity or potential and real ethical dilemmas is a key component of the professional nature of the HHN.

# HOME HEALTH NURSING CARE

HHNs work within their scope of practice according to local health authority policies and procedures or provincial legislation, nursing evidence and best practice, and doctors' orders. Home care workload depends on the client condition and the nursing care required. Nursing service may be provided on a visit or shift basis. On average, most HHNs have a caseload of 8–12 clients per day with a broad range of conditions, circumstances, and care requirements. The HHN's clients may include individuals of all ages—from infants to the very elderly.

HHNs provide care based on competencies that encompass disease prevention, restoration, maintenance, and treatment of conditions that may require chemotherapy; infusion therapy, including IV pumps and PICC lines; post-hospital medical and surgical care; chronic disease management; ventilator and tracheostomy care; services for older adults or children; enterostomal therapy; and wound care (CHCA, 2010). It is estimated that one-third (Baich, Wilson, & Cummings, 2010) to one-half of all home care clients (McIsaac, 2007) have wound care needs. Wound care can range from basic to very complex care and is related primarily to six diagnoses, including venous leg ulcers, pressure ulcers, pilonidal sinuses, surgical wounds, and diabetic foot ulcers. The HHN also works with many clients living with a life-limiting illness or who are dealing with end-of-life issues. For those who have chosen to remain at home for their end-of-life care, the HHN provides palliative care and functions as the liaison between patient, family, and other healthcare providers on the team. HHNs provide support for pain and symptom management, medication review, emotional and psychosocial support for both the patient and caregiver, and work collaboratively with the interprofessional team (also see Chapter 3).

Another important role of the HHN is to assess the family's coping and its ability to provide ongoing care for the client. It continues to be an expectation that family and friends will provide care to supplement the publicly funded service. This can be challenging for families, particularly if they are geographically dispersed and occupied with work and child-rearing. Many family caregivers forfeit work responsibilities in order to provide the care that will help keep a family member at home (see Canadian Research Box 5.1). Concepts such as protected job leaves, caregiver allowance, and tax credits that were introduced in the Kirby Report (2002) have begun to take hold as provinces and territories shift to home-based care.

**CANADIAN RESEARCH BOX 5.1**

**Do home care interventions improve quality of life for clients?**

Markle-Reid, M., Browne, G., & Gafni, A. (2013). Nurse-led health promotion interventions improve quality of life in frail older home care clients: Lessons learned from three randomized trials in Ontario, Canada. *Journal of Evaluation in Clinical Practice, 19*(1), 118–131. doi:10.1111/j.1365-2753.2011.01782.x

A great focus is being placed on the frail older adult population due to their rising numbers and complex health needs. Not only is there a need to reduce the cost of hospitalization, but home is where most people want to be. This paper examined the lessons learned from three randomized controlled trials that included 498 community-living, frail older adults (65 years of age or more) using home health services in southern Ontario, Canada. Each study was designed to evaluate the effectiveness of different multicomponent, nurse-led health promotion and disease prevention (HPDP) interventions. The nurse-led HPDP interventions were 6- or 12-month multicomponent and evidence-based strategies addressing known risk factors for functional decline and frailty. Across the three studies, a common approach was used to measure the change in health-related quality of life (HRQOL) (Short Form-36) and the costs of health services (based on the Health and Social Services Utilization Inventory).

The main lesson learned from the three studies is that nurse-led HPDP interventions for frail older home care clients provide greater improvements in HRQOL compared with usual home care. Nurse-led HPDP approaches are very acceptable to the frail, older adult population and can be implemented using existing home care resources. Nurse-led HPDP interventions should include multiple home visits, multi-dimensional screening and assessment, multicomponent evidence-based HPDP strategies, intensive case management, interprofessional collaboration, providers with geriatric training and experience, referral to and coordination of community services, and theory use. The results of the three trials underscore the need to reinvest in nurse-led HPDP interventions in home care to optimize HRQOL and promote "aging in place" for frail older adults.

### Discussion Questions

1. Identify three potential areas of health teaching an HHN could consider in order to improve the quality of life for an older adult.

2. State how these interventions would improve the quality of life for the client.

**C-HOBIC IN HOME HEALTH NURSING**

The HOBIC initiative, including the community-specific outcomes (C-HOBIC), is a project funded by the Ontario Ministry of Health and Long-Term Care. It is the collection of standardized information that is reflective of nursing in acute care, complex continuing care, long-term care, and home care setting across Ontario and in other areas of Canada, such as Manitoba. The HOBIC database is housed at the Institute for Clinical Evaluative Sciences (ICES), enabling an understanding of practice across sectors.

*Source:* Doran, D. M. (2011). *Nursing outcomes: The state of the science* (2nd ed.). Sudbury, MA: Jones & Bartlett Learning.

## Outcomes of Home Health Nursing

Given the aging population, the desire for people to remain at home, and the use of more unregulated workers in the home (Berta, LaPorte, Deber, Baumann & Gamble, 2013), it is important to articulate the critical contribution of nurses in home care. Doran, Mildon, and Clarke (2011) reported on the efficacy of nursing-sensitive indicators that demonstrate nursing impact on client safety and quality outcomes. Over the last 10 years, nursing-sensitive outcomes for home care have been captured through **Health Outcomes for Better Information and Care** or **C-HOBIC** (Institute for Clinical Evaluative Sciences, 2011). A subset of the RAI-HC,* C-HOBIC includes assessment of functional status, symptoms, and therapeutic self-care (see box titled "C-HOBIC in Home Health Nursing") and is an important way to understand the needs of clients for links to community resources, safety equipment, social interaction, adequate nutrition, transportation, and ongoing connections with primary care providers.

While limited, and studied primarily in Ontario, there is evidence that HHNs play a major role in individualized health promotion and preventive care by providing health assessment, support, and access to resources through regular home visits (Byles, 2000; Elkan et al., 2001). A study by Markle-Reid (2002) suggests that a diversity of home visiting interventions carried out by HHNs can favourably affect health and functional status and mortality rates, and reduce depression. As well, recent studies in Ontario demonstrated that home health nursing resulted in enhanced quality of life for older adults through early identification and management of risks for adverse events (e.g., falls, polypharmacy, depression, and caregiver stress) and for those receiving wound and palliative care (Markle-Reid et al., 2006) at no additional expense (Markle-Reid, 2002).

## Where Do Home Health Nurses Work?

In 2008 an estimated 500 000 people across Canada purchased home care privately to support care requirements (Health Council of Canada, 2008).

HHNs work for regional health authorities or, in Ontario, for service provider organizations such as Saint Elizabeth Health Care, or the **Victorian Order of Nurses** (see Chapter 1). **Saint**

---

* The Resident Assessment Instrument-Home Care (RAI-HC) is a standardized, multi-dimensional assessment system for determining client needs, and includes quality indicators, client assessment protocols, outcome measurement scales, and a case mix system.

**Elizabeth Health Care** is a national not-for-profit healthcare organization that has been an active participant in the development of community health since 1908 see photos 5.1 and 5.2. An example of the type of nursing activities that Saint Elizabeth Health Care has undertaken to promote better home care is the development of community-based care for people living with HIV/AIDS. In the late 1980s, at a time when little was known about the disease, Saint Elizabeth was one of the first in Ontario to provide community-based care for people living with HIV/AIDS. Demonstrating leadership and compassion, these palliative care nurses became very involved in raising awareness and educating nurses both within the organization and outside about caring for clients with HIV/AIDS.

Today, other for-profit service provider organizations deliver care in Ontario, such as Paramed (www.paramed.com/homecare/services/nursing), the Visiting Housekeepers Association (VHA) (www.vha.ca/services/nursing), and Bayshore Home Health (www.bayshore.ca/what-we-do/nursing). In other provinces, although home health nursing services may be similar, care is delivered through the regional health authority (e.g., Winnipeg Regional Health Authority, www.wrha.mb.ca) rather than independent home healthcare organizations.

There has been much controversy regarding the role of not-for-profit and for-profit agencies in Canada's healthcare system. Principles of the system would suggest that only

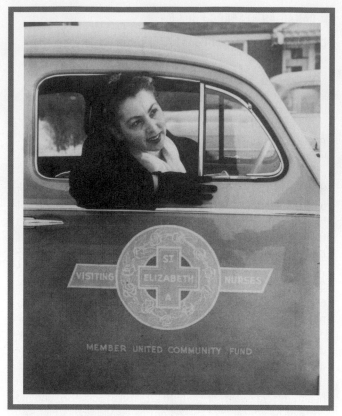

**PHOTO 5.2** Care was provided by Saint Elizabeth nurses not only in clinics as seen in Photo 5.1, but also by visiting clients and their families at home (n.d.).

*Source: Saint Elizabeth Health Care*

not-for-profit agencies funded by provincial and territorial governments should deliver care to Canadians. However, trade agreements with other countries foster open doors for investment from elsewhere. Thus, arguments can and have been made that for-profit agencies from within or outside of Canada should also have access to funding from government healthcare dollars and favourable tax status (Jackson & Sanger, 2003). Proponents of this stance point to increased access and timely care, as well as legal necessity, as rationales for inclusion, while the not-for-profit agencies counter that they provide both access and timely care, with better quality and cost control. Controversies such as this are mirrored in other healthcare sectors, such as same-day surgery and complex diagnostics (e.g., MRIs).

## ORGANIZATIONAL SUPPORTS FOR HOME HEALTH NURSING

Similar to other nursing care delivery models, HHNs require the support and infrastructure to maintain high-quality clinical care and a positive work environment. These supports include leadership, evidence-informed decision making and practice, ongoing professional development, and access to clinical supports and organizational infrastructure.

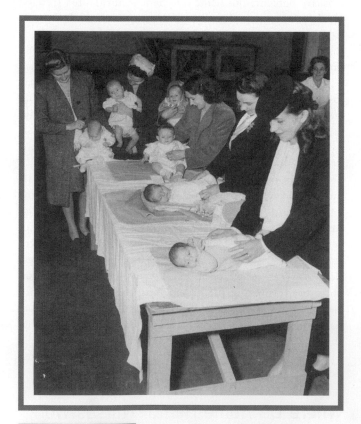

**PHOTO 5.1** The historical roots of Saint Elizabeth Health Care are based on providing care through the Archdiocese of Toronto to mothers and young children in an effort to ensure their health and well-being (1947).

*Source: Saint Elizabeth Health Care*

## Leadership

Research has shown that nurse managers play an important role in increasing staff nurses' job satisfaction, work productivity, and commitment to an organization (Udod, 2012) (see Chapter 2). Today there is greater emphasis on multidisciplinary care, cost containment, client safety, quality, and accountability. Often this means that leaders require different skill sets to collaborate with various stakeholders on ways to move initiatives forward. Achieving this requires knowledge, wisdom, and creativity at a time when resources are tight, the system is complex, and new technologies are being developed faster than ever before. Yet, most often HHNs do not work in the same location as organizational or local leaders but rather in groups, or teams, that cover large geographical regions. This makes it difficult for leaders to effectively communicate, build relationships, and be aware of the day-to-day challenges that HHNs face. A recent leadership intervention study for managers and clinical leaders in Ontario showed that leaders who had regular communication with staff, attended clinical practice meetings, and recognized staff efforts to change were more successful in implementing evidence-based guideline recommendations in home healthcare (see Canadian Research Box 5.2). Employee engagement is the foundation for achieving success, and leaders need to inspire their teams so that they will deliver unparalleled value to clients and other healthcare consumers.

### CANADIAN RESEARCH BOX 5.2

**Can leadership interventions improve HHNs' use of guidelines for care?**

Gifford, W., Davies, B., Graham, I., Tourangeau, A., Woodend, A. K., & Lefebre, N. (2013). Developing leadership capacity for guideline use: A pilot cluster randomized control trial. *World Views on Evidence-Based Nursing, 10,* 51–65. doi:10.1111/j.1741-6787.2012.00254.x. Copyright © by Wiley Publishing, Inc. Used by permission of Wiley Publishing, Inc.

This study was designed to examine the feasibility of a leadership intervention to impact home health nurses' use of guideline recommendations when caring for patients with diabetic foot ulcers. Four service delivery units with high populations of clients with diabetes were randomized to control or experimental groups. Clinical and management leadership teams participated in a 12-week leadership intervention that included face-to-face workshops as well as teleconferences. Participants learned about leadership strategies that included the use of chart audit results, feedback, and reminders. The strategies were then disseminated by the leaders to their respective staff. After three months, chart audits and interview data were examined to see if the protocol accomplished the goal, design, intervention, measures, and data collection procedures. This pilot demonstrated that some aspects of the study protocol were feasible while others require further development before expanding the study. Trial findings observed no significant difference in the primary outcome of use of guidelines in specific patient care. A significant increase was observed in the five-item outcome score chosen by intervention participants ($p = 0.02$), as well as the use of more relations-oriented leadership behaviours. Findings suggest that a leadership intervention has the potential to influence nurses' use of guideline recommendations, but further work is required to refine the intervention and outcome measures.

### Discussion Questions

1. The use of a leadership intervention to promote the use of evidence-based practice is an important part of providing high-quality home care. Given what you have learned about the current home care environment, what facilitators and barriers that are unique to this setting might there be for leaders?

2. Given that there are unique challenges in this setting due to the factors identified above, what strategies might be beneficial for leaders to engage nurses in evidence-based care?

## EVIDENCE-INFORMED DECISION MAKING/EVIDENCE-INFORMED PRACTICE

Evidence-informed decision making and practice (EIDM/EBP) has a long history in Canada and began with the Canadian Centre for Evidence-Based Nursing (CCEBN) started in 1998 by DiCenso and Ciliska from McMaster University (see Chapter 10). Since then, groups such as the **Joanna Briggs Institute** and the National Collaborating Centres for Public Health have assisted in accumulating research evidence upon which to base practice decisions. Evidence-informed decision making (EIDM) is an important part of the care delivered in home health. In the home care setting, a holistic approach to EIDM is required in order to actively partner with clients, to ensure care decisions match their individual preferences and unique situations. Although there are a number of successful EIDM models, one that has been successfully utilized in home care situations considers five aspects of clinical decision making—patient preferences and actions; healthcare resources; clinical state, setting, and circumstances; clinical expertise; and research evidence (DiCenso, Callum, & Ciliska, 2008)—and assists both clinicians and home care leaders to make decisions based on a holistic assessment and option possibilities.

Due to the complexity and autonomous nature of the home care environment, a variety of infrastructures are needed to support EIDM/EBP in this setting. For example, best practice guidelines such as those created by the Registered Nurses' Association of Ontario (RNAO) must be reviewed and priority areas that are unique for the home health sector identified. Topics such as person-centred care and establishing therapeutic relationships are the basis of all nursing care, although they are adapted in the home to ensure that the client decides on

**CASE STUDY**

**M**r. C is a 58-year-old man referred to a community nursing service provider organization with a primary referral diagnosis of a diabetic foot ulcer (DFU) associated with poorly fitting footwear. The home health nurse (HHN) who is admitting Mr. C completes a holistic health history and wound assessment. Based on the HHN's prior experience and education related to evidence-based practices specific to DFUs, the HHN identifies several interventions that may be appropriate, and collaborates with Mr. C to develop a plan of care.

### Discussion Questions

1. What information from the health history would be important for the HHN to consider when creating a nursing care plan?

2. What possible interventions should be considered for a client with a DFU?

3. What resources might the HHN consider exploring, discussing with, or advocating for with Mr. C?

4. What community health nursing standards does the HHN integrate into her practice with Mr. C?

the goals for care. To support the recommendations that are considered appropriate for the setting, professional development and clinical networks are needed to disseminate the knowledge to the point of care.

## PROFESSIONAL DEVELOPMENT

Self-regulation and the need for ongoing professional development is a high priority for nursing staff in all settings. However, this requirement is more challenging in home care as staff members are geographically dispersed and highly mobile. Further, the ability to readily consult with colleagues is more challenging, and education is sometimes provided through formal didactic educational or workshop sessions but more frequently through eLearning modules or other mobile learning options. Given the dynamic nature of the home care environment and the customized care required by each unique client receiving care, provider organizations foster a learning culture and an environment that supports knowledge and skill development and nurses as life-long learners.

## Clinical Networks and Organizational Infrastructures

Once knowledge is acquired, translation to practice is encouraged by organizational infrastructures and clinical experts or knowledge champions (Chaillet et al., 2006; Flodgren et al., 2011; Ploeg et al., 2010). Generally speaking, many home care or service provider organizations have several levels of clinical support, including a chief clinical executive or leader.

These leaders oversee general programs provided by home care organizations, such as population-based services for children, families, and older adults, or specialized programs such as wound care, palliative care, and home infusion. In some home care organizations, clinical program leaders or advanced practice nurses directly manage the programs to ensure that they are based on home health standards, evidence-based guidelines, and nursing competencies.

A clinical network of experts is typically available to provide timely clinical information, answer questions, and confirm policies and procedures. The network is available 24 hours a day, seven days a week to ensure that nurses have access to reliable and relevant information. In today's home care environment, this may take the form of information provided in person or through email, fax, cellphone, or Web-based sites. In some organizations, information is also available through eLearning products or knowledge repositories that make policies and procedures and other static information available for nurses to access anytime and anywhere online. In some home care organizations, this virtual support is complemented by champions who mentor nurses, through instruction or role modelling, on how to effectively provide client-centred care, establish therapeutic relationships, or manage complex conditions and at-risk situations (Chaillet et al., 2006; Flodgren et al., 2011).

As well, workflow methods or electronic "reminders" (Bywood, Lunnay, & Roche, 2008; Shojania et al., 2009) are positioned in the workflow and documentation processes to cue nurses for evidence-based care. To support the use of evidence in practice on an ongoing basis, audits through chart review and feedback from leaders on clinical outcomes are linked to the quality-improvement process, performance management, and ongoing review of each organization's reporting mechanisms.

## HOME HEALTHCARE NURSES: THE FUTURE

The future of home health nursing is bright, and given the predictions, a larger percentage of care will be delivered in the home in the coming years. A widely disseminated discussion document, "Vision 2020," predicted that by that year two-thirds of nurses will be working in the community versus the 30% that work there today (Villeneuve & MacDonald, 2006). Access to information has transformed the role of the client to enable collective decision making with healthcare providers that best suits their individual knowledge, circumstances, and values. Clients expect to be engaged in decision making related to their care, to receive timely information and options for care, and to focus on managing chronic disease and healthy living. So tomorrow's HHN will need to be technologically aware of the entirely new health "ecosystem" that will wrap around the client and client's family, and be able to manage multiple sources of data input, synthesize the information, and use it to benefit the client. But, undoubtedly, the essential role of the HHN will be to continue to be a professional in the home. For, although the future of home health nursing will see care moving beyond being person-centred to become "people powered," taking concepts such as empowerment and client decision making and combining them with care enabled by technology, the most important HHN role will still be to preserve the human experience.

## CONCLUSION

The role of the HHN will continue to increase as more and more people receive care in their home. This will mean that HHNs will need to develop innovative solutions quickly, customize care, and utilize technology. This will require ongoing leadership, including research into home health nursing care, new and innovative delivery models, alignment of the healthcare system, proficiency, and greater respect and work within interprofessional teams (Canadian Nurses Association, 2012).

## KEY TERMS

Canada Health Act   75
case management   p. 78
C-HOBIC   p. 81
Community Health Nurses of Canada (CHNC)   p. 80
Competencies for Home Health Nursing   p. 80
Elements of Home Health Nursing   p. 80
First Ministers Accord on Health Care Renewal   p. 76
Foundations of Home Health Nursing   p. 80
Health Outcomes for Better Information and Care
   (C-HOBIC)   p. 81
home care   p. 75
home health nurse   p. 75
Joanna Briggs Institute   p. 83
Kirby Report   p. 76
Quality and Professional Responsibilities   p. 80
Romanow Commission   p. 76
Saint Elizabeth Health Care   p. 82
Victorian Order of Nurses   p. 81

## STUDY QUESTIONS

1. How has the evolution of home care in Canada influenced nursing practice today?

2. What are the consequences to families of the expansion of home care within the health system?

3. How have social and societal expectations contributed to the evolution of home care in Canada?

4. Who qualifies to be a HHN?

5. List three roles of the HHN.

6. List the three main categories of home health nursing competencies.

7. What is the role of leadership in home health nursing?

8. What infrastructures are important to support evidence-informed practice in home health nursing?

9. What mechanisms are required for professional development in home health nursing?

After working through these questions, go to the MyNursingLab at www.pearsoned.ca/mynursinglab to check your answers.

## INDIVIDUAL CRITICAL-THINKING EXERCISES

1. What are the advantages or disadvantages of care delivered in the home?

2. What do you think the "lived experience" would be for people and their family living at home with a chronic disease such as diabetes?

## GROUP CRITICAL-THINKING EXERCISES

1. It has been a "perfect world" for the last six months! What is the one thing that has been different for you in home care? (Give a detailed explanation.)

2. Out of all the changes possible in Question 1, why is the one you chose significant for your group?

3. Based on your understanding of the significant factor you chose in Question 2, how will this affect hospital care? (or the healthcare system?)

## REFERENCES

Baich, L., Wilson, D., & Cummings, G. (2010). Enterostomal therapy nursing in the Canadian home care sector: What is its value? *Journal of Wound, Ostomy and Continence Nursing, 37*(1), 53–64. doi:10.1097/WON.0b013e3181c68d65

Berta, W., Laporte, A., Deber, R., Baumann, A., & Gamble, B. (2013). *The evolving role of health care aides in the long-term care and home and community care sectors in Canada*. Retrieved from http://www.human-resources-health.com/content/11/1/25/abstract

Byles, J. (2000). A thorough going over: Evidence for health assessments for older people. *Australia and New Zealand Journal of Public Health, 24*(2), 117–123. doi:10.1111/j.1467-842X.2000.tb00131.x

Bywood, P. T., Lunnay, B., & Roche, A. M. (2008). Strategies for facilitating change in alcohol and other drugs (AOD) professional practice: A systematic review of the effectiveness of reminders and feedback. *Drug and Alcohol Review, 27*(5), 548–558.

Canadian Home Care Association. (2008). *Portraits of Home Care in Canada, 2008*. Ottawa, ON: Author.

Canadian Home Care Association. (2013). *Portraits of Home Care in Canada, 2013*. Mississauga, ON: Author.

Canadian Hospice Palliative Care Association. (2013). *Valuing caregiving and caregivers: Family caregivers in the integrated approach to palliative care*. Ottawa ON: Author. Retrieved from http://www.hpcintegration.ca/media/37049/TWF-valuing-caregivers-report-final.pdf

Canadian Institute for Health Information. (2010). *Regulated nurses: Canadian trends, 2006 to 2010*. Ottawa, ON: Author.

Canadian Museum of Civilization. (1966). *The Medical Care Act, 1966*. Retrieved from http://www.civilization.ca/cmc/exhibitions/hist/medicare/medic-5h23e.shtml

Canadian Nurses Association. (2012). *The health of our nation, the future of our health system: A nursing call to action*. Ottawa, ON: Author.

Canadian Patient Safety Institute. (2013). *Safety at home: A pan-Canadian home care safety study*. Edmonton, AB: Author.

Chaillet, N., Dubé, E., Dugas, M., Audibert, F., Trouigny, C., Fraser, W. D., & Dumont, A. (2006). Evidence-based strategies for implementing guidelines in obstetrics: A systematic review. *Obstetrics & Gynecology, 108*(5), 1234–1245. doi: 10.1097/01.AOG.0000236434.74160.8b

Community Health Nurses of Canada. (2010). *Home health nursing competencies*. St. John's, NL: Author.

Community Health Nurses of Canada. (2010). *Home health nurse competencies (Version 1)*. St. John's, NL: Author.

Community Health Nurses' Initiatives Group. (2000). *Home health nursing—A position paper*. Toronto, ON: Registered Nurses' Association of Ontario.

DiCenso, A., Cullum, N., & Ciliska, D. (2008). Implementing evidence-based nursing: Some misconceptions. In N. Cullum, D. Ciliska, R. B. Haynes & S. Marks (Eds.), *Evidence-based nursing: An introduction*. Oxford, UK: Blackwell.

Doran, D. M. (2011). *Nursing outcomes: The state of the science* (2nd ed.). Sudbury, MA: Jones & Bartlett Learning.

Doran, D., Mildon, B., & Clarke, S. (2011). Towards a national report card in nursing: A knowledge synthesis. *Nursing Leadership, 24*(2), 38–57.

Elkan, R., Kendrick, D., Dewey, M., Hewitt, M., Robinson, J., Blair, M., . . . Eggar, M. (2001). Effectiveness of home based support for older people: Systematic review and meta-analysis. *BMJ, 323*(7315), 1–7.

Flodgren, G., Parmelli, E., Doumit, G., Gattellari, M., O'Brien, M. A., Grimshaw, J., & Eccles, M. P. (2011). Local opinion leaders: Effects on professional practice and health care outcomes. *Cochrane Database of Systematic Reviews, 8*(8).

Health Canada. (2003). *First Ministers' Accord on Health Care Renewal*. Retrieved from http://www.hc-sc.gc.ca/hcs-sss/delivery-prestation/fptcollab/2003accord/index-eng.php

Health Canada. (2004). *First Ministers' meeting on the future of health care 2004: A 10-year plan to strengthen health care*. Retrieved from http://www.hc-sc.gc.ca/hcs-sss/delivery-prestation/fptcollab/2004-fmm-rpm/index-eng php

Health Council of Canada. (2008). *Fixing the foundation: An update on primary health care and home care renewal in Canada*. Retrieved from http://www.healthcouncilcanada.ca/rpt_det.php?id=146

Humphrey, C., & Milone-Nuzzo, P. (1996). *Orientation to home care nursing*. Burlington, MA: Jones and Bartlett Learning.

Institute for Clinical Evaluative Sciences. (2011). *Health outcomes for better information and care (HOBIC)*. February 5, 2014. Retrieved from http://www.ices.on.ca/Research/Research-programs/Health-System-Planning-and-Evaluation/HOBIC.aspx

Jackson, A., & Sanger, M. (2003). *When worlds collide: Implications of international trade and investment agreements for non-profit social services*. Ottawa, ON: Canadian Centre for Policy Alternatives and Canadian Council on Social Development.

Kirby, M. J. L. (2002). *The health of Canadians—The federal role. Final report, volume six: Recommendations for reform*. The Standing Senate Committee on Social Affairs, Science and Technology. Retrieved from http://www.parl.gc.ca/content/sen/committee/372/soci/rep/repoct02vol6-e.htm#CHAPTER%20ONE

Li, P. S. (2000). *Cultural diversity in Canada: A social construction of racial differences. Strategic issues series*. Ottawa, ON: Department of Justice.

Markle-Reid, M. (2002). *Frail elderly home care clients: The effects and expense of adding nursing health promotion and preventive care to personal support services*. Retrieved from http://fhs.mcmaster.ca/slru/paper/S04-01.pdf

Markle-Reid, M., Browne, G., Weir, R., Gafni, A., Roberts, J., & Henderson, S. (2006). The effectiveness and efficiency of home-based nursing health promotion for older people: A review of the literature. *Medical Care Research and Review, 63*(5): 531–569. doi:10.1177/1077558706290941

Markle-Reid, M., Browne, G., & Gafni, A. (2013). Nurse-led health promotion interventions improve quality of life in frail older home care clients: Lessons learned from three randomized trials in Ontario, Canada. *Journal of Evaluation in Clinical Practice, 19*(1), 118–13.

McIsaac, C. (2007). Closing the gap between evidence and action: How outcome measurements inform the implementation of evidence-based wound care practice in home care. *Wounds, 19*(11), 299.

Mildon, B., & Underwood, J. (2010). *Competencies for home health nursing: A literature review*. Toronto, ON: Community Health Nurses of Canada.

Ontario Home Care Association. (2011). *Home care nursing in Ontario*. Retrieved from http://www.homecareontario.ca/docs/default-source/HHR/hc-nsg-in-ontario—mar-2011—final-rev.pdf?sfvrsn=8

Patterson, E., Hart, C., Bishop, S., & Purdy, N. (2013). Deciding if home care is right for me: The experience of the new graduate nurse. *Home Health Care Management & Practice, 25*(4), 147–154. doi:10.1177/1084822312473828

Ploeg, J., Skelly, J., Rowan, M., Edwards, N., Davies, B., Grinspun, D., . . . Downey, A. (2010). The role of nursing best practice champions in diffusing practice guidelines: A mixed methods study. *Worldviews on Evidence-Based Nursing, 4*, 238–251. doi:10.1111/j.1741-6787.2010.00202.x

Public Health Agency of Canada. (2007). *Core competencies for public health in Canada*: Release 1.0. Ottawa, ON: Author.

Registered Nurses' Association of Ontario. (2002). *Supporting and strengthening families through expected and unexpected life events*. Toronto, Canada: Author.

Registered Nurses' Association of Ontario. (2007). *Embracing cultural diversity in health care: Developing cultural competence*. Toronto, ON: Author.

InterRAI. (2014). *Home care*. Retrieved from http://www.interrai.org/home-care.html

Romanow, R. J. (2002). *Building on values—The future of health care in Canada, final report. Commission on the future of health care in Canada*. Ottawa, ON: Government of Canada.

Shojania, K., Jennings, A., Mayhew, A., Ramsay, C. R., Eccles, M. P., & Grimshaw, J. (2009). The effects of on-screen, point of care computer reminders on processes and outcomes of care. *Cochrane Database Syst Rev 3*. doi:10.1002/14651858.CD001096.pub2

Sneltvedt, T., Odlang, L.-H., & Sorlie, V. (2010). Standing on one's own feet: New graduate nurses' home health care challenges and work experience. *Home Health Care Management and Practice, 22*, 262–268. doi:10.1177/1084822309341256

Udod, S. (2012). Process of seeking connectivity: Social relations of power between staff nurses and nurse managers. *Nursing Leadership, 25*(4), 29–47.

Underwood, J., Mowat, D., Meagher-Stewart, D., Deber, R., Baumann, A., MacDonald, M., . . . Munroe, V. J. (2009). Building community and public health nursing capacity: A synthesis report of the National Community Health Nursing Study. *Canadian Journal of Public Health, 100*(5), 1–11.

Villeneuve, M., & MacDonald, J. (2006). *Toward 2020: Visions for nursing*. Ottawa, ON: Canadian Nurses Association.

Wagensteen, S., Johansson, I. S., & Nordstrom, G. (2008). The first year as a graduate nurse: An experience of growth and development. *Journal of Clinical Nursing, 17*, 1877–1885. doi:10.1111/j.1365-2702.2007.02229.x

## ABOUT THE AUTHORS

**Shirlee Sharkey**, RN, BScN, MHSc, President and Chief Executive Officer, Saint Elizabeth Health Care. As an award-winning and diversified not-for-profit, Saint Elizabeth delivers more than six million healthcare visits annually and employs 7000 people, providing nursing, rehabilitation, personal support, crisis intervention, research, and consulting. Shirlee's commitment to community advancement is evident in her leadership and involvement on many boards, ranging from health to education. Most recently, Shirlee was appointed to chair the Ontario Health Technology Advisory Committee, a standing committee for Health Quality Ontario.

**Nancy Lefebre**, RN, BScN, MScN, Chief Clinical Executive, and Senior Vice-President, Saint Elizabeth Health Care. Nancy is a registered nurse, a certified health executive, and a fellow of the Canadian College of Health Leaders. Nancy currently co-chairs the provincial home healthcare nursing practice committee in Ontario and is past president of the Academy of Canadian Executive Nurses. Nancy has more than 30 years of experience in the North American healthcare sector, working in long-term care, public health, and acute care with a long-term focus on home and community care.

**Karen L. Ray**, RN, BScN, MSc, is Manager of knowledge translation at Saint Elizabeth Health Care. In her current position Karen provides leadership, direction, and support for the creation, management, dissemination, and exchange of knowledge through participation in evidence to practice initiatives and research. As a home health leader, Karen has held a key role in enabling and operationalizing Saint Elizabeth Health Care's (SEHC's) activities as an RNAO "best practice spotlight" organization and also played an instrumental role in SEHC's partnership with the Queen's University Joanna Briggs Collaboration to establish the first evidence translation group in North America, focusing on home care.

**Kim Miller**, RN, BScN, MScN, is lead, educational program, at Saint Elizabeth Health Care. Most recently Kim has led the medical portfolio, a compilation of generalist areas such as medication, infusion therapy, bowel and bladder management, and enteral feeding, as well as the coordination of external educational services. Kim is a past president of the Community Health Nurses Initiatives Group (CHNIG), an interest group of the Registered Nursing Association of Ontario (RNAO) and past Ontario representative on the Community Health Nurses of Canada (CHNC) board of directors.

**Glen Chenard**, RN, BHSc, CDE, CCHN(C), CHPCN(C), CVAA(C), is an advanced Practice Consultant at Saint Elizabeth Health Care, where he provides clinical leadership for one of Canada's largest home health chronic disease management programs. Glen has practised in a variety of clinical, educational, and leadership roles in the home health sector and has developed a diverse portfolio, having led clinical programs in the areas of wound care, ostomy, continence, cardiorespiratory, diabetes, and dialysis. Glen's professional experience, including obtaining multiple specialty certifications and mentorship of other healthcare professionals preparing for certifications, has helped him to gain considerable expertise in understanding, integrating, and developing professional practice competencies.

# Advocacy, Ethical, and Legal Considerations

*Elizabeth Peter, Louise Sweatman, and Kathleen Carlin*

**After studying this chapter, you should be able to:**

1. Describe the central ethical values of Canadian nursing and how they relate to community health nursing.

2. Examine the attributes of social justice as they relate to advocacy, and to ethical and legal considerations for community health nursing.

3. Reflect critically on the central ethical issues in community health nursing.

4. Analyze the legal responsibilities of community health nurses.

5. Explain how capacity building is related to advocacy.

6. Analyze the political nature of ethical problems in the community.

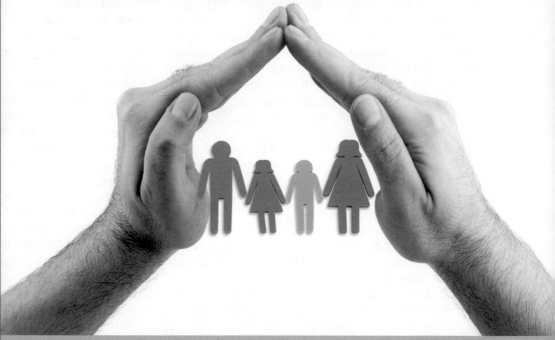

*Source: Edu_oliveros/Fotolia*

## INTRODUCTION

Community health nurses (CHNs) encounter ethical issues in all facets of their everyday work. Ethical nursing practice requires CHNs to be able to reflect critically upon their practice, make sound ethical decisions, and take appropriate action.

Community nursing practice must reflect the central values of Canadian nursing expressed in the Canadian Nurses Association's (CNA) (2008) "Code of Ethics for Registered Nurses." These values are listed in Table 6.1. The CNA code of ethics also recognizes ethical endeavours that address aspects of social justice related to broad societal issues in which nurses are asked to work toward eliminating social inequities.

The term "ethics" has been defined and used in numerous ways. For the purposes of this chapter, **ethics** refers to those values, norms, moral principles, virtues, and traditions that guide human conduct. Often, ideas that reflect what is good or right and what we ought and ought not to do are associated with ethics. Ethics is also a specialized area of philosophy. Moral philosophers study and reflect upon ethics and have developed formal ethical theories. These theories can be helpful in identifying, articulating, and analyzing ethical issues. The term **bioethics**, also known as healthcare ethics, refers to the study of ethical issues that are

| Table 6.1 | Canadian Nurses Association Nursing Values and Ethical Responsibilities |
|---|---|

**Providing Safe, Compassionate, Competent, and Ethical Care**

- Nurses provide safe, compassionate, competent, and ethical care.

**Promoting Health and Well-Being**

- Nurses work with people to enable them to attain their highest possible level of health and well-being.

**Promoting and Respecting Informed Decision Making**

- Nurses recognize, respect, and promote a person's right to be informed and make decisions.

**Preserving Dignity**

- Nurses recognize and respect the intrinsic worth of each person.

**Maintaining Privacy and Confidentiality**

- Nurses recognize the importance of privacy and confidentiality and safeguard personal, family, and community information obtained in the context of a professional relationship.

**Promoting Justice**

- Nurses uphold principles of justice by safeguarding human rights, equity, and fairness and by promoting the public good.

**Being Accountable**

- Nurses are accountable for their actions and answerable for their practice.

Source: From Code of Ethics for Registered Nurses. Copyright © 2008 by Canadian Nurses Association. Used by permission of Canadian Nurses Association.

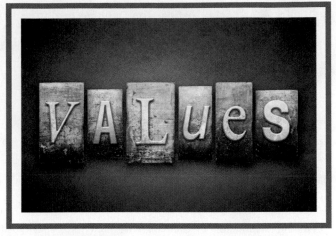

## SOCIAL JUSTICE

**Social justice** has been defined by the CNA (2006a) as "the fair distribution of society's benefits, responsibilities, and their consequences. It focuses on the relative position of one social group in relationship to others in society, as well as on the root causes of disparities and what can be done to eliminate them" (p. 7). It assumes that all societies experience broad, systematic oppression and inequities, such as racism, classism, sexism, and heterosexism, which affect some people more than others. Every individual contributes to oppression and inequity, even if unintentionally, and therefore is responsible also for contributing to the achievement of social, political, and economic parity. In this way, we are responsible not only for recognizing inequities and oppression, but also for taking responsible action (CNA, 2010).

The descriptor "social" in social justice places emphasis on the application of justice to social groups, such as the need to address population health and unjust social institutions and relationships. From this perspective, the experiences of individuals are embedded within larger political, economic, cultural, and social contexts (Reimer, Kirkham, & Browne, 2006). Fundamental to community health nursing is an understanding of the socio-environmental context of health, recognizing that basic resources and prerequisite conditions are necessary to achieve health (Community Health Nurses of Canada [CHNC], 2011, revised). Powers and Faden (2006) reinforce this notion by stressing that social justice is the foundational moral justification for public health as a social institution. A commitment is needed to address systematic disadvantage that severely limits the well-being of oppressed groups. Well-being involves multiple dimensions, including health, personal security, ability to reason, human attachment, and self-determination. Social justice strives to achieve sufficiently high levels in all these dimensions for everyone (Powers & Faden, 2006).

Social justice is also important when situating the ethical dimensions of healthcare policy within a broad, political understanding of the role of healthcare services in society. For example, Canadian home care services, because they are not covered by the Canada Health Act (1985), are often not

related to health and healthcare. Nursing ethics examines ethical issues in healthcare "from the perspective of nursing theory and practice" (Johnstone, 2008, p. 16).

Bioethics and nursing ethics have made use of a range of ethical theories and approaches, including deontology, utilitarianism, casuistry, principlism, virtue ethics, and feminist ethics. It is beyond the scope of this chapter to describe all these in a meaningful and comprehensive fashion. Instead, the chapter will be framed using several Canadian nursing documents that articulate the central ethical values and concepts used in community health nursing, including the CNA's "Code of Ethics for Registered Nurses" (2008) and "Social Justice . . . a Means to an End, an End in Itself" (CNA, 2010) (see Photo 6.1). Occasionally, insights from other perspectives such as utilitarianism and feminist ethics will be drawn in to add depth to the understanding of the complex issues CHNs face. Ultimately, this chapter, with its emphasis on social justice and everyday ethical and legal concerns, will assist nurses and nursing students in gaining the capacity to reflect critically on the multiplicity of ethical and legal dimensions inherent in community health nursing.

| Table 6.2 | Social Justice: Ten Defining Attributes |
|---|---|

Equity (including health equity) – Equity is based on the just treatment of all individuals, which includes equitable access and opportunity to meet health needs.

Human Rights (including the right to health) – These rights are defined by the United Nations Universal Declaration of Human Rights and the Canadian Charter of Rights and Freedoms.

Democracy and Civil Rights – These are outlined in the Canadian Bill of Rights. Democracy and civil rights exist when all have equal rights and power resides in the people and is not based on hereditary or arbitrary differences in privilege or rank.

Capacity Building – Capacity building refers to giving strength to individual and institutional skills, capabilities, knowledge, and experience through coaching, training, resource networking, and technical support.

Just Institutions – Just institutions engage in just practices and the fair treatment of all individuals in institutions.

Enabling Environments – Enabling environments support positive change, community empowerment, and policy development.

Poverty Reduction – The reduction of poverty through projects, programs, and structural reforms of an economic, social, or political nature increases the standard of living and the social and political participation of the poor.

Ethical Practice – The CNA code of ethics for registered nurses and ethics review boards define ethical practice for nurses.

Advocacy – Advocacy involves the active support of individual rights and positive policy or system change.

Partnerships – Partnerships that foster social justice are based on the equitable sharing of roles and responsibilities among institutions and individuals across sectors.

Source: Canadian Nurses Association. (2006a). Social justice . . . a means to an end, an end in itself." (February 2006a). @ Reprinted with permission. Further production prohibited.

adequately funded, leaving many vulnerable individuals without services. While most home care recipients are frail and elderly, increasingly children with complex medical problems are cared for in the home. This cost-shifting to the home and family has led to excessive demands on unpaid caregivers, especially women (Peter et al., 2007).

Social justice is not just a means to an end or an approach to evaluate current circumstances. It has attributes that are desired results, or ends. Ten such attributes have been identified (see Table 6.2). They comprise equity (including health equity), human rights (including the right to health), democracy and civil rights, capacity building, just institutions, enabling environments, poverty reduction, ethical practice, advocacy, and partnerships (CNA, 2010). When recognizing and acting on problems of inequity in Canadian society, CHNs strive to achieve these attributes in their communities.

It is also important to note three features of social justice approaches that are useful to consider when using social justice as a framework for everyday community nursing practice. These features tend to distinguish this type of approach from principle-focused ones typically used in bioethics. First, social justice approaches tend to be concerned with the ethical use of power in healthcare. Broad political and structural dimensions of problems in healthcare and also the day-to-day use of power by health professionals are examined. Power, in itself, is ethically neutral. How power is used, however, is of ethical significance. Worthley (1997) defines **professional power** as "the influence stemming from the professional position we hold. It is the ability to have an impact on the state of being of a person—physically, mentally, emotionally, psychologically, spiritually—in the context of the professional role" (p. 62).

Nurses and other health professionals can use their professional influence to improve the health and well-being of individuals, but they can also use this professional power to deny individuals the right to make choices regarding their health. This power can be exercised not only at the level of specific individuals but also can be used to address population-based inequities.

Second, a social justice approach, like feminist bioethics, tends to view persons as unique, connected to others, and interdependent; that is, vulnerable and unequal in power (Sherwin, 1998). It focuses on how persons are situated or positioned in society; that is, the entire context of their lives, including culture, history, politics, and socioeconomic status. This relational definition of persons is appropriate for community health nursing because CHNs often work with vulnerable individuals and groups who are socially disadvantaged. Through their work, CHNs also emphasize the importance of their relationships with the clients they serve as a means of caring and empowerment.

Third, attending to social justice tends to elicit concern for issues of everyday life and not primarily with crisis issues, like euthanasia. Not all ethical issues or problems are ethical or moral dilemmas. **Ethical dilemmas** "arise when there are equally compelling reasons for and against two or more possible courses of action, and where choosing one course of action means that something else is relinquished or let go" (CNA, 2008, p. 6). **Everyday ethics** in nursing refers to "how nurses attend to ethics in carrying out their daily interactions, including how they approach their practice and reflect on their ethical commitment to the people they serve" (CNA, 2008, p. 5). Everyday ethical concerns also can include those related to advocating for clients, working with limited resources, and relieving human suffering. Social justice expands the agenda of bioethics by examining broad healthcare issues that impact on everyday practice, such as the need to examine social inequities in Canada that prevent individuals from acquiring the determinants of health. It also recognizes that some perspectives, such as those of clients and nurses, have not been adequately brought into the dialogue and debate on ethical issues, nor have they been drawn upon fully in the development of bioethical theory.

## ETHICAL AND LEGAL ISSUES ARISING IN COMMUNITY HEALTH NURSING PRACTICE

A number of specific ethical and legal issues can arise in community health nursing practice. These will be identified and addressed as they pertain to broad areas of community practice such as health promotion, prevention and health protection, and health maintenance, restoration, and palliation. Specific areas of ethical and legal concern as they relate to capacity building, access and equity, and professional responsibility and accountability will also be addressed. The content that follows is organized according to the seven standards of practice for community health nursing. Refer to Chapter 3 for a discussion on the seven standards of practice.

## HEALTH PROMOTION: ETHICAL IMPLICATIONS

Liaschenko (2002) comments that much of the health promotion work that nurses have engaged in has not always focused on the material and sociopolitical conditions necessary for health. Instead there has been an overemphasis on individual behaviour patterns. She explains that this may be the result of nurses working within a biomedical system that primarily values repairing diseased or injured bodies and not the social fabric in which bodies live. CHNs are also not always in a position to directly influence sociopolitical factors, such as poverty, that they have identified as moral concerns in their work. There is a collective moral responsibility that goes beyond individual CHNs to bring about broad social and political change. Because we can be deeply connected as persons, it is possible to create social groups that can better address social injustices. Organized professional groups can generally advocate for social change in ways that are more effective than individuals alone might (Peter, 2011). For example, anti-poverty groups have brought greater public awareness of the problems facing many Canadians. Nevertheless, there are potential moral harms in health-promoting activities that need to be discussed. First, because health is a value-laden concept, CHNs can influence individuals to conform to social norms through health promotion strategies (Liaschenko, 2002). In other words, CHNs can unwittingly become agents of social control and medicalization.

**Social control** refers "to the social processes by which the behaviour of individuals or group is regulated. Since all societies have norms and rules governing conduct, all equally have some mechanisms for ensuring conformity to those norms and for dealing with deviance" (Scott & Marshall, 2009). The concept of **medicalization** is "the process of identification of an undesirable social condition or mental state as a medical problem subject to treatment. Studies of medicalization point to the historical and cultural specificity of many so-called 'diseases'" such as homosexuality, which historically was viewed as a disease (Calhoun, 2002).

Second, a possible moral harm of health promotion is its potential to create adversarial relationships between those who actively strive to improve their health and those who do not (Liaschenko, 2002). A danger exists that those who do not always try to enhance their health through diet, exercise, meditation, and so on may be viewed as morally weak and inferior. Taken to an extreme, if this type of adversarial relationship existed between CHNs and their clients it could compromise nurses' respect for the **dignity** of those they serve. The need for nurses to respect the inherent worth of the people they serve is a fundamental ethical responsibility of Canadian nurses (CNA, 2008). Ultimately, health promotion activities are powerful tools that must be used with careful reflection as to their consequences for the health and well-being of individuals and communities. CHNs must be mindful of the social and professional power they possess as respected and trusted health professionals. There exists an ethical responsibility to reflect upon whose good and whose conception of health is being promoted and why.

## Prevention and Health Protection: Ethical Implications

While preventive and health protective measures can greatly improve the well-being of populations, they also are not without their potential moral harms. Some of these harms are similar to those associated with health promotion in that they can further medicalization. Prevention and health protection information can weaken people's confidence and security in their health. Constant surveillance of one's body can provoke anxiety and can possibly lead to excessive diagnostic testing as well. These iatrogenic risks are an ethical concern because they can erode a person's sense of well-being (Vas & Bruno, 2003). For example, given the current emphasis on obesity, a large body size in women has come to symbolize self-indulgence and moral failure, which in turn may lead women to question their sense of self and right to good healthcare (Wray & Deery, 2008). CHNs must strive to find the right balance of providing information to protect their clients without unduly undermining their self-esteem, alarming them, or restricting their autonomous choices.

Without a conscious awareness of the sociopolitical and economic factors that underlie health and illness, it is possible that CHNs could too easily blame clients who do not heed health information and acquire a disease. Alternatively, CHNs could view these clients as powerless victims of their circumstances, thereby absolving them from any responsibility for their health and absolving CHNs from any responsibility to provide information or other support to assist them in making health choices. Either extreme would not respect the dignity of these clients and would not promote social justice.

A more helpful perspective would put together these explanatory frameworks in a way that does not eliminate the possibility of choice, but situates it. Sherwin (1998), a feminist ethicist, has developed the concept of relational autonomy that is helpful here. She describes how individuals are inherently social and relational beings who are significantly shaped by interpersonal and political relationships. Individuals exercise autonomy and choice within this web of interconnected and sometimes conflicting relationships. Options available to individuals are constrained by circumstances and the availability of resources. Pressure from significant others and social forces can also greatly influence decision making. For example, a young woman with limited financial means may engage in unprotected sexual intercourse with her male partner who refuses to wear a condom. She may understand the risk of unprotected sex, but "chooses" to have intercourse with him because she is financially dependent upon him and finds it difficult to say no to his requests for sex. While she makes a choice, this choice is limited by her economic dependency and perhaps also by societal expectations upon women to sexually satisfy their male partners. Nevertheless, it is possible that future partners will be more receptive to her request or her economic situation may improve. Having health information regarding disease prevention in such instances could assist her in making choices that protect her health.

It is important to recognize that efforts to prevent disease and injury restrict the liberty of individuals, thereby limiting their choice and autonomy. For example, seat-belt laws and speed limits restrict the liberty of individuals, but they are needed to protect health. Other strategies such as communicable disease surveillance and reporting can not only restrict liberty, but can also go against the ideals of confidentiality and privacy. Sound ethical reasons and legal authority must exist to impose these liberty-limiting strategies upon clients. In some instances, interventions are targeted to one group of people to protect another group's health, such as mandatory reporting of some communicable diseases (see Chapter 12). These interventions can be ethically justified if they fairly distribute benefits and burdens and limit burdens to the greatest extent possible.

The CNA (2006b) has adopted four utilitarian principles developed by Upshur (2002) for ethical decision making about public health interventions that are a form of social control. These are the **harm principle**, **least restrictive or coercive means**, **reciprocity**, and **transparency** (see Table 6.3).

The harm principle, developed by John Stuart Mill (1859–1974), establishes the initial justification for restricting the liberty of people in a democratic society (Mill, 1974). He states, "The only purpose for which power can be rightfully exercised over any member of a civilized community, against his will, is to prevent harm to others. His own good, either physical or moral, is not a sufficient warrant" (p. 68). For example, a CHN would only be justified in quarantining individuals if they had a harmful communicable disease, such as severe acute respiratory syndrome (SARS).

The second principle, least restrictive or coercive means, stipulates that the full force of governmental authority and power should not be used unless less-coercive methods are unavailable or have failed. Education, negotiation, and discussion should come before regulation and incarceration (Upshur, 2002). The CHN, therefore, would not incarcerate co-operative individuals exposed to SARS, but instead would provide instructions to them regarding quarantining themselves safely at home.

The third principle, reciprocity, indicates that if a public action is warranted, social entities, such as a public health department, are obligated to assist individuals in meeting their ethical responsibilities. In addition, because complying with the requests of the public health department may impose burdens on individuals, such as time and expense, the reciprocity principle demands that compensation be given (Upshur, 2002). Quarantined individuals, therefore, should be compensated for lost income and additional expenses, such as for childcare, and be assisted with things such as food while quarantined.

The fourth principle, transparency, refers to the way in which decisions are made. All relevant stakeholders should participate in decision making in an accountable and equitable fashion that is free of political interference or coercion (Upshur, 2002). For example, this principle indicates that the process of policy development for controlling infectious diseases such as SARS should include all potentially involved people, such as members of the public, healthcare professionals, hospital representatives, and public health and government officials.

## Health Maintenance, Restoration, and Palliation: Ethical and Legal Implications

This section of the chapter will address the ethical dimensions of several aspects of this multi-faceted CHN role, including community settings as sites of care, informed consent, family caregiving, and palliative care. Please see Chapter 3, Nursing Roles, Functions, and Practice Settings, for a more in-depth discussion.

**Community Settings as Sites of Care** Providing care in the community can be challenging because, unlike hospitals, many community settings were not designed primarily for the purposes of caregiving. Because of the variability of settings,

| Table 6.3 | Four Ethical Principles for Public Health Interventions |
|-----------|---------------------------------------------------------|
| 1. Harm principle | |
| 2. Least restrictive or coercive means | |
| 3. Reciprocity | |
| 4. Transparency | |

Source: Excerpt from Figure–Principles for the Justification of Public Health Intervention by R. E. G. Upshur in *Canadian Journal of Public Health*. Published by Canadian Public Health Association, © 2002.

CHNs must often adapt their approaches and procedures and they must often travel significant distances or use technology to reach their clients. For example, CHNs working for the Saskatchewan Cancer Agency provide mammography for First Nations women, who are an under-screened population for breast cancer, by travelling hundreds of kilometres on gravel roads in a mobile mammography bus (Griffin & Layton, 2008). Another example includes a home care program in the Northern Lights Health Region, which serves 20 communities across almost 200 000 square kilometres in Alberta through telemonitoring. The monitoring by nurses of clinical signs and symptoms has reduced emergency room and primary care visits, hospital admissions, and the number of home care visits (Canadian Home Care Association, 2009). The practices of these nurses are working toward social justice because their goals reveal a concern for health equity, the right to health and health services, the development of enabling environments, and advocacy.

Understanding the meaning and impact of various places or settings is central to community health nursing because CHNs deliver nursing services where clients live, work, learn, worship, and play (CHNC, 2011, revised), not in hospitals. Different places or settings accomplish different kinds of work; have different values, operational codes, and philosophies; and are influenced and structured by different kinds of knowledge and power. These factors combine to influence a person's moral agency within a particular place or environment (Peter, 2002). Nurses involved with the Supporting Frail Seniors to Stay Safely at Home Initiative from BC's Northern Health and Interior Health communities understand the importance of home for frail elders. This program has introduced a coordinated, multidisciplinary, planned, and client-centred care approach that has increased the quality of life and independence of frail elders (CHCA, 2008).

Thus, the experience of receiving and providing healthcare services cannot be overtly detached from the place in which it is received or provided (Andrews, 2002). Bioethics, including nursing ethics, has generally assumed that the hospital, not the community, is the setting of healthcare delivery, resulting in the neglect of many issues facing CHNs that are strongly shaped by the uniqueness of the settings or places in which they arise. Special ethical considerations arise when care is provided in the home because homes are highly significant and idealized places that are imbued with multiple meanings, including personal identity and autonomy, intimacy, normalcy, and security (Peter et al., 2007). As nursing services are increasingly offered in homes rather than hospitals, it is necessary for nurses to become mindful of the social and ethical implications of this change.

The potential unsuitability of homes for providing and receiving care raises ethical concerns. Anderson (2001) suggests that health policy assumes that we all have homes with family and friends readily available to provide care and that the necessary resources for care are there, such as bedding, laundry facilities, and others. The privileged middle class may possess these things, but many others do not. This potential barrier to the receipt of health services for large segments of our population is of serious ethical concern. Nurses should

aspire to promote social justice to ensure that all people receive health services and resources in proportion to their needs (CNA, 2008).

**Informed Consent** To meet their ethical and legal responsibilities, CHNs must support and respect the informed choices of their clients. In order for CHNs to assist clients in making informed choices, there are at least two elements that must be considered: the continuous exchange of information between the client and CHN and respect for the client's autonomy by accepting his or her decisions. These two elements are part of the concept of **informed consent**. Consent is a basic principle underlying the provision of care, and without it a case for assault, negligence, and professional misconduct can be made against the nurse. The process of consent includes CHNs disclosing, unasked, whatever a reasonable person would want and need to know in the client's position. CHNs must provide information about the nature of the treatment and procedures they are offering, including benefits and risks, alternative treatments, and consequences if the treatment is not given. The presentation of this information must consider the client's education, language, age, values, culture, disease state, and mental capacity. When clients provide their consent, it must be done voluntarily— that is, without being coerced—and they must have the capacity, or mental competence, to do so. Exceptions exist in which consent for treatment is not needed, such as in emergency situations and as required by law.

**Family Caregiving** The family's role in caregiving, or informal care, has greatly expanded as responsibility for the provision of healthcare services has progressively shifted from the state to the family or individual. Like formal, or paid, caregiving in the home, women also provide a disproportionate amount of informal care in the home (Canadian Policy Research Network, 2005; Duxbury, Higgins, & Schroeder, 2009; Keefe, 2011). The level of care provision is extraordinary, encompassing both personal and high-tech care. It can include assistance with activities of daily living, such as bathing, eating, cooking, laundry, cleaning, and transportation, and also the provision and management of medications, injections, IVs, catheterizations, dialysis, tube feeding, and respiratory care. While most informal caregivers want to provide care (Keefe, 2011), they are often responsible for 24-hour care with little public support and often with inadequate training for the responsibilities they assume (CPRN, 2005). Increased rates of emotional and physical strain among informal caregivers have been reported (Duxbury et al., 2009), along with significant out-of-pocket costs and lifelong income losses (Keefe, 2011).

The transfer of caregiving responsibilities to family caregivers raises a number of ethical concerns. CHNs have a responsibility to promote and preserve the health and well-being of their clients, but because persons are relational, nurses also have a similar responsibility to a client's family. At times, it may be difficult to determine who is or should be the focus of care. The evidence cited above illustrates that the health and well-being of clients may be threatened when caregivers are stressed and inadequately educated for their role.

Moreover, when delegating responsibilities to family caregivers who do not have adequate support or resources, CHNs may be compromising safe, competent, and ethical care. Choice is also limited because clients may have no other option than to provide and receive care at home. Ultimately, however, the source of these ethical problems lies outside of the nurse–client relationship. It is important to recognize that the situations of both CHNs and their clients are the result of broader political forces and agendas that have limited the availability of resources in order to reduce costs. The CNA code of ethics (2008) addresses the importance of nurses upholding principles of justice and equity to ensure that people gain access to a fair share of health services and resources that are of their choosing. Advocacy for clients is one way for CHNs to promote justice. Advocating change for clients would also improve the health and well-being of CHNs because it would lessen the frequency of nurses practising in a way that compromises their ethical ideals.

**Palliative Care** A very special and increasingly frequent part of a CHN's practice is palliative care. Although most deaths occur in institutions, many people are now spending the last days of their lives at home. While advances in Canada have been made, only 16 to 30% of dying Canadians have access to hospice palliative care, and 70% die in hospitals despite 80% of Canadians wanting to die at home (Canadian Council of Integrated Healthcare, 2012). Advocacy groups like the Quality End-of-Life Care Coalition of Canada (QELCCC) strive for change, believing that "all Canadians have the right to die with dignity, free of pain, surrounded by their loved ones, in a setting of their choice" (QELCCC, 2013).

The philosophy of palliative care is holistic and client-centred. The Canadian Hospice Palliative Care Nursing Standards of Practice (CHPCA) (CHPCA, 2009) guide nurses working in palliative care and complement the CNA (2008) code. The CHPCA standards emphasize the nurse's "respect for the personal meanings, specific needs and hopes of the person who is living in the last phase of his/her life and his/her family" (p. 11). While performing palliative care is extremely rewarding, it can also be stressful for the CHN, the client, and the family. This intimate area of practice is one in which respecting a client's dignity and right to choice may be difficult for some CHNs. Each CHN may hold his or her own values regarding end-of-life care practices, such as withholding cardiopulmonary resuscitation and other treatments, artificial nutrition and hydration, pain control, and assisted suicide or euthanasia. When the CHN's values do not match the choices made by clients or their families, ethical dilemmas may arise. Clients often have cultural and religious practices or rituals that are important to them around the time of death. For example, a Catholic client may ask for a priest to administer the Sacrament of the Sick and some religions have restrictions on who may care for the body after death. Respecting and facilitating these customs are part of the CHN's care (see Canadian Research Box 6.1).

One of the most important aspects of palliative care is relief of pain. Promoting the client's health and well-being includes providing for the client's comfort. Some CHNs may

have moral reservations about advocating for or administering adequate amounts of pain medication. They may worry that they are causing the client's death. Yet, ethically, giving comfort at the end of life is part of effective, dignity-preserving care. The Canadian Senate, in its report "Quality End-of-Life Care: The Right of Every Canadian" (2000), recognizes that providing pain control may also shorten life and recommends the clarification so that both the public and health professionals can learn that this is an acceptable and legal practice. The Senate also recommends increased training for healthcare professionals in pain control. It is up to CHNs working in this area of practice to keep up to date. Adequate pain control means not only an appropriate dosage of medication, but also having a plan in place so that the client gets the medication when it is needed; for example, not having to wait for a doctor's order or pharmacy delivery at the last minute.

While clients have the right to make informed choices about their care, as their illnesses progress they often become unable to make decisions. When a client cannot understand and appreciate the consequences of his or her choices, a substitute decision maker, usually the next of kin, steps in to make decisions for the person. The CHN needs to be aware of the laws in his or her province or territory regarding the process for substitute decision makers. When clients and their families or

---

### CANADIAN RESEARCH BOX 6.1

**How do meanings of home influence negotiations about care for Chinese immigrants with advanced cancer receiving palliative home care in Toronto, Canada?**

Nielsen, L. S., Angus, J. E., Gastaldo, D., Howell, D., & Husain, A. (2013). Maintaining distance from a necessary intrusion: A postcolonial perspective on dying at home for Chinese immigrants in Toronto Canada. *European Journal of Oncology Nursing, 17*(5), 649–656. doi:http://dx.doi.org/10.1016/j.ejon.2013.06.006

This ethnography drew on postcolonial theory to examine the circumstances of Chinese immigrants dying at home. Palliative home care was found to be an intrusion into the clients' and their families' everyday lives through its presence in the home and the domination of professional knowledge about dying at home. Yet, care recipients minimized these intrusions by keeping everyday routines, maintaining relationships with family and friends, and distancing themselves by expressing dissatisfaction. The authors suggest that while palliative home care is often idealized, it can be viewed as a necessary intrusion that centres on pain and symptom management. This perception is not ethno-specific, requiring providers to avoid stereotyping and recognize the individuality of care recipients.

#### Discussion Questions

1. How can the intrusion of palliative home care services be diminished?
2. How can the stereotyping of care recipients be avoided?
3. Why are intrusion and stereotyping ethical concerns?

substitute decision maker have discussed the client's preferences for treatment or withholding treatment, the substitute decision maker is able to make decisions based on what the client has wished. One of the ways that clients can communicate their wishes for care is by means of an **advance directive** (living will). An advance directive contains a person's wishes regarding future healthcare decisions. Advance directives are not only for people who are terminally ill. Anyone may stipulate what medical treatments he or she will accept or reject in certain situations, and it is used only if the person becomes incapable of making choices. The advantage of an advance directive is that it gives a person an opportunity to express wishes about treatments such as cardiopulmonary resuscitation (CPR), artificial feeding, and pain control while he or she is capable of doing so. Advance directives, however, cannot substitute for communication between patients, their families, and their caregivers.

An advance directive contains two sections. The instructional directive sets out wishes for treatment. For example, a person may state that if she becomes terminally ill, she does not want antibiotics for an infection. Another person may stipulate that in a crisis he does not want to be transferred to hospital. The second section, the proxy directive, is a power of attorney for personal care, by which a person designates one or more substitute decision makers for healthcare. This could be a family member or a friend but should be someone who knows the person well and is comfortable carrying out his or her wishes. Each section of an advance directive may exist separately; wishes concerning treatment may be set down without naming a proxy, or a proxy may be named without making any stipulations about treatment.

## Professional Relationships: Ethical Implications

In building professional relationships, CHNs must recognize the uniqueness of their own attitudes, beliefs, and values regarding health as well as those of their clients. They must also maintain professional boundaries while involving and trusting clients as full partners in the caring relationship. Maintaining professional boundaries can become particularly challenging in the home environment where nurse and clients often spend sustained periods of time together in relative isolation. The **professional boundary** in a nurse–client relationship has been defined as "the point at which the relationship changes from professional and therapeutic to non-professional and personal. Crossing a boundary means the care provider is misusing the power in the relationship to meet his/her own personal needs, rather than the needs of the client, or behaving in an unprofessional manner with the client" (College of Nurses of Ontario, 2009a, p. 4). In other words, the CHN must be cautious that the focus of the relationship remains on meeting the needs of the client and not on his or her own needs. Nevertheless, relationships need not be distant and entirely clinical, given that they are often developed in familial settings within home and community.

Insite, a supervised injection facility in Vancouver, exemplifies the importance of building relationships that involve caring, trust, and advocacy in the work of CHNs. These nurses work in a harm reduction setting to improve the health of individuals who use injection drugs. Relationship building is central to their activities, given that their clients experience barriers to accessing mainstream health services because often they face discrimination and lack financial resources and transportation. Without these nursing relationships, the role of these nurses in promoting health and reducing harm would not be possible. These roles involve a wide range of activities: needle exchange, primary nursing care, harm reduction education, referrals to health and social services, and addiction treatment (Lightfoot et al., 2009).

## Capacity Building: Ethical Implications

CHNs work collaboratively when building individual and community capacity. CHNs begin where individuals and communities are, helping them to identify relevant health issues and to assess their strengths and resources. CHNs use strategies that involve advocacy and empowerment (CHNC, 2011, revised). The World Health Organization (WHO) (2013, Track 1: Community Empowerment, para. 1) has described **empowerment** in the following way: "Community empowerment refers to the process of enabling communities to increase control over their lives . . . 'Empowerment' refers to the process by which people gain control over the factors and decisions that shape their lives. It is the process by which they increase their assets and attributes and build capacities to gain access, partners, networks and/or a voice, in order to gain control."

MacDonald (2013) argues that **advocacy** is the most common ethical orientation in public health nursing practice that embraces the character of WHO's perspective on empowerment. It takes a stand for the practices, aims, and reforms that are in line with the moral goals of public health, which have a strong social justice orientation: "The moral aim is to promote the health of the population as a social good that allows people to pursue other valued ends" (MacDonald, 2013, p. 399). Public health ethics tends to be distinct from traditional bioethics in its focus on the health of populations as opposed to individuals, and in its concern for the social determinants of health as opposed to individual agency and responsibility (Upshur, 2012). Therefore, there is an emphasis placed on advocacy activities that involve collective interventions to promote and protect the health of populations and that are sensitive to health inequities and to marginalized and vulnerable populations (Dawson & Verweiji, 2007; MacDonald, 2013).

Actions based on empowerment and advocacy foster the everyday ethical practice of CHNs. Empowerment and advocacy enhance the choices and health and well-being of communities because they draw on a community's fundamental strengths and needs without the values of others being imposed upon them. CHNs can exercise their professional power ethically—that is, in a manner that promotes, rather than restricts, the expression of community choices. For example, CHNs in a rural community near Edmonton, Alberta, initiated a project that through advocacy increased the number of community services accessed by pregnant women. These women were assessed by public health nurses who referred them to additional services as appropriate. Because prenatal anxiety, low self-esteem, and childcare stress are found to be predictors of postpartum depression, identifying and supporting women are important during pregnancy (Strass & Billay, 2008). With this initiative, these nurses are demonstrating some of the core competencies for public health by building partnerships, collaborating, and advocating for potentially vulnerable pregnant women. These competencies are essential for achieving social justice (Edwards & Davison, 2008).

Advocacy strategies can also involve broader political activities. For example, striving for environmental justice requires political involvement at a governmental level. Currently, disadvantaged communities do not benefit from the production and consumption sectors of society in the same way advantaged communities do in Canada, yet they experience the environmental impact of these sectors to a much greater extent through air and water pollution in the areas in which they live (Buzzelli, 2008). Initially, CHNs can address environmental injustices through voting, serving on a community board, or working on a local election campaign. Nurses can also move on to a more-involved political advocacy by running for local political office or becoming the spokesperson of an environmental justice group. At a deeper level, nurses can assume strategic positions in healthcare facilities, professional organizations, and government office. Through these positions, nurses can become engaged with policy development with respect to the health impact of production and consumption practices on disadvantaged groups (Boswell, Cannon, & Miller, 2005).

## Access and Equity: Ethical Implications

It is through facilitating access and equity that CHNs strive for social justice. CHNs must take into consideration that social factors such as age, sexual orientation, and socioeconomic status restrict equitable access and distribution of health services and determinants of health. Their activities can be at the local or global level and can involve promoting awareness and action regarding human rights, homelessness, poverty, unemployment, stigma, and so on (see Canadian Research Box 6.2).

Achieving social justice is extremely difficult. While access to healthcare services is highly important, income security, housing, nutrition, education, and the environment are essential in improving the health of vulnerable populations (Lantz, Lichtenstein, & Pollack, 2007). Addressing these concerns requires policy changes and radical social change.

The story of Workman Arts, a partner program at the Centre for Addiction and Mental Health (CAMH) in Toronto, is an example of community health professionals facilitating access and equity. Lisa Brown, a mental health nurse, is the founder and executive artistic director of Workman Arts. She was inspired and challenged by the talents of her clients and began to promote their creative expression through theatre. Workman Arts employs both professional actors and people who receive mental health services. The mission of Workman

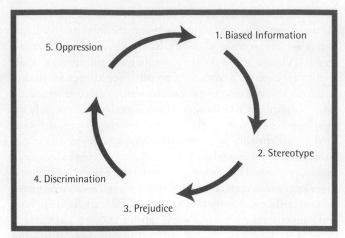

**FIGURE   6.1**   Cycle of Oppression

*Source:* McGibbon, E., Etowa, J., & McPherson, C. (2008). Healthcare access as a social determinant of health. *Canadian Nurse, 104*(7), 23–27.

Arts is "to support aspiring, emerging and established artists with mental illness and addiction issues who are committed to developing and refining their art forms, and to promote a greater understanding of mental illness and addiction through film, theatre, visual arts, music, and literary arts" (CAMH, 2013). The activities of Workman Arts foster social justice because they promote health equity by helping and advocating for people with mental illnesses, an often marginalized group, to access some of the determinants of health, such as employment and income. In doing so, they reduce poverty and build the capacity of vulnerable people.

McGibbon, Etowa, and McPherson (2008) describe a cycle of oppression that in both practice and policy can result in inequities in access to care. (See Figure 6.1.) When biased information based on stereotypes is used to inform decision making, nurses and others can become highly prejudiced and discriminate against people. This discrimination can ultimately lead to barriers in accessing needed healthcare services, which is ultimately a form of oppression and social injustice that can lead to poor health. The authors provide the example of how people receiving social assistance are often falsely perceived as lazy when instead they may be unemployed because they lack childcare and transportation. This prejudice can result in disrespect and a failure to provide referrals that would facilitate access to employment and, ultimately, better health.

### CANADIAN RESEARCH BOX 6.2

**What are the key dimensions of equity-oriented primary health care (PHC) organizations and what are strategies for operationalizing equity-oriented PHC services, particularly for marginalized populations?**

Browne, A. J., Varcoe, C. M., Wong, S. T., Smye, V. L., Lavoie, J., Littlejohn, D., . . . Lennox, S. (2012). Closing the health equity gap: Evidence-based strategies for primary health care organizations. *International Journal for Equity in Health, 11*(59), 1–15.

This research explored the key equity-oriented PHC services by interviewing patients and staff, using participant observation, and analyzing organizational documents at PHC centres in two of the poorest Canadian urban neighbourhoods. Four dimensions of equity-oriented PHC services were found: (a) inequity-responsive care, (b) trauma- and violence-informed care, (c) contextually tailored care, and (d) culturally competent care. Ten strategies were identified to guide organizations in enhancing the capacity of equity-oriented services:

1. Make an explicit commitment to equity in organizational policy statements.
2. Develop supportive structures, policies, and processes.
3. Revise the use of time to meet the needs of clients.
4. Attend to power differences in relationships among clients and teams.
5. Tailor care, programs, and services to context.
6. Actively counter the impact of oppression on health and access to care.
7. Promote community and patient participatory engagement.
8. Tailor care, programs, and services to individual and group histories.
9. Enhance access to social determinants of health.
10. Optimize the use of place and space.

### Discussion Questions

1. How do the strategies suggested relate to attributes of social justice?
2. How can power differences be diminished in PHC services?
3. Why would the researchers choose poor neighbourhoods to study?

## Professional Responsibility and Accountability: Ethical and Legal Implications

In demonstrating accountability, CHNs must adhere to regulatory standards, federal and provincial or territorial professional standards, laws, codes of ethics, and institutional policies. They have a responsibility to be knowledgeable and competent and must also help others around them, such as colleagues and students, to develop and maintain competence (CNA, 2008).

Increasingly, there has been attention given to the legal and ethical responsibility of nurses and other healthcare professionals to keep personal health information private and confidential. At both the federal and provincial or territorial levels, privacy legislation has been developed or is in the process of being developed. Because there are some variations across the country both in terms of the specifics of this legislation and its implementation within organizations, readers are urged to examine privacy regulations within their province or territory and employing organization.

The CNA (2008), however, has described nurses' responsibilities for maintaining privacy and confidentiality, and this description can provide CHNs with some direction. It emphasizes people's right to control their personal information and the potential harm that could come to individuals, families, and communities if privacy and confidentiality are not maintained. Therefore, nurses are required to disclose health information only on a need-to-know basis, using only the amount of information needed. They also must abide by relevant privacy legislation.

Health information is considered confidential to the client. CHNs must normally get consent before disclosing personal or health information and in a practice setting may share this information with other team members within their organization on a need-to-know basis.

However, there are exceptions in which information can be disclosed without consent. These exceptions include a court order, subpoena, police investigation, or an emergency situation to prevent serious harm or reduce significant risk to a person or a group of persons (CNO, 2009b). The most common exception for CHNs is the legal requirement to report child abuse and some infectious diseases. There are also less-common situations in which CHNs encounter individuals who disclose information revealing that a client is a threat to others. The general principle is that when nurses are aware that a client represents serious and probable danger to the well-being of another, they owe a duty of care to take reasonable steps to protect the individual in danger. This principle is supported in law and by the CNA code of ethics (2008), which indicates that nurses may disclose information if there is substantial risk of serious harm to someone.

## Negligence

When CHNs do not practise competently, allegations of negligence may be made against them. These situations are very stressful for nurses, and it is important to know what comprises negligence in Canadian law. There are four key elements that must be proven to make a finding of negligence: (a) that there was a relationship between the person bringing the claim (i.e., plaintiff; e.g., client, family) and the person being sued (i.e., defendant; e.g., nurse), (b) that the defendant breached the standard of care, (c) that the plaintiff suffered a harm, and (d) that the harm suffered was caused by the defendant's breach of the standard of care.

A nurse–client relationship usually exists from the instant the nurse offers assistance and the client accepts it. A duty of care is established when a nurse owes a duty to another—the nature and extent will depend on the circumstances. The standard of care has been legally defined as bringing a reasonable degree of skill and knowledge and exercising a degree of care that could reasonably be expected of a normal prudent practitioner of the same experience and standing (Keatings & Smith, 2010). The standard of care determination is often based on professional standards, such as those set by regulatory bodies.

**CASE STUDY**

Jane was recently hired by a visiting nurses agency. She is providing overnight nursing care for five-year-old Anthony who is ventilator-dependent. Anthony lives with his mother, Susan, and two siblings, aged six months and three years. Susan asks Jane if she could care for all three children while she goes to buy groceries at a 24-hour grocery store. Although the children are all sleeping, Jane is reluctant to assume care for Anthony's siblings. She explains to Susan that she cannot. Susan then becomes upset, stating that she cannot afford to pay for a babysitter and that the other nurses have no problem looking after all of the children for short periods of time. Jane does not know what to do.

### Discussion Questions

1. What ethical and legal issues are raised by this situation?

2. What sociopolitical factors situate these issues?

3. How could Jane help Susan in ways that do not violate professional and ethical standards?

Breaches of standard of care often stem from an action the nurse should have done (i.e., an omission) or an action that the nurse did negligently (i.e., a commission). The mere breach of the standard of care, however, is insufficient to support a negligence claim. There must be harm suffered from the breach that was reasonably foreseeable and there must be a causal connection between the harm suffered and the nurse's conduct.

CHNs, either individually or in partnership with others, also have the responsibility to take preventive and corrective action to protect clients from unsafe or unethical practice or circumstances. This action may entail reporting to appropriate authorities instances of unsafe or unethical care provided by family or others to children or vulnerable adults (CNA, 2008). In every Canadian jurisdiction there is legislation that permits disclosure where there is a reasonable belief of real or suspected physical or sexual abuse of someone, in situations where a child's welfare is at risk, and when there is information related to communicable and sexually transmitted diseases. These circumstances are supported by a legislated duty to report, as the protection of the individual and community take priority over the confidentiality of the client.

## CONCLUSION

In this chapter, common ethical and legal considerations in community health nursing were discussed. The CNA (2006a) framework on social justice, and the CNA (2008) code of ethics were introduced as relevant ethical perspectives to articulate and address these considerations. The unique responsibilities of CHNs and the variable settings in which they work raise particular ethical concerns that must be understood sociopolitically. Health promotion and protection activities can enhance the well-being of clients, but they also can be means of social control that can compromise client choice and confidentiality. Legislation can often provide guidance to CHNs in these instances. In many instances, CHNs are in a position to advocate for social justice so that the health and well-being of their clients can be protected. Although Canada is a developed nation, many Canadians do not have access to the determinants of health.

The health and well-being of CHNs and clients may be threatened when community settings are not suitable for providing care and when informal caregivers do not have the necessary resources for caregiving. CHNs providing palliative care to clients in their homes must possess an excellent knowledge of the ethical and legal considerations regarding end-of-life care, such as advance directives, pain control, and DNR ("do not resuscitate"). Like nurses in all settings, CHNs are required ethically to develop caring relationships with their clients that remain within the limits of professional boundaries. They must also be accountable for their work and must adhere to provincial or territorial and national ethical, legal, and professional standards.

## KEY TERMS

advance directive    p. 95
advocacy    p. 95
bioethics    p. 88
dignity    p. 91
empowerment    p. 95
ethical dilemmas    p. 90
ethics    p. 88
everyday ethics    p. 90
harm principle    p. 92
informed consent    p. 93
least restrictive or coercive means    p. 92
medicalization    p. 91
professional boundary    p. 95
professional power    p. 90
reciprocity    p. 92
social control    p. 91
social justice    p. 89
transparency    p. 92

## STUDY QUESTIONS

1. Identify and define the seven central ethical values of Canadian nurses.

2. What are the 10 defining attributes of social justice?

3. List and define the four principles for a public health intervention.

4. What does the process of informed consent involve? What information must the CHN provide and what factors must he or she take into consideration?

5. How can biased information about clients lead to oppression?

6. What are the four key elements that must be proven to make a finding of negligence?

> After working through these questions, go to the MyNursingLab at www.pearsoned.ca/mynursinglab to check your answers.

## INDIVIDUAL CRITICAL-THINKING EXERCISES

1. How are power and ethics related in community health nursing?

2. What aspects of community health nursing bring about social control? Can these be ethically justified? How?

3. How are nurse–client relationships in the community different from those in hospitals? What are the ethical implications of these differences?

4. What ethical responsibilities must community nurses consider when working with dying clients?

5. How can the CHN promote health and well-being of family caregivers?

## GROUP CRITICAL-THINKING EXERCISES

1. Identify a group in your community that experiences inequities that constrain their ability to meet their health needs. Discuss strategies that would promote social justice.

2. Ask each group member to write down his or her definition of health and then share it with the group. How are these definitions similar and different? How do they reflect different values?

3. Identify a nursing leader in your community who is promoting social justice. How is he or she accomplishing this?

## REFERENCES

Anderson, J. M. (2001). The politics of home care: Where is "home"? *Canadian Journal of Nursing Research, 33*(2), 5–10.

Andrews, G. J. (2002). Towards a more place-sensitive nursing research: An invitation to medical and health geography. *Nursing Inquiry, 9*(4), 221–238.

Boswell, C., Cannon, S., & Miller, J. (2005). Nurses' political involvement: Responsibility versus privilege. *Journal of Professional Nursing, 21*(1), 5–8.

Buzzelli, M. (2008). *Environmental justice in Canada—it matters where you live*. Ottawa, ON: CPRN.

Calhoun, C. (2002). Medicalization. In *Dictionary of the social sciences*. Oxford University Press. Retrieved from http://www.oxfordreference.com.myaccess.library.utoronto.ca

Canada Health Act. 1985, C.6, s.1.

Canadian Council of Integrated Healthcare. (2012). *Dying with dignity in Canada*. Toronto, ON: Author.

Canadian Home Care Association. (2008). *High impact practices*. Ottawa, ON: Author.

Canadian Home Care Association. (2009). *High impact practices*. Ottawa, ON: Author.

Canadian Hospice Palliative Care Association (CHPCA). (2009). *Hospice palliative care nursing standards of practice*. Ottawa, ON: Author. Retrieved from http://www.chpca.net

Canadian Nurses Association. (2006a). *Social justice . . . a means to an end, an end in itself* (1st ed.). Ottawa, ON: Author.

Canadian Nurses Association. (2006b). *Public health nursing practice and ethical challenges*. Ottawa, ON: Author.

Canadian Nurses Association. (2008). *Code of ethics for Registered Nurses*. Ottawa, ON: Author.

Canadian Nurses Association. (2010). *Social justice . . . a means to an end, an end in itself* (2nd ed.). Ottawa, ON: Author.

Canadian Policy Research Network. (2005). *A healthy balance: Caregiving policy in Canada*. Ottawa, ON: Author.

Canadian Senate Subcommittee to Update of Life and Death. (2000). *Quality of end-of-life care: The right of every Canadian*. Ottawa, ON: Author. Retrieved from http://www.parl.gc.ca

Centre for Addiction and Mental Health. (2013). *Workman Arts Project of Ontario*. Used by permission. Retrieved from http://www.camh.ca/en/hospital/about_camh/other_camh_websites/Pages/guide_asc_workman.aspx

College of Nurses of Ontario. (2009). *Practice standard: The therapeutic nurse–client relationship*. Toronto, ON: Author.

College of Nurses of Ontario (CNO). (2009). *Confidentiality and privacy—Personal health information*. Toronto, ON: Author.

Community Health Nurses of Canada. (2011, revised). *Canadian community health nursing standards of practice*. Retrieved from http://www.chnc.ca/nursing-standards-of-practice.cfm

Dawson, A., & Verwiji, M. (2007). *Ethics, prevention and public health*. New York, NY: Oxford University Press.

Duxbury, L., Higgins, C., & Schroeder, B. (2009). *Balancing paid work and caregiving responsibilities: A closer look at family caregivers in Canada*. Ottawa, ON: Canadian Policy Research Networks.

Edwards, N. C., & Davison, C. M. (2008). Social justice and core competencies for public health. *Canadian Journal of Public Health, 99*(2), 130–132.

Griffin, S., & Layton, B. (2008). Bringing care closer to home. *The Canadian Nurse, 104*(6), 12–13.

Johnstone, M.-J. (2008). *Bioethics: A nursing perspective* (5th ed.). Sydney, AU: Harcourt Saunders.

Keatings, M., & Smith, O. (2010). *Ethical and legal issues in Canadian nursing* (3rd ed.). Toronto, ON: Elsevier.

Keefe, J. (2011). *Supporting caregivers and caregiving in Canada*. Montreal, QC: Institute for Research on Public Policy.

Lantz, P. M., Lichtenstein, R. L., & Pollack, H. A. (2007). Health policy approaches to population health: The limits of medicalizaton. *Health Affairs, 26*(5), 1253–1257.

Liaschenko, J. (2002). Health promotion, moral harm, and the moral aims of nursing. In L. E. Young & V. E. Hayes (Eds.), *Transforming health promotion practice: Concepts, issues and applications* (pp. 136–147). Philadelphia, PA: F. A. Davis.

Lightfoot, B., Panessa, C., Sargent, H., Thumath, M., Goldstone, I., & Pauly, B. (2009). Gaining Insite: Harm reduction in nursing practice. *Canadian Nurse, 105*(4), 16–22.

MacDonald, M. (2013). Ethics of public health. In J. Storch, P. Rodney, & R. Starzomski (Eds.), *Toward a moral horizon: Nursing ethics in leadership and practice* (2nd ed., pp. 398–429). Don Mills: Pearson Education Canada.

McGibbon, E., Etowa, J., & McPherson, C. (2008). Health-care access as a social determinant of health. *Canadian Nurse, 104*(7), 23–27.

Mill, J. S. (1974). *On liberty*. London, UK: Penguin Books. (Original work published 1859).

Peter, E. (2002). The history of nursing in the home: Revealing the significance of place in the expression of moral agency. *Nursing Inquiry*, 9(2), 65–72.

Peter, E., Spalding, K., Kenny, N., Conrad, P., McKeever, P., & Macfarlane, A. (2007). Neither seen nor heard: Children and home care policy in Canada. *Social Science & Medicine*, 64, 1624–1635.

Peter, E. (2011). Fostering social justice: The possibility of a socially connected model of moral agency. *Canadian Journal of Nursing Research*, 43(2), 11–17.

Powers, M., & Faden, R. (2006). *Social justice: The moral foundations of public health and health policy*. New York, NY: Oxford University Press.

Quality End-of-Life Care Coalition of Canada. (2013). Used by permission of Canadian Hospice Palliative Care Association. Retrieved from http://www.qelccc.ca

Reimer Kirkham, S., & Browne, A. J. (2006). Toward a critical theoretical interpretation of social justice discourse in nursing. *Advances in Nursing Science*, 29(4), 324–339.

Scott, J., & Marshall, G. (2009). Social control. In *A dictionary of sociology*. Oxford University Press. Retrieved from http://www.oxfordreference.com.myaccess.library.utoronto.ca/views

Sherwin, S. (1998). A relational approach to autonomy in health care. In S. Sherwin (Ed.), *The politics of women's health: Exploring agency and autonomy* (pp. 19–47). Philadelphia, PA: Temple University Press.

Strass, P., & Billay, E. (2008). A public health nursing initiative to promote antenatal health. *Canadian Nurse, 104*(2), 29–33.

Upshur, R. E. G. (2002). Principles for the justification of public health intervention. *Canadian Journal of Public Health, 93*(2), 101–103.

Upshur, R. E. G. (2012). Setting the stage: Population and public health ethics. In Canadian Institutes of Health Research—Institute of Population and Public Health, *Population and public health ethics: Cases from research, policy, and practice*. Toronto: University of Toronto Joint Centre for Bioethics.

Vas, P., & Bruno, F. (2003). Types of self-surveillance: From abnormality to individuals "at risk." *Surveillance & Society*, 1(3), 272–291.

World Health Organization. (2013). 7th Global *Conference on Health Promotion*. Used by permission of World Health Organization. Retrieved from http://www.who.int/healthpromotion/conferences/7gchp/track1/en/index.html

Worthley, J. A. (Ed.). (1997). *The ethics of the ordinary in health care: Concepts and cases*. Chicago, IL: Health Administration Press.

Wray, S., & Deery, R. (2008). The medicalization of body size and women's healthcare. *Health Care for Women International, 29*, 227–243.

## ABOUT THE AUTHORS

**Elizabeth Peter**, RN, BScN, BA, MScN, PhD, is an Associate Professor at the Lawrence S. Bloomberg Faculty of Nursing, University of Toronto. Dr. Peter's scholarship reflects her interdisciplinary background in nursing, philosophy, and bioethics. She has written extensively in nursing ethics, focusing her work on ethical concerns in community nursing, with a special emphasis on home care. Theoretically, she locates her work in feminist healthcare ethics and has explored the epistemology of nurses' moral knowledge, using the work of Margaret Urban Walker. Elizabeth is currently the chair of the Health Science Research Ethics Board at the University of Toronto, a member of the Joint Centre for Bioethics, and a faculty member on the Nurse Faculty Mentored Leadership Academy of Sigma Theta Tau International. During her studies, she worked for many years at the Queen Street Mental Health Centre in Toronto as both a staff nurse and a nursing coordinator.

**Louise R. Sweatman**, RN, BScN, LLB, MSc, is a Nurse Lawyer. She received her bachelor of nursing and master of science with a focus on ethics from the Faculty of Nursing, University of Toronto. She worked as a psychiatric nurse and then went back to school for a law degree from Osgoode Hall Law School, York University in Toronto. She has worked in various provincial, national, and international organizations, including the Ontario Nurses Association, the Canadian Nurses Association, the International Council of Nurses, Assessment Strategies Inc., and the Canadian Medical Association. She is the founder and past chair of the Canadian Network of National Associations of Regulators. She is co-manager of the Canadian Gerontological Nursing Association and of the Professional Regulators Network.

**Kathleen Carlin**, RN, MSc, PhD, specializes in healthcare ethics. She is currently an instructor in the Department of Philosophy at Ryerson University. She has been consultant to the ethics committee at St. Joseph's Healthcare, Centre for Mountain Health Services (formerly Hamilton Psychiatric Hospital) in Hamilton, Ontario, and has consulted in ethics for community agencies and long-term care institutions. With Louise Sweatman, she co-founded an annual community health ethics workshop day, which ran for several years at the University of Toronto's Victoria College. She was the lead author of the chapter on ethics in *A Guide to End-of-Life Care for Seniors* and has consulted on Ethics in Practice documents for the Canadian Nurses Association. She has given numerous presentations on ethics at conferences and to community and professional groups.

# Theoretical Foundations of Community Health Nursing

*Claire Betker, Marjorie MacDonald, Mary E. Hill, and Megan Kirk*

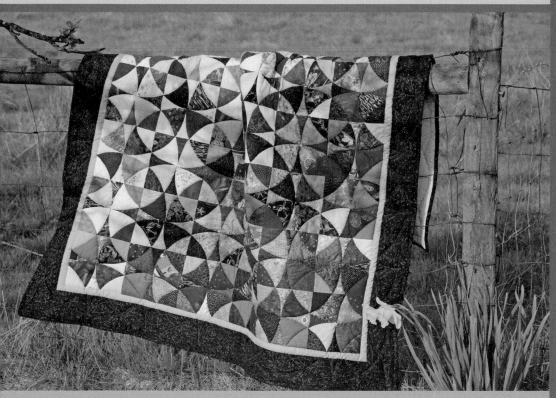

*Source: Courtesy of Mary E. Hill*

## LEARNING OUTCOMES

**After studying this chapter, you should be able to:**

1. Explain why an understanding of theory is important to community health nursing.

2. Discuss the historical development of nursing theory relevant to community health nursing.

3. Examine the theoretical foundations of community health nursing, including a variety of philosophies, conceptual models, frameworks, and theories useful to guide community health nursing.

4. Illustrate how theory-informed practice in community health nursing is important to clients, the health system, the profession, and research.

## INTRODUCTION

Our focus in this chapter is on the theories, **conceptual models**, **conceptual frameworks**, and on the **theoretical foundations** and **philosophical foundations** of knowledge that guide community health nursing. The broad scope of practice and the **values** and principles underlying community health nursing require diverse and extensive **knowledge** that is grounded in theory, research, and practice, all of which are interconnected.

**Theory** provides roots that anchor both practice and research in the nursing discipline (Falk-Rafael, 2005a). Research, in turn, produces evidence to guide the practice of the **community health nurse (CHN)** in educational, administrative, policy making, and practitioner roles. At the same time and in reciprocal fashion, the research and practice of nurses working in diverse community roles and settings contribute to community health nursing **theory development**. Thus, theory, research, and practice are integrated.

Community health nursing is often described as synthesizing or integrating public health science and nursing theory to promote and protect the health of populations (Keller, Strohschein, & Schaffer, 2011). In fact, in the Community Health Nurses of Canada (CHNC) standards of practice (2011, revised), the theoretical foundation of community health nursing practice is described as combining "**nursing theory** and knowledge (including **social sciences** and **public health science**) with home health and primary health care principles" (p. 6).

# WHAT IS THEORY AND WHY IS IT IMPORTANT?

"A theory is an organized, coherent, and systematic articulation of a set of statements related to significant questions in a discipline and communicated as a meaningful whole" (Meleis, 2012, p. 29). Nurses have been heard to say that theory is not always relevant in practice. Kurt Lewin, the father of action research, long ago said, "there is nothing more practical than a good theory" (1951, p. 169). In fact, many theories used by CHNs are grounded in the practice experiences of nurses and the life experiences of clients, which make these theories both relevant and practical.

Nurses often have their own ideas about the cause of a particular issue or problem for a client, or about the best way to work with individuals, families, or communities to address that issue. These ideas are actually "**informal theories**" or "theories in use" about the problem and the solution (Argyris & Schön, 1974). There are times when these informal theories may be inadequate or inappropriate. Nurses can select and integrate theory with past practice and experience to see and address issues in new ways. An intentional and systematic approach to using theories by CHNs can contribute to meeting the standards of practice (CHNC, 2011, revised) and achieving better results for the people and communities with whom they work.

One way of understanding theory is to describe **phenomena** (objects, events, experiences), explain relationships among phenomena, predict consequences, and prescribe nursing care or actions (Meleis, 2012). As such, theory can assist practitioners, decision makers, educators, and researchers to explain what they see and experience, inform their actions and decisions, and articulate possible outcomes. Sometimes, particularly in community health nursing, there is no rigorous research-based evidence available to guide practice in specific situations. In the absence of evidence, theory can be very useful in informing practice in a way that provides a firmer foundation than that of just "doing what we have always done." Nursing scholars and researchers have developed many nursing theories that can guide community health nursing. In fact, nursing theories are integrated with theories developed in public health and the social sciences to guide the practice, research, and education of CHNs.

The story of Jason is used throughout this chapter to demonstrate how theory and related ideas could be useful to guide community health nursing practice. Learn about Jason's story by going to the following link: www.youtube.com/watch?v=DtU_W4FeTno. Jason is a young indigenous boy who comes to the emergency department with a seriously infected cut on his leg. He lives in a neighbourhood where multiple factors such as unemployment, poverty, substandard housing, racism, discrimination, and classism contributed to circumstances that played a role in his injury. His situation provides an opportunity for those involved to question why he was injured in the first place.

The core **concepts, patterns of knowing**, and different levels of theoretical knowledge in nursing are important foundations for understanding theory and how it can be used. We begin by describing these foundations. A short history of theory development in community health nursing is then presented, which will provide a context for understanding the current state and use of theory by CHNs. An organizing framework, adapted from the Community Health Nurses of Canada **professional practice model** (CHNC, 2013) introduced in Chapter 3, is re-introduced to provide a structure for discussing the diverse theoretical foundations of community health nursing, ranging from the very abstract to the more concrete. The chapter concludes with a discussion of the breadth and range of the theoretical foundations for community health nursing practice, education, and research, highlighting the need for further community health nursing theory application and development.

# CORE CONCEPTS

Key public health concepts that contribute to the practice of public health nursing include "**social justice**, a **population focus**, reliance on **epidemiology**, **health promotion** and **prevention**, the greater good [or common good], and long-term commitment to community" (Keller et al., 2011, p. 251). Other concepts such as **health equity**, **determinants of health**, **capacity building**, **a strengths-based approach**, **caring**, **cultural safety**, and **collaboration** are important for community health nursing in Canada (CHNC, 2011, revised; CPHA, 2010). These concepts are addressed in other chapters throughout this textbook, so they are not elaborated on here. The glossary included in the document "Public Health – Community Health Nursing Practice in Canada: Roles and Activities" (CPHA, 2010) defines these and other core concepts.

# PATTERNS OF KNOWING

Before considering theories, it is important to think about the various patterns or ways of knowing that CHNs use. CHNs integrate multiple types of knowledge into their practice (CHNC, 2008). Carper (1978) identified four fundamental patterns of knowing in nursing, including aesthetic knowing, or the art of nursing that is actually feeling the experience with another; personal knowing, of oneself and the experiences that influence one's perspectives; ethical knowing, or a commitment of service with respect to human life and our moral obligations to society; and empirical knowing, which is using scientific processes and rigorous methodologies. White (1995) added sociopolitical knowing, which includes society's knowledge of nursing, and nursing's knowledge of society and its politics. This pattern of knowing called for nurses to find the "intersections between the health-related interests of the public and nursing and . . . become involved and active participants in these interests" (p. 85). The sociopolitical environment is multi-layered, and influences on health include the social context of the person and family as well as the sociopolitical context of the larger community. Building on White's work, Chinn and Kramer (2008) described an emancipatory pattern of knowing that places the practice of nursing within the broader social, political, and economic context.

Over time, a CHN working in Jason's neighbourhood to address the health and safety of local children will need to consider the sociopolitical environment. This is especially important when working with community members and organizations to facilitate community action. Emancipatory knowing is the capacity of the CHN "to recognize social and political problems of injustice or inequity, to realize that things could be different, and to piece together complex elements of experience and context to change a situation as it is to a situation that improves people's lives" (Chinn & Kramer, 2011, p. 64). This pattern of knowing requires CHNs to consider the concept of equity and what it means.

Health inequities are health differences between population groups—defined in social, economic, demographic, or geographic terms—that are unfair and avoidable (National Collaborating Centre for Determinants of Health, 2013). Health equity, on the other hand, means that all people are able to reach their full health potential and are not disadvantaged because of circumstances such as age, race, ethnicity, gender, or social class (Whitehead & Dalgren, 2006). It "involves the fair distribution of resources needed for health, fair access to the opportunities available, and fairness in the support offered to people when ill" (p. 5). Thus, emancipatory knowing encourages CHNs to think beyond the simple treatment of Jason's wound, to engage the community, challenge locally held attitudes, question existing laws and regulations, develop and advocate for strategies to prevent further injuries, and promote a healthier environment for children in that neighbourhood.

Together, all five ways of knowing provide a basis for the development of knowledge to guide community health nursing practice, research, education, policy, and administration.

## LEVELS OF THEORETICAL KNOWLEDGE IN COMMUNITY HEALTH NURSING

Theories are only one type of knowledge that provides direction for CHNs who seek ways to improve the health and quality of people's lives (Fawcett & Desanto-Madeya, 2013). Several important types of nursing knowledge that inform community health nursing can be organized by the level of abstraction (Fawcett & DeSanto-Madeya, 2013). The level of abstraction refers to the degree of complexity inherent in the knowledge component; the higher the level of abstraction, the less detail in the component. Starting with the most abstract, the types of knowledge are the community health nursing **metaparadigm**, philosophies, conceptual models and frameworks, and theories (Fawcett & DeSanto-Madeya, 2013). Later in this chapter, these are defined and elaborated on, and examples are provided. Briefly, a metaparadigm contains the global concepts essential to the practice of community health nursing. A philosophy is an abstract statement about what is believed to be true in terms of the development of knowledge and what is valued in terms of practice (Fawcett & DeSanto-Madeya, 2013). A conceptual model or framework contains abstract concepts and statements (or propositions) about their relationship, and provides a way to organize and visualize these (Fawcett & DeSanto-Madeya, 2013). Theories are more concrete and can be derived from conceptual frameworks and from practice. Middle range theories are concrete enough to be empirically tested (Fawcett & DeSanto-Madeya, 2013). See Table 7.1 for a list of many of the philosophies, theories, and conceptual models and frameworks that have been used to guide community health nursing practice.

| Table 7.1 | Examples of Philosophies, Theories, and Conceptual Frameworks used by CHNs |
|---|---|

This table, adapted from Appendix E of the Canadian Community Health Nursing Standards of Practice document (CHNC, 2011, revised) and supplemented from other sources, includes over 80 examples of philosophies, theories, and conceptual frameworks that could be used by CHNs in different aspects of their work. The examples have been placed in a category that best aligns with the level of abstraction of the theory or model. As some theories and models were named before there was consistency in defining and labelling them, there is not always agreement about which is a theory and which is a model. As a result, some theories are listed as frameworks or models, some models and frameworks are called theories, and there are even several models listed as grand theories. In this chapter, we discuss and define various types of theoretical foundations for nursing. Such a list will always be evolving and we know there are many more theories and models that are not included in the table.

| Category | Example |
|---|---|
| Nursing philosophies | – Florence Nightingale (1946) |
| | – Virginia Henderson (1966) |
| | – Watson's philosophy and science of caring (Watson, 1979, 2012) |

(continued)

| Table 7.1 | Continued |

| Category | Example |
| --- | --- |
| Broad theoretical perspectives | – Complexity theory (Capra, 1996) (Cilliers, 1998) (Gambino, 2008) (Castellani & Hafferty, 2009) (Byrne & Callaghan, 2014) |
| | – Critical social theory (Held, 1980) (Stevens & Hall, 1992) |
| | – Feminist theory (various) |
| | – Intersectionality (Walby, Armstrong, & Strid, 2012) |
| | – Postcolonial theory (various) |
| | – Ecological systems theory (Bronfenbrenner, 1979) |
| | – Systems theory (Von Bertalanffy, 1972) |
| Conceptual models, frameworks, and practice models | – Albrecht nursing model for home healthcare (Albrecht, 1990) |
| | – Calgary family assessment model (Wright & Leahey, 2012) |
| | – Canadian community as partner (Vollman, Anderson, & McFarlane, 2012) |
| | – Canadian community health nursing professional practice model (CHNC, 2013) |
| | – Community health promotion model (Yiu, 2008, 2012) |
| | – Comprehensive multi-level nursing practice model (Ferketich, Phillips, & Verran, 1990) |
| | – Dimensions model of community health nursing (previously known as the epidemiologic prevention process model) (Clark, 1999) |
| | – Empowerment holosphere (Labonte, 1993) |
| | – Health literacy model (Koh, Brach, Harris, & Parchman, 2013) |
| | – Health promotion model (Pender, 1996) |
| | – Integrative model for holistic community health nursing (Laffrey & Kulbok, 1999) |
| | – Interactive and organizational model of community as client (Kuehnert, 1995) |
| | – Intervention wheel (Minnesota Department of Health) (Keller, Strohschein, Schaffer, & Lia-Hoagberg, 2004b) |
| | – McGill model (Gottlieb & Rowat, 1987) |
| | – Multiple interventions for community health framework (Edwards, Mill, & Kothari, 2004) |
| | – Neuman's systems model (Neuman, 1995) |
| | – Population health promotion model (Hamilton & Bhatti, 1996) |
| | – Prince Edward Island circle of health framework (Munro et al., 2000) |
| | – Public health nursing model (Kuss, Proulz-Girouard, Lovitt, Katz, & Kennelly, 1997) |
| | – Public health nursing practice model (Los Angeles County Health Department of Health Services) (Smith & Bazini-Barakat, 2003) |
| | – Transitional care model (University of Pennsylvania School of Nursing) (Lopez-Cantor, 2012) |
| | – Vulnerable populations conceptual model (Flaskerud & Winslow, 1998) |
| Nursing theories | |
| • Grand nursing theories | – Interpersonal relations (Peplau, 1952) |
| | – Model of health (Newman, 1986) |
| | – Roy's adaptation model (Roy, 1987) |
| | – Science of unitary human beings (Rogers, 1983) |
| | – Self-care deficit model of nursing (Orem, 1985) |
| | – Theory of human becoming (Parse, 1992) |
| | – Transcultural/cultural care diversity and universality (Leininger, 1978) |
| | – Watson's human caring science (Watson, 1979, 2012) |

| Table 7.1 | Continued |
|---|---|
| • Middle range nursing theories | – Theory of bureaucratic caring (Ray, 1989)<br>– Critical caring (Falk-Rafael, 2005b)<br>– Relational inquiry (Hartrick Doane & Varcoe, 2005)<br>– Strengths-based theory (Gotlieb & Gotlieb, 2013)<br>– Translational environmental research in rural areas framework (TERRA) (Butterfield & Postma, 2009) |
| • Practice or substantive nursing theories | – Theory of collaborative decision making  (Dalton, 2003)<br>– Community energy theory (Helvie, 1981)<br>– Construct for public health nursing (White, 1982)<br>– Theory of hope (Duggleby et al., 2007)<br>– Theory of maternal engagement (Jack, DiCenso, & Lohfeld, 2005)<br>– Model of family caregiver relationships with home health providers (Funk & Stajduhar, 2011)<br>– Neal theory of home health nursing practice (Neal, 1999)<br>– Theory of peaceful end of life (Ruland & Moore, 1998)<br>– Supportive care model (Davies & Oberle, 1990) |
| Other public health and social science theories, models, and frameworks | – Adult learning theory (Knowles, 1978)<br>– Assets and strengths theory (Kretzman & McKnight, 1993)<br>– Attachment theory (Bowlby, 1969)<br>– Communications theory (various)<br>– Community mobilization  theory (Minkler, 2005)<br>– Community organization theory (Lindeman, 1923)<br>– Diffusion of innovation theory (Rogers, 2002, 2004)<br>– Epidemiology theory (Krieger, 2001)<br>– Health belief model (Strecher & Rosenstock, 1977)<br>– Health literacy skills framework (Squires, Peinado, Berkman, Boudewyns, & McCormack, 2012)<br>– Life course theory (Elder, 1996)<br>– Leadership theory (various)<br>– Management theory (various)<br>– Organizational change (various)<br>– Theory of planned behaviour and reasoned action (Ajzen, 1991)<br>– Reducing social inequities in health through settings-related interventions—a conceptual framework (Shareck, Frohlich, & Poland, 2013)<br>– Social cognitive theory/self-efficacy theory (Bandura, 1977)<br>– Social norms theory (Perkins, 2003)<br>– Social ecological theory (Stokols, 1992, 1996)<br>– Transtheoretical stages of change (Prochaska & DiClemente, 1985, 1992)<br>– Web of causation (Krieger, 1994) |

# HISTORY OF COMMUNITY HEALTH NURSING THEORY DEVELOPMENT AND USE

To gain an understanding of the current context of theory development and use in community health nursing, it is important to consider the history of theory in community health nursing. Over the past three decades, many nurses have written about the lack of theory development in community health nursing, particularly theories in which the community is the explicit focus of practice (Bigbee & Issel, 2012; Clarke, 1998; Falk-Rafael, 2000; Hamilton & Bush, 1988; Kulig, 2000; Laffrey & Craig, 2000; McKnight & Van Dover, 1994; Sills & Goeppinger, 1985; Stewart, 2000). The problem is that nursing models and theories originally developed for practice with individuals and families within an illness context in clinical settings have been adapted for practice in the community, rather than being developed explicitly for the broad practice of community health nursing (Falk-Rafael, 2000). Thus, there can be a lack of fit between these theories and the demands of practice in and with the community.

This same issue has not been raised in the home healthcare nursing literature, in part because nursing theories may be a better fit for home healthcare nursing practice than for public health nursing. For example, Orem's self-care deficit theory has been used to guide home health nursing practice (LaFerriere, 1995; Rice, 1994). Home health nursing focuses primarily on individuals and families dealing with illness, whereas public health nursing focuses on communities and populations from a health promotion perspective.

Theories with an illness focus directed at individual or family care can be relevant for CHNs who work primarily at that level (e.g., home healthcare nurses, primary care nurses, or even for public health nurses in some aspects of their practice), but these theories provide limited guidance for the broad practice of community health nursing. This is particularly true for those aspects of practice aimed at promoting or maintaining the health of communities and populations. Furthermore, these adaptations have only been partially successful because they have not addressed social justice, social determinants of health, distribution and use of power, value systems, health equity, advocacy, and political processes essential to understanding and working with communities and populations (McKnight & Van Dover, 1994; Sheilds & Lindsey, 1998).

In 1987, Schultz argued that nursing theories often depict individuals' problems as isolated events rather than as representative of a pattern of responses in a community or population. This argument remains valid today. Most nursing theories do not acknowledge that communities and populations can exhibit a pattern of responses in health and illness, nor do they explain relationships among such patterns and the environment or social context. For this reason, they have not provided much guidance for CHNs in their efforts to take action on these larger patterns at the community or population level.

Fortunately, some theoretical development is occurring in which a community or population focus and an emphasis on health promotion and prevention are evident. Not only are general nursing theories being adapted for work in communities (e.g., Falk-Rafael, 2000; Green, 2013) but conceptual frameworks and models specific to community health nursing are being developed as well (e.g., Cohen & Reutter, 2007; Edwards et al., 2004; Keller, Strohschein, & Briske, 2012; Vollman et al., 2012). A few theories specific to community health nursing practice are beginning to emerge in the literature (Falk-Rafael, 2005b; Falk-Rafael & Betker, 2012a, 2012b). Some of these will be discussed in the next section of this chapter. Despite these developments, the Association of Community Health Nursing Educators (2010) in the United States identified theory development as a research priority for community health nursing, and it is a priority in Canada as well.

# THEORETICAL FOUNDATIONS OF COMMUNITY HEALTH NURSING

As already discussed, despite significant theory development in nursing there has actually been very little theory developed in, of, and for community health nursing that takes into account the specific focus and concerns of community health nursing practice. As a result of such limited specific community health nursing theory, it is important to consider a wider range of theoretical knowledge, such as broad theoretical perspectives, conceptual models, and frameworks. Not only can these types of knowledge provide the theoretical foundation for new community health nursing theory development, but in the absence of relevant theory, they can provide a solid grounding for practice, research, and education.

The ideas that make up the theoretical basis of community health nursing are difficult to represent visually in a way that illustrates their interconnectedness. The CHNC professional practice model graphic (CHNC, 2013) is used to organize the discussion of CHN's foundations (see Figure 7.1). Each component in the CHNC model called "theoretical foundations" is described. Using a fan graphic (Figure 7.2), the most important types of theoretical knowledge in community health nursing are presented. These include the community health nursing metaparadigm; philosophies that encompass values, beliefs, and ethics central to the unique focus of community health nursing; broad theoretical perspectives used in community health nursing; conceptual models and frameworks; and grand, middle range, and practice theories. The theoretical concepts inherent in various theories, models, and frameworks are listed around the theoretical foundations model, and as mentioned earlier, some of the core concepts are described in detail in this chapter. Of course, not all elements in this framework are always used to guide community health nursing practice or develop theory, but they represent important components of theory and theory development. In the next sections, each element of our organizing framework shown in Figure 7.2 is described, highlighting how each relates to other elements in the framework, and illustrated with Jason's story.

# LEVELS OF PRACTICE

As reflected in the centre of the CHNC professional practice model (Figure 7.1), community health nursing theory, practice, and research, informed by all of the elements listed above, is directed at multiple **levels of practice**, either separately or in concert. Practising in diverse settings, including homes, clinics, schools, organizations, community spaces, and the street, CHNs support the health and well-being of individuals, families, groups, communities, systems, and populations (CHNC, 2011, revised). Individual-level practice involves working with people to change knowledge, attitudes, practices, and behaviours. When working with individuals, CHNs consider families as both context and influence on individual-level health. They also consider families as the unit of care and use interventions that promote the health of the whole family. Families, of course, make up a healthy neighbourhood and community. Although Jason and his family are one small unit in

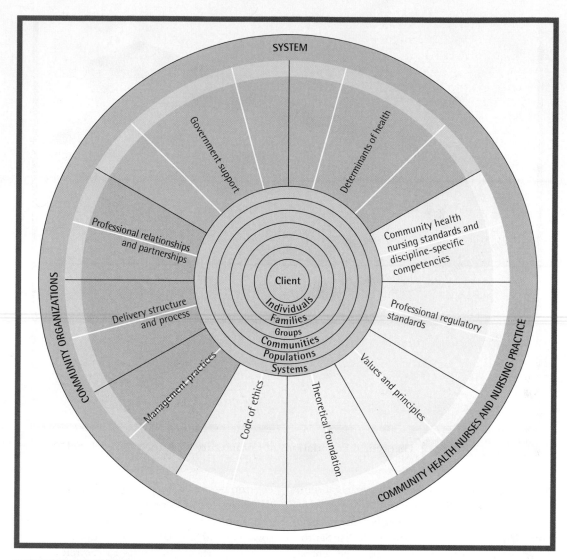

SYSTEM

Government support

Determinants of health

Professional relationships and partnerships

Community health nursing standards and discipline-specific competencies

Delivery structure and process

Professional regulatory standards

COMMUNITY ORGANIZATIONS

Management practices

Code of ethics

Theoretical foundation

Values and principles

Client

Individuals
Families
Groups
Communities
Populations
Systems

COMMUNITY HEALTH NURSES AND NURSING PRACTICE

**FIGURE 7.1** Canadian Community Health Nursing Professional Practice Model

*Source:* Community Health Nurses Association of Canada. (2013). *Canadian community health nursing professional practice model.* Copyright © 2013 by Community Health Nurses Association of Canada. Used by permission of Community Health Nurses Association of Canada. Retrieved from chnc.ca/documents/ CanadianCommunityHealthNursingProfessionalPracticeCompoments-E.pdf

their neighbourhood, other families would likely share the concerns for safe play areas for their children. Community-level practice looks to change community norms, attitudes, behaviours, and practices to promote the health of its members. Interventions are directed toward entire populations, or to sub-populations "under threat" (McGibbon, 2012), and require partnership, intersectoral collaboration, and community engagement.

CHNs might work with Jason's family to educate them about safe play while at the same time supporting families in Jason's neighbourhood in approaching their local government to raise awareness and advocate for improvements. Systems-level practice is aimed at society-wide change and works to change laws, organizations, policies, or power structures in the community that influence health. Advocacy is an important strategy for CHNs at the broader societal level. The Canadian Nurses Association (CNA) defines advocacy as "engaging others, exercising voice and mobilizing evidence to influence policy and practice.

It means speaking out against inequity and inequality. It involves participating directly and indirectly in political processes and acknowledges the important roles of evidence, power and politics in advancing policy options" (2015). Consider all levels of community health nursing practice as the theoretical foundations are explored in more detail in the next sections.

## THE COMMUNITY HEALTH NURSING METAPARADIGM

Over the years, there has been dialogue about the domains and boundaries of knowledge in nursing, which has implications for the definition of community health nursing as a synthesis of nursing, public health, and social science. Early theoretical work in nursing focused on identifying and describing the concepts that defined nursing and that could provide the basis

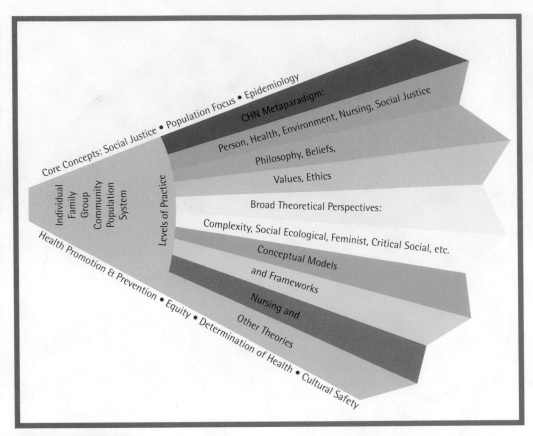

**FIGURE 7.2** Theoretical Foundations of Community Health Nursing Model

for theory development in nursing science. A metaparadigm, the most abstract level of knowledge, identifies the phenomena of central concern to a discipline and describes the concepts and the relationships among them (Fawcett & De Santo-Madeya, 2013). There is general agreement that the central concepts in nursing include person or client, environment, health, and nursing. Although a nursing theorist may conceptualize each term somewhat differently, when these concepts are considered together they provide the broad parameters of nursing and help to articulate what the work is about (Fawcett & De Santo-Madeya, 2013).

It is difficult to see the focus of community health nursing practice reflected in the early writing on the metaparadigm and in the descriptions of the defining concepts. However, conceptual work that took place in the 1980s and 1990s extended these foundational concepts to encompass the focus of community health nursing. For example, Schultz (1987) discussed the client as being "more than one." Most nursing theorists tended to focus on client, or person, as an individual, which did not take into account a focus on a "community as client." Chopoorian (1986), Stevens (1989), and Kleffel (1991) extended the foundational concept of environment and challenged nursing's narrow conceptualization of it as "the immediate surroundings or circumstances of the individual or family or as an interactional field to which individuals adapt, adjust, or conform" (Kleffel, 1991, p. 42). Finally, many theories do not include in their definition of nursing those actions taken by nurses to influence change in the larger social, political, and economic environment. Thus, a reconceptualizion of the scope and definition of nursing was required to take into account community, population, and societal levels of practice, and sociopolitical or emancipatory knowing.

Given these challenges to the relevance of the nursing metaparadigm for community health nursing, Shim, Benkert, Bell, Walker, & Danford (2007) reconceptualized these concepts from a community health nursing perspective and added social justice as a new metaparadigm concept (see Figure 7.3).

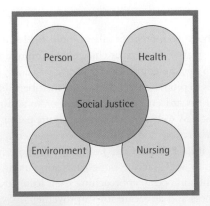

**FIGURE 7.3** Key Aspects of Nursing Knowledge (Metaparadigm)

*Source:* Canadian Public Health Association. (2010). *Public health– Community health nursing practice in Canada: Roles and activities.* Ottawa, ON: Author. Retrieved from http://www.cpha.ca/ uploads/pubs/3-1bk04214.pdf

They argued that because health inequities can only be addressed by consistently pursuing change at the system and population levels using political and economic solutions, social justice must be the central concept and philosophy that guides community health nursing.

The Community Health Nurses of Canada (CHNC, 2011, revised) and the Canadian Public Health Association (CPHA, 2010) draw on this work in defining the theoretical basis for community health nursing in Canada. Social justice is explicitly named as a value of community health nursing and is incorporated into each of the seven standards (CHNC, 2011, revised). Social justice is defined and discussed throughout this book (e.g., Chapters 3 and 8) in the context of ethics, and draws on work of the CNA (2006). Social justice is a central concept in the CNA code of ethics for registered nurses (2008). CNA (2006) identified 10 defining attributes of social justice, and include equity, human rights, enabling environments, and poverty reduction among them. These attributes of social justice are integrally related to other important theoretical concepts in community health nursing (e.g., social determinants of health).

Equity and inequity are discussed earlier in this chapter, and the social determinants of health are defined in Chapter 3 and Chapter 8. However, these are central concepts to consider in a discussion of community health nursing theory and theory development. There is strong evidence that the conditions of our lives influence our health, and the term "social determinants of health" refer to the social conditions that "interact to influence our health and well-being and affect how vulnerable we are to disease and injury" (National Collaborating Centre for Public Health, 2012, p. 1). The World Health Organization (2010) defined the social determinants of health as "the circumstances in which people are born, grow up, live, work and age, and the systems put in place to deal with illness" (p. 1). These circumstances influence health at global and national levels but also at the local level where Jason and his family live and play.

How can these broader notions of social justice, equity, and social determinants of health be applied by CHNs? In Jason's story, the concept of social justice takes centre stage. With no safe place for children to play, the likelihood of further injuries is significant. Taking an upstream (i.e., a prevention or health promotion) approach, and viewing the situation from the perspective of critical social justice, the CHNs in Jason's area might engage with local politicians, businesses, religious leaders among others to initiate a community development process to work toward safer and more stimulating environments for children who have limited resources. Social justice is informed by theories about the equitable or fair distribution of resources, including power, wealth, assets, privileges, and advantages, and includes a vision of a community that is equitable and in which all members are safe and secure. Using this perspective, a CHN in Jason's neighbourhood would consider the information about injuries and play space, engage with members of the community to consider solutions, and together take action at multiple levels to build capacity and ensure safety (Browne et al., 2012; Levy & Sidel, 2006).

# NURSING PHILOSOPHY, VALUES, BELIEFS, AND ETHICS

The second major component of our model of the theoretical foundations of community health nursing is nursing philosophy. This encompasses **values**, **beliefs**, and **ethics** and is central to the unique focus of community health nursing. Philosophy is about the nature of reality, knowledge, and knowing (Chinn & Kramer, 2011). Philosophies "communicate what the members of a discipline believe to be true in relation to the phenomena of interest to that discipline" (Fawcett & DeSanto-Madeya, 2013, p. 8). Philosophy provides an outline of basic beliefs about a subject and offers guiding principles. It challenges us to consider or to engage in inquiry and reflection about questions we face in daily practice; questions about issues such as power, equity, social justice, oppression, and racism. It is philosophy that stands behind the CHN's decision to walk away from Jason and his injury or to stay and consider how to make a difference within the neighbourhood and for a larger population of children.

Critical inquiry and the examination of beliefs and meaning are the processes of philosophy. Philosophies make a significant contribution to nursing knowledge in that they provide a broad understanding of nursing and provide a basis for theory development. Philosophy is more than a statement of beliefs; it is also the application of those beliefs to situations that are both known and unknown (Poliferoni, 2011). Florence Nightingale, known as the founder of modern nursing, developed a very early and enduring philosophy of nursing when she wrote *Notes on Nursing: What It Is and What It Is Not* in 1859 (1946). In this small book, Nightingale sought to describe nursing and the general rules for nursing practice (Masters, 2011). What Nightingale described in the mid-1800s reflects community health nursing today and our emphasis on illness and injury prevention, health promotion, and social justice (Pfettscher, 2010). Nightingale identified a key strategy for promoting health, which is to make health issues visible to the public and to politicians. Nightingale's perspective on nursing, social justice, and our role in advocacy and addressing the broader determinants of health informed "critical caring," a **middle range theory** developed by Canadian scholar Dr. Adeline Falk-Rafael described later in this chapter and featured in Canadian Research Box 7.1.

An important philosophical value in community health nursing is to promote the common good (Keller et al., 2011). Canadian feminist ethicists, in their relational perspective on public health ethics, state that the common good refers to the pursuit of shared human interests in survival, safety, and security for the good of all (Baylis, Kenny, & Sherwin, 2008). There are problems in the application of general nursing theory to community health nursing because most nursing theories reflect the value of individualism (Browne, 2001; Browne, 2004; Williams, 1989). Implicit in this is the notion that the interests of the individual should take precedence or be valued over the interests of the community or population. This is not necessarily a value shared by community health nursing (MacDonald, 2013). Not only is individualism an implicit value in most areas of nursing but it is a predominant value in

Western society at large (MacDonald, 2001; Minkler, 1989). This is particularly true in the United States where, historically, much of our nursing literature and theory originates. It should be no surprise then that the value of individualism is inherent in most nursing theories (Browne, 2001; Browne, 2004). An individualist ethic or value has been less apparent in Canada, at

---

### CANADIAN RESEARCH BOX 7.1

**How is critical caring theory reflected in current PHN practice? How does the theory need to be modified and further developed?**

Falk-Rafael, A., & Betker, C. (2012a). Witnessing social injustice downstream and advocating for health equity upstream: "The trombone slide" of nursing. *Advances in Nursing Science, 35*(2), 98–112.

Falk-Rafael, A., & Betker, C. (2012b). The primacy of relationships: A study of public health nursing practice from a critical caring perspective. *Advances in Nursing Science, 35*(4), 315–332.

These articles report the findings of a study that examined the relevance of critical caring theory to the practice of expert public health nurses (PHNs). A hybrid middle range theory, critical caring, was proposed by Dr. Adeline Falk-Rafael, a Canadian nurse scholar, in 2005 as a framework to guide PHN practice. It is a nursing theory informed by the ethics of caring and social justice and, as such, is considered an appropriate framework to guide nursing actions directed toward taking up the challenge by the Commission on the Social Determinants of Health to "close the gap" in health equity.

There were 26 PHNs who participated in this study: 10 in one-on-one interviews and 16 in two subsequent focus groups. Using a feminist, multi-site, comparative, and collective case study design, the study examined specific aspects of the theory. This design was chosen as it is useful for examining and refining theory, as comparisons are made across cases (i.e., individual nurses).

Three themes emerged in the findings. The themes "moral imperative" and "in pursuit of social justice," illustrate the public health nurses' caring and social justice moral centre, and how their practice is informed and guided by it. This supports PHNs as being ideally suited to take up the challenge to reduce health inequities through working with others to effect change in the social, cultural, economic, political structures, systems, and policies that create social injustice. A third theme, "barriers to moral agency," raised issues about PHNs ability to meet the challenge of reducing health inequities due to barriers reported by the participants. Barriers to moral agency that were identified included funding priorities, organizational policies and structures, and leadership that was not congruent with social justice. Government policies and politics also contributed to these barriers. The result for the nurses was ethical dilemmas and, at times, moral distress where there was a perceived inability to take action. In these articles,

critical caring theory is put forward as having the potential to be a "tool of resistance" that could be used to counter the forces that limit PHNs from working to their full scope of practice and fulfilling their potential in the challenge to close the health equity gap.

### Discussion Questions

1. As a CHN, you and your team have experienced frustration in developing the capacity to address the social determinants of health in your community. How can critical caring theory assist you to articulate the roles you could play?

2. What factors have you observed that would contribute to your team's frustration?

3. How could critical caring theory assist your team to give voice to the role of nurses in this important area? What would support your team to use this theory?

---

least until recently, where people are more likely to support government programs and regulation (e.g., healthcare and the Canada Health Act) in the public interest. Canada's healthcare system is based on principles of universality, accessibility, and public administration (Government of Canada, 1985), and reflects Canadians' greater support of a collectivist ethic. This is evident in the widely shared belief among Canadians (Romanow, 2002) that all of us are entitled to healthcare that is available to all regardless of ability to pay, accessible wherever one lives in the country, and administered without profit by a public institution. These principles oppose an individualist ethic. Nonetheless, individualism is still a value held by many Canadians that goes counter to the basic philosophy of community health nursing practice, which reflects collectivist values and the notion of the common good (MacDonald, 2013).

An example of individualism is to prioritize the right of individual nurses to refuse flu vaccination over the rights of an entire group of patients and the larger community to avoid risk imposed by others, nurses in particular. A collectivist value is reflected in policies that require vaccination, or some other mechanism to prevent viral transmission. Another example of collectivist values would be legislation requiring the use of seat belts or bicycle helmets. In this case, the common good is prioritized over an individual's right to choose to engage in risky behaviour.

These conflicting values in nursing make population-focused practice a real challenge for some nurses who have been educated and socialized to focus on individuals. As Laffrey and Craig (1995) pointed out, "There is constant tension between nursing's concern for human beings as individuals and their concern with the larger community and the aggregates of which it is composed" (p. 126). Theories to guide practice with individuals and families in communities are necessary, and the lack of theory to guide community health nursing practice at the other levels—community, population, systems, and society—is problematic.

# BROAD THEORETICAL PERSPECTIVES

The third aspect of the theoretical foundations model (Figure 7.2) identifies some broad theoretical perspectives that have been used to inform community health nursing theory, research, and practice. A theoretical perspective encompasses a variety of theories that differ in significant ways from each other but share some core concepts. These perspectives originate outside of nursing but contribute to a CHN's knowledge synthesis. They are also interconnected in part by including many of the same concepts that are discussed throughout this chapter (e.g., social justice, health equity, a population focus). Each perspective can provide a framework for incorporating more concrete and specific theories. This will become clear where an overview of six perspectives is provided in this section. Others are described in Table 7.2.

| Table 7.2 | Broad Theoretical Perspectives Relevant to Community Health Nursing | | |
|---|---|---|---|
| **Theory** | **Unique Features** | **Similarities and Differences to Other Theories** | **Relationship to Community Health Nursing Standards of Practice and Examples from CHN Practice** |
| Complexity science theory | The view that in any given situation there are numerous and diverse parts interacting with the potential to evolve to a new situation. There is no single complexity theory or approach to complexity. Some of the core concepts include interconnectedness, non-linearity, self-organization, and co-evolution. | Complexity moves away from linear cause-and-effect dynamics. It encourages CHNs to think differently about complex public health problems. Complexity theory is similar to intersectionality in that there may be overlapping influences; however, intersectionality does not consider the characteristics of the changing relationships. | All of the CHNC standards of practice reflect issues ranging from very simple to very complex, and occasionally to chaotic. Complexity theory can be useful at any of the practice levels, from an individual perspective to a systems perspective. |
| Social ecological theory | The health of individuals, communities, and populations is influenced by the interplay between people and their environment. | Like complexity and intersectionality, social ecological theory recognizes the impact of many different influences and the overlap among them. | CHNs engage in health promotion activities and consider the array of factors affecting the health of the client and family; e.g., well-child clinics. CHNs consider broad determinants of health, such as income, education, employment opportunities, physical environment, and support systems. |
| Critical social theory | Considers the multiple social and economic forces resulting in power differentials within society. | Places equity issues in the foreground. From this perspective a CHN challenges the status quo and engages with the problems of society. | Whether implementing strategies at the individual level or a broad population level, CHNs need to appreciate the multiple intersecting forces at play shaping the lives and well-being of those cared for. |
| Feminist theory | Focuses on the role of sexism and oppression in creating inequities. | Feminism is a component part of intersectionality. | This may come into play at multiple levels of practice. Feminist theory is a consideration for all of the seven CHNC standards of practice. |
| Intersectionality theory | Considers the multiple oppressive forces at play. | Similar to complexity, critical social, and social ecological theories with multiple influences; however, intersectionality has more of a focus on feminism as well as other "isms" such as racism and classism, and the compounding effect of the overlap among them. | As with feminism, intersectionality affects all levels of community health nursing practice, and all of the seven CHNC standards of practice. |

| Table 7.2 | Continued | | |
|---|---|---|---|
| **Theory** | **Unique Features** | **Similarities and Differences to Other Theories** | **Relationship to Community Health Nursing Standards of Practice and Examples from CHN Practice** |
| Postcolonial theory | Considers the role of race and history in creating inequities. | Similar to feminist theory with the focus of oppression in causing inequities in health. | Working with many different groups in the community, CHNs need to be aware of the influence and expectations of the dominant culture, what impact that could have on the local community, and their place within it. |

## Complexity Science Theory

Complexity science is a relatively recent addition to nursing's theoretical toolbox. It has a diverse range of interconnected disciplinary and theoretical roots but an elaboration of these is beyond the scope of this chapter. Complexity science is sometimes equated with and referred to as "complexity theory" or "complex adaptive systems theory," but these are only a small component of the broad map of complexity science (see www.art-sciencefactory.com/complexity-map_feb09.html). The evolution of complexity science has proceeded along several parallel yet interconnected paths. Much of the healthcare application of complexity science, including nursing applications (e.g., Anderson, Crabtree, Steele, McDaniel, & Reuben, 2005; Davidson, Ray, & Turkel, 2011) has been originally derived from systems theory. Examples include King's theory of goal attainment (1981) and Neuman's systems model (1972), which are based on the notion that human beings are open systems that interact constantly with their environments.

In general, the environments and structures within which CHNs practice can be considered complex adaptive systems (CAS), which are "a collection of individual agents with freedom to act in ways that are not always totally predictable and whose actions are interconnected" (Plsek & Greenhalgh, 2001, p. 625). Although there is no single complexity theory or approach to complexity, there are concepts central to any complexity science approach. These include interconnectedness or interdependency, non-linearity, self-organization, emergence, and co-evolution, which have been well described in the nursing literature (e.g., Anderson et al., 2005).

Interconnectedness occurs as agents in the system interact locally and exchange information to create new connections that allow information to spread through the system. Interactions at the local level give rise to global patterns. Relationships in the system are non-linear in that there is a disproportionate relationship between cause and effect; a small change might result in a very large effect, and vice versa. In self-organization, people mutually adjust their actions to cope, and adapt to changing environmental or contextual circumstances. This self-organization arises through the interrelationships and interdependencies of the agents in the system. Emergence occurs through the processes of self-organization and non-linear interactions, whereby there is an emergence of system-level properties that are distinct from the properties of the interacting agents. Herd immunity is an excellent example of a system-level property that arises from immunization

of only some members of the system (MacDonald, 2004). Finally, co-evolution means that because a CAS is open, agents within the system interact with others beyond the system so that both the CAS and the world beyond evolve and change in relation to each other.

Complexity theory helps nurses to understand their relationship to the systems within which they work, and the theoretical principles have implications for their practice (Ray, Turkel, & Cohn, 2011). For example, from a complexity science perspective, rigid rules and protocols have limited application or may even be counterproductive. In an era of standardization and protocols in nursing, complexity requires consideration of whether a one-size-fits-all approach to policy and practice is appropriate. Each situation and community is unique and may require a unique solution. In a complex system, the success of a given action or practice is dependent on the context, so success on one occasion does not mean there will be success the next time. Understanding phenomena requires us to see the whole in the part and the part in the whole (MacDonald, 2004), which is, of course, very congruent with notions of holism and eco-centric approaches in nursing (Kleffel, 1996). In complexity science, the essence of a phenomenon exists in the interrelationships and interdependencies among people, events, actions, and experiences (Westley, Zimmerman, & Patton, 2007). It is the interconnectedness of people and their environments that is a primary focus in complexity science. It is these notions of relationship and connection that are consistent with nursing values and all the theoretical perspectives discussed in this chapter.

Looking at Jason's story through a complexity lens enables the CHN to see the many influences on his current situation. With this in mind, the nurse can work on an individual basis with Jason as well as with his family, and at a community level. Complexity theory pushes us to consider the web-like influences at play in any situation and the interrelationships among the multiple agents in the system. Focusing on these relationships and how they are connected to each other will assist the CHN in ensuring that he or she is engaging appropriate actors in the process. The notion of emergence helps the CHN recognize that multiple smaller actions by many actors in concert across the various levels can result in a significant positive outcome. The concept of co-evolution guides the CHN to note unintended consequences in a related system as a result of actions in one system. As in Jason's story, what appears as a simple problem (a cut on the leg) is now seen as a much more complex problem involving poverty or racism. With a complexity approach, interconnected actions and solutions are considered.

## Social Ecological Theory

The fundamental theoretical assumption in social ecological theory is that health is influenced by the interplay among individuals or communities and their surroundings—family, community, culture, and physical and social environment (Stokols, 1992). Social ecology "pays explicit attention to the social, institutional, and culture contexts of people–environment relations, and draws on both large-scale preventive strategies of public health and individual-level strategies of behavioural sciences" (McLaren & Hawe, 2005, p. 12). Social ecology draws on systems concepts of adaptation (what people do to adapt to the demands of context), succession (interventions are influenced by the history of the setting with its norms, values, policies, and social structures), cycling of resources (interventions must build on existing strengths of individuals, groups, communities, and institutions), and interdependence (settings are systems, and changes in one aspect of the setting influences other aspects) (Stokols, 1996). The socio-environmental approach to health promotion described in Chapter 8 of this text is a social ecological perspective.

As mentioned, a social ecological perspective can encompass specific theories at each ecological level, which range from the individual level at the core to the societal level. For example, Gregson and colleagues (Gregson et al., 2001) used a range of theories at each level of their social ecology model to address nutrition education and social marketing programs with low-income audiences. At the individual level, theories such as stages of change (Prochaska, DiClemente, & Norcross, 1992) and the health belief model (Strecher & Rosenstock, 1997) were incorporated. Diffusion of innovations or organizational changes theories guided interventions at the organizational level of the system. At the community level, theories of community organizing, partnership, and social marketing were relevant. Finally, at the systems or political level, theories of policy change and political advocacy were used to inform action (Gregson et al., 2001).

The social ecological perspective is also reflected in the field of social epidemiology, one of the important sciences that informs the synthesis in community health nursing (Keller et al., 2011) and has been referred to as an "eco-social" perspective or a "social ecological systems" perspective (Krieger, 2001). Social epidemiology seeks to uncover and explain social inequalities in health and how these are distributed in the population. As in all ecological perspectives, the influences on health are multi-level and interconnected.

In relation to Jason's story, a CHN working in this community from a social ecological perspective would need to consider the various determinants of health, at multiple levels, to address preventable injury of youth in this neighbourhood. For instance, a CHN in collaboration with concerned community members could advocate at the political level for legislation around adequate funding to ensure proper disposal of unsafe materials on neighbourhood streets. As well, the CHN could work with community members and other community organizations to create a safe playground for local children. A CHN could also work at the individual and family levels to encourage children to stay clear of unsafe garbage on neighbourhood streets and to play on the designated playground being built in their community. At the highest ecological level, the political structure, CHNs can be involved in activities that are far upstream from the immediate determinants of injury but which address the societal conditions (e.g., poverty) that create inequity that resulted in injuries among particular segments of the population, such as children like Jason.

A social ecological approach to health promotion by CHNs addresses several of the CHNC standards of practice (CHNC, 2011, revised). Statements within the health promotion and prevention standards that relate to collaboration with individuals, families, communities, systems, and populations, and that require CHNs to consider sociopolitical issues, do reflect a social ecological approach. Demonstrating knowledge of the social determinants of health and implementing multiple health promotion and prevention strategies at all levels is also congruent with this perspective. As well, it is evident that an ecological perspective is reflected in the CHNC standards related to capacity building, professional relationships, and access and equity (2011, revised).

## Critical Social Theory

The need to address the underlying power differentials and social inequities that affect health leads us to consider another broad theoretical perspective. Critical social theory is one perspective that has been used by CHNs to inform their work with population groups who have been disadvantaged by social circumstances (Allen, 1985; Butterfield, 1990; Cohen & Reutter, 2007; Kleffel, 1991; Stevens & Hall, 1992). CHNs are committed to promoting the health of marginalized groups and populations "under threat" (McGibbon, 2012). This requires nurses to work not only with individual clients and families but also collaboratively with other sectors to influence public policy and address the structural and systemic determinants of health. Although others often use the term "vulnerable" to describe groups experiencing social disadvantage, McGibbon has moved away from the notion of vulnerability, and instead uses the term "under threat" to indicate that the source of oppression and marginalization is not within the individuals themselves but in the social and political structures that create systematic disadvantage.

Critical social theory provides a vantage from which to examine issues of community health practice and policy to see what is possible within the current situation. This perspective challenges the status quo and assumes a deliberate engagement with the problems of society and the processes of social transformation. In Jason's situation one can see that the simple act of attending to his leg wound alone misses the underlying factors that led to his injury in the first place. Asking "why" illuminates various social and community issues. This provides an opportunity for CHNs to engage with local policies and services to work toward improvements benefitting the larger community. Critical social theory takes the historically situated sociopolitical perspective, analyzes it, and then challenges the social inequities and injustices that resulted from it (Chinn & Kramer, 2011). Critical social theory "takes the stance that some values are better than others and makes an explicit commitment to social justice" (Strega, 2005, p. 207).

## Feminist Theory

Feminism encompasses the perspectives and methods committed to political and social changes that improve the lives of women and, in turn, the lives of all people (Chinn & Kramer, 2011). Feminism is defined by hooks (2000) as "a movement to end sexism, sexist exploitation, and oppression" (p. viii). Although there are multiple perspectives, debates, and disagreements within feminist theory, there are some commonalities among them. In general, feminism is focused on equity, oppression, and justice, which are central concerns in public health (Rogers, 2006) and community health nursing. Feminist theory sees inequality as based in social oppression rather than individual misfortune (McGibbon & Etowa, 2009). Lack of power, diminished opportunities, discrimination, and oppression are some of the less-noticeable aspects of inequality (Rogers, 2006). While equity is considered key to public health, a feminist perspective on equity suggests that simply being female is also a risk factor for increased inequity (Rogers, 2006).

Because much of the work of community health nursing is directed toward reducing the effects of poverty, their activities have the potential to make a difference in the lives of women and children who are over-represented in the population of the disadvantaged (Rogers, 2006). As well, women as family care providers are traditionally the ones most often mediating the preventive aspects of diet, exercise, and other aspects of health within the household (Rogers, 2006). Very often it is these women that CHNs work with individually, in families, and in groups. CHNs advocate for their clients in ways that promote health, empowerment, justice, and equality (Leipert, 2001).

It is interesting to consider that women form the majority of care providers for the aged, and that these two groups are significantly affected by funding decisions and allocation of health and other resources (Rogers, 2006). This has an impact on CHNs themselves, as most of them are women practising in a women's profession (Leipert, 2001). Feminism then aims to empower not only clients, but CHNs themselves (Leipert, 2001).

Reading between the lines in Jason's story, it is possible to see that issues of injustice and oppression are likely present. A CHN working in this community would want to consider how plans for improving health could be informed by a feminist perspective. This would start by considering the perspectives of the local population, building on their strengths, offering a range of options, and supporting efforts for change (Leipert, 2001). In working with the population under threat in Jason's neighbourhood, the CHN would develop closer connections and co-operation with community members and recognize needs identified by this group while taking into consideration cultural and economic diversity as well as the perceived power of his or her own position as a CHN and health expert (James, 1996, as cited in Leipert, 2001). Feminist theory assists CHNs in taking a stand with groups that experience conditions creating vulnerability; questioning oppressive situations; facilitating strategies developed by the group; and dealing with the broader social, political, and economic roots of poor health (Leipert, 2001). Through collaboration with families, groups, and communities, and by identifying the root causes of inequities in health, a feminist perspective is strongly linked with CHNC's (2011, revised) first standard, related to health promotion, as well as to standards three, four, five, and six.

## Intersectionality Theory

Another broad theoretical perspective, intersectionality, provides a way to understand how multiple social identities such as gender, race, disability, socioeconomic status, and other inequalities intersect at the level of the individual and reflect social constructions of oppression and privilege (Bowleg, 2012). Intersectionality examines difference and the influence of power on an individual or group who have their own histories within the context of their current surroundings (Corbin & Tomm Bonde, 2012). Like roads that meet at an intersection, the interweaving of multiple social determinants and mechanisms offers a more inclusive look at the factors of sexism, racism, as well as other "isms" that come together as oppression, which negatively impacts the health of individuals and populations.

Intersectionality has been described as a framework that accounts for the synergistic or amplifying influence of multiple forms of oppression (McGibbon, 2008). Yet, it has been noted that intersectionality has been defined and represented in a number of ways (McGibbon & Etowa, 2009). For instance, within nursing, intersectionality has been discussed as a useful paradigm for approaching research (e.g., Van Herk, Smith, & Andrew, 2011). It has also been used to better understand social justice for nursing action, education, practice, research, and policy (e.g., Pauly, MacKinnon, & Varcoe, 2009). As well, intersectionality has been used within a framework for guiding and providing ethical nursing care related to many facets of health (McGibbon & Etowa, 2009). For another example of intersectionality within nursing, turn to Chapter 28, Violence in Societies of this textbook.

In Jason's case, the combination of his Indigenous heritage, his poor economic situation, and the impoverished neighbourhood in which he lives culminates in the lack of a safe environment for children to live and play. CHNs need to be aware of how these factors may intersect to deepen the disadvantage experienced by Jason and his family as they struggle to ensure a safe environment in the context of racism, discrimination, and poverty. Nurses need to keep these in mind as they work with Jason, his family, and community partners to improve safety, prevent injuries, and ultimately to improve the health of the community.

## Postcolonial Theory

Postcolonial theory, as a broad theoretical perspective, challenges us to consider oppressive structures that assume a view reflecting dominant discourse and culture, and to give "voice to subjugated and indigenous knowledge, especially non-Western voices" (Reimer-Kirkham, Varcoe, et al., 2009, p. 155). A postcolonial theoretical perspective can contribute to "understanding how continuities from the past shape the present context of health and health care" (Browne, Smye, & Varcoe, 2005, p. 19). A better understanding of historical influences on the current experiences of those receiving care allows an appreciation of the lasting consequences of colonization on identity, race, and health. Postcolonial theory is an important theoretical perspective to draw on in community health nursing practice; it challenges our assumptions through encouraging self-reflection and exploration of the forms of oppression at play within any given nurse–client or nurse–community interaction.

Postcolonial theory is not only a useful theoretical perspective for frontline nurses, but it is also beneficial for nurse researchers in guiding the research process. For instance, it informs research question development, study design, and data analysis. Canadian nurse researchers have used postcolonial theory extensively in working with local Indigenous peoples, families, and communities (e.g., Smith, Edwards, Martens, & Varcoe, 2007; Smith, Varcoe, & Edwards, 2005; Van Herk, Smith, & Tedford Gold, 2012). As well, nurse researchers' interest in gender analysis in postcolonial theory has led to the use of postcolonial feminist theory to get at the root causes of racialized and gendered inequities (Reimer-Kirkham, Baumbusch, Schultz, & Anderson, 2009).

Postcolonial theory is important and useful within community health nursing research and practice to challenge the privileging of knowledge within Canada, but it is also useful within a global health context. For instance, in Chapter 33, Global Health, postcolonial theory may explain the differences between international health, global health, and public health, and lead to questions regarding the dominance and authority of Western knowledge in nursing practice throughout the world.

Thus, no matter a nurse's location, it is important to become aware of and question our ways of thinking and being. For instance, a CHN coming from a white middle-class background needs to be aware of the importance of cultural safety when working with Jason and his family, who have been identified as Aboriginal, by providing care and assisting in a way that fits with their cultural values and norms. Assumptions about ways to address health issues may not always fit with the standardized view of the dominant culture. Care needs to be given in a way that respects both cultural differences and acceptable solutions found for issues.

# CONCEPTUAL MODELS AND FRAMEWORKS

As the fourth blade in the theoretical foundations of community health nursing model (Figure 7.2), conceptual models and frameworks are the "scaffolding" for theories. Much of the development of theory in community health nursing has been in conceptual models and frameworks. A conceptual model or framework is defined as a set of relatively abstract and general concepts, the propositions that describe those concepts, and the general relations between the concepts. As discussed earlier in the section on broad theoretical perspectives, a model or framework can integrate theories. This was illustrated with the social ecological perspective already discussed. Similarly, the community health nursing models and frameworks discussed in this section incorporate specific middle range and practice or substantive theories.

Although the terms "framework" and "model" are often used interchangeably, some theorists suggest that a framework is less formal than a conceptual model and it does not usually contain propositions (Fawcett & De Santo-Madeya, 2013). In this chapter, conceptual frameworks and models are categorized together. For a list of several conceptual models and frameworks that are particularly relevant to community health nursing, refer to Table 7.3. The next section describes some conceptual models or frameworks that have been developed and used widely to guide community health nursing practice.

## Canadian Community as Partner

This community process model is based on Betty Neuman's systems model (Neuman, 1972) and was adapted specifically to inform community health nursing. It began as "Community as

| Table 7.3 | Conceptual Models and Frameworks | |
|---|---|---|
| **Conceptual Model or Framework** | **Key Points** | **Relationship to Community Health Nursing Standards of Practice and Examples from CHN Practice** |
| Canadian community as partner Vollman, Anderson, & McFarlane, 2003, 2012 | This conceptual model depicts the community as a dynamic system that interacts with its environment and moves iteratively through the phases of community assessment, analysis, diagnosis, planning, intervention, and evaluation. It sees interventions as primary, secondary, or tertiary preventive levels, and is consistent with the broad determinants of health. | CHNC standards 1 and 2, health promotion, and prevention, and health protection, are incorporated in this model, as are standards 3, 5, and 6. An example from practice is a local community demand for birth control services for teens, and the subsequent involvement of CHNs with teens and community partners to establish accessible and welcoming clinic services. |
| Community health promotion model Yiu, 2008, 2012 | This conceptual model guides CHNs to use collaborative community actions to improve sustainable health outcomes for the community. This is done by employing health promotion strategies at the community level. The nursing process and primary health care are integral to how this model is applied. | CHNC standards 1–7 may be demonstrated through the use of this model. An example from practice includes identifying all of the factors at play and how this informs the most appropriate action for a young mothers who are feeding their children a diet high in carbohydrates. |

*(continued)*

| Table 7.3 | Continued | |
|---|---|---|

| Conceptual Model or Framework | Key Points | Relationship to Community Health Nursing Standards of Practice and Examples from CHN Practice |
|---|---|---|
| Population health promotion: An integrated model of population health and health promotion<br><br>Hamilton & Bhatti, 1996 | This widely used Canadian model demonstrates the link between population health and health promotion at various levels of action. The model is used to identify specific actions as well as demonstrate how to combine various actions to create a comprehensive action strategy. Attention is directed to individual, family, and community levels. | An example of a specific health concern might be the development of community support groups for young parents. This model fits well with public health nursing discipline-specific competencies 3, 4 and 5 (CHNC, 2009), as well as CHNC standards 1, 2, 4, 5, and 6. |
| Multiple interventions for community health framework<br><br>Edwards et al., 2004 | This Canadian model is based on the assumption that interrelated social, cultural, political, and economic factors influence the health of individuals. Multiple intervention programs are based in a socioecological framework where a combination of interventions are used to target individual, community, and political levels, as well as different sectors such as education, transportation, housing, health, and others. It considers nested determinants of health and recognizes that effects may change over time with changing players and leadership, both locally and politically. | In Duncan, B.C., CHNs improved breastfeeding rates within their community by promoting the WHO's "Ten Steps" with colleagues in acute care. CHNs were involved in the development of health authority and school board policies to support breastfeeding. CHNs worked with local grocery stores and food banks to reduce formula promotions. They initiated photo contests, breastfeeding calendars, World Breastfeeding Day events, and parent support groups to change the local culture related to breastfeeding. CHNC standards 1, 2, 4, and 5 are closely linked to this framework. |
| Health promotion model<br><br>Pender, 1996 | This American nursing conceptual model focuses on health-promoting behaviour directed toward positive health outcomes at an individual level. It identifies how a range of individual experiences and characteristics affect the health-promoting behaviour of individuals. It is particularly useful in changing personal health especially in home healthcare, but less so for changing social determinants as it does not address the broader population. | CHNs develop a smoking cessation clinic after community assessments indicated higher-than-average smoking rates in the perinatal population. CHNs use motivational interviewing to assist clients in resolving health issues and refer to other community resources as needed. Although it has some connections with all of the CHNC standards, this model relates particularly well with standards 1, 3, and 5. |
| Calgary family assessment model<br><br>Wright & Leahey, 2012 | The Calgary family assessment model is an integrated, multi-dimensional frame-work based on systems, cybernetics, communication, and change theory. This is a model that can be used to assess a family or as an organizing framework for clinical work with individual families. It focuses on the interaction among all individuals within a family and is inclusive of past, present, and future family members. | A home health nurse can use this model, for example, with a family experiencing a major illness or facing death, to assess the relationships within the family support network. This model relates especially well to CHNC standards 3 and 5. |

| Table 7.3 | Continued | |
|---|---|---|
| **Conceptual Model or Framework** | **Key Points** | **Relationship to Community Health Nursing Standards of Practice and Examples from CHN Practice** |
| An integrative model for community health nursing<br><br>Laffrey & Kulbok, 1999 | This American model outlines nursing care for the individual, family, and community. CHNs practising in different settings will have different areas of practice and require different kinds of expertise. Multi-level practice is described within a population-centred perspective. An integrated approach supports the broad scope of practice in the community and provides a basis for collaboration and partnership. | CHNC standards related to this model include 1, 2, 3, and 5 in particular, although the remaining standards are also relevant. A practice example is the home health nurse who may be initially involved with a client recovering from an injury. The nurse soon recognizes the challenges inherent within the family and the community and connects with the public health nurse to follow up with the broader issues, planning together what could be done with the community to prevent similar injuries. |
| Intervention wheel<br><br>Keller & Strohschein, 2012 | Also known as the Minnesota intervention wheel, this model demonstrates the relationships between interventions and outcomes for different levels of practice. It depicts how PHNs improve population health through interventions with individuals, families, and communities, as well as the systems that impact on the health of communities. It considers the determinants of health and emphasizes health promotion and prevention interventions to improve population health. | A PHN might focus on ways to improve breastfeeding and immunization rates while working with a population of vulnerable, perinatal women. This may be accomplished through individual contact with moms, as well as by engaging with local partners to shift the prevailing community culture. CHNC standards 1, 2, 4, 5, and 6 fit particularly well with this model. |

Client" (Anderson & McFarlane, 1988) to reflect the unique focus of public health nursing practice on communities as a whole. The title shifted to "Community as Partner" in the second edition (Anderson & McFarlane, 1996) to signal the evolving concern for public participation in health decision making (Vollman et al., 2012). The Canadianization of Community as Partner grounded it more explicitly in health promotion, drawing on the Ottawa Charter (Vollman et al., 2012) (see Figure 7.4).

Consistent with Neuman's theory, the emphasis is on understanding the community as a dynamic system that interacts with its environment (Vollman et al., 2008, p. xiii). The model assists users in moving iteratively through the phases of community health nursing: assessment, analysis, diagnosis, planning, intervention, and evaluation. Assessment is guided by the assessment wheel (see Figure 7.4), with the people of the community whose health is affected by and affects various subsystems at its core. The authors explain that the subsystems are consistent with the broad determinants of health (see Chapter 8), an important aspect of community health nursing practice. For example, the education subsystem in the wheel parallels the education determinant of health.

Keep in mind Jason's neighbourhood as the phases of the community health nursing process are considered. Through analysis of the data gathered in the assessment phase (in partnership with the community), a community diagnosis is made about the priority issues to address. The CHN engages local partners in planning interventions to reduce or limit the community stressors and build community resilience. Using the model, interventions are conceptualized as primary (to prevent disease from occurring), secondary (early detection of disease), or tertiary (to slow or reduce disease processes). CHNs can intervene with activities directed at one or more levels of prevention, which progress from health promotion before disease processes have begun to reducing the symptoms or progress of a disease. Thus, theories of health promotion are relevant within this model. In fact, in the Canadian Community as Partner text (Vollman et al., 2012), discussion is built around intervention strategies from the five action areas of the Ottawa Charter (see Chapter 8). Each action area points to the need for specific theories to guide practice. For example, in the action area "strengthening community action," theories and principles of community development would be relevant. Once implemented, these interventions are evaluated. This process of assessment, analysis, planning, intervention, and evaluation is reflected in each of the seven standards of practice (CHNC, 2011, revised).

Using this model, a CHN would begin by collecting information about the number and nature of childhood

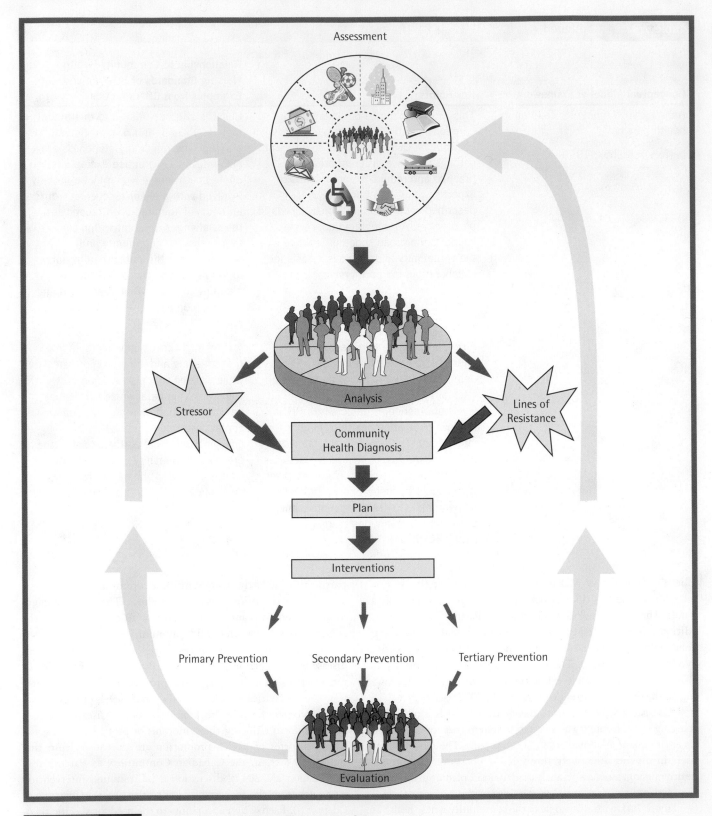

Assessment

Analysis

Stressor

Lines of Resistance

Community Health Diagnosis

Plan

Interventions

Primary Prevention    Secondary Prevention    Tertiary Prevention

Evaluation

**FIGURE    7.4**    Canadian Community as Partner Model

*Source:* Vollman, A. R., Anderson, E. T., & McFarlane, J. (2012). *Canadian community as partner: Theory and multidisciplinary practice* (3rd ed.). Philadelphia, PA: Republished with permission of Wolters Kluwer Health/Lippincott, Williams & Wilkins; permission conveyed through Copyright Clearance Center, Inc.

injuries in Jason's neighbourhood. The CHN might also gather local information and stories about individual events to illustrate the effects on families and the community, all the while working with community members to raise awareness of the issues. Through this process the CHN demonstrates caring, communication, and a commitment to the community through the development of relationships that facilitate the achievement of collaboratively identified health goals.

## The Community Health Promotion Model

The goal of the community health promotion model is to improve sustainable community health outcomes. This is done by using the critical thinking skills of the nursing process to apply various community level health promotion strategies. It uses a holistic approach to promoting the health of communities and populations to decrease inequities and improve the quality of life of communities. This is done by examining the interplay of the determinants of health on various community health issues. Chapter 13 provides an in-depth discussion of the community health promotion model.

## The Intervention Wheel

The intervention wheel (Figure 7.5) is an evidence-based, widely tested, and validated public health nursing conceptual model (Keller, Strohschein, Lia-Hoagberg, & Schaffer, 1998). The intervention wheel depicts how public health nursing improves population health through interventions with individuals, families, and communities, as well as with the systems that affect community health. It incorporates evidence that demonstrates the relationships between interventions and outcomes for different levels of practice.

The model was inductively derived from the practice of public health nurses and some home care nurses. The authors used grounded theory research method to identify 17 core public health nursing interventions that were common to the work of PHNs. Later, these interventions were subjected to an extensive, systematic review of evidence to support their effectiveness. Each intervention is accompanied by a set of steps and recommended best practices that are grouped together in coloured wedges of the wheel. Each colour represents a different class of PHN intervention.

The model is population-based in that—at all levels of practice, even the individual level—interventions are carried out in the service of improving population health. Using this model, it is possible to imagine how a CHN in Jason's neighbourhood can work at various levels to make a difference in his community. Drawing on the interventions in the orange wedge of the wheel (collaboration, coalition building, and

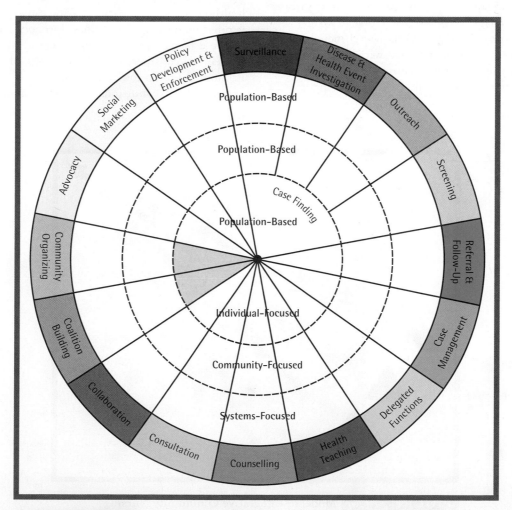

**FIGURE 7.5** The Intervention Wheel

*Source:* Public Health Interventions Applications for Public Health Nursing Practice, March 2001. Copyright © 2001 by Minnesota Department of Health. Used by permission of Minnesota Department of Health.

community organizing), the CHN can raise awareness of the issue of safety and injury prevention with community organizations and begin to collaborate with them, building a coalition to advocate (yellow wedge) for improvements in safety. By advocating with local municipal government officials on the issue of safe play, and other sectors like education and housing, CHNs in collaboration with others can initiate a conversation and set in motion the wheels of action for change. The intervention wheel specifically incorporates the first three CHNC (2011, revised) practice standards (health promotion; prevention; and health maintenance, restoration, and palliation), although it also reflects the importance of the remaining standards through the activities it includes.

Although this model is focused on the practice of PHNs, there are situations in which other CHNs will engage in public health functions and carry out interventions. For example, a home health nurse might follow Jason after his visit to the hospital to assist with his wound care, and may engage in one or more of the interventions at the individual or family level (Keller, Strohschein, Lia-Hoagberg, & Schaffer, 2004a; Keller et al., 2004b). A home health nurse might enact interventions in the blue wedge of the wheel: health teaching, counselling, and consultation. She or he might also use advocacy strategies (yellow wedge), screen for diseases (red wedge), or engage in collaboration (orange wedge) with others in the community. Because the wheel includes individual and family levels of practice within a population focus, which may include health promotion and disease prevention, these interventions would be quite appropriate for a home health nurse.

## An Integrative Model for Community Health Nursing

This model provides an integrated and holistic approach to community health nursing across settings and goes beyond the traditional nursing focus on the individual and family levels to include group and community levels (Laffrey & Kulbok, 1999). The model is conceptualized within a holistic and eco-centric perspective (Kleffel, 1996) in which the "human and non-human are one within the same organic system" (p. 4). Practice is conceptualized within a primary health care framework (Laffrey & Craig, 2000), and multi-level practice is described within a population-centred perspective (Kulbok, Laffrey, & Chitthathairattm, 2008). Primary health care is described in detail in Chapter 8.

This model (Figure 7.6) contains two dimensions: (1) the "client system" (individual, family, group, and community) and (2) the "focus of care," which encompasses health promotion at the core, including prevention of illness, disease, injury, and disability, as well as illness care. The fact that care is directed at different levels of clients and different foci of practice means that the model can be used to conceptualize the broad and diverse practice of CHNs. For example, home health nurses who primarily provide care for individuals and families might emphasize illness care, but could also incorporate a focus on prevention. There are various levels of prevention considered in the delivery of CHN services. Primordial prevention aims to impede the development of environmental conditions, such as economic, social, and

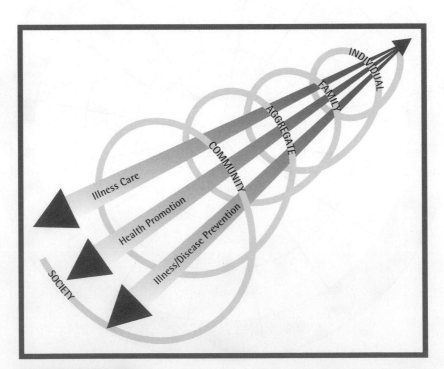

**FIGURE** 7.6 **Model of Integrative Community Nursing**

*Source:* Laffrey, S. C., & Kulbok, P. A. (1999). An integrative model for holistic community health nursing. *Journal of Holistic Nursing, 17*(1), 88–103. p. 92. Published by American Holistic Nurses Association, © 1999.

cultural factors that increase the risk of disease (Porta, 2008) and that may contribute to health inequities. Primary prevention addresses more immediate ways to prevent disease or injury from actually occurring. This is sometimes referred to as "upstream" prevention. Secondary prevention relates to early detection of disease, while tertiary prevention aims to slow or reduce disease processes. Quaternary prevention endeavours to prevent inappropriate or unnecessary medical interventions to minimize the suffering of a chronically ill client; for instance, the promotion of a healthy death (Last, 2007). CHNs use interventions directed at one or more levels of prevention, progressing from health promotion before disease processes have begun to reducing the symptoms and progress of a disease. Levels of prevention are also discussed throughout this book.

In Jason's situation, the home health nurse may have been initially involved in his wound care, but recognizing the challenges inherent within the family and the community, that nurse might have connected with the public health nurse to follow up with the broader issues, planning together about what could be done with the community to prevent further such injuries. The authors emphasize that no single practitioner can do everything, so collaboration and coordination across teams of nurses and other providers is essential in maintaining the integrity of the model.

This integrative model frames the practice of any CHN, allowing her or him to address fully the standards of practice (CHNC, 2011, revised). The model specifically addresses the first three standards (health promotion; prevention; and health maintenance, restoration, and palliation) because these map directly onto the model's three foci of practice. Because the aim of the model is to provide a basis for collaboration, it also addresses the fourth standard related to professional relationships. CHNs can also address standards 5 and 6, to build capacity and facilitate access and equity (CHNC, 2011, revised). Thus, this model is one of the few available in the literature that can be used by nurses working across diverse community health nursing–client systems and foci of practice. The model fully encompasses the holistic and integrative vision of CHNC (2011, revised) that CHNs collectively share a common history, values, skills, traditions, and beliefs, and that their distinctive practices are complementary within a shared philosophical base.

# NURSING AND OTHER THEORIES

The last blade of the theoretical foundations of community health nursing model (Figure 7.2) considers nursing theories as well as theories from public health and the social sciences. Nurses in all areas of practice know about and have used a range of theories, models, and frameworks to guide their practice both from within and outside of nursing. Theories contain relatively concrete and specific concepts (e.g., caring, self-care, adaptation) and propositions that define those concepts and their relationships. Nursing theories, like the broad range of knowledge components in this chapter, can be categorized by the degree of abstraction, ranging from fairly concrete and situation-specific **practice theory**, through middle range theory, to more abstract **grand theories**. Exemplar theories in each of these categories that have either been developed for community health nursing or adapted for use in community health nursing practice, education, and research are highlighted and briefly described in the following sections.

# GRAND NURSING THEORIES

Grand theories are broad in their scope, and the concepts are described in abstract terms. As such, they can be used in a broad range of practice situations and provide high-level guidance to practice and research. A brief summary of several grand nursing theories is included in Table 7.4. Two theories that relate particularly well to community health nursing are examined more closely.

## Human Caring Science

In the development of this grand nursing theory, Jean Watson focused on the concept of caring (Watson, 2012). Her work reflects the influences of some non-nursing theories, such as physics, psychology, and education (Falk-Rafael, 2000). Although initially aimed at the relationship between a nurse and an individual, Watson also considers the determinants of health (Watson, 1979), health promotion, and the health of communities (Falk-Rafael, 2000). This theory reflects the socio-environmental context of community health nursing, and recognizes the interdependence of the health of individuals and

| Table 7.4 | Grand Nursing Theories Relevant to Community Health Nursing | |
| --- | --- | --- |
| **Grand Theory** | **Key Points** | **Relationship to CHNC (2011, revised) Standards of Practice and Examples from CHN Practice** |
| Roy's adaptation model<br><br>Roy, 1987 | This grand nursing theory focuses on the interaction between individuals and their environment. Roy identified four modes of adaptation to achieve health, including physiological, self-concept, role function, and interdependence. The purpose of this theory is to explain how nurses can facilitate the change process toward an individual's intended goals. | In practice, a CHN might work with an elderly person recovering from a hip fracture who wishes to achieve mobility and independent living. The CHN works collaboratively with clients and their families to identify resources and provide support in adapting to a new level of ability. This connects with all of the CHNC standards of practice. |

(continued)

| Table 7.4 | Continued | |
|---|---|---|
| **Grand Theory** | **Key Points** | **Relationship to CHNC (2011, revised) Standards of Practice and Examples from CHN Practice** |
| Watson's human caring science<br><br>Watson, 1979 | Human caring science is based on 10 carative processes that reflect a deep respect for life and the power of human caring. It recognizes that human-to-human environmental and ecological associations are important, and it values the subjective experience of both the individual and the nurse and the relationship between them. | This theory reflects the socio-environmental context of community health nursing, and recognizes the interdependence of the health of individuals and the health of a community. CHNs working with vulnerable families in the perinatal period recognize the importance of their relationship with those families and their connections with the community. Whether working with individuals or families, communities or co-workers, the importance of developing a relationship is an important part of all of the CHNC standards. |
| Self-care deficit theory of nursing<br><br>Orem, 1985 | The self-care model aims to facilitate the client–nurse interaction to preserve the integrity of human beings through self-care by offering 10 self-care actions. The agency and capacity of the client are enhanced by strategies directed at controlling, maintaining, and motivating actions toward self-care. Orem explains the need for nursing as the inability to provide self-care due to situations of personal health. | The importance of the client–nurse interaction is an essential component of each of the seven CHNC standards of practice. |
| Theory of human becoming<br><br>Parse, 2003 | Three principles comprise this theory. The first is that people structure and knowingly choose the meaning of their reality. The second is that people create patterns in their life, which convey meaning and value. The third principle is that people continuously change in life as they engage with and choose from an infinite range of possibilities. Parse's theory of human becoming fits well with the work of CHNs. The ebb and flow of relationships, altered by changing environmental or personal circumstances, make up the fabric of the work CHNs engage in. Understanding and using Parse's approach helps in moving toward desired outcomes from the client's perspective, and guides nurses to practise in a wholly respectful way. | Parse's approach is apparent when CHNs use motivational interviewing as an aspect of client-centred care, or by engaging in self-reflection after caring for a palliative patient, assessing one's own awareness and assumptions that influence the care of the client. Whether working with individuals, families, or communities, an important aspect of CHN work is the development of relationships, and this is clearly reflected in each of the seven CCHN standards of practice. |

the health of a community. Watson (2012) describes caring as "a truly life-giving presence of being open and giving from the heart, receptive with respect, compassion, and dignity, creating a trusting relationship that is human-to-human" (p. 45). She describes 10 carative processes reflected by nurses in a caring relationship with clients, including, for example, practising loving kindness, being authentically present, seeking creative solutions, and creating a healing environment (Watson, 2012).

Watson emphasizes the role of nurses helping individuals to gain more self-caring, self-knowledge, self-control, and inner healing regardless of their health condition (2012). CHNs working with individuals, families, and communities recognize the importance of such a relationship in the development of prevention and health promotion activities. Without a caring relationship, CHNs would not be invited back

into homes to continue working with families, nor would they be identified as valuable and trusted resources in the community.

In the example of Jason, when a CHN followed up with Jason and his family after their encounter in the emergency department, being authentically present and working together with the family to seek creative solutions to prevent further injuries would make a significant difference in the way the family accepts the nurse's support. Developing a trusting relationship with Jason's family facilitates next steps to begin working with friends and neighbours in the local community to find solutions for safe play areas for children. Whether working with individuals or families, communities or co-workers, the importance of developing a relationship is an important part of all of the CHNC standards of practice (2011, revised).

## Self-Care Deficit Nursing Theory

Another relevant grand theory used in community health nursing practice is Dorothea Orem's "self-care deficit nursing" theory. Comprising three interrelated theories—theory of self-care, theory of self-care deficit, and theory of nursing systems—the central focus of Orem's work is the self-care needs of individuals and the nurse–client interaction aimed at preserving or improving client self-care. Orem (1985) outlined the need for nursing care when an individual is unable "to maintain continuously that amount and quality of self-care which is therapeutic in sustaining life and health" (p. 55).

Even though nursing practice guided by Orem's principles is most often directed at individual self-care abilities and deficits, Orem (1985) also considers how nurses provide care for individuals who are part of larger units, such as families, groups, and communities. Consequently, Orem's work has been used to guide CHN practice in family nursing (Reutter, 1984; Taylor, 2001) and hospice care (LaFerriere, 1995), and as the basis in developing a community nursing model (Taylor & McLaughlin, 1991).

Reutter (1984) uses Orem's theory of self-care to develop a family assessment guide that is useful for CHNs, and that explains how "the presuppositions underlying the self-care philosophy have been embraced by community health nursing for years, and indeed are necessary when working with individuals in the area of health promotion (p. 3)". Within this theory, clients are conceptualized as active participants in maintaining health and reaching health goals that are congruent with aims of community health nursing practice. Similarly, within a palliative care home setting, CHNs can find guidance in Orem's theory of self-care deficit, assisting clients and their families to manage care deficits in hopes of enhancing quality of life of those involved (LaFerriere, 1995). All of the seven CHNC (2011, revised) standards are mirrored in Orem's theories.

Using this grand theory, a CHN could assist Jason's family to identify their needs and desires in relation to the unsafe debris left on neighbourhood streets. In addition to assisting Jason's family to identify their self-care needs, a CHN could help this family connect with other concerned community members to build capacity, and partner with local agencies to address adequate clean-up of their neighbourhood streets and proper disposal of harmful debris. In this way, the CHN is helping to surface and address the needs of Jason, his family, and the broader community to protect neighbourhood children from unsafe debris on local streets. This theory does not provide guidance to intervene at the level of the broader social and political context of Jason and his family.

## MIDDLE RANGE THEORIES

Middle range theories contain a limited number of variables or concepts, are fairly narrow in their scope, and have a lower level of abstraction than either grand theories or conceptual models. These characteristics increase their usability for theory-based practice and research (Peterson, 2009). Middle range theories not only provide direction for practice, they are used to generate testable hypotheses for research. Knowledge generated through middle range theory development and validation has contributed to the maturation of the larger nursing discipline (Smith, 2003), which, in turn, contributes to more effective practice, enhanced impact, and improved health outcomes for individuals, families, and communities. The generation of more middle range theories in community health nursing would be helpful in developing the specialty of community health nursing. An outline of several middle range theories is included in Table 7.5. Critical caring theory, as one that was developed specifically for community health nursing in Canada, will be examined more closely.

| Table 7.5 | Middle Range Theories | |
|---|---|---|
| **Middle Range Theory** | **Key Points** | **Relationship to CHNC (2011, revised) Standards of Practice and Examples from CHN Practice** |
| Critical caring theory (Falk-Rafael, 2005b) | Canadian nurse scholar Falk-Rafael identifies seven carative health-promoting processes that reflect the core of public health nursing. This middle range theory uses a broad definition of client to encompass communities and populations. The carative health-promoting processes include the process of teaching and learning, the creation of supportive and sustainable environments, social justice, building capacity, and honouring local belief systems. | This theory connects with all of the CHNC standards of practice. An example of this is found in the approach taken by PHNs in the Nurse-Family Partnership/Healthy Connections program implemented in the province of B.C. in 2012, with the goal of developing and maintaining helping and trusting relationships with vulnerable families. |
| Strengths based theory (Gottlieb & Gottlieb, 2013) | This Canadian approach incorporates thinking about the positives, the things that work well, and what holds potential. It is about finding the balance between focusing on client strengths while at the same time dealing with problems. It is oriented to the individual, family, and community levels of intervention. | This approach is highlighted by CHNC standard 5, capacity building. An example would be CHNs who offer a chronic disease management clinic by providing support and strategies to manage and improve health for adults in low-income housing who have experienced a recent cardiac event. |

*(continued)*

| Table 7.5 | Continued | |
|-----------|-----------|--|
| **Middle Range Theory** | **Key Points** | **Relationship to CHNC (2011, revised) Standards of Practice and Examples from CHN Practice** |
| Relational inquiry (Hartrick Doane & Varcoe, 2005, 2007, 2008) | These Canadian nurse scholars explain how relational practice focuses on the way that personal, interpersonal, and contextual elements shape people's experiences and life situations. This approach considers how capacities and socio-environmental limitations influence people's health and illness experiences, decision making, and the various ways of managing health and illness. It recognizes that health, illness, and experiences are shaped by social, economic, cultural, family, historical, and geographical contexts as well as by biology, gender, age, and ability. | This theory particularly addresses CHNC standards 4 and 5: professional relationships and capacity building. An example from practice is work that CHNs do with vulnerable families living in poverty, and the importance of developing a trusting and respectful relationship with individuals and families, as well as with the larger community. |

## Critical Caring Theory

Critical caring, a middle range theory, "integrates critical feminist theories into nursing science and builds on previous work that linked caring science and empowered caring to public health nursing practice" (Falk-Rafael, 2005b, p. 47). It transforms the caritas processes, or caring practices described in Jean Watson's caring science (Falk-Rafael, 2000), a grand nursing theory, into seven carative health promoting processes that "form the 'core' of public health nursing practice and reflect the legacy and reality of public health nursing practice" (Falk-Rafael, 2005b, p. 38). Further, critical caring is proposed as a way of being (ontology), knowing (epistemology), choosing (ethics), and doing (praxis) (Falk-Rafael, 2005b).

Critical caring "root(s) public health nursing practice in an expanded nursing caring science that reincorporates the social justice agenda" (Falk-Rafael, 2005b, p. 38). Falk-Rafael used the metaphor of a tree (practice) anchored by its roots (theory) to describe the reciprocal relationship between theory and practice, where "theory that is nourished by practice is a living and growing entity that provides support for practice while dynamically defining the characteristics and parameters of practice" (p. 39).

This theory connects to all of the CHNC standards of practice (2011, revised) and would be very useful in working with Jason's family and his community. The seven carative health promoting processes described by Falk-Rafael help CHNs to consider the knowledge they bring to the situation, the importance of a helping-trusting relationship, and the value of reflexive practice. This theory also considers the process of teaching and learning, the creation of supportive and sustainable environments, building capacity, and honouring local belief systems. Falk-Rafael (2005b) notes that these processes have been identified as the core of community health nursing practice. It is a caring relationship based on these elements that a CHN brings when engaging with members of Jason's community to begin to work together toward positive change. Falk-Rafael (2005a) describes community health nursing practice as being "at that intersection where societal attitudes, government policies, and people's lives meet. Such privilege creates a moral imperative not only to attend to the health needs of the public but also, like Nightingale, to work to change the societal conditions contributing to poor health" (p. 219)—that is, to engage in social justice.

CHNs are "leaders of changes to systems in society that support health, and they play key roles in disease, disability and injury prevention, as well as in health promotion" (CPHA, 2010, p. 6). Reducing health inequities and ensuring access to health and healthcare is clearly within nursing's mandate. Reutter and Kushner (2010) called upon CHNs to take up the challenge to "close the gap" posed by the World Health Organization's (WHO) Commission on the Social Determinants of Health, which demonstrated that "social injustice is killing people on a grand scale" (WHO, 2008, p. 26). Reutter and Kushner further advocated for public health nurses to use a critical caring theory to guide their work of promoting health equity. Using this nursing theory as a guide, CHNs will be better able to understand the social, political, economic, and historical context of health inequities; provide sensitive empowering care through informed action; and work to change the underlying social conditions that result in and perpetuate health inequities (Reutter & Kushner, 2010).

## PRACTICE OR SUBSTANTIVE THEORIES

Practice or substantive theories are the least complex, contain fewer concepts, and refer to specific, well-defined phenomena. Practice theories tend to be prescriptive and thus provide direction for practice (McEwen, 2011). For example, Funk and Stajduhar (2011) developed a practice theory that considers the relationship between home health nurses and families when providing end-of-life care. This practice theory is discussed further in Canadian Research Box 7.2. A number

**CANADIAN RESEARCH BOX 7.2**

**What are the family caregivers' accounts of their relationship with and experiences with home care nurses? Describe how to enhance caregivers' relationship and satisfaction with home health services?**

Funk, L., & Stajduhar, K. (2013). Analysis and proposed model of family caregivers' relationships with home health providers and perceptions of the quality of formal services. *Journal of Applied Gerontology, 32*(2), 188–206.

This Canadian study explores family caregivers' accounts of relationships with home care nurses. The findings, combined with previous research, were used to inform the "Model of Family Caregivers' Relationships with Home Health Providers and Perceptions of the Quality of Formal Services." Using ethnography, qualitative interviews were carried out with 26 bereaved caregivers in a western Canadian regional health authority. The caregivers were asked to describe their relationships with home care nurses. Data was analyzed using symbolic interactionism. While the caregivers acknowledged the reciprocal nature of the relationships and their role in building the relationship, the behaviours of the home care nurse were influential to the relationship. The findings showed that the frequency and continuity of contact as well as the length of contact between the nurse and the family caregiver were factors that influenced the quality of the relationship. Conversation, socializing, and sharing information were also important. Nurses who demonstrated affection, acknowledgment, respect, commitment, knowledge, and understanding were appreciated.

The results of this study identify that the concept of relationship takes into consideration a view of competent delivery of appropriate care as well as the caregiver's feelings of trust, familiarity, comfort, and security. The resultant conceptual model links relationship preconditions (i.e., time and frequency of contact) and relational demonstrations (i.e., affection, respect, and knowledge) with perceived quality of the relationship and perceived quality of care.

### Discussion Questions

1. Identify key descriptors and dimensions of effective relationships and discuss the importance of these in a CHN's daily practice.

2. Describe ways in which the CHN can develop or support the development of these relational qualities.

3. Identify how organizational systems and structures could promote or prevent the development of the relationships and how that would impact the perceived quality of care.

of Canadian substantive theories that provide guidance and direction for some specific areas of community health nursing are included in Table 7.6. This table provides information about the nature of these substantive theories as well as some practice examples to illustrate them, and their links to the CHNC (2011, revised) standards of practice. One substantive theory is highlighted.

## A Theory of Maternal Engagement with Public Health Nurses and Family Visitors

This grounded theory was developed by a group of Canadian nurses and epidemiology researchers Jack, DiCenso, and Lohfeld (2005). They describe the process by which mothers identified as being at risk of poor parenting practices engage with PHNs. This theory helps PHNs identify client perceptions about the provision of home visits and highlights the importance of developing a trusting relationship between mothers and the public health nurse. Mothers often cope with feelings of vulnerability and powerlessness during the initial phase of engagement with an unfamiliar nurse, working to protect their families and limit their vulnerability. This involves moving through the phases of *overcoming fear*, *building trust*, and *seeking mutuality*. To increase the effectiveness of home visiting and to establish a connected relationship, this theory guides the CHN to understand and assimilate the perspectives of mothers as they move through the above three phases in establishing a relationship. The CHNC standard 4, professional relationships (2011, revised), is supported by this substantive theory.

## Theories Originating in Other Disciplines

As discussed previously, CHNs often use theories from other disciplines to inform their practice; for example, the stages of change (Prochaska, DiClemente, & Norcross, 1992). This theory considers the various stages of change that individuals progress through, such as precontemplation, contemplation, determination, action, and maintenance, in dealing with addictive or other problem behaviours (Prochaska et al., 1992). In Jason's situation, it might be that his parents recognize that their addiction to smoking not only affects the health of their family but also places an additional economic strain on the household. They may have tried unsuccessfully to quit in the past, but using this approach, the CHN may help them to anticipate and work through the challenges of quitting.

The theory of diffusion of innovation by Rogers has also been used by CHNs in assisting community members to take up new approaches. This theory is described as "the process through which an innovation, defined as an idea perceived as new, spreads via certain communication channels over time among the members of a social system" (Rogers, 2004, p. 13). In an effort to improve the availability of fresh fruits and vegetables in Jason's impoverished neighbourhood, a CHN might facilitate the establishment of a "good food box" system in the hope that it would benefit not only Jason's family but many other families in the area as well. CHNC standards (2011, revised) relating to health promotion and health maintenance reflect both of these theories. See the last section of Table 7.1 for a long but not exhaustive list of theories from other disciplines that CHNs might use.

| Table 7.6 | Practice or Substantive Theories | |
|---|---|---|
| **Practice Theory** | **Key Points** | **Relationship to CHNC (2011, revised) Standards of Practice and Examples from CHN Practice** |
| Theory of maternal engagement with public health nurses and family visitors (Jack et al., 2005) | This grounded theory, developed by Canadian nurses and epidemiology researchers, describes the process by which mothers identified as being at risk of poor parenting practices engage with public health nurses (PHNs). This theory helps PHNs to identify client anxieties and perceptions related to the provision of home visits. It highlights the importance of the development of a trusting relationship between mothers and the PHNs. | CHNC standards 4 and 5 are particularly relevant to this theory. Home visits are a key strategy for PHNs in providing support for parents of young children. To increase the effectiveness of home visiting and to establish a relationship, it is essential for nurses to engage in a process of building trust, seeking mutuality, and understanding the perspectives of mothers. |
| Supportive care model (Davies & Oberle, 1990) | This Canadian model of support in palliative nursing considers six dimensions of nursing care: valuing, maintaining integrity, connecting, empowering, doing for, and finding meaning. This model focuses on CHN practice at the individual and family levels. | This model aligns well with CHNC standard 3, health maintenance, restoration, and palliation; with standard 4, professional relationships; and with standard 5, building capacity. The palliative care work that home health nurses do involves individuals as well as their families. |
| Theory of hope (Duggleby & Wright, 2005) | This Canadian theory describes the process through which palliative patients live with hope and acknowledge life as it is. This theory discusses how health status can be assessed and mutual plans developed among nurse, client, and family in order to maximize the abilities of the individual and family within the context of the community. | Home health nurses working with patients requiring palliative care consider how individuals and families endure and cope with suffering. This model aligns with CHNC standard 3, health maintenance, restoration, and palliation; standard 4, professional relationships; and standard 5, building capacity. |
| Model of family caregiver relationships with home health providers (Funk & Stajduhar, 2011, 2013) | This Canadian model considers the relationship between home health nurses and families, particularly during end-of-life experiences, and looks at ways to enhance those relationships and the satisfaction with those services. | This model is particularly relevant to home health nurses in their work with palliative patients, and it connects directly to CHNC standard 3, health maintenance, restoration, and palliation. |

## CASE STUDIES

Below are two case studies that reflect common situations CHNs could be confronted with in their practice. A brief summary of each case study is followed by a description and application of a theory used to guide community health nursing practice. Also included is a brief discussion of how some of the components of our organizing framework are reflected in each case. The first story is about a young family struggling to get by. The second story presents the struggle of two people who are married, both of whom are living with chronic conditions. A link to each case study is provided to learn more about each story.

### Case Study #1: Della's Story

Watch Della's story at the following link: www.saskatoonpoverty2possibility.ca/The-starting-point.html.

A working poor family from Saskatoon living in a run-down neighbourhood struggles with the demands of life. Social and economic conditions are known to affect health status, increasing the risk of poorer mental and physical health outcomes for the family members living in these conditions. Inequalities lead to health disparities between neighbourhoods and populations. When these differences are avoidable, unfair, and systematic (National Collaborating Centre for Determinants of Health, 2013), they are considered inequities and require intervention at multiple levels. However, when a CHN enters into a situation with disadvantaged families with young children, the nurse needs to keep in mind that not everyone may be open to sharing personal aspects of their life. A CHN needs to realize that a trusting and open relationship with a mother may take time to establish.

One theory addressing relationship is the theory of maternal engagement with PHNs and family visitors (Jack et al., 2005). This theory was developed by Canadian nurse and epidemiology researchers and describes the process by which mothers identified as being at risk of poor parenting practices engage with PHNs. The theory highlights the importance of developing a trusting relationship as well as the need for nurses to continually be aware of the quality of those relationships especially in the initial phase of engagement with a nurse.

The middle range nursing theory of critical caring is also useful and informative to the nurses working with this family. One element of this theory is the preparation of self for interactions with clients and families. It is important to take the time to be aware of yourself as a CHN and of your planned approach to any given individual, family or community situation. See Canadian Research Box 7.1 for more information about this theory.

Another way to approach this situation is through relational inquiry. Canadian nurses Gweneth Hartrick Doane and Colleen Varcoe (Hartrick Doane & Varcoe, 2005) describe relational inquiry as one with roots in complexity theory and in which the relationships among individuals, situations, contexts, processes, and environments continually connect and affect each other. Using this approach to family nursing encourages CHNs to recognize and relate to differences between themselves as nurses and the people with whom they are working. To promote health and healing, the nurse fosters a therapeutic relationship by facilitating an atmosphere in which individuals, families, or community members feel comfortable, secure, and valued enough to express themselves freely.

While all of the details about Della's circumstances are not known, issues of oppression and sexism are likely at play. These are key components of feminist theory, which is a critical theoretical perspective and which attends closely to the injustices and unfair circumstances experienced by women. Oppression and sexism are also social determinants of health (McGibbon, 2012). A CHN visiting Della's family might incorporate all seven CHNC standards of practice (2011, revised), including health maintenance, restoration, and palliation, to address Della's immediate health needs. When nurses and families do not have the same priorities, tensions that might surface include resistance to involvement with the CHN despite the supports and resources that are available. In this situation the CHN works with the family to access the most appropriate community resource available and, when unavailable, advocates for consideration to develop it in collaboration with the community. PHNs are often confronted with the tension between the health of an individual and population health. Core concepts in this situation are many and include cultural safety, health promotion, and a strengths-based approach.

### Discussion Questions

1. What role do you think the public health nurse could take if it turned out that Della was pregnant again?

2. What other oppressive forces could be at play in Della's situation?

3. How do you think these circumstances will affect the future of Della's children?

#### Case Study #2: A Story about Care

This is a palliative and end-of-life care story illustrative of home health nursing. Please go to this link www.youtube.com/watch?v=GhhAo-MiVVs and watch the video entitled "A story about care." In this vignette, Jim Mulcahy shares his experience with end-stage lymphoma and that of his wife Sarah who is living with Huntington's disease. He talks about how meaningful a simple and genuine touch is. Jim's story demonstrates the power of a caring relationship with healthcare providers who can see the person and not merely the disease. After viewing this video, consider how a CHN working with home health could relate to the individuals and families with whom she or he works, and see people holistically, as complex individuals who have a life outside and apart from their medical history.

Canadian nurse scholars Betty Davies and Kathy Oberle developed the supportive care model for palliative nursing that consists of six central dimensions of nursing care (Davies & Oberle, 1990). The first of these dimensions is valuing or the attitude that a nurse brings toward the person she or he is caring for. The second dimension is maintaining integrity of the nurse in terms of psychological, moral, and emotional well-being. Following that is connecting, which relates to establishing a relationship. Empowering involves helping people to identify and develop their inner strength to do what they need or would like to do. "Doing for" comprises the physical care provided to individuals. And finally, finding meaning involves making personal sense of what is happening or has happened. This enables CHNs to feel that they are doing the best they can to contribute to the healing of a patient.

In the same vein, Duggleby and Wright (2005) offer a theory of hope related to elderly palliative patients—how they endure and cope with suffering. This theory describes the process through which these patients live with hope and acknowledge life as it is. Both models align with CHNC standard 3, health maintenance, restoration, and palliation, and with standard 4 regarding professional relationships (2011, revised). These theories reflect the way in which health status can be assessed and mutual plans developed among nurse, client, and family that maximize the abilities of the individual and family within the context of the community. Core community health nursing concepts that are significant in this case study and in the supportive care model include caring, a strengths-based approach, hope, well-being, relationships, and empowerment.

A broad theoretical perspective that is reflected in this example is socialecological theory, in that the nurse needs to consider the multiple influences at play, which have an impact on the health and well-being of patients and their families.

As healthcare has changed, greater focus has been placed on tasks, doing of procedures, and "doing for" clients even in the home setting. However, this model urges nurses to maintain a focus of care on people as whole persons and not solely on procedures and administrative aspects of care. With that being said, there are challenges that could confront a home health nurse, including a heavy caseload, time constraints, or other unexpected events. However, a key aspect of promoting health is the development of a therapeutic relationship throughout the course of care.

### Discussion Questions

1. How would you ensure that you are prepared to develop a relationship with a palliative patient?

2. In addition to providing direct care to Jim, how will you support the family?

3. How will you support Jim to live with hope, recognizing that you have limited time to spend given your heavy caseload?

# CONCLUSION

In this chapter the importance of theory in guiding community health nursing practice and research is emphasized. There has been limited development of theories, however, that are specific to the phenomena that concern CHNs. Clearly, more theory development is needed so that the work of CHNs at the community and population levels is informed by theories that explicitly reflect our concerns and do not have to be adapted from theories developed in an illness context for the care of individuals. At the same time, while there are few community health nursing theories per se, there has been a considerable amount of theoretical development in community health nursing that reflects a broad synthesis of knowledge from the public health sciences, social sciences, and nursing. This development was illustrated in an organizing framework which drew on the CHNC professional practice model graphic (theoretical foundations).

Drawing on nursing's metaparadigm, CHNs have developed a unique metaparadigm that defines the concepts in ways that reflect their phenomena of concern, explains the levels of practice, and places social justice at the core. CHNs' work has been informed for many years by theoretical perspectives such as social ecological theory, feminism, and critical social theory and more recently by emerging perspectives such as complexity science, postcolonial theory, and intersectionality. CHNs have also developed a range of models and frameworks to guide research and practice that (a) draw from the core theoretical concepts of community health nursing, (b) reflect CHNs' values base, (c) direct action at the multiple levels of intervention for CHNs, ranging from the individual to society, and (d) encompass the full range of community health nursing competencies across the continuum of care, including health promotion, disease prevention, health maintenance and restoration, and palliation.

Through Jason's story, it is evident that the core concepts of community health nursing and the kinds of actions that might be taken to address community health issues are related and interconnected as well as common to all the theoretical perspectives, models, frameworks, and theories discussed in this chapter. Jason's story demonstrates how the living conditions in which people are born, live, and play influence their health and increase the chances of preventable injury. These unfair and avoidable circumstances are commonly referred to as the social determinants of health, where an imbalance of money, resources, opportunity, and power result in health inequities between people in society. Actions to address these conditions that ensure access to health (versus access to healthcare) take place at multiple levels, and CHNs work at all of these levels. CHNs do not work solely with individuals to help them address the problems they encounter after they occur, but they work upstream to prevent them from occurring—not only for the individuals concerned but for the communities of which they are members. CHNs collaborate and work with families, communities, and populations as well as at the political level to build capacity for people to take action on improving their own health, advocating for the determinants of health in order to promote equity and social justice.

Finally, community health nursing has a very broad scope of practice, and the values and principles underlying community health nursing practice require a diverse and extensive knowledge base grounded in theory, research, and practical experience,

all of which are intimately interconnected. Theory informs the conduct of community health nursing research, which produces the evidence used to guide the practice of CHNs in educational, administrative, and practitioner roles. At the same time, in an iterative fashion, research and the practical experience of nurses working in diverse community roles and settings contribute to community health nursing theory development.

# KEY TERMS

beliefs    p. 109
capacity building    p. 102
caring    p. 102
collaboration    p. 102
community health nurse (CHN)    p. 101
concepts    p. 102
conceptual frameworks    p. 101
conceptual models    p. 101
cultural safety    p. 102
determinants of health    p. 102
epidemiology    p. 102
ethics    p. 109
grand theory    p. 121
health equity    p. 102
health promotion    p. 102
informal theories    p. 102
knowledge    p. 101
levels of practice    p. 106
metaparadigm    p. 103
middle range theory    p. 109
nursing theory    p. 102
patterns of knowing    p. 102
phenomena    p. 102
philosophical foundations    p. 101
population focus    p. 102
practice theory    p. 121
prevention    p. 102
professional practice model    p. 102
public health science    p. 102
social justice    p. 102
social sciences    p. 102
strengths-based approach    p. 102
theoretical foundations    p. 101
theory development    p. 101
theory    p. 101
values    p. 101, 109

# STUDY QUESTIONS

1. Which of the following elements make up the CHN metaparadigm?

    a. Health, healing, person, environment, and nursing

    b. Person, environment, nursing, health, and social justice

    c. Person, health, nursing, and environment

    d. Communities, nursing, prevention, equity, and environment

2. Which of the following components contribute to the theoretical foundations of community health nursing?

a. Determinants of health, prevention, health inequities

b. Practical experience, research

c. Grand nursing theories

d. Social ecological theory, feminist theory, complexity theory

e. Values, beliefs, and ethics

f. All of the above

3. How are theory, research, and practice integrated?

4. What key concepts in CHN practice are drawn from public health?

5. Name the key Canadian documents that support and inform CHN practice.

6. Why is the individual-based approach to community health nursing so widespread? How is the individual-based approach to health promoted in current theories?

> After working through these questions, go to the MyNursingLab at www.pearsoned.ca/mynursinglab to check your answers.

## INDIVIDUAL CRITICAL-THINKING EXERCISES

1. The Canadian Public Health Association (CPHA, 2010) states that "The public/CHN combines knowledge from public health science, primary health care (including the determinants of health), nursing science, and the social sciences" (p. 8). Given this statement, what aspects of nursing science do nurses bring to the practice of community or PHN?

2. In order to enhance cultural safety, it is important for healthcare providers to reflect on and consider their own values, beliefs, and biases. Reflect on the influences in your life that might shape your approach to client care.

3. Some nurses believe that theory is not relevant to nursing practice. What do you think about this statement, and why? What factors contribute to this belief about the relevance of theory to practice?

4. What kind of theory might you use as a CHN working with a family with multiple health problems? What would support you in the use of that theory?

5. When a PHN provides immunizations to an individual, how does this contribute to population health? What is one conceptual model that helps to explain this?

## GROUP CRITICAL-THINKING EXERCISES

1. Some portions of the population tend to experience greater health inequities than others; for example, First Nations populations or families living in poverty. Discuss with your group how a postcolonial perspective might help you to view this situation differently.

2. Discuss how a social ecological view might influence health promotion activities related to improving childhood immunization rates in a small community.

3. Using critical social theory, brainstorm and then discuss strategies you would use to address Jason's situation. How would you go about advocating for policies that would help to address preventable injuries in Jason's community (i.e., what would be your first steps)?

## REFERENCES

Ajzen, I. (1991). The theory of planned behavior. *Organizational Behavior and Human Decision Processes, 50,* 179–211.

Albrecht, M. N. (1990). The Albrecht model for home health care: Implications for research, practice, and education. *Public Health Nursing, 7*(2), 118–126.

Allen, D. G. (1985). Nursing research and social control: Alternative models of science that emphasize understanding and emancipation. *Image: The Journal of Nursing Scholarship, 17*(2), 58–64.

Anderson, E. T., & McFarlane, J. M. (1988). *Community as client: Application of the nursing process.* Philadelphia, PA: J.B. Lippincott Company.

Anderson, E. T., & McFarlane, J. M. (1996). *Community as partner: Theory and practice in nursing* (2nd ed.). Philadelphia, PA: Lippincott.

Anderson, R. A., Crabtree, B. E., Steele, D. J., McDaniel, J., & Reuben, R. (2005). Case study research: The view from complexity science. *Qualitative Health Research, 15*(5), 669–685.

Argyris, C., & Schön, D. (1974). *Theory in practice: Increasing professional effectiveness.* San Francisco, CA: Jossey-Bass.

Association of Community Health Nursing Educators. (2010). Research priorities for public health nursing. *Public Health Nursing, 27*(1), 94–100.

Bandura, A. (1977). Self-efficacy: Toward a unifying theory of behavioral change. *Psychological Review, 84*(2), 191–215.

Baylis, F., Kenny, N., & Sherwin, S. (2008). A relational account of public health ethics. *Public Health Ethics, 1*(3), 196–209.

Bigbee, J. L., & Issel, M. (2012). Conceptual models for population focused public health nursing interventions and outcomes: State of the art. *Public Health Nursing, 29*(4), 370–379.

Bowlby, J. (1969). *Attachment and loss: Vol. 1 Attachment.* New York, NY: Basic Books.

Bowleg, L. (2012). The problem with the phrase "women and minorities": Intersectionality—an important theoretical framework for public health. *American Journal of Public Health, 102*(7), 1267–1273.

Bronfenbrenner, U. (1979). *The ecology of human development: Experiments by nature and design.* Cambridge, MA: Harvard University Press.

Browne, A. J., Varcoe, C. M., Wong, S. T., Smye, V. L., Lavoie, J., Littlejohn, D., . . . Lennox, S. (2012). Closing the health equity gap: Evidence-based strategies for primary health care organizations. *International Journal for Equity in Health, 11*(59), 1–15.

Browne, A. J. (2001). The influence of liberal political ideology on nursing science. *Nursing Inquiry, 8*(2), 118–129.

Browne, A. J. (2004). Response to critique of "The influence of liberal political ideology on nursing science." *Nursing Inquiry, 11*(2), 122–123.

Browne, A. J., Smye, V. L., & Varcoe, C. (2005). The relevance of postcolonial theoretical perspectives to research in Aboriginal health. *Canadian Journal of Nursing Research, 27*(4), 16–37.

Butterfield, P. G. (1990). Thinking upstream: Nursing a conceptual understanding of the societal context of health behavior. *Advances in Nursing Science, 12*(2), 1–8.

Butterfield, P., & Postma, J. (2009). The TERRA framework: Conceptualizing rural environmental health inequities through an environmental justice lens. *Advances in Nursing Science, 32*(2), 107–117.

Byrne, D., & Callaghan, G. (2014). *Complexity theory and the social sciences: The state of the art.* New York, NY: Routledge.

Canadian Nurses Association. (2006). *Social justice . . . a means to an end, an end in itself.* Ottawa, ON: Author.

Canadian Nurses Association. (2008). *Code of Ethics for Registered Nurses.* Ottawa, ON: Author.

Canadian Nurses Association. (2015). *Advocacy.* Reprinted with permission. Further reproduction prohibited. Retrieved from https://www.cna-aiic.ca/en/advocacy

Canadian Public Health Association. (2010*). Public health – Community health nursing practice in Canada: Roles and activities*. Ottawa, ON: Author. Retrieved from http://www.cpha.ca/uploads/pubs/3-1bk04214.pdf

Capra, F. (1996). *The web of life: A new synthesis of mind and matter*. London, UK: HarperCollins.

Castellani, B., & Hafferty, F. W. (2009). *Sociology and complexity science: A new field of inquiry*. Berlin, Germany: Springer.

Carper, B. (1978). Fundamental patterns of knowing in nursing, *Advances in Nursing Science, 1*(1), 13–23.

Chinn, P. L., & Kramer, M. K. (2008). *Integrated theory and knowledge development in nursing* (7th ed.). St. Louis, MO: Elsevier, Mosby.

Chinn, P. L., & Kramer, M. K. (2011). *Integrated theory and knowledge development in nursing.* (8th ed.). St. Louis, MO: Elsevier, Mosby.

Chopoorian, T. J. (1986). Reconceptualizing the environment. In P. Moccia (Ed.), *New approaches to theory development.* New York, NY: National League for Nursing.

Cilliers, P. (1998). *Complexity and postmodernism: Understanding complex systems*. London, UK: Routledge.

Clark, M. J. (1999). *Nursing in the community: Dimensions of community health nursing*. Stamford, Conn: Appleton & Lange.

Clarke, P. N. (1998). Nursing theory as a guide for inquiry in family and community nursing. *Nursing Science Quarterly, 11*(12), 47–48.

Cohen, B., & Reutter, L. (2007). Development of the role of public health nurses in addressing child and family poverty: A framework for action. *Journal of Advanced Nursing, 60*(1), 96–107.

Community Health Nurses of Canada. (2008). *Canadian community health nursing standards of practice.* Toronto, ON: Author.

Community Health Nurses of Canada. (2011, revised). *Canadian community health nursing: Professional practice model & standards of practice.* St. John's, NL: Author. Retrieved from https://www.chnc.ca/documents/ CHNC-ProfessionalPracticeModel-EN/index.html.

Community Health Nurses of Canada. (2013). *Canadian community health nursing professional practice model.* Toronto, ON: Author.

Corbin, J., & Tomm Bonde, L. (2012). Intersections of context and HIV/AIDS in sub-Saharan Africa: What can we learn from feminist theory? *Perspectives in Public Health, 132*(8), 8–9.

Dalton, J. M. (2003). Development and testing of the theory of collaborative decision-making in nursing practice for triads. *Journal of Advanced Nursing, 41*(1), 22–33.

Davidson, A. W., Ray, M. A., & Turkel, M. C. (Eds.). (2011). *Nursing, caring, and complexity science: For human-environment well-being.* New York, NY: Springer Publishing Co.

Davies, B., & Oberle, K. (1990). Dimensions of the supportive role of the nurse in palliative care. *Oncology Nursing Forum, 17*(1), 87–94.

Duggleby, W., & Wright, K. (2005). Transforming hope: How elderly palliative patients live with hope. *Canadian Journal of Nursing Research, 37*(2), 70–84.

Duggleby, W., Wright, K., Williams, A., Degner, L., Cammer, A., & Holtslander, L. (2007). Developing a living with hope program for caregivers of family members with advanced cancer. *Journal of Palliative Care, 23*(1), 24–31.

Edwards, N., Mill, J., & Kothari, A. (2004). Multiple intervention research program in community health. *Canadian Journal of Nursing Research, 36*(1), 40–55.

Elder, G. H. (1996). Human lives in changing societies. In R. B. Cairns, G. H. Elder, & E. J. Costello (Eds.), *Developmental science* (pp. 31–62). Melbourne, Australia: Cambridge University Press.

Falk-Rafael, A. R. (2000). Watson's philosophy, science, and theory of human caring as a conceptual framework for guiding community health nursing practice. *Advances in Nursing Science, 23*(2), 34–49.

Falk-Rafael, A. R. (2005a). Speaking truth to power: Nursing's legacy and moral imperative. *Advances in Nursing Science, 28*(3), 212–223.

Falk-Rafael, A. R. (2005b). Advancing nursing theory through theory-guided practice: The emergence of a critical caring perspective. *Advances in Nursing Science, 28*(1), 38–49.

Falk-Rafael, A. R., & Betker, C. (2012a). Witnessing social injustice downstream and advocating for health equity upstream: "The trombone slide" of nursing. *Advances in Nursing Science, 35*(2), 98–112.

Falk-Rafael, A. R., & Betker, C. (2012b). The primacy of relationships: A study of public health nursing practice from a critical caring perspective. *Advances in Nursing Science, 35*(4), 315–332.

Fawcett, J., & DeSanto-Madeya, S. (2013). *Contemporary nursing knowledge: Analysis and evaluation of nursing models and theories* (3rd ed). Philadelphia, PA: F. A. Davis Co.

Ferketich, A. L., Phillips, L. R., & Verran, J. A. (1990). Comprehensive Multi-Level Nursing Model for Rural Hispanics. (Agency for Health Care Policy and Research Grant HSO 6801-01). Bethesda, MD: Agency for Health Care Policy and Research.

Flaskerud, J., & Winslow, B. (1998). Conceptualizing vulnerable populations health related research. *Nursing Research, 47*(2), 69–78.

Funk, L., & Stajduhar, K. (2011). Analysis and proposed model of family caregivers' relationships with home health providers and perceptions of the quality of formal services. *Journal of Applied Gerontology, 32*(2), 188–206.

Gambino, M. (2008). Complexity and nursing theory: A seismic shift. In C. Lindberg, S. Nash, & C. Lindberg (Eds.), *On the edge: Nursing in the age of complexity* (pp. 49–72). Bordentown, New Jersey: PlexusPress.

Gottlieb, L. N., & Gottlieb, B. (2013). *Strengths-based nursing care: Health and healing for person and family*. New York, NY: Springer Publishing Company.

Gottlieb, L., & Rowat, K. (1987). The McGill model of nursing. *Advances in Nursing Science, 9*(4), 51–61.

Government of Canada. (1985). *Canada Health Act*. Retrieved from http://laws-lois.justice.gc.ca/eng/acts/C-6

Green, R. (2013). Application of the self-care deficit nursing theory: The community context. *Self-Care, Dependent-Care and Nursing, 20*(1), 5–15.

Gregson, J., Foerster, S. B., Orr, R., Jones, L., Benedict, J. Clarke, . . . Zotz, K. (2001). System, environmental and policy changes: Using the social-ecological model as a framework for evaluating nutrition education and social marketing programs with low-income audiences. *Journal of Nutrition Education, 33*, S4–S15.

Hamilton, N., & Bhatti, T. (1996). *Population health promotion: An integrated model of population health and health promotion*. Ottawa, ON: Public Health Agency of Canada.

Hamilton, P. A., & Bush, H. A. (1988). Theory development in community health nursing: Issues and recommendations. *Scholarly Inquiry for Nursing Practice, 2*(2), 145–160.

Hartrick Doane, G., & Varcoe, C. (2005). *Family nursing as relational inquiry: Developing health-promoting practice*. Philadelphia, PA: Lippincott Williams & Wilkins.

Hartrick Doane, G., & Varcoe, C. (2007). Relational practice and nursing obligations. *Advances in Nursing Science, 30*(3), 192–205.

Hartrick Doane, G., & Varcoe, C. (2008). Knowledge translation in everyday nursing: From evidence-based to inquiry-based practice. *Advances in Nursing Science, 31*(4), 283–295.

Held, D. (1980). *Introduction to critical theory: Horkheimer to Habermas*. Berkeley, CA: University of California Press.

Helvie, C. O. (1981). *Community health nursing: Theory and practice*. New York, NY: Harper & Row.

Henderson, V. (1966). *The nature of nursing: A definition and its implications for practice, research, and education*. New York, NY: McMillan.

hooks, b. (2000). *Feminist theory: From margin to center* (2nd ed). London, UK: Pluto Press.

Jack, S. K., DiCenso, A., & Lohfeld, L. (2005). A theory of maternal engagement with public health nurses and family visitors. *Journal of Advanced Nursing, 49*(2), 182–190.

Keller, L. O., & Strohschein, S. (2012). Population-based public health nursing practice: The intervention wheel. In M. Stanhope & J. Lancaster (Eds.), *Public health nursing: Population-centered health care in the community* (8th ed., pp. 186–215). Maryland Heights, MO: Elsevier.

Keller, L. O., Strohschein, S., & Schaffer, M. A. (2011). Cornerstones of public health nursing. *Public Health Nursing, 28*(3), 249–260.

Keller, L. O., Strohschein, S., Lia-Hoagberg, B., & Schaffer, M. (2004a). Population-based public health interventions: Practice-based and evidence supported. Part 1. *Public Health Nursing, 21*(5), 453–468.

Keller, L. O., Strohschein, S., Schaffer, M., & Lia-Hoagberg, B. (2004b). Population-based public health interventions: Innovation in practice, teaching and management. Part II. *Public Health Nursing, 21*(5), 469–487.

Keller, L. O., Strohschein, S., Lia-Hoagberg, B., & Schaffer, M. (1998). Population-based public health nursing interventions: A model from practice. *Public Health Nursing, 15*(3), 207–215.

Keller, L. O., Strohschein, S., & Briske, L. (2012). Population-based public health nursing practice: The intervention wheel. In M. Stanhope & J. Lancaster (Eds.), *Public health nursing – Revised reprint: Population-centered health care in the community* (8th ed.). Maryland Heights, MO: Elsevier.

King, I. M. (1981). *A theory for nursing: Systems, concepts, process*. New York, NY: Wiley & Sons.

Kleffel, D. (1991). Rethinking the environment as a domain of nursing knowledge. *Advances in Nursing Science, 14*(1), 40–51.

Kleffel, D. (1996). Environmental paradigms: Moving toward an ecocentric perspective. *Advances in Nursing Science, 18*(4), 1–10.

Knowles, M. S. (1978). Andragology: Adult learning theory in perspective. *Community College Review, 5*(3), 9–20.

Koh, H. K., Brach, C., Harris, L. M., & Parchman, M. L. (2013). A proposed "health literate care model" would constitute a systems approach to improving patients' engagement in care. *Health Affairs, 32*(2), 357–367.

Kretzmann, J. P., & McKnight, J. L. (1993). *Building communities from the inside out: A path toward finding and mobilizing a community's assets*. Chicago, IL: ACTA Publications.

Krieger, N. (1994). Epidemiology and the web of causation: Has anyone seen the spider. *Social Science & Medicine, 39*(7), 887–903.

Krieger, N. (2001). Theories for social epidemiology in the 21st century: An ecosocial perspective. *International Journal of Epidemiology, 30*(4), 668–677.

Kuehnert, P. L. (1995). The interactive and organizational model of community as client: A model for public health nursing practice. *Public Health Nursing, 12*(1), 9–17.

Kulbok, P. A., Laffrey, S. C., & Chitthathairatt, S. (2008). Integrating muiltilevel approaches to promote community health. In M. Stanhope & J. Lancaster, (Eds.), *Public health nursing: Population-centered health care in the community* (7th ed.). St. Louis, MO: Mosby Elsevier.

Kulig, J. (2000). Community resiliency: The potential for the development of community health nursing theory. *Public Health Nursing, 17*(5), 374–385.

Kuss, T., Proulx-Girouard, L., Lovitt, S., Katz, C. B., & Kennelly, P. (1997). A public health nursing model. *Public Health Nursing, 14*(2), 81–91.

Labonte, R. (1993). Health promotion and empowerment: Practice frameworks. *Centre for Health Promotion, HP-10-0102*.

Laferriere, R. H. (1995). Orem's theory in practice: Hospice nursing care. *Home Healthcare Nurse, 13*(5), 50–54.

Laffrey, S. C., & Craig, D. M. (1995). Health promotion for communities and aggregates: An integrated model. In M. Stewart (Ed.), *Community nursing: Promoting Canadians' health* (pp. 125–145). Toronto, ON: W. B. Saunders.

Laffrey, S. C., & Kulbok, P. A. (1999). An integrative model for holistic community health nursing. *Journal of Holistic Nursing, 17*(1), 88–103.

Laffrey, S. C., & Craig, D. M. (2000). Health promotion for communities and aggregates: An integrative model. In M. Stewart (Ed.), *Community nursing: Promoting Canadians' health* (pp. 105–125). Toronto, ON: W. B. Saunders.

Last, J. M. (Ed.). (2007). *A dictionary of public health*. New York, NY: Oxford University Press.

Leininger, M. (Ed.). (1978). *Transcultural nursing: Concepts, theories, and practice*. New York, NY: John Wiley & Sons.

Leipert, B. D. (2001). Feminism and public health nursing: Partners for health. *Scholarly Inquiry for Nursing Practice, 15*(1), 49–62.

Levy, B. S., & Sidel, V. W. (2006). The nature of social injustice and its impact on public health. In B. S. Levy & V. W. Sidel (Eds.), *Social injustice and public health* (pp. 5–24). New York, NY: Oxford University Press.

Lewin, K. (1951). *Field theory in social science: Selected theoretical papers by Kurt Lewin*. D. Cartwright (Ed.). Oxford, England: Harpers.

Lindeman, E. C. (1923). Aspects of community organization in relation to public policy. *Annals of the American Academy of Political and Social Science, 105*, 83–87.

Lopez-Cantor, M. T. (2012). Transitional care. In F. Chiappelli, X. M. C. Brant, & C. B. Cajulis (Eds.), *Comparative effectiveness and efficacy research and analysis for practice (CEERAP)* (pp. 165–180). New York, NY: Springer.

MacDonald, M. (2004). From miasma to fractals: The epidemiology revolution and public health nursing. *Public Health Nursing, 21*(4), 380–391.

MacDonald, M. (2001). Health promotion: Historical, philosophical and theoretical perspectives. In L. E. Young & V. E. Hayes (Eds.), *Transforming health promotion practice: Concepts, issues, and applications* (pp. 22–45). Philadelphia, PA: F. A. Davis Co.

MacDonald, M. (2013). Public health ethics. In J. Storch, P. Rodney, & R. Starzomski (Eds.), *Toward a moral horizon: Nursing ethics for leadership and practice* (pp. 398–429). Toronto, ON: Pearson.

Masters, K. (2011), Models and theories focused on nursing goals and functions. J. B. Butts & K. L. Rich (Eds.), *Philosophies and theories for advanced nursing practice* (pp. 383–412). Sudbury, MA: Jones & Bartlett Learning.

May, K. M., Phillips, L. R., Ferketich, S. L., & Veraan, J. A. (2003). Public health nursing: The generalist in a specialized environment. *Public Health Nursing, 20*(4), 252–259.

McEwen, M. (2011). Overview of theory in nursing. In M. McEwen & E. M. Wills (Eds.), *Theoretical basis for nursing* (3rd ed.). Philadelphia, PA: Lippincott, Williams & Wilkins.

McGibbon, E. A. (2008). Health and health care: A human rights perspective. In D. Raphael (Ed.), *Social determinants of health: A Canadian perspective*. Toronto, ON: Canadian Scholars' Press.

McGibbon, E. A. (2012). People under threat. In E. A. McGibbon (Ed.), *Oppression: A Social Determinant of Health*. Halifax, NS: Fernwood Publishers.

McGibbon, E. A., & Etowa, J. (2009). *Anti-racist health care practice*. Toronto, ON: Canadian Scholars' Press.

McKnight, J., & Van Dover, L. (1994). Community as client: A challenge for nursing education. *Public Health Nursing, 11*(1), 12–16.

McLaren, L., & Hawe, P. (2005). Ecological perspectives in health research. *Journal of Epidemiology and Community Health, 59*, 6–14.

Meleis, A. I. (2012). *Theoretical nursing: Development and progress*. (5th ed.). Philadelphia, PA: Lippincott Williams & Wilkins.

Minkler, M. (1989). Health education, health promotion, and the open society. *Health Education and Behavior, 16*(1), 17–30.

Minkler, M. (Ed.). (2005). *Community organizing and community building for health*. New Brunswick, NJ: Rutgers University Press.

Munro, M., Gallant, M., MacKinnon, M., Dell, G., Herbert, R., MacNutt, G., . . . Roberston, K. (2000). The Prince Edward Island conceptual model for nursing: A nursing perspective of primary health care. *Canadian Journal of Nursing Research, 32*(1), 39–55.

National Collaborating Centre for Determinants of Health. (2013). *Let's talk: Health equity*. Antigonish, NS: NCCDH, St. Francis Xavier University.

National Collaborating Centre for Public Health. (2012). *What are the Social Determinants of Health?* Retrieved from http://www.nccph.ca/docs/NCCPHSDOHFactsheet_EN_May2012.pdf

Neal, L. J. (1999). The Neal theory: Implications for practice and administration. *Home Healthcare Nurse, 17*(3), 181–187.

Neuman, B. N. (1972). A model for teaching total person approach to patient populations. *Nursing Research, 21*(3), 264–269.

Neuman, B. (1995). *The Neuman sytems model* (3rd ed.). Norwalk, CT: Appleton & Lange.

Newman, M. A. (1986). *Health as expanding consciousness*. St. Louis, MO: Mosby.

Nightingale, F. (1946). *Notes on nursing*. Philadelphia, PA: Edward Stern & Company. (Original work published 1859).

Orem, D. E. (1985). *Nursing: Concepts of practice* (3rd ed.). New York, NY: McGraw Hill.

Parse, R. R. (1992). Human becoming: Parse's theory of nursing. *Nursing Science Quarterly, 5*, 35–42.

Parse, R. R. (2003). *Community: A human becoming perspective*. Sudbury, MA: Jones & Bartlett Learning.

Pauly, B. M., MacKinnon, K., & Varcoe, C. (2009). Revisiting "Who gets care?" Health equity as an arena for nursing action. *Advances in Nursing Science, 32*(2), 118–127.

Pender, N. J. (1996). *Health promotion in nursing practice* (3rd ed.). Stamford, CT: Appleton & Lange.

Peplau, H. E. (1952). *Interpersonal relations in nursing*. New York, NY: G. P. Putnam's Sons.

Perkins, H. W. (Ed.). (2003). *The social norms approach to preventing school and college age substance abuse: A handbook for educators, counselors, and clinicians*. San Francisco, CA: Jossey-Bass.

Peterson, S. J. (2009). Introduction to the nature of nursing knowledge. In S. J. Peterson & T. S. Bredow (Eds.), *Middle range theories: Application to nursing research* (2nd ed., pp. 3–45). Philadelphia, PA: Lippincott Williams & Wilkins.

Pfettscher, S. (2010). Florence Nightingale 1820–1910: Modern nursing. In M. R. Alligood & A. M. Tomey (Eds.), *Nursing theorists and their work* (7th ed., pp. 71–90). St. Louis, MI: Mosby Elsevier.

Plsek, P., & Greenhalgh, T. (2001). The challenge of complexity in health care. *British Medical Journal, 323*(7313), 625–628.

Poliferoni, E. C. (2011). Philosophy of science: An introduction. In J.B. Butts & K. L. Rich (Eds.), *Philosophies and theories for advanced nursing practice* (pp. 3–18). Sudbury, MA: Jones & Bartlett Learning.

Porta, M. (2008). *Dictionary of epidemiology*. New York, NY: Oxford University Press.

Prochaska, J. O., & DiClemente, C. C. (1985). Common processes of change in smoking, weight control, and psychological distress. In S. Shiffman & T. Wills (Eds.), *Coping and substance abuse* (pp. 345–363). San Diego, CA: Academic Press.

Prochaska, J. O., DiClemente, C. C., & Norcross, J. C. (1992). In search of how people change: Applications to addictive behaviors. *American Psychologist, 47*(9), 1102–1114.

Ray, M. (1989). The theory of bureaucratic caring for nursing practice in the organizational culture. *Nursing Administration Quarterly, 13*(2), 31–42.

Ray, M. A., Turkel, M. C., & Cohn, J. (2011). Relational caring complexity: The study of caring and complexity in health care hospital organizations. In A. W. Davidson, M. A. Ray, & M. C. Turkel (Eds.), *Nursing, caring, and complexity science: For human-environment well-being* (pp. 95–117). New York, NY: Springer Publishing.

Reimer-Kirkham, S., Varcoe, C., Browne, A. J., Lynam, M. J., Khan, K. B., & McDonald, H. (2009). Critical inquiry and knowledge translation: Exploring compatibilities and tensions. *Nursing Philosophy, 10*, 152–166.

Reimer-Kirkham, S., Baumbusch, J. L., Schultz, A. S. H., & Anderson, J. (2009). Knowledge development and evidence-based practice: Insights and opportunities from a postcolonial feminist perspective for transformative nursing practice. In P. G. Reed & N. B. Crawford Shearer (Eds.), *Perspectives on nursing theory* (5th ed., pp. 349–364). Philadelphia, PA: Wolters Kluwer Health; Lippincott Williams & Wilkins.

Reutter, L., & Kushner, K. (2010). Health equity through action of the social determinants of health: Taking up the challenge in nursing. *Nursing Inquiry, 17*(3), 269–280.

Reutter, L. (1984). Family health assessment—An integrated approach. *Journal of Advanced Nursing, 9*, 391–399.

Rice, R. (1994). Conceptual framework for nursing practice in the home: The Rice model of dynamic self-determination. *Home Healthcare Nurse, 12*(2), 51–53.

Rogers, E. M. (2002). Diffusion of preventive innovations. *Addictive Behaviors, 27*, 989–993.

Rogers, E. M. (2004). A prospective and retrospective look at the diffusion model. *Journal of Health Communication, 9*, 13–19.

Rogers, M. E. (1983). Science of unitary human beings: A paradigm for nursing. In I. W. Clements & F. B. Roberts (Eds.), *Family health: A theoretical approach to nursing care* (pp. 219–227). New York, NY: John Wiley & Sons.

Rogers, W. A., (2006). Feminism and public health ethics. *Journal of Medical Ethics, 32*, 351–354. doi:10.1136/jme.2005.013466

Romanow, R. (2002). *Building on values: The future of health care in Canada, final report*. Commission on the Future of Health Care in Canada: National Library of Canada.

Roy, C. (1987). Roy's adaptation model. In R. R. Parse (Ed.), *Nursing science: Major paradigms theories and critiques* (pp. 35–45). Philadelphia, PA: W. B. Saunders.

Ruland, C. M., & Moore, S. M. (1998). Theory construction based on standards of care: A proposed theory of the peaceful end of life. *Nursing Outlook, 46*(4), 169–175.

Shareck, M., Frohlich, K. L., & Poland, B. (2013). Reducing social inequities in health through settings related interventions – a conceptual framework. *Global Health Promotion, 20*(2), 39–52.

Schultz, P. R. (1987). When client means more than one: Extending the foundational concept of person. *Advances in Nursing Science, 10*(1), 71–86.

Sheilds, L. E., & Lindsey, A. E. (1998). Community health promotion nursing practice. *Advances in Nursing Science, 20*(4), 23–36.

Shim, S., Benkert, R., Bell, S., Walker, D., & Danford, C. (2007). Social justice: Added metaparadigm concept for urban health nursing. *Public Health Nursing, 24*(1), 73–80.

Sills, G., & Goeppinger, J. (1985). The community as a field of inquiry in nursing. *Annual Review of Nursing Research, 3*, 1–57.

Smith, D., Varcoe, C., & Edwards, N. (2005). Turning around the intergenerational impact of residential schools on Aboriginal people: Implications for health policy and practice. *Canadian Journal of Nursing Research, 37*(4), 38–60.

Smith, D. A., Edwards, N. C., Martens, P. J., & Varcoe, C. (2007). Making a difference: A new care paradigm for pregnant and parenting Aboriginal people. *Canadian Journal of Public Health, 98*(4), 321–325.

Smith, K., & Bazini-Barakat, N. (2003). A public health nursing practice model: Melding public health nursing principles with the nursing process. *Public Health Nursing, 20*(1), 42–48.

Smith, M. J. (2003). Evaluation of middle range theories for the discipline of nursing. In M. J. Smith & P. R. Liehr (Eds.), *Middle range theory for nursing* (pp. 189–211). New York, NY: Springer Publishing.

Squires, L., Peinado, S., Berkman, N., Boudewyns, V., & McCormack, L. (2012). The health literacy skills framework. *Journal of Health Communication: International Perspectives.* doi:10.1080/10810730.2012.713442

Strecher, V. J., & Rosenstock, I. M. (1997). The health belief model. In A. Baum, S. Newman, J. Weinman, R. West, & C. McManus (Eds.), *Cambridge handbook of psychology, health and medicine* (pp. 113–116). New York, NY: Cambridge University Press.

Strega, S. (2005). The view from the poststructural margins: Epistemology and methodology reconsidered. In L. Brown & S. Strega (Eds.), *Research as resistance: Critical, indigenous and anti-oppressive approaches* (pp. 199–236). Toronto, ON: Canadian Scholars' Press.

Stevens, P. E. (1989). A critical social reconceptualization of environment in nursing: Implications for methodology. *Advances in Nursing Science, 11*(4), 56–68.

Stevens, P. E., & Hall, J. M. (1992). Applying critical theories to nursing in communities. *Public Health Nursing, 9*(1), 2–9.

Stewart, M. (2000). Framework based on primary health care principles. In M. Stewart (Ed.), *Community nursing: Promoting Canadians' health* (pp. 58–82). Toronto, ON: W. B. Saunders.

Stokols, D. (1992). Establishing and maintaining healthy environments: Toward a social ecology of health promotion. *American Psychologist, 47*(1), 6–22.

Stokols, D. (1996). Translating social ecological theory into guidelines for community health promotion. *American Journal of Health Promotion, 10*, 282–298.

Taylor, S. G., & McLaughlin, K. (1991). Orem's general theory of nursing and community nursing. *Nursing Science Quarterly, 4*(153), 153–160.

Taylor, S. G. (2001). Orem's general theory of nursing and families. *Nursing Science Quarterly, 14*(7), 7–9.

Van Herk, K. A., Smith, D., & Andrew, C. (2011). Examining our privileges and oppressions: Incorporating an intersectionality paradigm into nursing. *Nursing Inquiry, 18*(1), 29–39.

VanHerk, K. A., Smith, D., & Tedford Gold, S. (2012). Safe care spaces and places: Exploring urban Aboriginal families' access to preventive care. *Health and Place, 18,* 649–656.

Vollman, A. R., Anderson, E. T., & McFarlane, J. (2003). *Canadian community as partner.* Philadelphia, PA: Lippincott Williams & Wilkins.

Vollman, A. R., Anderson, E. T., & McFarlane, J. M. (2008). *Canadian community as partner: Theory and practice in nursing.* Philadelphia, PA: Lippincott Williams & Wilkins.

Vollman, A. R., Anderson, E. T., & McFarlane, J. (2012). *Canadian community as partner: Theory and multidisciplinary practice* (3rd ed.). Philadelphia, PA: Wolters Kluwer; Lippincott Williams & Wilkins.

Von Bertalanffy, L. (1972). The history and status of general systems theory. *Academy of Management Journal, 15*(4), 407–426.

Walby, S., Armstrong, J., & Strid, S. (2012). Intersectionality: Mulitple inequalities in social theory. *Sociology, 46*(2), 224–240.

Watson, J. (1979). *Nursing: The philosophy and science of caring.* Boston, MA: Little, Brown & Co.

Watson, J. (2012). *Human caring science.* Sudbury, Massachusetts: Jones & Bartlett.

Westley, F., Zimmerman, B., & Patton, M.Q. (2007). *Getting to maybe: How the world is changed.* Toronto, ON: Vintage Canada.

White, J. (1995). Patterns of knowing: Review, critique and update. *Advances in Nursing Science, 17*(4), 73–86.

White, M. S. (1982). Construct for public health. *Nursing Outlook, 30,* 527–530.

Whitehead, M., & Dahlgren, G. (2006). *Concepts and principles for tackling social inequities in health: Levelling up* (Part 1). Geneva, Switzerland: World Health Organization.

Williams, D. M. (1989). Political theory and individualistic health promotion. *Advances in Nursing Science, 12*(1), 14–25.

Wodak, A. (1999). What is this thing called harm reduction? *International Journal of Drug Policy, 10,* 169–171.

World Health Organization. (2010). *Backgrounder 3: Key concepts.* Used by permission of World Health Organization. Retrieved from http://www.who.int/social_determinants/final_report/key_concepts_en.pdf

World Health Organization Commission on Social Determinants of Health. (2008). *Closing the gap in a generation: Health equity through action on the social determinants of health.* Geneva, Switzerland: Author.

Wright, L. M., & Leahey, M. (2012). *Nurses and families: A guide to family assessment and intervention* (6th ed.). Philadelphia, PA: F. A. Davis Co.

Yiu, L. (2008). Community care. In L. L. Stamler & L. Yiu (Eds.), *Community health nursing: A Canadian perspective* (2nd ed., pp. 176–195). Toronto, ON: Pearson Canada Inc.

Yiu, L. (2012). Community care. In L. L. Stamler & L. Yiu (Eds.), *Community health nursing: A Canadian perspective* (3rd ed., pp. 213–235). Toronto, ON: Pearson Canada Inc.

## ABOUT THE AUTHORS

**Claire Betker**, RN, BN, MN, PhD(c), CCHN(C), has worked as a registered nurse in community health for more than 30 years at local, regional, provincial, and national levels in mental health, home health, primary health care, and public health. Most recently she was the Senior Knowledge Translation Specialist with the National Collaborating Centre for Determinants of Health. Claire has been very involved with the Community Health Nurses of Canada in Manitoba and nationally, participating in several standing committees and serving as president and past president. Claire served on the board of directors of the Canadian Nurses Association (2010–2014) as the representative for the Canadian Network of Nursing Specialties. In 2010, Claire was awarded the Canadian Public Health Association and the Public Health Agency of Canada's Human Resources Individual Award for her contribution to public health workforce development in Canada. She is currently a PhD candidate at the University of Saskatchewan, College of Nursing, where her interest is in theory and its contribution to public health nursing practice and leadership development.

**Marjorie MacDonald**, RN, PhD, is a Professor with the School of Nursing at the University of Victoria Faculty of Human and Social Development. Marjorie's research interests include public health nursing, public health policy and practice, health services research related to public health services and systems renewal, primary health care,

adolescent health promotion, smoking and drug use prevention, adolescent health literacy, and advanced practice nursing, particularly in a public health context. Marjorie is the president of the B.C. Public Health Association.

**Mary E. Hill**, RN, BScN, PhD(c), MEd, was formerly a manager of Child, Youth, and Family Services with the Vancouver Island Health Authority in the Cowichan Valley as well as in Langford, Ladysmith, and Nanaimo. She has over 35 years of experience in public health nursing and community health services management. She has maintained a particular interest in perinatal services, breastfeeding supports, and tobacco prevention activities. Currently, she is a full-time student in the doctoral program in nursing at the University of Victoria, where she is exploring the effectiveness of PHN practice with vulnerable perinatal women.

**Megan Kirk,** RN, PhD(c), MSc, BScN, is currently a nursing doctoral student at the University of Victoria. She has been interested in the area of prevention within both of her graduate degrees. In her master's thesis, she explored the influence of work hours on the cardiovascular health of female hospital employees. Now, in her doctorate, she is focusing on the work of public health nurses and elucidating the impact of their efforts on the health and well-being of individuals, families, communities, and populations. She hopes to highlight the difference that public health nurses make in the communities they serve.

# Health Promotion

*Candace Lind, Melanie Lind-Kosten, and Sylvia Loewen*

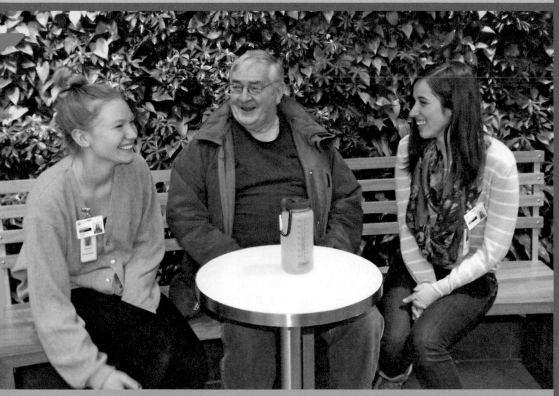

*Source: Courtesy of Nikita Baker*

## LEARNING OUTCOMES

**After studying this chapter, you should be able to:**

1. Define and describe the concepts of health and health promotion.

2. Identify key issues that have blocked implementation of recommendations from the seven global health promotion conferences.

3. Describe the origins and characteristics of the population health promotion model.

4. Identify and discuss nursing interventions that exemplify the three levels of prevention: primary, secondary, and tertiary.

5. Describe the differences between upstream and downstream approaches to addressing health issues in a population.

6. Describe the concept of primary health care and identify its values, principles, and elements.

7. Define social marketing and discuss the "four Ps" of marketing.

8. Describe values, beliefs, and attitudes that guide community health nursing practice and promote a collaborative partnership approach to health promotion.

## INTRODUCTION

Canada is credited with being a birthplace of the worldwide **health promotion** movement. Health promotion is a complex social and political process that has been the focus of much international discussion over the last few decades; however, many of the large-scale potential benefits of health promotion have yet to be realized. Numerous complex factors have affected the advancement of health promotion, which are discussed in this chapter. The chapter starts with an overview of health, including definitions of health, health promotion, and primary health care. The history of primary health care and health promotion, including the Ottawa Charter and subsequent international or global charters for health promotion, are presented. Population health promotion and the population health promotion model are introduced and discussed. The sections that follow include risk communication, population health indicators, levels of prevention, upstream approaches to promoting health, harm reduction, the health belief and other social-behavioural models, and social marketing. The chapter closes with a focus on the important nursing values, beliefs, and attitudes necessary for health-promoting practice, relationship development and partnership approaches to practice, nursing advocacy and activism, and future directions for health promotion.

# DEFINITIONS OF HEALTH

**Health** is a difficult concept to define. The Oxford etymological dictionary (Hoad, 1996) describes health as a state of sound body, mind, and spirit; a state of wholeness. The traditional Euro-Canadian understanding of health and healthcare rests within the biomedical model where health has been understood as the absence of disease and illness, rather than a state of wholeness. From a biomedical perspective, to achieve health one needs only attend to physical pathology (Kaplan, 2000). However, health is more than a static biomedical concept. Health is a dynamic process with multiple assumptions and understandings that evolve over time and evolve with varying professional perspectives and purpose. Although the practice of medicine views health mainly through the biomedical model, nursing has defined the concept of health as an evolving, holistic human experience, informed by multiple professions, recognizing the medical definition is just one aspect of health (Payne, 1983).

Promoting health is the foundation of nursing practice (Canadian Nurses Association, 2009). Nurses work alongside multiple professions (in interprofessional teams) to promote, support, maintain, and restore health in individuals, families, and communities. The international concept of health had been disease focused until 1946, when the World Health Organization (WHO) broadened the definition from just the absence of disease to "a state of complete physical, mental and social well-being and not merely the absence of disease or infirmity" (WHO, 1948, para. 1). This change in the conceptualization of health shifted the understanding of health away from disease control to include more comprehensive aspects of being human. This broad definition of health has been adopted as a foundational understanding to inform many professions concerned with the health of humans and societies. With a need to expand on the notion of health as a state of complete well-being, health-related professions have adapted the WHO's definition to create definitions tailored to inform and guide their unique practices. Nursing, anthropology, sociology, and social work are some professions that have adopted the WHO's definition, adding their own unique views of health to meet the needs of their professional focus. For example, anthropology (the study of human societies and cultures) defines the concept of health as being bound within the political, economic, and religious domains of a society (Kleinman & Petryna, 2001). Within the practice of sociology, person-centred care (PCC) is a movement to expand healthcare's definition of health to include human capabilities, such as the ability to use imagination and senses to enjoy everyday experiences (Frank, 2013). This movement identifies the value of social factors, capabilities, and strengths of a person, as well as the quality of the healthcare provider–client relationship, as important considerations of a person's overall health (Frank, 2013; Venkatapura, 2013). The profession of social work considers health within the broad context of integrating services to improve function, longevity, and access to quality care (Fisher & Elnitsky, 2012).

These broad concepts of health have been adopted to guide nurses to help people in living up to their full potential mentally, physically, spiritually, and socially, so they can experience a life worth living. CHNs define health as "a resource for everyday life that is influenced by circumstances, beliefs and the determinants of health" (Community Health Nurses Association of Canada, 2008, p. 10). Founded on the principles of social justice, community health nurses strive to promote and protect the health of individuals, families, and communities regardless of where they live, work, or play (CHNAC, 2008). Nursing's holistic view of health acknowledges that it can be a unique experience for individuals, families, and communities. Individuals or families may view health through a lens aligned with their immediate needs: being able to socialize with friends during rapidly declining health, having a supportive family in the face of crisis or life-altering illness, having a warm meal and place to sleep on a cold night, or having the right to happiness as well as the freedom and autonomy to live life one's own way. Community members hold values and preferences that differ from mainstream society, where being healthy may mean living without fear of persecution. Within the broad and inclusive lens of social justice, health may mean living in a just and fair society where equitable distribution of resources can support universal education, access to equitable healthcare, and the freedom to contribute as a full member of society with equal rights, privileges, and rewards (CNA, 2010). Health might be described as having support to live to one's full potential within a family, community, or society that can love, support, and care for its members.

# DEFINITIONS OF HEALTH PROMOTION

Health promotion has a long history in Canada and globally; however, its full implementation continues to be challenging. Health promotion is still sometimes narrowly used or conceptualized as the equivalent of health education. Health education is a common information-sharing health promotion strategy used to increase people's knowledge, and oftentimes used to assist with individual behavioural change or to help produce more healthful environments. However, health education is only one of several key components and action areas of health promotion, as illustrated in the Ottawa Charter and the population health promotion model (PHPM) below. What is health promotion? According to the WHO,

> **Health promotion** is the process of enabling people to increase control over, and to improve, their health. To reach a state of complete physical, mental and social well-being, an individual or group must be able to identify and to realize aspirations, to satisfy needs, and to change or cope with the environment. Health is, therefore, seen as a resource for everyday life, not the objective of living. Health is a positive concept emphasizing social and personal resources, as well as physical capacities. Therefore, health promotion is not just the responsibility of the health sector, but goes beyond healthy lifestyles to well-being. (2009a, p. 1)

This definition is the most widespread in use and remains unchanged since the landmark 1986 **Ottawa Charter for Health Promotion** was written, as an outcome from the

First International Conference on Health Promotion. The WHO's health promotion glossary of terms adds that health promotion represents a comprehensive social and political process. Therefore, health promotion actions must go beyond simply strengthening people's skills and abilities to manage their own health and instead move toward action to change social, environmental, and economic conditions to alleviate their impact on public and individuals' health (WHO, 1998). People are helped to increase control over the determinants of their health as the means of improving their health. Health promotion should be an integral part of nursing practice in any setting. Nurses must work together with people to understand their needs from their perspectives and work within those perspectives to set up the conditions to facilitate healthy change—and help people feel empowered to create the changes that will help themselves. In recent years, the increased need for political advocacy, investment in strategies that address the determinants of health, building health promotion capacity, and partnership development have been deemed critical for dealing with the challenges of living in an increasingly global world (Smith, Tang, & Nutbeam, 2006). Health promotion is often viewed as a process or a framework in which people work together to create conditions that sustain health and address broader social and economic conditions that affect a population's health (Fawcett et al., 2010) by applying a wide range of activities and approaches to achieve outcomes (Raphael, 2010). In essence, health promotion seeks to enhance people's ability to exercise control over the environmental, social, and behavioural conditions that affect their quality of life. Health promotion strategies encourage citizen engagement in improving the determinants of health and well-being, which improves quality of life (Raphael, 2010). Health promotion therefore goes well beyond simply addressing healthy lifestyles, to improve overall well-being. Health promotion is an amalgamation of values and practices that promote health. Health promotion has also been described as a combination of educational, political, regulatory, or organizational activities or conditions of living that are conducive to the health of individuals or communities (McKenzie, Neiger, & Thackeray, 2013). Partnerships and community involvement have been described as the main contributing factors that achieve long-term impacts (Franco-Paredes, Zeuli, Hernandez-Ramos, & Santos-Preciado, 2010).

Raeburn and Rootman (2007) stated that health promotion has a positive and action-oriented nature, whereby it builds healthiness rather than just focuses on prevention or treatment of illness and other conditions. Ultimately, "health promotion aims to reduce differences in health status and vulnerability, and to ensure equal opportunities and resources to enable all people to achieve their fullest health potential and quality of life" (Frankish, Moulton, Rootman, Cole, & Gray, 2006, p. 176). Therefore, "health promotion represents a comprehensive social and political process, it not only embraces actions directed at strengthening the skills and capabilities of individuals, but also action directed toward changing social, environmental and economic conditions so as to alleviate their impact on public and individual health" (Hills, Carroll, & Vollman, 2007, p. 330).

Nurses act upon many levels and across many sectors of society to promote the health of people. The **social determinants of health** are just as important, and often can be even more important than the biological or physical determinants of a person's health. Therefore, although caring for people when they are sick or injured is an important component of nursing work, nursing practice is not just focused on looking after people in hospitals or in their homes when they are ill, or focused on teaching them about health. Nursing must also be involved in activism, advocacy, and other ways of creating social change to improve people's health. Cathy Crowe's multifaceted work to raise awareness and address the issues of homelessness and Cheryl Forchuk's work advocating for discharged mental health patients' safe integration into communities are Canadian examples of nursing activism efforts to raise awareness and create change to improve people's health.

# PRIMARY HEALTH CARE

Health promotion is a component of **primary health care (PHC)**. PHC is defined as

> essential health care based on practical, scientifically sound and socially acceptable methods and technology made universally accessible to individuals and families in the community through their full participation and at a cost that the community and country can afford to maintain at every stage of their development in the spirit of self-reliance and self-determination. It forms an integral part both of the country's health system, of which it is the central function and main focus, and of the overall social and economic development of the community. It is the first level of contact of individuals, the family and community with the national health system bringing health care as close as possible to where people live and work, and constitutes the first element of a continuing health care process." (WHO, 1978, pp. 2–3)

**Primary care** is sometimes confused with PHC; however, primary care is a narrower concept that refers to a person-centred comprehensive approach (often biomedical) to care delivery at the point of entry into the healthcare system (WHO, 2008). For example, nurse practitioners working in the community provide primary care services to clients, and their practices may also be informed by the values and principles of PHC.

The WHO describes PHC as the route to better health for all, with five key elements required to achieve that goal:

- reducing exclusion and social disparities in health (universal coverage reforms);
- organizing health services around people's needs and expectations (service delivery reforms);
- integrating health into all sectors (public policy reforms);
- pursuing collaborative models of policy dialogue (leadership reforms); and
- increasing stakeholder participation (WHO, 2013a, p.1).

# Primary Health Care Values, Principles, and Elements

The underlying values of PHC are social justice and equity. Social justice refers to the fair distribution of society's benefits and responsibilities, and focuses on eliminating the root causes of inequities (CNA, 2010), leading to equality of opportunities for health. Equity refers to the fair distribution of resources for health. Philosophically, PHC permeates all of society and social justice, and equity directs nursing's focus toward improving the health of the most disadvantaged, thereby giving all people the same opportunities for health and quality of life. Strategically, PHC strategies may focus on developing strengths or assets; offering opportunities for change to address deficits or needs; maximizing the involvement of the community; including all sectors that impact the determinants of health (but avoiding duplication of services); and using only health methods and technologies that are accessible, acceptable, affordable, and appropriate for each situation (University of Saskatchewan, 2011).

There are five principles of PHC: accessibility, public participation, health promotion, appropriate technology, and intersectoral collaboration or co-operation. Accessibility means that healthcare is universally available to all people regardless of geographic community and is delivered in a timely manner. This means the distribution of healthcare providers must include rural, remote, and urban communities. However, barriers to accessibility go well beyond geographic barriers—they can also refer to barriers created by healthcare providers' assumptions about, or biases against, certain groups of people. For example, if a healthcare provider refuses to provide sexually transmitted infection screening to a lesbian couple because of a belief that sexually transmitted infections occur primarily through heterosexual transmission, this is an accessibility barrier. Additionally, healthcare providers who actively stigmatize vulnerable populations (such as people living with homelessness, people with addictions, or people involved in the sex trade) by the way they treat them in emergency departments are also creating barriers to accessible healthcare service. People who feel discriminated against may avoid seeking healthcare when needed because of fear of stigmatization.

The second principle of PHC is public participation. This means people are actively encouraged to participate in making decisions about their own health and in identifying the health needs of their communities. The design and delivery of healthcare must be flexible, responsive, and ensure respect for diversity. Through health promotion, people build understandings about the social determinants of health and develop skills to improve and maintain their own health and well-being.

Appropriate technology means that the appropriate modes of care are available based on a society's social, economic, and cultural development. Equity is an important component of appropriate technology. Appropriate technology does not mean an MRI in every village; rather, it means that alternatives to high-cost or high-technology services must be developed in many environments. Appropriate models of healthcare must be developed and tested before implementation.

Intersectoral collaboration or co-operation means that because health and well-being are linked to economic and social policy, intersectoral collaboration is needed to establish national and local health goals, healthy public policies, and planning and evaluation of health services. Providers from different health professions and sectors of society must collaborate and function interdependently to meet the needs of the public. They must all also participate in government policy formation that impacts the health and well-being of people in their society.

Optimal PHC approaches involve full participation of the community of people they will impact. Community involvement includes development, coordination, delivery, and evaluation of initiatives and should include laypeople, community leaders, and practitioners with primary health care implementation experience and expertise. The WHO has outlined eight essential components of PHC, and these are used as guiding principles to set direction and measure success:

1. *Education about health problems and prevention techniques.* Education serves the purpose of identifying and preventing (or controlling) dominant health challenges for a target population. A solid understanding of primary health care and the health challenges for the target population is necessary before the first steps are taken to create healthier populations. Research and application of knowledge occur throughout the process.

2. *Promotion of food supply and proper nutrition.* This element includes the provision of an appropriate, nutritious food supply. In developing nations the focus is on providing an adequate food supply for the population, whereas in developed countries such as Canada, strategies focus more on obesity and nutrition (Canadian Obesity Network, 2013).

3. *Adequate supply of safe water and basic sanitation.* Basic sanitation includes removal of garbage and safe disposal of bodily waste products.

4. *Maternal and child healthcare, including family planning.* Evidence shows that adequate and quality health services are associated with improvements in maternal, perinatal, neonatal, and child mortality rates and health outcomes. In 2010, worldwide approximately 287 000 women died of pregnancy- and childbirth-related complications and most of these could have been avoided if the pregnant women had access to quality skilled care before, during, and after childbirth (WHO, 2013b).

5. *Immunization against major infectious diseases.* If the vaccines currently available were widely administered, two million deaths per year could be averted among children under five years old (WHO, 2009b).

6. *Prevention and control of locally endemic diseases.* Endemic diseases are those that are prevalent in people in a particular group, community, or region, but in relatively low numbers. A Canadian example of an endemic disease is tuberculosis in northern

Canada populations. A multifaceted PHC approach is required to eradicate this endemic disease (Health Canada, 2012).

7. *Appropriate treatment of common diseases and injuries using the PHC principle of appropriate technology.* Appropriate technology means using the right intervention or initiative, at the right time, so that the needs of the entire population are met. It is based on the best scientific evidence demonstrating effectiveness. It also includes using the right resources and the right healthcare providers, based on the local economy, using the PHC value of equity.

8. *Provision of essential drugs* (WHO, 2013c). Drugs sustain and can improve life in the case of many chronic illnesses, providing an otherwise unattainable higher quality of life for many people.

Implementation of the PHC elements may be hampered by numerous factors, such as political will, cultural values (including race, age, or gender biases), lack of resources, or inadequate infrastructure. Poor outcomes of PHC initiatives may also result from misguided but well-intended decisions that reflect the values and norms of the dominant culture rather than those that involve the target population in all levels and aspects of decision making, from resource allocation to the parameters of projects or initiatives. In recognition of this type of bias, the Canadian Institutes of Health Research (2013) developed the Institute of Aboriginal Peoples' Health to better understand why Aboriginal morbidity and mortality rates are significantly worse than non-Aboriginal Canadians' rates, and to promote innovative research that will serve to improve the health of Aboriginal people in Canada. Before receiving research funding, researchers must have demonstrated a good relationship with the Aboriginal community they seek to work with, including consultation, information sharing, partnering with Aboriginal community members, and demonstrating respect for the community.

# HISTORY OF PRIMARY HEALTH CARE AND HEALTH PROMOTION

Canada is considered an international leader in the **health promotion movement, population health,** and PHC (Canadian Public Health Association, 2010). Almost immediately after Canada became a country in 1867, Canadians began lobbying for improvements to the determinants of health, such as safe water and sewage disposal systems, and for the government to take action on overcrowded and slum housing, poverty, malnutrition, and unsafe food and milk supplies (Canadian Public Health Association, 2010). An early example of the principles of PHC arose in the 1940s in Canada. Members of the Co-operative Commonwealth Federation (CCF) political party in Saskatchewan (under Tommy Douglas's leadership) were concerned that the poorest people in the province could not afford hospital services. They implemented a provincial hospital insurance program in 1947. Eliminating exclusion from healthcare services based on

inability to pay for services was also the rationale for introducing a national hospital insurance program in 1957, a program which paid hospitalization fees for all Canadians. Despite this program, the inability to pay a doctor's fees remained common. Therefore, in 1966 Canada instituted a national medicare program that would pay for costs incurred for treating people in hospital, clinics, and doctors' offices (Canadian Health Coalition, 2009). Healthcare service is one component of PHC. Addressing the needs of the poor ensured that they could receive healthcare services, and this became a precursor to future PHC initiatives.

From 1974 to 1994 the Canadian federal government played a large part in establishing Canada as a leader in health promotion. This began with the release of "A new perspective on the health of Canadians" in 1974 written by Marc Lalonde, then Minister of National Health and Welfare, Canada, currently called Health Canada. Four elements of the health field concept were presented: human biology, environment, lifestyle, and healthcare organization. The purpose of this working document was to unfold a new perspective on the health of Canadians and stimulate interest in future health programs for Canada. However, it achieved much more. It shifted national thinking toward health promotion, albeit mainly focused on lifestyles, and led to the establishment of Canada as an initiator and world leader in health promotion. Participaction, a well-known program encouraging individual exercise and healthy living, was launched in the 1970s as one initiative resulting from the Lalonde Report (Participaction Archive Project, n.d.).

In Canada, the health promotion programs that arose from the Lalonde Report were under-resourced, and the public face of health promotion became focused on lifestyle programs such as tobacco, alcohol, drugs, and nutrition. What was not taken forward well from the report was the call for a focus on environment as one of the causes of ill health. Lalonde had identified environmental risks as those that include the physical and social environments. He stated, "One of the most important but least understood environmental problems is the effect of rapid social change on the mental and physical health of Canadians . . . [and] the number of economically deprived Canadians is still high, resulting in a lack of adequate housing and insufficient or inadequate clothing. All the foregoing environmental conditions create risks which are a far greater threat to health than any present inadequacy of the healthcare system" (Lalonde, 1974, p. 18). In 1974, Lalonde stated that the healthcare system is mainly oriented to treating illness, which, unfortunately, remains the case today. Most healthcare dollars are still allocated for acute care or hospital treatment.

The Lalonde Report received international attention, helping stimulate the WHO to convene a meeting of member countries to address the disparities in health status between developed and undeveloped countries. In 1978, an international conference on PHC resulted in the Declaration of Alma-Ata (WHO, 1978). An important component of the declaration was the statement that health "is a fundamental human right and that the attainment of the highest possible level of health is a most important worldwide social goal whose realization requires the action of many other social and economic sectors in addition to the health sector" (WHO, 1978, p. 1). This declaration drew attention to the inequalities in healthcare status between high-income and low-income countries and stated that interventions should be practical, scientifically sound, socially acceptable, and universally accessible to individuals and families in the community, at a cost the people and country could afford. Community participation at all levels of intervention should, as much as possible, use local resources, including educating and hiring indigenous healthcare professionals.

In 1978 Canada established a Health Promotion Directorate, the first of its kind in the world. This directorate formed a comprehensive national program of public information on lifestyle issues, promoting a social climate supportive of healthy lifestyles, supported self-help, and citizen participation. The Health Promotion Directorate also promoted the adoption of health promotion programs within healthcare, social welfare, and other programs.

In 1984 the WHO wrote a small discussion document on the concept and principles of health promotion, introducing the principles of involving the population as a whole and directing action to the determinants of health. This was taken up in a 1985 Canadian federal policy review initiated by federal bureaucrats and supported by Honourable Jake Epp, the Federal Minister of Health at the time. In 1986 the minister released a report titled "Achieving Health for All: A Framework for Health Promotion," more commonly called the Epp Report. This report defined the three mechanisms of health promotion as (a) self-care, (b) actions people take to help each other cope, and (c) healthy environments (Epp, 1986). As a part of setting a new direction, Minister Epp agreed to host the First International Conference on Health Promotion in Ottawa, Ontario, in collaboration with the WHO and the Canadian Public Health Association. The conference representatives built on the Epp Report, creating the Ottawa Charter for Health Promotion, which contributed to establishing Canada as a leader in PHC—in addition to leadership in health promotion. Although the Alma-Ata declaration stated that the spirit of social justice is important in attaining health for all through PHC, the Ottawa Charter emphasized social justice more strongly when it stated that the prerequisites for health included peace, shelter, education, food, income, a stable ecosystem, sustainable resources, social justice, and equity (WHO, Health and Welfare Canada, & CPHA, 1986). The Ottawa Charter is still used worldwide today, and its continuing value has been reaffirmed repeatedly during a further seven international conferences on health promotion.

## THE OTTAWA CHARTER FOR HEALTH PROMOTION

The **first international conference on health promotion** was held in Ottawa, Ontario, in November 1986 with 212 participants from 38 countries (WHO et al., 1986). This conference resulted in the production of the Ottawa Charter for Health Promotion. The document was intended to be a worldwide charter for action, presenting strategies and approaches for health promotion that were considered vital for major progress toward individual and collective commitment to an ambitious goal of "Health for All by the Year 2000" in a movement toward a "new public health."

A logo that represented this call for action was developed to include the following key components in a schematic representation (see Figure 8.1). The main graphic elements of the health promotion logo are one outer circle, one inner circle, and three wings that originate from this inner circle, one of which is breaking the outside circle. The logo incorporates five key action areas for health promotion:

a. Building healthy public policy. This means health must be on the agenda of policy makers across all sectors and levels of society—not just the health sector.

b. Creating supportive environments for health. The way that society is organized (e.g., living and working conditions) must be addressed, as health cannot be separated from other goals.

c. Strengthening community action. At the heart of this action strategy is community empowerment—for communities to have a greater sense of ownership and control over their own endeavours and destinies. Community development is an important component of this strategy.

d. Developing personal skills. Enhancing people's life skills enables them to exercise more control over their own health. Education and institutional action are required.

e. Reorienting health services toward preventing diseases and promoting health. The responsibility for health promotion in health services is one that is shared by all citizens; we must work together toward creating a healthcare system that contributes to the pursuit of health. (WHO et al., 1986).

The outside circle represents the goal of building healthy public policies, symbolizing the need for policies to "hold things together." The three wings inside the circle symbolize the need to address all key action areas of health promotion identified in the Ottawa Charter in an integrated and complementary manner. The upper wing that is breaking the outer circle suggests that society and communities, as well as individuals, are constantly changing and, therefore, the policy sphere has to constantly react and develop to reflect these changes to enable building healthy public policies. The inner circle of the logo represents the three basic strategies for health promotion: enabling (strategies that ensure equal opportunity for people to achieve health), mediating (strategies that mediate between different sectors of society), and advocating (strategies that aim to make social and other conditions favourable for health), which are needed and applied to all health promotion action areas. Overall, the logo (Figure 8.1) is a visual representation of a comprehensive, multi-strategy approach to health promotion. Health promotion applies diverse strategies and methods in an integrated manner for effective action. Since 1986, the WHO has kept this symbol as the health promotion logo. It has undergone some visual modifications for

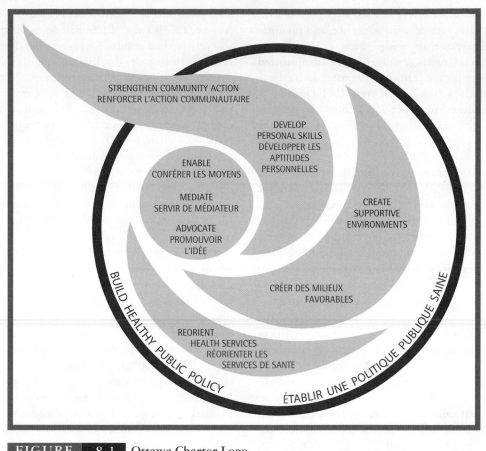

FIGURE 8.1 Ottawa Charter Logo

*Source:* World Health Organization, Health and Welfare Canada, & Canadian Public Health Association. (1986). *Ottawa charter for health promotion.* Ottawa, ON: Author.

subsequent health promotion conferences, but its essence has remained the same.

The Ottawa Charter remains the key policy document of the international health promotion movement (Lindstrom & Eriksson, 2009). Although the Ottawa Charter included social justice as a key prerequisite for health, it has more recently been criticized from the perspective of low-income or resource-poor countries for not having been explicit in the need to access human rights (Perkins, 2009).

## Other Charters for Health Promotion

To date, there have been eight global conferences on health promotion. The **second international conference on health promotion** was held in Adelaide, South Australia, in 1988. Health was asserted as a human right and a sound social investment; therefore, health is a fundamental social goal (WHO, 2009a). Recommendations arose for people's involvement in health policy creation and co-operation between sectors of society (WHO, 2009a). In 1991 the **third international conference on health promotion** was held in Sweden. At the time of this conference, public concern about global environmental threats had grown and the need for a focus on sustainable development was highlighted (WHO, 2009a). The call for action that arose from this conference

included addressing inequities and social justice, with millions of people living in extreme poverty and deprivation in increasingly degraded environments. Women were particularly highlighted as a population that remains oppressed in much of the world, with sexual exploitation and discrimination hampering their meaningful contributory capacity in creating supportive environments for health (WHO, 2009a). Education was declared a basic human right and a key catalyst to causing the political, economic, and social change required to ensure health. Military expenditure was identified as causing much more than deaths and disability to populations; it was also recognized as the cause of new forms of **"ecological vandalism"** (WHO, 2009a).

The **fourth international conference on health promotion** was held in Jakarta, Indonesia, in 1997. This was the first such conference held in a low-income country and involving the private sector in supporting health promotion (WHO, 2009a). Health promotion action was declared to have a marked impact on the social determinants of health and was the path to improving human rights and reducing inequities in health status. Poverty was identified as the greatest threat to health (WHO, 2009a). Clear evidence was identified that comprehensive approaches to health development are the most effective, participation is essential to sustain efforts, and access to education and information fosters participation (WHO, 2009a). New partnerships for health must arise between and across different sectors at all levels of a society's government. For example, additional resources for education and housing, not just for the health sector, are needed. New investments for health should reflect the needs of vulnerable or marginalized groups, such as older people, children, women, indigenous peoples, and populations living in poverty (WHO, 2009a). Empowering principles were woven throughout the declaration, and it was noted, particularly, in the declaration that "health promotion is carried out by and with people, not on or to people" (WHO, 2009a, p. 20).

The **fifth global conference on health promotion** in Mexico in 2000 led to the Mexico Ministerial Statement for the Promotion of Health, and strategies to move ideas to action (WHO, 2009a). The ministerial statement acknowledged promotion of health and social development as a central duty and responsibility of governments (WHO, 2009a). New and emerging diseases threatened the worldwide progress in health outcomes. Once again, the declaration stated that there is ample evidence that health promotion strategies are effective. But this had been stated before, so it appeared that the issue was no longer a lack of evidence of the effectiveness of health promotion, but rather that the problems lie elsewhere; for example, in political will to change. The ministerial statement was signed by 88 countries, including Canada and the United States.

The **sixth global conference on health promotion**, held in Thailand in 2005, led to the **Bangkok Charter for Health Promotion in a Globalized World** (WHO, 2009a). This charter affirmed that policies and partnerships to empower communities and improve health and equity should be at the centre of global and national development (WHO, 2009a). Health promotion is based on the critical human right to have the highest attainable standard of health, without discrimination. The charter recognized that, worldwide, the vulnerability of children and exclusion of marginalized populations has increased, with increasing inequities within and between countries (WHO, 2009a). Although progress had been made in placing health at the centre of development, progress in the areas of political action, broad participation, and sustained advocacy had not occurred and many proven-effective health promotion strategies had not been fully implemented (WHO, 2009a). A commitment to health for all still required advocacy, investment, capacity development, regulation and legislation, and partnerships and alliances across society and governments to create sustainable actions, as well as needing to be an integral part of domestic and foreign policies (WHO, 2009a). Health is a major determinant of social, economic, and political development. Therefore, governments must give priority to investments in health (WHO, 2009a). The issues were summed up as the need to close the implementation gap:

> Since the adoption of the Ottawa Charter, a significant number of resolutions at national and global levels have been signed in support of health promotion, but these have not always been followed by action. (p. 28)

The **seventh global conference on health promotion** was held in the Republic of Kenya in 2009, and its findings were published in a document entitled "**The Nairobi Call to Action**" (WHO, 2009b). In this document, health promotion was affirmed as remaining the core and most cost-effective strategy to improve health and quality of life, and reduce health inequities and poverty worldwide. The Ottawa Charter was also affirmed as remaining as relevant then for leading health promotion efforts as it had been in 1986. The **eighth global conference on health promotion** took place in Helsinki, Finland, in 2013. Leaders in health promotion came together to discuss how political decisions related to health are implemented in the form of practical actions. The **Helsinki Statement on Health in All Policies** that resulted from conference deliberations affirmed the importance of considering the health implications of decisions across sectors of government (WHO, 2013c). A "health in all policies" approach seeks synergies across government sectors in order to improve population health. Unfortunately, reaffirming the values, principles, and action strategies has yet to result in effective changes for populations. Implementation gaps still exist in policy, practice, governance, and political will, resulting in the continuation of avoidable illness and suffering for individuals, as well as various social and economic implications for populations (WHO, 2009c). The issue is not lack of evidence of the effectiveness of health promotion interventions, but it is multi-factorial, stemming from deeper issues and mandates that drive policies and practices. Issues and barriers may be related to the difficulties inherent in situating health promotion responsibilities beyond just those of the health sector, and in understanding that health promotion goes far beyond just promoting healthy lifestyles. Putting health on the agendas of policy makers, governments, social and economic sectors, industry, the media, and voluntary organizations, as outlined in the Ottawa Charter, is a daunting task. Navarro (2009) reflected on the root cause of this continuing lack of progress in health promotion, which he attributes to the continuation of neo-liberal government policies that accentuate and promote class dominance and class alliances based on power. The result is a continuation of poverty as the major determinant of health of people in most countries (both low income and high income), so the "urgent public health project is to recover the representativeness of political institutions and make them accountable to the large sections of the population that have been disenfranchised . . . [as] disease is a social and political category imposed on people within an enormously repressive social and economic capitalist system" (p. 15). This statement was not new. Rudolf Virchow (a pathologist) had been contracted by the Polish government to survey the 1848 typhus epidemic and submit a report for recommendations. He concluded in a now-famous statement: "Medicine is a social science, and politics nothing but medicine on a grand scale" (Taylor & Rieger, 1985, p. 548). Virchow's recommendations included improving income, employment, housing, and nutrition for the citizens, calling for political reforms in the areas of democracy, universal education, disestablishment of the church, taxation reform, and others. His recommendations were unacceptable to the government and he was suspended in 1849 and left the political sphere for 11 years (Taylor & Rieger, 1985).

Programs aimed at changing individual behaviour have limited effectiveness; therefore, health strategies must be broadened to include political, economic, social, and cultural interventions, with the empowerment of people to engage in public policy changes as one of their main objectives (Navarro, 2009). Even Lalonde (1974) had identified the important role of governments in improving the health of Canadians, along with individual citizens, healthcare professionals, and institutions. He acknowledged, however, that "this fragmentation of responsibility has sometimes led to imbalanced approaches, with each participant in the health field pursuing solutions only within his [sic] area of interest" (Lalonde, 1974, p. 33). In 1985, Taylor and Rieger stated, "the social origins of illness are no longer disputed, yet 130 years after the publication of the Virchow's Report, governments are still unwilling to accept the corollary; that is, that socioeconomic improvements are more necessary than medical ones" (1985, p. 557). What are our governments' priorities today? What are their areas of interest, if they follow a neo-liberal agenda (a political agenda that includes reduced government involvement in and funding for social and other services, and favours privatization and a market economy)? How does that affect their view of health, and whose responsibility is it to create the conditions for a healthy society?

Reflecting the continuing global issues in health promotion, challenges in implementing health promotion in Canada continue. In partnership with the Canadian Health Services Research Foundation (CHSRF), the Canadian Nurses Association (CNA) commissioned a research report to analyze public policy and programming focused on the determinants of health and health outcomes in Canada (Muntaner, Ng, & Chung, 2012). The issue is that all levels of governments (federal to municipal) have taken minimal action to narrow health inequalities by focusing on social determinants of health and public policy, even though income, housing, food insecurity, and social exclusion form the major modifiable social determinants of health over the life course (Muntaner et al., 2012). A scoping review of the literature indicated a clear central finding of a large, negative, and statistically significant association between the social determinants of health and health inequalities in Canada (Muntaner et al., 2012). Although the social determinants of health have been recognized as important to nursing practice for many years, this review suggests specific action nurses can take to address this pressing issue. Action includes nursing collaboration with government, civil, and health sectors, with roles in advocacy, policy analysis, and political activities—that is, to become active social change agents. A call for nurses to refocus practice on social justice (characteristic of early public health nursing) has led to CHNs in Canada calling for practice focused on reducing health and social inequalities to become a standard and core competency of nursing practice (Muntaner et al., 2012). Nurses must focus on the root causes of health inequalities, identify which determinants of health require action, implement the principles of social justice, and engage in advocacy for the most disadvantaged groups in society (Muntaner et al., 2012). Policy recommendations include initiatives to reduce child and adult poverty (through financial assistance and social wages), increases in minimum wages to a "living wage" necessary for supporting housing and food needs, campaigns and social movements for the rights of socially excluded groups, advocacy for intersectoral action on health inequalities across levels of government to coordinate social determinant of health policies, support for political candidates who are receptive to taking action on social determinants of health, and encouragement for greater workplace democracy to protect and increase worker bargaining power (Muntaner et al., 2012).

# POPULATION HEALTH PROMOTION

Health promotion involves a comprehensive, multi-strategy approach, applying diverse strategies and methods in an integrated manner. This characteristic is one of the preconditions for health promotion to be effective. Health promotion addresses the key action areas identified in the Ottawa Charter in an integrated and coherent manner.

**Population health promotion** is a process of taking action on the interrelated conditions (i.e., social determinants of health) that affect a population's health, to create healthy change. Population health promotion focuses on maintaining or improving the health of populations and reducing disparities in health status between people, evident in the health issues that those with inadequate income face. A health promotion approach to health reduces inequities and increases opportunities for empowerment of people so that they can increase control over their life events and their health. In population health promotion, population health concepts are integrated with the principles that guide action on health promotion. The population health promotion model (PHPM) (Flynn, 1999) explains the relationship between population health and health promotion. It shows how a population health approach can be implemented through action on the full range of health determinants by using the multiple health promotion strategies outlined in the Ottawa Charter for Health Promotion.

There remains debate about the use of evidence in health promotion practice. However, an evidence base for health promotion practice does exist (Juneau, Jones, McQueen, & Potvin, 2011). If a narrow view of evidence prevails among practitioners, such as a belief that it consists solely of rigid empirical research, then the evidence base may appear to be slim. However, if an expansion into multiple styles of research is valued, then there is much research evidence that practitioners can (and do) use. There is a current trend away from individual-centred health promotion interventions toward those that target groups or entire populations, which reflects a long-awaited evolution of the field of health promotion from lifestyle-based health education to environmental and social justice oriented health promotion (Juneau et al., 2011). Local relevance is now understood to be paramount in planning health promotion, and examples of participatory research projects are now emerging in the health promotion literature (Potvin, Junea, Jones, & McQueen, 2011) as some of the best examples of improving local interventions. This approach to health promotion holds promise, whereas decades of attempts to change individuals' behaviour have met with little or no long-term health-promoting results.

A "think tank" involving public health experts and health system stakeholders was held in Alberta in 2003 to discuss the future of public health in Canada. It was concluded that, in general, Canadians are healthy but there are major inequities in the health status of different groups. These inequities are rooted in social, economic, cultural, and environmental determinants of health (Frank, Di Ruggiero, & Moloughney, 2004). Some participants argued that there has been insufficient attention given to social determinants of health and the need for public health action in this area, and that there is a need for public health policy analysis to better understand why public health has received little attention from decision makers (Frank et al., 2004). Suggestions for action included using a lobbyist who understands high-level government decision making, and seeking broad partnerships beyond traditional partners to advocate for system change (Frank et al., 2004).

Health promotion, not public health, has been described as our best link to social justice, social change, and social reform, because of its focus on the reduction of disparities that have an impact on health. This was espoused originally in the Ottawa Charter and this focus has remained since then (Dupere et al., 2007). As Marie-Claude Lamarre (2011) of the International Union for Health Promotion and Education put it,

> Health promotion does not exist as a single and universal concept but rather as a multi-dimensional concept engraved in the history of public health, within local political, cultural, social, and economic conditions. What creates a link between these visions is that we agree to address health as a social enterprise through a set of strategies led jointly to attain a common objective including advocacy, education, training, research, legislation, coordination of policies and community development, no matter what the problems, concerned populations, contexts and life settings are. Another common link is that of targeting the determinants of health and associating health achievement to structural adjustments brought about by political, economic and social changes.

> . . . values and principles form the habits of mind that in turn provide a common basis for the practice of health promotion. These include: a socioecological model of health that takes into account the cultural, economic, and social determinants of health; a commitment to equity, and social justice; a respect for cultural diversity and sensitivity; a dedication to sustainable development; and a participatory approach to engaging the population in identifying needs, and setting priorities for action, and to planning, implementing, and evaluating practical and feasible solutions. (p. 3)

## The Population Health Promotion Model

The **population health promotion model (PHPM)** is a Canadian-developed model (visually represented in the form of a cube) for understanding the who, what, how, and why of intervention or action on multiple levels across a society to create healthy change. Nancy Hamilton and Tariq Bhatti from the Health Promotion Development Division of Health Canada developed this model in 1996, and Larry Flynn from Health Canada revised (streamlined) the model in 1999. In order to promote the health of populations we need to understand what the determinants of health are, which goes well beyond an understanding based on genetics or biology. We also need to understand what people's needs are, develop action strategies for promoting health, look at where action should be targeted (i.e., at one level or across multiple levels), and understand the foundation and evidence base for helping guide nurses in choosing what interventions to implement. What are our decisions based on? Evidence includes research, evaluation, experiential learning, values, and assumptions, which are at the base of this cube because they are the foundations of professional decision making that create the frame of possibilities a nurse will view—what she or he may be limited by or opened up toward considering for interventions. All of the components of the cube, and the decisions that have to be made, arise from this foundation for evidence-based decision making (Figure 8.2).

The PHPM incorporates a number of values and assumptions: comprehensive action needs to be taken on all the determinants of health; multiple entry points for planning and implementing are essential; health problems may affect some groups more than others; solutions to problems involve changing social values and structures; one's health is a result of a combination of one's own health practices plus the impact of social and physical environments in which we live, work, and play; health-promoting opportunities arise in environments with social justice and equity and where relationships are built on mutual respect and caring (rather than on power and status); and meaningful participation of community members is needed. Understanding one's own values and assumptions is important as this may create openings to listening to and valuing other perspectives, realizing that you do not hold the one "truth" and there may be multiple perspectives on a situation. Self-understanding creates the opportunities for working in true partnerships with others, especially if they feel you are willing to listen and include them in a non-token manner. The PHPM addresses the root causes of problems people face, and therefore suggests areas where the most powerful interventions to create healthy change should occur.

The social determinants of health include economic and social conditions that shape the health of individuals, communities, and societies (Raphael, 2010). Health problems may affect certain groups more than others. If it is the responsibility of society as a whole to take care of its members, then solutions to problems might necessitate changing social values and structures.

**Explanation of the Four Sides of the Cube** The PHPM is a four-sided cube. The sides of the cube include social determinants of health, levels of action, action strategies, and the foundations of the cube become the fourth side. The intent of this model is to help guide actions to improve health, asking the following: On what should we take action, how should we take action, and with whom should we act? (Public Health Agency of Canada, 2001). The social determinants of health on the PHPM cube consist of income and social status, social environments, work and working conditions, education, social support networks, genetic endowment, personal coping skills, health services, healthy child development, culture, physical environments, and gender.

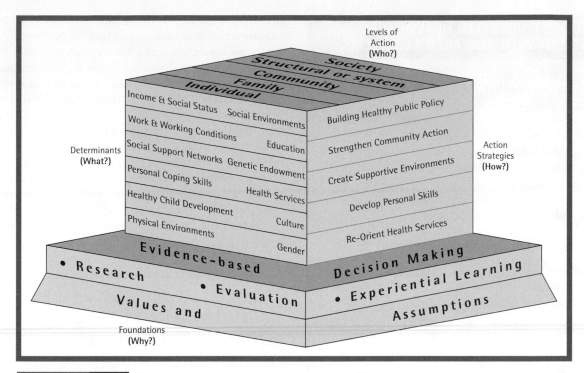

**FIGURE   8.2   The Population Health Promotion Model**

*Source:* Flynn, L. (1999). *Population health promotion model*. Revised from original model developed by N. Hamilton and T. Bhatti, Health Promotion Development Division, Health Canada, 1996. Winnipeg, MB: Health Canada, Manitoba/Saskatchewan Region. Adapted and reproduced with permission from the Minister of Health, 2015.

The side of the cube called "levels of action" draws attention to the fact that action must be taken at various levels within society, including at the individual, family, and community levels, including people linked by a common interest or by geographic setting; at the structural or system level (e.g., housing or education sectors); and within society as a whole (PHAC, 2001).

A comprehensive set of action strategies derived from the Ottawa Charter comprises the side of the cube called "action strategies." These include (a) build healthy public policy, (b) strengthen community action, (c) create supportive environments, (d) develop personal skills, and (e) re-orient health services. The base of the model provides a foundation giving direction for action on population health that is grounded in evidence-based decision making, research, evaluation, experiential learning, values, and assumptions.

## Social Determinants of Health: Variations in the Literature

Social determinants of health pre-date the PHPM, with its origins attributed to the discussion of the impact of physical and social environments in the Lalonde Report and expanded upon in 1996 by Tarlov to include housing, education, social acceptance, employment, and income (Raphael, 2009). These determinants of health were developed out of attempts to understand why members of different socioeconomic groups experience different health outcomes (Raphael, 2009). The CNA has understood for some time that it is critical for nurses to assess the multitude of factors that affect their clients' health. For example, ask an individual where their position is in their workplace hierarchy; "those lower in the [job] hierarchy experienced three times the risk of

death from heart disease, stroke, cancer, gastrointestinal disease, accident, and suicide compared with those at the top of the hierarchy. These differences could not be explained by differences in medical care" (CNA, 2005, p. 1). It is paramount that nurses understand that serious illness and early death related to poverty are connected to low social standing. Poor health and early death then are linked to social determinants of health, not just to accessibility to healthcare.

Poverty can have a hugely negative effect on people's health, extending across and highlighting the interconnectedness of many of the social determinants of health, such as social environments, social support networks, educational attainment, gender, employment status, and income and social status. Stewart et al. (2009) compared experiences of social isolation and perceptions of belonging among low-income and higher-income people in two Canadian jurisdictions. They found that low-income people experienced greater isolation and a lower sense of belonging than did higher-income people. Poverty was also closely connected to a sense of feeling prejudged, stigmatized, avoided, and isolated, preventing some lower-income people from becoming involved in community activities, thereby leading to further distancing and self-isolating behaviours (Stewart et al., 2009). This internalized marginalizing process can further magnify a person's feelings of disempowerment and worthlessness and lead to other detrimental effects on emotional, mental, and physical health. Stewart et al. (2009) suggest that programs and policies to reduce income inequalities by tackling the root causes of poverty may help increase a sense of belonging and decrease the social isolation of vulnerable populations.

Various authors have added to or modified the social determinants of health. The Public Health Agency of Canada (PHAC) has retained the 12 determinants already described but expanded

## WHICH TIPS FOR BETTER HEALTH ARE CONSISTENT WITH RESEARCH EVIDENCE?

The messages given to the public by governments, health associations, and health workers are heavily influenced by the ways in which health issues are understood. Contrast the two sets of messages provided below. The first set is individually oriented and assumes individuals can control the factors that determine their health. The second set is societally oriented and assumes the most important determinants of health are beyond the control of most individuals. Which set of tips is most consistent with the available evidence on the determinants of health?

### The Traditional Ten Tips for Better Health

1. Don't smoke. If you can, stop. If you can't, cut down.
2. Follow a balanced diet with plenty of fruit and vegetables.
3. Keep physically active.
4. Manage stress by, for example, talking things through and making time to relax.
5. If you drink alcohol, do so in moderation.
6. Cover up in the sun, and protect children from sunburn.
7. Practice safer sex.
8. Take up cancer screening opportunities.
9. Be safe on the roads: follow the Highway Code.
10. Learn the First Aid ABCs: airways, breathing, circulation. (Donaldson, 1999)

### The Social Determinants Ten Tips for Better Health

1. Don't be poor. If you can, stop. If you can't, try not to be poor for long.
2. Don't have poor parents.
3. Own a car.
4. Don't work in a stressful, low-paid manual job.
5. Don't live in damp, low quality housing.
6. Be able to afford to go on a foreign holiday and sunbathe.
7. Practice not losing your job and don't become unemployed.
8. Take up all benefits you are entitled to, if you are unemployed, retired, or sick or disabled.
9. Don't live next to a busy major road or near a polluting factory.
10. Learn how to fill in the complex housing benefit/asylum application forms before you become homeless and destitute. (Gordon, 1999; personal communication)

*Source:* Raphael, D. (2009). *Social determinants of health* (2nd ed.). Toronto, ON: Canadian Scholars' Press. Used by permission of Canadian Scholars' Press.

determinants of health in the future. Raphael (2009) more recently added food security and housing but stated that these really just echo the Ottawa Charter's prerequisites of health, which include peace, shelter, education, food, income, stable ecosystem, sustainable resources, social justice and equity.

In a recent Chief Public Health Officer's report on the State of Public Health in Canada, Butler-Jones (2012) stated that the determinant of health factors include income and social status, social support networks, education and literacy, employment and working conditions, social environments, physical environments, personal health practices and coping skills, healthy child development, biology and genetic endowment, health services, gender, and culture; all of which affect Canadians throughout their lifecourse. These are very similar to the original 12 listed in the cube model.

## CANADIAN NURSES ASSOCIATION ROLE IN THE SOCIAL DETERMINANTS OF HEALTH

The CNA stated that the landmark Ottawa Charter for Health Promotion was developed in response to growing expectation of a new global public health movement, but its principles are as true today as they were when the charter was launched years ago. "When it was developed, the charter focused on action to achieve 'Health for All by the Year 2000 and beyond.' It pointed out that many conditions are needed for good health, including an adequate healthcare system, peace, shelter, education, food, income, a stable ecosystem, sustainable resources, social justice, and equity. These prerequisites have become a strong component of the practice of health promotion for nurses across the continuum of care" (Ashley, 2011, p. 20).

In 2011, CNA president Judith Shamian and several CNA staff members attended a commemorative event in Ottawa to celebrate a quarter century of the Ottawa Charter and met the charter's Canadian (Irving Rootman) American (David McQueen) and European (Ilona Kickbusch) pioneers. These leaders described how the charter changed our definition of health care so that it focused on social justice and "offered three challenges to health professionals globally: to continue to focus on the social determinants of health to build the capacity for health promotion within individuals, communities, and society as a whole; to reaffirm our commitment for a more equitable world; and to encourage investment in public health through public support and working beyond the health sector with education and private industry" (Ashley, 2011, p. 20).

Nurses have the opportunity to reduce social inequalities and inequities and positively influence the health of Canadians through engaging in politics and policy analysis and acting as advocates. By upholding the principles of social justice, nurses can ensure the most marginalized and disadvantaged groups in society have access to services that address multiple determinants of health, which, once accessed, have positive benefits for the quality of health and living for all Canadians (Muntaner et al., 2012). Examples of opportunities to have a

on some: education and literacy, employment or working conditions, personal health practices and coping skills, biology and genetic endowment (PHAC, 2011). Newer additions to the social determinants of health have included more specific, or narrowed areas, such as housing and Aboriginal status. War or conflict and hope have been put forward and are being considered as positive influence on the health outcomes of Canadians include the following nursing actions:

- supporting initiatives that reduce child and adulthood poverty levels by increasing financial assistance and social wages (SDOH provided through public funds);
- supporting initiatives that increase minimum wages to "living wages," to ensure that economic security, stable housing, and food needs are met;
- supporting campaigns and social movements that advocate for progressive taxation (where tax rate is based on income), the right to food security and affordable housing, and the enforcement of laws that protect the rights of socially excluded groups;
- advocating for intersectoral action on health at municipal, provincial or territorial, and federal levels of government to coordinate action undertaken by sectors outside the health sector;
- supporting political parties at provincial or territorial and federal levels of government that are receptive to taking action on SDOH (such as those that are pro-labour or pro-redistribution of wealth); and
- encouraging greater workplace democracy to increase the number of unionized workplaces since labour unions are important determinants of generous welfare states, narrower social inequalities and better population health (Muntaner et al., 2012, p. 3).

To address health inequalities and the social determinants of health for all Canadians, the CNA (2013) recognizes the need for nurses to advocate for improvements in social and physical environments, adequate housing, early childhood support, education, equitable access to healthcare, and social supports, all as necessary approaches to address the disparities in physical and mental health outcomes for Canadians across the lifespan. The profession of nursing has a vast body of knowledge and experience and holds the potential to offer a strong and powerful voice for change, augmented by large numbers of nurses across the country. Collectively, nurses are the largest group of healthcare professionals in Canada. Nurses have a professional and social responsibility to become a significant part of re-shaping Canada's healthcare system into one that addresses the social determinants of health for all Canadians, rather than simply standing by and watching a re-shaping of healthcare focused on meeting the requirements of institutions (CNA, 2012).

## Toronto Charter on the Social Determinants of Health

A national conference called "Social Determinants of Health across the Lifespan: A Current Accounting and Policy Implications" was held at York University in Toronto in 2002. The conference focused on a discussion and analysis of the state of the social determinants of health in Canada. Policy implications to strengthen the social determinants of health were discussed and a **Toronto Charter on the Social Determinants of Health** was written (Raphael, 2009). This charter suggested

the social determinants of health should include Aboriginal status, early life, education, employment and working conditions, food security, gender, healthcare services, housing, income and its distribution, a social safety net, social exclusion, and unemployment and employment security (Raphael, 2009). These determinants closely parallel the PHPM determinants of health, with specific differences including identification of Aboriginal status as a separate determinant of health in Canada (as it is related to poor health outcomes), and with the issues of food security and housing meriting their own stand-alone determinant status as well.

At the York University conference, health policy experts and health professionals discussed the rising social and economic inequalities among Canadians, including the social and economic costs they create. The health status of Canadians is profoundly impacted by the quality of the social, physical, and economic environments they live in, and as the quality of these environments deteriorates, so do people's health. At the conference, the above 12 proposed social determinants of health of the Toronto Charter were examined as focal points for efforts to promote health and social justice for all Canadians by improving the quality of the determinants of health. The Toronto Charter recognized that Canadian women, Aboriginal people, Canadians of colour, and new Canadians were significantly more at risk than others when there is deterioration in the quality of any of the determinants of health (Raphael, Bryant, & Curry-Stevens, 2004; "Strengthening the Social Determinants," 2003).

The Community Health Nurses of Canada (CHNC) expanded the list to include 20 determinants of health: income and income distribution, education and literacy, unemployment and job security, employment and working conditions, early childhood development, food insecurity, housing, environment, biology and genetic endowment, healthy child development, social exclusion, social status, social safety networks, health services, personal health practices and coping skills, Aboriginal status, gender, culture, race, and disability (CHNC, 2011, revised).

Other determinants of health could include mental health and obesity (International Association for the Study of Obesity, Canadian Obesity Network, & Centre for Addiction and Mental Health, 2012). Action strategies have been developed. The "Toronto Charter for Physical Activity" (2010) advocates for governments, organizations, and communities to create environments to support physical activity for whole populations, as it "promotes well-being and mental health, prevents disease, improves social connectedness and quality of life, provides economic benefits and contributes to environmental sustainability" (Global Advocacy Council of Physical Activity & International Society for Physical Activity and Health, 2010, p. 1). Physical activity is identified as a powerful way to decrease non-communicable diseases and improve the health of Canadians and people worldwide. Policies and practices throughout societies influence whether or not physical activity becomes socially acceptable, physically achievable, or remains unattainable. Urban design, school policies, accessibility to public transportation, and the media profoundly influence whether or not individuals have the opportunity to engage in healthy daily physical activity. Non-communicable diseases such as heart disease, stroke, diabetes, and many cancers are directly linked to physical inactivity, making it the fourth leading cause of death worldwide. Since the factors that influence physical inactivity are complex and multi-sectoral, multiple sectors of society should be included in the search for feasible solutions to the issue of inactivity. For governments and policy makers ready to motivate, inspire, and support communities and individuals to become participants in physical activity, a complementary document was developed with seven recommended "best investments" to increase population levels of physical activity:

1. "Whole-of-school" programs. This investment advocates for highly active activities for children, as well as opportunities for staff and families to participate in physical activities.

2. Transportation policies and systems that prioritize walking, cycling, and public transportation. This investment helps to improve air quality and ease traffic congestion.

3. Urban design regulations and infrastructure that provide for equitable and safe access to recreational physical activity, and opportunities for transport-related walking and cycling, targeted for people across the life course.

4. Physical activity and non-communicable disease prevention integrated into PHC systems. Healthcare workers, including nurses and physicians, have the opportunity to screen for potential issues and educate a large portion of the population on the importance of incorporating physical activity into daily life.

5. Public education, including using mass media to reach people to raise awareness and change social norms on physical activity.

6. Community-wide programs involving multiple settings and sectors, and that mobilize and integrate community engagement and resources. To successfully implement this investment in population health, whole-community approaches are more successful at encouraging physical activity than are single-program delivery approaches.

7. Sports systems and programs that promote "sport for all" and encourage participation across the lifespan. This investment promotes adapting sports programs to reduce financial and social barriers; to appeal to women, men, girls, and boys of all ages; and to be accessible and inclusive for people with mental and physical disabilities (GAPA & ISPAH, 2011).

## JASON'S STORY

The following story is offered as an example that shows the complex interplay of factors that determine the health of Canadians:

Why is Jason in the hospital?

Because he has a bad infection in his leg.

But why does he have an infection?

Because he has a cut on his leg and it got infected.

But why does he have a cut on his leg?

Because he was playing in the junk yard next to his apartment building and there was some sharp, jagged steel there that he fell on.

But why was he playing in the junk yard?

Because his neighbourhood is kind of run down. A lot of kids play there and there is no one to supervise them.

But why does he live in that neighbourhood?

Because his parents can't afford a nicer place to live.

But why can't his parents afford a nicer place to live?

Because his dad is unemployed and his mom is sick.

But why is his dad unemployed?

Because he doesn't have much education and he can't find a job.

But why . . . ?

(Federal, Provincial, and Territorial Advisory Committee on Population Health, 1999, p. vii)

Jason's story shows the cascade of societal inequities that contributed to a young boy's injury and hospitalization. As this story indicates, the health of Canadians may be determined more by societal values than by individual lifestyle and behaviour. The most appropriate question to ask should not be "why doesn't Jason play somewhere other than a junk yard?" but rather, "why is there a junkyard and not a safe playground in Jason's neighbourhood?" (Photo 8.1) The condition of the places where we live, work, and play directly affects the psychological and physical health of all the Jasons of the world, and also of their families, friends, neighbours, and the broader community (Mikkonen & Raphael, 2010). Without some form of post-secondary education, people like Jason's father are not likely to work for much more than minimum wage, thereby restricting the options of where a family can afford to live. Low-cost housing often exists in high-density population neighbourhoods, which may not have safe green spaces and parks for children and families to relax and play in.

The health of Canadians is largely determined by the social conditions people live within, and many of these social conditions are out of their reach or control as they are related to the distribution of income and societal wealth, affordable

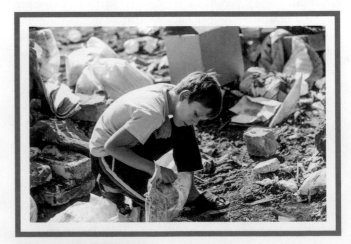

**PHOTO 8.1** Boy playing in junkyard

*Source: Maxim Ibragimov/Shutterstock*

post-secondary education, employment status and working conditions, high-quality affordable housing, safe neighbourhoods, the availability and accessibility of healthcare, affordable medications, and the availability of social services during times of need (Mikkonen & Raphael, 2010). Nursing actions that would help promote Jason's health include addressing the root causes of poverty and an unjust society (Lind, Loewen, & Mawji, 2012). It does very little to change Jason's outcome to simply tell him to play somewhere else when the environment he lives in provides no other options for him and society does little to support the necessary social changes to make his living environment healthy (Frankish et al., 2006). Because they work closely with individuals, families, and communities, CHNs see opportunities to address health promotion issues as well as advocate for and support vulnerable communities to move toward self-empowerment, and to work to create change through social action.

The Canadian Nurses Association (CNA) encourages all nurses to support the health of society by promoting public policies that address the social determinants of health. Nurses are in an opportune position to act as advocates, as nurses have more contact time with the population than any other healthcare professional (Mildon, 2013a). Because of this contact time and their educational preparation, nurses have a collective wealth of experience and knowledge. By participating in health research, nurses can also add to what is known about the relationship between the determinants of health and the state of health of Canadians (CNA, 2009), and use that knowledge to inform their work as agents of social change. Perhaps by changing the unhealthy environments and social conditions that a large number of Canadians have little choice but to live within, stories like Jason's would become less common.

## RISK COMMUNICATION

**Risk communication** refers to the transmission of information about an existing or imminent health or environmental risk, the anticipated severity of the risk, and the percentage of people it will impact. Communication of risk is vital because in our current social environment risks changes rapidly with the introduction of new and varied technologies. Providing people with timely information is the single most influential way to shape their decision making and subsequent behaviour. Communication has to be strategic, appropriate for the target audience, and grounded in evidence from both social and physical science (Health Canada, 2006). Contact tracing is a form of risk communication that is discussed further in Chapter 12.

Risk management refers to the broad collection of activities involved in addressing health or safety risks. Risk management within health promotion identifies subpopulations or target populations that have a unique health concern or similar risk factors that can lead to several different health concerns. The subpopulation may have social, cultural, economic, or geographic commonalities. Risk factors can then be targeted in a way that is most effective for that population, where a generalized approach may have been too diluted and not specific enough to create a measurable change. Additionally,

this approach is often more amenable to implementing several different concurrent strategies to address multiple determinants of health. It is easier to identify and involve community leaders, and the evaluation process is simpler (PHAC, 2013a). One example would be smoking cessation strategies that specifically target pregnant women rather than targeting the population in general.

## POPULATION HEALTH AND POPULATION HEALTH INDICATORS

Population health is an approach used to understand and improve the health of an entire population or subpopulations, such as children, the elderly, or newcomers to Canada. Linked to health promotion that is not focused on individual people, a **population health approach** identifies and takes action to improve the root causes of health issues that impact the health of the overall population (PHAC, 2013b). Health inequities are addressed through research to determine the primary factors that influence health at the population level and strategies are subsequently developed, implemented, and evaluated to address influential and modifiable risk factors (Vollman, Anderson, & McFarlane, 2012). The factors that influence a population's health are usually interrelated conditions that occur over the life course. Applications of knowledge from past interventions can make a measurable difference to the health of populations.

**Population health indicators** are used to measure the health of populations as well as the progress made toward creating healthier citizens. Health indicators are closely related to the determinants of health, and examples of indicators include self-rated well-being surveys, life expectancy, number of people with a specific diagnosis or type of injury (e.g., lung cancer, hip fractures), number of hospitalization days per injury or diagnosis, death rate, potential years of life lost, and number and reason for emergency room visits, to name a few. Many of these measurement indicators are collected and collated annually to allow healthcare professionals to compare data, track changes, and identify areas of success and areas for improvement. Health status indicators can be found in Statistics Canada publications, community health profiles, census data, and health status reports (Health Canada, 2014) as well as in other reports and publications from government and large organizations.

To further understand a population's health, it is necessary to have additional information on the protective factors and risk factors specific to that population (Kindig & Stoddart, 2003). Assessments could include a community's levels of physical activity, breastfeeding practices, diet, tobacco use, alcohol and illegal drug usage, living and working conditions, number of crosswalks and safe places to cross busy streets, schools and their entrance requirements, number and condition of playgrounds and green spaces, presence of recreational centres, and pollution levels.

Environmental scans are reports that summarize changes or noteworthy data in health status indicators and include current and emerging issues in order to support healthcare decision making. They are used to identify trends that influence health and changes to healthcare services, such as urbanization, globalization, rapid technological changes, or social security in a larger societal context. To help identify trends and issues, health professionals or government decision makers may include a limited literature search, key informant interviews, surveys to obtain public opinion (or to obtain data not available through health status indicators) or even a summary of newspaper articles on a specific topic for a predetermined and specified period of time. Windshield surveys (walking or driving visual scans) are another useful tool if a topic or issue is limited to a geographical area or to structures, such as playground equipment. Overall, the goal of an environmental scan is not to conduct an exhaustive search but to facilitate good decision making by providing necessary information on a specific topic using reasonable efforts exerted within a short time frame.

**Population health interventions** include policy and program development to address social, economic, and physical environment factors that influence people's decision making (Hawe & Potvin, 2009). Developing a population health intervention may begin by obtaining information from other health providers regarding past successful and unsuccessful strategies. Information gathered from online searches, literature reviews, and key informant interviews will help prevent duplication of unsuccessful interventions and may encourage health professionals to build on interventions that have been successful elsewhere. The population health approach coupled with the PHPM (Flynn, 1999) provides a framework to plan how to target the health of a population and develop interventions. An identified population could be either geographically located or an aggregate of people with commonalities such as age, interests, diagnosis, culture, or religious affiliation. Population health interventions may be implemented at community, sector, or societal levels. Strategies developed to change the health of a population are generally different from those used to work with individuals. Development of personal skills at a population level is facilitated by **social marketing** interventions, which may include use of websites; bus, billboard, or television advertisements; and radio interviews or newspaper columns. Many people do not change their behaviour based solely on knowledge of what is best for their health. For example, smokers may believe smoking is bad for their health but because it is an addiction they continue to smoke. As a result, multiple action strategies to improve population health frequently include building healthy public policies that legislate healthy behaviour (e.g., tobacco bylaws, seat belt laws, speed limits) or create supportive environments (e.g., tobacco cessation programs, soft playground surfaces, safe bike paths) for health.

Developing and implementing successful population health strategies that will make a positive and measurable difference in a population's health is challenging even when healthcare professionals have information identifying the social, economic, and physical forces impacting the health concern. Achieving health promotion goals can take years, oftentimes requiring multiple health promotion strategies implemented at various levels (ranging from individual to society) while simultaneously addressing multiple determinants

of health. For example, one group may be lobbying government to pass healthy public policies while another is working with community members to develop personal skills at an individual level. Tobacco cessation initiatives are an example of a successful multifaceted population health intervention strategy. Over 60 years ago tobacco was identified as a cause of lung cancer, and in 1959 the Canadian Public Health Association began an anti-tobacco educational campaign targeting smokers. Over the following decades multiple strategies were implemented to move toward creating a tobacco-free society. Approaches used to build healthy public policy included (a) increasing taxes on tobacco to make it less affordable (especially for children and teens), (b) leveraging substantial penalties for selling tobacco products to those under 18 years of age, (c) lobbying efforts that resulted in bylaws that decreased second-hand smoke exposure, and (d) banning tobacco advertising. Efforts implemented simultaneously focused on developing personal skills through campaigns to raise the awareness of the dangers of tobacco use and provided strategies smokers could use to assist them to quit smoking. Targeted strategies for disadvantaged and high-risk groups with significantly higher smoking rates included reorienting health services to offer increased numbers and types of cessation services for individuals and included strengthening community groups to take action in creating environments where smoking behaviour was less convenient, along with **social marketing campaigns** that de-normalized smoking (Cancer Council Australia, 2013; CPHA, 2011; Gilmore, Tavakoly, Taylor, & Reed, 2013). In Canada smoking rates have decreased from approximately 30% of the general population in 1996/97 to 21% in 2009. Nevertheless more population interventions are required as approximately 37 000 preventable annual deaths are still attributed to tobacco (CPHA, 2011).

## "AT-RISK" POPULATIONS

"**At risk**" is a term often used to describe a group or population that has a higher risk of a particular illness (morbidity) or negative life outcome (such as mortality) than might be experienced by other populations (Kozier et al., 2014; Roach, 2000). Although offering useful awareness of issues for prevention to focus upon, this approach can also devolve into creating or perpetuating stigmas such as racism, sexism, ageism, and other prejudices that affect healthcare professionals' assumptions about particular groups and their behaviours toward them, potentially leading to oppressive behaviours directed toward people considered to be at risk. For example, a common assumption made about social assistance recipients is that they are lazy and choose to be unemployed. If healthcare practitioners hold this stereotyped view of recipients, they may discriminate against them while developing care plans, and minimize their full access to competent and compassionate healthcare and resources. Similarly, another population at risk of further stigma by this labelling is Aboriginals. Although many morbidity (e.g., rates of diabetes) and mortality (e.g., deaths related to disease and suicide) statistics are higher for Aboriginal groups, a deficit-driven approach situates the problems as lying within individuals rather than serving as a reflection of the wider social and historical contexts and inequities (Adelson, 2005). Discriminatory practices based on racism make the healthcare system unsafe for many Aboriginal people (Health Council of Canada, 2012). See Chapter 22 on Aboriginal health for more in-depth discussion.

As described by Roach (2000), dangerous assumptions could occur, "if the basis for the excess mortality among certain racial groups is an intrinsic characteristic of the group, some might consider this a sign of 'racial inferiority'" (p. 261), and act accordingly. However, to believe the causes are solely external to that particular group may not be welcomed by politicians or other decision makers, because "if the excess mortality rate is entirely due to various types of social injustices (such as racism and discrimination, resulting in a lack of education, underemployment, and poor access to care, resulting in a fatalistic self-destructive lifestyle), the moral and financial implications would be staggering" (Roach, 2000, p. 261).

Labelling a group of people "at risk" may be a double-edge sword, with either or both good and bad implications or outcomes. For example, this labelling can bring attention to and address the causes of health inequities, consider longer-term risk exposure, provide easier access to resources to address issues, and bring public and political attention and support to an issue. The downside of labelling a group at risk is that this practice may further marginalize and stigmatize a group, expanding societal assumptions of their incapacity or incompetence, and providing a continuing justification of oppressive practices. This may lead to nurses making paternalistic assumptions that drive actions directed toward a group, as nurses may be rendered blind and deaf to that group's decision-making capabilities and voice.

Many traditional research approaches or programs for a population that has been labelled at risk have included interventions to prevent disease or promote health that focus exclusively on requiring those people to learn the facts and then change their own high-risk behaviour. These interventions have been less successful than those that have targeted government regulation or action (i.e., clean water, adequate sewage, housing standards, highway safety, or occupational safety) (Syme, 2000). The multiple risk factor intervention trial (MRFIT) has been described as one such classic failure by its own lead researcher (Syme, 2000). This was a multi-million dollar, randomized control trial conducted across 20 cities in the United States. The research focused on reducing the death rate from heart disease in men by lowering men's risk through behavioural change. Interventions with 6428 men targeted tobacco reduction, diet change, and control over hypertension. The men were closely followed by clinic staff and counsellors over a 6- to 8-year period. They found that the men in the intervention group did not have better results than those men in the control (non-intervention) group (Syme, 2000). In addition to postulating why this and other trials had failed, Syme realized that the focus of health promotion interventions must shift. "In trials like MRFIT, nothing is done to change the distribution of disease in the population because such programs do not address the forces in society that caused the problem in the first place" (p. 80). He concluded, "it is . . . social, economic, organization, or political situations that are at the root of most problems" (p. 92). However, multiple levels for interventions are also important, and the most important of these may be the necessity of empowering individuals as a first step in the movement toward societal change (Syme, 2000).

## THREE LEVELS OF PREVENTION

When nurses look at health promotion and the levels of prevention, they widen their lenses beyond disease prevention to include injury prevention, thereby capturing a broad area to promote the health of individuals, families, and communities. **Prevention interventions** can occur at primary, secondary, or tertiary levels (Offord, 2000). In these levels, actions are directed at either preventing injury or illness from occurring (primary), early identification and treatment to stop a disease process or mitigate its potential negative outcomes (secondary), or if injury has already occurred (or advanced disease is detected), the goal is to prevent further harm and restore maximum function (tertiary), whether to an individual or to a community (Allender & Spradley, 2005; Hitchcock & Bartfay, 2010).

**Primary prevention** promotes health through an **upstream approach** using the identification of potential risk factors and the mobilization of policy and public awareness to avoid injury or illness. Primary prevention is the avoidance of illness or injury through health promotion activities and protective actions; disease or injury has not yet occurred in the population. Strategies are aimed at preventing or reducing the risk of disease or injury from occurring; for example, by improving or maintaining health, boosting the immune system, or preventing injury. Some nursing interventions at this level include (a) promoting the use of seat belts, (b) promoting properly installed CSA-approved car seats to transport newborn babies home, (c) advocating for smoke-free public spaces, and (d) public education to help stop the spread of sexually transmitted infections (STIs) in all age groups. Safe housing, sanitation, and nutrition are other initiatives. Included at this level are immunizations against childhood diseases as well as nurse-managed mass immunization clinics against the influenza virus (CHNC, 2012).

The value of primary prevention is visible in Canada's history with the influenza virus. At the end of World War I, in 1918, Canadian soldiers returned home unwittingly transporting the Spanish influenza with them. From 1918 to 1919 the influenza virus spread quickly, becoming a worldwide epidemic that took the lives of an estimated two million people. The Canadian death toll from the four-year war was 60 000, but in sharp contrast, the Canadian death toll from the one-year Spanish influenza epidemic was 50 000 people. Many who succumbed were young, healthy people who died within a day of contracting the virus. In an attempt to control this epidemic, many non-essential services throughout the country were shut down, quarantines were imposed by each province, and face masks were required to be worn in all public spaces. As a direct result of this epidemic, in 1919 a department of health was created in Canada (Canadian War Museum, n.d.). Primary prevention interventions such as yearly mass immunizations against influenza have helped to prevent a repeat epidemic of such magnitude and devastation. Primary prevention actions have also minimized the spread of preventable childhood diseases, minimized the risk of injuries from car crashes, and helped to slow the spread of many communicable diseases, thereby helping to preserve the health of all Canadians.

**Secondary prevention** promotes health through the early identification of diseases and conditions and timely treatment of them. At this level, the focus is to halt an illness if possible and perhaps effect a cure, or at least slow the progression of a disease through therapeutic treatments and medications. Examples of secondary prevention include (a) screening measures such as examining skin for signs of melanoma, (b) blood tests for diabetes, (c) testicular self-exam, (d) yearly cholesterol tests, and (e) colonoscopies. A remarkable example of successful secondary prevention was the advent of the Papanicolaou (Pap) smear. Used to screen for early detection of cervical cancer, the routine use of Pap smears has had a significant impact on women's deaths from this cancer. Since the 1950s the use of Pap smears has decreased the number of deaths by over 70% (Daley et al., 2013). The availability of and easy access to blood pressure machines throughout communities (i.e., in local grocery or drug stores) is an example of self-monitored secondary prevention. Individuals can become active participants in monitoring their cardiovascular health in part by checking their own blood pressure. When an unusual blood pressure reading arises, individuals can arrange to have their blood pressure assessed more thoroughly by a healthcare provider, potentially preventing damage from undetected and untreated hypertension.

**Tertiary prevention** is initiated once an individual becomes symptomatic, or disease or injury is evident. The focus is on maintaining or restoring function and preventing further disability from the disease or injury. The goal of tertiary prevention is to limit disability and to rehabilitate or restore the affected person to the maximum possible capability, maximize their quality of life, and meet their self-identified goals. Examples of tertiary prevention include rehabilitation for people who have experienced a stroke or counselling for a rape victim. Nurses identify potential complications and implement strategies to help a person adapt, considering their vulnerabilities, strengths, and preferences. Nurses may provide education, monitor treatment effectiveness, or address adverse side effects. An example of nursing interventions using tertiary prevention is described in Chapter 32, Emergency Preparedness. In cases of a disaster such as the 2013 floods in Calgary and southern Alberta that left thousands of people homeless, CHNs may intervene at multiple different levels. These can include providing a range of services such as door-to-door first aid in the disaster zone, emotional support, safety and sanitation education, assessing individual and family needs, and connecting people with basic necessities such as housing, food, and medications. Community-level tertiary interventions include consultation and collaboration with community partners to focus on helping restore a community to its prior level of function.

# UPSTREAM AND DOWNSTREAM APPROACHES TO PROMOTING HEALTH

McKinlay (1994) offers a story as an example of health promotion offering upstream and **downstream approaches** to improving the health of populations. What follows is an adaptation of that story.

Imagine a town situated in a valley where the river provides most of the drinking water. Despite its idyllic appearance, every year many people experience episodes of diarrhea, vomiting, and dehydration, with the most severely impacted including young children, the vulnerable, and the elderly. The town health department has implemented many strategies to help people stay well, such as boiled water advisories advertised on television, radio, billboards, and posters. There are a few wells that have clean drinking water, but these have low flow rates with only enough clean water for the few families who can afford it. The town health department has enough funds to provide antibacterial pills to the people most impacted and pay for medications such as antibiotics for the people who get sick. However, despite all these yearly efforts the morbidity and mortality rates in this town due to gastrointestinal infections remain 10 times the national average. What is not well known is that upstream is a factory that dumps unfiltered sewer into the river (Photo 8.2). The factory owner obtained

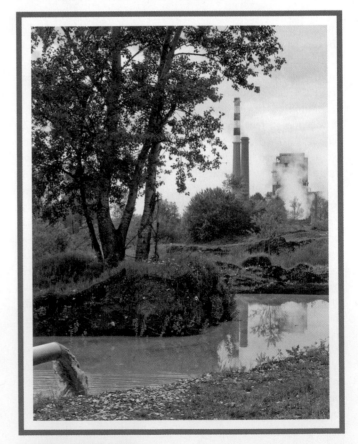

**PHOTO 8.2** Dirty water stems from pipe polluting the river

*Source: Dragana Gerasimoski/Shutterstock*

approval to dump years ago because the products being discarded into the river are organic and biodegradable. However, in recent years the number and size of factory operations have increased dramatically. One day a group of public health nurses received permission to do a community assessment and environmental scan to investigate the problem. They tested the river water and learned the bacterial count was much higher than recommended. From municipal and district reports they learned it had been 15 years since the policies regarding sewage dumping into the river had been addressed. Driving upstream they observed the factory sewage pipes steadily dumping large quantities of waste products into the river. Coming back to their town they encouraged the town health department to take action upstream to ensure that the water the town people were drinking downstream was cleaner. However, town council replied that due to the high cost of treating the ill townspeople, providing antibacterial products to clean the water, and the cost of providing boiled water advisories, there was no money left over to address the upstream issues.

The upstream story may sound bizarre but there are many similar situations in Canada where there is less-than-adequate healthcare funding available for prevention and promotion strategies due to the high cost of providing acute care services. Acute care services are usually tertiary prevention measures, are focused on individual treatment and cure, and are considered downstream interventions. Upstream approaches are oftentimes prevention and promotion strategies focused on policy interventions that benefit the whole population, or PHC interventions that focus on people's well-being by addressing and taking action on the root causes of preventable diseases and injuries. Examples of upstream approaches could include nursing actions that advocate for safer environments—those that encourage safe and affordable exercise, such as walking, running, inline skating, and biking—or lobbying for higher tobacco taxes that encourage people to quit or reduce tobacco use (CPHA, 2011; PHAC, 2013b). Upstream approaches usually extend beyond addressing individual behaviours and identify programs, policies, and environmental changes that will impact the health of a population. The earlier examples of creating environments that encourage exercise and increase the cost of tobacco make it easier for people to make healthy lifestyle choices. Policies such as adding fluoride to municipal water supplies (to prevent dental caries), adding iodine to salt, or vitamin D to milk are upstream interventions made by elected officials to improve the health of the populations they represent.

## HARM REDUCTION

**Harm reduction** is a philosophy and approach to healthcare delivery, programs, or policies, implemented with a goal to protect the health of, and reduce secondary harm for, individuals who engage in high-risk activities that are associated with poor health outcomes. The goal is not cessation of the high-risk behaviour, but rather it is to reduce the more immediate and related harms arising from engaging in that behaviour. A harm reduction approach ensures access to evidence-based

information for individuals to make informed decisions about their lives and health and equal access to promotive healthcare services. Harm reduction requires a non-judgmental stance that focuses on reducing potential harm from high-risk activities while treating individuals with respect and dignity. It is a health-promoting strategy whereby individuals who engage in high-risk lifestyles and behaviours can receive specialized healthcare services to address their concerns and minimize potential negative health outcomes and harms (International Harm Reduction Association, 2010; Pauly, 2007). These individuals may have difficulty accessing healthcare for a wide variety of reasons, including negative past experiences or fear of being judged.

Harm reduction strategies seek to address health inequities and bring meaningful healthcare to those who might otherwise be marginalized by some healthcare providers. Nurses working within this philosophy understand that the goal of care is to protect health by reducing harm but also recognize that complex social issues form the root causes of many high-risk behaviours (Pauly, 2007). Harm reduction seeks to ensure there is equitable access to promotive healthcare, medical care, counselling, and social services for marginalized persons. Harm reduction is not concerned with fixing problems or offering solutions; it is about meeting people "where they are at," providing non-judgmental, compassionate care with the goal of reducing the secondary harm people might experience from engaging in particular high-risk behaviours (International Harm Reduction Association, 2010; Pauly, 2007; Taylor & Caine, 2013). Abuse of illegal and prescription drugs or alcohol; engaging in unsafe, unprotected sexual activities; and limiting exposure to second-hand tobacco smoke are examples of behaviours that harm reduction safety nets address. Providing at-risk individuals with products and healthcare services while they are actively engaging in harmful behaviours not only promotes health and reduces overall negative health outcomes, but it ensures that the universal right to healthcare is accessible to some of the most marginalized, vulnerable Canadians (Taylor & Cain, 2013). As a philosophy, harm reduction recognizes the deeply complex relationship between root causes, social determinants of health, social justice, and health inequities that exist among different socioeconomic groups (Pauly, 2007). Nursing values, beliefs, and attitudes necessary to practise the philosophy of harm reduction with clients are discussed further in more detail later in this chapter.

Harm reduction programs benefit the health of the public as well as the individual by helping to control the spread of communicable diseases like human immune deficiency virus (HIV), hepatitis C, STIs, and preventable lung diseases. For example, tobacco smoke causes physical harm to smokers, but second-hand smoke also harms bystanders who are exposed to it in locations where tobacco use is not regulated (e.g., personal cars and homes). One harm-reduction alternative to smoking is the use of electronic cigarettes. For individuals who are unable or unwilling to abstain from smoking, electronic cigarettes provide the means to continue the habit under a model of tobacco harm reduction (THR) (Phillips & Rodu, 2013). Electronic cigarettes and other alternatives for THR, such as smokeless tobacco (oral snuff) and nicotine patches, do not create smoke that harms others. These are examples of harm reduction that benefits a community as the risk is reduced to only the user.

Examples of other harm reduction programs that nurses participate in include promoting the use of helmets with bicycles, distributing condoms to help control the spread of STIs, and promoting clean needle exchange programs to reduce the incidence of needle sharing and subsequent spread of blood-borne illnesses within the intravenous drug (IVD) user community. At the individual level, harm reduction models provide a safety net that mitigates the potential harm individuals may be exposed to. Nurses practice harm reduction in part by ensuring individuals have access to clean IVD supplies, access to safe disposal for used syringes, and supportive services to promote physical and mental safety for both the individual and the public. Harm reduction in the context of STIs is discussed further in Chapter 31.

## Safe Injection Sites

Vancouver's "Insite" is North America's first and only safe injection facility, operated by nurses. Operating from a harm reduction model, Insite opened in 2003 in Vancouver's Eastside. IVD use in the area was high, as were mortality rates among that community. Prior to the opening of Insite's 12-booth safe injection sites, users self-injected in alleys where they were at a high risk of experiencing theft, violence, arrest, or accidental overdose. After the opening of Insite, the fatal overdose rate decreased by 35% in and around the area, compared to a fatal overdose rate decrease of only 9.3% in the rest of the city (Marshall, Millroy, Wood Montaner, & Kerr, 2011). In this nurse-run clinic (employing nurses, counsellors, and support staff), clients who were traditionally hard to reach now had a safe place to inject, in addition to access to healthcare, addiction treatment, mental health counselling, social support, and a way to connect with outside services (Bard, 2011). At Insite, clients are given clean needles and supplies, can exchange dirty needles, are monitored for potential overdose while they inject, and are provided with emergency care if an overdose happens. There they can have their health concerns addressed and learn about the importance of using only clean supplies to protect themselves and others against the spread of blood-borne diseases (Jozaghi & Andresen, 2013). Expanded well beyond offering a needle exchange program, Insite addresses the need for health services and a way to connect people with other support services, mental, and physical care.

Insite's harm reduction IVD program has demonstrated its value by saving taxpayers $1.9 million a year in HIV and accidental overdose-related healthcare costs (Pinkerton, 2011). Nurses are instrumental in providing harm reduction services to Insite as well as to many other harm reduction programs and have been at the forefront of the movement to protect Insite from closure. In 2011, the Supreme Court of Canada ruled against the federal government's attempts to have the safe injection site permanently closed. Nursing organizations across Canada supported the program and its nurses

during the long court battle (Keepnews, 2011). Nurses argued that "people at risk of addiction or people dealing with an addiction have a constitutional right not to be denied access to health services that reduce the risk of morbidity and mortality related to addiction" (Lynkowski, 2011, para. 4). The nurses' legal argument advocating for the constitutional rights of this marginalized group of citizens influenced the outcome of the Supreme Court's decision to keep North

### CASE STUDY

Benita Cohen

One of the key roles of the CHN working in a public health setting is to support the family in the first year of the life of a new child. This includes assisting parents in their new role(s), promoting optimal child development, and connecting the family with appropriate community resources.

Imagine that you are a CHN who has been given a postpartum referral from the local hospital. The referral contains the following information: first-time mother, 17 years old; newborn male born at 36 weeks' gestation, weighing six pounds; unclear if infant's father is involved; very little contact with the healthcare system prior to giving birth; receiving social assistance; has no phone. You arrive at the address, which is located in a low-income neighbourhood, and find the mother alone with her infant in a tiny one-bedroom apartment on the third floor of a poorly maintained building without an elevator. You observe that the apartment has very few furnishings, dirty dishes piled in the sink, empty junk food wrappers and containers everywhere, and a strong smell of cigarette smoke. The mother quickly becomes tearful, stating that she doesn't have enough money to pay the rent, and she has no family and few friends in the community.

Using the population health promotion model as a guide, answer the discussion questions.

#### Discussion Questions

1. What information do you already know and what additional information do you need to obtain about the determinants of health affecting this family?

2. Give specific examples of one or more health promotion strategies that you as the CHN could use at the individual, family, or community level to address each of the following determinants of health affecting this family. Consider other health professionals or workers in other disciplines or sectors with whom you might collaborate in these strategies:

   a. income and social status

   b. social support networks

   c. personal health practices and coping

   d. healthy child development

   e. access to health services

3. What knowledge, skills, or attitudes does the CHN require in order to effectively promote the health of this family?

America's only supervised injection facility open (Lynkowski, 2011). At the heart of the court battle was the drive to ensure the health and safety of a marginalized, vulnerable group of Canadian citizens. It became the responsibility of nurses to speak out against the closure of Insite and protect these vulnerable people by addressing immediate issues as well as confronting the social forces that create an environment of health inequity. The Canadian Nurses Association has tirelessly advocated for supervised injection sites, as shared by the president of CNA: "We presented to the provincial/territorial health ministers on harm reduction; called on the federal government to replace Bill C-65 with a new bill based on the principles of harm reduction, established best practices and sound research; and appeared before the media to further drive home the message" (Mildon, 2013b, p. 4).

Nursing's roles in harm reduction include developing, managing, operating, and promoting harm reduction programs; advocacy work to educate governments and society about the foundational principles and positive benefits of harm reduction programs; and reducing barriers to accessing healthcare that exist for homeless people, people who abuse substances, sex trade workers, or others whose lifestyles place them at risk for increased morbidity and mortality (Pauly, 2007). At a political level, nurses address harm reduction by confronting and addressing the underlying root causes of harmful behaviours: (a) poverty, (b) inequity, and (c) social injustice. Nurses act as advocates and are activists for social change to address the root causes that determine the health of Canadians. Nurses lobby governments and sectors across society to provide safe neighbourhoods, affordable housing, food security, fair working conditions and remuneration, safe and affordable educational childcare programs for working parents, timely psychological support for survivors of trauma or abuse, and the rights of women and children to be full members of society.

## Community Health Application Example

Leonard Syme shared a story about an issue with high rates of hypertension and stress in San Francisco bus drivers. The bus company was looking for a program to teach drivers better coping skills so they could deal more effectively with their stress levels. They even suggested including nutrition and exercise programs, and encouraging employees to seek medical attention for their high blood pressures. However, after extensive research and working in a partnership approach to explore the issues with the drivers themselves, Syme's team discovered the bus drivers were experiencing multiple health-related issues in addition to hypertension, and that the root cause of the issue was not their personal behaviours; rather, it was a brutal and unrealistic bus schedule over which they had no control (Syme, 2000). The bus drivers' lack of control over harmful working conditions was causing their multiple health issues (Photo 8.3). Bus drivers were mobilized to press for changes through their union, and once the company understood an individualistic approach was not going to solve the larger issues, they then became open to structural and organi-

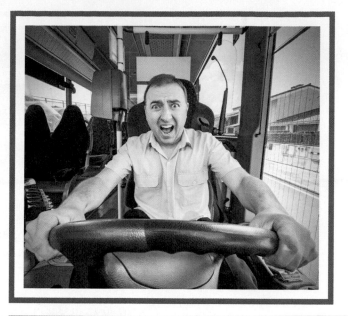

**PHOTO** **8.3** Bus driver stressed over bus schedule

*Source: Leonardo2011/Shutterstock*

zational change. This story exemplifies community health nursing concepts of **empowerment** and **community development** that played key roles in addressing the root causes of this pervasive health issue and success for bus drivers gaining a measure of control over their workplace environments.

## HEALTH BELIEF AND OTHER MODELS

The **health belief model** (Figure 8.3) is a common model used to promote health, with its origins dating back to social theory research completed by Rosenstock in the 1960s. Rosenstock investigated the reasons why people did not adopt healthy lifestyles or participate in preventative healthcare measures, with a goal of improving population health (Rosenstock, 1966). The health belief model that arose from this area of research suggests there is a greater probability of people making healthy choices if they believe that (a) they have a high risk of getting the disease, (b) the consequences of the disease are serious, (c) taking action to minimize the risk will benefit them, and that (d) there are relatively few obstacles or challenges to making the behaviour or lifestyle change, (e) they are prompted or reminded to perform the behaviours, and (f) they believe they can execute the behaviour (self-efficacy) (Champion & Skinner, 2008).

The health belief model has become a focus of widespread education, programming, and research. Carpenter (2010) completed a meta-analysis of the literature on the effectiveness of the health belief model variables in predicting behaviour, and found that increasing an individual's perception of the severity of a disease was not highly effective in changing behaviour; however, the belief that taking action would produce positive outcomes produced consistently positive outcomes. Perceptions of benefits and perceptions of

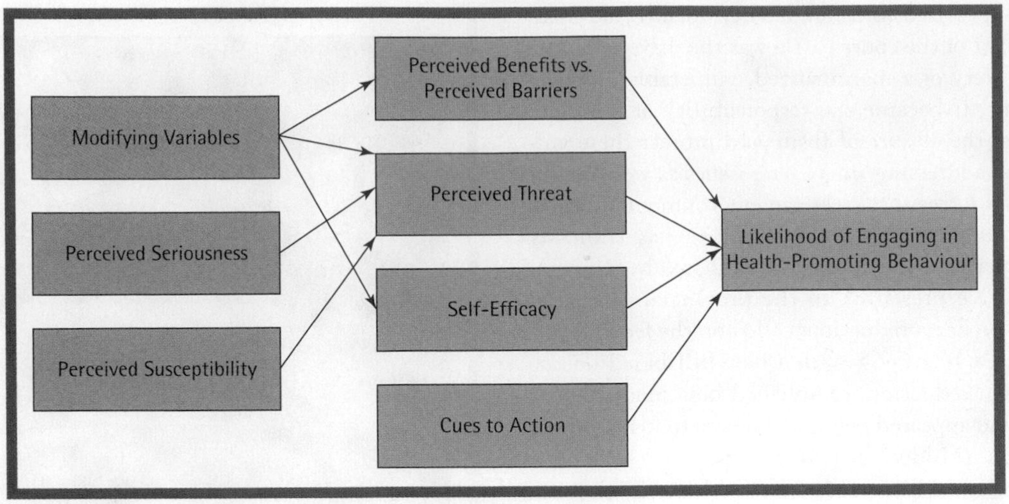

FIGURE 8.3 The Health Belief Model

*Source:* Champion, V. L., & Skinner, C. S. (2008). The health belief model. In K. Glanz, B. K. Rimer, & K. Viswanath (Eds), *Health behavior and health education: Theory, research, and practice* (4th ed., pp. 45–64). San Francisco, CA: Jossey-Bass.

barriers to performing a healthy lifestyle action were the strongest predictors of behaviour. There is a tendency for nurses, and other healthcare professionals, to believe individuals and populations will change their behaviour based solely on an understanding of how serious the consequences may be. Many marketing campaigns are developed based on this belief. An example is placing graphic pictures of lung cancer tumours on cigarette packages. However, this approach has little or no impact on people who smoke unless it is linked with reducing the barriers and promoting the benefits of change to them. Strategies or interventions focused on the relationship between risks and benefits and those that make it easier for people to make healthy choices have resulted in numerous successful health promotion interventions (Sohl & Moyer, 2007). The health belief model is directed at individuals rather than populations, but community, sector, or societal level involvement is also necessary to increase the population's awareness of issues, to educate about benefits and risks, to create environments that make a healthy choice the easy choice, to reduce real or perceived barriers to making a lifestyle change, and to provide a means to cue individuals to participate in a healthy behaviour or stop unhealthy behaviours. Advertising campaigns may popularize suggested cues, such as to change the batteries on your smoke detector when you adjust your clocks to and from daylight savings time. The health belief model is effective when used in combination with PHC, the population health promotion model, change theory, and models that address self-efficacy.

## Other Models

There are a number of other models that are used to predict or change health behaviours, ranging from those that target individual health behaviours to those that target groups and communities. Examples of other models focused on individuals include the theory of reasoned action, the theory of planned behaviour (Montano &

Kasprzyk, 2008), the PRECEDE-PROCEED model (Gielen, McDonald, Gary, & Bone, 2008), and the transtheoretical model and stages of change (Prochaska, Redding, & Evers, 2008). Ecological models are described as those that emphasize environmental and policy effects on behaviour, acknowledging that there are multiple levels of influence that affect individuals' behaviours (Sallis, Owen, & Fisher, 2008).

A shift away from an individual focus to include broader multi-level and social change models are emerging, representing a paradigm shift in understanding what the targets of effective interventions need to be (Orleans, 2008). Examples of these emerging models include community-building approaches (Minkler, Wallerstein, & Wilson, 2008) and a number of theories of organizational change (Butterfoss, Kegler, & Francisco, 2008; Whitney & Trosten-Bloom, 2003).

## SOCIAL MARKETING

Social marketing is a term that was introduced in 1971 to describe the use of marketing principles and techniques to advance a social cause, idea, or behaviour (Kotler & Roberto, 1989). Social marketing is a strategy that uses proven concepts and techniques from the commercial sector to promote changes in social behaviours. The goal of social marketing is to encourage health-promoting behaviours, or to eliminate or significantly reduce behaviours that negatively impact a population's health. It has been described as a health intervention approach (Gordon, McDermott, Stead, & Angus, 2006). Used appropriately, social marketing holds enormous potential to create healthy change and influence social issues (Andreasen, 1995). Examples of successful long-running social marketing campaigns include Participaction (see Figure 8.4), with exercise promotion strategies. Other examples include promotions to increase breastfeeding or to decrease unprotected sex. Social marketing is most effective for populations that are considering change or have been unsuccessful when they try to change. Social marketing is also used when health promoters have a goal of improving the health of communities or populations that are not easy to reach via other methods. For example, it could be fairly easy to intervene with children who attend school as they are a "captive audience," but to reach other audiences, such as working adults, social marketing is one of the few successful strategies. Even though similar approaches may be used, social marketing campaigns are not education campaigns where the objective is just to create awareness of an issue. The objective of social media campaigns is to promote "socially beneficial behaviour change" (Grier & Bryant, 2005, p. 319). Although social marketing can be highly effective, one caution is that it is not always appropriate to use. Social marketing would be ineffective for people who actively resist change or who are entrenched in a particular behaviour with no interest in change. Alternate strategies may be required. For example, legislative intervention (passing a law that required everyone to comply) was required to achieve high percentages of seat-belt use in Canadian populations.

Six essential benchmarks of a successful social marketing intervention (see Table 8.1) have been described as (a) voluntary behaviour change with measurable objectives; (b) consumer research, whereby the intervention is derived from knowledge of consumers' values and needs; (c) segmentation and targeting, where different variables are considered for a more focused selection of target groups; (d) a marketing mix that uses the

"Four Ps" described in Table 8.1; (e) exchange, meaning the target group feels it receives a reward (tangible or intangible); and (f) competition, whereby competing behaviours are identified and strategies are developed to minimize competing forces to the targeted behaviour change (Gordon et al., 2006).

Before initiating a social marketing strategy, nurses must have a clear understanding of their target audience and what specific behaviour they want that group to change or adopt, and there must be a clear and concise statement of the desired

| Table 8.1 | Andreasen's Benchmarks of a Successful Social Marketing Intervention |
|---|---|
| **Benchmark** | **Explanation** |
| 1. Behaviour Change | Intervention seeks to change behaviour and has specific measurable behavioural objectives. |
| 2. Consumer Research | Intervention is based on an understanding of consumer experiences, values, and needs. Formative research is conducted to identify these. Intervention elements are pre-tested with the target group. |
| 3. Segmentation and Targeting | Different segmentation variables are considered when selecting the intervention target group. Intervention strategy is tailored for the selected segment(s). |
| 4. Marketing Mix | Intervention considers the best strategic application of the "marketing mix." This consists of the four Ps of "product," "price," "place," and "promotion." Other Ps might include "policy change" or "people" (e.g., training is provided to intervention delivery agents). Interventions that only use the promotion P are social advertising, not social marketing. |
| 5. Exchange | Intervention considers what will motivate people to engage voluntarily with the intervention and offers them something beneficial in return. The offered benefit may be intangible (e.g., personal satisfaction) or tangible (e.g., rewards for participating in the program and making behavioural changes). |
| 6. Competition | Competing forces to the behaviour change are analyzed. Intervention considers the appeal of competing behaviours (including current behaviour) and uses strategies that seek to remove or minimize this competition. |

Source: Adapted from McDermott et al., 2005a.

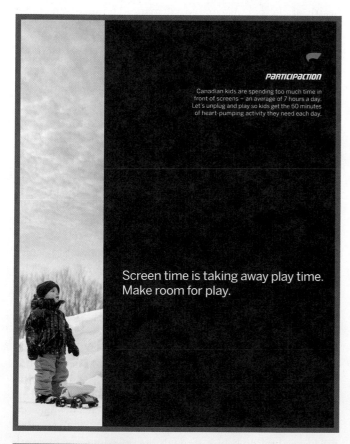

**FIGURE 8.4** Participaction Social Marketing Poster

*Source:* Courtesy of ParticiPACTION

- What is the nature and scope of the issue your program is trying to resolve? (Why this, why now?)
- What are the solutions and approaches you plan to implement? Have they been tried and tested in conditions similar to your own? You are strongly encouraged to review existing literature and interview colleagues on their relevant experiences.
- Based on your answers to the previous questions, which target audiences should you try to influence? You may have more than one target audience. Your target audiences may be internal (employees, board of directors, committee members, and volunteers) or external (population segments, decision-makers, professionals, politicians, partners, etc.). Include any potential partners on your list. Do not automatically assume that they will form partnerships with you. Specify what you want each of your target audiences to "do" in an "observable" way. This is the most important issue when analyzing target audiences.

| Target audiences | What you want them to "do" |
| --- | --- |
|  |  |
|  |  |
|  |  |
|  |  |
|  |  |

**FIGURE 8.5** Worksheet 1: Change Objectives

*Source:* Lagarde, F. (2004). Worksheets to introduce some basic concepts of social marketing principles. *Social Marketing Quarterly, 10*(1), 36–41.

change. Most health promotion practitioners have many important messages they want delivered to a target audience. It is usually challenging to determine which one is the highest priority and which is most likely to achieve measurable change. An important question to ask is therefore, "if the target population follows the suggested action, will I achieve my program goal?"

Social marketing is based on the Four Ps of commercial marketing, which include offering the right product, at the right price, presented in the right time and right place, and promoted in the right way. The product being "sold" is an idea or behaviour related to better health—a social practice or a tangible object, with service or support offered to assist the target audience to adopt the desired behaviour. Examples of products could be weight loss or tobacco cessation programs. An important concept in social marketing is having a clear call to action. A call to action is not suggesting that a smoker quits or a sedentary person exercises but, rather, is giving them the next step toward attaining that goal, such as a phone number to call for help.

The price refers to the cost to the target audience. The target audience has to accept this cost, and while it is not necessarily a financial cost it means that sometimes they will have to forfeit or forego something else if they make the desired change. For example, the price of quitting alcohol or tobacco use may be incurring withdrawal symptoms, loss of a comfortable coping strategy, or change in familiar socialization patterns. The unhealthy behaviour is the competition for the health-producing behaviour. If the target audience perceives that the price is too high they will either not attempt change or will quickly return to the competition, which is the familiar or habitual harmful behaviour. If the price is deemed high the campaign must consider what type of product will help reduce the cost to the target market. A campaign planner who has reviewed the literature about fears associated with quitting alcohol consumption may be led to include images of a similar population socializing in a coffee shop instead of in a bar. This is also called an **exchange intervention**, where a coffee with friends is exchanged for alcoholic beverages. To improve the health of the population, social marketers must remember that the healthy option must be made more attractive than the unhealthy option.

The right time and place refers to considering the timing for, and means by which, the social product is delivered to the target audience. The timing of a message can be maximized to dovetail with an issue a community identifies, as there may be a readiness for change at that point and an opportunity for an intervention. For an example of right time and place, to encourage increased exercise for parents of growing children, campaign developers would first need to recognize many parents are very busy and have little time to meet their own needs. However, if an exercise program could occur while their children are engaged in an activity at the same location, these timing and place considerations may incorporate parents' lifestyle needs.

Finally, the right promotion refers to the means by which the product is promoted or advertised to the audience. This means the campaign reaches the audience, the audience understands what you are offering them, and the action you want them to take is very clear. The action may be a phone number to call, a website to visit, or a product to purchase. It delivers a short, clear message of what the target audience should do.

Consumer research uses an analysis of the target audience, which includes their perceptions of barriers (price), social norms impacting the issue, and the competition. The competition refers to what else (other than the desired behaviour) may satisfy the same need in the group. For example, if the goal or product is healthy babies through breastfeeding, the competition may be formula feeding (Grier & Bryant, 2005). This information can be learned through completing interviews and focus groups with people who have and those who have not adopted a desired behaviour. It is also important to learn as much as possible about what incentives have made it possible for people with similar characteristics to change and what has deterred others from making the change. An environmental scan can assist in understanding the social norms of a community and help gain a better understanding of the settings in which people live, work, commute, and play, as these contribute to social behaviour. Including the social determinants of health from the population health promotion model can provide a larger-scale understanding about what impacts the health of a community and whether social marketing is the most appropriate strategy for a particular issue. Consumer research often results in further segmentation of the target group. For example, a local fetal alcohol network wanted to reach young women who drank alcohol in pregnancy. Focus groups revealed social drinking in young women is highly influenced by their peers and partners. Therefore, the campaign was further segmented to reach the young women's circles of friends.

Careful assessment and planning are necessary to determine the key message, the characteristics of the target audience, the

barriers and facilitators to change, and the place and promotional approaches to use. This may include completing literature reviews, consulting key stakeholders, collecting census information such as income and educational levels of the target population, completing focus groups, or conducting surveys (Lagarde & Gendron, 2011). Selecting a social marketing approach is based on the availability of resources and on the characteristics of the target audience, including its size, age range, education levels, income, employment status and occupations, geographic location (inner-city, suburban or rural), languages spoken, culture, and any other distinctive characteristic. For example, mailing postcards to a target population is only an effective strategy if you have accurate mailing information and the target group can read. Posters in bathroom stalls may be the choice for campaigns to reduce sexually transmitted infections. Television, Internet, and bus advertisements are more expensive but often the method of choice for scattered populations (Lagarde, 2004).

After extensive research has been done and a preliminary campaign has been developed, you must pilot test it on a small subset of the target population. These people should be able to easily identify what you are asking them to do and how you are

---

Worksheet 2 can be photocopied and filled out for each audience identified in Worksheet 1. Remember that:

- There is not necessarily a direct or obvious link between needs and desired behaviours;
- Benefits refer to the adoption of the desired behaviours or actions from the target audience's perspective—not from the perspective of experts on the issue;
- Barriers may be perceived or real;

- Influencers refer to people or groups that can have favourable (+), neutral (=), or unfavourable (−) influences;
- You need to identify locations, groups, events or media where you can potentially reach the target audience; and
- In gathering information about the audience, be sure to distinguish between those who have already adopted the behaviour and those who have not. This will help with the segmentation process.

Audience:

What you want them to do (see Worksheet 1):

| | Those who have adopted the behaviour | Those who have *not* |
|---|---|---|
| Demographic data (number, age, sex, level of education, family status, income, occupation, urban or rural population, languages, and other cultural characteristics) | | |
| Overall needs | | |
| Benefits of adopting the behaviour | | |
| Real or perceived barriers to adopting the behaviour | | |
| Stage(s) of change | | |
| Influencers | | |
| Media habits and participation in events | | |
| Membership in groups and places where target audience can be reached | | |

Segmentation: Among those who have not yet adopted the behaviour, can you identify specific segments based on demographic, behavioural, or lifestyle data? Please explain.

**FIGURE 8.6** Worksheet 2: Abridged Audience Analysis

*Source:* Lagarde, F. (2004). Worksheets to introduce some basic concepts of social marketing principles. *Social Marketing Quarterly, 10*(1), 36–41.

going to help them do it. They should also tell you whether the campaign makes the desired change more attractive than other competing social messages that may exist (e.g., if you come drink at our bar we'll guarantee you'll meet new friends). For further help, Lagarde (2004) developed worksheets (Figures 8.5 and 8.6) to introduce basic concepts of social marketing practices, recommending that students and novice practitioners use these sheets to help guide this complex process and increase the effectiveness of a social marketing campaign.

## APPROACHES TO CREATING AND SUPPORTING HEALTH IN SOCIETY

### Nursing Values, Beliefs, and Attitudes Necessary for Health-Promoting Practice

Nursing values, beliefs, and attitudes affect practice behaviour. As every nurse is first a human being who comes with a history and personal culture, it is important to examine what drives practice, aside from skills and knowledge. Values, beliefs, and assumptions lie beneath our foundation of evidence-based decision making, research evaluation, and experiential learning in the base of the PHPM. Self-knowledge starts with examining where one's own values come from. Oftentimes they come from one's family of origin, but also from one's culture, society, peers, and workplaces. Values are enduring beliefs or attitudes about the worth of a person, object, idea, or action; sometimes these are unconsciously held. Examples of nursing values include social justice, altruism, autonomy, human dignity, and integrity (Kozier et al., 2014). Beliefs are opinions, interpretations, or conclusions that we accept as true; sometimes these are based more on faith than on fact. An example of a belief is that if one works harder, then one will be able to get better pay. Attitudes are a mental position or feelings toward a person, object, or idea; these often last over time (Kozier et al., 2014). Examples of attitudes valued in nursing practice include acceptance, openness, and compassion. Assumptions often operate unconsciously; these are beliefs that are taken for granted and remain unexamined. One example is that nursing is women's work. Although incorrect, this general societal assumption still seems to be commonplace and may restrain some very competent men from entering nursing.

A case study in the form of a simulation mannequin developed in a faculty of nursing shows another example of how understanding one's values, beliefs, and attitudes can affect practice behaviour. Imogene Henderson is a mannequin dressed up and moulaged to represent a battered sex trade worker and then introduced to undergraduate nursing students in their community health theory class (Mawji & Lind, 2013). Students are asked to look at Imogene's injuries and speculate what might have happened to her, and then to identify what health issues she may be at risk for. Following this class discussion, students are told Imogene's life story, which includes childhood poverty, abuse, trauma, and subsequent life on the streets. Students are asked to discuss how she is likely viewed and treated by society, and to provide a rationale for their answer to the question of whether or not it is okay that her life has turned out this way (Mawji & Lind, 2013). This exercise has proved to be an eye-opening experience for some students who had thought they held non-judgmental attitudes but, when faced with her profession, discovered they held beliefs and attitudes that would potentially negatively affect their behaviour and approach to working with a person like Imogene.

## Collaborative Partnership Approaches

Collaborative and partnership approaches are effective community-development and relationship-building strategies employed by CHNs. Relationships are built with individuals, families, communities, and key decision makers working within systems or structures that have an impact on the health of communities. Human beings are social creatures and relationship-building skills are critical to developing trust, building bridges, forming partnerships, sharing power, building respect, achieving reciprocity, and focusing on strengths-based approaches when working with communities. Developing a relational practice environment requires the development of trust and rapport, good listening skills, an effective and inclusive communication style, shared commitment, **resilience** and flexibility (having a "plan B" in your back pocket), and working from a mindset of partnering with clients and communities. These are also conditions that facilitate community development, a concept discussed in Chapter 7. This community development occurs in part because of the relational practice environments nurses set up with others within a community. The focus is on developing relationships with others as a means of partnering effectively with them to address health promotion strategies for their identified health challenges or concerns. As an outcome of this approach to practice, social capital may be built within a community. Social capital is described as a resource that a community acquires when co-operation for mutual benefit leads to the achievement of goals and results from a process in which trust, reciprocity, and civic engagement are built between community members (Minkler et al., 2008).

Developing collaborative relationships with communities is quite different from traditional hierarchical relationships in healthcare. Traditional hierarchical relationships tend to be more authoritative, paternalistic, unilaterally top-down, "power-over" approaches that arise from a "treatment mentality" toward nursing practice—a perspective that suggests the healthcare professional is the expert with the knowledge and power to treat and cure disease, and the role of the client or patient is to comply with the professional's plan. This value is much like a parent–child relationship where the parent knows best. On the other hand, a collaborative partnership approach arose from the health promotion movement. It is based on reciprocal relationships, participatory practices, and mutual

| Table 8.2 | Comparison of Traditional and Strengths-Based Problem-Solving Approaches |
|-----------|---------------------------------------------------------------------------|
| **Traditional Problem-Solving Steps** | **Strengths-Based Appreciative Approach** |
| 1. "Felt need" identification of problem | 1. Appreciating and valuing the best of what exists in the present |
| 2. Analysis of causes | 2. Envisioning the potential based on existing strengths |
| 3. Analysis of possible solutions | 3. Dialoguing what could be done |
| 4. Action planning (treatment) | Underlying assumptions: |
| Underlying assumptions: | The community can address its problems |
| The community is a problem to be fixed | Community knows best |
| Experts know best | Asset model |
| Deficit model | |

Source: Lind, C., & Smith, D. (2008). Analyzing the state of community health nursing: Advancing from deficit to strengths-based practice using appreciative inquiry. *Advances in Nursing Science, 31*(1), 28–41.

relationships. Rooted in an ethos of caring based on an egalitarian system of values, the nurse's role is to help the other person (or community) grow and develop, and it supports the client's efforts to make decisions and assume responsibility for themselves. Mutual respect and joint decision making are at the base of this approach to care so that it resembles more of an adult-to-adult relationship wherein each partner has comparable status and power. Both the nurse and the client have knowledge and expertise, albeit different, that can be shared in a mutual approach and joint responsibility for decision making. Mutual respect is visible in this approach to care.

Why do nurses build partnerships with people through public participation? As Raeburn and Rootman (2007) stated, "other than policy development and advocacy, community development/capacity building is arguably the most important single approach available to health promotion practitioners, one that fully embodies the central health promotion principles of empowerment, participation, and a sense of control by ordinary people" (p. 25). How do nurses build partnerships with people? Working from within the population health promotion perspective, building trusting relationships and rapport, building personal confidence and skills through valuing clients' expertise and knowledge, engaging in empowering educational strategies, connecting to broader social networks, and tapping into clients' strengths are all ways in which nurses build partnerships (Aston, Meagher-Stewart, Edwards, & Young, 2009).

## Resilience or Strengths-Based Approach

Capacity-building approaches are discussed in Chapter 7, Theoretical Foundations of Community Health Nursing. Resiliency approaches are those that focus on strengths of a group, rather than on deficits, and build upon those to create health promotion initiatives. Working from a strengths-based approach does not negate or overlook the fact that individuals, communities, and populations have health issues and problems. Rather, it is a way to engage people in co-creating a healthier future by first focusing on what they are doing well, what works well, and what their strengths are, and then building upon these strengths to create a healthier future (Table 8.2). Resilience-creating, appreciative, strengths-based approaches are health-promoting approaches to nursing practice, which can move policies and programs toward more socially just practices congruent with community health nursing values (Lind & Smith, 2008). When people feel they are listened to and that their ideas are valued in an appreciative approach to practice, this is both a health-promoting and empowering strategy that can challenge a deficit orientation regarding a group's capabilities and create openings for improving health (Lind & Smith, 2008).

## NURSING HEALTH PROMOTION RESEARCH FOR ACTION

Nurses provide care for people from conception to death and in a variety of settings ranging from acute-care institutions to community-based settings and people's homes with the goal of helping people achieve and maintain their maximum level of health and wellness. Many of the people nurses care for have health conditions, illnesses, or injuries that could have been prevented with early intervention or prevention strategies, so nurses are well aware that an "ounce of prevention is worth a pound of cure." Nurses work closely with individuals, which results in an appreciation of the challenges that illness and injury cause, not only for the individual but also for their families, communities, and the larger society. They repeatedly hear about the chain of events that lead to life-threatening or life-altering outcomes for individuals and families. Nursing passion for health promotion and prevention activities results from knowledge of the effects of real-life situations on real people. The following Canadian Research Boxes 8.1 to 8.3 are some examples of nursing research and action that seek to promote the health of individuals and communities. These examples demonstrate the diversity of health promotion research projects and how nurses have applied health promotion principles in a variety of settings. In each situation there was a team that worked together with community members and key stakeholders; each project occurred over a lengthy time period; and the changes were approved of and valued by the targeted communities.

### CANADIAN RESEARCH BOX 8.1

**Among frail older adults eligible for publicly funded home care services, does a multi-component, nurse-led HPDP (health promotion and disease prevention) strategy, when compared with usual home care, (1) improve HRQOL (health-related quality of life)? (2) have a favourable effect on risk factors for frailty and functional decline? (3) reduce expenditures for other health and social service utilization from a societal perspective? and (4) benefit some subgroups of older adults more than others?**

Markle-Reid, M., Browne, G., & Gafni, A. (2013). Nurse-led health promotion interventions improve quality of life in frail, older home care clients: Lessons learned from three randomized trials in Ontario, Canada. *Journal of Evaluation in Clinical Practice, 19*(1), 118–131.

The goal of this research was to evaluate the effectiveness of different multi-component, nurse-led HPDP interventions in three trials. The research included 498 community-living, frail, older adults (homecare clients 65 years or older) living in southern Ontario. The authors noted that people over the age of 65 are the fastest-growing population in Canada and this population lives with the highest rates of disability and illness. Nevertheless, many older adults are choosing to age in their own homes. Markle-Reid, Browne, and Gafni saw an opportunity to implement health promotion strategies to assist frail seniors living in their homes and improve the quality of the seniors' (and their caregivers') lives. They implemented and evaluated 6- or 12-month-long multi-component evidence-based strategies targeting risk factors for functional decline and frailty. These included strategies to promote health, prevent disability, and support independence by proactively identifying and addressing unrecognized problems and linking them to the appropriate services or support. The impact on home care services was measured afterward and showed there was no difference in costs incurred between the clients who were on the health-promoting program and those who were not. However, the clients on the program showed improved quality of life as measured by improvement in mental health, physical functioning, and social support.

#### Discussion Questions

1. How does promoting the health of frail older adults impact their ability to live independently?

2. How could a resilience or strengths-based approach to nursing care influence the health outcomes of frail older adults living independently?

3. Using the population health promotion model as a guide, with a group of fellow students discuss potential interventions to support the population of older adults who choose to age in place.

### CANADIAN RESEARCH BOX 8.2

**How do we create messages to increase young women's awareness that cigarette smoking and second-hand smoke increase the risk of being diagnosed with breast cancer?**

Haines, R. J., Bottorff, J. L., McKeown, S. B., Ptolemy, E., Carey, J., & Sullivan, K. (2010). Breast cancer messaging for younger women: Gender, femininity and risk. *Qualitative Health Research, 20*(6), 731–742.

A nurse-led health promotion research team in British Columbia conducted a mixed methods study to understand how to best create messages to increase young women's awareness that cigarette smoking and second-hand smoke increase the risk of being diagnosed with breast cancer (Haines et al., 2010). The preparatory work included completing an environmental scan of social marketing campaigns with messages addressing breast cancer and young women. The researchers were disturbed by social marketing campaigns using messages or a strategy that "sexually objectifies young women's breasts and bodies" (p. 731). They questioned why images of slim young women with exposed breasts were required for young women to understand or "hear" the message. Focus groups were completed with young women to assess their reactions to current breast cancer education and social marketing messages, and to help design effective messaging linking breast cancer and tobacco exposure within a holistic context that ensures dignity and valuing of young women's bodies, minds, and abilities. Findings from the research identified that stereotypical representations of femininity sexually objectify young women's bodies, providing the message that beauty and appearance are more valued than physical health and well-being. Current breast cancer preventative campaigns that use images of women with perfect bodies and beautiful faces can create harm by alienating young women who do not identify with that representation of gender and beauty. The researchers identified the importance of including young women's feedback and input in the design of campaigns that will resonate with how young women view age, gender, and health issues in relation to breast cancer risk.

#### Discussion Questions

1. The initial research intent was to create a social marketing campaign to increase young women's awareness of the potential harm associated with cigarette smoke. What preliminary information did the researchers collect that caused them to be concerned?

2. Other health-promoting groups had approved and paid for social marketing strategies that sexually objectified women's breasts in smoking cessation advertisements. What nursing values or education may have contributed toward this research team's identification of the potential risks of sexual objectification?

3. What other unique contributions could a nursing perspective bring to social marketing?

CANADIAN RESEARCH BOX 8.3

Research study goals included "to assess changes when a combined action research and setting-based health promotion approach was used by students and organizational leaders working in partnership" (p. 4). The focus was to jointly design and take action to create health-promoting changes relevant to student-identified health priorities.

Budgen, C., Callaghan, D., Gamble, D., Wiebe, R., Feddersen, M., Dunn, S., Johnson, R., McHugh, N., Morrison, H., Sullivan, K., & Cull, I. (2011). Creating a healthier campus community using action research and health promotion strategies: Students and organizational leaders as partners. *International Journal of Health, Wellness and Society, 1*(3), 155–175.

This nurse-led study on a university campus combined community-based participatory action research with settings-based health promotion strategies and a youth–adult partnership approach. Students and organizers worked together as co-researchers to identify health issues and create health-promoting change. Researchers collected data using field notes and document review as well as surveys. Student researchers from the university community used photovoice method, which involved using digital cameras to photograph campus life and activities related to health (to help identify areas of strengths and concern), later recording the changes they saw. Photographs were analyzed and themes about potential issues arose that directed the creation of survey questions. Survey questions focused on gathering students' ideas on what makes a campus healthy, what makes their campus healthy or unhealthy, and what could make their campus healthier. The final survey question shared the issue areas compiled from analysis of photographs and asked participants to choose the top three issues for action. Campus food was one of the top priorities identified for improvement. The research team engaged in multiple levels of health promotion activity based on the Ottawa Charter including finding common ground between the health promotion project and university food vendors, both of which wanted to increase student satisfaction with campus food. An evaluation at the end of the two-year study indicated that students had more access to healthy food and their satisfaction with campus food had increased. Though health promotion strategies helped attain results from this research, other community health skills were required to maintain interest, form egalitarian partnerships, recruit and mentor team members, and form new relationships as some student co-researchers left the study and new students entered.

### Discussion Questions

1. Were you surprised that students on this campus were more satisfied with healthier food? Why or why not?

2. A focus of this study was to identify health issues and help create a healthier university campus. Ultimately, the area of action was specific and targeted—to provide students with healthier food. Why is this a good example of a health promotion study? Why would ongoing planning and action be necessary?

3. How is the WHO definition of health promotion exemplified in this research study?

# ADVOCACY AND ACTIVISM IN HEALTH PROMOTION PRACTICE

The profession of nursing has a history of **social action** and **activism**. This includes leaders such as Florence Nightingale, who shaped the profession of nursing as a social movement intent on reform, and Lillian Wald. Early in the 20th century, Lillian Wald used activism as a public health intervention to effect change for the people living in poverty in the College Settlement on Henry Street in New York City. Her lobbying work led to changes for child labour and the development of a federal Children's Bureau (De Leeuw & De Leeuw, 1961). Lavinia Dock was at the forefront of the fight for women's right to vote, and Margaret Sanger, credited with creating the term "birth control," was indicted and jailed for her efforts to distribute birth control information to women. Although social activism is a component of nursing's past, nurses have not used the route of social expression on a major scale since the days of Lillian Wald. In recent history, because more nurses practise in an environment that gives preference to the individual, they are not perceived as social activists but more as patient advocates. It is the attention to society as a whole that makes advocacy a social justice issue and a mandatory component of public health and community nursing practice. Nursing practice settings are already starting to shift from hospitals to work based more in community settings in Canada (Bartfay, 2010), which will create more opportunities for nursing practice focused on health promotion and different forms of advocacy and activism.

Ignoring the political realities of health, particularly health inequities, is one way of habituating them and rendering them invisible. We do not see what we have become used to, and worse, we make assumptions that normalize certain situations. Health professionals have an important and necessary role to play in countering this process through objective debate. To remain silent over injustices is an unacceptable—and political—act. According to the CNA (2000), the primary determinants of health and illness are social, political, and economic in nature. "To be concerned with health is to be concerned with the social context, and that nursing is, indeed, a political act" (CNA, 2000, p. 1). Nurses have the ability to see the bigger picture and this is where the roots of political activism lie. To be advocates for clients, patients, or communities may require becoming political activists. A rhetorical question can help nurses reflect personally on this issue: Should I focus on helping people adapt to poverty or focus on helping people learn how to influence the environment that has contributed to their situation of poverty? Which is most likely to lead to lasting change?

If nurses use upstream approaches to engage in health-promoting practice with communities, it means they must move away from patching societal wounds with ineffective programs and instead look for the structural and foundational changes required to effect change on the social determinants of health. Structural changes arise from policy changes that direct the focus of interventions. Nursing action could include support for political action to modify the environment and strengthen resources for healthy living, reinforce social networks and social support within a community, and develop the material resources and economic base available to the community. In Jason's story, using community development principles (see Chapter 7), one example of an effective nursing intervention could include a focus on mobilizing support by creating awareness of unsafe play spaces, and lobbying for the resources for building a safe playground for Jason and other neighbourhood children.

## CONCLUSION

Concerns about poverty in Canada—visible in the widening gaps between the rich and the poor—are increasing, generating a pressing need to conduct assessment and intervention research to reduce health disparities in vulnerable groups. New approaches to research on reducing health disparities are needed (Stewart et al., 2008). Stewart et al. (2008) suggested that research using participatory strategies may be one such approach that not only studies the issues but simultaneously promotes empowerment, reduces distrust, and engages stakeholders, such as vulnerable people, in the analysis process and solution creation for reduction of health disparities. However, one caution is that engaging such stakeholders in an assessment and analysis process that then encounters inflexible policy or government decision makers must also address other strategies to effect change so that these research projects do not become a disempowering process in themselves. Strategies such as lobbying for change, influencing policy and other decision makers, or supporting communities' initiatives that they cannot carry out on their own are all examples of other areas where practitioners and researchers can support changes to the root causes of poverty, inequity, and health disparities.

Today, primary health care has shifted the focus from what individuals can to do improve their own health to what communities, organizations, society, and governments can do to improve the health of the people. Traditional goals often encouraged health professionals to determine what creates health and predetermine strategies and services to correct problems, or they led to strategies whereby people from developed countries would parachute into developing countries to "fix" local problems. The objectives of PHC and health promotion are to bolster and strengthen the capacity of local people, work with their leadership, and increase their capacity to create environments and services that promote health and make healthy choices the easier choices to make. The WHO (2013d) defines this as people-centred care, an approach that focuses on the health needs and health-related expectations of the target population rather than on diseases. People-centred care shapes health policy and health service, operating from a foundation that health is created where people live, play, and work, and from a belief that health is a resource for everyday living (WHO et al., 1986).

Health promotion planning and programming will always include multiple levels in which nurses can and must take action. Individual-level interventions will likely always include key components such as nutrition and lifestyle teaching; however, they will remain simply not enough if we wish to create better health for whole populations. This means that the social determinants of health must play a key part in all

interventions if we wish to have any lasting changes occur. It is not enough to teach people about the hazards of smoking and implement stop-smoking programs; for every adult who quits smoking, there is a child somewhere who starts smoking. What stops us from addressing the root causes and engaging in primary prevention efforts? Often we implement band-aid solutions in a downstream approach when what is really needed are large-scale structural, systemic, and societal changes. These are the types of changes that require political will and political intervention, as expressed over and over again throughout the international health promotion charters. Nursing's scope of practice includes advocacy, which can be translated as the need for social action and activism on a larger scale, similar to the earlier pioneer nursing work of Lillian Wald and Margaret Sanger. To remain silent, refuse to act, or refuse to even acknowledge that nursing practice addresses root causes of the health issues faced by people is to remain part of the problem and to condone the status quo. Do we want to continue to provide ineffectual band-aids for all the Jasons who become entrapped in a revolving door of health risks they may not be able to change?

## KEY TERMS

activism   p. 163

at risk   p. 150

Bangkok Charter for Health Promotion in a Globalized World   p. 142

community development   p. 155

downstream approaches   p. 152

ecological vandalism   p. 141

eighth international conference on health promotion   p. 142

empowerment   p. 155

exchange intervention   p. 158

fifth international conference on health promotion   p. 142

first international conference on health promotion   p. 140

fourth international conference on health promotion   p. 141

harm reduction   p. 153

health   p. 136

health belief model   p. 155

health promotion   p. 135

health promotion movement   p. 139

Helsinki Statement on Health in All Policies   p. 142

The Nairobi Call to Action   p. 142

Ottawa Charter for Health Promotion   p. 136

population health   p. 139

population health approach   p. 149

population health indicators   p. 149

population health interventions   p. 150

population health promotion   p. 143

population health promotion model (PHPM)   p. 144

prevention interventions   p. 151

primary care   p. 137

primary health care (PHC)   p. 137

primary prevention   p. 151

resilience   p. 160

risk communication   p. 149

second international conference on health promotion   p. 141

## STUDY QUESTIONS

1.  Describe the differences and similarities among PHC, population health, and health promotion.

2.  Define harm reduction.

3.  Define PHC and describe its two values, five principles, and eight elements.

4.  What is the limitation of using an approach to health promotion that focuses exclusively on behaviour change?

5.  What are three ways that nurses can play an important role in addressing social determinants of health?

6.  What are the elements necessary to creating a relational practice environment?

7.  Define the "four Ps" of social marketing.

8.  Define primary, secondary, and tertiary levels of prevention.

9.  Describe potential helpful and harmful results from labelling a community or population "at risk."

10. Describe the health belief model.

> After working through these questions, go to the
> MyNursingLab at www.pearsoned.ca/mynursinglab to
> check your answers.

## INDIVIDUAL CRITICAL-THINKING EXERCISES

1.  How do you define your own health?

2.  Prior to reading this chapter, what did the term "health promotion" mean to you? Has your initial interpretation changed, and if so, how?

3.  Think about the community you live in. What are the main issues affecting your community's health? How could you use the population health promotion model to begin to develop interventions?

4.  You are a CHN in a community where there appears to be an increasing number of obese children in the elementary school you visit. Describe an upstream approach to community health promotion in this situation.

5.  Visit the website of your provincial/territorial nursing association. Search for policy or position statements on PHC. Look for descriptions of activities that influence healthcare reform. Discuss the initiative with your peers and colleagues. Identify opportunities for CHNs to participate in the initiative. Reflect on how you can become involved.

## GROUP CRITICAL-THINKING EXERCISES

1.  Discuss your answers to Individual Critical-Thinking Exercise 2 with one or more partners. How do your responses compare? What factors influenced your original understanding of health promotion? How are these different from those of your partners?

2.  What is the definition of health promotion that the World Health Organization uses and why is this the definition that CHNs use?

3.  With a partner, interview a CHN in your community. Ask the following questions: What does the term "health promotion" mean to you? What are the main health issues in your area? Describe some of the health promotion activities in your practice. What are the barriers to engaging in health promotion activities? Analyze the responses with your partner. How would you summarize this CHN's approach to health promotion?

## REFERENCES

Adelson, N. (2005). The embodiment of inequity: Health disparities in Aboriginal Canada. *Canadian Journal of Public Health, 96*(2), S45–S61.

Allender, J. A., & Spradley, B. W. (2005). *Community health nursing: Promoting and protecting the public's health* (6th ed.). Philadelphia, PA: Lippincott Williams & Wilkins.

Andreasen, A. (1995). *Marketing social change.* San Francisco, CA: Jossey-Bass.

Ashley, L. (2011). Health promotion charter rings true after 25 years. *Canadian Nurse, 107*(7), 20. Copyright © 2011 by Canadian Nurses Association. Used by permission of Canadian Nurses Association.

Aston, M., Meagher-Stewart, D., Edwards, N., & Young, L. M. (2009). Public health nurses' primary health care practice: Strategies for fostering citizen participation. *Journal of Community Health Nursing, 26*(1), 24–34.

Bard, R. (2011). Let's not lose Insite. *Canadian Nurse, 107*(4), 3.

Bartfay, W. J. (2010). A brief history of community health nursing in Canada. In J. E. Hitchcock, P. E. Schubert, S. A. Thomas, & W. J. Bartfay (Eds.), *Community health nursing: Caring in action* (1st Canadian ed., pp. 11–22). Toronto, ON: Nelson Education.

Butler-Jones, D. (2012). *The Chief Public Health Officer's report on the state of public health in Canada, 2012: Influencing health – The importance of sex and gender.* Retrieved from http://publichealth.gc.ca/CPHOreport

Butterfoss, F. D., Kegler, M. C., & Francisco, V. T. (2008). Mobilizing organizations for health promotion: Theories of organizational change. In K. Glanz, B. K. Rimer, & K. Viswanath

(Eds.), *Health behavior and health education: Theory, research, and practice* (4th ed., pp. 335–361). San Francisco, CA: Jossey-Bass.

Canadian Health Coalition. (2009). *The history of health care.* Retrieved from http://medicare.ca/main/the-facts/the-history-of-medicare

Canadian Institutes of Health Research. (2013). *About Institute of Aboriginal Peoples' Health.* Retrieved from http://www.cihr-irsc.gc.ca/e/8172.html

Canadian Nurses Association. (2000). Nursing is a political act – The bigger picture. *Nursing now: Issues and trends in Canadian nursing, 5*(8), 1–4.

Canadian Nurses Association. (2005). *Social determinants of health and nursing: A summary of the issues.* Retrieved from http://www.cna-aiic.ca/~/media/cna/page%20content/pdf%20en/2013/07/26/10/38/bg8_social_determinants_e.pdf

Canadian Nurses Association. (2009). *Determinants of health.* Ottawa: Author.

Canadian Nurses Association. (2010). *Social justice ... a means to an end, an end in itself* (2nd ed.). Retrieved from http://www2.cna-aiic.ca/CNA/documents/pdf/publications/Social_Justice_2010_e.pdf

Canadian Nurses Association. (2012). *A nursing call to action: The health of our nation, the future of our health system.* Retrieved from http://www2.cna-aiic.ca/CNA/documents/pdf/publications/nec/NEC_Report_e.pdf

Canadian Nurses Association. (2013). *2012 Annual Report.* Retrieved from http://www.cna-aiic.ca/~/media/cna/page%20content/pdf%20en/2013/07/26/09/24/cna_annual_report_2012_e.pdf

Canadian Obesity Network. (2013). *Creating a credible community for change.* Retrieved from http://www.obesitynetwork.ca/about

Canadian Public Health Association. (2010). *Canada's leadership in addressing the social determinants of health.* Retrieved from http://www.cpha.ca/en/programs/history/achievements/01-sdh/leadership.aspx

Canadian Public Health Association. (2011). *The winnable battle: Ending tobacco use in Canada.* Retrieved from http://www.cpha.ca/uploads/positions/position-paper-tobacco_e.pdf

Canadian War Museum. (n.d.). Retrieved from http://www.warmuseum.ca/cwm/exhibitions/guerre/influenza-e.aspx

Cancer Council Australia. (2013). *National cancer prevention policy: Tobacco control.* Retrieved from http://wiki.cancer.org.au/prevention/Tobacco_control/Effective_interventions

Carpenter, C. J. (2010). A meta-analysis of the effectiveness of health belief model variables in predicting behavior. *Health Communication, 25,* 661–669.

Champion, V. L., & Skinner, C. S. (2008). The health belief model. In K. Glanz, B. K. Rimer, & K. Viswanath (Eds.), *Health behavior and health education: Theory, research, and practice* (4th ed., pp. 45–64). San Francisco, CA: Jossey-Bass.

Community Health Nurses Association of Canada. (2008). *Canadian community health nursing standards of practice.* Retrieved from http://www.chnc.ca/documents/chn_standards_of_practice_mar08_english.pdf

Community Health Nurses of Canada. (2011, revised). *Canadian community health nursing: Professional practice model & standards of practice.* St. John's, NL: Author. Retrieved from https://www.chnc.ca/documents/CHNC-ProfessionalPracticeModel-EN/index.html

Community Health Nurses of Canada. (2012). *Public health nursing: Primary prevention of chronic diseases.* Retrieved from http://www.chnc.ca/documents/2012maychnccdreport.pdf

Daley, E., Perrin, K., Vamos, C., Hernandez, N., Anstey, E., Baker, E., . . . Ebbert, J. (2013). Confusion about Pap smears: Lack of knowledge among high risk women. *Journal of Women's Health, 22*(1), 67–74. doi:10.1089/jwh.2012.3667

De Leeuw, A., & De Leeuw, C. (1961). *Nurses who led the way.* Racine, WI: Whitman.

Dupere, S., Ridde, V., Carroll, S., O'Neill, M., Rootman, I., & Pederson, A. (2007). Conclusion: The rhizome and the tree. In M. O'Neill, A. Pederson, S. Dupere, & I. Rootman (Eds.), *Health Promotion in Canada: Critical perspectives* (2nd ed., pp. 371–388). Toronto, ON: Canadian Scholars' Press.

Epp, J. (1986). *Achieving health for all: A framework for health promotion.* Ottawa, ON: Minister of Supply and Services Canada.

Fawcett, S., Abeykoon, P., Arora, M., Dobe, M., Galloway-Gilliam, L., Liburd, L., & Munodawafa, D. (2010). Constructing an action agenda for community empowerment at the 7th Global Conference on Health Promotion in Nairobi. *Global Health Promotion, 17*(4), 52–56.

Federal, Provincial, and Territorial Advisory Committee on Population Health. (1999). *Towards a healthy future: Second report on the health of Canadians.* Charlottetown, PEI: Author.

Fisher, M. P., & Elnitsky, C. (2012). Health and social services integration: A review of concepts and models. *Social Work in Public Health, 27*(5), 441–468. doi:10.1080/19371918.2010.525149

Flynn, L. (1999). *Population health promotion model.* Revised from original model developed by N. Hamilton and T. Bhatti, Health Promotion Development Division, Health Canada, 1996. Winnipeg, MB: Health Canada, Manitoba/Saskatchewan Region.

Frank, J., Di Ruggiero, E., & Moloughney, B. (2004). Think tank on the future of public health in Canada. *Canadian Journal of Public Health, 95*(1), 6–11.

Frank, L. (2013). Person centered care, autonomy, and the definition of health. *The American Journal of Bioethics, 13*(8), 59. doi:10.1080/19371918.2010.525149

Frankish, C. J., Moulton, G., Rootman, I., Cole, C., & Gray, D. (2006). Setting a foundation: Underlying values and structures of health promotion in primary health care settings. *Primary Health Care Research and Development, 7*(2), 172–182.

Franco-Paredes, C., Zeuli, J., Hernandez-Ramos, I., & Santos-Preciado, J. I. (2010). Preserving idealism in global health promotion. *Global Health Promotion, 17*(4), 57–60.

Gielen, A. C., McDonald, E. M., Gary, T. L., & Bone, L. R. (2008). Using the PRECEDE-PROCEED model to apply health behaviour theories. In K. Glanz, B. K. Rimer, & K. Viswanath (Eds.), *Health behavior and health education: Theory, research, and practice* (4th ed., pp. 407–433). San Francisco, CA: Jossey-Bass.

Gilmore, A. B., Tavakoly, B., Taylor, G., & Reed, H. (2013). Understanding tobacco industry pricing strategy and whether it undermines tobacco tax policy: The example of the UK cigarette market. *Addiction, 108*(7), 1317–1326.

Global Advocacy Council for Physical Activity, & International Society for Physical Activity and Health. (2010). *The Toronto charter for physical activity: A global call to action.* Used by permission of Global Advocacy Council for Physical

Activity, International Society for Physical Activity and Health. Retrieved from http://www.activecanada2020.ca/background-documents/toronto-charter

Global Advocacy Council for Physical Activity, & International Society for Physical Activity and Health. (2011). *Non Communicable Disease Prevention: Investments that Work for Physical Activity.* Retrieved from http://www.activecanada2020.ca/backgrounddocuments/toronto-charter

Gordon, R., McDermott, L., Stead, M., & Angus, K. (2006). The effectiveness of social marketing interventions for health improvement: What's the evidence? *Public Health, 120*(12), 1133–1139.

Grier, S., & Bryant, C. A. (2005). Social marketing in public health. *Annual Review of Public Health, 26,* 319–330. doi: 10.1146/annurev.publhealth.26.021304.144610

Hawe, P., & Potvin, L. (2009). What is population health intervention research? *Canadian Journal of Public Health, 100*(1), I8–I14.

Health Canada. (2006). *Strategic risk communications framework.* Retrieved from http://www.phac-aspc.gc.ca/publicat/2007/risk-com/pdf/ris-comm_e.pdf

Health Canada. (2012). *First Nation & Inuit health: Tuberculosis.* Retrieved from http://www.hc-sc.gc.ca/fniah-spnia/diseases-maladies/tuberculos/index-eng.php

Health Canada. (2014). *Health indicators.* Retrieved from http://www.hc-sc.gc.ca/hcs-sss/indicat/index-eng.php

Health Council of Canada. (2012). *Empathy, dignity, and respect: Creating cultural safety for Aboriginal people in urban health care.* Toronto, ON: Author.

Hills, M., Carroll, S., & Vollman, A. (2007). Health promotion and health professions in Canada: Toward a shared vision. In M. O'Neill, A. Pederson, S. Dupere, & I. Rootman (Eds.), *Health promotion in Canada: Critical perspectives* (2nd ed., pp. 330–346). Toronto, ON: Canadian Scholars' Press.

Hitchcock, J. E., & Bartfay, W. J. (2010). Frameworks for assessing families. In J. E. Hitchcock, P. E. Schubert, S. A. Thomas, & W. J. Bartfay (Eds.), *Community health nursing: Caring in action* (1st Canadian ed., pp. 239–283). Toronto, ON: Nelson Education.

Hoad, T. F. (Ed.). (1996). *The concise Oxford dictionary of English etymology.* Oxford, UK: Oxford University.

International Association for the Study of Obesity, Canadian Obesity Network, & Centre for Addiction and Mental Health. (2012). *Toronto charter on obesity & mental health.* Retrieved from http://www.worldobesity.org/site_media/uploads/Toronto_Charter_on_Obesity_Mental_Health.pdf

International Harm Reduction Association. (2010). *What is harm reduction?* Retrieved from http://www.ihra.net/files/2010/08/10/Briefing_What_is_HR_English.pdf

Jozaghi, E., & Andresen, M. A. (2013). Should North America's first and only supervised injection facility (In Site) be expanded in British Columbia, Canada? *Harm Reduction Journal, 10*(1), 1–9. doi:10.1186/1477-7517-10-1

Juneau, C.-E., Jones, C. M., McQueen, D. V., & Potvin, L. (2011). Evidence-based health promotion: An emerging field. *Global Health Promotion, 18*(1), 79–89.

Kaplan, R. M. (2000). Promoting wellness: Biomedical versus outcomes models. In M. S. Jamner & D. Stokols (Eds.), *Promoting human wellness: New frontiers for research, practice, and policy* (pp. 44–77). Berkeley, CA: University of California.

Keepnews, D. M. (2011). Canada's Insite decision: A victory for public health. *Policy, Politics, & Nursing Practice, 12*(3), 131–132. doi:10.1177/1527154411431154

Kindig, D., & Stoddart, G. (2003). What is population health? *American Journal of Public Health, 93*(3), 380–383.

Kleinman, A., & Petryna, A. (2001). Health, anthropological aspects. In *International encyclopedia of the social & behavioral sciences.* New York, NY: Elsevier.

Kotler, P., & Roberto, E. L. (1989). *Social marketing: Strategies for changing public behavior.* New York, NY: The Free Press.

Kozier, B., Erb, G., Berman, A., Snyder, S. J., Buck, M., Yiu, L., & Stamler, L. L. (2014). *Fundamentals of Canadian nursing: Concepts, process, and practice* (3rd Canadian ed.). Toronto, ON: Pearson.

Lagarde, F. (2004). Worksheets to introduce some basic concepts of social marketing principles. *Social Marketing Quarterly, 10*(1), 36–41.

Lagarde, F., & Gendron, M. (2011). Reaching the hard-to-reach with hope and help. *Social Marketing Quarterly, 17*(2), 98–101.

Lalonde, M. (1974). *A new perspective on the health of Canadians: A working document.* Ottawa, ON: Government of Canada.

Lamarre, M.-C. (2011). 2011 . . . a year of celebrations. *Global Health Promotion, 18*(4), 3–4. Copyright © 2011 by Sage Publications Ltd. (UK). Used by permission of Sage Publications Ltd. (UK).

Lind, C., Loewen, S., & Mawji, A. (2012). Health promotion. In D. D'Amico, C. Barbarito, C. Twomey, & N. Harder (Eds.), *Health & Physical Assessment in Nursing* (Canadian ed., pp. 22–36). Toronto, ON: Pearson Canada.

Lind, C., & Smith, D. (2008). Analyzing the state of community health nursing: Advancing from deficit to strengths-based practice using appreciative inquiry. *Advances in Nursing Science, 31*(1), 28–41.

Lindstrom, B., & Eriksson, M. (2009). The salutogenic approach to the making of HiAP/healthy public policy: Illustrated by a case study. *Global Health Promotion, 16*(1), 17–28.

Lynkowski, D. (2011). CPHA applauds Supreme Court decision on Vancouver's supervised injection facility. *CPHA Health Digest, 35*(3). Copyright © 2011 by Canadian Public Health Association. Used by permission of Canadian Public Health Association. Retrieved from http://www.cpha.ca/en/about/digest/xxxv-3/xxxv-3-02.aspx

Marshall, B. D. L., Millroy, M.-J., Wood, E., Montaner, J. S. G., & Kerr, T. (2011). Reduction in overdose mortality after the opening of North America's first medically supervised safer injecting facility: A retrospective population based study. *Lancet, 377,* 1429–1437. doi:10:1016/S01406736(10)62353-7

Mawji, A., & Lind, C. (2013). Imogene: A simulation innovation to teach community health nursing. *Clinical Simulation in Nursing, 9*(11), e513–e519. doi:http://dx.doi.org/10.1016/j.ecns.2013.03.004

McKenzie, J. F., Neiger, B. L., & Thackeray, R. (2013). *Planning, implementing & evaluating health promotion programs: A primer* (6th ed.). Boston, MA: Pearson.

McKinlay, J. (1994). *An annotated bibliography of works held in the library of Australiasia.* Adelaide, Australia: Royal Geographical Society of Australasia, South Australian Branch.

Mikkonen, J., & Raphael, D. (2010). *Social determinants of health: The Canadian facts.* Toronto, ON: York University School of Health Policy and Management.

Mildon, B. (2013a). Turning awareness into advocacy. *Canadian Nurse, 109*(8), 4.

Mildon, B. (2013b). A force for social good. *Canadian Nurse, 109*(9), p. 4.

Minkler, M., Wallerstein, N., & Wilson, N. (2008). Improving health through community organization and community building. In K. Glanz, B. K. Rimer, & K. Viswanath (Eds.), *Health behavior and health education: Theory, research, and practice* (4th ed., pp. 287–312). San Francisco, CA: Jossey-Bass.

Montano, D. E., & Kasprzyk, D. (2008). Theory of reasoned action, theory of planned behaviour, and the integrated behaviour model. In K. Glanz, B. K. Rimer, & K. Viswanath (Eds.), *Health behavior and health education: Theory, research, and practice* (4th ed., pp. 67–96). San Francisco, CA: Jossey-Bass.

Muntaner, C., Ng, E., & Chung, H. (2012). *Better health: An analysis of public policy and programming focusing on the determinants of health and health outcomes that are effective in achieving the healthiest populations.* Ottawa, ON: Canadian Health Services Research Foundation.

Navarro, V. (2009). What we mean by social determinants of health. *Global Health Promotion, 16*(1), 5–16.

Offord, D. R. (2000). Selection of levels of prevention. *Addictive Behaviours, 25*(6), 833–842.

Orleans, C. T. (2008). Foreword. In K. Glanz, B. K. Rimer, & K. Viswanath (Eds.), *Health behavior and health education: Theory, research, and practice* (4th ed., pp. xiii–xv). San Francisco, CA: Jossey-Bass.

Participaction Archive Project (n.d.). *Historic timeline.* Retrieved from http://scaa.sk.ca/gallery/participaction/english/structure/timeline.html

Pauly, B. (2007). Harm reduction through a social justice lens. *International Journal of Drug Policy, 19*, 4–10. doi:10.1016/j.drugpo.2007.11.005

Payne, L. (1983). Health: A basic concept in nursing theory. *Journal of Advanced Nursing, 8*, 393–395.

Perkins, F. (2009). A rights-based approach to accessing health determinants. *Global Health Promotion, 16*(1), 61–64.

Phillips, C. V., & Rodu, B. (2013). Tobacco harm reduction: opportunity and opposition. *Drugs and Alcohol Today, 13*(2), 73–78. doi:10.1108/DAT-032013-0015

Pinkerton, S. D. (2011). How many HIV infections are prevented by Vancouver Canada's supervised injection facility? *International Journal of Drug Policy, 22*(3), 179–183. doi: 10:1016/j.drugpo.2011.03.003

Potvin, L., Juneau, C.-E., Jones, C. M., & McQueen, D. V. (2011). How is evidence used for planning, implementation and evaluation of health promotion? A global collection of case studies, *Global Health Promotion, 18*(1), 7–8.

Prochaska, J. O., Redding, C. A., & Evers, K. E. (2008). The transtheoretical model and stages of change. In K. Glanz, B. K. Rimer, & K. Viswanath (Eds.), *Health behavior and health education: Theory, research, and practice* (4th ed., pp. 97–121). San Francisco, CA: Jossey-Bass.

Public Health Agency of Canada. (2001). *Population health promotion: An integrated model of population health and health promotion.* Retrieved from http://www.phac-aspc.gc.ca/ph-sp/php-psp/php3-eng.php#Developing

Public Health Agency of Canada. (2011). *What determines health?* Retrieved from http://www.phac-aspc.gc.ca/ph-sp/determinants/index-eng.php

Public Health Agency of Canada. (2013a). *Health promotion.* Retrieved from http://www.phac-aspc.gc.ca/hp-ps/index-eng.php

Public Health Agency of Canada. (2013b). *What is the population health approach?* Retrieved from http://www.phac-aspc.gc.ca/ph-sp/approach-approche/appr-eng.php

Raeburn, J., & Rootman, I. (2007). A new appraisal of the concept of health. In M. O'Neill, A. Pederson, S. Dupere, & I. Rootman (Eds.), *Health promotion in Canada: Critical perspectives* (2nd ed., pp. 19–31). Toronto, ON: Canadian Scholars' Press.

Raphael, D. (2009). *Social determinants of health* (2nd ed.). Toronto, ON: Canadian Scholars' Press.

Raphael, D. (2010). Setting the stage: Why quality of life? Why health promotion? In D. Raphael (Ed.), *Health promotion and quality of life in Canada: Essential readings* (pp. 1–13). Toronto, ON: Canadian Scholars' Press.

Raphael, D., Bryant, T., & Curry-Stevens, A. (2004). Toronto Charter outlines future health policy directions for Canada and elsewhere. *Health Promotion International, 19*(2), 269–273.

Roach, M. (2000). Race and health: Implications for health care delivery and wellness promotion. In M. S. Jamner & D. Stokols (Eds.), *Promoting human wellness: New frontiers for research, practice, and policy* (pp. 258–293). Berkeley, CA: University of California Press.

Rosenstock, I. M. (1966). Why people use health services. *Milbank Memorial Fund Quarterly, 44*, 94–127.

Sallis, J. F., Owen, N., & Fisher, E. B. (2008). Ecological models of health behavior. In K. Glanz, B. K. Rimer, & K. Viswanath (Eds.), *Health behavior and health education: Theory, research, and practice* (4th ed., pp. 465–485). San Francisco, CA: Jossey-Bass.

Smith, B. J., Tang, K. C., & Nutbeam, D. (2006). WHO health promotion glossary: New terms. *Health Promotion International Advance Access, 1*–6. doi:10.1093/heapro/dal033

Sohl, S. J., & Moyer, A. (2007). Tailored interventions to promote mammography screening: A meta-analysis review. *Preventative Medicine, 45*(4), 252–261. doi:10.1016/j.ypmed.2007.06.009

Stewart, M. J., Makwarimba, E., Barnfather, A., Letourneau, N., & Neufeld, A. (2008). Researching reducing health disparities: Mixed-methods approaches. *Social Science & Medicine, 66*(6), 1406–1417. doi:10.1016/j.socscimed.2007.11.021

Stewart, M. J., Makwarimba, E., Reutter, L. I., Veenstra, G., Raphael, D., & Love, R. (2009). Poverty, sense of belonging and experiences of social isolation. *Journal of Poverty, 13*(2), 173–195. doi:10.1080/10875540902841762

Strengthening the Social Determinants of Health: The Toronto Charter for a Healthy Canada (2003). Retrieved from http://depts.washington.edu/ccph/pdf_files/Toronto%20Charter%20Final.pdf

Syme, S. L. (2000). Community participation, empowerment, and health: Development of a wellness guide for California. In M. S. Jamner & D. Stokols (Eds.), *Promoting human wellness: New frontiers for research, practice, and policy* (pp. 78–98). Berkeley, CA: University of California Press.

Taylor, M., & Caine, V. (2013). Exploring practices of harm reduction. *Alberta RN, 68*(4), 17–19.

Taylor, R., & Rieger, A. (1985). Medicine as social science: Rudolf Virchow on the typhus epidemic in upper Silesia. *International Journal of Health Services, 15,* 547–559.

The Toronto charter for physical activity (2010). Retrieved from http://www.activecanada2020.ca/background-documents/toronto-charter

University of Saskatchewan (2011). Definition of primary health care. College of Medicine, Primary Health Care Group. Retrieved from http://www.medicine.usask.ca/research/health-research-groups/primary-health-care-research-group-1/definition-of-primary-health-care

Venkatapuram, S. (2013). Health, vital goals, and central human capabilities. *Bioethics, 27*(5), 271–279. doi: 10.1111/j.1467-8519.2011.01953.x

Vollman, A. R., Anderson, E. T., & McFarlane, J. (2012). *Canadian community as partner: Theory & multidisciplinary practice* (3rd ed.). Philadelphia, PA: Wolters Kluwer/Lippincott Williams & Wilkins.

Whitney, D., & Trosten-Bloom, A. (2003). *The power of appreciative inquiry: A practical guide to positive change.* San Francisco, CA: Berrett-Koehler.

World Health Organization. (1948). Preamble to the Constitution of the World Health Organization as adopted by the International Health Conference, New York, 19–22 June, 1946; signed on 22 July 1946 by the representatives of 61 States (Official Records of the World Health Organization, no. 2, p. 100) and entered into force on 7 April 1948.

World Health Organization. (1978). Reprinted from *Declaration of Alma-Ata.* Retrieved from http://www.who.int/publications/almaata_declaration_en.pdf

World Health Organization. (1986). Reprinted from *The Ottawa charter for health promotion.*

World Health Organization. (1998). *Health promotion glossary.* Geneva, Switzerland: Author.

World Health Organization. (2008). *Primary health care: Now more than ever.* Geneva, Switzerland: Author. Retrieved from www.who.int/entity/whr/2008/en

World Health Organization. (2009a). *Milestones in health promotion: Statements from global conferences.* Geneva, Switzerland: Author.

World Health Organization. (2009b). *State of the world's vaccines and immunization.* Retrieved from http://www.unicef.org/media/files/SOWVI_full_report_english_LR1.pdf

World Health Organization. (2009c). *The Nairobi call to action for closing the implementation gap in health promotion.* Geneva, Switzerland: Author.

World Health Organization. (2013a). *Primary health care.* Retrieved from http://www.who.int/topics/primary_health_care/en

World Health Organization. (2013b). *Maternal, newborn, child and adolescent health.* Retrieved from http://www.who.int/maternal_child_adolescent/documents/countries/indicators/en

World Health Organization. (2013c). *The Helsinki statement on health in all policies.* Retrieved from http://www.who.int/healthpromotion/conferences/8gchp/8gchp_helsinki_statement.pdf

World Health Organization. (2013d). *Health systems strengthening glossary.* Retrieved from http://www.who.int/healthsystems/hss_glossary/en/index8.html

World Health Organization, Health and Welfare Canada, & Canadian Public Health Association. (1986). *Ottawa charter for health promotion.* Ottawa, ON: Author.

## ABOUT THE AUTHORS

**Candace Lind** is an RN with a BN, MN, and PhD in Nursing from the University of Calgary and a completed post-doctoral fellowship in Community Health Nursing from the University of Ottawa. She is an Associate Professor in the Faculty of Nursing at the University of Calgary, where her program of research focuses on child and adolescent health promotion and encompasses research that is relationship-based, informs interprofessional practice and policy development, and addresses the ways in which adolescents are conceptualized in society. Her research and community health undergraduate teaching are informed by the attributes of social justice and the social determinants of health, and she is particularly interested in strengths-building, health-promoting approaches to practice and research.

**Melanie Lind-Kosten** is an RN with a BScN from the University of Victoria and an MEd from the University of Calgary. She is a Nursing Instructor in the Faculty of Nursing at the University of Calgary, where she teaches community health practice and theory. Melanie's nursing career practice experience spans Canada and the United States, and includes women's surgery, hemodialysis, palliative homecare, working with homeless populations, and seniors' care facility design.

**Sylvia Loewen** is an RN with a BN, University of Manitoba and an MN, University of Calgary. Her career focus is the growing family, a primarily in community settings as a public health nurse, a pediatric clinical nurse specialist in home care, and a manager in health promotion. Sylvia is currently a Senior Instructor for the Faculty of Nursing, University of Calgary. Her teaching expertise is in pediatrics and community health, and she is the faculty coordinator for students' final practice placements.

# Cultural Care

*Kathryn Edmunds*

LEARNING OUTCOMES

**After studying this chapter, you should be able to:**

1. Identify the assumptions, meanings, and characteristics underlying the concept of culture.

2. Explain the intersections among culture, multiculturalism, diversity, race, and ethnicity.

3. Describe the current state of migration to Canada for permanent and temporary residents, and refugees.

4. Examine the relationship between culture and health.

5. Evaluate the similarities and differences between cultural competence and cultural safety, and the implications for community health nursing practice.

6. Articulate how cultural beliefs and values shape your personal interactions and the interactions between nurses and clients.

7. Develop the knowledge, attitudes, sensitivity, processes, and skills needed to provide cultural care with communities.

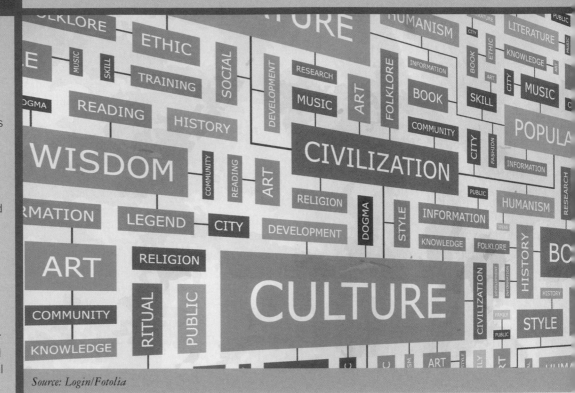

*Source: Login/Fotolia*

## INTRODUCTION

Canadian nurses have a long history of providing care to all people and communities while adapting to local contexts and resources and advocating for change. This is congruent with nursing's tradition of conceptualizing clients as holistic beings inseparable from their environments, as well as being concerned with issues of individual and collective marginalization, inequity, and social justice. The Canadian Nurses Association (CNA) recognizes that in order for optimal client outcomes to occur for our increasingly diverse society, care must be provided that "is the application of knowledge, skills, attitudes or personal attributes required by nurses to maximize respectful relationships with diverse populations of clients and co-workers" (2010, p. 1).

Valuing multiple ways of knowing, engaging in reflective practice, facilitating access and equity, empowering clients through partnerships, and providing culturally appropriate care in multiple settings are all expectations embedded in the standards of practice of the Community Health Nurses of Canada [CHNC] (2011, revised). Within the standard of access and equity, some particularly relevant expectations for the community health nurse (CHN) providing cultural care are as follows:

- collaborates with individuals, families, groups, communities, populations, or systems to identify and provide programs and methods of delivery that are acceptable to them and responsive to their needs across the lifespan;
- provides culturally sensitive care in diverse communities and settings;
- supports the individual, family, group, community and population's right to choose alternate healthcare options; and
- advocates for equitable access to health and other services and equitable resource allocation (p. 20).

In this chapter, we will explore some of the assumptions, meanings, and characteristics of the concept of culture and the intersections among culture, multiculturalism, diversity, race, and ethnicity. Current trends in migration to Canada will be explored. The relationship between culture and health will be discussed, as will how constructions of culture shape nurse–client interactions. The knowledge, attitudes, sensitivity, and skills that are needed to provide care, and the similarities and differences between cultural competence and cultural safety will be described, including implications for community health nursing practice with all residents of Canada.

## CONCEPT OF CULTURE

"'Culture,' is one of the two or three most complicated words in the English language" (Williams, 1983, p. 87). Madeline Leininger (2006) founded transcultural nursing, which evolved from her nursing practice blended with post-graduate studies in anthropology. For Leininger, care was the central and unifying focus of nursing. Her definition of **culture** was "the learned, shared, and transmitted values, beliefs, norms, and lifeways of a particular culture that guides thinking, decisions, and actions in patterned ways and often intergenerationally" (p. 13). The purpose of her theory of **Culture Care Diversity and Universality** was to discover, explain, and predict factors that influence care meanings and practices from both the client's and nurse's perspectives, and to discover care similarities and differences across cultures in order to guide nursing practice (see Leininger's "Sunrise Enabler to Discover Culture Care" in MyNursingLab). Leininger's transcultural care decisions and actions provide a framework for planning nursing care with individuals, families, and communities. Strengths of Leininger's theoretical approach include flexibility with an emphasis on in-depth assessment, meaning, and care within the context of culture; the inclusion of diverse health contexts; and the generation of nursing knowledge and interventions (Andrews & Boyle, 2012a).

However, Gustafson (2005) contends that transcultural nursing rests on a broadly defined concept of culture that is narrowly applied. The focus is on individual identity within an understanding of culture that "essentializes" or emphasizes the similarities of experiences and simplifies differences. The culture of origin is accentuated and often perceived to be static, rather than recognizing the multiple identities and the relational processes involved in all our encounters, as well as changes that occur through migration (Gray & Thomas, 2006; Williamson & Harrison, 2010).

Transcultural nursing has also been criticized for a lack of clarity in conceptual definitions (such as cultural competence), and for the assumption that knowledge and understanding of other cultures leads to tolerance, respect, and changes in discriminatory behaviours (Andrews & Boyle, 2012a), with little attention as to how to address and reconcile differing perspectives. The focus on the individual who is "different" makes it easy to disregard the cultures of healthcare professionals and institutions, and perpetuates existing assumptions, boundaries, and social relations.

Current conceptualizations of culture recognize that it is more complex and nuanced when compared to traditional understandings of culture as a system of shared beliefs, values, expressions, and meanings. According to Browne et al. (2009), culture is a "dynamic, power laden process created by people in relation to one another, their environments, and sociopolitical and historical contexts" (p. 173). Culture is grounded in history, yet is situated and constructed in the current location, reflecting underlying power relationships (Gray & Thomas, 2006). Being open to and aware of multiple ways of knowing and experiencing the world leads to the recognition that actions can take place in different contexts. Identification with a particular culture can lead to **ethnocentrism**, which is the belief that one's own culture is the best or most desirable. Nursing itself is a cultural phenomenon shaped by societal values and assumptions about health, illness, and caring (Dreher & Skemp, 2011). Nurses who believe that the culture and practices of nursing are the only or "best" way to interpret what the client is expressing and to achieve improvements in health are being ethnocentric (see the guide "Questions for Reflection and Building Awareness in Community Practice" in MyNursingLab).

## ASSUMPTIONS AND CHARACTERISTICS OF CULTURE

Culture is more than beliefs, practices, and values (Aboriginal Nurses Association of Canada, 2009). What we have learned to value represents our assumptions about how to perceive, think, and behave in acceptable, appropriate, and meaningful ways within existing social, historical, and political contexts. The focus on individuals when providing care reflects the dominant North American value and assumption of personal autonomy, which can deemphasize issues of power and oppressive systems. Not surprisingly, the nursing profession in North America illustrates this value by stressing the care of individuals and families. An almost exclusive focus on the individual has implications for CHNs, providing "little or no guidance for addressing how we act as a community, the duties and obligations, and the mutual and disparate moral interests of individuals, families, and communities" (Shirley, 2007, p. 14). The CHNC (2011, revised) standards and competencies as well as the Canadian Public Health Association's (CPHA) (2010) guidelines for public health and community health nursing practice reveal a greater and more explicit emphasis on assumptions regarding the importance of culture in the contexts of broader structural issues, social justice, and the determinants of health.

Culture is learned, shared, changes, and is embedded in all aspects of our lives. Culture is expressed in groups, professions, organizations, communities, and societies. There are characteristics shared by all cultures (Allender, Rector, & Warner, 2014):

■ *Culture is socially constructed.* Cultural norms, behaviours, and values are learned through socialization within the family and community. However, culture is interpreted and shaped individually as well as being situated, negotiated, and transformed within complex social and power relations and the broader structural forces that affect us. Behaviours that the nurse may assume are universal will differ across *and within* cultures.

■ *Culture is an integrated system* embedded in everyday life. Beliefs and healthcare practices are usually consistent with the overall paradigms that are used to make sense out of the world.

■ *Culture is shared.* Beliefs that have meanings and are shared by a group are called cultural values. These values are transmitted within a group and imparted over time. Values shared by people form cultural stability and security. They guide members about what to believe and how to act. However, it is important to remember that individuals may not share, or may even find constraining, the values of their cultural groups or their communities.

■ *Culture is largely implicit and tacit.* This means it shapes us at an unconscious level. Most of the time, we do not stop to consider the assumptions and expectations that ground our behaviours and decisions. Culture is one aspect that shapes the way we do things in our everyday lives.

■ *Culture is fluid and dynamic.* Culture is always adapting and changing, especially with increased global migration and access to technology. Consider the changes to Canadian culture that have occurred in the past few decades. Minority cultures have certainly been influenced by the dominant Canadian culture; however, growing diversity and global interconnectedness have influenced the Canadian culture in return.

■ *Culture is expressed and intersects* with other social constructs such as race, gender, ethnicity, class, language, and disability. People with both visible and invisible disabilities may consider themselves to be sharing common cultural identities and experiences, rather than having a "pathological" disorder (Marks, 2007). The historical and current importance of French language rights in Quebec is an outward expression of cultural identity. In particular, culture is often conflated with, or seen to represent, ethnicity and race in ways that reduce very complex situations and ways of being and relating to sets of static behaviours and "cultural" attributes.

## INTERSECTIONS

**Diversity** refers to variety and differences of attributes among, between, and within groups. We all have attributes that give us membership in certain groups, yet we are all diverse and intersect with others in many ways. Diversity can refer to both the preservation and value of traditions, and to adaptation leading to creativity and innovation. However, focusing on diversity may have the result of reinforcing differences between groups when diversity is seen as linked to a fixed heritage (Schim, Doorenbos, Benkert, & Miller, 2007). Diversity also includes characteristics and constructs such as gender, language, sexual orientation, and disabilities. Like culture, diversity is a process of change, affecting people in similar and different ways.

**Ethnicity** is a way of describing social identity with a group that is based on a shared heritage, language, social structure, and beliefs and values. However, the dominant culture tends not to define itself in terms of ethnicity; it is usually minority groups that are viewed as ethnic. Cultural and ethnic diversity has always existed in Canada, though at the time of Confederation in 1867, formal recognition for linguistic, religious, and legal diversity based on ethnicity was restricted to the English and French. **Race** is often thought of as an objective biological distinction, usually based on visible differences such as skin colour. However, the concept of race has no scientific basis and has been described as "a social construction involving the classification of individuals into arbitrary groups and the assignment of disparate meaning and value to those constructed groups" (Etowa & McGibbon, 2012, p. 73). **Racism** is interrelated with socioeconomic status, employment opportunities, discrimination, and marginalization. **Racialization** is a term that calls attention to the significant consequences of assigning racial designations. Historically, labels of race have been used to maintain dominant power and social orders and this continues to occur today. The use, significance, and meanings of the concepts of ethnicity and race are inconsistent in nursing research literature, often disregarding the power dynamics involved (Varcoe, 2006).

In 1971, federal **multiculturalism** policy recognized and acknowledged cultural pluralism as an essential and valued contribution to Canadian culture. This was a response to the previous focus on French and English biculturalism. More recently still, debate about the assumptions, benefits, and barriers of multiculturalism has occurred as the meaning of this policy and legislation in Canada has gone through phases and changes of interpretation. Currently, the focus of multiculturalism is the integration of practices of diversity, tolerance, and respect for multiple ways of knowing and being, with issues of equity and social justice (Srivastava, 2007). This is seen to benefit the entire population. Canada was the first country to enshrine multiculturalism in federal law and the Canadian Multiculturalism Act of 1988 states,

> The Constitution of Canada . . . recognizes the importance of preserving and enhancing the multicultural heritage of Canadians; . . . [and] the government of Canada recognizes the diversity of Canadians as regards race, national or ethnic origin, colour and religion as a fundamental characteristic of Canadian society and is committed to a policy of multiculturalism designed to preserve and enhance the multicultural heritage of Canadians while working to achieve the equality of all Canadians in the economic, social, cultural and political life of Canada. (Government of Canada, 1988)

However, there are issues of power inherent in multiculturalism and CHNs should not assume that all residents of Canada perceive multiculturalism in such a constructive and beneficial light. Power relations are evident when we struggle within and across communities to reconcile valuing and acceptance of cultural diversity with practices that may perpetuate injustice or may be perceived as not in accordance with the larger society. There have been recent controversies regarding the use of alternative justice systems based on culture or religion for those reasons. Multiculturalism can be considered to be a public policy that suppresses the need to tackle ingrained inequities (Varcoe, 2006) and there has been little research that supports cultural sensitivity as a mechanism leading to increased tolerance or respect for ethnic and racialized groups (Yiu Matuk & Ruggirello, 2007).

International movement in migration will continue to dynamically influence the Canadian identity in terms of racial, ethnic, religious, and linguistic diversity. **Transnationalism**, which refers to the enduring and frequent connection with their countries of origin for migrants residing in a new country, has shifted the ways in which relocation is perceived (Isaacs, 2010). As our understanding of culture broadens to include workplace and professional cultures, the concept of multiculturalism is becoming increasingly complex. This is reflected in the embeddedness of Canadian society in our interconnected global world, and that people have layered identities and flexible and multiple links within and across socially constructed labels. Open and honest discussion needs to take place regarding which residents of Canada are considered to be multicultural and why, who is considered to be "truly" Canadian, and the meanings and consequences of these social definitions.

## CANADIAN DIVERSITY

Immigration has had a considerable impact on the growth and diversity of Canada's population.

With more than 200 ethnic origins reported in the Canadian census of 2011, all regions of the country are diverse, reflected in different ways across our provinces and territories. The number of people reporting multiple ethnic identities, including being Canadian, continued to increase to 42.1% of the population (Statistics Canada, 2013). The most commonly reported ethnic origin was Canadian, either alone or with other origins, and more than one million people identified 13 different ethnic origins. The list of ethnic origins included the diverse Aboriginal population (see Chapter 22): "just over 1 369 100 people reported having First Nations (North American Indian) ancestry, while 447 700 reported Métis and 72 600 reported Inuit" (Statistics Canada, 2013, p. 14). In 2011, Canadian census data showed that 6.8 million people (20.6% of the total population) were born outside the country; this was the highest proportion among the G8 countries and second to Australia globally (see Figure 9.1). Three-quarters of the foreign-born population in Canada are proficient in more than one language (Statistics Canada, 2013).

Migrants may share some similarities (e.g., language barriers, and adjustment and adaptation to Canada). Yet there can also be significant differences both within and across their diverse cultures and migration experiences. The term **immigrant** refers to those who are eligible for permanent residency; this includes people accepted in the categories of economic immigrants (people selected for their skills and ability to contribute to Canada's economy), family class immigrants (people sponsored by a Canadian citizen or permanent resident), and government-assisted and privately sponsored refugees (Citizenship and Immigration Canada [CIC], 2015).

According to Statistics Canada (2013), prior to 1971, more than 75% of immigrants to Canada were from Europe. Currently, the top source countries for immigrants are the Philippines, China, and India. Factors that have caused this shift include changes to federal immigration policies in the 1960s, which ended discriminatory immigration policies

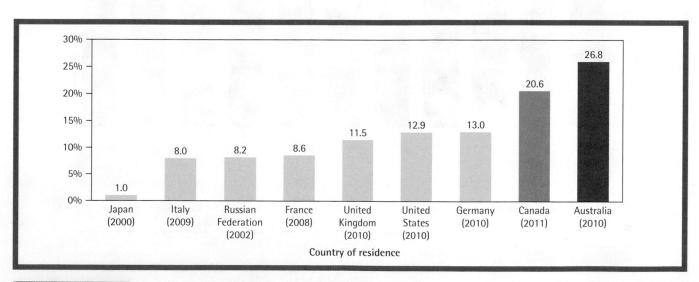

**FIGURE 9.1** Foreign-born Population, as a Proportion of the Total Population, G8 Countries and Australia

*Source:* Cited in Statistics Canada (2013). *Immigration and ethnocultural diversity in Canada: National household survey 2011.*(Government No. 99-010-X2011001). Ottawa, ON: Author, p. 7.

based on race, religion, and nationality, and increasing global migration. Canada receives immigrants from over 200 countries; however, recent immigrants from Asia (including the Middle East) comprised 57% of all immigrants from 2006 to 2011, and 60% of all immigrants from 2001 to 2005.

The number of permanent residents admitted to Canada has remained fairly stable at around 250 000 people per year for the past 10 years. A total of 260 404 permanent residents were admitted in 2014, of whom 23 286 were refugees (CIC, 2015). The median age of newcomers in 2011 was younger (31.7 years) compared to the Canadian-born population (37.3 years). Canada's visible minority population is increasing at a faster growth rate than the total population, largely because of the high proportion of recent immigrants (78%) belonging to visible minorities (Statistics Canada, 2013). In 2006, 16.2% of the total population identified themselves as belonging to a visible minority group, increasing to 19.1% in 2011. Since 2006, South Asians (people citing ethnic origins from countries such as India, Pakistan, Sri Lanka, and Bangladesh) have been the largest visible minority group, exceeding Chinese (Statistics Canada, 2013).

The vast majority of newcomers live in large urban areas and 95% settle in Ontario, British Columbia, Quebec, and Alberta. Canada's largest cities, such as Toronto, Vancouver, and Montreal, became home to 63.4% of recent immigrants in 2011. Greater numbers of newcomers settled in Montreal, Calgary, Edmonton, and Winnipeg in 2011 compared to 2006, and fewer in Toronto (Statistics Canada, 2013).

Provincial and territorial settlement diversity is reflected in Figure 9.2. Quebec controls its own immigration policy and requires commitment to living in a francophone society for acceptance. This reinforces Quebec's sovereignty and is a mechanism to preserve French as the dominant language in that province, while welcoming newcomers (Blad & Couton, 2009). A higher proportion of people from Africa and the Middle East, which include French-speaking countries, immigrate to Quebec compared to Canada as a whole (48.3% vs. 23.9%) (CIC, 2015).

## Temporary Residents

**Temporary residents** are people with temporary work permits, international students, and refugee claimants who are awaiting decisions regarding their applications seeking asylum in Canada. The two largest groups of temporary residents are foreign workers (279 939 in 2013) and international students (304 876) (CIC, 2014). While the rate of immigration for permanent residents has remained stable, the numbers of people with temporary work permits and international students have increased almost 300% and 200% respectively since 2004. The number of temporary workers present in Canada in 2013 greatly exceeded the number of permanent residents admitted for work that year (148 154) (CIC, 2015, 2014). Most of the skilled temporary workers entering Canada are from the United States and Europe. Workers in low-skilled

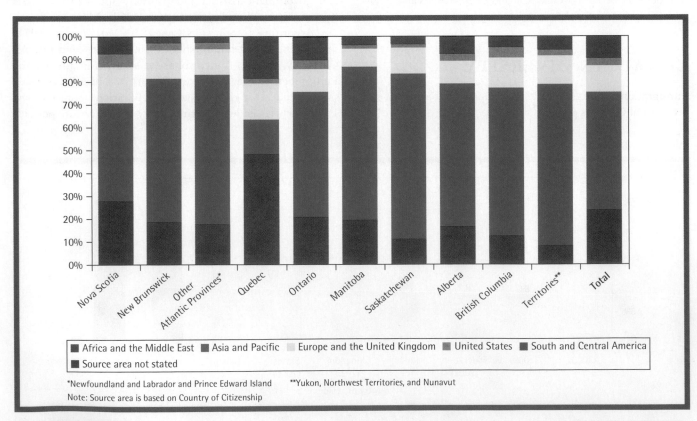

**FIGURE 9.2** Canada – Permanent Residents by Province or Territory and Source Area, 2014

*Source:* Citizenship and Immigration Canada. (2015). *Canada facts and figures 2014: Immigration overview – permanent residents, p. 44.* Retrieved from http://www.cic.gc.ca/english/pdf/2014-Facts-Permanent.pdf

classifications come from countries such as Mexico, the Caribbean (mainly men), and the Philippines (mainly women), and compete for jobs that are poorly paid and considered to be less desirable (Boyd & Pikkow, 2008). Women temporary migrants are more likely to be streamed into lower skilled categories compared to men. Overall, the three top source countries for foreign workers in Canada are the United States, the Philippines, and Mexico; the three top source countries for international students are China, India, and Korea (CIC, 2015).

Recurring migration for employment, reflecting the intersection of economic globalization and local necessity, is becoming progressively widespread. At the same time that increasing numbers of Canadian citizens are migrating internally in search of work, there is growing dependence on temporary foreign workers in sectors where it can be difficult to find local people who will work for low wages in often isolated and hazardous circumstances, and where the work is not mobile, such as agriculture, construction, caregiving, and hospitality services (Preibisch, 2007).

Temporary residents are not eligible for many of the government settlement services, such as language classes and comprehensive healthcare, that are available to permanent residents. There has been limited research in Canada exploring the health of temporary residents. A significant barrier has been that temporary residents are not included in the comprehensive and longitudinal immigrant health surveys that have been conducted by the federal and provincial governments (Edmunds, Berman, Basok, Ford-Gilboe, & Forchuk, 2011).

# NEWCOMER HEALTH

Immigrants bring significant strengths, such as determination, resilience, and diversity, yet they can also experience significant challenges, some of which arise from differing migration pathways. New immigrants to Canada rate their health more highly than the Canadian born. Reasons for this include that immigrants are required to have medical screening before their acceptance and entry into Canada, and non-refugees often have healthier pre-migration lifestyles. However, health status declines quickly after arrival, though in variable ways (Kim, Carrasco, Muntaner, McKenzie, & Samuel, 2013). Factors associated with increased risks of health decline include low income, unemployment, lack of language skills in French or English, gender, age, place of birth, experiences of discrimination, and barriers to accessing healthcare services (Fuller-Thomson, Noack, & George, 2011). Foreign-born visible minority women have reported the greatest health decline after 10 years in Canada (Spitzer, 2012).

Language acquisition is challenging and underlies many aspects of recent immigrants' lives. Though limitations in English or French fluency affect job attainment, there are other factors that influence obtaining secure employment. Immigrants' credentials and previous employment may not be recognized in Canada (Spitzer, 2012); they lack Canadian work experience and frequently do not have business networks or contacts to facilitate job acquisition. Recent women immigrants had a lower probability of having their previous work experience recognized compared to men; members of a visible minority were less likely to have previous experience recognized compared to members of non-visible minority groups, and refugees had the lowest rate of all (Houle & Yssaad, 2010). The process for internationally educated professionals (e.g., nurses, physicians, engineers, etc.) to obtain Canadian registration is complex, lengthy, and costly.

Limited social support, especially for those without extended families, can be another challenge for recent immigrants. Social isolation, experiences in refugee camps, and awareness of hardships experienced by family members remaining in the country of origin result in the potential for post-traumatic stress disorder. Canadian agencies, such as health units, frequently encourage families to access resources in the community to assist them in developing a support network. Social networks of families and friends provide psychological and emotional support, much-needed information and orientation to a new country, and can facilitate establishing economic stability (Fuller-Thomson et al., 2011).

All these challenges affect the overall health for newcomers to Canada. There may be waiting periods of three months in order to be eligible for provincial health coverage. New Canadians often have difficulty finding a family doctor; thus, the health services they receive often are limited to episodic treatment rather than comprehensive care. In 2012, changes were made to Canadian healthcare eligibility for refugees through the Interim Federal Health (IFH) program. Instead of receiving comprehensive healthcare, most refugee claimants, who are considered to be temporary residents, received limited healthcare services, often only when their disease was considered a danger to public health. After protest and advocacy from health and social service providers, including a successful Federal Court challenge, some of the reductions in IFH services were reversed in 2014. However, many barriers to access remain (Canadian Council for Refugees, 2015). Changes to IFH coverage highlight the role of government policy and ideology in determining who is deserving of what types of immigration classification and which services of publicly funded healthcare.

Issues such as immigration status, precarious employment, insecure housing, and lack of knowledge about the Canadian healthcare systems can be complicated by language barriers and differing cultural meanings regarding health, illness, and care practices. Building trust is an essential first step to building relationships, and often interpreters are necessary. Family members, especially spouses or children, should not be asked to interpret. It is important for CHNs (and student nurses) to be aware of the policies related to working with interpreters and the services available in their institutions and clinical placements. (The resources "Working with Interpreters and Strategies for Working Effectively with Interpreters" can be found in MyNursingLab.)

The CHN working with migrant populations must be aware of their needs related to immigration and settlement.

While there are certainly unique challenges for migrants, nurses must also be aware that many of the issues vary little from issues faced by the general Canadian-born population. Nurses also need to remember that despite the preceding emphasis on challenges, migrants have considerable and important skills and strengths. They have demonstrated significant resiliency through the act of immigration itself.

Recent immigrants are healthier than resident Canadians, have numerous positive and health-promoting cultural values and practices, and many are highly educated; almost 45% of all immigrants in 2008 had a university degree (Houle & Yssaad, 2010). As with all clients, effective CHN care builds on collaboration in the context of existing strengths and supports. (See Canadian Research Box 9.1.)

### CANADIAN RESEARCH BOX 9.1

**How are immigrant and refugee women's postpartum depression experiences of seeking help influenced by gender?**

O'Mahony, J. M., & Donnelly, T. T. (2013). How does gender influence immigrant and refugee women's postpartum depression help-seeking experiences? *Journal of Psychiatric and Mental Health Nursing, 20,* 714–725. doi:10.1111/jpm.12005. Copyright © 2013 by John Wiley & Sons, Ltd. Used by permission of John Wiley & Sons, Ltd.

Migration is a risk factor for depression during pregnancy and postpartum. Increasing numbers of immigrants and refugees to Canada are from non-European countries, and these women experience many barriers to healthcare services and care for postpartum depression (PPD). Healthcare providers need to know how to support migrant women to adjust to life in Canada and cope with PPD. The purpose of the research was to investigate how the interaction between cultural, political, social, and economic factors as well as race, gender, and class shaped the help-seeking strategies and experiences of migrant women with PPD.

For this critical ethnography, in-depth qualitative interviews were conducted with 30 non-European immigrant and refugee women who had been residing in Canada for less than 10 years. Nine of the participants had been diagnosed with PPD. Based on screening, the other participants had been at high risk for PPD within the past 5 years. Two major themes were identified: the influence of structural barriers related to immigration status, and barriers related to gender roles.

It was a common finding that many of the participants were sponsored as a family member, usually by their husbands, which meant that their permanent immigration status was not assured.

Some of the women felt they were in a precarious situation and were reluctant to draw attention to themselves by seeking help for PPD. As new mothers, traditional gender roles intensified their isolation, dependency, and vulnerability. Poverty, discrimination, and poor spousal or family relationships contributed to the complexity of their lives and could contribute to the risk for PPD.

### Discussion Questions

1. How do current immigration policies negatively affect women?

2. What role do the cultural values of migrant women have in planning cultural care? What is being missed if that is the only focus?

3. How would you support the strengths these women have?

## CULTURE, COMMUNITY, AND HEALTH

Considering culture in the context of diversity, multiple intersections also means being aware of culture and its relationships among the social determinants of health. As described by the World Health Organization (WHO) (2008), "the structural determinants and [social] conditions of daily life constitute the social determinants of health and are responsible for a major part of health inequities between and within countries" (p. 1). These determinants of health, such as culture, income, education, social support, and access to healthcare are significant for all individuals, families, and communities. According to Allender et al. (2014), culture is possibly the most relevant social determinant of community health. The underlying premise for culture as a determinant of health is defined by the Public Health Agency of Canada (2013) as "some persons or groups may face additional health risks due to a socioeconomic environment, which is largely determined by dominant cultural values that contribute to the perpetuation of conditions such as marginalization, stigmatization, loss or devaluation of language and culture, and lack of access to culturally appropriate healthcare and services." The emphasis in this statement is on the role of the dominant culture in maintaining conditions damaging to those who are considered to be different from the mainstream. Yet this emphasis remains largely ignored in how we demonstrate being culturally aware and sensitive in our day-to-day practice, where the focus becomes helping those who are different integrate into systems and structures that may be detrimental to their health.

As culture is individually and collectively defined and expressed, so is health. Many immigrants and temporary residents define health, healthcare, and health promotion very differently from the dominant culture in their host country. This can lead to the perception on the part of healthcare providers that people "don't care" or are "non-compliant" about their health or the health of their families. However, people will continue to use healthcare practices and resources from their cultures of origin in ways that are meaningful to them.

Yet many of the needs of migrants are the same as for other Canadians. Determinants influencing health such as precarious employment, literacy, lack of housing, and food security affect many residents of Canada, though newcomers and those with language barriers may need more assistance with very practical strategies in their daily lives (e.g., banking, shopping, adjusting to a Canadian climate, childcare, etc.). CHNs need to assess the values, beliefs, and needs of all their clients in order to probe further in their assessments; to provide more comprehensive, anticipatory, and preventive care; and to advocate and collaborate with all people.

Culture is not a problem to be solved and "cultural barriers" often have more to do with the limitations of our organizations, systems, and focus on a disease orientation than on the "different" cultural values, beliefs, and practices of our clients! Diverse perspectives and insights can enhance community action and change. "Capacity-building, civic engagement, inclusion, and participation are keys to health promotion and social transformation within communities. The [cultural] lens through which individuals, organizations, and communities see each other informs their response to health and social problems as well as their action in building community" (Racher & Annis, 2012, p. 174).

# CULTURAL COMPETENCE AND CULTURAL SAFETY

First described by Leininger, **cultural competence** was seen as the mechanism to address culturally specific health needs. The concept of cultural competence integrates the knowledge, attitudes, and skills that nurses would use in order to plan effective and appropriate interventions. In her concept analysis of cultural competence, Dudas (2012) identified three dimensions: *awareness*, which means having some knowledge of cultural similarities and differences combined with self-reflection; *attitudes*, which include sensitivity, openness, being non-judgmental, and respecting differences; and *behaviours*, which require creativity while providing care through a "cultural lens." Camphina-Bacote (2002) described five constructs that inform the *process of cultural competence*: cultural awareness (self-examination), cultural knowledge, cultural skill (collecting and assessing data), cultural encounters (the process of relationships), and cultural desire (motivation of the healthcare provider).

Current conceptualizations of cultural competence acknowledge that is a lifelong process of approaching relationships with openness and humility rather than focusing on "knowing" specific cultures. "Abandoning a desire for certainty, closure, and control in relationships and replacing it with efforts to be tentative, experimental, and open-ended is useful in community practice. . . . Building bridges to connect diverse worlds is not merely a set of strategies but is an all-encompassing 'way of being' that comes from an ethic of care" (Racher & Annis, 2012, p. 171). The CHN is the learner, and the course of culturally competent care emerges from the interaction between providers and recipients (Schim et al., 2007). However, in practice there continues to be a focus on an individual client with "cultural" needs. In their review of the cultural competency literature, Renzaho, Romios, Crock, and Sønderlund (2013) identified as a major limitation the lack of research evidence exploring if patient outcomes are improved with increased healthcare provider knowledge and awareness of culture. In addition to individual resources and skills, it is necessary to recognize and integrate the role of institutional resources and structures (such as interpreters, continuing education, and organizational commitment and policies), which

support culturally competent practices (Racher & Annis, 2012; Registered Nurses' Association of Ontario, 2007; Srivastrava, 2007), as well as the importance of the social determinants of health in shaping people's lives. As affirmed by Ludwig-Beymer (2012), "cultural competency cannot live in one or two nurses; it must be systematic. It must involve all layers of the organization: the policy-making level, the administrative level, the management level, and the provider level. In addition, an organization must have a mutually beneficial relationship with the community it serves to achieve cultural competence" (p. 239). Table 9.1 lists key themes identified by the RNAO (2007) for cultural competence at all levels.

The concept of *cultural safety* arose in New Zealand in response to issues raised by Maori nurses. It has some elements in common with cultural competence; however, cultural safety makes explicit issues of power. **Cultural safety** is defined as effective nursing practice with clients from another culture, as determined by those clients. Some examples of culture are age, gender, sexual orientation, socioeconomic status, ethnic origin or migrant experience, religion, and disability. Nurses need to question what client values and behaviours they may be

| Table 9.1 | Key Themes for Building and Maintaining Cultural Competence |
|---|---|

**1. Practitioner skill set**

Cultural competence is a mandatory skill set for all healthcare providers.

**2. Workforce diversity**

Recruiting and retaining staff to achieve diversity in the workforce can benefit not only the healthcare professional in the delivery of culturally competent care but also minority groups in the care they access and receive.

**3. Systems and supports**

Embedding cultural competence processes and practices within organizational structures and curricula will promote the development of cultural competence.

**4. Decision support systems and practice improvement**

Utilizing indicators related to an organization's diversity climate is critical to measuring success and determining accountability for embracing diversity.

**5. Education and training**

Undergraduate and graduate education and life-long learning within practice settings must embed the principles of cultural competence throughout the learning process.

**6. Collaboration**

Organizations that promote collaboration and work collaboratively with each other will improve services for culturally diverse populations and contribute to a work environment that embraces diversity.

Source: Registered Nurses' Association of Ontario. (2007). *Embracing cultural diversity in health care: Developing cultural competence.* Toronto, ON: Author, p. 25.

defining as "cultural" and how they may be supporting the cultural practices of their institutions that sustain inequities. "Unsafe cultural practice comprises any action which diminishes, demeans, or disempowers the cultural identity and well-being of an individual" (Nursing Council of New Zealand, 2011, p. 7). The emphasis is on the experience of clients receiving nursing care; supporting the capacity of clients, including communities, to shape and contribute to their health experiences and outcomes; and the recognition of the context of power relations.

Strengths of a cultural safety approach include drawing our attention more explicitly to addressing inequities, supporting CHNs in the following:

- improve healthcare access for patients, aggregates, and populations;
- acknowledge that we are all bearers of culture;
- expose the social, political, and historical contexts of healthcare;
- enable practitioners to consider difficult concepts, such as racism, discrimination, and prejudice;
- acknowledge that cultural safety is determined by those to whom nurses provide care;
- understand the limitations of "culture" in terms of having people access and safely move through healthcare systems and encounters with care providers; and
- challenge unequal power relations (Aboriginal Nurses Association of Canada, 2009, p. 2).

Proponents of cultural safety consider cultural awareness, sensitivity, and competence as providing a starting place for comprehending cultural complexities, and that cultural safety is particularly congruent with advocacy (Aboriginal Nurses Association of Canada, 2009). Canadian nurse theorists and researchers have contributed much to the discussion about cultural safety in a multicultural environment (Williamson & Harrison, 2010). However, similar to cultural competence, the concept of cultural safety has been criticized for being inadequately understood and utilized in practice, and lacking research with regard to client outcomes (Johnstone & Kanitsaki, 2007; Williamson & Harrison, 2010).

## CULTURAL ASSESSMENTS

A variety of cultural assessment guides for individuals and families have been developed (Andrews & Boyle, 2012b; Giger, 2013; Higginbottom et al., 2011; Leininger, 2006; Purnell, 2013; Spector, 2012). Useful guides need to provide a format with open-ended questions that facilitate descriptive responses and building a relationship between clients and nurses. (See "A Guide to Transcultural Assessment" in MyNursingLab.) The intention of cultural assessments is to discover meanings and experiences of health and illness through the frame of culture. Cultural assessment guides share the classification and identification of important cultural domains so that culturally informed care can be provided.

However, the limitations of current assessment guides are shared as well, whereby the collection of cultural data becomes the focus, the relational processes are de-emphasized, and it can be difficult to separate data specific to the client from cultural generalizations (Giger, 2013).

When participating in cultural assessments, the CHN must be careful not to focus on how the client differs from the nurse or healthcare institutions, which we often assume to be the "norm." Knowledge of shared cultural characteristics and patterns can be useful as a beginning; however, individual experiences and meanings vary as everyone participates in multiple cultures, has many layers of identity, and is influenced by the dominant social order. Generalizations can be useful in providing background information about meanings of care and health practices but must be used with caution and sensitivity. Clients, whether they are individuals, families, or communities, may or may not share or value generalizations about their culture that are known to the nurse. There is continuous interplay between making use of background information the nurse may have and checking that information with every client. Background information about cultural values and practices that is never confirmed with clients and assumed to be true for all becomes a **stereotype**.

Most often, cultural assessments are conducted with individuals and families. Yet clients are always embedded in and influenced by their larger societies. Thus, it is important to assess the culture(s) of communities. (See Table 9.2, Community

| Table 9.2 | Community Cultural Assessment |
|---|---|

The following are some questions to assess the culture of a community:

- How would you describe what culture means to your community?
- With which culture(s) do you identify?
- What are some shared cultural values for your community?
- Are there some differing cultural values?
- Are there any aspects of your community's culture that are beneficial to your life and health?
- Are there any aspects of your community's culture that "get in the way" of your health?
- What are some of the other areas of your everyday life in your community that enhance or create barriers for your health?
- How is diversity reflected in your community?
- How does your community support inclusion of its members? Are there factors that exclude community members from full participation?
- What would you like nurses to know about your community's culture(s)?
- How would you like nurses to work with you in order to improve health in your community?

Source: From *Embracing Cultural Diversity in Health Care: Developing Cultural Competence.* Copyright © 2007 by Registered Nurses' Association of Ontario. Used by permission of Registered Nurses' Association of Ontario.

Cultural Assessment.) CHNs need to be aware of the interactions between the cultural assessments of individuals and families and the population focus necessary for a community assessment. Questions relating to culture should be integrated within the community assessment phase of the community health nursing process (see Chapter 13). Culture should be interpreted broadly and not limited to descriptions of ethnicity. Some examples of questions to ask are in Table 9.2. Other valuable considerations can be found in "Touchstones for Working with Diverse Communities" in MyNursingLab, in Andrews and Boyle's *Transcultural Nursing Guide for Groups and Communities* (Andrews & Boyle, 2012b), and in Dreher and Skemp (2011). Adding a cultural component to a community nursing assessment strengthens the base upon which everything follows, as both shared and diverse cultural experiences contribute to and shape every community's characteristics and uniqueness (Boyle & Baird, 2012).

## IMPLICATIONS FOR COMMUNITY HEALTH NURSING PRACTICE

It would not be possible to have comprehensive knowledge of every culture, nor is it necessary. CHNs need to have the assessment, interviewing, and collaborative skills in order to be open to the processes of discovery and self-reflection required for providing effective care with all clients. These skills are also needed with other healthcare providers, and community agencies and organizations. CHNs work with unique individuals, families, and communities for the mutual construction of actualized and potential solutions at downstream and upstream levels of care. Planning and implementing nursing care is not based on how different (or similar) someone might seem; it is based on bringing assessment and relational skills to every encounter so that values and beliefs can be discovered and strengths supported.

As an example of providing cultural care in the community, Table 9.3 illustrates how CHNs could provide care based on the levels of prevention in order to promote influenza immunization in a neighbourhood with a large immigrant population from a variety of countries (primary, secondary, and tertiary levels of prevention are discussed in Chapters 3 and 7).

How would the cultural care you provide be different in a neighbourhood that did not have a large immigrant population? The answer is it would not be! Perceptions, values, and meanings are culturally based and require exploration in every encounter. Specific interventions may vary, such as the need for translated fact sheets in different languages, but the processes of assessment, building respectful relationships, and collaborating in the development of interventions are the same. Clients are often left out of evaluating outcomes, yet their voices are critical in knowing if our involvement has been culturally safe.

Both nurses and clients bring multiple cultures to their interactions. Nurses need to be aware of how their personal culture(s), the culture of nursing, and the culture of their institution have shaped them. Clients (individuals, families, communities, populations) are shaped by their personal cultures, professional values, and unique life experiences as well. While discovering the clients' values, beliefs, and assumptions, nurses need to avoid focusing on the clients'

| Table 9.3 | Increasing Low Influenza Immunization Rates with Immigrant Population |
|---|---|
| Primary Prevention | Meet with local community and healthcare provider groups to discuss |
| | 1. perceptions, values, and meanings of the immunization program from recipient and provider perspectives; |
| | 2. barriers to receiving and providing immunization, such as location, transportation, time of day, need for verbal and written information, and interpretation and translation services; and |
| | 3. facilitating engagement of the community and providers in planning appropriate and innovative ways to promote and provide immunizations. |
| Secondary Prevention | Meet with local community and healthcare provider groups to discuss |
| | 1. perceptions and meanings of possible adverse reactions to immunization, such as redness, swelling, and rare serious reactions; |
| | 2. the primary care services available for assessment and follow-up if needed, and barriers to those services; and |
| | 3. planning to reduce barriers and promote services. |
| Tertiary Prevention | Meet with local community and healthcare provider groups to discuss |
| | 1. assessing and evaluating what strategies and interventions supported increased immunization rates and what was less successful; |
| | 2. advocating for needed changes to policies and service delivery; and |
| | 3. implementation of changes to sustain and improve immunization rates. |

cultures in a way that promotes stereotyping and excludes reflection regarding issues of power, professional and organizational cultures, and personal self-awareness (see the guide "Questions for Reflection and Building Awareness in Community Practice" in MyNursingLab). The keys to understanding and providing effective cultural care lie in approaching relationships with humility, appreciating the diversity within and among all of us, and acknowledging influences such as the effects of dominant cultures, including health care systems, and the social determinants of health. (See Canadian Research Box 9.2.)

---

### CANADIAN RESEARCH BOX 9.2

**What are the relational nursing practice patterns in palliative home care?**

Ward-Griffin, C., McWilliam, C., & Oudshoorn, A. (2012). Negotiating relational practice patterns in palliative home care. *Journal of Palliative Care, 28*(2), 97–104.

Palliative care in the home is challenging for all involved as complex and changing relationships develop among clients, their families, and professional caregivers. Focusing on the perspectives of nurses providing care to Canadian seniors with advanced cancer, the purpose of this ethnography was to explore the sociocultural context of home-based palliative care. During a six- to eight-month time frame, 19 in-depth interviews were conducted with three palliative care nurses and participant observation occurred in four households.

Three relational practice patterns were discovered: making time–forfeiting time, connecting–separating, and enabling–disabling. Within each theme there were conflicting tensions in the provision of palliative care that the nurses had to navigate. The nurses perceived "making time" as essential to the development of relationships with clients and their families. However, time was also something that had to be forfeited in the context of limited home care services. The practice pattern of connecting–separating related to the importance of connecting to clients, yet at the same time, nurses needed to maintain professional boundaries. Enabling–disabling reflected the potential for collaboration and supporting empowerment strategies with clients and families and the limited ability to deliver health-promotive care due to nurses' increasing caseloads and staff shortages. The culture of home-based palliative nursing revealed that time was both a resource and a limitation in providing holistic and relational care. The larger system constraints such as lack of funding, lack of time, and a focus on physical tasks were identified as major barriers.

#### Discussion Questions

1. What cultures are being explored in this research? What is identified as the dominant culture?

2. How would you use this research to provide direction for practice, policy, and research?

3. What insight does this research provide to clients, families, and communities?

---

### CASE STUDY

You are a CHN in a rural town of 15 000 people. In recent years there has been an increase in the numbers of new immigrants and temporary migrant workers who are "visibly" different. Prior to this, the population of the community had remained fairly constant. You are aware of comments circulating in the community, such as "These people are changing our town, it doesn't look the same anymore," and "Why should we be providing services to newcomers and people who are only here to work? Our grandparents started from nothing when they came to Canada."

You have been asked to join a community committee sponsored by the local social planning council to assess and address settlement needs such as translation services and improving available resources, as well as concerns regarding isolation and work safety of the temporary workers. The social planning council has the mandate to assess needs, provide services, and make recommendations for the entire community.

#### Discussion Questions

1. Which people representing which groups should be on the committee? Why?

2. How would you contribute to constructive discussion, exploring viewpoints and perspectives?

3. What could be some achievable outcomes from the committee work? How long would this take?

## CONCLUSION

This chapter has explored the concept of culture and the intersections among culture, multiculturalism, diversity, race, and ethnicity. Canadian experiences of diversity and multiculturalism were discussed, as were the relationships among culture, health, and the social determinants of health. The culturally competent and culturally safe sensitivities and skills that are needed to provide care during nurse–client interactions were described, including implications for community health nursing practice with all residents of Canada.

A culturally competent and culturally safe approach requires commitment to personal reflection and growth, an understanding of the layers of cultural identity that shape us all, and the development of knowledge and relationship-building skills. This is so that in every interaction the nurse strives to discover the values and meanings of health for the client in the context of structural forces and power relations. CHNs must nurture our common humanity and social responsibilities while also addressing systemic inequities. This means listening for history and context, not only to understand clients, but also in order to comprehensively change policy and practice. Culturally relevant community-based services are developed through "collaboration and partnerships between community leaders, health consumers, and healthcare providers. When community residents or health consumers are involved as partners, community-based services are more likely to be responsive to locally defined needs, are better used, and are sustained through local action" (Boyle & Baird, 2012, p. 278).

## KEY TERMS

cultural competence   p. 177
cultural safety   p. 177
Culture Care Diversity and Universality   p. 171
culture   p. 171
diversity   p. 172
ethnicity   p. 172
ethnocentrism   p. 171
immigrant   p. 173
multiculturalism   p. 172
race   p. 172
racialization   p. 172
racism   p. 172
stereotype   p. 178
temporary residents   p. 174
transnationalism   p. 173

## STUDY QUESTIONS

1. Describe the characteristics of culture.

2. Define and describe the links among culture, diversity, ethnicity, race, and multiculturalism.

3. What is the relationship between culture and health?

4. Describe the similarities and differences between cultural competence and cultural safety. What are the implications of these similarities and differences for CHN practice?

5. Describe how cultural beliefs and values shape the interactions between nurses and clients.

6. Describe the knowledge, attitudes, sensitivity, and skills needed to provide nursing care framed by culture to all residents of Canada.

> After working through these questions, go to the MyNursingLab at **www.pearsoned.ca/mynursinglab** to check your answers.

## INDIVIDUAL CRITICAL-THINKING EXERCISES

1. What implications does the Canadian Charter of Rights and Freedoms (1982) have on nursing practice when working with culturally diverse families?

2. In your work as a public health nurse you meet a family new to Canada at a community health fair. Communicating using very limited English, the parents tell you that money is very scarce, the mother is pregnant with her fifth child, the family does not have permanent residence status in Canada, and they are uncertain whether they will be allowed to stay. They are worried they will be deported to their country of origin. What community supports and services would you assist this family to access in order of priority and why?

3. What are the key differences between healthy cultural identification and ethnocentrism?

4. How would you assess whether the nursing model or theory you are using is helping you deliver culturally competent and culturally safe care?

5. How does culture influence health and illness within diverse communities? What roles do the social determinants of health and public policies play?

## GROUP CRITICAL-THINKING EXERCISES

1. How would you go about gaining and demonstrating the skills and behaviours needed for culturally competent and culturally safe practice?

2. In pairs, do a cultural assessment ("A Guide to Transcultural Nursing Assessment" can be found in MyNursingLab). What have you learned about your own culture? What have you learned about your partner's culture? What did you discover about the process?

3. Are the members of your nursing class representative of your community's population? Why or why not?

4. Discuss as a group the similarities and differences between your understandings of diversity and multiculturalism.

## REFERENCES

Aboriginal Nurses Association of Canada. (2009). *Cultural competence and cultural safety in nursing education: A framework for First Nations, Inuit and Métis nursing*. Ottawa, ON: Author. Used by permission of Aboriginal Nurses Association of Canada. Retrieved from http://www.anac.on.ca/Documents/Making%20It%20Happen%20Curriculum%20Project/FINALFRAMEWORK.pdf

Allender, J. A., Rector, C., & Warner, K. (2014). *Community health nursing: Promoting and protecting the public's health* (7th ed.). Philadelphia, PA: Lippincott, Williams & Wilkins.

Andrews, M. M., & Boyle, J. S. (2012a). Theoretical foundations of transcultural nursing. In M. M. Andrews & J. S. Boyle (Eds.), *Transcultural concepts in nursing care* (6th ed., pp. 3–16). Philadelphia, PA: Wolters Kluwer/Lippincott Williams & Wilkins.

Andrews, M. M., & Boyle, J. S. (2012b). *Transcultural concepts in nursing care* (6th ed.). Philadelphia, PA: Wolters Kluwer/Lippincott Williams & Wilkins.

Blad, C., & Couton, P. (2009). The rise of an intercultural nation: Immigration, diversity and nationhood in Quebec. *Journal of Ethnic and Migration Studies, 35*(4), 645–667. doi:10.1080/13691830902765277

Boyd, M., & Pikkow, D. (2008). Finding place in stratified structures: Migrant women in North America. In N. Piper (Ed.), *New perspectives on gender and migration: Livelihood, rights and entitlements* (pp. 19–58). New York, NY: Routledge.

Boyle, J. S., & Baird, M. B. (2012). Culture, family, and community. In M. M. Andrews & J. S. Boyle (Eds.), *Transcultural concepts in nursing care* (6th ed., pp. 277–315). Philadelphia, PA: Wolters Kluwer/Lippincott Williams & Wilkins.

Browne, A. J., Varcoe, C., Smye, V., Reimer-Kirkham, S., Lynam, J., & Wong, S. (2009). Cultural safety and the challenges of translating critically oriented knowledge in practice. *Nursing Philosophy, 10,* 167–179.

Camphina-Bacote, J. (2002). The process of cultural competence in the delivery of healthcare services: A model of care. *Journal of Transcultural Nursing, 13*(3), 181–184. Retrieved from http://tcn.sagepub.com.proxy1. lib.uwo.ca:2048/cgi/reprint/13/3/181

Canadian Council for Refugees. (2015). *Refugee health survey by province and by category.* Retrieved from http://ccrweb.ca/sites/ccrweb.ca/files/ccr-refugee-health-survey-public.pdf

Canadian Nurses Association. (2010). *Position statement: Promoting cultural competence in nursing.* Ottawa, ON: Author. Used by permission of Canadian Nurses Association. Retrieved from http://www.cna-aiic.ca/~/media/cna/page-content/pdf-en/ps114_cultural_competence_2010_e.pdf?la=en

Canadian Public Health Association. (2010). *Public health – community health nursing practice in Canada: Roles and activities* (4th ed.). Ottawa, ON: Author. Retrieved from http://www.chnc.ca/documents/PublicHealth-CommunityHealthNursinginCanadaRolesandActivities2010.pdf

Citizenship and Immigration Canada. (2014). Canada facts and figures 2013: Immigration overview – temporary residents. Retrieved from http://www.cic.gc.ca/english/pdf/2013-Facts-Temporary.pdf

Citizenship and Immigration Canada. (2015). Canada facts and figures 2014: Immigration overview – permanent residents. Retrieved from http://www.cic.gc.ca/english/pdf/2014-Facts-Permanent.pdf

Community Health Nurses of Canada. (2011, revised). *Canadian community health nursing: Professional practice model and standards of practice.* St. John's, NL: Author. Retrieved from http://www.chnc.ca/documents/chnc-standards-eng-book.pdf

Dreher, M., & Skemp, L. (2011). *Healthy places healthy people: A handbook for culturally informed community nursing practice* (2nd ed.). Indianapolis, IN: Sigma Theta Tau International.

Dudas, K. I. (2012). Cultural competence: An evolutionary concept analysis. *Nursing Education Perspectives, 33*(5), 317–321.

Edmunds, K., Berman, H., Basok, T., Ford-Gilboe, M., & Forchuk, C. (2011). The health of women temporary agricultural workers in Canada: A critical review of the literature. *Canadian Journal of Nursing Research, 43*(4), 68–91.

Etowa, J. B., & McGibbon, E. A. (2012). Race and racism as determinants of health. In E. A. McGibbon (Ed.), *Oppression: A social determinant of health* (pp. 73–88). Halifax, NS: Fernwood.

Fuller-Thomson, E., Noack, A. M., & George, U. (2011). Health decline among recent immigrants to Canada: Findings from a nationally-representative longitudinal survey. *Canadian Journal of Public Health, 102*(4), 273–280.

Giger, J. N. (2013). *Transcultural nursing: Assessment and intervention* (6th ed.). St. Louis, MO: Mosby Elsevier.

Government of Canada. (1988). Canadian *Multiculturalism Act: R.S.C., 1985, c. 24 (4th Supp.)* Ottawa, ON: Author. Used by permission of Department of Justice Canada. Retrieved from http://laws.justice.gc.ca/eng/acts/C-18.7/page-1.html

Gray, D. P., & Thomas, D. J. (2006). Critical reflections on culture in nursing. *Journal of Cultural Diversity, 13*(2), 76–82.

Gustafson, D. L. (2005). Transcultural nursing theory from a critical cultural perspective. *Advances in Nursing Science, 28*(1), 2–16.

Higginbottom, G. M. A., Richter, M. S., Mogale, R. S., Ortiz, L., Young, S., & Mollell, O. (2011). Identification of nursing assessment models/tools validated in clinical practice for use with diverse ethno-cultural groups: An integrative review of the literature. *BMC Nursing 10*(16), 1–11. Retrieved from http://www.biomedcentral.com/1472-6955/10/16

Houle, R., & Yssaad, L. (2010). *Perspectives: Recognition of newcomers' foreign credentials and work experience.* Ottawa, ON: Statistics Canada. Catalogue no. 75-001-X. Retrieved from http://www.statcan.gc.ca/pub/75-001-x/2010109/pdf/11342-eng.pdf

Isaacs, S. (2010). Transnational cultural ecologies: Evolving challenges for nurses in Canada. *Journal of Transcultural Nursing, 21*(1), 15–22.

Johnstone, M.-J., & Kanitsaki, O. (2007). An exploration of the notion and nature of the construct of cultural safety and its applicability to the Australian health care context. *Journal of Transcultural Nursing, 18*(3), 247–256. doi:10.1177/1043659607301304

Kim, I.-H., Carrasco, C., Muntaner, C., McKenzie, K., & Samuel, N. (2013). Ethnicity and post migration health trajectory in new immigrants to Canada. *American Journal of Public Health, 103*(4), 96–104.

Leininger, M. (2006). Culture care diversity and universality theory and evolution of the ethnonursing method. In M. Leininger & M. R. McFarland (Eds.), *Culture care diversity and universality: A worldwide nursing theory* (2nd ed., pp. 1–41). Boston, MA: Jones and Bartlett.

Ludwig-Beymer, P. (2012). Creating culturally competent organizations. In M. M. Andrews & J. S. Boyle (Eds.), *Transcultural concepts in nursing care* (6th ed., pp. 211–242). Philadelphia, PA: Wolters Kluwer/Lippincott Williams & Wilkins.

Marks, B. (2007). Cultural competence revisited: Nursing students with disabilities. *Journal of Nursing Education, 46*(2), 70–74.

Nursing Council of New Zealand. (2011). *Guidelines for cultural safety, the Treaty of Waitangi and Maori health in nursing education and practice.* Wellington, NZ: Author. Retrieved from http://nursingcouncil.org.nz/Publications/Standards-and-guidelines-for-nurses

Preibisch, K. L. (2007). Local produce, foreign labour: Labour mobility programs and global trade competitiveness in Canada. *Rural Sociology, 72*(3), 418–449.

Public Health Agency of Canada. (2013). *Underlying premises and evidence table.* Retrieved from http://www.phac-aspc.gc.ca/ph-sp/determinants/determinants-eng.php#evidence

Purnell, L. D. (2013). *Transcultural health care: A culturally competent approach* (4th ed.). Philadelphia, PA: F. A. Davis.

Racher, F. E., & Annis, R. C. (2012). Honouring culture and diversity in community practice. In A. R. Vollman,

E. T. Anderson, & J. McFarlane (Eds.), *Canadian community as partner: Theory and multidisciplinary practice* (3rd ed., pp. 154–176). Philadelphia, PA: Wolters Kluwer/Lippincott Williams & Wilkins.

Registered Nurses' Association of Ontario. (2007). *Embracing cultural diversity in health care: Developing cultural competence.* Toronto, ON: Author. Retrieved from http://rnao.ca/sites/rnao-ca/files/Embracing_Cultural_Diversity_in_Health_Care_-_Developing_Cultural_Competence.pdf

Renzaho, A. M. N., Romios, P., Crock, C., & Sønderlund, A. L. (2013). The effectiveness of cultural competence programs in ethnic minority patient centered health care—a systematic review of the literature. *International Journal for Quality in Health Care, 25*(3), 261–269. doi: 10.1093/intqhc/mzt006

Schim, S., Doorenbos, A., Benkert, R., & Miller, J. (2007). Culturally congruent care: Putting the puzzle together. *Journal of Transcultural Nursing, 18*(2), 103–110. doi:10.1177/1043659606298613

Shirley, J. (2007). Limits of autonomy in nursing's moral discourse. *Advances in Nursing Science, 30*(1), 14–25.

Spector, R. E. (2012). *Cultural diversity in health and illness* (8th ed.). Upper Saddle River, NJ: Pearson Prentice Hall.

Spitzer, D. (2012). Oppression and immigrant health in Canada. In E. A. McGibbon (Ed.), *Oppression: A social determinant of health* (pp. 113–122). Halifax, NS: Fernwood.

Srivastava, R. (2007). *The health care professional's guide to clinical cultural competence.* Toronto, ON: Mosby.

Statistics Canada. (2013). *Immigration and ethnocultural diversity in Canada: National household survey 2011.* (Government No. 99-010-X2011001). Ottawa, ON: Author. Retrieved from http://www12.statcan.gc.ca/nhs-enm/2011/as-sa/99-010-x/99-010-x2011001-eng.pdf

Varcoe, C. (2006). Doing participatory action research in a racist world. *Western Journal of Nursing Research, 28*(5), 525–540. doi:10.1177/0193945906287706

Williams, R. (1983, revised). *Keywords: A vocabulary of culture and society.* New York, NY: University Press.

Williamson, M., & Harrison, L. (2010). Providing culturally appropriate care: A literature review. *International Journal of Nursing Studies, 47*(6), 761–769.

World Health Organization. (2008). *Closing the gap in a generation: Health equity through action on the social determinants of health.* Geneva, Switzerland: Author. Retrieved from http://whqlibdoc.who.int/publications/2008/9789241563703_eng.pdf

Yiu Matuk, L., & Ruggirello, T. (2007). Culture connection project: Promoting multiculturalism in elementary schools. *Canadian Journal of Public Health, 98*(1), 26–29.

## ABOUT THE AUTHOR

**Kathryn Edmunds**, RN, BN (University of Manitoba), MSN (Wayne State University, with a specialization in transcultural nursing), PhD(c), is currently a doctoral candidate in the Arthur Labatt Family School of Nursing at Western University. She has been a faculty member in Nursing at the University of Windsor and has extensive experience as a public health nurse with the Windsor-Essex County Health Unit working in rural southwestern Ontario. Current theoretical and research interests include the relationships among uprootedness, displacement, gendered migration, culture, and health, and the current critiques in the nursing literature of the concept of culture from critical theoretical perspectives.

# Research

### Rebecca Ganann and Donna Ciliska

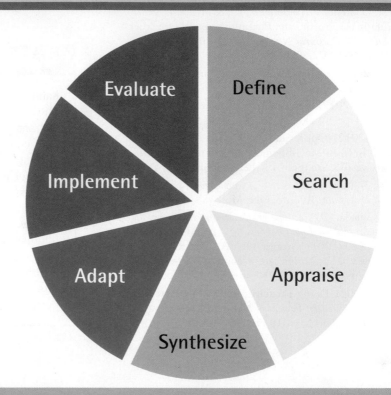

*Source:* Adapted with permission from *A Model of Evidence-Informed Decision Making in Public Health* (2012), a fact sheet created by and available from the National Collaborating Centre for Methods and Tools.

## INTRODUCTION

The professional practice model (introduced in Chapter 3) indicates that community health nurses (CHNs) participate in knowledge generation and knowledge translation and integrate knowledge and multiple ways of knowing; they engage in evidence-informed decision making (Community Health Nurses of Canada, 2011, revised). CHNs participate in research and have opportunities, frequently unrecognized, for improving their practice by utilizing high-quality research. As part of their critical thinking, CHNs often ask important questions that impact their nursing practice. The following list provides some examples of how CHNs may pose questions related to their practice:

■ There are many opportunities for CHNs to promote health during the perinatal period. As one example, CHNs may provide support for maternal mental health as part of their role, but they may not be sure about the **effectiveness** of their interventions. Are there any **interventions** that have been shown to decrease postpartum depression and anxiety? Can proactive peer telephone support help to prevent postpartum depression in new mothers? (Dennis, Hodnett, & Reisman, 2009)

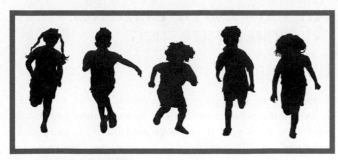

**PHOTO 10.1** The school years are formative for healthy lifestyle development.

*Source: Srnicholl/Fotolia*

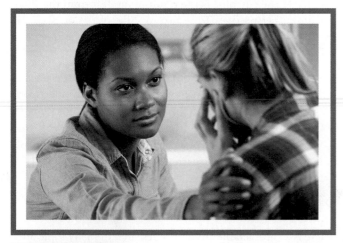

**PHOTO 10.2** Parenting stress is commonly experienced by families of children with developmental disabilities.

*Source: Monkey Business/Fotolia*

- School-aged children are a population group that CHNs may work with. A key time period to teach healthy lifestyle habit development is during the formative school years (see photo 10.1). The local school board is concerned that there is too little time to teach the required curriculum, so they are considering reducing the time spent in physical activity. At the same time, the region is concerned about the increasing numbers of overweight children. Are school-based physical activity programs effective in improving activity duration in children? (Dobbins, Husson, DeCorby, & LaRocca, 2013) (see Canadian Research box 10.1 for the evidence).
- Parents of developmentally delayed children experience considerable stress (see photo 10.2). Can parenting programs reduce their psychological distress? (Singer, Ethridge, & Aldana, 2007)

CHNs are faced with questions like these every day. After graduation, how can nurses continue to be educated critical thinkers whose practice is based on high-quality research evidence? How can busy nurses keep current with the research findings? How can nurses meet the provincial nursing standards for using evidence in practice, the national public health core competencies (Public Health Agency of Canada, 2008), or the national Community Health Nursing Standards of Practice

(Community Health Nurses of Canada, 2011, revised)? This chapter highlights strategies that CHNs can use to develop and sustain **evidence-based nursing** (EBN) practice.

## WHAT IS EVIDENCE-BASED NURSING?

The term "evidence-based nursing" has evolved from the initial work done in evidence-based medicine. EBN is defined as the conscientious, explicit, and judicious use of current best evidence in making decisions about the care of individual patients. Evidence-based practice means integrating individual clinical expertise with the best available external clinical evidence from systematic research (Sackett, Rosenberg, Gray, & Haynes, 1996). In evidence-based practice, research utilization is integrated with other information that might influence the management of health issues and problems, such as clinical expertise, preference for alternative forms of care, and available resources. In Figure 10.1, elements in evidence-informed decision making are presented. Each element in the model appears to have equal weight; however, the process of evidence-based practice may be more complicated in reality. For example, peer maternal mental health supporters have the skills to provide effective telephone-based support and make appropriate referrals. We know from the research evidence that the peer support intervention for maternal mental health is effective (Dennis et al., 2009). However, some new mothers may see the peer support person as intrusive and not be open to receiving support via telephone.

Evidence-based practice may have been misunderstood in the past to mean the application of research findings to a decision, regardless of the context or patient preferences. In an effort to overcome this type of confusion, some authors now call the process "**evidence-informed practice**," particularly in relation to the use of evidence in policy making (Canadian Health Services Research Foundation, 2004). We have conceptualized evidence-informed practice as broader in context than research utilization. For those who work in public health, the following schemata of the steps of evidence-informed public

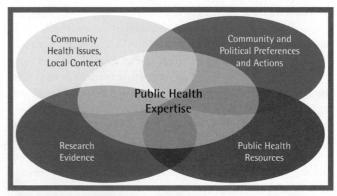

**FIGURE 10.1** A Model for Evidence-Informed Decision Making in Community Health

*Source:* Adapted with permission from *A model of evidence-informed decision making in public health* (2012), a fact sheet created by and available from the National Collaborating Centre for Methods and Tools.

health process have been developed; the process is the same for evidence-informed nursing. This process is circular in nature, beginning with *defining* the question and moving through various phases (see Figures 10.2–10.4 and Figures 10.6–10.9). Because this is an iterative process, when the evaluation phase is complete, you proceed to build on previous work and define a new question to move through the cycle with. Engaging in this iterative process assists in building an evidence-informed practice as CHNs. What difference does the use of research make? Heater, Becker, & Olson (1988) conducted a **meta-analysis** to determine the contribution of research-based practice to client **outcomes**. They found 84 nurse-conducted studies involving 4146 patients and reported that clients who received research-based nursing care made "sizeable gains" in behavioural knowledge and physiological and psychosocial outcomes compared with those receiving routine nursing care. The same review would be a massive undertaking today, as there are so many more studies that would need to be included.

## Why Don't All Nurses Base Their Practice on Evidence?

Even though awareness has improved over the last few decades, nurses lack the knowledge and skills to be able to find, access, and interpret the best available research evidence, and then apply, implement, and evaluate its impact (Alspach, 2006; Melnyk et al., 2004). In addition, organizational and system barriers may contribute to some inability to use research evidence (Squires, Moralejo, & LeFort, 2007). Estabrooks, Chong, Brigidear, & Profetto-McGrath (2005) surveyed nurses across seven units in four different Canadian hospitals regarding their preferred knowledge sources for clinical practice. While education differed across the units, the pattern of preferred knowledge sources was consistent: nurses used personal experience, colleagues, and patients for information before going to textbooks or journals. These findings were also consistent across two earlier Canadian studies. The more-current research has switched focus from measuring use of research to understanding the factors that determine research utilization, such as personal characteristics of the health professional, characteristics of the organization, and characteristics of the change to be implemented (Dobbins, Davies, Danseco, Edwards, & Virani, 2005; Farmer et al., 2008; Graham et al., 2006).

The sheer volume of research currently available is more than any nurse can manage. Nurses working individually could only hope to find and read a small proportion of the research that is published each year. This is compounded by the fact that much of the research relevant to community health nursing is published in non-nursing journals. In addition to barriers faced by individual nurses, multiple political, cultural, economic, and other environmental barriers must be overcome in order to practise in an evidence-based way. Furthermore, there is a substantial time lag of 8 to 15 years between the time technical information is generated and the time it is used in actual practice (Lomas, 1991; Utterback, 1974). The following section will describe the process of evidence-informed nursing. We hope that you will use this process to help guide your nursing practice in community health.

# THE PROCESS OF EVIDENCE-INFORMED NURSING

## 1. Define

Nurses need to maintain inquiring minds in order to evaluate interventions and consider options for other interventions. In order to find relevant research, clinical questions need to be structured, usually consisting of the **situation**, the intervention, and the outcomes (Flemming, 1998). The situation is the patient, client, population, or problem being addressed; the intervention is the action that is under consideration for some health promotion, disease prevention, or treatment effect; and the outcome is the result of interest from the client or clinical perspective. To return to some of the questions in the "What Is EBN?" section, the phrasing of the questions might be as follows:

- For new mothers (situation), does a structured peer mental health telephone support program (intervention) affect post-partum depression and anxiety in new mothers (outcomes)?
- Is glucosamine (intervention) effective in reducing pain and increasing functional ability (outcomes) in people with osteoarthritis (situation)?

## 2. Search

There is a considerable amount of research in many topic areas of community health. In practice, CHNs need skills to be able to find high-quality relevant information quickly. An Internet search engine may overwhelm you with the number of "hits." It is important to note that literature from search results on the Internet appear in order of the frequency of other people choosing them as opposed to any quality criteria. However, there are several free-access databases that either contain articles that have already been critically appraised or will allow

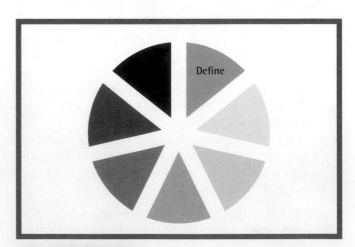

**FIGURE   10.2** Define

*Source:* Adapted with permission from *A model of evidence-informed decision making in public health* (2012), a fact sheet created by and available from the National Collaborating Centre for Methods and Tools.

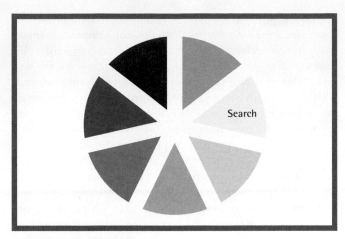

FIGURE 10.3 Search

*Source:* Adapted with permission from *A model of evidence-informed decision making in public health* (2012), a fact sheet created by and available from the National Collaborating Centre for Methods and Tools.

you to use quality filters, such as limiting by study design. When you conduct a literature search, you can consider synonymous terms for the situations, interventions, and outcomes. For example, for the patient or population, new mothers might be found under other search terms, such as postpartum, maternal, primipara, or multipara. The same process is followed for the interventions and outcomes. This will allow you to find all the possible search terms, leading to a more efficient search. The most effective search may done with the assistance of a health sciences librarian. Taking the original question, the list of synonyms for each component of the question, and any articles already found on the subject will allow the librarian to see how this type of article is indexed in the relevant databases. It is also important to be clear about the purpose of finding this literature. Is the goal to find a guideline about a particular topic that would give direction regarding management or policy and procedure decisions? For example, should sexually active teens be screened for cervical cancer? The answer to this question is likely to be a policy decision at the provincial or regional level. What are the Canadian recommendations? You can go to the Canadian Task Force on Preventive Health Care and find the answer (http://canadiantaskforce.ca/guidelines/screening-for-cervical-cancer). Or is the goal to find a systematic review that will provide a synthesis of the individual studies on a topic (see the section "What Is a Systematic Review?" later in this chapter)? Or has a policy decision been made, and what you are looking for are the detailed interventions that nurses need to put into action? You are likely to find the answers to this question in more detail in the individual **intervention studies** rather than the systematic review. However, keep in mind that the systematic review would identify those individual studies for you. Not everyone has access to a librarian all of the time. The following will discuss how to access reputable information quickly.

The most time-efficient sources of good data are the websites that give you "pre-appraised" research, meaning they have selected the best articles through critically appraising, rating, and summarizing the research, thus giving you the "gold nuggets" of good-quality research. For CHNs in Canada, one "go-to" place for pre-appraised research is Health Evidence (www.healthevidence.org). This service searches databases broadly (e.g., Medline, Embase, Cochrane Library, Campbell Collaboration Library, and others) on a quarterly basis for systematic reviews that are relevant to community health in Canada. Any relevant reviews are entered into the Health Evidence database and rated for quality on a scale of one to ten, independently, by two different qualified raters. You can search by free text or by the narrowed categories or strategies they offer for different populations, different intervention types, and different intervention locations. Some of the high-quality reviews have a three- to four-page structured abstract that has a brief description of the background of the issue, results of the review, level of evidence for different outcomes, and implications for practice and policy. Levels of evidence is a categorization of quantitative study designs that go in descending order or strength (increasing potential for **bias**), from **systematic reviews** (with or without statistical summary, which is called meta-analysis), followed by **randomized controlled trials**, then **observational studies**. Using Health Evidence is of additional benefit, since reviews (particularly Cochrane reviews) may be 60 pages or more in length. By reading the summary statements, you will be able to assess whether or not the respective research is useful for your purposes. You may then decide if you would like to continue reading the entire document or move on to another. Another source of pre-processed information is Clinical Evidence (http://clinicalevidence.bmj.com). It is an evidence-based tool organized around common primary care and hospital-based problems. It provides concise accounts of the current state of knowledge, ignorance, and uncertainty about the prevention and treatment of a wide range of clinical conditions based on thorough searches of the literature. Clinical Evidence uses information from the Cochrane Library (see below) and the abstraction journals. However, it starts not with the journals, but with **clinical questions** such as prevention and treatment of pressure sores or management of acute stroke or acute myocardial infarction. This source may be more useful to those CHNs who work in home care (Chapter 5) or primary care (Chapter 8).

The Cochrane Collaboration is an international organization that aims to help people make informed decisions about health by preparing, maintaining, and ensuring the accessibility of rigorous, systematic, and up-to-date reviews (including meta-analyses where appropriate) of the benefits and risks of specific healthcare interventions (Jadad & Haynes, 1998). Examples of the Cochrane Collaboration's relevance to community health include smoking cessation in the workplace, parent training for improving maternal psychosocial health, and prevention of falls in the elderly. The Cochrane Library is the product of the Collaboration's work and includes reports and protocols; 4000 systematic reviews produced within the Collaboration; abstracts of more than 11 000 reviews summarized and critically appraised by the Centre for Reviews and Dissemination at the University of York, U.K.; and citations for more than 600 000 randomized controlled trials. You can search the Cochrane Library online (www.thecochranelibrary.com) without charge for abstracts of reviews, and through subscription for full access to their resources.

If no answer is found to the structured question within the pre-appraised literature, it is necessary to go to other databases. Free online access is available for PubMed (www.ncbi.nlm.nih.gov/pubmed), which can be searched with key words, setting limits for type of publication, year of publication, language, a nursing subset of journals, and so on. Another useful place to search is the Cumulative Index of Nursing and Allied Health Literature (CINAHL). Similar to PubMed, CINAHL allows for limits to be set and to search by author or key word. In all cases, there is a mixture of free access and pay-per-view access to full-text articles, unless you have access through an established library consortium.

## 3. Appraise

Once the articles are found and retrieved, you must decide if their quality is sufficient so that you can be confident in using them. Some healthcare research is too poor in quality to be used in decision making regarding practice. As previously stated, this is less critical with some of the pre-appraised sources of research. Several checklists for quality (validity) have been developed (Ciliska, Thomas, & Buffett, 2008) to help people acquire and hone **critical appraisal skills**; that is, the ability to decide if an article is of sufficient methodological quality that it warrants attention for decision making. With a little practice, these skills become easier and quicker to apply.

Outcomes or intervention research answers questions about effectiveness or harm and has a quantitative design. As stated in Chapter 11, Epidemiology, different research designs are best for answering particular types of questions. For example, questions about effectiveness or harms of certain interventions and prevention are best answered by randomized controlled trials in which the investigators have no control over who is placed in the intervention group versus the control group. The most efficient way to access evidence of this type that may inform your practice is a systematic review of randomized controlled trials. However, randomized controlled trials may be unethical, such as randomizing mothers to breastfeed or not to see if breastfeeding is associated with eczema, or randomizing preteens to smoke to see if it causes lung cancer. Also, trials are very expensive. If a trial cannot be done due to ethical or financial reasons, the next best design to answer the question is a **cohort design**, where at least two groups are compared before and after one group receives an intervention. (See Chapter 11 or a basic nursing research text for more information on study designs.)

Questions exploring perceptions, feelings, and experiences are best answered through a qualitative design such as **phenomenology** or **grounded theory**. Questions and interventions that evolve through partnerships between researchers and participants are best dealt with through **participatory action research (PAR)**. PAR is action-oriented research in which the researchers and participants are partners in developing the question, intervention, and evaluation. PAR helps to ensure that the group under study gets the questions that are most important to them asked and answered and that the information is immediately useable for them (see Canadian Research box 10.2 for an example of a PAR study with Aboriginal women). Research may be quantitative or qualitative and may involve triangulation of data from multiple sources (Grove, Burns, & Gray, 2012).

One principle when critically appraising articles is to ensure that the appropriate design was used to answer the question. More recently, researchers are realizing that healthcare topics are very complex and that **mixed methods research** may be most appropriate. Mixed methods include both quantitative and qualitative methods, either concurrently or sequentially. For example, a randomized controlled trial of the effectiveness of different forms of birth control for teens would be enhanced by an understanding of their preferences for a type of birth control.

The Additional Research Boxes in MyNursingLab discuss criteria for critical appraisal of systematic reviews, single intervention studies, and qualitative research and demonstrate the application of the criteria to actual research studies.

## Critical Appraisal of Intervention Studies (Treatment or Prevention)

It is likely that you will find several studies that relate to your question. The decision to use an intervention study (treatment or prevention) depends on the findings and the quality of the study design. The quality determines the level of confidence in the findings of the study. These are the major questions used to evaluate primary studies of interventions or prevention:

- Are the results valid?
- What were the results?
- Will the results help me in improving the health of clients? (Ciliska, Cullum, & Marks, 2001; Sackett, Strauss, Richardson, Rosenberg, & Haynes, 2000)

The following section discusses more specific critical appraisal criteria that help to answer these questions. You will have a chance to practise applying the critical appraisal criteria to an article (Ratner et al., 2004) in the case study found at the end of the chapter.

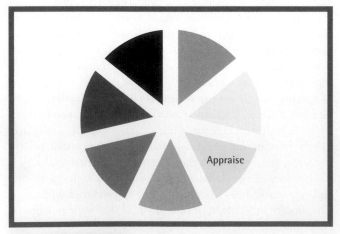

**FIGURE 10.4** Appraise

*Source:* Adapted with permission from *A model of evidence-informed decision making in public health* (2012), a fact sheet created by and available from the National Collaborating Centre for Methods and Tools.

**Are the Results Valid?** This question considers whether the reported results are likely to reflect the true size and direction of the treatment effect. Was the research designed to minimize bias and lead to accurate findings? (See the box "Questions Used to Critically Appraise Intervention Studies [Treatment or Prevention].")

*Was the assignment of participants to treatment groups randomized, and was the randomization concealed?* The purpose of randomization is to remove any control over who is assigned to an intervention or control group. As well, groups should be similar in all respects, except for exposure to the intervention. Known and unknown factors (age, gender, socioeconomic status, disease severity) that could influence the outcome of the study are evenly distributed among the groups. Different methods, such as a table of random numbers or computer-generated random numbers, ensure that all participants have an equal chance of being in each of the study groups. The methods section of the article should tell if and how participants were randomized.

The person recruiting the participants into the study should not know to which group each person is allocated. This is called *allocation concealment.* Concealment could happen through a process of calling a central office to get the allocation of the participant or through the use of numbered, opaque, sealed envelopes. In this way, the recruiter does not know until after participants are registered to which group they will be assigned, and the participant does not know at all. This prevents the recruiter from exercising bias in recruitment.

*Was follow-up sufficiently long and complete?* The first of these two criteria has to be judged by the clinician reading the paper. The definition of appropriate length of follow-up varies with different practice questions. For example, success in weight loss measured at six months after a year-long intervention does not give a true picture of how many people are able to maintain the weight loss over time. A minimum expectation would be a one-year follow-up. Similarly, with early childhood interventions, follow-up for only two years may mean that some important outcomes that occur later in life for the child or family are missed.

The second part of these criteria relates to completeness of follow-up. Seldom are studies able to retain all participants until the end of the follow-up. If large numbers are lost, it reduces the confidence one can have in the results. To continue with the weight-loss example, large dropouts are usual during treatment and follow-up. If the author reports on only those who remained in the study, those participants are more likely to be doing well in terms of their weight loss. Participants who were unsuccessful with the intervention are more likely to drop out, thereby making the intervention look far more effective than it is in reality. A retention rate of 80% is considered good; however, this is somewhat topic dependent, as one would expect the dropout rates of a transient population (e.g., homeless individuals) to be much higher.

*Were participants analyzed in groups to which they were assigned?* This criterion relates to the fact that participants should be analyzed in the group to which they were randomized, regardless of whether or not they actually received the treatment or completed treatment as assigned. This is also used in relation to **intention-to-treat analysis.** If the participants who discontinued treatment—for example, due to unpleasant side effects—were omitted from analysis, we would be left only with participants who had better outcomes, making the treatment look more effective than it actually was. Intention-to-treat analysis includes data (often baseline) for all dropouts so the effect is no change in dropouts. This gives a more conservative estimate of the effect of the intervention, compared to the analysis that leaves them out and only includes those who completed the intervention.

*Were participants, clinicians, outcome assessors, and data analysts unaware of (blinded to or masked from) participant allocation?* Several of the groups involved in a trial have the potential to bias the outcomes if they know whether a participant is in the intervention or control group. **Bias** means any systematic tendency to produce an outcome that differs from the truth. It includes the tendency to look more carefully for particular outcomes or to probe more deeply for outcomes in one group and not the other, as well as for participants to more likely recall an event or exposure that could have an impact if they

---

### CANADIAN RESEARCH BOX 10.1

#### What is the evidence for school-based activity programs?

Dobbins, M., Husson, H., DeCorby, K., & LaRocca, R. L. (2013). School-based physical activity programs for promoting physical activity and fitness in children and adolescents aged 6 to 18. *Cochrane Database of Systematic Reviews 2013, Issue 2.* Art. No.: CD007651. doi:10.1002/14651858.CD007651.pub2

The purpose of this systematic review was to summarize the evidence of the effectiveness of school-based interventions in promoting physical activity and fitness in children and adolescents. Of the 16 219 titles identified and screened and 587 articles retrieved, 44 were relevant and included in the review. The authors conclude that there is moderate quality evidence that school-based physical activity interventions have a positive impact on physical activity, reduced television viewing, and increased $VO_2$ max (a test of maximum oxygen uptake that determines the body's maximal oxygen utilization capacity).

#### Discussion Questions

1. Some people naively look at systematic reviews and see that many titles were discarded; in the example above, they found 44 of the initial 16 219 titles. They then claim that not all studies get used; large numbers get thrown out, making a systematic review not really a look at all the available research. How would you respond?

2. Is this conclusion convincing—that school-based interventions can improve physical activity, increase $VO_2$ max, and reduce television viewing? Are these meaningful changes? Are they worth putting resources into school-based interventions?

3. What are the policy implications for the local school board and board of health?

have an adverse outcome than if they do not have an adverse outcome (Oxman, Guyatt, Cook, & Montori, 2002). Studies can be labelled single, double, or triple blinded depending on how many of the groups were unaware of the allocation of the participants. Authors should clearly state which groups were blinded or masked. For example, if participants know they are in the intervention group, they may have increased sensitivity to the good or bad effects of the treatment. Participant blinding is easier to do in drug trials where placebos can be made to look identical to the active drug. However, it is far more difficult in community nursing to blind participants to a nurse coming into their home or delivering a physical versus a primarily psychosocial intervention. It is often possible to minimize the potential bias by ensuring that the participant does not know the specific outcome(s) being examined. Similarly, clinicians who care for the participants and know the allocation may unconsciously alter the way they give care and may have a heightened awareness of positive outcomes or adverse outcomes in a way that biases the evaluation.

The most important group to be blinded is the one that measures the outcomes. Ideally, clinicians providing care are not assessing outcomes. The measurement of key outcomes can be unconsciously distorted by the clinicians' beliefs about the intervention and its side effects. Objective outcome measures, such as antibody titres for measles, are less subject to outcome assessor bias than self-report of full measles immunization. Similarly, data analyses should be done with coded data that do not allow for identification of treatment groups. Consequently, readers of randomized trials should look for reports of which groups were and were not blinded to the participant allocation. If blinding is not possible, the authors should report on steps taken to minimize possible biases.

*Were participants in each group treated equally except for the intervention being evaluated?* Randomization should ensure that the only difference between study groups is the treatment being evaluated. An important principle is that additional treatments, or extra care, should not be given. Readers of randomized trials should look carefully at the descriptions of interventions received by all groups, especially if the practitioners are not blinded to allocation.

*Were the groups similar at the start of the trial?* Randomization should ensure that the groups of study participants were similar at the beginning. Usually, a table of baseline characteristics is prepared and some analysis is done to check that randomization actually "worked." If the groups show statistically significant differences at the beginning, the impact of the intervention may be altered, which can affect the validity of the result. If imbalances do exist at baseline, adjustment in the analysis can be done with statistical techniques such as using baseline values as a covariate.

**What Were the Results?** Once you have determined that the results are valid, it important to understand what the results really mean. The questions discussed and explained below will guide you through this process.

*How large is the effect? Is it clinically important? How precise is the treatment effect?* The effects of treatment are measured using one or more outcome measures. They can be **dichotomous** (yes/no; alive/dead; pregnant/not pregnant) or **continuous** (weight, adjustment score, blood pressure, self-esteem). Different statistical tests are used for different types of data. Often statistical test results are reported as *p* **values**. The convention is that any *p* value less than 0.05 is considered statistically significant and means that the intervention has an effect on the outcome. More information may be gained about the extent of that difference by the use of other statistical tests, such as **relative risk reduction (RRR)** and **absolute risk reduction (ARR)**.

The RRR is the proportional reduction in rates of poor outcomes (e.g., death or readmission) between the experimental (better outcomes) and control (greater poor outcomes) participants. For example, an RRR of 50% means that there were 50% fewer deaths in the experimental group compared with the control group.

$$RRR = \frac{\text{Event rate in control group} - \text{Event rate in experimental group}}{\text{Event rate in the control group}}$$

---

## QUESTIONS USED TO CRITICALLY APPRAISE INTERVENTION STUDIES (TREATMENT OR PREVENTION)

1. **Are the Results of This Study Valid?**
   a. Was the assignment of participants to treatment groups randomized, and was the randomization concealed?
   b. Was follow-up sufficiently long and complete?
   c. Were participants analyzed in the groups to which they were assigned?
   d. Were participants, clinicians, outcome assessors, and data analysts unaware of (blinded to or masked from) participant allocation?
   e. Were participants in each group treated equally except for the intervention being evaluated?
   f. Were the groups similar at the start of the trial?

2. **What Were the Results?**
   a. How large is the effect? Is it clinically important?
   b. How precise is the treatment effect?

3. **Will the Results Help Me in Caring for My Clients?**
   a. Are my clients so different from those in the study that the results do not apply?
   b. Is the treatment feasible in our setting?
   c. Were all the clinically important outcomes (harms as well as benefits) considered?
   d. What are my clients' or community's values and preferences for both the outcomes we are trying to prevent and the side effects that may arise?

*Source:* Adapted from Cullum, N. (2001). Evaluation of studies of treatment or prevention interventions, part 2: Applying the results of studies to your patients. *Evidence-Based Nursing, 4*(1), 7–8. Reproduced with permission of the BMJ Publishing Group Ltd.

**Relative risk (RR)** is the proportion of participants experiencing an outcome in the intervention group divided by the proportion experiencing the outcome in the control group. However, RR does not take into account the number of people in the study who would have died anyway without the intervention. This is called the absolute risk reduction (ARR). For example, an ARR of 2% means that there were 2% fewer deaths in the experimental group than the control group.

$$ARR =$$
Event rate in control group – Event rate in experimental group

Yet another approach is to report the **number needed to treat (NNT)**. This describes the number of people who must be treated with the intervention in order to prevent one additional negative outcome (e.g., death) or promote one additional positive outcome (e.g., smoking cessation).

$$NNT = \frac{1}{ARR}$$

When researchers report statistical significance, it is imperative to ask if this is **clinically important** or meaningful. It is quite possible for results to be statistically significant but clinically unimportant. In a hypothetical example studying weight-loss interventions for obese women, the group with a more-intensive intervention lost a mean of five kilograms more than the group in the less-intensive intervention. Though the researchers found this statistically significant ($p = 0.03$), it was not personally meaningful to the morbidly obese women. Also, the researchers had predetermined that they would not consider weight loss to be clinically meaningful unless the participants reached 10% weight loss. Therefore, this five-kilogram weight loss was not a clinically meaningful result.

Precision of the results can never be absolute but is estimated by calculating **confidence intervals (CIs)** around the RRR or ARR. CIs are a range of values with a specified probability (usually 95%) of including the true effect, which can never be known absolutely. Wide CIs indicate less precision in the estimated effect of the intervention. There is no magic number of what constitutes wide or narrow CIs; that judgment takes exposure to many studies. Also, it involves being able to make the same clinical decision at the end of the confidence interval closest to no difference, as you would make from the overall results. Precision increases with larger sample sizes.

### Will the Results Help Me in Caring for My Clients?

■ Are my clients (individuals, families, communities, systems, or populations) so different from those in the study that the results do not apply?

■ Is the treatment feasible in our setting?

■ Were all the clinically important outcomes (harms as well as benefits) considered?

■ What are my clients' values and preferences for both the outcome we are trying to prevent and the side effects that may arise?

■ Are there implications of this study applicable at the broader policy level?

This set of questions is context dependent. That is, you as practitioner need an understanding of your client population needs and values, and an ability to value the benefits against the risks and costs to the client, population, and an agency. This is rarely a decision of an individual practitioner, and in community health it is more often an agency, government policy, or population-level decision.

In order to use the findings of a study, one needs to consider these questions and make judgments in relation to one's own client population. Consider how similar the characteristics of the study participants are to your own clients. Think about reasons why you should *not* apply the study results to your population, rather than looking for evidence that the clients are exactly the same as yours. Feasibility in your setting depends on factors such as cost, organizational resources, nursing skills, availability of special equipment, and acceptability to clients. Harms and benefits should be included in the reports by including various obvious outcomes such as health impacts but also other outcomes like quality of life and economics. In particular, negative effects or side effects should be included.

## Critical Appraisal of Systematic Reviews

A systematic review is a summary of research evidence that relates to a specific question. It could involve causation, diagnosis, or prognosis but more frequently involves effectiveness of an intervention. The terms "systematic review" and "overview" are often used interchangeably. Basing a practice decision on a single study may be a mistake, as the study may have an inadequate sample size to detect clinically important differences between treatments, leading to a false negative conclusion. Discrepant findings across studies of the same question may occur due to chance or subtle differences in study design or participants. Therefore, it is useful to look at a summary of all the research related to a single clinical question.

In a narrative review, authors may selectively pick articles that support their viewpoint and ignore those that do not, so that the conclusion is set before the articles are selected. Systematic reviews differ from an unsystematic narrative review in that they attempt to overcome possible biases by following a rigorous methodology of search, retrieval, relevance and validity (quality) rating, data extraction, synthesis, and report writing. Explicit pre-set criteria are used for relevance and validity. Two people conduct each stage independently and then compare results and discuss discrepancies before moving on to the next stage. Details of the methods used at every stage are recorded.

A meta-analysis is a type of systematic review in which the quantitative results of several studies are combined to get an overall summary statistic that represents the combined effect of the intervention across different study populations. The reviewers must decide whether the statistical combination (meta-analysis) is appropriate by using both clinical judgment and a statistical test for heterogeneity. The clinical judgment requires the reviewers to examine the methodologies and statistical tests completed in the studies under review and ascertain if it is reasonable to combine them in a meta-analysis. The statistical tests determine the extent to which the differences between results of individual studies are greater than one would expect if all studies were measuring the same underlying effect and the observed differences were due only to chance. The more significant the test of heterogeneity, the less likely that the observed differences are from chance alone and that some other factor, such as design, participants, intervention, or outcome, is responsible for the differences in the treatment effect across studies (Sackett et al., 2000). Readers must use their own expertise to decide whether the statistical combination is reasonable in terms of clinical and methodological sense. Systematic reviews help to answer clinical questions without having to access large numbers of research reports; they overcome the obstacles of lack of time and, sometimes, lack of skills necessary to conduct the critical appraisal. But can one be confident in using all reviews? A search may easily yield more than 200 reviews—are they all of equal value? What does one do if they give conflicting results?

Common misconceptions of systematic reviews are that many readers think they include *only* randomized trials, that they must adopt a biomedical model, and that they have to have some statistical synthesis (Petticrew, 2001). If these were true, there would be few reviews of interest in community health, as many community health questions have not been or cannot be addressed by randomized trials. Fortunately, review methods are improving to include non-randomized studies, such as cohort studies; to use a population health model; and to synthesize without necessarily including meta-analysis. The Cochrane Public Health Group (http://ph.cochrane.org) has been a leader in promoting the methods, conduct, and use of systematic reviews and meta-analyses in community healthcare. Many websites contain high-quality systematic reviews relevant to community health and resources for skill building in critical appraisal of reviews. (See MyNursingLab for additional resources.)

In this section, we look at how to critically appraise systematic reviews to decide if the methods have sufficient rigour that the results may be applied to client or management decisions. The same major questions used for evaluation of intervention studies can be used to evaluate systematic reviews (see the box "Questions Used to Critically Appraise Systematic Review Articles"). For an example of application, see Case Study A in MyNursingLab.

**Are the Results Valid?** *Is this a systematic review of randomized trials?* Questions about the effectiveness of treatment or prevention are best answered by randomized controlled trials if it is ethically possible to do so, whereas questions about harm or prognosis are best answered by cohort studies (Roberts & DiCenso, 1999). You should look to see if the authors used randomized trials (if ethically possible) or the next most rigorous design that included a comparison group (quasi-experimental or cohort analytic designs).

*Does the systematic review include a description of the strategies used to find all relevant studies?* Every systematic review grows from a focused question, through the development of the search

---

### QUESTIONS USED TO CRITICALLY APPRAISE SYSTEMATIC REVIEW ARTICLES

1. **Are the Results of This Systematic Review Valid?**
   a. Is this a systematic review of randomized trials?
   b. Does the systematic review include a description of the strategies used to find all the relevant articles?
   c. Does the systematic review include a description of how the validity of individual studies was assessed?
   d. Were the results consistent from study to study?

2. **What Were the Results?**
   a. How large was the treatment effect?
   b. How precise was the estimate of treatment effect?

3. **Will the Results Help Me in Caring for My Clients?**
   a. Are my clients so different from those in the study that the results do not apply?
   b. Is the treatment feasible in our setting?
   c. Were all the clinically important outcomes (harms as well as benefits) considered?
   d. What are my clients' values and preferences for both the outcomes we are trying to prevent and the side effects that may arise?

*Sources:* Adapted from Ciliska, D., Cullum, N., & Marks, S. (2001). Evaluation of systematic reviews of treatment or prevention interventions. *Evidence-Based Nursing, 4*(4), 100–104; Sackett, D. L., Strauss, S. E., Richardson, W. S., Rosenberg, W., & Haynes, R. B. (2000). *Evidence based medicine: How to practice and teach EBM.* London, England: Churchill Livingstone.

---

strategies and search terms for each database, to retrieval of studies. Explicit inclusion or exclusion criteria are predetermined, and the review should state that two people independently reviewed each article for inclusion. A thorough search for both published and unpublished studies should be done for a systematic review. The publication of research in a journal is more likely to occur in studies that have statistically significant results. Studies in which a new intervention is not found to be effective are frequently not published, a phenomenon known as publication bias. Systematic reviews that do not include unpublished studies may overestimate the effect of an intervention; that is, it will appear that the intervention is more effective than it really is. Therefore, in addition to searching through relevant databases such as CINAHL, MEDLINE, PsycINFO, ERIC, or Cochrane Library, researchers should hand-search relevant journals; review reference lists from retrieved articles; contact experts, authors, and relevant manufacturing companies; and review abstracts presented at relevant scientific meetings. For policy-related reviews it may be important that the authors have searched for unpublished studies, also known as "grey literature," such as an evaluation of local implementation of a policy conducted by a health region or authority. Unless the authors of the reviews tell us what they did to locate relevant studies, it is difficult to know if any were missed.

*Does the systematic review include a description of how the validity of individual studies was assessed?* A narrative review often reports on study findings without considering the methodological strengths of the studies. Differences in study quality often explain differences in results across studies, with those of poorer quality tending to overestimate the effectiveness of the interventions (Kunz & Oxman, 1998). Quality ratings are sometimes used in the analysis to compare outcomes across studies by study strength. Or, if there are many studies to consider, the authors may choose to apply a quality rating threshold for inclusion (i.e., include only high-quality studies) or give greater attention and weight to the stronger studies. This predefined quality checklist minimizes reviewer bias by helping to ensure that reviewers appraise each study consistently and thoroughly. Having two or more raters helps to reduce mistakes and bias and increases the reader's confidence in the systematic review. The quality rating tools usually include criteria such as those presented for evaluating interventions.

*Were the results consistent from study to study?* The reader would be most confident using the results of a review if the results were similar in all included studies; that is, showing the same direction of effect—all being positive, all negative, or all showing no effect. But what if the direction of effect differs across studies? Differences may be due to types of clients included; the timing, duration, and intensity of the intervention; the outcomes measured; and/or the ways in which the outcomes were measured. If there are differences in results, the reader may also consider if there are differences in the quality of the primary studies that could influence the effect estimates (as discussed earlier).

**What Were the Results?** *How large was the treatment effect? How precise was the estimate of treatment effect?* Comparing a simple count of studies that helped, harmed, or showed no difference in treatments would assume that all studies had equal validity, power of the sample size to detect a difference, and duration and intensity of interventions and follow-up. Meta-analysis, when appropriate, can assign different weights to individual studies so that those with greater precision or higher quality make a greater contribution to the summary statistic. Summary statistics usually used include **odds ratio (OR)**, relative risk (RR, defined earlier), and **weighted mean difference**. The odds ratio describes the likelihood of a participant in the experimental group having an event (e.g., pregnancy) divided by the likelihood of a participant in the control group having the event. In a study such as prevention of pregnancy, one would consider that an RR or OR of less than 1 represents a beneficial treatment. Weighted mean difference is the mean of the difference found between control and intervention groups across studies entered into a meta-analysis. Both OR and RR are used for dichotomous data (dead/alive, pregnant/not pregnant), while weighted mean difference is used for continuous data (blood pressure, blood glucose, stress measurement scale). (For more information on OR and RR, see Chapter 11.)

The precision of the results is estimated by calculating confidence intervals (CI, defined earlier) around the summary statistic. The CI is useful for decision making because we can

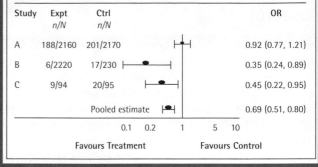

Each study is shown as a horizontal line with the OR for that study as the point on the line. The ends of the line show the 95% CIs. The numbers of participants are shown to the left of the line, and to the right are the numerical OR and 95% CIs. If a CI touches or crosses the vertical line of 1, that result is not statistically significant. The horizontal line just above the x-axis is the summary of the studies (the meta-analysis) that shows the combined impact of the intervention.

| Study | Expt n/N | Ctrl n/N | OR |
|-------|----------|----------|-----|
| A | 188/2160 | 201/2170 | 0.92 (0.77, 1.21) |
| B | 6/2220 | 17/230 | 0.35 (0.24, 0.89) |
| C | 9/94 | 20/95 | 0.45 (0.22, 0.95) |
| | Pooled estimate | | 0.69 (0.51, 0.80) |

0.1   0.2   1   5   10

Favours Treatment          Favours Control

**FIGURE 10.5** Example of Meta-Analysis Display

look at both extremes of the effect. If the lower extreme is 1 or close to it, the effect of the intervention is quite small and probably not worthwhile. A hypothetical display is shown in Figure 10.5 to demonstrate how output tables are read. The summary odds ratio of the three studies in Figure 10.5 is 0.69 (95% CI: 0.51–0.90), which indicates that the treatment was effective in producing the desired outcome.

### Will the Results Help Me in Caring for My Clients?

- Are my clients so different from those in the study that the study results do not apply?
- Is the treatment feasible in our setting?
- Were all the clinically important outcomes (harms as well as benefits) considered?
- What are my clients' values and preferences for both the outcome we are trying to prevent and the side effects that may arise?

As with the critique of individual studies, the questions listed above are all context dependent; that is, you need an understanding of your client population and their preferences, resources in your setting, and an ability to value the benefits against the risks and costs to the client, population, and agency. For example, feasibility in a school-based multifaceted sexual health program intervention would relate not only to the skills of the nurses and resources of the health department to complete such an intervention, but also to the ability of the school board to withstand the parental pressures for abstinence programs. In addition, researchers try to look for all outcomes of interventions, both positive and negative, that might affect the participants and the healthcare system. Outcomes might include mortality, morbidity, costs, quality of life, and participant satisfaction. Participant and family values must be considered. If, in the example above, families are unwilling to have their children exposed to multifaceted sexual health education programs, the students must be given an alternative during that school time.

Where possible, decisions should not be made on the basis of a single study. Systematic reviews allow for much more confidence in the research evidence. This is particularly important for consideration at the policy level.

## Critical Appraisal of Qualitative Research

**Qualitative research** is important for the development of nursing knowledge. Qualitative research describes, explores, and explains phenomena and is concerned with the process or experience rather than outcomes. Done for the purpose of obtaining rich data, sampling is purposive as opposed to the random or probability sampling in quantitative research. Data collection is done in many ways, but the most common are observation and group or individual interviews. Data analysis is completed using codes, themes, and patterns, not by statistical techniques, and it produces rich, deep descriptions rather than numbers. Qualitative research does not allow inference to a population as a whole, but allows the researcher to generalize to a theoretical understanding of the phenomena being studied (Grove et al., 2012).

Major types of qualitative research used in nursing include (a) phenomenology, (b) grounded theory, (c) **ethnography**, (d) case study, (e) qualitative description, and (f) PAR. The first three are the most common. Phenomenology seeks to describe the lived experiences of people (Creswell, 2012), such as the experience of people returning home after a stroke. Grounded theory generates theories or models of the phenomena being studied (Creswell, 2012), such as the development of a model of coping used by family caregivers of people who have HIV. Ethnography describes a culture (Creswell, 2012) and answers questions such as what it is like to be a pregnant teen trying to continue with school. Reading qualitative research deepens our understanding of the perceptions and actual experiences of people we work with and has the potential to enrich our interactions and care through a more complete understanding of their situation and experiences. When researchers want to explore a program, activity, or event in detail, they use case study design. This method involves multiple modes of in-depth data collection over a sustained period of time (Creswell, 2012). The purpose of qualitative descriptive studies is to provide a comprehensive summary of events in everyday terms. The methods of sampling, data collection, and analysis can vary, but researchers stay close to the data (Sandelowski, 2000). As stated earlier, action-oriented research questions and interventions that evolve through partnerships between researchers and participants are best dealt with through PAR (Grove et al., 2012).

The questions used to evaluate primary treatment studies or systematic reviews can be used to evaluate qualitative research (see the box titled "Questions Used to Critically Appraise Qualitative Research Reports"). For application of these criteria to Canadian studies, see Case Study B about a grounded theory study and Case Study C about participatory action study in MyNursingLab.

**Are the Findings Valid?** *Is the research question clear and adequately substantiated?* This question will determine whether the qualitative study will be read or not. The article should clearly establish the question and what is already known about the topic.

*Is the design appropriate for the research question?* On a grand level, it is important to determine that the authors used the appropriate method that fits the purpose of the study (e.g., that phenomenology is used to explore experience and meaning for clients following colostomy, rather than using an ethnographic approach). A more sophisticated appraisal considers the fit of the philosophical background of a particular perspective with the purpose of the study.

*Was the method of sampling appropriate for the research question?* The study should report on how participants were selected. Many different types of sampling are used in qualitative research, including theoretical sampling or purposeful sampling for maximum variation, typical cases, extreme cases, or critical cases.

*Were data collected and managed systematically?* The study should try to define the breadth (variation, multiple perspectives) and depth (numbers and types of data collected). Also, has each investigator kept track of the process—data collection, exploring hunches, decision making, and data analysis procedures—through the use of journaling and memos?

*Were the data analyzed appropriately?* The researcher should report on how the data were organized and reduced in order to identify patterns. Are there clear links between the data (e.g., the narrative and quotes) and the themes that were developed out of the data? Often the analysis identifies further areas for data collection and analysis. Usually, the researcher uses other team members to assist in the analysis, providing various interpretations of the data. Member checking (taking the results

---

### QUESTIONS USED TO CRITICALLY APPRAISE QUALITATIVE RESEARCH REPORTS

1. **Are the Findings Valid?**
   a. Is the research question clear and adequately substantiated?
   b. Is the design appropriate for the research question?
   c. Was the method of sampling appropriate for the research question?
   d. Were data collected and managed systematically?
   e. Were the data analyzed appropriately?

2. **What Were the Findings?**
   a. Is the description of findings thorough?

3. **Will the Results Help Me in Caring for My Clients?**
   a. What meaning and relevance does the study have for my practice?
   b. Does the study help me understand the context of my practice?
   c. Does the study enhance my knowledge about my practice?

*Source:* Adapted from Russell, C. K., & Gregory, D. M. (2003). Evaluation of qualitative research studies. *Evidence-Based Nursing, 6*(2), 36–40. Reproduced with permission of the BMJ Publishing Group.

back to the participants or people associated with the issue under study) is often done to validate the findings, assess for resonance of findings with participant experience, and gather alternative interpretations of the analysis.

**What Were the Findings?**  *Is the description of findings thorough?* Qualitative research is difficult to write within the word limit of standard journals. It is difficult to fit the rich description of results and analysis into one publication. It is expected that authors have used direct quotations of the participants to illustrate the descriptions and conceptualizations.

### Will the Results Help Me in Caring for My Clients?

■ What meaning and relevance does the study have for my practice?

■ Does the study help me understand the context of my practice?

■ Does the study enhance my knowledge about my practice?

As with the other critical appraisal tools, this final section has to be contextualized to the specifics of the population, the agency, and the individual practitioners. The authors should establish the need for and relevance of the research while arguing why they conducted the research and discussing the results. Readers must use their critique of the study as well as the information presented in the report to decide if any parts of the research findings are potentially transferable to their own practice and policy decisions at the local, provincial, or national level.

## 4. Synthesize

The synthesis stage requires that you (a) consider the evidence found, (b) determine how to deal with conflicting results in different studies, and (c) identify which evidence you will use for decision making. The first criteria for deciding which evidence to use would be to use the study that you have appraised to be of highest quality. The second criteria would be the date

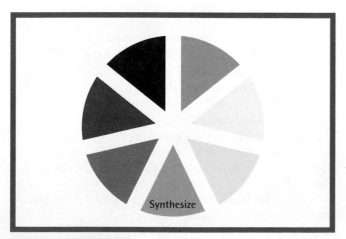

**FIGURE** **10.6** **Synthesize**

*Source:* Adapted with permission from *A model of evidence-informed decision making in public health* (2012), a fact sheet created by and available from the National Collaborating Centre for Methods and Tools.

of publication; particularly for systematic reviews, you would want a review that was been done within the past two years (otherwise the studies are old). Alternatively, for an older review, you can replicate the search and find studies that have come out since the search in that review ended. If there are conflicting results from reviews or individual studies of equal quality, then your third criteria to apply would be to consider relevance to your population, and lastly, the resources required to implement the intervention.

Each case study in MyNursingLab shows high-quality evidence around the clinical scenario and practice question. We encourage you to study them carefully. In community health nursing, many decisions to implement a change in practice or policy are beyond the individual; they are decided by a team. In every case, the decision involves all of the five aspects of Figure 10.1: the research evidence, community health issues and local context, community and political preferences and actions, public health resources, and public health expertise. Furthermore, if the decision goes beyond individual clients or small groups, political and organizational elements become involved. This is particularly evident in the final decision of the example of an intervention around school-based sexual health education. The students, parents, and high school would all have to be involved in the decision if there is any chance for a school-based intervention for sexual health to be successful.

What does one do if no research evidence is found during the database search? Or if the research that comes up is of consistently poor quality? In those cases, expert opinion or usual practice is the standard for decision making. One may be able to find practice guidelines on the topic. These depend on a thorough literature review and then consensus meetings with expert panels in order to make practice decisions, particularly where research evidence does not exist (Registered Nurses' Association of Ontario, 2010; U.S. Department of Health and Human Services, Agency for Healthcare Research and Quality, 2010). Similarly, "best practice" documents describe programs or interventions that seem to be effective but may not yet have been rigorously evaluated.

Caution must be exercised when implementing interventions for which there is no good evaluation. Rationale for decisions needs to be documented. CHNs must be particularly vigilant in observing for effects, both positive and negative, then ensuring that they are documented. Unfortunately, many effects are not evident until years after the intervention when no one is observing any longer! Areas of clinical interest where evaluation does not exist are prime research questions that should receive priority attention from funding agencies.

## 5. Adapt

Once your team makes a decision on the research evidence to use, you have to consider all the population and political factors involved in making a program or policy decision. A tool was developed, based on a literature review, that helps you to consider a multitude of factors, in addition to the research results. It is called the *Applicability and Transferability Tool*, by Buffett, Ciliska, and Thomas (2011), and may be found at www.nccmt.ca/pubs/A&Trevised-startEN.pdf. In the decision-making process, the tool prompts team members to

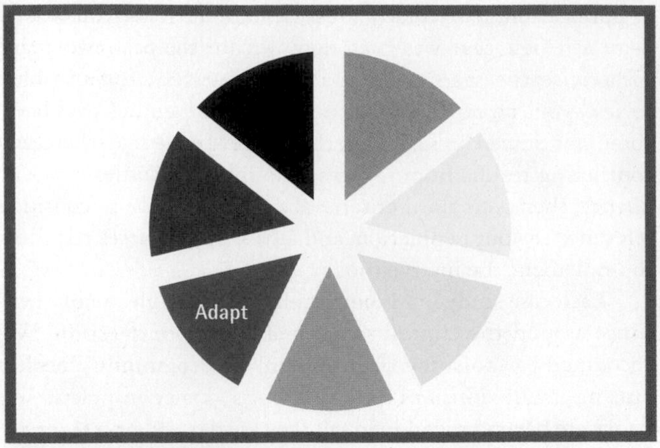

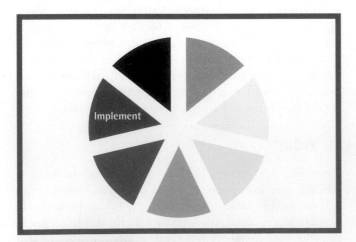

FIGURE 10.7 Adapt

*Source:* Adapted with permission from *A model of evidence-informed decision making in public health* (2012), a fact sheet created by and available from the National Collaborating Centre for Methods and Tools.

think about how the intervention needs to be adapted to the local population. Factors that need to be considered include the magnitude of the issue in your population, the social acceptability of the program or policy you are considering implementing, the political acceptability of your intervention, and the ability to garner resources for the program or policy you have chosen to implement.

## 6. Implement

Once a decision to change practice and organizational support is achieved, a comprehensive plan has to address how the others who work within the organization will be informed of the proposed change. Changing the practice of healthcare professionals has been studied extensively with mixed and unclear results. The "Effective Practice and Organization of Care" review group (www.epoc.cochrane.org/en/index.html) within the Cochrane

FIGURE 10.8 Implement

*Source:* Adapted with permission from *A model of evidence-informed decision making in public health* (2012), a fact sheet created by and available from the National Collaborating Centre for Methods and Tools.

Collaboration conducts systematic reviews of educational, behavioural, organizational, financial, and regulatory interventions related to changing the practice of healthcare professionals or the organization of healthcare. One review studied strategies for guideline dissemination and implementation (Grimshaw et al., 2004). This review included 235 studies of 309 comparisons. They found that the median absolute improvements in performance across interventions was 14.1% in comparisons of reminders, 8.1% in comparisons of dissemination of educational materials, 7.0% in comparisons of audit and feedback, and 6.0% in comparisons of multifaceted interventions involving educational outreach. This is somewhat surprising, as you might expect that there would be enhanced performance improvements with multiple interventions.

It is recommended that a "diagnostic analysis" be done to identify factors likely to help and hinder the proposed change (University of York, NHS Centre for Reviews and Dissemination, 1999). For example, opinion leaders have been shown to be effective in some studies with physicians, but not other studies (University of York, NHS Centre for Reviews and Dissemination, 1999), and they were not successful as an intervention with nurses (Hodnett et al., 1996). Thus, evidence of the use of opinion leaders as a strategy of change has been inconclusive (Flodgren et al., 2011).

The diagnostic analysis (environmental scan) must consider barriers and supports in relation to the characteristics of the innovation (the change being introduced), the client (individual, families, communities, systems, or populations), the practitioners, the organization, and the environment so that barriers can be reduced and supports strengthened. It is important to consider characteristics of the innovation, such as the resources it will require (will it cost more or actually be time/resource saving?) and how different it is from current practice. Relevant characteristics of individual practitioners include such issues as level of education, years of experience, and general acceptance or resistance to change. Organizational characteristics include affiliation with an academic setting, size, level of care, funding sources, organizational structure, research participation, research orientation, and usual valuing of research findings. The environment includes factors such as rural or urban setting, economic status of the community, and health issues valued by the community (Dobbins, Ciliska, Cockerill, Barnsley, & DiCenso, 2002). Few studies have formally evaluated organizational change (Flodgren, Rojas-Reyes, Cole, & Foxcroft, 2012; Parmelli et al., 2011).

Important stakeholders must be identified. They may include the nurses, medical staff, clients, and accounting staff. Each group should attend a different meeting to hear a tailored message about the proposed change, rationale, and timelines. The goal of each meeting is to get support for the practice change from each stakeholder group. A champion may be needed with the enthusiasm and energy to push for this practice change. Identifying opinion leaders and influencing their understanding and attitudes about the proposed practice change is another strategy worth pursuing, despite the inconclusiveness (mentioned above) that this strategy is effective. Interventions to promote dissemination, uptake, and utilization of research results is an area that requires further focused research in order to complete the cycle of evidence-based practice, from question identification to implementation and evaluation.

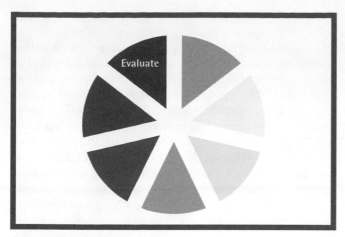

**FIGURE 10.9** Evaluate

*Source:* Adapted with permission from *A model of evidence-informed decision making in public health* (2012), a fact sheet created by and available from the National Collaborating Centre for Methods and Tools.

## 7. Evaluate

After implementing a practice or policy change, an evaluation period is needed to see if it is working for both providers and clients. This does not mean replicating the original study that was used as a basis for the practice change. It does, however, mean a period of data collection to ensure that the desired outcomes are similar to the rates of those in the original study and to assess participation rates to understand client (individual, family, community, system, or population) acceptability. It is also significant to note if any potential negative outcomes are similar to those listed in the study. Finally, it is important to let others who work with similar populations know about what you did and how it worked. This dissemination can be done through formal mechanisms (e.g., conference presentations and papers, educational meetings), or informally through dialogue within networks and online forums.

## USING RESEARCH FOR MANAGEMENT DECISIONS AND POLICY DEVELOPMENT

While research evidence is useful for individual practitioners working with individual clients, it is also important that management decisions be evidence based. Decisions regarding the implementation of a new intensive intervention in a community are usually made where there is no additional funding coming to an agency for the new program. Therefore, if the organization wishes to begin such a program, it needs to find the resources within what currently exists. This may mean taking staff away from some other programs or activities to dedicate their time to the new initiative. Reviewing the research evidence for both the proposed activity and any existing programs helps managers to make those decisions. For example, following a string of four adolescent suicides, one school requested that the health department offer suicide prevention interventions at the school the following fall. During the

summer, the health department conducted a systematic review of the effectiveness of school-based suicide prevention programs for teens. They found that the available research was of poor quality and no evidence supported the decision to implement the suicide prevention programs; furthermore, some studies indicated that there was harm to adolescent males who experienced such a program in that they were more likely to engage in negative coping behaviours and to commit suicide (Ploeg et al., 1996). The management team, therefore, decided to present this information to the school and to offer instead a comprehensive "healthy school" initiative, which would also be evaluated.

The actual conduct (as opposed to the search and discovery) of systematic reviews has contributed to their use by clinicians and policy-level decision makers. From the chapter authors' experiences with the Effective Public Health Practice Project (www.ephpp.ca), potential review questions are sought from the policy, management, and front-line clinician perspectives. The groups that conducted the reviews included the methodological experts along with the community practitioners who were chosen for their content expertise and their understanding of the context, and relevance to community health. They assisted in identifying and refining the priority questions, rating articles

---

### CANADIAN RESEARCH BOX 10.2

**How can PAR change participation in cervical cancer screening by Aboriginal women?**

Maar, M., Burchell, A., Little, J., Ogilvie, G., Severini, A., Yang, J. M., & Zehbe, I. (2013). A qualitative study of provider perspectives of structural barriers to cervical cancer screening among First Nations women. *Women's Health Issues, 23*(5), e319–e325. doi:10.1016/j.whi.2013.06.005

In 11 First Nations communities in rural Ontario, the researchers studied factors that influence participation in cervical cancer screening by Aboriginal women using a PAR method, as is consistent with Canadian guidelines for research with Aboriginal people. Health and social services providers, many of whom were First Nations women, participated in in-depth interviews to explore community attitudes about cancer, cervical screening, and both barriers and facilitators to screening. Participants identified a shortage of appropriately trained healthcare providers; a lack of recall system; lack of transportation, education, and socioeconomic inequalities; generational effects; and a colonial legacy as barriers to cervical cancer screening. Practitioners felt that strategies to increase cervical cancer screening rates in Aboriginal communities need to go beyond individual level educational and behavioural approaches to remove structural barriers to participation.

#### Discussion Questions

1. As a nurse working in a primary health care centre with Aboriginal women, how would you use this information in practice? What value can it add to your work?

2. What components would you argue should be a part of your cancer screening program?

3. What policies would you consider implementing?

## CASE STUDY

### Critical Appraisal of an Intervention Study

Ratner, P. A., Johnson, J. L., Richardson, C. G., Bottorff, J. L., Moffat, B., Mackay, M., Fofonoff, D., Kingsbury, K., Miller, C., . . . & Budz, B. (2004). Efficacy of a smoking-cessation intervention for elective-surgical patients. *Research in Nursing and Health, 27*(3), 148–61.

*Scenario:* You community has higher-than-provincial rates of smoking. Smoking prevention and cessation is a population priority set by a joint committee of local citizens and the health authority. Your local hospital has contacted your community health agency to see if there could be any assistance for setting up a smoking cessation program for people scheduled to undergo elective surgery. Your agency is happy to partner on this initiative, and you volunteer to help the hospital team consider the program options. At your first meeting, you ask if there is any research on the topic. Since no one remembers seeing any such literature, they ask you to do a search and report back at the next meeting. You decide to try the search skills you learned at a recent seminar, which should allow you to find high-quality primary studies in a short time. You go to PubMed (www.pubmed.gov), and click "Clinical Queries" on the left side, under "PubMed Services." A screen comes up that allows you to search by "Clinical Study Category," "Systematic Reviews," or "Medical Genetics." You first try Find Systematic Reviews and enter the words "smoking cessation pre-surgical." There are no articles, so you repeat under Clinical Study Category using the category of "therapy." Three articles come up—one is a trial by Ratner and colleagues on the efficacy of smoking cessation for elective surgical patients (2004). You retrieve the full document.

In the article you retrieved by Ratner et al., the procedure section reports that the participants were randomized to receive either usual care or the smoking-cessation intervention. After recruitment, the study personnel opened a sealed envelope containing a computer-generated, randomly determined group allocation. Thus, participants were randomized, but we are not sure that allocation was concealed (by opaque envelopes) from personnel prior to recruitment. The intervention consisted of specially trained nurses who did three aspects of the intervention. The first was a 15-minute face-to-face counselling session in the pre-assessment clinic (1–3 weeks before surgery), followed by a review of progress in hospital within 24 hours after surgery, then telephone counselling starting about one week after the in-hospital session, which continued weekly for one month and then biweekly for the second and third months. All encounters built on advice to stop smoking at least 24 hours before surgery, skill building and strategies to quit smoking, and a telephone hotline number.

The control group received "usual care" in which participants were managed by the usual pre- and postoperative teaching, which may have included discussion about smoking cessation although there was no formal protocol to do so.

Of the 418 people who met eligibility criteria, 57% agreed to participate. Though this is not as high as you would normally like for most interventions, you realize that it is probably a good participation rate for smokers. Follow-up lasted for one year, probably a reasonable length of time to assess an intervention like this for smoking cessation. Follow-up at one year was 71.3%; again this is less than you would hope to see, yet higher than follow-up for many smoking cessation studies. Intention-to-treat analysis was done. Outcome assessors were blinded; participants and clinicians were not, and could not be in an intervention like this. There were no differences between the two groups in demographic or smoking-related characteristics at baseline.

Smoking abstinence for at least 24 hours before surgery and 6- and 12-month abstinence rates were the primary outcomes. For presurgery, 73% of those in the intervention group abstained before surgery compared with 53% in the control group. This was statistically significant ($p < 0.003$). In fact, the control group was more likely to increase the amount smoked before surgery (25.4% versus 9.9% in the control group, $p < 0.004$). At 6 months and 12 months, the authors used intention-to-treat analysis, attributing positive smoking status to participants lost to follow-up. In that analysis, there were no significant differences in smoking status at either measurement time. For example, the odds ratio for abstinence in the intervention group at 12 months was 0.92 (95% CIs 0.47 to 1.78). The odds ratio is close to 1, indicating little difference in rates between the two groups, and also the confidence interval crosses 1, indicating no statistical significance.

If the effect had been significant over time, the last area of the critique is to see if the article described the participants in enough detail to see if they might be similar to the population of interest. In this case, Ratner et al. gave details about the type of surgery and demographics. You could probably make a judgment about applicability to your population based on their description. You take this critique to the next committee meeting, and together you decide to explore other smoking-cessation programs, as pre-surgical abstinence is probably not enough to justify the expense of the program. You go back to the search phase!

### Discussion Questions

1. Will you present this study to your committee next meeting? Should this study inform your program?

2. Let's say on your next search, you found several other interventions that had statistically significant findings at one-year follow-up. How would you use the research to argue for resources to be reallocated from the hospital pre-op programs and directed to a smoking cessation intervention described? Role play that you are the nurse and your classmates are the committee to whom you are reporting.

3. When it is difficult or impossible to randomize people (e.g., when a media or city/community-wide intervention is to be done), what is the next most rigorous design after a randomized controlled trial?

for relevance to the question, reviewing drafts, and helping to write clinical, management, and policy implications. This process has also been used in Alberta by the Alberta Heritage Foundation for Medical Research. Similarly, people working at institutional or government policy levels are increasingly aware of and value the need for research evidence, yet they face other competing factors (e.g., public opinion and pressures, fiscal restraints) when making policy decisions.

## Participating in Community Health Research

CHNs are involved in many different types of research, the most common being program evaluation using process outcomes such as numbers of clients, numbers of groups, hours spent, and reasons for home visits. These types of data are important for tracking uses of services and how resources are spent within the agency. Client outcome measurement is the next most likely information collected; for example, client mortality, morbidity, immunization status or coverage, communicable disease outbreak, goals met, or adolescent pregnancies after a school program. CHNs are usually asked to log these data, at least in formal records. They also may be required to report it in other formats, or the agency may conduct periodic chart reviews or database summaries. These local data often feed into provincial and national databases and registries of statistics. Some of these databases are available to regions within the provinces so that local rates can be followed.

## CONCLUSION

In this chapter, we reviewed evidence-informed practice as it relates to community health nursing. While evidence can be observations made by the nurse, expert "gut hunches," or advice of colleagues, we too often ignore the evidence from research (Estabrooks et al., 2005). Therefore, this chapter focused on research evidence—finding, critiquing, and using it. Particular detail was presented in relation to critical appraisal of research articles on effectiveness questions (primary studies or systematic reviews) or qualitative research to judge whether they should be utilized in practice, management, or policy decisions. The process of using quality research evidence does not end with the critical appraisal and individual decisions to implement with clients. In community health nursing, evidence-informed practice more often involves getting organizational "buy-in" and changing policies and procedures or interventions. We presented information about understanding the barriers to utilizing research to change community health nursing practice, management practice, and policy making.

Research, in the form of process evaluation, currently takes place daily in every community organization in Canada. Therefore, CHNs have many opportunities to become involved in research. Further, as the valuing of research evidence increases in community health nursing, the critical attitude to practice will increase so that healthcare professionals will more frequently ask relevant practice questions. Since there is not a research-based answer for every practice question within community health, the need to conduct research in community health will continue. CHNs will find they are asked to participate in research by collecting data, providing interventions, or developing research proposals.

## KEY TERMS

absolute risk reduction (ARR)   p. 190
bias  p. 189
clinical questions   p. 187
clinically important   p. 191
cohort design   p. 188
confidence intervals (CIs)   p. 191
continuous   p. 190
critical appraisal skills   p. 188
dichotomous   p. 190
effectiveness   p. 184
ethnography   p. 194
evidence-based nursing (EBN)   p. 185
evidence-informed practice   p. 185
grounded theory   p. 188
intention-to-treat analysis   p. 189
intervention studies   p. 187
interventions   p. 184
meta-analysis   p. 186
mixed methods research   p. 188
number needed to treat (NNT)   p. 191
observational studies   p. 187
odds ratio (OR)   p. 193
outcomes   p. 186
participatory action research (PAR)   p. 188
phenomenology   p. 188
*p* values   p. 190
qualitative research   p. 194
randomized controlled trials   p. 187
relative risk (RR)   p. 191
relative risk reduction (RRR)   p. 190
situation   p. 186
systematic reviews   p. 187
weighted mean difference   p. 193

## STUDY QUESTIONS

1. Identify four factors to consider for evidence-informed decision making.

2. What attitude provides the basis for the EIDM to begin?

3. In what ways might you conduct research as part of your daily role in community health nursing?

4. Why would you seek out systematic reviews to answer clinical questions?

5. Name the four major categories of factors to consider when planning to implement a clinical practice or policy change. Give a few examples under each category.

6. Give examples of client-related questions that would most appropriately be answered by phenomenology, grounded theory, and ethnography.

After working through these questions, go to the MyNursingLab at www.pearsoned.ca/mynursinglab to check your answers.

## INDIVIDUAL CRITICAL-THINKING EXERCISES

1. Pick an intervention that has been shown to be effective and discuss how you would plan to implement that practice change in a nursing agency. What factors would you assess? What processes would you use?

2. Answer the following using Figure 10.5.
   a. How many studies were involved in this meta-analysis?
   b. Which of those studies had statistically significant findings?
   c. How would you interpret the result? Is the intervention effective? Is it statistically significant? Is it precise?

3. In a randomized trial about physical activity for obese middle-aged women, the intervention group (diet and exercise) lost 2.4% of their original weight, versus the control group who lost 1% of their original weight. This was statistically significant (p 0.05). Is this a clinically important outcome? Would you use this study to advocate for diet and exercise for weight loss?

4. In a study of an intervention to increase school students' use of helmets when in-line skating, the intervention consisted of an in-school educational video plus free helmets, versus the video alone. The odds ratio for observed helmet use was 3.85 in favour of the video plus free helmets (CI 3.05 to 4.11). Was this a statistically significant result? Put the results into words using the odds ratio.

## GROUP CRITICAL-THINKING EXERCISES

1. Select an article that evaluates an intervention relevant to community health nursing. Use the criteria in the first text box titled "Questions Used to Critically Appraise Intervention Studies (Treatment or Prevention)" to critically appraise the article and come to a decision about using the intervention in your own practice.

2. As in question 1, critically appraise a systematic review article using the criteria in the second text box titled "Questions Used to Critically Appraise Systematic Review Articles."

3. As in question 1, critically appraise an article on qualitative research using the criteria in the third text box titled "Questions Used to Critically Appraise Qualitative Research Reports." If it is a valid study, discuss what the study findings contribute to your understanding of the issue that was explored.

## REFERENCES

Alspach, G. (2006). Nurses' use and understanding of evidence-based practice: Some preliminary evidence. *Critical Care Nurse, 26*(6), 11–12.

Buffet, C., Ciliska, D., & Thomas, H. (2011). *It worked there. Will it work here? Tool for assessing applicability and transferability of evidence (A: When considering starting a new program)*. Hamilton, ON: National Collaborating Centre for Methods and Tools.

Canadian Health Services Research Foundation. (2004). *What counts? Interpreting evidence-based decision-making for management and policy*. Report of the 6th CHSRF Annual Invitational Workshop. Ottawa, ON: Author. Retrieved from http://www.cfhi-fcass.ca/migrated/pdf/event_reports/2004_workshop_report_e.pdf

Ciliska, D., Cullum, N., & Marks, S. (2001). Evaluation of systematic reviews of treatment or prevention interventions. *Evidence-Based Nursing, 4*(4), 100–104.

Ciliska, D., Thomas, H., & Buffett, C. (2008). *A compendium of critical appraisal tools for public health practice*. Hamilton, ON: National Collaborating Centre for Methods and Tools. Retrieved from http://www.nccmt.ca/tools/index-eng.html

Community Health Nurses of Canada. (2011, revised). *Canadian community health nursing: Professional practice model & standards of practice*. St. John's, NL: Author. Retrieved from https://www.chnc.ca/documents/CHNC-ProfessionalPracticeModel-EN/index.html

Creswell, J. W. (2012). *Qualitative inquiry and research design: Choosing among five approaches*. Thousand Oaks, CA: Sage Publications.

Dennis, C. L., Hodnett, E., & Reisman, H. M. (2009). Effect of peer support on prevention of postnatal depression among high risk women: Multisite randomized controlled trial. *British Medical Journal, 338*, a3064.

Dobbins, M., Ciliska, D., Cockerill, R., Barnsley, J., & DiCenso, A. (2002). A framework for the dissemination and utilization of research for health care policy and practice. *Online Journal of Knowledge Synthesis in Nursing, 9*(7), 149–160. doi:10.1111/j.1524-475X.2002.00149.x

Dobbins, M., Davies, B., Danseco, E., Edwards, N., & Virani, T. (2005). Changing nursing practice: Evaluating the usefulness of a best-practice guideline implementation toolkit. *Nursing Leadership, 18*(1), 34–45.

Dobbins, M., Husson, H., DeCorby, K., & LaRocca, R. L. (2013). School-based physical activity programs for promoting physical activity and fitness in children and adolescents aged 6 to 18. *Cochrane Database of Systematic Reviews, 2*. Art. No.: CD007651. doi:10.1002/14651858.CD007651.pub2

Estabrooks, C. A., Chong, H., Brigidear, K., & Profetto-McGrath, J. (2005). Profiling Canadian nurses' preferred knowledge sources for clinical practice. *Canadian Journal of Nursing Research, 37*(2), 118–40.

Flemming, K. (1998). Asking answerable questions. *Evidence-Based Nursing, 1*, 36–37.

Farmer, A. P., Légaré, F., Turcot, L., Grimshaw, J., Harvey, E., McGowan, J. L., & Wolf, F. (2008). Printed educational materials: Effect on professional practice and health care outcomes. *Cochrane Database Systematic Reviews, 16*(3), Art. No.: CD004398.

Flodgren, G., Parmelli, E., Doumit, G., Gattellari, M., O'Brien, M. A, Grimshaw, J., & Eccles M. P. (2011). Local opinion leaders: Effects on professional practice and health care outcomes. *Cochrane Database of Systematic Reviews, 8*. Art. No.: CD000125. doi:10.1002/14651858. CD000125.pub4.

Flodgren, G., Rojas-Reyes, M. X., Cole, N., & Foxcroft, D. R. (2012). Effectiveness of organisational infrastructures to promote evidence-based nursing practice. *Cochrane Database of Systematic Reviews, 2.* Art. No.: CD002212. doi:10.1002/14651858.CD002212.pub2

Graham, I. D., Logan, J., Harrison, M. B., Straus, S. E., Tetroe, J., Caswell, W., & Robinson, N. (2006). Lost in knowledge translation: Time for a map? *Journal of Continuing Education in the Health Professions, 26*(1) 13–24.

Grimshaw, J. M., Thomas, R. E., MacLennan, G., Fraser, C., Ramsay, C. R., Vale, L., . . . Donaldson, C. (2004). Effectiveness and efficiency of guideline dissemination and implementation strategies. *Health Technology Assessment, 8*(6), 1–72. doi:10.3310/hta8060

Grove, S. K., Burns, N., & Gray, J. (2012). *The practice of nursing research: Appraisal, synthesis and generation of evidence.* St. Louis, MO: Elsevier.

Heater, B. S., Becker, A. M., & Olson, R. (1988). Nursing interventions and patient outcomes. A meta-analysis of studies. *Nursing Research, 37*(5), 303–307.

Hodnett, E. D., Kaufman, K., O'Brien-Pallas, L., Chipman, M., Watson-MacDonell, J., & Hunsburger, W. (1996). A strategy to promote research-based nursing care: Effects on childbirth outcomes. *Research in Nursing and Health, 19*(1), 13–20.

Jadad, A. R., & Haynes, R. B. (1998). The Cochrane collaboration: Advances and challenges in improving evidence-based decision making. *Medical Decision Making, 18*(1), 2–9.

Kunz, R., & Oxman, A. (1998). The unpredictability paradox: Review of empirical comparisons of randomized and non-randomized clinical trials. *BMJ, 317,* 1185–1190.

Lomas, J. (1991). Words without action? The production, dissemination, and impact of consensus recommendations. *Annual Review of Public Health, 12*(1), 41–65.

Melnyk, B., Fineout-Overholt, E., Feinstein, N. F., Li, H., Small, L., Wilcox, L., & Kraus, R. (2004). Nurses perceived knowledge, beliefs, skills, and needs regarding evidence-based practice: Implications for accelerating the paradigm shift. *Worldviews on Evidence-Based Nursing, 1*(3), 185–193.

Oxman, A., Guyatt, G., Cook, D., & Montori, V. (2002). Summarising the evidence. In G. Guyatt & D. Rennie (Eds.), *Users' guides to the medical literature: A manual for evidence-based clinical practice* (pp. 155–173). Chicago, IL: AMA Press.

Parmelli, E., Flodgren, G., Schaafsma, M. E., Baillie, N., Beyer, F. R., & Eccles, M. P. (2011). The effectiveness of strategies to change organisational culture to improve healthcare performance. *Cochrane Database of Systematic Reviews, 1.* Art. No.: CD008315. doi:10.1002/14651858.CD008315.pub2

Petticrew, M. (2001). Systematic reviews from astronomy to zoology: Myths and misconceptions. *BMJ, 322,* 98–101.

Ploeg, J., Ciliska, D., Dobbins, M., Hayward, S., & Thomas, H. A. (1996). Systematic overview of adolescent suicide prevention programs. *Canadian Journal of Public Health, 87,* 319–324.

Public Health Agency of Canada. (2008). *Core Competencies for Public Health. 1.0.* Ottawa, ON: Author. Retrieved from http://www.phac-aspc.gc.ca/ccph-cesp/index-eng.php

Ratner, P. A., Johnson, J. L., Richardson, C. G., Bottorff, J. L., Moffat, B., Mackay, M., . . . Budz, B. (2004). Efficacy of a smoking-cessation intervention for elective-surgical patients. *Research in Nursing and Health, 27*(3), 148–161.

Registered Nurses' Association of Ontario. (2010). *Best practice guidelines.* Toronto: ON: Author. Retrieved from www.rnao.org

Roberts, J., & DiCenso, A. (1999). Identifying the best research design to fit the question, part 1: Quantitative designs. *Evidence-Based Nursing, 2*(1), 4–6.

Sackett, D. L., Rosenberg, W., Gray, J. A. M., & Haynes, R. B. (1996). Evidence-based medicine: What it is and what it isn't. *British Medical Journal, 312*(7050), 71–72.

Sackett, D. L., Strauss, S. E., Richardson, W. S., Rosenberg, W., & Haynes, R. B. (2000). *Evidence based medicine: How to practice and teach EBM.* London, England: Churchill Livingstone.

Sandelowski, M. (2000). Whatever happened to qualitative description? *Research in Nursing & Health, 23,* 334–340.

Singer, G. H. S., Ethridge, B. L., & Aldana, S. I. (2007). Primary and secondary effects of parenting and stress management interventions for parents of children with developmental disabilities: A meta-analysis. *Mental Retardation and Developmental Disabilities Research Reviews, 13,* 357–369. doi:10.1002/mrdd

Squires, J. E., Moralejo, D., & LeFort, S. M. (2007). Exploring the role of organizational policies and procedures in promoting research utilization in registered nurses. *Implementation Science, 2*(1), 17.

University of York, NHS Centre for Reviews and Dissemination. (1999). Getting evidence into practice. *Effective Health Care, 5*(1). Retrieved from http://www.york.ac.uk/media/crd/ehc51.pdf

U.S. Department of Health and Human Services, Agency for Healthcare Research and Quality. (2010). *National guideline clearinghouse.* Retrieved from www.ahrq.gov

Utterback, J. M. (1974). Innovation in industry and the diffusion of technology. *Science, 183*(4125), 620–626.

## ABOUT THE AUTHORS

**Rebecca Ganann**, RN, MSc, is an Assistant Clinical Professor and doctoral student in the School of Nursing, McMaster University. Her research interests include community health, knowledge translation, immigrant women's perinatal health, primary health care, and health services research.

**Donna Ciliska**, RN, PhD, is a Professor Emeritus at the School of Nursing, McMaster University, and senior knowledge translation advisor to the National Collaborating Centre for Methods and Tools. Her research interests include community health, obesity, eating disorders, and research dissemination and utilization.

# CHAPTER 11

# Epidemiology

*Lynnette Leeseberg Stamler*

## LEARNING OUTCOMES

**After studying this chapter, you should be able to:**

1. Describe the theoretical underpinnings of the epidemiologic process and its historical and present value to community health nurses (CHNs).

2. Differentiate between association and causality and explain some of the criteria that suggest a causal relationship.

3. Differentiate between screening and surveillance, and give local examples of each.

4. Discuss the various measurements used in epidemiologic research and reports and their meaning for CHNs.

5. Describe the research study designs commonly used in epidemiologic research and link the research question with the appropriate design.

6. Discuss how epidemiology has expanded to the study of disease and health promotion.

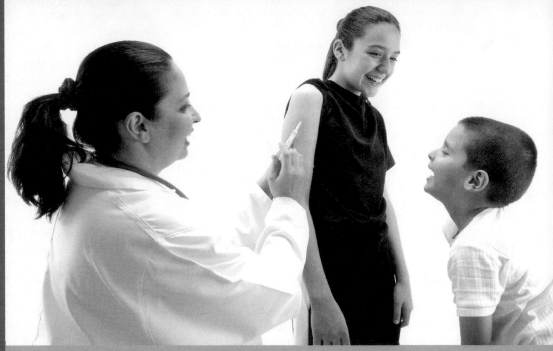

*Source: Levent Konuk/Shutterstock*

## INTRODUCTION

Throughout history, humans have ascribed different causes for disease. During the religious era, disease was thought to be a consequence of divine intervention. The environment was the next general cause of disease, which was attributed to miasmas (vaporous atmospheres) or other physical forces. It was not until the 1870s that specific bacteria were recognized as causing disease. During the past century, health professionals have come to understand that there are multiple factors or influences on many diseases and health challenges. In addition to learning the many causes of disease, health researchers are working to discover the factors that promote health.

In this chapter you will learn the basics of the science of epidemiology, understand the types of data used in community health nursing, and begin to acquire the skills to identify and ask questions, using epidemiologic data to find some of the answers.

## WHAT IS EPIDEMIOLOGY?

**Epidemiology** is defined as "the study of the occurrence and distribution of health-related states or events in specified populations, including the study of the determinants influencing such states and the application of this knowledge to control the health problem"

(Porta, 2008, p. 81). The most well-known of these would be public health epidemiology (or infectious disease epidemiology). Some authors stratify the concept with sub-definitions, such as exposure-oriented (e.g., nutritional, environmental), and disease-oriented (e.g., cancer, injury).

Friis and Sellers (2014) note that the purpose of epidemiology is to describe, explain, predict, and control challenges to population health. Epidemiologists first seek to describe health-related events by answering the questions who, what, when, and where, and by following trends in the population. Further explorations expand descriptions by answering the questions how and why, and by examining causality and modes of transmission. From this information come predictions that guide interventions and the use of healthcare resources. Finally, controls are implemented to prevent new illness; cure, if possible, those who are ill; and rehabilitate or prevent complications for those with a chronic disease.

## Historical Background of Epidemiology

Though large-scale, focused epidemiologic studies are a relatively new phenomenon, the basis of understanding for such studies has been noted throughout history. Hippocrates is credited with being the first to notice and record a possible relationship between the environment and the health or disease of people.

He suggested that physicians study "the mode in which the inhabitants live and what are their pursuits, whether they are fond of eating and drinking to excess, and given to indolence, or are fond of exercise and labor, and not given to excess in eating and drinking" (Hippocrates, 400 BCE).

Though history has recorded the existence and duration of epidemics such as the plague or the Black Death, few large-scale efforts were made to accurately record data that would increase the understanding of these epidemics. By the 1600s, statistics such as numbers of births and deaths were being recorded in London, England, and a haberdasher, John Graunt, was the first to study these statistics. He noted, for instance, gender differences in births (more males than females), seasonal variations in deaths, and high levels of infant deaths.

It was not until 1839 that Dr. William Farr initiated a more complete gathering of statistical data in England. With these data he was able (among other things) to compare death rates among workers in different types of jobs, and between prison inmates and the rest of the population. During a cholera epidemic in the mid-1850s, Dr. John Snow noticed an apparent relationship between the number of cholera deaths in various neighbourhoods and the source of the drinking water. He clearly demonstrated that people who lived in areas or homes served by particular water companies had much higher death rates from cholera than those in neighbourhoods served by other water companies.

Florence Nightingale, a contemporary of Snow and Farr, was also convinced of the effect of the environment on disease and death. When she arrived at Scutari during the Crimean War, she discovered horrendous conditions and a lax method of recording deaths and their causes. She stressed accurate recording of these statistics and used them to explain and publicize the reality of the situation. Her polar diagrams, for instance, clearly demonstrated that in January 1855, 2761 soldiers died from contagious diseases, 83 from wounds, and 324 from other causes. It became clear that without ongoing recruitment, the entire army could have been wiped out from disease alone (Cohen, 1984). It was through her influence and her record-keeping that she was able to persuade authorities to allow her to implement sanitation practices that significantly decreased the death rates during and after the war.

In the 1900s, it became evident that although vital statistics of death and illness were important, following populations for a period of time to ascertain the progression of various diseases and their treatments was also important. As well, new research methodologies were developed to gather and compare data appropriately. As medical scientists discovered and implemented new treatments, the primary causes of death changed over time from predominantly contagious diseases to chronic diseases that were influenced by lifestyle behaviours. For instance, between the 1920s and the 1970s, death rates from health challenges such as cardiovascular and renal diseases rose, while death rates for diseases such as tuberculosis and influenza decreased (see Figure 11.1). In 1949, the first cohort study—the Framingham Heart Study—was begun, followed in 1950 by the publication of the first case-control studies of smoking and lung disease. Four years later, the Salk polio vaccine field trial was conducted. Modern epidemiologic studies have all been developed from these pioneering works.

## Basic Building Blocks in Epidemiology

Several concepts and processes are the basic building blocks of the science of epidemiology. These include the epidemiologic model, the concept of susceptibility, modes of transmission, the natural history or progress of disease, association and causation, and the web of causation. Modern CHNs use these concepts and processes to determine and test appropriate interventions.

**Epidemiologic Model** The classic epidemiologic model contains the elements of host, agent, and environment. The model is frequently presented as a triangle. The **host** is the human being in which the disease occurs. The **agent** is the contagious or non-contagious force that can begin or prolong a health problem. Agents include bacteria and viruses, as well as "stimuli" such as smoking or the absence of vitamin C. The **environment** is the context that promotes the *exposure* of the host to the agent. The **epidemiologic model** posits that disease is the result of the interaction among these three elements.

Some authors have included other elements in the epidemiologic model. For example, Gordis (2009) included the vector as an additional concept. He defined **vector** as a factor (such as a deer tick) that moves between the agent and the host, assisting the movement of the disease between the other two elements. Timmreck (1998), on the other hand, added the concept of time to the model. Harkness (1995) noted that

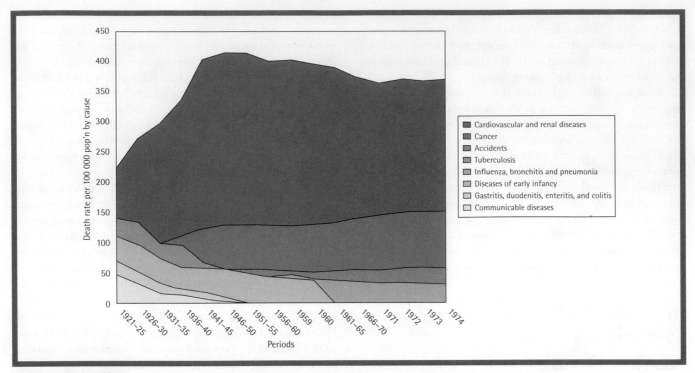

**FIGURE  11.1**  Comparisons of the Most Common Causes of Death of Canadians over Time

*Source:* Statistics Canada. www.statcan.ca/english/free[in/11-516-XIE/sectionb/sectionb.htm. Reproduced with permission.

Adapted from Table B35-50: Average annual number of deaths and death rates for leading causes of death, Canada, for five-year periods, 1921 to 1974. Available from http://www.statcan.gc.ca/pub/11-516-x/sectionb/b35-50-eng.csv

Fraser, R. D. (1983). Section B: Vital Statistics and Health. In Statistics Canada, *Historical statistics of Canada* (2nd ed.). Available from http://www.statcan.gc.ca/pub/11-516-x/11-516-x1983001-eng.htm

using a **Venn diagram** instead of the classic triangle emphasized the interrelatedness within the model. With the Venn diagram, overlaps do exist (see Figure 11.2).

**Epidemiologic Variables**  In order to completely and accurately describe the patterns of health challenges, the descriptive variables of epidemiology are used. These are named person, place, and time (Friis & Sellers, 2014). Within each variable are factors or characteristics that further describe the event. For instance, under the variable of person, one might look at age differences, sex, ethnicity, genetic predisposition, immune status, marital status, place of birth, and immigration. Other environmental influences for the person such as education level, socioeconomic status, and occupation are also important pieces of information. Lastly, individual lifestyle characteristics such as dietary practices, use of alcohol or tobacco, and physical activity may be helpful.

The variable of time considers such characteristics as cyclic or seasonal variation of a health event, health challenges following specific events (such as postpartum depression), or time trends (increase of chronic disease over time) (Friis & Sellers, 2014). The variable of place can include variation between regions, countries, or continents; population density; rural/urban; or specific geographical characteristics, such as working in a particular building or living close to a cataclysmic

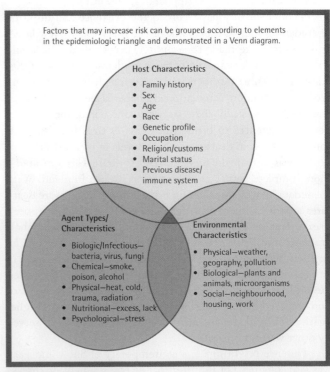

**FIGURE  11.2**  Epidemiologic Triangle as a Venn Diagram

event such as Chernobyl (Friis & Sellers, 2014). During the beginning identification of AIDS, careful documentation of person, time, and place assisted health professionals to accurately describe the health challenge.

**Susceptibility** One might think that if a group of people were all exposed in the same manner to the same disease, all would get the disease to the same degree. However, the combination of characteristics of each individual within that host group, interacting with the factors present or absent in the other elements of the epidemiologic triangle, determines the risk (or degree of **susceptibility**) of each person to a particular agent. Susceptibility and **risk** can also be described as vulnerability, which determines the individual host response. The answers to the person, place, and time questions, while pointing to group susceptibility, can also point to group protection. For instance, we may discover that one or more of the characteristics studied (such as age or physical activity) may in fact mitigate some of the effects of other characteristics.

Within each element of the epidemiologic triangle are factors or characteristics that may increase or decrease the risk or susceptibility of the host to the disease. Figure 11.2 identifies some of these factors or characteristics. It is evident that some factors (e.g., lifestyle behaviours) may be changed or modified by the individual, while others (e.g., age, gender, genetic makeup) are not under the control of the individual.

**Modes of Disease Transmission** A **mode of transmission** is one way in which a disease moves to a new host. **Direct transmission** involves contact between the person with the disease and another person. This may be accomplished through touching with contaminated hands, skin-to-skin contact, or sexual intercourse. **Indirect transmission** involves a common vehicle or vector that moves the disease to the new host. An example of a common vehicle is a contaminated water supply or lake. A mosquito can also function as a common vector in disease transmission. Indirect transmission may be airborne (droplets or dust), water-borne, vector-borne, or vehicle-borne (contaminated utensils, hygiene articles, or clothing). Different **pathogens** (microorganisms or other substances that cause disease) are viable under different conditions; therefore, one needs to ascertain the potential mode of transmission for each disease.

Because a given disease may have more than one mode of transmission, understanding those modes is central to controlling the disease. For example, when AIDS first became recognized as a threat to public health, the mode of transmission was greatly misunderstood: it was not known whether the disease could be contracted through everyday contact, such as by using a toilet seat used by someone with AIDS or by shaking that person's hand. It soon became clear that such minimal contact did not result in disease transmission. However, the fear of AIDS greatly increased the use of universal precautions by health professionals—a positive outcome. More recently we have seen efforts to ensure our understanding of the spread of Ebola, and strategies to contain it are, in fact, correct and effective.

**Natural History/Progression of a Disease** A disease in a human host should be seen as a process rather than as a single incident. In 1965, Leavell and Clark plotted the natural progression of the disease process and identified prevention and health promotion strategies that could be employed at each stage. As illustrated in Figure 11.3, the first stage in the disease process is the **prepathogenesis** period. During prepathogenesis, the human host may be exposed to a variety of agents through several modes of transmission. Depending on the unique characteristics of the prospective host, repeated exposure or a combination of additional stressors may be required for the host to become susceptible to the agent and the disease to begin. **Stressors** are events or situations that cause discomfort to a person, such as chronic fatigue or a poor diet. During the prepathogenesis period (also called the **incubation** period), **primary prevention** activities, or "measures designed to promote general optimum health" (Leavell & Clark, 1965, p. 20) are used by health professionals and the general public alike.

When the human host begins to react to the agent (or stimulus), the period of **pathogenesis** begins. Depending on the disease, the host may or may not experience symptoms, but microscopic changes take place that indicate the presence of the disease. Pathogenesis ends with recovery, disability, or death. Two categories of health promotion activities are used during the period of pathogenesis. The first category is early diagnosis and treatment, which occurs early in the pathogenesis period. For instance, screening mammography is used for early detection of breast cancer, and the Pap test screens for cervical cancer. The second category, disability limitation, occurs later in the pathogenesis period, when the disease is active or there are recognizable symptoms. During this period, health promotion activities are aimed at preventing complications; for example, ongoing examination and care of the feet in persons living with diabetes. Early diagnosis and disability limitation may also be called **secondary prevention**.

**Tertiary prevention** is the term given to the last health promotion category and occurs during the latter phases of the pathogenesis period. At this stage, health promotion activities might include client and family education to understand the chronicity of the disease, to adapt to sequelae of the disease process, or to maximize the health of the individual through use of aids such as a walker or adapted eating utensils. Figure 11.3 identifies this period as rehabilitation, but it may also be the time when palliative care and assistance for the individual and family to move toward a dignified death would be appropriate. It is important to recognize that the presence of chronic diseases or health challenges in individuals also increases their vulnerability or susceptibility to additional health challenges. This has become increasingly evident as more and more of our population lives longer due to enhanced medical care and health practices. Disease processes that would have ensured a speedy death only a few decades ago are now managed with little ongoing medical care. CHNs can use their knowledge of the progression of a disease and the levels of prevention to plan and implement interventions at the individual, family, aggregate, and population levels.

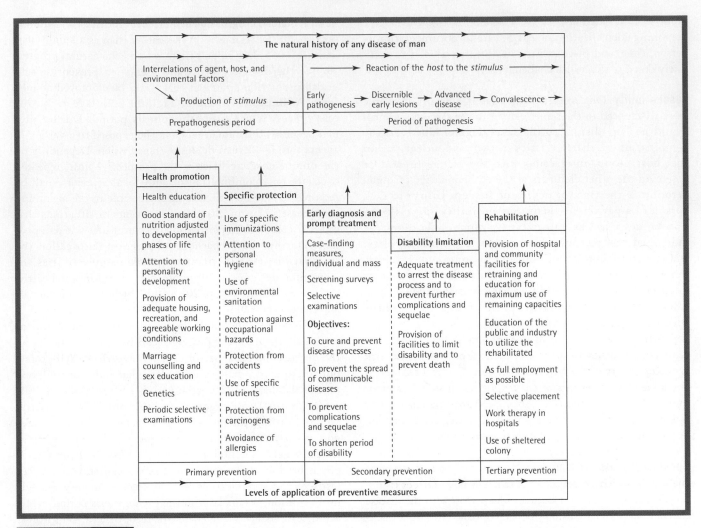

**FIGURE 11.3** Natural History of a Disease

*Source:* Leavell, H. F., & Clark, E. G. (1965). *Preventive medicine for the doctor in his community: An epidemiologic approach.* New York, NY: McGraw-Hill, p. 21. Reproduced with permission of The McGraw-Hill Companies.

## Screening and Surveillance

Screening and surveillance are tools that CHNs and other public health officials use to assist them in preventing or controlling certain diseases. These concepts can be difficult for new practitioners to understand. Diagnostics is the use of tests to ascertain if an individual with a symptom has a disease that can be diagnosed and treated. For example, a person who had fallen and had limb pain may undergo an x-ray to look for a fracture. The testing of individuals who do not have symptoms is called **screening** (Weiss, 2008). An example of this would be a colonoscopy to look for signs of rectal cancer. Screening or diagnostic tests need to be constantly examined to ensure they have both validity (they test what you want them to test) and reliability (they are consistent in their results over time and populations). As new knowledge about a disease is uncovered, the diagnostic or screening tests or policies may change. An example of this is the teaching and use of breast self-examination, which has become more controversial over the last decade or so.

**Surveillance** is the constant watching or monitoring of diseases to assess patterns and quickly identify events that do not fit the pattern. Gathering and analyzing the number and type (age, gender) of individuals of persons diagnosed with influenza in a certain geographic location (province) over a period of time to ascertain if public health interventions need to be initiated is an example of surveillance. Here a sudden spike in the incidence may signal the beginning of an epidemic. In the case of infectious diseases, such as sexually transmitted infections (e.g., HIV), surveillance may also include the monitoring of people with the disease, and their contacts as well as the general population. In the case of diseases with a genetic component, data may be collected to track the disease through extended family relationships. In all cases, the data must be reliable so that appropriate decisions can be made and effective interventions can be planned and implemented.

**Association and Causation** Before planning interventions that prevent or ameliorate a disease or health problem, one has to clearly understand the how and why of the disease or health problem. Two terms are used to describe the relationship between a stressor and a disease: association and causation. An **association** occurs when there is reasonable evidence that a connection exists

**CASE STUDY**

**Based on:**

Jaeger, V., Shick-Porter, M., Moore, D., Grant, D., & Wolfe, V. (2011). GotFlu Channel: An online syndromic surveillance tool supporting college health practice and public health work. *Journal of American College Health 59*(5), 415–418. doi:10.1080/07448481.2010.521961

Savage, R., Chu, A., Rosella, L. C., Crowcroft, N. S., Varia, M., Policarpio, M. E., . . . Johnson, I. (2011). Perceived usefulness of syndromic surveillance in Ontario during the H1N1 pandemic. *Journal of Public Health, 34*(2), 195–202.

To maximize scarce resources within the healthcare facility of a university, Brock University established a surveillance tool for the second wave of H1N1 influenza during September to December 2009. In collaboration with the information technology department, a website was launched where students could sign in and record their symptoms, self-identify as having the flu based on the symptoms, learn about self-care and when and where to seek help, and come back to the site to communicate the later absence of further symptoms, thus triggering a medical excuse note. By utilizing this website, health services staff could follow up with students who did not indicate reversal of symptoms, and spend significant time on students who were in need of additional medical care. As a comparison, they saw 376 students with influenza in this time period compared to 14 in the same period in 2008. This allowed limited health services staff to adequately manage during a pandemic period.

### Discussion Questions

1. What were the primary advantages of such a syndromic surveillance system?
2. Do you think this could be used in a larger population? (Hint: See Savage et al., 2011, above.)

between a stressor or environmental factor and a disease or health challenge (see Canadian Research Box 11.2). For example, a CHN might notice that many patients who exhibit a certain condition spent their childhoods in a particular geographic location. Thus, the relationship is first noticed through observation. Based on these observations, the CHN or epidemiologist examines the data to see if the relationship or association is strong or weak—is it all patients or just a few? If the association appears strong from the limited data sample, then a larger, more comprehensive exploration might be conducted. Such investigations often generate data from several sources.

When a relationship or association has been confirmed beyond doubt, **causation** (or causality) is said to be present. In other words, causality occurs when one can state that there is a definite, statistical, cause-and-effect relationship between a particular stimulus and the occurrence of a specific disease or health challenge, or that the occurrence could not happen by chance alone.

In some ways, causation was simpler when the majority of diseases were infectious, as they were more likely to have only one cause. For example, streptococcus bacteria produce strep infection. Two important concepts in establishing causality are "necessary" and "sufficient." "Necessary" refers to the notion that a particular stressor *must* be present before a given effect can occur. For example, exposure to *Mycobacterium tuberculosis* is required before a person becomes ill with tuberculosis. "Sufficient" refers to the amount of exposure required to result in the disease. For instance, some people exposed to *Mycobacterium tuberculosis* only once (minimal dose) become ill, and some do not become ill unless exposed several times (larger dose).

In the past 40 years, several authors have identified factors or criteria that researchers and practitioners could use to assess a causal relationship between a stimulus and the occurrence of a disease (Hill, 1965). The most commonly cited criteria of causation are summarized in Table 11.1 (Bhopal, 2008; Friis & Sellers, 2014; Gordis, 2009; Merrill & Timmrick, 2006). The criteria may be used for individual health challenges as well as population events.

Though strict adherence to these criteria is perhaps the purview of researchers, CHNs can use them as well. When reading research that examines a particular nursing practice or new intervention, it is prudent to examine the presented results or recommendations in light of the criteria in Table 11.1. Similarly, when CHNs observe a recurring phenomenon that appears to have a relationship with a human or environmental factor, a close examination of the data in light of the criteria may assist them in planning subsequent observations.

**Web of Causation** Previous chapters have introduced the concept of determinants of health. In contrast to the time when each illness was thought to have a unique and specific cause, it is now recognized that many health problems have multiple causal factors, both direct and indirect. For instance, issues of

| **Table 11.1** | **Illustrations of Causation Criteria** |
|---|---|

*Temporal relationship* – A person does not get the disease until after exposure to the cause

*Strength of association* – Exposure to a specific stressor or cause is most likely to bring on the disease

*Dose-response* – Persons who are most exposed to the contaminated food (e.g., ate the most) are the most ill

*Specificity* – The cause is linked to a specific disease (e.g., *Mycobacterium tuberculosis* does not result in chickenpox)

*Consistency* – Everyone who eats contaminated food gets the illness. If other food in another time and place is contaminated with the same bacteria, the same illness occurs

*Biologic plausibility* – Consistent with the biologic/medical knowledge that is known (new discoveries may precede biologic plausibility)

*Experimental replication* – Several studies done by different scientists in different places produce the same or similar results

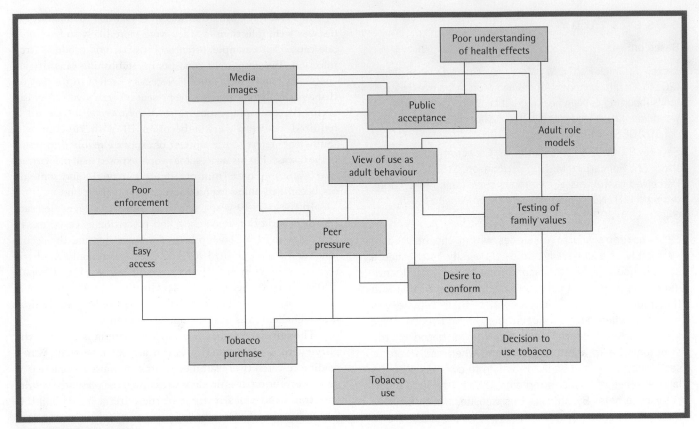

**FIGURE 11.4** Web of Causation for Adolescent Tobacco Use

*Source:* From *Community health nursing: Advocacy for population health* (5th ed.), by Mary J. Clark, © 2008, p. 66. Reprinted and electronically reproduced by permission of Pearson Education, Inc., New York, NY.

poverty, education, and environment (e.g., pollution) have been shown to be influential in many health challenges. It is in looking for the causes of today's health challenges and assessing for the presence or absence of particular determinants of health that the CHN is well served by partnering with practitioners from a variety of disciplines. For instance, in addition to other health professionals, the CHN looking at population influences might look to the disciplines of sociology, anthropology, genetics, psychology, geography, and economics. As well, working with experts in social trends and public policy could bring additional understanding to the specific issue at hand.

A model called a **web of causation** can be helpful to CHNs in visualizing the relationships among the many causes or influences of a given health challenge. Within that model, the relationship between the direct and indirect causes can be hypothesized, at which point research studies can be designed to test the hypotheses suggested by the web of causation.

Figure 11.4 illustrates a web of causation for adolescent tobacco use. Obviously, the most direct causes or factors of adolescent tobacco use are the decision to use tobacco and the actual purchase or acquisition of tobacco. However, behind those primary causes are several other causal factors possessing various levels of influence. For instance, the decision to use tobacco can be influenced both by peer pressure and the testing of family values.

At any one time, each individual is subjected to multiple agents delivered through many modes of transmission. If one compared webs of causation for several common health challenges,

some specific health promotion activities would appear to serve more than one purpose. Conversely, there may be a health promotion activity that is helpful for one challenge but contributes to susceptibility for another challenge. CHNs must examine all possible benefits and consequences of an intervention.

# MEASUREMENT IN EPIDEMIOLOGY

To determine the extent of a disease process or health challenge and its final effects on a population, data must be collected and analyzed. However, for the resulting measurements to be useful to the CHN, the raw data or crude numbers must be presented in conjunction with other factors, such as population, time frame, or human characteristic (e.g., gender, race, age). These numbers, expressed as fractions, are known as **rates**. The numerator of each fraction is generally the crude count of the disease in question, and the denominator is generally the size of the population in question. In each case, the population or subpopulation of the numerator and denominator of the fraction are the same. For example, a rate of teen pregnancies might look like this:

$$\text{Rate} = \frac{\text{Number of live births delivered to teen mothers in the population}}{\text{Total number of teen women in the population}}$$

| Table 11.2 | Commonly Used Rates in Epidemiology |
|---|---|
| **Rate** | **Formula** |
| Crude mortality rate | $\dfrac{\text{Total deaths from any cause in a given year in a population}}{\text{Average total population for the same year}}$ |
| Specific mortality rate | $\dfrac{\text{Total deaths from a specific cause in a given year in a population (subgroup)}}{\text{Average number of population (subgroup) for the same year}}$ |
| Infant death rate | $\dfrac{\text{Total deaths of infants in given year in population}}{\text{Total number of live births in same year in population}}$ |
| Prevalence rate | $\dfrac{\text{Number of people with given disease in given population at one point in time}}{\text{Total in given population at same point in time}}$ |
| Incidence rate | $\dfrac{\text{Number of new cases of given disease in population in given time (one year)}}{\text{Average total population in same time}}$ |
| Relative risk | $\dfrac{\text{Incidence rate of disease in exposed population}}{\text{Incidence of disease in unexposed population}}$ |

This fraction, or rate, is usually expressed for a set number of the population (e.g., per 100 000 people, per 100 cases, or per 1000 births) so that different-sized populations can be compared. Table 11.2 presents the formulae for commonly used rates, and the following section describes these rates, how they are calculated, and how they might be used by CHNs.

## Mortality (Death) Rates

Healthcare providers are legally required to complete death certificates for all deaths and file them with the government authorities. Thus, death or **mortality rates** are generally complete and easily obtainable. Mortality rates can be crude or specific in nature. **Crude mortality rates** compare the number of deaths from a specific cause within the entire population, while **specific mortality rates** compare the number of deaths from a specific cause in a particular subgroup with that whole subgroup. For example, if one examined all deaths from motor vehicle collisions and compared them with the total population, one would have a crude mortality rate. However, if one examined only teenage male deaths from motor vehicle collisions, one would compare that with the number of male teens driving at that time, a specific mortality rate. Mortality rates from a specific cause are often different when different subgroups (e.g., teenage males, children aged 4–8, elderly persons) are examined. For example, Figure 11.5 illustrates the age-specific suicide rates for Canada for 2011, stratified (divided) by gender. Note the line that represents the specific total mortality rate for each age group. If only these data were presented, it would be statistically correct but fail to inform the reader that the rate for

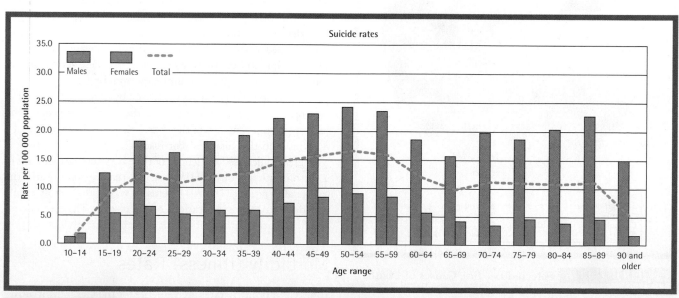

**FIGURE 11.5** Suicide Rates by Age and Gender, Canada, 2011

*Source:* Statistics Canada. www.statcan.gc.ca/tables-tableaux/sum-som/l01/cst01/hlth66d-eng.htm; www.statcan.gc.ca/tables-tableaux/sum-som/l01/cst01/hlth66e-eng.htm; www.statcan.gc.ca/tables-tableaux/sum-som/l01/cst01/hlth66f-eng.htm

males is significantly higher than for females in each age group. These stratified data would lead one to conclude that males are more susceptible (or at least more successful) than females to death by suicide.

**Proportional mortality rates** can be used to stratify crude mortality rates. The number of deaths from a specific cause in a given population for a particular time period is compared with the total number of deaths in that same population and time period. A common use of proportional mortality rates is to state that *x*% of the deaths in a given year were due to breast cancer or motor vehicle collisions (see Figure 11.6). Note that two causes of death, cancers and diseases of the heart, account for over half the deaths.

Historically, the health of a population has been exemplified by maternal and infant mortality rates. Families used to have many children, partly because few were expected to live past the first years of life (assuming the mother and child survived the birth and neonatal period). With the advent of better hygiene as well as prenatal and postnatal care, maternal and infant mortality rates decreased. CHNs often compare infant mortality rates across developing and developed countries, the assumption being that lower maternal and infant mortality rates are indicative of a healthier population. When looking at these statistics, it is particularly important to determine the stage (e.g., perinatal vs. infant) that has been studied so that the comparisons are accurate. The following definitions are used in maternal and infant mortality statistics. In all but the perinatal rate,

the denominator is the number of live births in that year in that population.

- Maternal or puerperal death rate: any deaths of the mother resulting from pregnancy-related causes;
- Perinatal death rate: fetal deaths occurring during the last few months of pregnancy and during the first seven days of life. Here the denominator includes both live births and fetal deaths;
- Neonatal death rate: deaths occurring in infants in their first 28 days of life; and
- Infant death rate: deaths occurring in the first year of life

A more recent way of presenting mortality statistics is in terms of **potential years of life lost (PYLL)**. This has arisen from the assumption that a person who dies early in life has lost greater potential than has a person who dies much later in life. PYLL statistics give CHNs additional information on which health challenges or diseases result in the greatest lost potential to the population. While this may raise some ethical issues in terms of where a society or country chooses to place its resources, PYLL statistics are certainly a part of the picture that must be heeded.

## Survival (Prognosis) Rates

**Survival rates** are often used to describe the effect of a given disease (e.g., cancer) and are also referred to as prognosis rates. Survival rates partially answer the common client question, "How bad is it?" Survival rates can also be used to compare the efficacy of various treatments for a specific disease. For diseases such as cancer, and its treatments, the prognosis or survival rate most frequently used is the five-year survival rate. This is determined by calculating the percentage of persons with the disease who are alive five years after diagnosis. While five years is a convenient time period to use for comparing the effect of various treatments, it is easy for clients and health professionals alike to fall into the trap of somehow equating five-year survival with a decreased risk of future mortality from that disease. One of the arguments presented in favour of widespread breast screening is early detection of the disease. While it is hoped that early detection coupled with prompt treatment will increase the survival time, there is still conflicting evidence that these actions in fact contribute to decreased mortality rates from breast cancer.

The **case-fatality rate** is calculated by dividing the number of people who die from a disease by the number of people who have the disease, answering the question, "How likely is it that I will die from this disease?" For instance, while recent advances have greatly increased the length of time between the diagnosis of a person with a positive HIV test and that person's death, the case-fatality rate for HIV/AIDS remains very high, as most people will die from the complications of the disease. The case-fatality rate for a person with arthritis, for instance, is much lower.

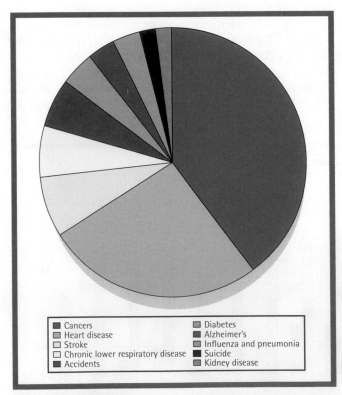

**Legend:**
- Cancers
- Heart disease
- Stroke
- Chronic lower respiratory disease
- Accidents
- Diabetes
- Alzheimer's
- Influenza and pneumonia
- Suicide
- Kidney disease

**FIGURE 11.6** Selected Leading Causes of Death, Canada, 2011

*Source:* Statistics Canada. http://www.statcan.gc.ca/tables-tableaux/sum-som/l01/cst01/hlth36a-eng.htm

## Morbidity (Illness) Rates

Illness or morbidity rates are valuable for the CHN. **Morbidity rates** give a picture of a population and a disease or health challenge over time, suggesting questions about the susceptibility of the population or subpopulation and the effectiveness of either health promotion or treatment strategies. Two types of rates are commonly used to describe morbidity in a population. The first is **prevalence**, which provides a picture of a specific disease process in a population at one given point in time. The second is **incidence**, which describes the identification of new cases of a disease in a population over time. Together with mortality rates and survival rates, they present a fairly complete picture of the population's response to a disease or health challenge.

If the disease is short-lived, such as measles or the flu, the prevalence does not reveal much. However, CHNs might use this rate in epidemic situations to plan for extra staff to deal with increased inquiries or clinic visits from concerned clients, for example during the H1N1 crisis. If the disease is short-lived, resulting in few deaths, the incidence and prevalence rates are very similar. If, on the other hand, the health challenge is chronic in nature, the incidence rate (number of new cases) stays fairly static over time, while the prevalence rate increases as more people live with the disease. If the disease is long-term with complications, such as diabetes or multiple sclerosis, the prevalence rate over time informs CHNs about the need for community and institutional support for the future. This is very important in terms of public and community health planning.

The population in question is usually the population at risk for the disease. For instance, when calculating the incidence of prostate cancer, the number of cases is compared with the population of males rather than with the whole population. Incidence rates, when calculated within the same population over several years, show whether the population seems more or less susceptible to the disease in question. For example, the number of motor vehicle collisions in a given year involving teenage drivers might change over time in response to changes in the legal drinking age.

When CHNs test for a specific cause of a health challenge, they compare the incidence of that health challenge in a population exposed to the identified cause with the incidence of the same health challenge in a population not exposed to the same cause. If the suspected cause were indeed a factor, one would expect the incidence rates to be quite different. For example, one would expect the incidence of lung cancer to be much greater in smokers than in non-smokers. If the cause being examined is not the *only* cause of the disease (e.g., lung cancer), one might find that the incidence rates are more similar than expected. Such results might lead the CHN to explore other factors (e.g., second-hand smoke) to explain the incidence rates.

One frequently asked question is, "Are some populations more at risk of or vulnerable to a specific disease than others?" To find the answer to that question, a statistic known as **relative risk** is used. This measure divides the incidence of a given problem or disease in a population exposed to a given risk factor by the incidence of the same problem in a population not exposed to the same risk. For example, CHNs might compare the incidence of childhood asthma in a population exposed to a certain air pollutant with the incidence in a population not exposed to that pollutant. If the resulting number is 1.0, it means that both groups have the same risk of the health problem, and most likely the risk factor in question makes little or no difference. If the resulting number is >1.0, it indicates that the risk in the exposed group is higher than the risk in the unexposed group, and the risk factor in question is at least one of the significant risk factors for the problem or disease. Should the relative risk ratio be <1.0, the given risk factor is probably not significant for the problem or disease. However, such results may indicate that the factor in question has a protective effect; for example, a population where the physical activity is high may have a lower relative risk for diabetes.

Incidence and prevalence rates can be further stratified to increase the descriptiveness of the statistic. Data are frequently obtained through interviewing members of the population, also known as self-reporting. For instance, the question, "Do you currently smoke?" elicits data that could contribute to a **point prevalence** statistic of smokers in the population. This statistic describes the situation only for that particular point in time. The question, "Have you smoked within the last six months?" gives us data that could be useful for **period prevalence** statistics. However, asking, "Have you ever smoked?" gives the researcher data that could be used for **cumulative** or **lifetime incidence** statistics. This demonstrates why it is important for researchers to clearly state their methods and sources of data in journal articles and reports, and why it is equally important for CHNs reading those articles to critically examine the evidence presented.

# RESEARCH IN EPIDEMIOLOGY

## Sources of Epidemiologic Data

Surveillance and other epidemiologic analyses and research are only as good as the data on which they are based. Thus, CHNs need to ensure that they use consistent and accurate sources of data. One of the largest sources of epidemiologic data is the government. Canada has several sources of government or government-funded data, such as the Public Health Agency of Canada, Health Canada, Statistics Canada, and the provincial government health ministries. As birth and death statistics are required by law to be filed with the appropriate government agency, they are generally very accurate. Birth and death statistics can be teamed with the census data reported by Statistics Canada for further detail. Statistics Canada data can be found in their daily newsletter (*The Daily*), which reports on recent data and analysis and often provides a historical trend analysis for the disease (e.g., breast cancer) or issue (e.g., family structure in Canada). Statistics Canada also has a website where more detailed information such as profiles of individual communities and archived newsletters can be found.

In the wake of Walkerton and SARS, it was recognized that a stronger emphasis on public health by the government was required. In response, the Public Health Agency of Canada (PHAC) was formed. Many of the reports and statistics previously reported by Health Canada may now be found at the PHAC website. These include information on surveillance of

**reportable diseases** (diseases that are required to be reported by law; for example, tuberculosis, sexually transmitted infections, AIDS) as well as surveillance data on cancer, chronic disease, and cardiovascular diseases. Health Canada remains a source of information on many disease states, including epidemiologic data and links to other sites. All provinces also maintain health websites that provide information for the province in question. Specifically, many of the provincial health ministry websites provide birth and infant mortality statistics.

The Canadian Institute for Health Information (CIHI) is also an excellent source for data. A non-governmental organization, CIHI collects and collates information from many sources to provide analyses that can inform policy. The epidemiologic data that it reports includes data from hospital sources and from the various provincial health plans. Thus, this organization may provide information on incidence and prevalence of non-reportable diseases.

In addition, there are agencies that focus solely on specific disease issues. For example, the Canadian Diabetes Association or the Heart and Stroke Foundation of Canada are sources for statistics relative to those diseases. When using information found on the Internet, the CHN needs to examine the source of the data to ensure it is from a reputable organization.

For the CHN wanting to compare data between Canada and the United States, the Centers for Disease Control and Prevention website is a valuable resource. For international data, the World Health Organization's website is very helpful. In addition to websites, many organizations produce a variety of reports that are frequently found in university and college libraries or are available for download or purchase in print.

The final source of data is to gather data oneself. Although this can result in accurate data that deal with the specific question being asked, the cost of creating a survey instrument that is clear and understood by all respondents, choosing an appropriate sample (especially a national sample), and gathering the data often is beyond the financial reach of most researchers. If this is the case, researchers may be able to add questions to a survey being conducted by a community health-care centre or agency.

## Types of Epidemiologic Research

Research is one method of finding answers to questions. It is critical that CHNs have a clear understanding of research methodologies in order to understand, participate in, and conduct research. This is because the study design is strongly linked to the research question—if an inappropriate study design is chosen, the results will not provide answers.

Different authors categorize types of epidemiologic research in different ways. For example, Grobbee and Hoes (2009) viewed it from a medical perspective and categorized in terms of diagnostic, etiologic, prognostic, and intervention research, each contributing different kinds of evidence to use in clinical practice. Conversely, Bhopal (2008) used the types of research designs as the categories—case series/population case, cross-sectional, case-control, cohort, and trial. The first four can also be termed observational or descriptive research, because they are concerned with the variables of time, person, and place and answer the basic questions of who, when, and where. Analytic observational research adds the techniques of comparison and attempts to answer the questions of how and why. Trial or intervention research is considered experimental research, where the researcher manipulates selected variables and, for example, examines the efficacy of a new treatment, tests for causality, or compares communities in terms of a public health intervention. In the following section, each of the research designs will be considered.

**Case series** studies are counts of selected variables within a specific population. Through this data collection the researcher determines morbidity and mortality rates, and through analysis of the various factors, looks for evidence of association and causality. Case series studies are often the basis of higher level studies, and provide the researcher with data to generate hypotheses to be tested. Examples of research questions that could be answered include the following: Are mortality rates for cardiac disease higher for men than for women? Does age at diagnosis or geographic residence affect survival rates for persons with multiple sclerosis? What are the current incidence rates for HIV in young homosexual males compared with 5, 10, or 20 years ago? Frequently, factors that increase risk may be used as a variable of interest; for example, gender may be considered to be a risk factor for heart disease.

**Cross-sectional studies** are snapshots of the present and may also be called prevalence studies. Cross-sectional data may be collected as baseline data for planning and implementing

---

### CANADIAN RESEARCH BOX 11.1

**Does participation in school sports during adolescence affect mental health later in life?**

Jewett, R., Sabiston, C. M., Brunet, J., O'Loughlin, E. K., Scarapicchia, T., & O'Loughlin, J. (2014). School sport participation during adolescence and mental health in early adulthood. *Journal of Adolescent Health, 55*, 640–644. doi:10.1016/j.adohealth.2014.04.018

Prior research has indicated that mental health issues that begin in adolescence tend to remain during early adulthood. In this longitudinal study (part of the Nicotine Dependence in Teens study), 853 adolescents completed self-report surveys regarding participation in sports every three months for five years beginning in Grade 7. Three years later, they completed a mailed survey regarding depressive symptoms, perceived stress, and mental health status. Those who participated regularly in sport during secondary school years were found to have lower scores on all three indicators three years later. While these data do not indicate that participation in sport is a preventative factor for future mental health issues, an association between these variables is demonstrated, signalling the need for further research, including intervention.

#### Discussion Questions

1. How might you, as a CHN, use this study in your community?

2. What research design might you use for future research, and why?

interventions, or to measure change. (See Canadian Research Box 11.1.) For example, CHNs may be concerned about the age of initiation of smoking behaviours relative to a specific planned health curriculum. The CHNs may work with the community to develop an anonymous survey that asks about smoking behaviours, and administer it to students in various grade levels within the school district. The results of the survey may indicate that more than one-third of students in Grade 6 have already tried smoking, suggesting that beginning health education about smoking in Grade 6 is too late. The CHNs and teachers decide to move their initial anti-smoking education to Grades 1 and 2, in which fewer than 3% of the students have tried to smoke. A time series of cross-sectional studies could also be used with a particular group of students to assess the effectiveness of the intervention. After implementing the new curriculum in Grades 1 and 2, Grade 6 classes would be tested in subsequent years. The data would be compared with those from the present Grade 6 students, who did not receive the intervention, to ascertain if the program made a difference in the future smoking behaviours of students.

In **case-control** studies, the individuals in the group with the disease are matched with individuals who are similar in some characteristics (e.g., age, gender, time, geographic residence) but who have not manifested the disease in question. The health histories or characteristics of the individuals in both groups are then obtained. These data are compared and the common factors and differences between the two populations are identified.

A case-control study of children with type 2 diabetes would include children with the disease in one group and children without the disease in the other group. The two groups would be matched for age and geographic location. The epidemiologist might search for common and different factors such as amount of physical activity, obesity, and family history of diabetes. In each case, the researcher would expect to find some similarities and differences between the two groups that could contribute to theories of causality.

The relative risk ratio compares the risk for a particular disease between two populations: one exposed to a stressor and one not exposed to the stressor. Case-control studies also involve two groups: one group composed of individuals who have the disease and one of individuals who do not have the disease. Relative risk cannot be calculated here because neither the incidence nor the prevalence is known. The **odds ratio** provides epidemiologists with an estimate of the relative risk factor. To demonstrate the calculation of this statistic, consider the following example. A hypothetical community health centre practice has 200 male patients between the ages of 45 and 65; 50 of them have lung cancer and 150 do not. Thirty-five of the patients with lung cancer are smokers, while 15 patients without lung cancer are smokers. Table 11.3 illustrates the calculation of the odds ratio for this example. See Canadian Research Box 11.2.

In **cohort studies**, the researcher examines the individual histories of a group of people manifesting a particular disease to find out what factors they share and what differences can be discerned. Cohort studies may be retrospective or prospective. **Retrospective studies** are studies that begin in the present and search the past for information to explain the present. **Prospective studies** (or longitudinal studies) begin in the present and follow the subjects into the future or make predictions about the future that can be tested at a later date. These studies focus on individuals exposed to a particular health problem or potential stressor over time. For a prospective study, it is important to measure the incidence of the problem at various times. For instance, a group of people with high exposure to a stressor (e.g., occupational stress) may be matched with a group of people with low exposure to the problem, and both are followed for a period of time. The incidence levels of the health problem being studied (e.g., hypertension or myocardial infarction) in the two groups are compared at each measuring time.

Prospective studies have several unique issues:

- The sample size must be very large at the beginning to allow for attrition as people move, die, or lose interest.
- It is evident that health problems generally increase with increased age. By its very nature, a longitudinal study follows

| Table 11.3 | Calculation of Odds Ratio | | |
|---|---|---|---|
| **Risk Factor** | **Persons with Lung Cancer** | **Persons without Lung Cancer** | **Total** |
| Smokers | 35 (*a*) | 15 (*b*) | 55 |
| Non-smokers | 15 (*c*) | 135 (*d*) | 145 |
| Total | 50 | 150 | 200 |

$$\text{Odds ratio} = \frac{\text{Exposed persons with the disease/unexposed persons with the disease}}{\text{Exposed persons without the disease/unexposed persons without the disease}}$$

$$\text{OR} = \frac{a/c}{b/d} = \frac{ad}{bc} = \frac{(35)(135)}{(15)(15)} = \frac{4725}{225} = 21$$

The odds ratio for these data is 21. As with the relative risk ratio, a number >1.0 means that the persons exposed to the risk factor are more likely to develop the disease than those who are not exposed. In this example, male smokers are 21 times as likely to develop lung cancer as men who do not smoke. For a further example, please see Canadian Research Box 11.2.

---

**CANADIAN RESEARCH BOX 11.2**

**Does cellphone use during driving really cause accidents?**

Asbridge, M., Brubacher, J. R., & Chan, H. (2013). Cellphone use and traffic crash risk: A culpability analysis. *International Journal of Epidemiology, 42*(1), 259–267.

These authors used data from the Insurance Corporation of British Columbia Traffic Accident System. They compared accidents where the police identified the drivers as using a cellphone (n = 312) with those where the police reports did not indicate cellphone use by the driver (n = 936). An association was found between cellphone use and accident culpability. The odds ratio was calculated, and it was found to be 1.70 (95% confidence interval, 1.22-2.36, P = 0.022). Data were examined to find out if there were any further links with male drivers, drivers aged 26–65 years old, and unimpaired drivers. Middle-aged drivers were found to be particularly at risk.

### Discussion Questions

1. How could the CHN use these data for public awareness programs?

2. How might the CHN answer when teenagers point to the high risk for middle-aged drivers rather than teenagers?

---

a group of people who are aging. Thus, a method to control for the effects of aging must be applied to any results.

- Outside factors may affect the different groups differently. For instance, researchers may decide to compare hypertension in Canadian and U.S. executives who live in large cities and experience long commutes to work. The cities chosen are Toronto, Montreal, Chicago, and New York. The time frame is 1995–2015. Might the events of September 11, 2001, have an effect on the data and results?

In trials or experimental studies, the researcher manipulates some of the variables in order to ascertain the effect of the manipulation. **Manipulation** means to change something that is happening to some or all of the subjects within the study, rather than only observing what is present. In healthcare, the manipulation usually involves a new treatment or the encouragement of a new behaviour. The researcher believes that the new treatment or behaviour will positively affect the health of the subjects and uses the research to test that belief or hypothesis.

The "gold standard" of experimental study design is the **randomized controlled trial** (RCT). In fact, some scientists consider this the only valid form of experimental design. In an RCT design, individuals are assigned randomly either to a group that receives the new treatment or to a group that does not receive the new treatment. The latter is known as the control group. After a period of time, specific variables are measured in each group and compared. Frequently, neither the researchers nor the subjects are aware of which group they are part of until the end of the study. This is known as a blind RCT.

In community nursing and health promotion, the treatment or intervention studied may be a new health education or social marketing protocol (e.g., new advertisements for breast screening) or a change in policy (e.g., adding fluoride to drinking water for a community). In the example of new marketing for screening, the outcome examined could be the increase or decrease in the number of persons participating in the screening. In the case of adding fluoride to the drinking water, the outcome measured might be the number of dental cavities found in six-year-olds.

In the examples above, randomized control groups would be almost impossible. One variation of this might be that several communities may be compared, with one or more serving as treatment groups and the others serving as control groups. Another variation may be that the community might serve as its own control group—measuring the outcome of interest (e.g., participation in screening) before and after the treatment (e.g., advertising for breast screening clinics).

**Ethical Concerns** Ethical concerns during observational studies such as case, cross-sectional, case-control, or cohort are rare but possible because of the nature of those studies. The researcher is not manipulating the variables, but is systematically collecting and analyzing observations to make inferences and predictions. However, CHNs must always remember that most people are interested in participating in any study that they perceive will help someone else with a health problem. If a researcher has no intention of *using* the data (e.g., to plan interventions that are intended to be carried out), it is unethical to collect them. Ethics approval must be sought for any study where data are collected about or from humans. In any trial or experimental study, the competing issues of strong scientific experimental design and ethical considerations must be addressed. The first ethical concern is how the human subjects are approached. Most healthcare agencies and university research centres have an ethics committee that reviews research proposals to ensure that humans are treated fairly, the information is gathered and used in a confidential manner, and the privacy of the subjects is protected. However, ethical questions also arise about the design of the research. For instance, is it ethical to withhold a treatment that is felt to be beneficial from people who need it because a research design with a control group would be more scientific? Researchers must consider these questions and consult with appropriate sources for advice when designing scientific and ethical research studies.

## CONCLUSION

In this chapter, the science of epidemiology, its historical influences, and the evolution of its theoretical underpinnings were examined. The theories have been presented with modern examples, illustrating how the historical continues to have influence in the present. The notions of agent, host, and environment have been discussed, as well as modes of transmission and the natural history of disease.

Measurement is an important concept in epidemiology, and mortality, morbidity, and survival rates were each presented. The notion of risk or susceptibility was examined both theoretically and statistically. The importance of accurate sources for epidemiologic data was noted, as well as sources for Canadian data. Observational and experimental research designs were presented, with the caution that it is very important that the research design should fit the research question. Causality as a societal belief as well as a statistical conclusion was noted, and causality criteria that the CHN can use to examine observations as well as published research were included. The notion of the web of causation was presented to coincide with the current belief in multiple direct and indirect causes for most health challenges.

The science of epidemiology is an important one for the CHN. Community health professionals are confronted with increasingly complex health challenges that were unheard of just a few short decades ago, such as type 2 diabetes in children. It is becoming increasingly evident that Hippocrates had it right more than two millennia ago: nurses must look at what the person eats, what the person does, and what the person's habits are. Health practitioners face the task of using the results of epidemiologic research to influence citizens to change or enhance their activities of daily living to actively promote maximum health, while recognizing that the individual and group environment may well influence people in other directions.

Modern CHNs, while facing more complex challenges, also have the advantages of access to strong data, government and societal interest in health, and a better-educated populace. The science of epidemiology is but one of their tools.

## KEY TERMS

agent   p. 203
association   p. 206
case-control   p. 213
case series   p. 212
case-fatality rate   p. 210
causation   p. 207
cohort studies   p. 213
cross-sectional studies   p. 212
crude mortality rates   p. 209
cumulative or lifetime incidence   p. 211
direct transmission   p. 205
environment   p. 203
epidemiologic model   p. 203
epidemiology   p. 202
host   p. 203
incidence   p. 211
incubation   p. 205
indirect transmission   p. 205
manipulation   p. 214
mode of transmission   p. 205
morbidity rates   p. 210
mortality rates   p. 209
odds ratio   p. 213
pathogens   p. 205
pathogenesis   p. 205
period prevalence   p. 211
point prevalence   p. 211
potential years of life lost (PYLL)   p. 210
prepathogenesis   p. 205
prevalence   p. 211
primary prevention   p. 205

proportional mortality rates   p. 210
prospective studies   p. 213
randomized controlled trial   p. 214
rates   p. 208
relative risk   p. 211
reportable diseases   p. 212
retrospective studies   p. 213
risk   p. 205
screening   p. 206
secondary prevention   p. 205
specific mortality rates   p. 209
stressors   p. 205
surveillance   p. 206
survival rates   p. 210
susceptibility   p. 205
tertiary prevention   p. 205
vector   p. 203
Venn diagram   p. 204
web of causation   p. 208

## STUDY QUESTIONS

1. Identify and define five criteria for causality.

2. Differentiate between mortality and morbidity rates. How does each inform the CHN?

3. Name and define three types of observational studies relating to CHN practice. Using different examples from those in the chapter, suggest two research questions that might be answered with each of the types.

4. Identify the three elements of the epidemiologic triangle and define each.

5. Differentiate between incidence and prevalence. What does it mean when the incidence and prevalence rates for a given health problem are very different? What does it mean when they are very similar?

6. Describe prospective and retrospective studies and give two examples of research questions that could be answered with each.

> After working through these questions, go to the MyNursingLab at www.pearsoned.ca/mynursinglab to check your answers.

## INDIVIDUAL CRITICAL-THINKING EXERCISES

1. Select a health problem. Using Figure 11.3 as a guide, suggest five CHN actions for each level of prevention. Include actions for individuals as well as populations. How might CHNs collaborate with other health professionals to implement the actions?

2. Discuss the pros and cons of having national registries for disease processes such as tumours, diabetes, and HIV/AIDS. Did your discussion differ according to the statistics available regarding incidence and prevalence? What about possible social stigma?

3. One of the more recent mortality statistics is PYLL. Suicide is one health problem that is examined in terms of PYLL. Using the data in Figure 11.5, at what age group would you target your prevention interventions? Why? How did the concept of PYLL influence your decision?

4. How might CHNs use their knowledge of surveillance and epidemiologic data for their community to influence their practice? How can CHNs be involved in epidemiologic research and/or the collection and analysis of epidemiologic data?

5. Why are infant and child mortality rates used as a measure of the health of a population? Using the national and provincial infant mortality rates (www.statcan.gc.ca/tables-tableaux/sum-som/l01/cst01/health21a-eng.htm), what do you discern about provincial disparities? Are you surprised? What factors might influence the rates noted? Where might you go to find further evidence?

## GROUP CRITICAL-THINKING EXERCISES

1. Select a condition that you are familiar with (e.g., type 2 diabetes, asthma, heart attack). From two different provinces' health websites and the PHAC website, compare the mortality and morbidity rates for that condition. Are they similar or different? What factors might influence the rates in those jurisdictions?

2. As a group, discuss the pros and cons of using an epidemiologic approach to planning CHN actions.

3. Physical activity is recognized as a protector of health for all humans, regardless of age and current health status. Using the tables found at www40.statcan.gc.ca/l01/cst01/health78b-eng.htm; www.statcan.gc.ca/tables-tableaux/sum-som/l01/cst01/health77a-eng.htm; and www.statcan.gc.ca/tables-tableaux/sum-som/l01/cst01/health77b-eng.htm, consider how you might design a national campaign aimed at increasing physical activity. Which groups would be most important to target? Why?

## REFERENCES

Bhopal, R. (2008). *Concepts of epidemiology: Integrating the ideas, theories, principles and methods of epidemiology.* New York, NY: Oxford University Press.

Cohen, I. B. (1984). Florence Nightingale. *Scientific American, 3,* 128–137.

Friis, R. H., & Sellers, T. A. (2014). *Epidemiology for public health practice* (5th ed.). Sudbury, MA: Jones and Bartlett.

Gordis, L. (2009). *Epidemiology* (4th ed.). Philadelphia, PA: W. B. Saunders.

Grobbee, D. E., & Hoes, A. W. (2009). *Clinical epidemiology: Principles, methods and applications for clinical research.* Sudbury, MA: Jones and Bartlett.

Harkness, G. A. (1995). *Epidemiology in nursing practice.* St. Louis, MO: Mosby.

Hill, A. B. (1965). The environment and disease: Association or causation? *Proceedings of the Royal Society of Medicine, 58,* 295–300.

Hippocrates. (400 BCE). *On airs, waters and places.* The Internet classics archive, Part 1. Retrieved from http://classics.mit.edu/Hippocrates/airwatpl.1.1.html

Leavell, H. F., & Clark, E. G. (1965). *Preventive medicine for the doctor in his community: An epidemiologic approach.* New York, NY: McGraw-Hill.

Merril, R. M., & Timmreck, T. C. (2006). *An introduction to epidemiology.* Sudbury, MA: Jones and Bartlett.

Porta, M. S., & International Epidemiological Association. (2008). *A dictionary of epidemiology* (5th ed.). Oxford, UK: Oxford University Press.

Savage, R., Chu, A., Rosella, L. C., Crowcroft, N. S., Varia, M., Policarpio, M. E., . . . Johnson, I. (2012). Perceived usefulness of syndromic surveillance in Ontario during the H1N1 pandemic. *Journal of Public Health 34*(2), 195–202. doi:10.1093/pubmed/fdr088

Timmreck, T. C. (1998). *An introduction to epidemiology.* Sudbury, MA: Jones and Bartlett.

Weiss, N. S. (2008). Clinical epidemiology. In K. J. Rothman, S. Greenland, & T. L. Lash (Eds.), *Modern epidemiology* (pp. 641–651). Philadelphia, PA: Wolters Kluwer Health.

### ABOUT THE AUTHOR

**Lynnette Leeseberg Stamler**, RN, PhD, FAAN, is Professor and Associate Dean for academic programs at the University of Nebraska Medical Center, College of Nursing. From 1984 to 2012 she taught in Canadian schools of nursing and was a VON nurse prior to her teaching career. She completed her BSN at St. Olaf College, Minnesota, her MEd in health education at the University of Manitoba, and her PhD in nursing at the University of Cincinnati.

Her research interests include patient/health education, diabetes education, nursing education, and quality care. She is active in national and international nursing organizations, including Sigma Theta Tau International and the Nursing Honor Society, and was president of the Canadian Association of Schools of Nursing from 2008 to 2010. In 2011 she was inducted into the American Academy of Nursing.

# Communicable Diseases

*Marianna Ofner-Agostini*

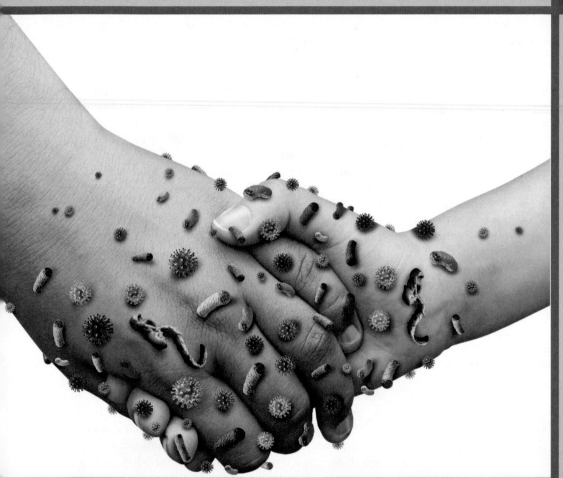

*Source: Freshidea/Fotolia*

## INTRODUCTION

**Communicable diseases** are illnesses caused by a "specific infectious agent, or its toxic products that arise through transmission of that agent, or its products from an infected person, animal or inanimate source to a susceptible host; either directly or indirectly through an intermediate plant or animal host, vector or the inanimate environment" (Heymann, 2008, p. 704). As long as history has been recorded, communicable diseases have been identified as part of our lives. However, with the turn of the century came a decline in morbidity and mortality due to improved sanitation, implementation of infection control procedures and programs, the development of vaccines to prevent certain illnesses, and the discovery of antibiotics to treat bacterial infections. Along with these developments came a change in the way society and public health authorities viewed communicable diseases. Public health authorities shifted away from a "response and treatment" focus to one with more emphasis on prevention, control, and early detection of outbreaks. Changes in communicable diseases have impacted other societal facets as well, including both tourism and trade. This was evident during the **SARS** outbreak of 2003 when the city of Toronto "shut down" as thousands of people were placed in quarantine and hundreds more were hospitalized. Tourism to the city and the Toronto Stock Exchange (TSX) were significantly impacted at that time. Another example of how communicable diseases affect more than just individual health occurred in Canada and the United Kingdom, where sales of beef were extensively affected by bovine spongiform encephalopathy, or "mad cow disease." Consumers of beef feared acquiring the human form of this disease called new variant **Creutzfeldt-Jakob disease**. Cattle farming provinces in Canada were severely impacted by this emerging disease, while to date only one case has ever been identified in Canada, and that case appeared to have been infected in the U.K. (Public Health Agency of Canada, 2009a; PHAC, 2011).

Communicable diseases occur in every society, from rural areas to cities, in all countries, and without discrimination between rich and poor. With advances in technology and modern medicine, the severity of the illnesses associated with many of these diseases has been reduced. However, with increasing population mobility due to efficient transportation systems, and with lifestyle and environment changes, communicable diseases know no boundaries and are now seen in previously untouched areas across the world. Community health nurses (CHNs) must have a sound knowledge base of communicable diseases in order to prevent or limit the transmission of these diseases and protect the health of the public. This chapter will offer a historical perspective of communicable diseases; the host-agent-environment model; different classification methods, including the nature and types of communicable diseases; and the roles of international, national, provincial or territorial, and local governments. The role of CHNs in the field of communicable diseases will also be discussed in terms of primary, secondary, and tertiary prevention.

# COMMUNICABLE DISEASES: A HISTORICAL PERSPECTIVE

For many centuries, communicable diseases such as tuberculosis (TB), smallpox, leprosy, cholera, scarlet fever, typhoid fever, diphtheria, and poliomyelitis have caused many casualties and threatened the health of humankind. The first recorded worldwide threat from a communicable disease occurred in the 14th century, causing an estimated 50 million deaths. The bubonic plague, also known as the "Black Death," had half of its cases in Africa and Asia and the other half in Europe, where one-quarter of the population succumbed (World Health Organization, 2014a). The influenza pandemic (Spanish flu) in 1918–1919 was a major global threat, resulting in at least 20 million deaths worldwide (Heymann, 2008). Many communicable diseases were brought to Canada with the arrival and migration of early settlers in the 16th century. Since Aboriginals had not had exposure to these diseases, and therefore no opportunity to develop natural immunity, they had

little or no resistance. Aboriginal people were severely affected by the infectious and parasitic diseases carried by the settlers.

Since the mid-1800s, advances in scientific and medical knowledge and in public health measures have contributed to declining mortality and morbidity among Canadians from communicable diseases. The development of microscopes, germ theories, vaccines, and the improvement of nutrition, sanitation, and living conditions have been instrumental in this decline. In 1967, 60% of the world's population was at risk for contracting smallpox. At that time, health professionals from the World Health Organization (WHO) launched the highly successful smallpox eradication program. The last known case of smallpox was in Somalia in 1977, and by 1980 the world was declared smallpox free (WHO, 2010). The documented success of the smallpox eradication program opened up the doors for the WHO's Expanded Program on Immunization in 1974. Initially, the program targeted diphtheria, whooping cough, tetanus, measles, poliomyelitis, and tuberculosis. In 1977, as part of the WHO's strategy to achieve health for all by 2000, global policies for immunization were established with the hope of providing universal immunization for all children by 1990 (WHO, 2013a). By 2010, approximately 85% of infants around the world had received at least three doses of the DTP (diphtheria, tetanus, and polio) vaccine (WHO, 2013a). Most countries have added hepatitis B and haemophilus influenzae type b (Hib) vaccines to their routine infant immunization schedules. The importance of adding pneumococcal conjugate vaccine and rotavirus vaccines is also being recognized (WHO, 2013a). Immunization is accepted as the most successful health intervention. As a result, the Global Vaccine Action Plan (GVAP) was endorsed by 194 member states of the WHO Assembly in May 2012. The GVAP is a framework to improve access to existing vaccines for all people, regardless of where they are born, who they are, and where they live (WHO, 2013b).

Public health professionals continue their efforts to combat infectious diseases, such as malaria, TB, and parasitic diseases, which can cause life-long disabilities and have socioeconomic consequences (WHO, 2009a). As a result of recent developments in vaccine production and disease control, infectious diseases such as TB and influenza now have less of an impact on morbidity and mortality in Canada. However, newly emerging and re-emerging infectious diseases are increasingly challenging the public health system worldwide. Some more recent notifiable infectious diseases in Canada that fit this description are Invasive group A Streptococcus disease, *Clostridium difficile* associated diarrhea, and West Nile virus infection.

When treatment protocols to cure TB were developed in 1948, it was anticipated that the disease would be eradicated by 2000. Ironically, TB has now re-emerged as an increased public health threat because of multi-drug-resistant strains and clients' non-compliance with chemoprophylaxis. TB affects vulnerable populations such as older adults, those with immune deficiencies, many Aboriginal communities, and those that are socioeconomically disadvantaged (Government of Canada, 2014a). Today's global travel and trade, climate change, poverty, inconsistent healthcare resources, the challenges of vector control programs, overuse of antibiotics, and changing lifestyle practices can lead to rapid transmission of infectious diseases. Determinants of health, such as income, education, and housing, have been shown to globally affect the incidence of TB in the Aboriginal and homeless populations, where the incidence of TB is higher than in the general population (PHAC, 2014a).

Due to the availability of vaccines and antiviral drugs, existing diseases, such as influenza, are less of a threat than was true historically. However, the advent of new strains of influenza also taxes the healthcare system during the vaccine development period, with the medical system waiting to obtain strain-specific vaccines for primary prevention. The WHO has become increasingly vigilant with mechanisms for international **disease surveillance**, which has reduced the delay in recognizing global communicable disease threats. One of the very positive outcomes of increased vigilance was demonstrated in the 2009 **H1N1 influenza pandemic**. Unlike SARS, there was a relatively short period between the first cases of the 2009 H1N1 pandemic influenza in Mexico and notification of international public health agencies about the potential threat.

In Canada, in part as a response to the SARS outbreak in 2003, the Government of Canada recognized the need to strengthen Canada's capacity to protect Canadians from infectious diseases and other threats to their health. This resulted in the creation of the Public Health Agency of Canada (PHAC). Established in September 2004, the agency was confirmed as a legal entity in December 2006 (PHAC, 2008).

As mentioned in Chapter 4, Public Health Nursing, the role of the PHAC is to:

- promote health,
- prevent and control chronic diseases and injuries,
- prevent and control infectious diseases,
- prepare for and respond to public health emergencies,
- serve as a central point for sharing Canada's expertise with the rest of the world,
- apply international research and development to Canada's public health programs, and
- strengthen intergovernmental collaboration on public health and facilitate national approaches to public health policy and planning (PHAC, 2014b).

As part of its role, the PHAC publishes a weekly, bilingual, peer-reviewed, open-access online scientific journal called the *Canada Communicable Disease Report* (CCDR). This publication is one way to provide timely and practical information on infectious diseases to clinicians, public health professionals, and policy makers to inform various health interventions in terms of practice; program development, implementation, and evaluation; and policy development (PHAC, 2014c).

# TRANSMISSION OF COMMUNICABLE DISEASES

As previously stated, communicable diseases are illnesses caused by a "specific infectious agent, or its toxic products that arise through transmission of that agent, or its products from an infected person, animal or inanimate source to a susceptible host; either directly or indirectly through an intermediate plant or animal host, vector or the inanimate environment" (Heymann, 2008, p. 704). There are many ways of classifying communicable diseases and the categorization varies depending on the purpose and use for the classifications. One way to classify communicable diseases is by the **epidemiologic triangle**, as discussed in Chapter 11. The epidemiologic triangle is used to describe the dynamics of the **agent, host**, and **environment**. In order for an infectious disease to be acquired, three elements are needed: an infective agent, a susceptible host, and a supportive environment. To prevent the disease, it is necessary to modify one or more of the elements on the corners of the triangle. For example, one could immunize the host, disinfect a room to eliminate the agent, or develop a protective environment by wearing personal protective equipment, like a mask, when caring for a patient with a respiratory infection.

Figure 12.1 displays the different ways in which communicable diseases can be classified. The classification is dependent on what you are using the categories for, and in what setting. For example, in a hospital setting you may want to categorize the disease by its means of transmission, particularly if you are trying to determine which infection control precautions need to be put in place.

A communicable disease may occur as an individual case or a group of cases, known as an outbreak. An **outbreak** occurs when the new cases of a disease exceeds the normal occurrence

| Clinical Characteristics Classification | Microbiologic Classification | Means of Transmission Classification | Reservoir in Nature Classification | Public Health Programs Classification |
|---|---|---|---|---|
| Diarrheal | Bacterial | Contact | Human | Vaccine preventable |
| Respiratory | Viral | Food or water borne | Animals (zoonoses) | Respiratory |
| Central nervous system | Fungal | Air borne | Soil | Enteric, food borne, and water borne |
| Cardiovascular | Parasitic | Vector borne | Water | Sexually transmitted and blood borne |
| Sepsis | Prion | Perinatal | | Zoonotic and vector borne |

**FIGURE 12.1** Classification of Communicable Diseases

during a given period of time. For example, TB and invasive pneumococcal disease are common outbreaks in under-housed populations in winter and spring seasons in Canada. **Endemic** refers to the constant presence of a disease or infectious agent within a given geographic area or population group. For example, malaria is always present in some countries. Occasionally, the occurrence of a disease is in excess of what would normally be expected; this is called an **epidemic**. For instance, while influenza may be a constant presence (endemic), it has the potential to become an epidemic during some times of the year. More rarely, a **pandemic** occurs over a very wide area and usually affects a large proportion of the population (e.g., pandemic [H1N1] 2009 influenza, and acquired immune deficiency syndrome [AIDS]) (Last, 1988). **Syndemic** is an uncommon term, but it is significant in today's emerging changes for infectious diseases. Syndemic refers to the synergistic interaction of two or more coexistent diseases and the resultant excess in burden of disease. This became evident in Canada when AIDS was emerging. As AIDS became more and more prominent, so did the AIDS-indicative disease of TB. TB became a syndemic disease that occurred as a result of an altered immune system, which made human immunodeficiency virus (HIV) persons vulnerable to TB infections, thereby increasing the incidence of TB (Ofner, 1993). This syndemic effect is likely also seen with most sexually transmitted infections, where open sores in the genital area due to one infection makes an individual more susceptible to other sexually transmitted infections they may be exposed to.

"Communicable diseases kill more that 14 million people each year mainly in the developing world. In these countries, approximately 46% of all deaths are due to communicable diseases, and 90% of these deaths are attributed to acute diarrheal and respiratory infections of children, AIDS, tuberculosis, malaria, and measles" (Heymann, 2008, p. 12). Preventing transmission is key to controlling the number of people infected with an organism. Understanding the infectious agent's characteristics is paramount to assisting healthcare personnel to prevent, diagnose, control, and manage a communicable disease. The communicable diseases that are discussed in the following sections have been categorized into the following classifications: (a) vaccine-preventable infections, (b) sexually transmitted and blood-borne infections, (c) enteric, food-borne, and water-borne infections, (d) zoonotic and vector-borne infections, (e) respiratory infections, and (f) healthcare-associated infections. These terms have been used in order to match the Canadian Notifiable Diseases Surveillance System Report.

# VACCINE-PREVENTABLE DISEASES

"The impact of vaccination on the health of the world's people is hard to exaggerate. With the exception of safe water, no other modality, even antibiotics, has had such a major effect on mortality reduction and population growth" (Plotkin & Orenstein, 2008, p. 1). The goal of the immunization program in Canada is the elimination of vaccine-preventable diseases (PHAC, 06a). Smallpox (globally) and poliomyelitis (in developed ries) have been eradicated through successful immunization s. **Measles, mumps, and rubella** have been dramatically

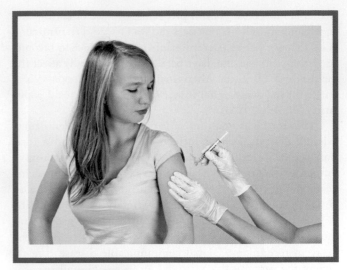

PHOTO 12.1  Girl getting a flu shot

*Source: Elenathewise/Fotolia*

reduced in some countries. **Diphtheria, haemophilus influenzae type b, hepatitis B, human papillomavirus (HPV), influenza,** measles, **meningococcal disease,** mumps, **pertussis, streptococcus pneumoniae (pneumococcus),** poliomyelitis, rubella, **tetanus,** and **varicella** are all vaccine-preventable diseases (see Photo 12.1). The recommended **immunization** for infants and children in Canada is provided in Figure 12.2. Depending on resources and the burden of illness in the specific province, this schedule, developed by the **National Advisory Committee on Immunization (NACI)** and the **Public Health Agency of Canada (PHAC),** can be modified.

New vaccines licensed in Canada since June 2006 include the human papillomavirus (HPV) vaccine and the **rotavirus** vaccine. HPV is mainly transmitted by sexual contact, and the vaccine is available to prevent an infection that occurs years before but is associated with the appearance of cervical cancer. The rotavirus vaccine would decrease rotaviruses consistently involved in acute gastrointestinal illnesses in children. Vaccines against West Nile virus (Drebot & Artsob, 2006) and malaria are also in development. NACI is instrumental in developing guidelines for any newly licensed vaccines in Canada. It also provides general guidelines for the most desirable immunization practices to assist CHNs and other healthcare providers in critically examining their standards of practice related to immunization.

Three additional immunization schedules are available for people not immunized in early infancy, for those aged less than 7, between 7 and 17 years, and those 18 years and older. These schedules can be found in the seventh edition of the Canadian Immunization Guide 2006 (www.naci.gc.ca). Additional vaccines were added to this schedule in 2013, and include the human papillomavirus (HPV) with HPV2 vaccine for girls at months 0, 1, and 6; HP4 vaccine for boys at months 0, 2, and 6; and the rotovirus vaccine (RV) (PHAC, 2014d).

**Herd immunity** is one major public health advantage of a vaccination program. Both the vaccinated and unvaccinated are protected from disease through herd immunity. If one is vaccinated one typically does not contact the disease and hence does not spread it to others. Even when vaccinated people do become ill their symptoms are often milder and, hence, they are

| Age at vaccination | DTaP-IPV | Hib | MMR | Var | HB | Pneu-C-7 | Men-C | Tdap | Inf |
|---|---|---|---|---|---|---|---|---|---|
| Birth | | | | | Infancy 3 doses ★ | | | | |
| 2 months | ⊙ | ✦ | | | | ⧓ | ⊙ | | |
| 4 months | ⊙ | ✦ | | | | ⧓ | (⊙) | | |
| 6 months | ⊙ | ✦ | | | | ⧓ | ⊙ or | | 6–23 months ⊖ 1–2 doses |
| 12 months | | | ■ | ● | or | ⧓ 12–15 months | ⊙ if not yet given | | |
| 18 months | ⊙ | ✦ | ■ | | | | | | |
| 4–6 years | ⊙ | | or ■ | | | | | | |
| 14–16 years | | | | | Pre-teen/teen 2–3 doses | | ⊙ if not yet given | ▲ | |

The following abbreviations are the agreed upon standards for use in Canada:

DTaP-IPV-Hib: diphtheria toxoid, tetanus toxoid, acellular pertussis, polio, *Haemophilus influenzae* type b, pediatric formulation; Tdap: tetanus toxoid, diphtheria toxoid, acellular pertussis, adult formulation; Men – meningococcus; Pneu – pneumococcus; HB: hepatitis B; Chol-Ecol-O: cholera – E.coli

IPV – poliomyelitis vaccine; Inf: influenza; HA: hepatitis A; Rab: rabies; JE: Japanese encephalitis; Typh-I: typhoid – injection; Typh-O: Typhoid – Oral; TBE; tickborne encephalitis

MMR: measles, mumps, rubella; Var: varicella; YF: yellow fever; BCG: Bacilles Calmette-Guérin

**FIGURE 12.2** Canadian Routine Immunization Schedule for Infants and Children

*Source:* The National Advisory Committee on Immunization (NACI). (2006). *Canadian Immunization Guide 2006 – Table 1.*

less likely to spread the infection. In Figure 12.3, the top box represents a group of individuals in which no one is vaccinated and an outbreak occurs. In the middle box, a portion of the population is vaccinated but not enough to give it "herd immunity." The last box represents a population in which a significant enough number of the population is vaccinated, which then protects many of the other members of that population.

# SEXUALLY TRANSMITTED INFECTIONS AND BLOOD-BORNE INFECTIONS

## Sexually Transmitted Infections

**Sexually transmitted infections (STIs)** are infections that are spread through insertive and receptive sexual practices (vaginal, anal, or oral) with an infected person. In addition, some viral STIs such as **genital herpes** and human papillomavirus can be transmitted by intimate skin-to-skin contact (Government of Alberta, 2012).

Different types of sexual activity may result in greater risk of acquisition of an infection. Receptive anal intercourse and vaginal intercourse carry the highest risk of acquiring an STI (Royce, Sena, Cates, & Cohen, 1997). STIs are different from other infections since their risk of acquisition is primarily determined by behavioural factors. STI incidence is highest among adolescents and young adults. **Chlamydia** is the most commonly reported notifiable infection in Canada. From 2000 to 2012, the chlamydia rate increased from 149.7 to 298.7 per 100 000 persons (PHAC, 2014e). Chlamydia may be asymptomatic in up to 70% of females and 1–25% of males. Due to the high frequency of asymptomatic chlamydia infections, the likelihood of participating in unprotected sex will lead to further transmission. Refer to Chapter 31 for more specific information on STIs.

The most important clinical care items for all STIs by CHNs are to reinforce the use of condoms (primary prevention); ensure that screening and diagnostic testing be performed on high-risk, sexually active groups (secondary prevention); and ensure timely and adequate treatment of infections (tertiary prevention). This is significant since some STIs may have pathogens resistant to standard treatment and therefore require additional testing of the laboratory sample. Antimicrobial sensitivity testing would then need to be performed in order to identify the most appropriate antibiotic treatment. One example of this is cephalosporin-resistant gonorrhea.

## Blood-borne Infections

**Blood-borne infections** are infections that are carried and transmitted by blood (PHAC, 2010a). The most common examples of blood-borne infections are **HIV**, hepatitis B, **hepatitis C**, and **viral haemorrhagic fevers**. Diseases that are not usually transmitted directly by blood contact, but rather by insect or some other vector, are more usefully classified as vector-borne diseases, even though the causative agent can be found in blood. Vector-borne diseases will be discussed as a separate category in this chapter.

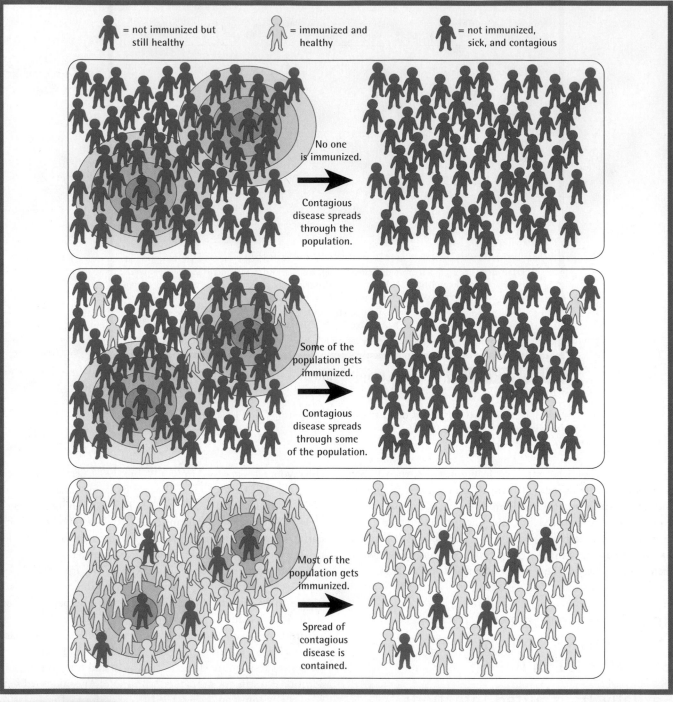

= not immunized but still healthy

= immunized and healthy

= not immunized, sick, and contagious

No one is immunized.

Contagious disease spreads through the population.

Some of the population gets immunized.

Contagious disease spreads through some of the population.

Most of the population gets immunized.

Spread of contagious disease is contained.

**FIGURE** **12.3** Understanding Herd Immunity

*Source:* From *Community immunity ("herd" immunity)*. National Institute of Allergy and Infectious Diseases. Copyright © 2013 by U.S. Department of Health and Human Services. Used by permission of U.S. Department of Health and Human Services.

As our scientific knowledge and surveillance abilities have increased, potential indirect contact modes of transmission in some diseases have been identified, such as donor organs and blood products that are transplanted or transfused. Changes to screening practices were subsequently made to organ and blood donor screening and testing practices as well as the clinical use of donated organs and blood. **Canadian Blood Services** (2009) now screens all blood products for \_\_\_wn infectious diseases, such as HIV, **syphilis**, hepatitis B \_\_ and **West Nile virus**. Please refer to Chapter 31 for \_\_\_ormation about blood-borne pathogens.

A more recent concern among the blood-borne pathogens has been the 2014 outbreak of Ebola in West Africa. The WHO reports as follows:

The Ebola virus causes an acute, serious illness which is often fatal if untreated. The current outbreak in West Africa, (first cases notified in March 2014), is the largest and most complex Ebola outbreak since the Ebola virus was first discovered in 1976. There have been more cases and deaths in this outbreak than all others combined. It has also spread between countries starting in Guinea then spreading across land borders to Sierra

Leone and Liberia, by air (one traveller only) to Nigeria, and by land (one traveller) to Senegal. On August 8, the WHO Director-General declared this outbreak a Public Health Emergency of International Concern.

It is thought that fruit bats of the Pteropodidae family are natural Ebola virus hosts. Ebola is introduced into the human population through close contact with the blood, secretions, organs or other bodily fluids of infected animals such as chimpanzees, gorillas, fruit bats, monkeys, forest antelope and porcupines found ill or dead or in the rainforest.

Ebola then spreads through human-to-human transmission via direct contact (through broken skin or mucous membranes) with the blood, secretions, organs or other bodily fluids of infected people, and with surfaces and materials (e.g. bedding, clothing) contaminated with these fluids.

Healthcare workers have frequently been infected while treating patients with suspected or confirmed EVD. This has occurred through close contact with patients when infection control precautions are not strictly practiced. (WHO, 2014b)

# ENTERIC, FOOD, AND WATER-BORNE INFECTIONS

## Enteric Infections

**Enteric infections** are infections that enter the body through the mouth and intestinal tract (Centers for Disease Control and Prevention, 2013a). This primarily occurs through eating, drinking, and digesting contaminated foods or liquids. Direct contact with contaminated feces or vomit is a secondary method of acquiring an infection. Infections acquired through ingestion of food are called food-borne infections and those by water are called water-borne infections. Infections acquired through feces are enteric infections acquired through person-to-person or contaminated object-to-person transmission. An example would be a hepatitis A infection. Hepatitis A is typically acquired through the ingestion of fecal contaminated food or water sources. Examples include ingesting raw or undercooked shellfish from contaminated waters (polluted with sewage), drinking contaminated water, and eating food that has been in contact with a contaminated food handler (i.e., someone who does not wash his or her hands after using the washroom).

## Food-borne Infection and Food-borne Intoxication

**Food-borne infection** and **food-borne intoxication** are illnesses acquired through the consumption of contaminated food. Riemann and Cliver (2006) noted that *infections* occur when people consume food containing pathogenic microorganisms, which multiply in the gastrointestinal tract; *intoxications* occur when bacteria multiply in food and produce a toxin that is poisonous to the person ingesting the food. The most common causes of food-borne illnesses include the following:

- toxins released by bacterial growth in food before consumption (e.g., *Clostridium botulism*, *Staphylococcus aureus*, and *Bacillus cereus*) or in the intestines (*Clostridium perfringens*);
- bacterial, viral, or parasitic infections (brucellosis, campylobacter enteritis, diarrhea caused by Escherichia coli, hepatitis A, listeriosis, salmonellosis, shigellosis, toxoplasmosis, viral gastroenteritis, trichinosis); and
- toxins produced by harmful algal species (shellfish poisoning).

Food-borne infections can usually be recognized by illness that occurs within a variable but usually short time frame after a meal. **Food-borne outbreaks** are identified when illness presents among individuals who have consumed common foods. For example, a community food-borne outbreak of E. coli O157:H7 was identified in 2008 in Ontario, when over 350 persons who all consumed food from the same fast-food establishment became ill. Fifty persons in this outbreak had lab-confirmed disease (North Bay Parry Sound District Health Unit, 2009). Food-borne outbreaks can be community-based or have a much more widespread impact depending on food distribution patterns. For example, a food-borne outbreak with national impact occurred in 2008 when listeria was associated with contaminated meat. Another food-borne outbreak with provincial impact occurred in 2005 in Ontario when bean sprouts were found to be associated with salmonella disease. Thorough and prompt collection and testing of implicated foods is essential, as is laboratory testing of stool samples obtained from cases. Many cases are often unreported to health authorities, and outbreaks are often unrecognized.

Food-borne diseases can be prevented and controlled by (a) avoiding food contamination, (b) destroying contaminants (e.g., meat irradiation is one option), and (c) eliminating spread or multiplication of the contaminants. Ultimately, prevention rests on educating food handlers about proper practices in cooking and storage of food and personal hygiene. This includes (a) keeping clean, (b) separating raw and cooked, (c) cooking thoroughly, (d) keeping food at safe temperatures, and (e) using safe water and raw materials (WHO, 2009b).

## Water-borne Diseases

**Water-borne pathogens** usually enter water supplies through fecal contamination from animals or humans to cause enteric illnesses (e.g., cholera, typhoid fever, dysentery, some types of salmonella, shigellosis, vibrio, and various coliform bacteria including E. coli O157:H7). An **outbreak of water-borne disease** is usually defined as two cases that are epidemiologically linked by time, location of water exposure, and that experience similar symptoms after consuming water from a common source (CDC, 2013b). Municipal water systems that have appropriate filtration and chlorination have decreased diseases such as amebic dysentery and giardiasis. Effective filtration devices are needed for control of protozoa because they do not respond to traditional chlorine treatment because do enteric and coliform bacteria. Outbreaks of cryptosporidium in North Battleford, Saskatchewan (PHAC, 2001), and E. coli in Walkerton, Ontario (PHAC, 2000), have raised awareness of the importance of safe municipal water systems across Canada. Public health inspectors and public health nurses work closely with the local medical officer of health to investigate, track, and determine linkages between cases. Provincial databases such as the integrated Public Health Information System (PHAC, 2007a) allow tracking of disease occurrence and its source, if known.

## Parasitic Diseases

**Parasitic diseases** are categorized with enteric infections since the primary mode of transmission in Canada typically is water and secondarily is person-to-person spread through contaminated feces. When associated with water, they tend to be acquired by drinking from unfiltered surface-water sources or shallow wells, or swimming in bodies of fresh water. Large community outbreaks have occurred from drinking treated but unfiltered water. Smaller outbreaks have resulted from contaminated food, person-to-person transmission in daycare centres, and contaminated recreational waters (including swimming and wading pools). An outbreak in 1993 of cryptosporidiosis occurred in the Kitchener-Waterloo area of Ontario, and was believed to have affected between 23 900 and 100 000 residents. These residents were drinking from the municipal water system that likely was contaminated by the stools of cattle that during an unusually large rain season leached into rivers that fed the city's water treatment plant. Large supplies of water were pushed through the water system too quickly to allow time for the larger cryptosporidial oocysts to settle, and traditional chlorine disinfection likely did not work. This resulted in the oocysts entering the city's water supply. Residents of the city who used that water supply as their source became ill while other residents who had other sources for their water supply did not become ill.

## ZOONOTIC AND VECTOR-BORNE DISEASES

## Zoonotic Infections

**Zoonotic infections** are diseases transmissible between animals and humans; however, they do not need humans to maintain their life cycles. Transmission occurs by bites, inhalation, ingestion, direct contact, and arthropod intermediaries. Rabies, hantavirus pulmonary syndrome, salmonellosis, listeriosis, and brucellosis are examples of zoonotic diseases.

## Rabies

**Rabies** has the highest case-fatality rate of any known human infection—essentially 100%. In 2013, the major carriers of rabies in Canada were bats, foxes, and skunks (Government of Canada, 2014b). The virus is transmitted through a bite, scratch, or pre-existing open wound, and attacks the central nervous system (Government of Canada, 2014b). The best prevention is the vaccination of animals against rabies and pre-exposure vaccination of animal workers. **Post-exposure prophylaxis (PEP)** is available after an exposure and occurs in consultation with public health officials. Determination of the need for

follow-up by a CHN requires critical assessment of the endemic rates. For example, an animal exposure in Newfoundland would require further investigation to determine the history of the animal's habitation, since rabies is not usually present in the animal population in Newfoundland. Rabies could be introduced by an animal brought from, or that migrated from, a rabies-endemic area. An exposure in eastern Ontario, where raccoon rabies is prevalent, would require follow-up. Often CHNs recommend or administer rabies immune globulin (RIG), with the dosage calculation based on client weight, with a series of rabies vaccine. The animal, if located, should be kept in a confined area for a period of 10 days in order to determine if the animal was infectious with rabies at the time of the exposure. Most infected animals will succumb to rabies within a five-day period, but 10 days is used to avoid any possible exceptions. If the animal exhibits signs and symptoms of rabies or dies during the isolation period, the exposed person is started on PEP as soon as possible. If the animal is deceased immediately following the exposure, rabies testing of brain tissue is conducted at a national laboratory and the exposed individual is offered PEP based on the findings. If a client is started on PEP and animal testing indicates that the rabies virus was not present, the PEP can be stopped prior to completion (PHAC, 2006a).

## Hantavirus

**Hantavirus** is a viral disease found in the droppings, urine, and saliva of infected rodents, and humans can contact the virus from breathing in airborne particles or from being bitten. In Canada, although the risk of exposure is low, when it happens, the disease can be very severe (Government of Canada, 2014b). Humans can inhale the virus, which may lead to hantavirus pulmonary syndrome (HPS). The earliest documented case of HPS in Canada was contracted in Alberta in 1989 (Alberta Health Services, 2012). Since then, there have been over 70 confirmed cases. Most of the cases occurred in western Canada (Manitoba, Saskatchewan, Alberta, and British Columbia). Hantavirus infections contracted by Canadians outside the country have also been recognized, including two fatal cases from South America (PHAC, 2009b). HPS is extremely serious, since 38% of cases are fatal (Alberta Health Services, 2012). Primary prevention strategies taken by those at risk, such as workers in agricultural or rural settings or hikers and campers, include keeping woodpiles away from dwellings, keeping items off the floor to prevent rodent nesting, trapping rodents, wet-mopping areas where droppings are located to prevent aeration of feces, and not camping near rodent-infected areas.

## Vector-borne Infections

**Vector-borne infections** are caused by viruses, bacteria, and parasites that living creatures carry and pass on to other living creatures. Disease carriers, called "vectors," are usually mosquitoes, ticks, and mammals. For example, mosquitoes carry the infectious agents that cause malaria (see Photo 12.2) and West Nile virus. Other vector-borne diseases include Lyme disease, avian influenza, and rabies (British Columbia

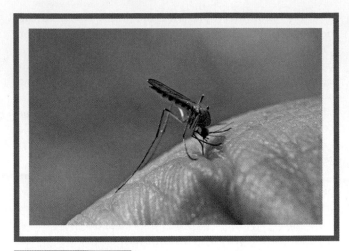

PHOTO 12.2 Mosquito biting skin

Source: Matauw/Fotolia

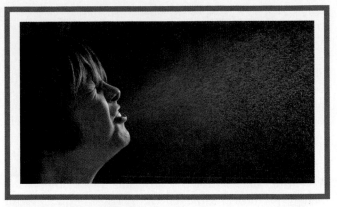

PHOTO 12.3 Respiratory secretion spread when sneezing

Source: Maartje van Caspel/E+/Getty Images

Ministry of Health, n.d.). Climate change has a potential impact on the distribution of various diseases. Vector-borne diseases most commonly seen in Canada include Eastern equine encephalitis, Lyme disease, and West Nile virus.

## Lyme Disease

**Lyme disease** is transmitted by black-legged ticks carried by migratory birds, mice, squirrels, rodents, and other small animals that can carry the bacterium. While black-legged ticks (also called deer ticks) can be found in all areas of Canada, only about 10% are infected with Lyme disease. Areas of concern include parts of southern Ontario, Lunenburg County in Nova Scotia, and parts of southern British Columbia. Malaria and dengue fever, also vector-borne diseases, are seen in travellers who have contracted these diseases in other countries from the bite of an infected mosquito.

## West Nile Virus

West Nile virus (WNV) is carried and spread by mosquitoes. WNV can cause severe neurological complications. Personal protection against this vector and reducing areas where mosquitoes breed are important in its control.

## DISEASES TRANSMITTED BY RESPIRATORY ROUTES

In a large percentage of patients with acute respiratory infections, the causative organism is not known. Most infections within the respiratory system are caused by viruses. Bacteria are another source of acute respiratory infections, but at a lesser frequency. Typically, upper viral respiratory infections are caused by rhinoviruses (30–50%) or coronaviruses (5–20%). The remaining infections (30–65%) are due to influenza viruses, parainfluenza viruses, respiratory syncytial virus, adenoviruses, and certain enteroviruses (Berman et al., 1983; Reed, 1981).

## Influenza

Human influenza is a respiratory infection caused by influenza virus and is spread by droplets through coughing or sneezing (see Photo 12.3). Vaccination against influenza lasts four to six months, and is routinely given on an annual basis at the onset of the influenza season, typically starting in October or November. Each year the influenza vaccine contains three influenza strains predicted by WHO to be the most common circulating strains. Due to the significant morbidity, mortality, and societal costs associated with influenza, vaccinations are recommended for everyone six months or older, especially those with chronic illness; people aged 65 and over; residents in chronic care and nursing homes; healthcare service providers; and pregnant women (PHAC, 2014f). The spread of **avian influenza H5N1** (or bird flu) throughout Southeast Asia and Europe had generated much discussion on the implications for human health. However, in April 2009 a novel strain of influenza H1N1 was recognized in Mexico, causing a cluster of illness with the potential to become a pandemic. On June 11, 2009, the WHO raised the pandemic alert level to 6, indicating that a novel strain of influenza was rapidly spreading from human to human and across international jurisdictions. Globally, many nations declared an influenza pandemic. This event moved public health activity from the planning phase to action at local, provincial, and federal levels throughout Canada.

## Tuberculosis

In Canada, **tuberculosis (TB)** statistics are collected nationally through the Canadian Tuberculosis Reporting System (CTBRS). In 2011, there were 1607 new active and re-treatment TB cases. The incidence rate of TB has been declining over the past decade, with a low overall rate of 4.7 per 100 000 population. Canada's provinces with the largest populations—British Columbia, Ontario, and Quebec—have the largest total number of TB cases, representing 70% of TB cases. In 2011 TB was also disproportionately distributed among specific sub-populations, with 67% of all cases occurring among foreign-born individuals, 19% among Canadian-born Aboriginals, 12% among Canadian-born non-Aboriginals, and 2% with unknown origins (Public Health Agency of Canada, 2014a).

**Pulmonary TB** accounts for 68% of the reported cases, followed by TB of the peripheral lymph nodes at 11%. Drug resistance to traditional treatment has been seen in 8% of the Canadian cases, with 7% monoresistant and 1% having resistance to two or more drugs with no cases of extensively drug-resistant TB (XDR-TB) reported in 2008.

Community health nurses caring for patients with pulmonary tuberculosis need to adhere to strict infection prevention and control practices and direct observation therapy protocols. Although the PHAC "Guidelines for preventing the transmission of tuberculosis in Canadian healthcare facilities and other institutional settings" (1996) is old, the procedures remain the same. A more recent and full description of the care of patients with TB, including diagnosis, treatment, and prevention, is included in the Ontario Lung Association report entitled "Tuberculosis: Information for Health Care Professionals" (4th edition), available for download at www.on.lung.ca.

# HEALTHCARE-ACQUIRED AND HEALTHCARE-ASSOCIATED INFECTIONS

**Healthcare-associated (HCA) infections**, such as Methicillin-resistant *Staphylococcus aureus* (MRSA), are acquired as a result of being admitted to or attending a healthcare facility where exposure can take place. HCA infections typically occur in patients who are admitted to hospital, but others who visit or work within the facility may also be susceptible to such infections. For example, HCA infections can be acquired through outpatient clinics or healthcare facility day treatment programs (e.g., dialysis clinic, doctors' office visit, or outpatient cancer treatments).

Effective **surveillance systems, infection-control programs,** and education for nurses in hospitals and community settings, including long-term care homes, are essential in controlling the spread of infections to vulnerable clients. Screening patients who are at risk for healthcare-acquired infections will ensure early identification and appropriate infection control procedures, and mitigate transmission to other patients. Typical healthcare-associated organisms are either identified as a colonization or an infection. **A colonized patient** is one who is colonized with the organism but shows no signs or symptoms of infection. This type of person, if swabbed (a specimen sample is taken from the nose, rectum, or peritoneal area), it grows the organism. Colonized patients are treated with appropriate medication as if they had an infection. Colonized and **infected patients** may receive similar care including more stringent **infection control practices**, being put in isolation, or cohorted with other similar patients, and appropriate treatment.

**Hand hygiene** is the most effective way of preventing the spread of healthcare-associated infections by direct contact with hands, surfaces, or objects that have been contaminated by an infected person. Routine precautions are taught and their use encouraged by all healthcare faculty employees. Nurses in particular need to be vigilant since they are the healthcare professionals with the most "hands-on" time with patients and, therefore, more likely to transmit or acquire these types of organisms.

The four priority antibiotic-resistant organisms found within hospitals in Canada are **Methicillin-resistant *Staphylococcus aureus* (MRSA)**, vancomycin-resistant *enterococci* **(VRE)**, *Clostridium difficile*, and carbapenamase-producing organisms (e.g., enterobacteriaceae). The **Canadian Nosocomial Infection Surveillance Program (CNISP)** monitors healthcare-associated infections within **sentinel hospitals** throughout Canada (PHAC, 2007b). CNISP was established in 1994, with the overall objective of providing rates and trends of healthcare-associated infections at Canadian healthcare facilities, thus enabling comparison of rates (benchmarks) and provision of data that can be used in the development of national guidelines on clinical issues related to healthcare-associated infections. At present, 54 sentinel hospitals from 10 provinces participate in the CNISP network (PHAC, 2012a).

The practice of infection control and familiarity with infection control policies and practices within facilities are essential for CHNs. Nurses are at the front line of defence against transmission. Using routine precautions with every patient prevents transmission of organisms that cause infections. This figure is a summary of the elements of routine infection prevention and control practices. The Public Health Agency of Canada has developed additional **guidelines** for infection control and prevention listed in Table 12.1. These guidelines are listed in Table 12.1 and can be found at http://publications.gc.ca/collections/collection_2013/aspc-phac/HP40-83-2013-eng.pdf.

| Table 12.1 | **List of Infection Prevention and Control Guidelines Currently Available** |
|---|---|

**Public Health Agency of Canada Guidelines for Infection Prevention and Control**

- Routine Practices and Additional Precautions for Preventing the Transmission of Infection in Healthcare Settings (2013)
- *Clostridium difficile* Infection—Infection Prevention and Control Guidance for Management in Long-term Care Facilities **(New: January 2013)**
- *Clostridium difficile* Infection—Infection Prevention and Control Guidance for Management in Acute Care Settings **(New: January 2013)**
- Seasonal Influenza—Infection Prevention and Control Guidance for Management in Home Care Settings **(New: December 2013)**

| Table 12.1 | Continued |
| --- | --- |

- Infection Prevention and Control Guideline for Flexible Gastrointestinal Endoscopy and Flexible Bronchoscopy
- Guidance: Infection Prevention and Control Measures for Healthcare Workers in Acute Care and Long-term Care Settings for Seasonal Influenza (2010)
- Guidance: Infection Prevention and Control Measures for Healthcare Workers in All Healthcare Settings—Carbapenem-resistant Gram-negative Bacilli (2010)
- Infection Prevention and Control Guidelines for the Prevention of Healthcare Associated Pneumonia (2010)
- Essential Resources for Effective Infection Prevention and Control Programs: A Matter of Patient Safety—A Discussion Paper (2010)
- Classic Creutzfeldt-Jakob Disease in Canada, Quick Reference Guide (2007)
- Classic Creutzfeldt-Jakob Disease in Canada (2002)
- Advisory Notice: Infection Control for Creutzfeldt-Jakob Disease (1996)
- Foot Care by Health Care Providers (1997)
- Hand Washing, Cleaning, Disinfection and Sterilization in Health Care (1998)
- Preventing Infections Associated with Indwelling Intravascular Access Devices (1997)
- Construction-related Nosocomial Infections in Patients in Health Care Facilities (2001)
- Prevention and Control of Occupational Infections in Health Care (2002)
- Guidelines for Preventing the Transmission of Tuberculosis in Canadian Health Care Facilities and Other Institutional Settings (1996)

CHNs should become familiar with the different infection control and prevention guidelines, and utilize the ones that are most appropriate in their scope of practice. "The Routine Practices and Additional Precautions for Preventing the Transmission of Infection in Healthcare Settings, 2012" (PHAC, 2012b) publication should be the foundation for all interactions within the healthcare system (Figure 12.4). Figure 12.5 displays the elements

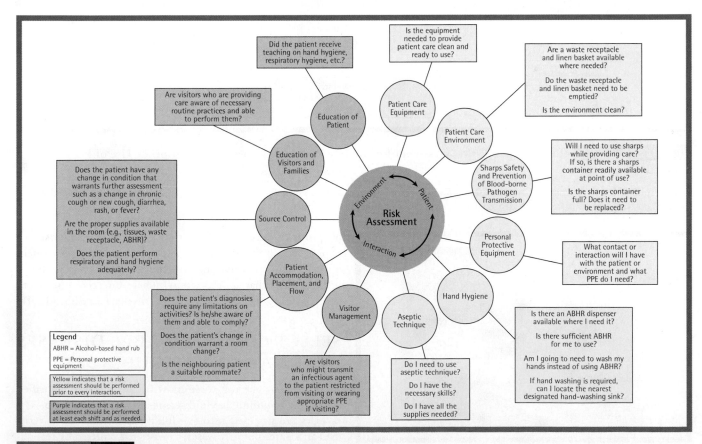

**FIGURE 12.4** Elements of Routine Practices Summary

*Source:* Public Health Agency of Canada. (2012). *Routine practices and additional precautions assessment and educational tools.* Reproduced with permission from the Minister of Health, 2015. © All rights reserved.

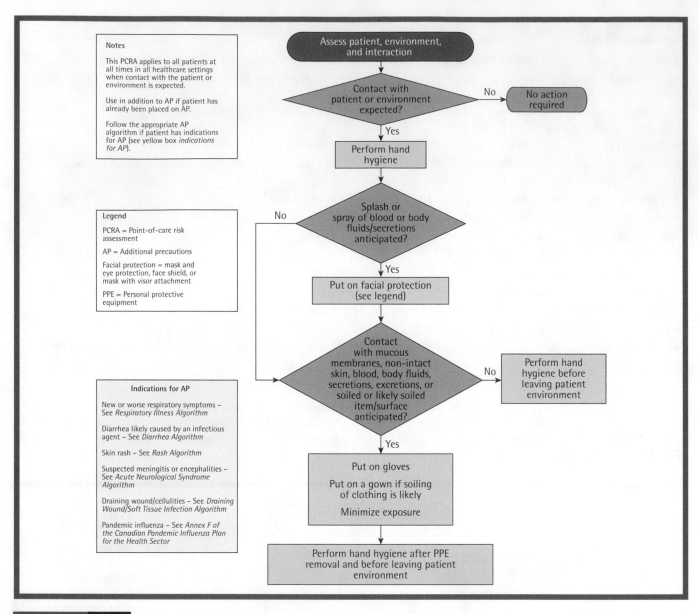

**Notes**

This PCRA applies to all patients at all times in all healthcare settings when contact with the patient or environment is expected.

Use in addition to AP if patient has already been placed on AP.

Follow the appropriate AP algorithm if patient has indications for AP (see yellow box *indications for AP*).

**Legend**

PCRA = Point-of-care risk assessment

AP = Additional precautions

Facial protection = mask and eye protection, face shield, or mask with visor attachment

PPE = Personal protective equipment

**Indications for AP**

New or worse respiratory symptoms – See *Respiratory Illness Algorithm*

Diarrhea likely caused by an infectious agent – See *Diarrhea Algorithm*

Skin rash – See *Rash Algorithm*

Suspected meningitis or encephalities – See *Acute Neurological Syndrome Algorithm*

Draining wound/cellulities – See *Draining Wound/Soft Tissue Infection Algorithm*

Pandemic influenza – See *Annex F of the Canadian Pandemic Influenza Plan for the Health Sector*

**FIGURE** **12.5** Point-of-Care Risk Assessment for Routine Practices Algorithm: Appropriate Use of Personal Protective Equipment

*Source:* Public Health Agency of Canada. (2012). *Routine practices and additional precautions assessment and educational tools.* Reproduced with permission from the Minister of Health, 2015. © All rights reserved.

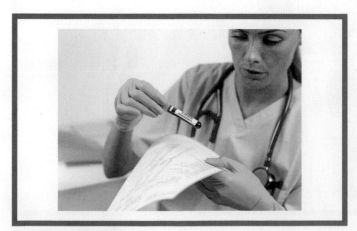

**PHOTO** **12.4** Using Personal Protective Equipment

*Source: Tek Image/Science Source*

of "**point-of-care**" **practice**, in which every encounter with a patient within the healthcare system entitles a risk assessment of the patient, the environment, and the interaction within it to determine what appropriate personal protective equipment (e.g., gloves, gowns, masks, etc.) are needed (see Photo 12.4).

## SELECT COMMUNICABLE DISEASES IN CANADA BY GROUPINGS

In Table 12.2, the top three most frequent newly identified (incidence) communicable diseases are listed by group. The diseases are grouped into the following categories: enteric, food and water-borne diseases; diseases transmitted by respiratory routes; healthcare-acquired infections; vaccine-preventable diseases; sexually transmitted and blood-borne pathogens; and zoonotic and vector-borne diseases.

| Table 12.2 | Select Communicable Diseases in Canada | | | | | |
|---|---|---|---|---|---|---|
| Disease | Infectious Agent | Mode of Transmission | Incubation Period | Clinical Presentation | Period of Communicability | Control Measures |
| **Enteric, Food- and Water-borne Diseases** | | | | | | |
| 12.2.1 CAMPYLO-BACTER ENTERITIS or CAMPYLO-BACTERIOSIS | *Campylobacter jejuni* and less commonly *Campylobacter coli* | Ingestion of the organisms in undercooked meat, particularly poultry, other contaminated food and water, or raw milk; and from contact with infected pets, farm animals, or infected infants. Person-to-person transmission appears to be uncommon. | Usually 2–5 days, with a range of 1–10 days, depending on dose ingested. | An acute zoonotic bacterial enteric disease of variable severity characterized by diarrhea, abdominal pain, malaise, fever, nausea, and/or vomiting. | Throughout the course of infection; usually several days to several weeks. | Isolation: enteric precautions for hospitalized patients. Concurrent disinfection: cleaning of areas and articles soiled with stools. |
| 12.2.2 SALMONELLOSIS | Nearly all *Salmonella* isolated from ill persons are serotypes of *S. enterica* subsp. *enterica*. Approximately 2500 serotypes of *Salmonella* have been identified. | Ingestion of the organism in food derived from infected animals, or contaminated by feces of an infected animal or person. | From 6 to 72 hours, usually about 12 to 36 hours. | A bacterial disease commonly manifested by acute enterocolitis, with sudden onset of headache, abdominal pain, diarrhea, nausea, and sometimes vomiting. | Throughout the course of infection, extremely variable, usually several days to several weeks. | Proper hand washing should be stressed. Enteric precautions when handling feces and contaminated clothing and bed linen: – concurrent disinfection of feces and articles soiled therewith – culture stools of household contacts and those who are involved in food handling, direct patient care, or care for young children or elderly people in institutional settings |

*(continued)*

**Table 12.2** Continued

| Disease | Infectious Agent | Mode of Transmission | Incubation Period | Clinical Presentation | Period of Communicability | Control Measures |
|---|---|---|---|---|---|---|
| 12.2.3 GIARDIASIS | *Giardia lamblia* (*G. intestinalis, G. duodenalis*), a fragellate protozoan | Person-to-person transmission occurs by hand-to-mouth transfer of cysts from the feces of an infected individual, especially in institutions and daycare centres. This is probably the principal mode of spread. Anal intercourse also facilitates transmission. | Usually 3–25 days or longer; median 7–10 days. | A protozoan infection, principally of the upper small intestine, it can (a) remain asymptomatic; (b) bring on acute, self-limited diarrhea; and (c) lead to intestinal symptoms such as chronic diarrhea, steatorrhea, abdominal cramps, bloating, frequent loose and pale greasy stools, fatigue, malabsorption (of fats and fat-soluble vitamins), and weight loss. | Entire period of infection, often months. | Enteric precautions: – concurrent disinfection of feces and articles soiled therein – microscopic examination of feces of household members and other suspected contacts, especially if symptomatic |

**Diseases Transmitted by the Respiratory Route**

| Disease | Infectious Agent | Mode of Transmission | Incubation Period | Clinical Presentation | Period of Communicability | Control Measures |
|---|---|---|---|---|---|---|
| 12.2.4 INVASIVE PNEUMOCOCCAL DISEASE OR PNEUMOCOCCAL PNEUMONIA | *Streptococcus pneumoniae* (pneumococcus) | Droplet spread. Person-to-person transmission of the organisms in common but illness among casual contacts and attendants is infrequent. | Not well determined; may be as short as 1–3 days. Infection is thought to be preceded by asymptomatic colonization. | Include sudden onset, high fever, rigors, pleuritic, chest pain, dyspnea, tachypnea, and cough productive of "rusty" sputum. | Presumably until discharges of mouth and nose no longer contain sufficient numbers of pneumococci, which usually occurs within 24 hours of initiation of effective antibiotic therapy. | Respiratory isolation may be warranted for hospitalized patients with highly antibiotic-resistant infection, who may transmit it to patients of high risk of pneumococcal disease. Hand hygiene and cough etiquette. No practical value to investigation of contacts or source of the infection. |
| 12.2.5 INVASIVE GROUP A STREPTOCOCCAL DISEASE | Group A Beta-hemolytic Streptococci | Large respiratory droplets or direct contact with patients or carriers, extremely rarely through indirect contact through objects. | Short, usually 1–3 days, rarely longer. | Clinical presentation varies and depends on where the invasive disease occurs. Examples of the types of invasive disease include streptococcal toxic shock syndrome (STSS), necrotizing fasciitis (NF), pneumonia, and bacteremia. Symptoms will vary depending on primary site of infection. | In untreated, uncomplicated cases, 10–21 days; in untreated conditions with purulent discharges, weeks or months. With adequate penicillin treatment, transmissibility of group A streptococcal disease generally ends in 24 hours. | Disinfection of purulent discharges and all articles soiled therewith. Terminal cleaning. Critical assessment of adherence to infection control practices should be undertaken in group A streptococcal outbreaks in facilities housing highly vulnerable populations (e.g., nursing homes and acute and long-term rehabilitation facilities). |

| Table 12.2 | Continued | | | | |
|---|---|---|---|---|---|
| **Disease** | **Infectious Agent** | **Mode of Transmission** | **Incubation Period** | **Clinical Presentation** | **Period of Communicability** | **Control Measures** |
| | | | | | Drainage and secretion precautions may be terminated after 24 hours effective antibiotic therapy. | |
| 12.2.6 PULMONARY TUBERCULOSIS (TB, TB DISEASE) | *Mycobacterium tuberculosis* | Exposure to tubercle bacilli in airborne, aerosolized droplet nuclei, that measure 1–3 microns in diameter, and are produced by persons with pulmonary or high respiratory tract tuberculosis (e.g., laryngeal) during forceful expiratory efforts (e.g., coughing, singing, or sneezing). The droplet nuclei are inhaled by a vulnerable contact into the pulmonary alveoli. Here, the aerosolized particles containing *M. tuberculosis* are ingested by alveolar macrophages, initiating a new infection. | Two to 10 weeks from infection to demonstrable primary lesion or significant TB skin test (TST) reaction and positivity of interferon-gamma release assays (IGRA). Latent infection may persist for a lifetime. | Cough, fatigue, fever, night sweats, weight loss, and pleuritic pain are common signs and symptoms associated with pulmonary TB disease. Most children (less than 5 years) with TB are asymptomatic at presentation. Older children and adolescents are more likely to experience adult-type disease and often present with a classic triad of fever, night sweats, and weight loss. Degree of communicability depends on number of bacilli discharged, virulence of bacilli, adequacy of ventilation, exposure of bacilli to sun or UV light, and opportunities for aerosolization through coughing, sneezing, talking, or singing or during aerosolized procedures. | Theoretically, as long as viable tubercle bacilli are discharged in the sputum. Effective antimicrobial chemotherapy usually eliminates communicability within 2–4 weeks.<br><br>Effective antimicrobial chemoprophylaxis usually eliminates communicability within 2–4 weeks. | Isolation until antibiotic treatment of a minimum of 2 weeks has been completed.<br><br>Contact tracing and TB skin testing of all vulnerable contacts.<br><br>Screening with tuberculin testing/x-rays among the at-risk populations.<br><br>Provide adequate anti-TB chemotherapy and prophylactic treatments.<br><br>Patients in a congregated setting should be placed in airborne infection isolation rooms with negative pressure ventilation. Persons entering the room should wear N95 face respirators.<br><br>Hand washing and good housekeeping practices must be maintained according to policy.<br><br>Recently, with the emergence of highly drug-resistant forms of TB (MDR-TB, XDR-TB), quarantine measures may be warranted to enforce isolation.<br><br>Investigation of potentially exposed contacts is recommended at the time of diagnosis. TST or IGRA tests for all household members and other close contacts are recommended. |

*(continued)*

| Table 12.2 | Continued | | | | | |
|---|---|---|---|---|---|---|
| **Disease** | **Infectious Agent** | **Mode of Transmission** | **Incubation Period** | **Clinical Presentation** | **Period of Communicability** | **Control Measures** |
| **Vaccine-Preventable Diseases** | | | | | | |
| 12.2.7 CHICKENPOX/ HERPES ZOSTER (varicella) | Varicella-zoster virus | Airborne through respiratory secretions or direct or indirect contact from vesicle fluid of person with varicella-zoster. | 10–21 days | Low-grade fever, maculopapular rash on trunk, face, scalp, mucous membrane of mouth, then changes to vesicular for 3–4 days. Herpes zoster is a local manifestation of reactivation of latent varicella infection in the dorsal root ganglia. | From 2–5 days before onset of rash and until skin lesions have crusted. | Exclude from childcare, school, work, and public places at least 5 days until all vesicles become crusted. Avoid contact with immunosuppressed persons. Varicella-zoster immunoglobulin (IG) within 96 hours of exposure in susceptible close contacts of cases. |
| 12.2.8 MEASLES (Rubeola, Hard measles, Red measles, Morbilli) | Measles virus, a member of the genus Morbillivirus of the family paramyxoviridae | Airborne by droplet spread, or direct contact with nasal or throat secretions of infected persons; less commonly by articles freshly soiled with nose and throat secretions. Measles is one of the most highly communicable infectious diseases. | About 10 days, but may be 7–18 days from exposure to onset of fever, usually 14 days until rash appears; rarely, as long as 19–21 days. | Prodromal fever, conjunctivitis, coryza, cough, and small spots with white or bluish-white centres on an erythematous base on the buccal mucosa (Koplik spots). A characteristic red blotchy rash appears on the 3rd to 7th day; the rash begins on the face, then becomes generalized, lasts 4–7 days, and sometimes ends in brawny desquamation. Leukopenia is common. The disease is more severe in infants and adults than in children. | From 1 day before the beginning of the prodromal period (usually about 4 days before rash onset). | Children should be kept out of school for 4 days after the appearance of the rash. Immunization of contacts previously not immunized within 72 hours of exposure. |
| 12.2.9 INFLUENZA | Influenza A, B, and C viruses | Large droplet is the primary means of transmission through coughing and sneezing by infected person. | Average 2 days (range 1–4). | Fever, cough (usually dry), headache, myalgia, prostration, coryza, and sore throat. | In adults, 3–5 days and in children 7–10 days. | Education about basic personal hygiene (hand hygiene). Yearly immunization for the immunocompromised, those with chronic conditions, the |

| | **Table 12.2** | **Continued** | | | |
|---|---|---|---|---|---|
| **Disease** | **Infectious Agent** | **Mode of Transmission** | **Incubation Period** | **Clinical Presentation** | **Period of Communicability** | **Control Measures** |
| | | | | | | elderly, and those who might spread infection (health personnel). |
| | | | | | | Antivirals available to the unimmunized and to residents in institutions. |
| | | | | | | Cohort ill persons from well persons in institutions and at home, if possible. |
| **Sexually Transmitted Infections and Blood-Borne Pathogens** | | | | | | |
| 12.2.10 CHLAMYDIA (genital infections) | *Chlamydia trachomatis* | Sexual intercourse | Poorly defined, probably 7–14 days or longer | In males primarily as a urethritis, this includes moderate or scanty macropurdent discharge, urethral itching, and burning on urination. In females as a cervical infection, with symptoms that include mucopurulent endocervical discharge with edema, erythema, and easily induced endocervical bleeding. | Unknown-infected individuals presumed to be infectious. Without treatment, infections can persist for months. Relapses are probably common. | Health and sex education. Presumptive treatment of sexual partners. Clients encouraged to wear condoms during intercourse. |
| 12.2.11 HEPATITIS B | Hepatitis B virus (HBV) | Sexual, perinatal, and percutaneous exposure through blood, serum, and vaginal fluids. | Usually 60–90 days; range 45–180 days. | Insidious onset of symptoms, nausea, vomiting, anorexia, lethargy, abdominal discomfort, jaundice. | Many weeks before onset of symptoms, may persist for life. | Pre-exposure vaccination to at-risk populations; vaccination to susceptible sexual contacts. Give HBIG treatment to contacts as needed. Universal precautions to prevent exposure to blood and blood products. |

*(continued)*

**Table 12.2** Continued

| Disease | Infectious Agent | Mode of Transmission | Incubation Period | Clinical Presentation | Period of Communicability | Control Measures |
|---------|------------------|----------------------|-------------------|-----------------------|---------------------------|------------------|
| 12.2.12 HEPATITIS C | Hepatitis C virus (HCV) | Parenterally; less frequently are sexual and mother to child. | 6–9 weeks | Insidious, with anorexia, nausea, vomiting, lethargy, abdominal discomfort, jaundice. Progression to jaundice less frequent than hepatitis B (90% asymptomatic). | From one or more weeks before onset of symptoms. Persists in most people indefinitely. | No available vaccine. Routinely screen blood products. Education. Interferon treatment for active disease. |
| **Zoonotic and Vector-Borne Diseases** | | | | | | |
| 12.2.13 MALARIA | *Plasmodium falciparum, P. vivaz, P, ovale,* and *P. malariae.* | Most malaria is transmitted by the bite of an infective female *Anopheles sp.* mosquito. | Approximately 9–14 days for *P. falciparum;* 12–18 days for *P. vivaz* and *P. ovule,* and 18–40 days for *P. malariae.* | The early clinical manifestations of malaria are non-specific and similar enough among species to make differentiation impossible without laboratory studies. The first few days, patients experience febrile illness, chills, myalgias and arthralgias, headache, diarrhea, vomiting, and other non-specific signs. | | Insecticide-treated mosquito nets are the most universally useful measure. Indoor residual spraying with insecticides. Avoid being outdoors at dusk or dawn. Systemic use of insect repellent on exposed skin as well as clothing. Use screens over doors and windows. Before travel to endemic areas, the more appropriate chemoprophylactic antimalarial drugs for the destination(s) should be prescribed. |

| Table 12.2 | Continued | | | | |
|---|---|---|---|---|---|
| Disease | Infectious Agent | Mode of Transmission | Incubation Period | Clinical Presentation | Period of Communicability | Control Measures |
| 12.2.14 LYME DISEASE | *Borrelia burgdorferi* | Tick borne | From 3 to 32 days after tick exposure (mean 7–10 days), early stages of the illness may be unapparent and the patient may present with later manifestations. | Characterized by a distinct skin lesion, systemic symptoms and neurological, rheumatological, and cardiac involvements occurring in varying combinations over months to years. | | Avoid tick-infested areas when feasible. After being in an infested area, examine body for ticks and remove them. |
| 12.2.15 BRUCELLOSIS | *Brucella abortus* | Contact through breaks in the skin with animal tissue, blood, urine, vaginal discharges, aborted fetuses and especially placentas, and ingestion of raw milk and dairy products from infected animals. Airborne infection occurs in pens and stables for animals, and for humans in laboratories and abattoirs. | Variable and difficult to ascertain, usually 5–60 days; 1–2 months is commonplace and occasionally several months. | | | Educate public about the risk of drinking untreated milk or eating products made from unpasteurized or otherwise untreated milk. |

Sources: Heymann, D. L. (Ed.). (2008). *Control of communicable diseases manual* (19th ed.).
Government of Canada. (2013). (unpublished report). *Canadian Notifiable Diseases Surveillance System 2009–2011: National number and rate (per 100,000 population/per 100,000 live births) of reported cases by age group and sex.*
Government of Victoria, Australia. (2009). *Red book: 2009 Report of the Committee on Infectious Diseases* (28th ed.). Elk Grove Village, IL: American Academy of Pediatrics.

# DISEASES WITH MULTIPLE TRANSMISSION MODES

CHNs often are challenged with the need to manage cases of disease that do not fit one specific mode of transmission and, therefore, make case and contact follow-up complex and multifaceted. For example, hepatitis A can be transmitted through contaminated food and water or through sexual contact. Therefore, the CHN must identify contacts and recommend post-exposure prophylaxis based on all possible modes of transmission, and prevent further transmission by providing comprehensive education and exclusion.

# REPORTABLE/NOTIFIABLE DISEASES IN CANADA

## Legislation

In 2013, 50 notifiable diseases were reported by provinces and territories to the Public Health Agency of Canada. Diseases in Canada have been reported from provinces and territories since 1924, previously being reported to Health Canada. Public health and communicable disease surveillance is a shared responsibility, with local public health departments having the primary responsibility for detecting, monitoring and controlling, and reporting communicable diseases. Public health nurses within local public health offices do the majority of communicable disease work, alongside public health inspectors, who monitor water and food sources for potential public health threats to wellness.

## Nationally Notifiable Diseases

The list of nationally notifiable diseases is revised periodically. In 2006, the most recent list of nationally notifiable diseases was published in the *Canada Communicable Disease Report* (PHAC, 2006b). A set of 10 criteria are used to determine which diseases should be included on the list of notifiable diseases reportable in Canada. Examples of the criteria measures used include incidence, severity, communicability, and socioeconomic burden.

The terms *reportable* and *notifiable* diseases are commonly used interchangeably. A communicable disease is identified as a **notifiable disease** through the collaboration and consensus of experts in infectious disease. These experts from around the world study the impact of an identified disease by analyzing morbidity and mortality, and then recommend the need for notification. The morbidity and mortality impact may be in a small, defined area or on a worldwide scale. As a result, reporting of some communicable diseases is required within provinces and territories within Canada, and in some instances internationally, to the WHO.

In Canada, the list of notifiable diseases at the federal level is agreed upon by consensus among provincial and territorial and federal health authorities. The National Notifiable Diseases list helps to ensure uniformity among provincial and territorial efforts, conformity with international reporting requirements, and helps to facilitate both tracking and required control efforts by public health personnel (PHAC, 2009c). Because the epidemiology of infectious diseases changes, this necessitates a periodic review of and modification to the National Notifiable Diseases list (see Table 12.3).

## Reporting of Communicable Diseases

In Canada, both provincial/territorial and national guidelines and legislation dictate which diseases must be reported, who is responsible for reporting them, what the reporting format should be, and what the mechanism for reporting is to the national surveillance system. The list of reportable diseases is mandated by provincial or territorial legislation and, therefore, differs by province or territory, although the recommendations are provided by PHAC. Currently, some provinces and territories report within iPHIS, which stands for integrated Public Health Information System (PHAC, 2007a). It is the database used by public health units to report information on cases of reportable diseases. If there is a requirement for international health reporting, the PHAC reports to the WHO. The International Health Regulations (IHR) (WHO, 2009c) are the only legally binding instrument requiring the reporting of communicable diseases at the international level, and reporting is currently limited to cholera, plague, and yellow fever (Heymann, 2008). The WHO updates and revises the IHR to address the threat of new and re-emerging infections, and to accommodate new reporting sources. A number of diseases *under surveillance* by WHO (e.g., H5N1 and AIDS) are required to be reported at varied frequency, depending on the disease and the geographic area in which it has occurred (see Canadian Research Box 12.1).

---

### CANADIAN RESEARCH BOX 12.1

**How can HIV drug-resistance patterns in Canada help public health interventions?**

Brooks, J. I., Niznick, H., Ofner, M., Merks, H., & Angel, J. B. (2013). Local phylogenetic analysis identifies distinct trends in transmitted HIV drug resistance: Implications for public health interventions. *BMC Infectious Diseases, 13*(1), 509.

An HIV strain can develop resistance to anti-HIV medication and become drug resistant. This virus and the associated drug resistance (DR) can then be transmitted from patient to patient through any of the typical ways HIV is transmitted. This is referred to as transmitted drug resistance (TDR). Phylogenetic analysis is a laboratory method that looks at the genetics of the HIV strain in order to determine similarities or differences among viruses. If strains are genetically similar, one can assume that somewhere along the line the individuals shared a contact, either directly or indirectly, through other contacts that have similar encounters. Using phylogenetics to identify clusters of related HIV strains

| Table 12.3 | Diseases under National Surveillance, as of January 2009 | |
|---|---|---|
| Acquired Immunodeficiency Syndrome (AIDS) | Hantavirus Pulmonary Syndrome (HPS) | Pertussis |
| Acute Flaccid Paralysis (AFP) | Hepatitis A | Plague |
| Anthrax | Hepatitis B | Poliomyelitis |
| Botulism | Hepatitis C | Rabies |
| Brucellosis | Human Immunodeficiency Virus (HIV) | Rubella |
| Campylobacteriosis | Influenza, laboratory-confirmed | Salmonellosis |
| Chlamydia | Invasive *Haemophilus influenzae* type b (Hib) and non-b Disease | Severe Acute Respiratory Syndrome (SARS) |
| Cholera | Invasive Group A Streptococcal Disease | Shigellosis |
| *Clostridium difficile* Associated Diarrhea | Invasive Listeriosis | Smallpox |
| Congenital Rubella Syndrome (CRS) | Invasive Meningococcal Disease | Syphilis |
| Creutzfeldt-Jakob Disease (CJD), Classic and New Variant | Invasive Pneumococcal Disease | Tetanus |
| Cryptosporidiosis | Legionellosis | Tuberculosis |
| | Leprosy (Hansen's Disease) | Tularemia |
| Cyclosporiasis | Lyme Disease | Typhoid |
| Diphtheria | Malaria | Varicella (Chickenpox) |
| Giardiasis | Measles | Verotoxigenic *Escherichia coli* Infection |
| Gonorrhea | Mumps | Viral Haemorrhagic Fevers |
| Group B Streptococcal Disease of the Newborn | Norovirus infection | West Nile virus Infection |
| | Paralytic Shellfish Poisoning | Yellow Fever |

Source: Public Health Agency of Canada. (2010). *Diseases under national surveillance* (January, 2009). Reproduced with permission from the Minister of Health, 2015. Retrieved from http://www.phac-aspc.gc.ca/bid-bmi/dsd-dsm/duns-eng.php

can help public health in determining the behaviours most likely associated with that group of transmissions (e.g., unprotected sex, sharing of injection drug needles) and the demographics of those of whom to target public health intervention.

### Discussion Questions

1. How would the study results potentially inform a CHN's practice when investigating a cluster of HIV among a specific group?

2. What sensitivities need to be considered when working with patient populations that are vulnerable to stigmatization?

3. If contact tracing is difficult for sexually transmitted HIV acquisition due to people not being able to identify where they met their sexual partners, what other ways to find contacts can you think of?

While some infectious diseases are common and mild (such as the common cold or pediculosis), others are serious enough to be defined as notifiable diseases (such as hepatitis C and HIV/AIDS) and must be reported to the local health authority. Local public health personnel are mandated by the provinces and territories to report all notifiable diseases to their respective ministry or department of health. In addition, some diseases must also be reported at the federal level.

# CONTROL AND MANAGEMENT OF COMMUNICABLE DISEASES

The successful control and management of communicable diseases is integrally tied to using sound principles of epidemiology (see Chapter 11). **Surveillance** of a disease consists of "the process of systematic collection, orderly consolidation, analysis and evaluation of pertinent data with prompt dissemination of the results to those who need to know, particularly those who are in a position to take action" (Heymann, 2008, p. 713). Through data analysis, the investigator may uncover the cause or source of the disease (e.g., investigation of a case of salmonella infection may uncover a contaminated food item in a restaurant).

# SURVEILLANCE

## Active Surveillance

Monitoring of diseases, investigation of disease outbreaks, and observation of patterns of disease are responsibilities of the local health authorities. **Active surveillance** is the collection of data utilizing screening tools, interviews, and sentinel systems to identify disease occurrence in the community when individuals present with suggestive symptoms. Such surveillance depends on the creation of surveillance screening tools that heighten the awareness of healthcare practitioners in relation to a specific disease.

Active surveillance may be best illustrated by the screening created in response to the increasing risk across Canada of West Nile virus (WNV), first recognized as a threat in North America in 1999. When WNV was first reported, provincial and federal health authorities applied public health measures to identify the spread of this new communicable disease. WNV was detected for the first time in Canada in 2001, in birds and mosquitoes. In 2002, Canadian health authorities documented human WNV illness activity in five provinces: Nova Scotia, Quebec, Ontario, Manitoba, and Saskatchewan. In 2007, more than 2200 human cases were identified in Canada (PHAC, 2009d). The active surveillance activities during the early days of WNV infections in Canada were conducted partly through the availability of a screening tool. Similarly, a screening tool has been developed by the Ontario Ministry of Health and Long-Term Care for active surveillance of influenza-like illnesses (ILI). The ILI screening tool is utilized in emergency rooms and other acute care settings to provide consistent and early identification of respiratory illnesses, such as influenza and SARS, in order to facilitate the necessary control activities to decrease transmission risks in hospitals and other settings (see Canadian Research Box 12.2). It is also utilized to quickly detect and contain clusters and outbreaks, and helps to identify any new or virulent microorganism-caused respiratory infections (Ontario Ministry of Health and Long-Term Care, 2009).

---

**CANADIAN RESEARCH BOX 12.2**

**What are the actions and procedures that need to be done to decrease the possibilities of the development of healthcare-associated secondary infections within hospitals?**

Muscedere, J., Ofner, M., Kumar, A., Long, J., Lamontagne, F., Cook, D., . . . Fowler, R. For the ICU-FLU Group and the Canadian Critical Care Trials Group. (2013). The occurrence and impact of bacterial and fungal organisms: Complicating critical care illness associated with influenza A (H1N1) infection. *CHEST Journal, 144*(1), 39–47. doi:10.1378/chest.12-1861

In April 2009, the first deaths from a novel strain of H1N1 influenza A virus were reported in Mexico and the United States. The virus quickly spread to other countries, including Canada. As of July 2009, the WHO reported almost 100 000 confirmed cases of human infection worldwide and almost 500 deaths, including 25 in Canada. Many of the severe cases of H1N1 developed secondary infections while in hospital. These hospital-associated infections may lead to increased mortality among patients who may have survived had they not acquired this secondary infection. The two most common pathogens found in this study were coagulase negative staphylococci and *Staphylococcus aureus*. These two organisms are typically transmitted within hospital on the hands of healthcare workers.

---

**Discussion Questions**

1. What is the first line of defence against the transmission of healthcare-associated infections within a hospital environment, and particularly within an intensive care unit (ICU)?

2. Why is it important for healthcare providers to follow routine practices in infection prevention and control? Include examples for patient, staff, environment, and economic burden.

3. When a person with influenza develops a bacterial infection, what are some of the important clinical practices that need to be considered?

---

## Passive Surveillance

**Passive surveillance** occurs when a healthcare provider must notify the local health authority to report an identified case of a "reportable" disease. It is said to be "passive" since a case typically is presented to the healthcare provider and one is not actively going out and looking for sick individuals. Reportable diseases are identified in the public health act of each province or territory. Whenever a case of a reportable disease is identified, the collection of information to further describe the case is necessary. This includes information about the person, the symptoms and date of onset of the presenting illness, and his or her travel history, and may include social history, sexual history, diagnostic tests done to date, and prescribed treatment.

Surveillance, whether active, passive, or both, does not end with the notification of the disease case to the local health authority; rather, it initiates the next steps toward the control and management of the disease. Surveillance also plays a significant role in the management of reports of suspected cases of disease. CHNs provide guidelines to institutions, healthcare professionals, and others in relation to diagnostic tests and control measures to identify and manage a *suspected* case of disease in terms of transmission risk and potential community impact.

## OUTBREAKS AND CONTACT TRACING

**Contact tracing** is a response to a communicable disease report. After a notifiable communicable disease is reported to the local health authority, the infected person is interviewed by a CHN regarding **contacts**, that is, people exposed to the client during the incubation of the disease. The CHN must know the mode of transmission, incubation period, and infectious period of the particular disease in order to determine what constitutes a contact in each individual situation. The *initial contact definition* must be formulated based on signs and symptoms, and on place and time of exposure. A list of contacts must be collected from the first identified case. With this list, the local health authority proceeds with further assessment and investigation and follows up with recommendations for treatment or post-exposure chemoprophylaxis as deemed necessary.

Contacts are identified based on the possibility of transmission, where the window of risk can be very short or quite long. For example, when investigating a case of measles, the CHN would include in the contact list those people who were in contact with the infectious individual seven days prior to the onset of the rash; whereas, while investigating a case of TB, the CHN may identify not just recent contacts but contacts as far back as three months. The **degree of exposure** (the time spent with the infected person) and where the exposure took place are included in the collected data. Not all reportable diseases warrant the same type of contact tracing, because of varying degrees of burden of illness (e.g., varicella) or because of the nature of the communicability (e.g., TB).

The ease with which public health professionals are provided with comprehensive and inclusive lists of contacts will depend on how the individual or community comprehends the scope of the issue, or an individual's or community's experience with the disease in the past. For example, obtaining contacts from those who have had an experience with an adolescent dying from meningococcal disease is easier than obtaining a comprehensive list of contacts from an infected food service worker whose perception is that hepatitis A infection is not a serious disease. The report is only as reliable and accurate as the person relaying the information and the parameters required for reporting. That is, if the physician or nurse is unsure of the signs and symptoms of the disease, the need for reporting will go unrecognized and the surveillance and contact tracing may be delayed.

Ongoing education of healthcare professionals helps to ensure detailed disease reporting. The **integrated Public Health Information System (iPHIS)** (PHAC, 2007a) is an electronic system of reporting that allows jurisdictions within a province to communicate disease patterns and contacts with one another. As well, the **National Enteric Surveillance Program** (PHAC, 2015), an outbreak-specific electronic system, has been developed for healthcare professionals to communicate outbreaks of respiratory or enteric illnesses inter-provincially. It enables public health professionals to make links in person, place, and time for clients with similar presentation.

Contact tracing requires a confidential approach, since much of the information is disease and client specific. An exception to the confidential necessity and practice of contact tracing is occasionally required. During the SARS outbreak that occurred in Toronto during March through May of 2003, quarantine acts of the federal and Ontario ministries of health allowed health and safety authorities to conduct contact tracing in a public forum by naming those with SARS in the public media. Their purpose was to protect the public as well as to notify the contacts of those first infected persons in order to allow the contacts to self-identify and come forward for health assessment. Although contact tracing might be viewed as an infringement of a person's right to privacy, it is necessary to contain the spread of disease while providing ethically competent care (see Chapter 6).

Effective contact tracing requires comprehensive assessment of the infected individual and accurate disease reporting. While facilitating this process, the CHN is also assessing the individual as part of the community where they live, work, and play. For example, contact tracing conducted during an outbreak of TB in a homeless shelter required the local public health unit to become cognizant of the community defined by this unique population. This involved learning about the soup kitchens, drop-in centres, parks, and other areas where these individuals congregated. Local public health personnel could not achieve this task without the assistance of the ill individual (who provided information about the likely first case) and the community partners (who work closely with this population). These partners are not limited to healthcare providers but include all community agencies that provide services to the homeless. The result of the partnership was to develop a more focused and targeted screening of contacts. CHNs who work with marginalized populations, such as in street nursing programs across Canada, develop trusting relationships that facilitate contact tracing in these populations.

Contact tracing can involve identification of individuals who have not had any proximal contact with the case, and these individuals are called **indirect contacts**. In order to effectively manage cases of blood-borne disease with possible indirect contact modes of transmission, it is important in contact tracing to recognize that an individual infected with a disease may not be able to provide all contact information, as some contacts may be unknown to them. As noted earlier, blood products and solid organ implantation are now recognized as a significant disease transmission risk for recipients. For example, West Nile virus (WNV) was identified in four clients receiving organs from an asymptomatic donor in 2002 (Centers for Disease Control and Prevention, 2002). Other emerging diseases, such as Creutzfeldt-Jakob disease (CJD), necessitate that the CHN thoroughly understand modes of transmission in order to perform thorough history-taking in contact tracing. It would be important to know, for example, if instruments used in invasive procedures involving brain or neural tissue on a client diagnosed with CJD may have been contaminated.

**Response to Outbreaks** An **outbreak** can be identified when expected symptoms in the population exist at an increased level. These symptoms may exist in the general population or in institutions such as hospitals, long-term care homes, or daycare centres. An outbreak may not necessarily be a reportable disease but may initially be of unknown etiology, suggestive of a communicable disease. An outbreak can be identified when a group of persons present with similar signs and symptoms, such as fever, coughing, and malaise in the case of an outbreak of influenza-like illness. Generally, **outbreak reports** are communicated to public health authorities as soon as possible to allow investigation for a cause of illness. In addition, early notification facilitates early institution of appropriate control methods, such as cohorting (separation) of well and ill clients into separate areas.

The terms "case" and "index case" are used throughout any discussion of outbreaks. A **case** refers to a single ill individual. When an individual person is identified as the likely first case in an outbreak, this person is referred to as the **index case**. Often, the index case in an outbreak is identified after other persons become ill and all surveillance data indicates that the outbreak began with the identified individual. The purpose in identifying a common source (contaminated food) or an index case (infectious person) is two-fold: (a) to interrupt further transmission of the disease by identifying the route of transmission, and (b) to understand the cause of the outbreak by identifying the origin of the pathogen. The information that a CHN gathers to understand and define an outbreak is often like pieces of a puzzle and requires the CHN to possess critical-thinking and analytic skills.

**Steps in Managing an Outbreak** The initial investigation of an outbreak includes review of the signs and symptoms the ill clients have in common, the onset, whether some clients are recovering, the usual course of the illness, and the source of the outbreak (e.g., a contaminated air conditioning unit in a case of legionella outbreak or an infected person in the case of a pertussis, measles, or mumps outbreak). Heymann (2008) outlines six general steps in the management of an outbreak:

1. verifying the diagnosis,
2. confirming the existence of an outbreak,
3. identifying affected persons and characteristics,
4. defining and investigating the population at risk,
5. generating a hypothesis, and
6. containing the outbreak.

An outbreak report is usually generated after the outbreak is determined to be over, although in large outbreaks, reporting may occur throughout the course of the outbreak. Scientific study and learning is generated after each outbreak, as each presents differently. Debriefing sessions with all those involved in any aspect of the outbreak is an important and often missed learning opportunity. Efforts should be made to approach debriefing sessions with a structured format to avoid placing blame on individuals and to ensure behaviour change occurs to prevent similar outbreaks from happening again.

# ROLE OF THE COMMUNITY HEALTH NURSE

History has shown that communicable diseases are controlled through changes in practice or environment. Typhoid and cholera are two communicable diseases that can be transmitted via contaminated water. The sanitation of water is one of the public health triumphs that occurred in the early 1900s. Improved sanitation and the development of vaccines for typhoid and cholera have virtually eliminated these diseases from the developed world. These diseases still continue to plague low-income countries where water sanitation and vaccination programs are limited or not available (Heymann, 2008).

CHNs broke the chain of infection at the mode of transmission link by educating the public on personal hygiene and the importance of clean drinking water. Today, breaking the chain of infection is achieved through various methods, each one targeted at different links. For example, immunization programs (especially for children) modify the susceptible host into a resistant host, whereas prophylaxis can diminish or reduce the ability of the infectious agent to multiply after entry into the susceptible host. Sterilization of instruments, proper cleaning of food in restaurants, and **harm reduction** methods are strategies targeted at the **reservoir**, thereby altering the ability of the infectious agent to transmit from one host to another.

Mounting immunization campaigns, screening, ensuring that quarantine requirements are met, instituting isolation, providing prophylaxis, and acting as consultants on communicable disease to community groups are some of CHNs' service delivery activities. CHNs working with the medical officer of health are responsible for monitoring and reporting communicable disease occurrences in the community as reported by other healthcare providers, schools, childcare agencies, laboratories, the general public, and healthcare institutions.

## Levels of Preventive Measures

CHNs use the nursing process to implement primary, secondary, and tertiary prevention activities in controlling communicable diseases. As a reminder, *primary prevention* attempts to prevent the disease from occurring. *Secondary prevention* detects a disease or condition in a certain population, usually by screening or testing for the disease. *Tertiary prevention* involves the reduction of the extent and severity of the health problem in order to minimize the disability.

The main **primary prevention measures** for controlling communicable disease include

- promoting and implementing immunization programs, notifying contacts, and making referrals for follow-up diagnosis;
- providing chemoprophylaxis and antitoxins for prevention of disease;

- working with public health authorities and community partners concerning protective and control measures for communicable diseases; and
- educating the public on safe sexual practices, optimal nutrition, healthy environments for better air quality and sanitation, and use of preventive measures such as universal precautions.

**Secondary prevention measures** include

- screening, which includes case finding, referral, and mass screening for early detection;
- early diagnosis, which includes interpretation of diagnostic results;
- early treatment, which includes provision of antimicrobial medications for newly diagnosed contacts;
- teaching for medication and treatment compliance, including provision of supportive care such as diet, rest, and exercise, and teaching for side effects of medications; and
- advocacy for accessible diagnostic and treatment services for socially disadvantaged groups such as the poor, the underhoused, and people with language and cultural barriers.

**Screening** There are two reasons to test or screen for a communicable disease. The first is in response to the disease being identified in the community; epidemiological reports can reveal or identify a population that is at risk for disease. CHNs screen the population to validate these reports and to identify the at-risk individuals. The individuals being tested have not been identified in the contact screening but are part of the population at risk. For example, a student is diagnosed with TB and all students in his or her school, not just those with close contact to the index student, may be tested for TB. The list of exposures of the case must be analyzed to also identify the *index* or *first case*. As well, the history of the cases may help to determine the index case; that is, who first presented with the disease symptoms. The second and a more general strategy is testing and screening after broad immunization campaigns, which are done as a standard of practice (e.g., titres following a hepatitis B vaccination series). The **titres** check the efficacy of the immunization to ensure that those who received the vaccine now have antibodies to the disease. A random sample of those immunized is used as a strategy by pharmaceutical companies to demonstrate efficacy of vaccine by using **seroconversion rates**.

**Isolation and Quarantine** Isolation and quarantine are also secondary preventive measures. Treatment or management of some infectious agents includes isolation or quarantine to reduce the transmission and break the chain of infection. **Isolation** refers to separation of an *infectious person* for a period of time to prevent or limit the direct or indirect transmission of the infectious agent. **Quarantine** is the restriction of activities for a *well person* who has been exposed to an infectious agent. Generally, communicable diseases that are transmitted by direct or airborne routes require that the contacts be separated from other people and possibly placed in quarantine. The length of the isolation or quarantine period is specific to the incubation and communicable period of each disease (Heymann, 2008). For example, varicella is

considered to be most infectious two days before the onset of the rash and remains infectious until all lesions are dried and crusted, whereas hepatitis A is most infectious during the two weeks before onset of symptoms until one week after the appearance of jaundice. The communicable period is not always known for every disease, especially emerging diseases. SARS is considered to have an incubation period of up to 10 days (Heymann, 2008). During the SARS outbreak, it was uncertain when the infected person was most contagious or when the symptoms displayed by the patient equated to communicability. For this reason, contacts were placed in quarantine for a minimum of 10 days.

**Prophylaxis** Prophylaxis, a secondary preventive measure, is the utilization of chemoprophylaxic or immunoprophylaxic agents to prevent illness from a pathogen or infectious agent following a known or possible exposure. Prophylaxic agents may be prescribed for exposed vulnerable hosts such as pregnant women, infants, people who have an immune disorder or transplant, or anyone who had contact with a disease that has high morbidity and mortality rates or a disease that has significant long-term effects.

Immunoprophylaxic agents include both active and passive immunizing agents. **Active immunizing agents** are vaccines that stimulate the immune system to create antibodies. **Passive immunizing agents** include immune serum globulin, which is of human origin, and immune globulins that contain specific antibodies to a particular organism, such as hepatitis B immune globulin (HBIG) or rabies immune globulin (RIG).

Prophylaxis provides protection to the vulnerable hosts in the general population. The role of the CHN is to identify the vulnerable hosts, monitor the therapy if it is long term, and possibly administer or facilitate the administration of one-time prophylaxis. An example of the use of **chemoprophylaxis** includes the administration of isoniazid (INH) to children younger than six years of age who are identified as contacts in a TB outbreak despite having a negative response to the tuberculin skin test. These children are given this medication daily for three months. It is recognized that young children may not have the ability to fight the TB organism as well as an older child or adult. The medication provides the child with the ability to fight the organism, reduces bacterial load, and reduces the possibility of disseminated disease. A tuberculin skin test is repeated after three months, and if the result continues to be negative and no other immune disorder appears to exist, the INH can be discontinued. **Immunoprophylaxis** can be an appropriate choice if, for example, during an outbreak of varicella in the community, contact tracing reveals that one of the contacts is a pregnant woman; she may be a candidate for varicella-zoster immune globulin (VZIG). The VZIG will either protect the woman from acquiring varicella or lessen the symptoms if the disease occurs, thereby protecting the fetus.

**Tertiary prevention measures** aim to reduce the extent and severity of the health problems in order to minimize the complications by

- educating and monitoring treatment compliance to prevent complications, and
- monitoring effectiveness of treatment and identifying and referring for adverse effects.

Education of the public may be carried out at the individual, family, and community levels through community-based programs. Education is not directed at a single stage in the chain of infection; rather, it targets the whole chain and teaches measures that can be adopted into the individual's personal health habits. The goal is to help the client and the communities return to baseline functioning, or a new state of health. Examples include the administration of **direct observed therapy (DOT)**, which is a mechanism used to ensure TB clients take their prescribed medications. The nurse observes the clients taking the medications on a pre-set schedule. This is to prevent the risk of non-compliance and thereby reduce the possibility of drug-resistant TB, which could place communities at risk.

Through various levels of prevention activities, CHNs play major roles in education, health promotion, direct care, community development and mobilization, liaison, research, advocacy, program planning and evaluation, and policy formulation. All are essential skills in epidemiologic investigation for successful management and control of communicable diseases. Utilizing these skills is essential, as was shown by the role of CHNs in the H1N1 pandemic of 2009. Although the 2009 pandemic was considered to be mild, Canada was one of the few countries that had a pandemic plan in place well in advance of the H1N1 influenza virus outbreak. The overall goals of the Canadian Pandemic Influenza Plan were to minimize serious illness and overall deaths, and to minimize societal disruption caused by the pandemic. In the 2009 pandemic, there were 428 deaths and 8678 hospitalizations in Canada due to influenza A/H1N1 (PHAC, 2010b). Across Canada, recommendations for healthcare workers that were made by PHAC were followed by acute and community health workers on issues like infection control and occupational health, resource management, clinical care, and the distribution of antivirals and vaccines. Guidelines were followed by CHNs on addressing the outbreak, reinforcing the recommended infection control practices and public health measures. As a result, minimal illness occurred and societal disruption was kept to a minimum. Effective pandemic preparedness is essential to mitigate the effects of a pandemic, particularly if it becomes severe. CHNs play a pivotal role in planning with community partners to create policies, to enhance environmental supports, and to provide educational resources.

## CONCLUSION

This chapter has discussed the basic principles of communicable disease control, including vaccine-preventable diseases and the role of the CHN in dealing with them. The topic of communicable disease control is broad, and each day the world faces a new disease that may or may not find its way into any community. CHNs must be prepared to respond to the unexpected. They must work in partnership with the local, national, and global communities to develop effective surveillance methods and screening tools, to enhance emergency response mechanisms, and to implement public health measures in primary, secondary, and tertiary prevention for communicable disease control. It is imperative that CHNs possess a strong relationship with their community partners, a solid knowledge base of epidemiology and current information on communicable diseases, knowledge of available resources, and strong decision making and research skills. Integration of these skills will help the CHN to be successful in the role of protecting and promoting the health of Canadians.

## KEY TERMS

active immunizing agents    p. 241
active surveillance    p. 237
agent    p. 219
avian influenza H5N1    p. 225
blood-borne infections    p. 221
Canadian Blood Services    p. 222
Canadian Nosocomial Infection Surveillance Program (CNISP)    p. 226
carbapenamase-producing organisms    p. 226
case    p. 239
chemoprophylaxis    p. 241
chlamydia    p. 221
*Clostridium difficile*    p. 226
colonized patient    p. 226
communicable diseases    p. 217
contact tracing    p. 238
contacts    p. 238
Creutzfeldt-Jakob disease    p. 218
degree of exposure    p. 239
diphtheria    p. 220
direct observed therapy (DOT)    p. 241
disease surveillance    p. 219
endemic    p. 220
enteric infections    p. 223
environment    p. 219
epidemic    p. 220
epidemiologic triangle    p. 219
food-borne infection    p. 223
food-borne intoxication    p. 223
food-borne outbreaks    p. 223
genital herpes    p. 221
guidelines    p. 226
H1N1 influenza pandemic    p. 219
haemophilus influenzae type b    p. 220
hand hygiene    p. 226
hantavirus    p. 224
harm reduction    p. 240
healthcare-associated (HCA) infections    p. 226
hepatitis B    p. 220
hepatitis C    p. 221
herd immunity    p. 220
HIV    p. 221
host    p. 219
human papillomavirus (HPV)    p. 220
immunization    p. 220
immunoprophylaxis    p. 241
index case    p. 239
indirect contacts    p. 239

## STUDY QUESTIONS

1. What is the link between epidemiology and control of communicable diseases?

2. What are the modes of transmission of communicable diseases?

3. A high school student is diagnosed with tuberculosis. How would you conduct contact tracing?

4. A daycare centre has just notified you, a new CHN, that a child in its care has meningitis. The staff and parents of other children are very anxious. Describe your nursing interventions.

5. The local health authority has just hired you to work on hepatitis A management and control. Being new to the region, what would be your priority tasks?

6. What information would you need from the infectious individual and about his or her disease (e.g., HIV) to conduct comprehensive contact tracing?

After working through these questions, go to the MyNursingLab at www.pearsoned.ca/mynursinglab to check your answers.

## INDIVIDUAL CRITICAL-THINKING EXERCISES

1. You receive several laboratory reports for the same disease from the same geographical area. What steps are needed to differentiate between increased incidences and usual occurrence of the disease?

2. In Question 1, what would be your sources of information for the investigation?

3. You are working in a downtown clinic that provides services to marginalized/vulnerable persons. A client presents to the clinic with non-specific ailments. You are collecting the history. The client reveals addictions to crack cocaine and other substances, and that he has multiple sexual partners. Your recommendation is to have a full work-up for STIs. The client refuses. Discuss your nursing responsibilities.

4. Refer to Question 3; the client's HIV test shows a positive result. What should be your next steps?

5. You have been assigned a client who has active tuberculosis, and who has been on treatment in his or her home country and who has just arrived in Canada and does not understand English or the purpose of the treatment. How would you ensure an accurate nursing assessment for this client and how would you facilitate a supportive treatment environment for this client?

## GROUP CRITICAL-THINKING EXERCISES

1. Large numbers of immigrants come from regions where the prevalence of tuberculosis is high. This has resulted in the importation of a large burden of latent infection that can be expected to generate future active cases in aging immigrant populations. Discuss the implications for caring for the future active cases. Healthy public policy should be included in the discussion as opposed to local health authority policy.

2. AIDS can manifest after years of HIV-positive status; a positive HIV test may not occur until three months after the contact. Similarly, in tuberculosis, the skin test can be negative up to 12 weeks post-exposure, and the manifestations of the disease may occur sometime in the person's lifetime. Discuss the implications of contact tracing for these two diseases.

3. Emerging diseases, changes in antibiotic resistance, and threats of terrorism with biological agents have heightened the awareness of surveillance needs worldwide. Since September 11, 2001, the threats of smallpox and anthrax have been in the media. Discuss the information needed to control the spread of smallpox.

## REFERENCES

Alberta Health Services. (2012). *Public health notifiable disease management guidelines: Hanta Virus Pulmonary Syndrome.* Alberta: Author. Retrieved from http://www.health.alberta.ca/documents/Guidelines-Hantavirus-2012.pdf

Berman, S., Duenas, A., Bedoya, A., Constain, V., Leon, S., Borrero, I., & Murphy, J. (1983). Acute lower respiratory tract illnesses in Cali, Colombia: A two-year ambulatory study. *Pediatrics, 71*(2), 210–218.

British Columbia Ministry of Health. (n.d.). *Vector-borne diseases.* Vancouver, BC: Author. Retrieved from http://www.health.gov.bc.ca/protect/ehp_vector.html

Canadian Blood Services. (2009). *Testing.* Ottawa, ON: Author. Retrieved from http://www.bloodservices.ca/centreapps/internet/uw_v502_mainengine.nsf/page/testing?OpenDocument

Centers for Disease Control and Prevention. (2002, September 6). Public health dispatch: West Nile virus infection in organ donor and transplant recipients—Georgia and Florida, 2002. *Morbidity and Mortality Weekly Report, 51*(35), 790. Retrieved from http://www.cdc.gov/mmwr/preview/mmwrhtml/mm5135a5.htm

Centers for Disease Control and Prevention. (2013a). *Enteric Diseases Epidemiology Branch.* Atlanta, GA: Author. Retrieved from http://www.cdc.gov/ncezid/dfwed/edeb

Centers for Disease Control and Prevention. (September 6, 2013b). Surveillance for waterborne disease outbreaks associated with drinking water and other nonrecreational water— United States, 2009–2010. *Morbidity and Mortality Weekly Report (MMWR), 62*(35), 714–720. Retrieved from http://www.cdc.gov/mmwr/preview/mmwrhtml/mm6235a3.htm)

Drebot, M. A., & Artsob, H. (2006). West Nile virus: A pathogen of concern for older adults. *Geriatrics and Aging, 9*(7), 465–471.

Government of Alberta. (2012). *Alberta treatment guidelines for sexually transmitted infections (STI) in adolescents and adults.* Edmonton, AB: Author. Retrieved from http://www.health.alberta.ca/documents/STI-Treatment-Guidelines-2012.pdf

Government of Canada. (2014a). *Tuberculosis.* Ottawa, ON: Author. Retrieved from http://healthycanadians.gc.ca/diseases-conditions-maladies-affections/disease-maladie/tuberculosis-tuberculose-eng.php

Government of Canada. (2014b). *Rabies in Canada.* Ottawa, ON: Author. Retrieved from http://travel.gc.ca/travelling/health-safety/diseases/rabies

Heymann, D. L. (2008). *Control of communicable diseases manual: An official report of the American Public Health Association* (19th ed.). Washington, DC: American Public Health Association.

Last, J. M. (1988). *A Dictionary of Epidemiology.* New York, NY: Oxford University Press.

North Bay Parry Sound District Health Unit. (2009). *Investigative summary of the escherichia coli outbreak associated with a restaurant in North Bay, Ontario: October to November 2008.* (North Bay: NBPS-DHU, June 2009). Retrieved from http://www.myhealthunit.ca/en/partnerandhealthproviderresources/resources/InvestigativeSummaryoftheEcoliOutbreakJune2009.pdf

Ofner, M. (1993). *Tuberculosis and AIDS in Ontario—A record linkage.* Public Health and Epidemiology Report for Ontario (PHERO), 4:11.

Ontario Ministry of Health and Long-Term Care. (2009). Screening tool for influenza-like illness in the emergency department. Retrieved from http://www.health.gov.on.ca/en/pro/programs/emb/health_notices/ihn_screening_tool_042909.pdf

Plotkin, S. A., & Orenstein, W. A. (2008). *Vaccines* (5th ed.). Philadelphia, PA: W. B. Saunders.

Public Health Agency of Canada. (1996). Guidelines for preventing the transmission of tuberculosis in Canadian health care facilities and other institutional settings. *Canada Communicable Disease Report, 20*(SS1). Retrieved from http://www.collectionscanada.gc.ca/webarchives/20071120001332/http://www.phac-aspc.gc.ca/publicat/ccdr-rmtc/96vol22/22s1/index.html

Public Health Agency of Canada. (2000). Waterborne outbreak of gastroenteritis associated with a contaminated municipal water supply, Walkerton, Ontario. *Canada Communicable Disease Report, 26*(20), 170–173. Retrieved from http://www.phac-aspc.gc.ca/publicat/ccdr-rmtc/00vol26/index.html

Public Health Agency of Canada. (2001). *Waterborne Cryptosporidiosis outbreak, North Battleford, Saskatchewan. Canada Communicable Disease Report 27*(22), 185–192. Retrieved from http://www.collectionscanada.gc.ca/webarchives/20071122093556/; http://www.phac-aspc.gc.ca/publicat/ccdr-rmtc/01vol27/index.html

Public Health Agency of Canada. (2006a). *Canadian immunization guide* (7th ed.). Ottawa, ON: Government Services Canada.

Public Health Agency of Canada. (October 1, 2006b). Final report and recommendations from the National Notifiable Diseases Working Group. *Canada Communicable Disease Report, 32*(19). Retrieved from http://www.phac-aspc.gc.ca/publicat/ccdr-rmtc/06vol32/dr3219a-eng.php

Public Health Agency of Canada. (2007a). *Canadian Integrated Public Health Surveillance (CIPHS).* Ottawa, ON: Author. Retrieved from http://www.phac-aspc.gc.ca/surveillance-eng.php

Public Health Agency of Canada. (2007b). *The Canadian nosocomial infection surveillance program.* Ottawa, ON: Author. Retrieved from http://www.phac-aspc.gc.ca/surveillance-eng.php

Public Health Agency of Canada. (2008). *Who we are.* Ottawa, ON: Author. Retrieved from http://www.phac-aspc.gc.ca/cphorsphc-respcacsp/2008/fr-rc/cphorsphc-respcacsp06a-eng.php#2

Public Health Agency of Canada. (2009a). *Creutzfeldt-Jakob disease (CJD).* Ottawa, ON: Author. Retrieved from http://www.phac-aspc.gc.ca/hcai-iamss/cjd-mcj/index-eng.php

Public Health Agency of Canada. (2009b). *Hantaviruses.* Ottawa, ON: Author. Retrieved from http://www.hc-sc.gc.ca/hl-vs/iyh-vsv/diseases-maladies/hantavirus-eng.php

Public Health Agency of Canada. (2009c). *National notifiable diseases.* Ottawa, ON: Author. Retrieved from http://dsol-smed.phac-aspc.gc.ca/dsol-smed/ndis/list_e.html

Public Health Agency of Canada. (2009d). *West Nile virus MONITOR: Human surveillance (2002–2008).* Ottawa, ON: Author. Retrieved from http://www.phac-aspc.gc.ca/wnv-vwn/index-eng.php

Public Health Agency of Canada. (2010a). *Canadian guidelines on sexually transmitted infections.* Ottawa, ON: Author. Retrieved from http://www.phac-aspc.gc.ca/std-mts/sti-its

Public Health Agency of Canada. (2010b). *Surveillance: Deaths associated with H1N1 flu virus in Canada.* Ottawa, ON: Author. Retrieved from http://www.phac-aspc.gc.ca/alert-alerte/h1n1/surveillance-archive/20100128-eng.php

Public Health Agency of Canada. (2011). *Frequently asked questions about Variant Creutzfeldt-Jakob Disease (Variant CJD).* Ottawa, ON: Author. Retrieved from http://www.phac-aspc.gc.ca/cjd-mcj/vcjd-faq-03-eng.php#a11

Public Health Agency of Canada. (2012a). *The Canadian nosocomial infection surveillance program.* Ottawa, ON: Author. Retrieved from http://www.phac-aspc.gc.ca/nois-sinp/survprog-eng.php

Public Health Agency of Canada. (2012b). *Routine practices and additional precautions assessment and educational tools.* Ottawa, ON: Her Majesty the Queen in Right of Canada. Retrieved from http://www.ipac-canada.org/pdf/2013_PHAC-RPAP_Tools_eng.pdf

Public Health Agency of Canada. (2014a). *Tuberculosis in Canada, 2012 – pre-release.* Ottawa, ON: Author. Retrieved from http://www.phac-aspc.gc.ca/tbpc-latb/pubs/tbcan12pre/index-eng.php

Public Health Agency of Canada. (2014b). *About the Agency.* Ottawa, ON: Author. Public Health Agency of Canada, 2015. Adapted and Reproduced with permission from the Minister of Health, 2015. Retrieved from http://www.phac-aspc.gc.ca/about_apropos/index-eng.php

Public Health Agency of Canada. (2014c). *Canada communicable disease report (CCDR).* Ottawa, ON: Author. Retrieved from http://www.phac-aspc.gc.ca/publicat/ccdr-rmtc/dr-rm-ab-pr-eng.php

Public Health Agency of Canada. (2014d). *Canada immunization guide.* Ottawa, ON: Author. Retrieved from http://www.phac-aspc.gc.ca/publicat/cig-gci/p01-12-eng.php#tab1

Public Health Agency of Canada. (2014e). *Notifiable diseases on-line.* Ottawa, ON: Author. Retrieved from http://dsol-smed.phac-aspc.gc.ca/dsol-smed/ndis/index-eng.php

Public Health Agency of Canada. (2014f). *National Advisory Committee on Immunization (NACI): Statement on seasonal influenza vaccine for 2014–2015.* Ottawa, ON: Author. Retrieved from http://publications.gc.ca/collections/collection_2014/aspc-phac/HP40-114-2014-eng.pdf

Public Health Agency of Canada. (2015). *National Enteric Surveillance Program.* Retrieved from https://www.nml-lnm.gc.ca/NESP-PNSME/index-eng.htm

Reed, S. E. (1981) The etiology and epidemiology of common colds and the possibilities of prevention. *Clinical Otolaryngology, 6,* 379–387.

Riemann, C., & Cliver, D. (Eds.). (2006). *Foodborne infections and intoxications* (3rd ed.). New York, NY: Academic Press.

Royce, R. A., Seña, A., Cates, W. J., & Cohen, M. S. (1997). Sexual transmission of HIV. *New England Journal of Medicine, 336*(15), 1072–1078.

World Health Organization. (2009a). *Communicable diseases: Highlights of communicable disease activities, major recent achievements.* Geneva, Switzerland: Author. Retrieved from http://www.searo.who.int/EN/Section10.htm

World Health Organization (WHO). (2009b). *Five keys to safer food.* Geneva, Switzerland: Author. Reprinted with permission from World Health Organization. Retrieved from http://www.who.int/foodsafety/publications/5keysmanual/en

World Health Organization. (2009c). *International health regulations.* Geneva, Switzerland: Author. Retrieved from http://www.who.int/topics/international_health_regulations/en

World Health Organization. (2010). *Anniversary of smallpox eradication.* Geneva: Switzerland. Retrieved from http://www.who.int/mediacentre/multimedia/podcasts/2010/smallpox_20100618/en

World Health Organization. (2013a). *Immunization, vaccines and biologicals: The expanded programme on immunization.* Geneva: Switzerland. Retrieved from http://www.who.int/immunization/programmes_systems/supply_chain/benefits_of_immunization/en

World Health Organization. (2013b). *Global vaccine action plan 2011–2020.* Geneva, Switzerland: Author. Retrieved from http://www.who.int/immunization/global_vaccine_action_plan/GVAP_secretariat_report_2013.pdf

World Health Organization. (2014a). *Plague. Fact Sheet N°267.* Geneva, Switzerland: Author. Retrieved from http://www.who.int/mediacentre/factsheets/fs267/en

World Health Organization. (2014b). *Ebola virus disease. Fact Sheet N°103.* Geneva, Switzerland: Author. Reprinted with permission from World Health Organization. Retrieved from http://www.who.int/mediacentre/factsheets/fs103/en

## ABOUT THE AUTHOR

**Dr. Marianna Ofner-Agostini**, RN (Ontario), BScN (University of Windsor), MHSc and PhD (University of Toronto) is a Senior Advisor and Epidemiologist at the Public Health Agency of Canada and an Adjunct Professor in the Dalla Lana School of Public Health and the Bloomberg Faculty of Nursing at the University of Toronto. Marianna has worked at the local, provincial, and federal public health levels for over 25 years, primarily in communicable disease surveillance and outbreak investigations. Marianna was a key investigator during the SARS outbreak in Toronto and during H1NI. She is the former Program Director of the Canadian Field Epidemiology Training Program, a program that trains nurses, doctors, veterinarians, and epidemiologists in outbreak investigations and public health methods.

# CHAPTER 13

# Community Nursing Process

*Lucia Yiu*

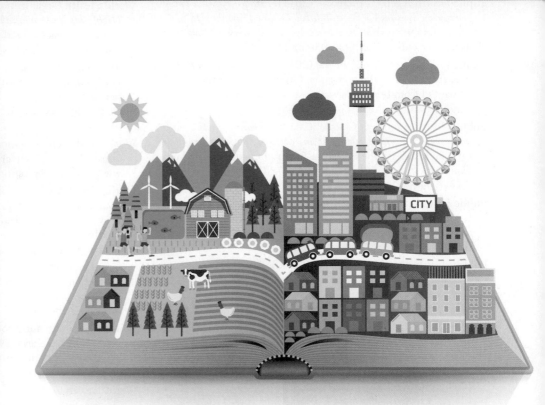

*Source: Pongsuwan/Fotolia*

## INTRODUCTION

Community health nurses (CHNs) care for people where they live, learn, play, and work. Their goal is to improve the health of the community by promoting, preserving, and protecting the health of individuals, families, aggregates, and populations. Their practice includes promoting health, building individual or community capacity, connecting and caring, facilitating access and equity, and demonstrating professional responsibility and accountability (Community Health Nurses of Canada, 2011, revised). When entering the practice of community health nursing, novice nurses often ask, "What does caring for a community mean?" "Where and how do I begin?" and "What is a healthy community?"

Unlike having clients in hospitals or acute-care settings who actively seek episodic care for their presenting problems, CHNs must determine *who* and *where* their clients are, and *why*, *what*, *when*, and *how* best to promote their health in the community. Today, as a result of early hospital discharges, clients in the community have more and more complex and acute health problems than before. Not only do CHNs need to attend to the post-hospital complex care for their clients, they must respond to the diversity and changing population demographics of their populations, who are aging rapidly with the rising rates of chronic illnesses. Additionally, CHNs must strive to work autonomously to build community partnerships that are based on a philosophy of primary health care to achieve health for all. This chapter provides an overview of the community health nursing process, including community assessment, selected community health practice models, population health promotion, community development, and community participatory tools.

## COMMUNITY CLIENTS VERSUS COMMUNITY PARTNERS

CHNs have always cared for the *community as their clients.* Historically, CHNs cared for sick and destitute individuals and families. Florence Nightingale cared for the soldiers in the Crimean War by improving sanitation and hygiene conditions to reduce infections and deaths among them. Lillian Wald established the Henry Street Settlement in New York to improve housing, nutrition, and sanitation for impoverished mothers and children (McKay, 2012). Today, CHNs continue to care for their clients in various community settings, healthy or sick, from homes to schools, workplaces, community centres, and clinics.

CHNs also work with the *community as partner*; they collaborate with multidisciplinary teams of healthcare providers, politicians, leaders, and the public at large to implement an affordable, accessible, and well-integrated primary health care system to meet the needs of their community. Through this intersectoral partnership, CHNs help strengthen the various social determinants of health and advocate for equity in health. (See Chapters 3, 5, and 8.)

## COMMUNITY DEFINED

Developing an understanding of a community is fundamental to providing competent community care. A **community** may be defined as a group of people who live, learn, work, and play in an environment at a given time. They share common characteristics and interests, and function within a larger social system such as an organization, region, province, or nation. The core of any community is its people, who are characterized by their age, sex, socioeconomic status, education level, occupation, ethnicity, and religion.

A community is also defined by its place or geopolitical boundaries, which often are used to determine the location of service delivery (Vollman, Anderson, & McFarlane, 2012). **Geopolitical boundaries** refer to both *geographic* boundaries such as mountains, rivers, or lakes, and *political* boundaries such as districts or areas of service delivery that are bounded by legal jurisdictions with real or imagined boundaries. **Aggregate communities** refer to groups of people with common interests, culture, beliefs, or goals. **Virtual communities** such as chat rooms, MySpace, blogs, Twitter, WhatsApp, and Facebook, are places where members share their common interests on the Internet.

## Community Functions

To sustain the day-to-day livelihood of their residents, all communities provide the following **community functions**:

- space and infrastructure for housing, schools, recreation, government, and health and social services;
- employment and income, including productivity and distribution through consumption of goods, trading, and economic growth;
- security, protection, and law enforcement to protect the public from crime;
- participation, socialization, and networking for all community members; and
- linkages with other community systems for opportunities for growth and capacity building.

## Community Dynamics

Community functions are supported by three interactive **community dynamics**: effective communication, leadership, and decision making (Clemen-Stone, Eigsti, & McGuire, 2002).

**Communication** Competent communities have strong and cohesive vertical, horizontal, and diagonal patterns of communication among the community key partners. *Vertical communication* links communities to larger communities or to those with higher decision-making power. *Horizontal communication* connects the community to work collaboratively with its own members, environment, and other service systems. *Diagonal communication* reinforces the cohesiveness and communication of all system components, both horizontally and vertically, and helps reduce the silo effects that occur when communication is done only vertically and horizontally.

**Leadership** Leaders lead their members by influencing the decision-making process using their status and position in the community. *Formal leaders* are elected official politicians, such as mayors, members of parliament, or the prime minister. *Informal leaders* are those with prominent positions in the community, such as religious leaders, executives or representatives of community organizations or professionals, elders of community groups, philanthropists, celebrities, or local heroes.

**Decision Making** Formal leaders use government policies to make decisions for the community, while informal leaders use their status to influence community groups and to effect change. Effective leaders collaborate with community groups to advocate for optimal change.

---

### HEALTHY COMMUNITIES

#### A Healthy Communities Process Involves

- Equitable community engagement
- Intersectoral partnerships
- Political commitment
- Healthy public policy
- Asset-based community development

#### Qualities of a Healthy Community Include

- Clean and safe physical environment
- Peace, equity, and social justice
- Adequate access to food, water, shelter, income, safety, work, and recreation for all
- Adequate access to healthcare services
- Opportunities for learning and skill development
- Strong, mutually supportive relationships and networks
- Workplaces that are supportive of individual and family well-being
- Wide participation of residents in decision making
- Strong local cultural and spiritual heritage
- Diverse and vital economy
- Protection of the natural environment
- Responsible use of resources to ensure long-term sustainability

*Source:* Ontario Healthy Communities Coalition. (n.d.). *What makes a community healthy?* Copyright © by Ontario Healthy Communities Coalition. Used by permission of Ontario Healthy Communities Coalition. Retrieved from http://www.ohcc-ccso.ca/en/what-makes-a-healthy-community

---

## HEALTHY COMMUNITIES

Competent community dynamics foster public participation, mutual support, and community action to promote community growth and, ultimately, healthy communities. What, then, is a healthy community? "**Healthy communities**" was a movement that began in the 1980s and became an international movement that promotes the health and well-being of members in the community. The guiding principles of healthy communities are based on the concepts of health and health promotion (see Chapter 8), and that community members from multiple sectors working together to create a sustainable and healthy community. See the box titled "Health Communities" for what constitutes healthy communities.

## SELECTED MODELS AND FRAMEWORKS OF COMMUNITY HEALTH NURSING PRACTICE

CHNs use models and frameworks to systematically collect data and analyze the relationships of various data components. The selected model or framework must be easy to use

and reflect one's practice philosophy. Most existing nursing models and frameworks focus only on individual and not community care. (See Chapter 7.) This section briefly describes those frameworks commonly used in community nursing practice.

## Community-as-Partner Model

Vollman et al. (2012) described community and nursing process as the two main attributes in their community-as-partner model. The *community attribute* is the **community assessment wheel**, which depicts the components of the community assessment: physical environment, education, safety and transportation, politics and government, health and social services, communication, economy, and recreation. At the core of this community assessment wheel are the community residents.

The *nursing process attribute* reflects Betty Neuman's stress adaptation model, which is derived from the general systems theory. Within the community are the *lines of resistance* or strengths that protect the community from harm or threats. Surrounding the community are the *normal lines of defence* that reflect the normal state of health attained by the community. *Flexible lines of defence* form the outer layer around the community to buffer stressors impacting the community. These stressors create tension-producing stimuli and may, in turn, penetrate the various lines of defence surrounding the community, affecting the system equilibrium. CHNs assess and analyze the degree of reaction to the stressors experienced by the community and implement purposeful primary, secondary, and tertiary interventions to promote client-optimal health. (See Chapter 7.)

## Epidemiologic Framework

CHNs may use the *epidemiologic triangle* (host–environment–agent) to examine the frequency and distribution of a disease or health condition in the population being studied. They determine *what* the community is, *who* is affected (host), *where* and *when* the condition occurred (environment), and *why* and *how* (agent) it occurred. They may also use the "web of causation" to study the chains of causation and their effects on a health problem. (See Chapter 11.)

## Community Capacity Approaches

**Capacity building** is a process to *strengthen* the ability of an individual, an organization, a community, or a health system to develop and implement health promotion initiatives and sustain positive health outcomes over time. It involves human resource and skills development, leadership, partnership, resource allocation, and policy formulation. Optimal capacity building is realized when the community is empowered to change and to overcome deficits to achieve a strong infrastructure to support its functions and dynamics (Minkler, 2012; Traverso-Yepez, Maddalena, Bavington, & Donovan, 2012).

**Community asset mapping** is used to outline the assets and capacity of the community and identify strengths and potential resources for program planning and interventions (Kretzmann & McKnight, 1993). An inventory of the community assets map may include skills and experiences of individuals and organizations, services, and physical and financial resources within and outside the community. CHNs evaluate the "assets" and build community capacity through activities such as strategic planning, community mobilization, and community development. (See examples of community asset maps at www.google.ca/search?q=community+asset+mappin g&newwindow=1&tbm=isch&tbo=u&source=univ&sa=X&e i=Z4U2UtKIO4S72wWutYHoBQ&ved=0CDQQsAQ&biw =1366&bih=652&dpr=1.)

## Community Health Promotion Model

The goal of the **community health promotion model** (CHPM) is to apply community health promotion strategies to achieve collaborative community actions and to improve sustainable health outcomes of the community. The CHPM (Figure 13.1) incorporates strategies from Epp's (1986) health promotion framework, the Ottawa Charter of Health Promotion (World Health Organization, Canadian Public Health Association, & Health and Welfare Canada, 1986), and primary health care principles (WHO, 1978) to guide community planning, intervention, and evaluation. (See Chapters 8 and 14.) Nursing process and primary health care are an integral part of the CHPM.

The CHPM provides a framework for purposeful and systematic community assessment, planning, implementation, and evaluation. It uses a holistic approach to promoting the health of the population to attain a higher quality of community life and health equity. The CHPM emphasizes the health of the population is influenced by the interplay of various social determinants of health in the environments they live in. These may include employment, housing, food, education, childhood years, workplace safety, social inclusion, and access to health systems. CHNs examine the impact and challenges of how people cope with their environment, with a goal of reducing health inequities among people of various social positions within and between communities and countries (Public Health Agency of Canada [PHAC], 2011). For example, a young single mother's decision to feed a high-carbohydrate diet to her children may not be her poor lifestyle choice but rather her inability to meet her children's nutritional needs is a result of her low education and income. Community health nursing process using the CHPM is described below.

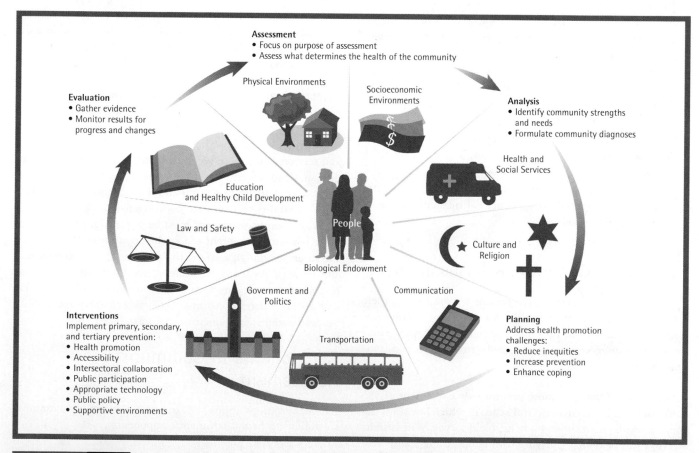

**FIGURE 13.1 Community Health Promotion Model**

*Source:* Community Health Promotion Model by Camillia F Matuk. Copyright © by Camillia F Matuk. Used by permission of Camillia F Matuk.

# COMMUNITY HEALTH NURSING PROCESS

The process of community health nursing is continuous and cyclical; it consists of four phases: assessment, planning, implementation, and evaluation. CHNs may enter at any of these phases while focusing on the purpose of their nursing involvement. This goal-oriented activity enables CHNs to collect relevant community data, critically analyze the problem or issue, make inferences on the implications of the problems or issues, formulate community nursing diagnoses, plan and implement the interventions, and evaluate the outcomes. The following sections focus on community assessment and common intervention tools.

## Community Assessment

**Community assessment** is an ongoing systematic appraisal of the community. It is a comprehensive process because the health of the community clients is affected by the complexity of community functions and dynamics and the various social determinants of health. Some key questions that guide the beginning steps of community assessment are as follows:

- What is the purpose of my community assessment? Why is it needed? Which social determinants of health are being affected?
- Who, where, and what are the characteristics of my target population? How is my population different from others in the region or the nation?
- Where is my community and what are its characteristics (e.g., community functions, process, and boundaries)?
- What information about the community do I need to know and where can I obtain this information?
- What would be the best approaches or techniques to collect my community data? Who, how, and when should I engage the community to do these?
- What are my resources or constraints to complete this community assessment (e.g., time, political environment, expertise, labour, and cost)?

## Purpose of Community Assessment

CHNs must be very clear on the reasons for conducting their community assessment. There are four types of community assessment that may be used alone or in a combination: environmental scan, needs assessment, problem investigation, and/ or resource evaluation.

**Environmental Scan** The most preliminary assessment of the community is an **environmental scan**, in which one scans the overall environment through a windshield survey. **Windshield surveys** can be done by driving, riding on public transportation, or walking around the neighbourhood. As with health inspection on individual clients, CHNs use their senses of sight, touch, hearing, and smell to gather information and form their preliminary assessment of their community. They

can see the people, the housing conditions, the geography, and the physical layout of various services in the community. During a walking tour, CHNs can listen to what languages people speak to one another and what concerns them during their daily conversations in their neighbourhood cafés or markets. They can smell the air quality or taste the water, and they can feel the temperature, humidity, or the oppression or friendliness of the people. By scanning the environment, CHNs can familiarize themselves with their work environment and connect people to the resources in the environment in which they live. Windshield surveys are best done at two different times of day and on different days of the week for data comparison purposes.

**Needs Assessment** Appropriate and cost-effective services that meet the health needs of the population are based on the community's *needs* or deficits, not on its unrealistic *wants* or *desires*. **Needs** are what the community experiences as the gap between its current situation and desired situation. To perform a needs assessment—for example, opening a teen health centre—CHNs must (a) investigate the nature of the needs, (b) determine if the expressed needs represent the opinions of the community, and (c) determine whether the community is willing and has the resources to take action for change.

**Problem Investigation** Problem investigations are conducted in response to a problem or concern. For example, with an outbreak of E. coli or measles in a community, CHNs investigate the occurrence and distribution of the disease, explore the roots or causes of the problems and their effects, and develop plans to respond appropriately.

**Resource Evaluation** Service providers aim to provide cost-effective, efficient, and seamless services through resource allocation and re-allocation. **Resource evaluation** involves the assessment and evaluation of existing community resources and services. This includes an examination of the adequacy of human, financial, and physical resources, community partnerships, service utilization, gaps and duplications, affordability, and accessibility to the target populations.

Community assessment must be purposeful and evidence-based, showing the intent of *who* the population (P) is, *what* is the intervention (I), *where* is the setting (S) for intervention, and the anticipated intervention *outcome* (O). In short, community assessment begins with a PISO statement. Tables 13.1A and 13.1B illustrate examples of how evidence-based PISO purpose statements or questions are formulated.

## Components in Community Assessment

All of the various approaches to assess a community examine the following basic assessment components:

**Community History and Perception** Understanding the past allows the CHN to build on existing strengths and avoid repeating the same failures. Areas for examination include the history of the issues of concern and community actions taken

| Table 13.1A | Formulating a Focus–Evidence–Purpose Statement/Question |
|---|---|

In this example, a CHN wants to address risky drinking on university campus by applying a harm reduction strategy. The aim is to decrease the incidence of negative consequences associated with excessive alcohol consumption.

PISO* statement: What **harm reduction strategies** are effective in **decreasing risky drinking and negative consequences** among **campus students** at the **University of Windsor**?

| | |
|---|---|
| **P**opulation | undergraduate students |
| **I**ntervention | harm reduction strategies |
| **S**etting | University of Windsor |
| **O**utcome | decreasing risky drinking and negative consequences |

*PISO is a term used in Albert, D., & Herrera, C. (2009, November 20). *Getting lost in the evidence? Part 1: Developing an evidence question and search strategy.* Fireside Chat Presentation. Ottawa, ON: University of Ottawa.

| Table 13.1B | Examples of PISO* Focus Evidence Questions |
|---|---|

| Type of Community Assessment | Population | Intervention/ Strategy | Setting | Outcome | Focus Evidence Question |
|---|---|---|---|---|---|
| Problem investigation | Campus students (17–22 yrs) | Harm reduction strategy | University of Windsor | Decrease risky drinking behaviour | What **harm reduction strategies** are effective in **decreasing risky drinking and negative consequences** among **campus students** at the **University of Windsor**? |
| Resource evaluation | Clients with low income | Program evaluation | Downtown area in Windsor | Use of Methadone clinic from January to June | How well do **low-income clients** living in the **downtown core of Windsor use the Methadone clinic** from **January to June**? |
| Environmental scan | Clients with disabilities | Community mapping and surveys | Windsor-Essex County | Transportation service for individuals with disabilities | Based on **community mapping and surveys**, how available are the **transportation services** for **rural clients with disabilities** living in **Windsor-Essex county**? |
| Needs assessment | Newcomers | Focus groups | Windsor-Essex County | Challenges and barriers to assessing breast health services | Through **focus groups discussions**, what are the **challenges and barriers to accessing breast health services** as experienced by **newcomers** living in **Windsor-Essex County**? |

*PISO is a term used in Albert, D., & Herrera, C. (2009, November 20). *Getting lost in the evidence? Part 1: Developing an evidence question and search strategy.* Fireside Chat Presentation. Ottawa, ON: University of Ottawa.

in the past; the attitudes of officials and local politicians; and the community's perceptions, attitudes, beliefs, and felt needs for health, education, and healthcare services. CHNs should explore reasons for any noted discrepancies between their and their clients' perceptions.

**Population** The core of any community is people. A **population** is a diverse group of people or aggregates residing within the boundaries of a community. A **group** refers to two or more people, while an **aggregate** is a group of people with common interests, demographics, cultural heritages, and socioeconomic and education levels. Population and aggregates are terms commonly used interchangeably. A **target population** refers to the population for whom nursing intervention is intended. **Population at risk** refers to a group of individuals who have a high probability of developing illness. People who are

disadvantaged, susceptible, or vulnerable to health inequity, injury, disease, or premature death are described as a **priority or vulnerable population**.

In addition to biology and genetic endowment, CHNs also examine the composition of the population by age distribution, sex, marital status, social class, occupation, birth rate, employment, religion, education level, family size, and other factors related to their developmental and situational needs. Community data such as trends in mortality rates (e.g., maternal and infant death rates and suicide rates), morbidity rates (e.g., common infectious diseases and chronic conditions), and life expectancy give indications regarding the health status of the population. CHNs study the rate of population growth or decline to examine the population trends and plan for anticipated services. For example, when noting the aging Canadian population in Figure 13.2 and the most recent hospital

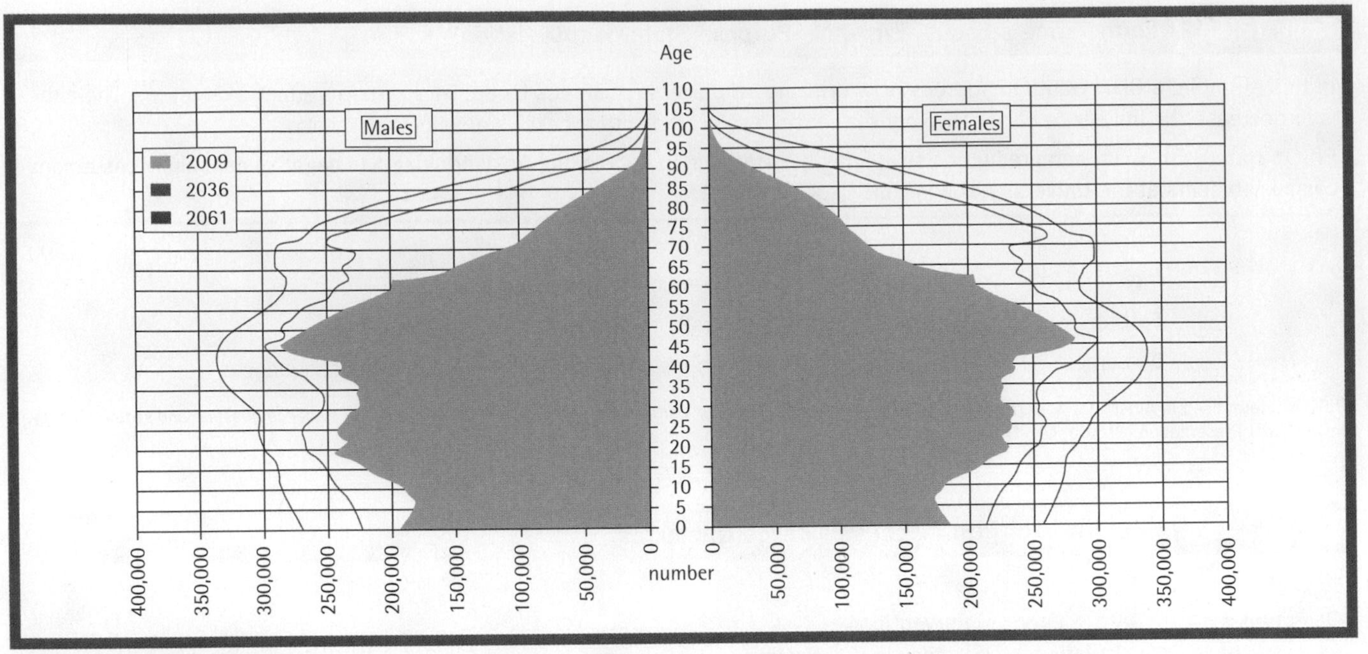

**FIGURE** **13.2** Age Pyramid (in Number) of the Canadian Population, 2009, 2036, and 2061

*Source:* Statistics Canada. (2012). *Age pyramid (in number) of the Canadian population, 2009, 2036, and 2061.* Demography Division, Chart 3.5. From http://www.statcan.gc.ca/pub/91-520-x/2010001/ct047-eng.htm. Modified December 21, 2012.

admission statistics, where about 56% of the unintentional fall–related hospital admissions were for people over 65 years of age (Canadian Institute for Health Information, 2013a), CHNs could anticipate chronic health conditions in the aging population will put more demands on home care services; they could also consider fall prevention programs as priority interventions, especially for frail elderly clients living alone in their homes.

People tend to reside in areas for a variety of reasons: proximity to their employment and extended family, accessibility to education, amenities, recreational facilities, crime rate, political reasons, and climate. The *density* of the population may shift with time and demographic makeup. For example, an influx of refugees or unemployed workers into a community may be driven by political or economic changes.

Communities are not static. The needs, characteristics, makeup, and health status of the population also change over time within its physical and social environments. For example, a surge in a community's unemployment rate may result in high family stress, a poor economy, and the relocation of many young people to other communities for work; strengthening community and social services for these communities would then become a health priority. Similarly, promoting healthy lifestyles and community support to combat social isolation and poverty is much needed in the remote northern communities because of their higher rates of smoking, obesity, suicide, and alcohol use compared to the nation's averages (Statistics Canada, 2013a).

**Boundaries** The boundary of the community refers to where the target population lives, works, plays, and learns. Healthy communities do not exist in isolation; they have permeable boundaries for the exchange of services among communities. Communities are separated from or connected to other communities by physical or artificial boundaries. **Physical boundaries** include geographic boundaries, such as mountains, valleys, roads, lakes, rivers, or oceans. **Artificial boundaries** include (a) *political boundaries*, which depict governance of various townships, counties, cities, and provinces; and (b) *situational boundaries*, which are governed by specific circumstances such as zoning for school children, traffic patterns, or smoking areas.

**Environments** Physical, chemical, biological, social, and psychosocial factors in the environment contribute to our quality of life. Air and water pollution may cause respiratory problems, digestive problems, cancer, and birth defects; geographic isolation may lead to poor access to health services, poverty, and depression (PHAC, 2011) (see Chapter 29). Physical environments include (1) *biological and chemical characteristics*: vegetation and forestry, animals and insects, bacteria and other microorganisms, food and water supply, chemicals, and toxic substances; and (2) *physical characteristics*: geography, climate, and natural resources such as soil, mountains, valleys, rivers, lakes, oceans, water, air, oil, and designs of communities, buildings, and roads.

**Socioeconomic Environments** The interaction between social and economic conditions of the community affects the health and well-being of individuals and populations. High employment rates, new housing, and business developments are common signs for communities with a healthy economy. In poor economic times, a community must have resources such as social services, housing, and food banks to assist those in need.

A strong social network within a community allows its residents to build relationships, share resources, and avoid potential risks to good health (PHAC, 2013).

**Income and Social Status** Income and education are the most important determinants of health (Senate of Canada, 2009). While income and social status are positively associated with education level, good health, and quality of life, upward or downward mobility can be seen in various social classes during economic turmoil (PHAC, 2013). Many low-income families are working poor with low education; they are in and out of poverty depending on job and housing availability and whether they have health issues. Common health issues they experience include mental illness, diabetes, substance-related disorders, and chronic obstructive pulmonary disease.

Income equality, employment, housing, and food security all affect people's health and their sense of well-being (PHAC, 2013). Only 47% of the low-income Canadians rated their health as very good or excellent, compared to 73% of those in the highest income bracket. Those who live in poverty have higher hospital admission rates and shorter life expectancy than those with higher incomes. New Canadian mothers living on low incomes were 20 times more likely to have multiple health problems than those living on high income; rising income could dramatically improve maternal and child health (O'Campo & Urquia, 2012). (See Canadian Research Box 13.1.)

**Employment and Working Conditions** Unemployment, underemployment, economic instability, and stressful or unsafe working conditions significantly affect not only people's physical, mental, and social health and general well-being, but their families and communities. People who are employed and work in a safe workplace experience less stress, live longer, and have fewer health problems (PHAC, 2013).

**Social Supports and Networks** Early hospital discharge, an aging population, and rising chronic diseases have led to the need for strong formal and informal social supports and networks from families, friends, and communities. Research shows a positive relationship between social support and health status and perceived health (Anuruang et al., 2013; PHAC, 2013).

**Diversity and Social Inclusion** Healthy communities embrace harmony, safety, and diversity as the social norm. For example, schools instill cultural awareness and sensitivity in young children, thereby reducing racism or bullying; service agencies provide classes to strengthen parenting skills and promote family relationships, which indirectly prevents family violence; and neighbourhood watch programs reduce crime rates. Social inclusion by gender, age, ability, sexual orientation, race, ethnicity, and religion will create a community where people feel they belong and so strive to reach their full potential as members (Linsay & McPherson, 2012; PHAC, 2013).

**Recreation** Recreation provides a form of socialization and a means for healthy physical and mental activity for people outside of their family, school, and work life. Healthy communities have accessible and affordable recreational facilities or activities for their residents of all ages to play or to spend time together after school or work.

**Education and Healthy Child Development** Education provides people the needed life skills and technical skills for their day-to-day living and, therefore, health and prosperity. Canadians with low literacy skills are more likely to be poor and unemployed, suffer from poor health, have low self-esteem, and miss opportunities for learning and community participation than those with higher levels of education (Mitic & Rootman, 2012; PHAC, 2013).

## CANADIAN RESEARCH BOX 13.1

### What are the predictors of smoking during pregnancy in Canada?

Cui, Y., Shooshtari, S., Forget, E. F., Clara, I., & Cheung, K. F. (2014). Smoking during pregnancy: Findings from the 2009–2010 Canadian Community Health Survey. *PLoS One, 9*(1), e84640. doi:10.1371/journal.pone.0084640

The purpose of this secondary analysis from Canadian Community Health Survey (CCHS) was to study the prevalence of smoking during pregnancy in relation to the social determinants of this behaviour. Data were collected on two provinces and two territories between 2009 and 2010. Results showed that the prevalence of smoking during pregnancy was 23% higher among women in the Northern Territories (59.3%) than those in Alberta (34.8%) and Ontario (18.5%). When comparing to women under 25 years old, the smoking rate was higher among those with low income (59.6%), with less than university education (18.8%), not having a regular medical doctor (50.5%), having poor perception of health (43.1%), having at least one mental disease (35.3%) and one chronic disease (23.2%), and who were regular alcohol drinkers (27.8%). Results were statistically significant in that the odds of smoking during pregnancy were lower among women of increased maternal age and having the highest level of family income, a regular medical doctor, and good to excellent self-perceived health. Mothers who reported to having at least one chronic disease and one mental illness, including depression and anxiety, had greater odds of smoking during pregnancy. The researchers concluded that it was important to know the population's lifestyle characteristics that are associated with smoking during pregnancy, and urged healthcare providers and policy makers to implement population health promotional strategies to achieve healthy pregnancy outcomes.

### Discussion Questions

1. What information would you need to consider when promoting smoking cessation among pregnant women?
2. List some of the population health promotion strategies that could be used to prevent smoking during pregnancy and to promote the health of pregnant women.

Healthy physical, cognitive, and emotional development in children is determined by effects ranging from preconception health and prenatal care to the quality of parental nurturing and supervision (see Chapter 16). Poor early childhood developmental characteristics, such as low birth weight or poor nutrition, can delay language or brain development and compromise physical and mental health through to adulthood.

Schools are ideal settings in which children can learn to adopt societal norms and health behaviours in their early years. Disadvantaged and low-income children tend to not perform well in school; they are at greater risk for poor health. Youth with positive assets such as parental nurturing and monitoring, school engagement, and peer connections are more likely to have high self-worth and healthy lifestyles (PHAC, 2013) (see Chapter 17). CHNs can advocate for adequate social policy surrounding issues such as parental leaves, national childcare policy, unemployment benefits, and social assistance to meet the health and social needs of families and children.

**Culture and Religion** Canada is second to Australia in having a vast number of people of different races or ethnic groups, colours, and religions. One in every five Canadians is foreign-born and belongs to a visible minority group, with 58% from Asia and the Middle East; 67.3% were Christians and Catholics, while others were Muslim, Hindu, Sikh, or Buddhist (Statistics Canada, 2014). **Religion** offers a form of spiritual support for many people, especially those in crisis; it can also frame individuals' healthcare practices. For example, Jehovah's Witnesses refuse blood transfusions and Muslims need adjustment of family, school, and work routines during their religious celebrations and prayers.

**Culture** is the way we think, live, act, believe, and feel. Various ethnocultural groups in many Canadian communities strive to preserve their heritage through their own social activities and language classes. Visible minorities and new Canadians with language and cultural barriers are often alienated from the mainstream society and experience inequities in health from poverty, social isolation, bullying, and poor access to services (e.g., high unemployment or underemployment rates in newcomers and a high incidence of suicide and diabetes in Aboriginal people) (Cornelson, 2011). Consequently, many ethnic groups tend to live and work in their own ethnic communities to avoid marginalization. CHNs must address the diversity, cultural competence and safety and societal tolerance as they work with this population. (See Chapter 9.)

**Health and Social Services** Most people, whether sick or healthy, seek health services at some time in their lives. *Health services* include primary, secondary, and tertiary care, ranging from promotion and protection of health to hospital, rehabilitative, and palliative care services. *Social services*, including welfare, unemployment benefits, mothers' allowance, and disability pensions, are examples of assistance for those who are single parents, unemployed, or have physical or mental disabilities. An infrastructure of a wide range of health and social services can help people emerge from their crises. CHNs who are knowledgeable about various community resources can refer or coordinate these services efficiently to meet their clients' needs.

Territorialism and unwillingness to share information or resources among community agencies for fear of losing program funding often result in fragmentation or duplication of services. CHNs assess what and how health and social services are used and delivered to their communities, and whether service gaps, unmet needs, duplications, and strengths exist. They work with the community to facilitate better coordination and more accessible and affordable services to the people in need.

**Transportation** A reliable and affordable transportation system is necessary to ensure that community members have access to the essential services they need. CHNs attend to the transportation needs for rural clients, the poor, the frail elderly, and those with physical limitations; and they mobilize resources to meet their needs (e.g., reduced taxi fare or volunteer drivers for seniors or those with disabilities).

**Communication** Effective and efficient communication is crucial for building supportive and collaborative relationships. Conveying clear messages, the methods, location, and timing of which are pivotal in communicating how to deliver quality care to the community members. The common modes of formal and informal communication for community members include the local newspapers, newsletters, emails, radio, television, flyers, Twitter, Facebook, and community forums.

**Governments and Politics** Governments set policies to deliver essential services to meet the basic needs and goals of the community. They provide formal leadership to communities and reinforce compliance to their policies (e.g., smoke-free regulations, service agreements). While formal leaders hold authority in making decisions, informal leaders and community members often have the power to influence change.

CHNs must be aware of the existing government policies, work with both formal and informal leaders, and be involved in the decision-making process. They assess the relationships and the degree of cooperation or conflict between the community and other agencies or decision-making bodies.

**Law and Safety** Governments set rules and regulations as law. Crimes such as homicides, assaults, and thefts are symptoms of family and community response to stress (e.g., family violence, unemployment, and drug use). Safety is a prerequisite to quality of life. Communities grow and prosper economically in peaceful times. Peace is achieved when society has law and order. CHNs assess whether residents are feeling safe by examining the occurrences of crimes (i.e., types, rates, and locations) and collaborating with the police in crime prevention to create a safe place for people to live.

## Community Data Collection

Communities have multi-system components; thus, collecting community data can be abundant and complex. It is essential for CHNs to be very clear on the purpose of their community assessment and to use credible and appropriate sources and techniques to collect valid community data. One or a multiple methods may be used to collect the needed community data. Generally, existing data should be examined before gathering new data. New data can be gathered from surveys and meetings with community residents and leaders or other key informants.

There are two main types of community data: (1) *quantitative data*, such as facts and figures shown in population statistics or health status reports, and (2) *qualitative data*, such as statements or opinions gathered from windshield surveys, focus groups, forums, key informants, or public or town hall meetings.

## Sources of Community Data

The following are common community data sources:

- Participant observation
  - windshield survey, walking tours
- Literature review
  - published studies including systemic reviews help validate the community needs and show evidence of best practices for interventions
- Demographic and epidemiologic data
  - Statistics Canada (e.g., census data, trends, and vital statistics)
- National and local policy data
  - Public Health Agency of Canada (e.g., diseases, injuries, and other threats to public health)
  - Canadian Institute for Health Information (e.g., statistics related to determinants of health and diseases, health-care occupations, spending, and hospitalizations)
  - local, provincial, and federal health departments and municipal planning departments (e.g., local census, housing, and business and industrial developments)
  - Environment Canada (e.g., environmental indices)
  - local organizations, such as hospitals, school boards, and agencies (e.g., annual reports on services delivered)
  - municipal traffic departments and provincial transportation departments (e.g., traffic accidents, resulting injuries, and deaths)
  - Workers' Compensation Board (e.g., work-related injuries and deaths)
  - other social data from Juristat (for crime statistics and trends, victim services, and court statistics) and Citizenship and Immigration Canada (for immigration-related statistics)
- Community surveys
  - Canadian Community Health Survey (e.g., health profiles and indicators, mortality, and census information)
  - key informant surveys (e.g., focus groups, community forums)

## Methods for Community Data Collection

The extent of community data collection is often determined by the resources available and the time constraints. In addition to the various data collection methods mentioned in the previous paragraph, this section specifically focuses on community surveys, community forums, and focus groups.

**Community Surveys** Community surveys are a series of questions addressing the issue(s) or population(s) being studied. They capture a broad range of data from a representative sample population in a short period of time. They can be conducted via regular mail, Internet, telephone, or face-to-face interviews. The data collected provide a *snapshot* of the population being studied at that particular time and may be generalized to describe the larger population. National surveys are usually done every 5 to 10 years to examine changes in behaviours over time. The Canadian Community Health Survey was conducted biannually from 2001 to 2007 and now is conducted annually.

**Community Forums** Community forums are public meetings in which community members discuss issues of concern and share their experiences and opinions with their community leaders or decision makers. A community forum is an inexpensive way to collect community data. The people who attend these meetings are either directly involved in or affected by the topic being discussed (e.g., the impact of a school closure, service restructuring in a community, or crime reduction in a neighbourhood). CHNs should note that when opinions are expressed by one person or a few people who dominate the discussions, their opinions may not represent the majority's view and the purpose of the forum may be derailed. Community forums should be conducted by trained facilitators to elicit maximum public response.

**Focus Groups** Focus groups are small group discussions with an average of 8 to 12 people that usually last one to two hours. There may be a series of focus groups on the same topic across the community, region, province, or nation. They may be conducted by trained facilitators. Similar to the community forums, focus groups are smaller in scale and the participants are more homogeneous in their characteristics or experience related to the issue or topic being discussed. Focus groups and community forums are useful for collecting more in-depth information, such as qualitative data when surveys fail to serve this purpose. (See the box titled "Conducting a Focus Group or Community Forum.") They are not a place for debate or confrontation.

CHNs use multiple strategies to collect the needed data as no single source or method can provide all the assessment data on a community. Epidemiological and research skills are particularly important for analyzing and interpreting vital statistics and figures. (See Chapters 10 and 11.) Collecting community data can be an overwhelming experience, but it need not be a time-consuming process. The key is to focus on the purpose of the assessment and to understand what determines the health of the community client, and where and how to collect meaningful data.

## CONDUCTING A FOCUS GROUP OR COMMUNITY FORUM

**Prior to the Meeting:**

■ Determine the purpose and goals of the meeting. Develop four to six open-ended questions, focusing on the problem or need to be addressed, and ways to encourage discussion and idea sharing. Allot time for each question.

■ Arrange for an effective facilitator to conduct the meeting and a recorder to record or take notes of the meeting discussions.

■ Identify and recruit participants who are representative of the community and who can offer insights and unbiased opinions.

■ Select a convenient, comfortable, private, and well-equipped location. Prepare refreshments, nametags, paper, and pens within the allowed budget. Review the meeting itineraries, and prepare a meeting agenda.

**At the Meeting:**

■ Welcome and thank participants for their attendance. (5 min)

■ Introduce yourself and the facilitator. Explain the purpose of the meeting and the ground rules (e.g., stay on topic, no one will dominate the conversation), how the meeting discussion will be conducted and recorded, and the information used. (5–10 min)

■ Introduce the topic of discussion. Ask the participants (individually or in small groups) to discuss one question at a time. Invite their ideas. Listen to their ideas, remain non-judgmental, and ask for clarification as needed. Record their responses. Ensure that all members participate in the discussion. Stay on topic; discourage anyone from dominating the discussion. (30–60 min)

■ Before ending the session, invite participants to offer further comments. Summarize main themes discussed at the meeting. Explain how the meeting information will be used and disseminated and thank participants for their participation. (5–10 min)

**Immediately after the Meeting:**

■ Record your observations of group participation or typical questions asked. Transcribe and summarize discussions and comments recorded at the meeting.

■ Analyze findings, extract themes and ideas, draw conclusions, and prepare report. Share results with the group and translate results to action where applicable.

## Population Health

Population health builds on the traditional practice of health promotion and public health with a focus on preventive activities and disease management. **Population health** is "an approach to health that aims to improve the health of the entire population and to reduce health inequities among population groups. . . . it acts upon the broad range of factors and conditions that have a strong influence on our health" (PHAC, 2012, para. 4). Federal, provincial, territorial, and local governments play a leadership role to implement population health policies and set clear program goals and targets (Senate of Canada, 2009).

Healthy populations contribute to the overall productivity and quality of life in the community, and to a sustainable and equitable healthcare system. Based on this belief, the Public Health Agency of Canada (2002) developed a **population health template** with eight key elements and corresponding action steps for health practitioners, educators, and researchers: (1) focus on the health of population, (2) address the determinants of health and their interactions, (3) base decisions on evidence, (4) increase upstream investments, (5) apply multiple strategies, (6) collaborate across sectors and levels, (7) employ mechanisms for public involvement, and (8) demonstrate accountability for health outcomes. There are also international *health indicators* that measure quantifiable information on the health of the population and the healthcare system: (1) health status, (2) non-medical determinants of health, (3) health system performance, (4) community and health system characteristics, and (5) equity (CIHI, 2013b; Statistics Canada, 2013b).

Promoting the health of the populations in their community is not new to CHNs. To excel in this, CHNs must overcome personal and systemic barriers that impede their care. Community organizations need to provide an infrastructure that supports population health promotion. CHNs also need to develop competent knowledge and skills on community health nursing, with an emphasis on leadership, community partnership, policy development, and advocacy skills (Schofield et al., 2009).

**Risk Assessment** It will be impossible for CHNs to work with every member in the community. Thus, CHNs assess the conditions of risks and benefits that apply to the entire population or to its significant aggregates, and deliver health services only to those who are at risk. **Risk** refers to the probability or likelihood that healthy persons exposed to a specific factor will acquire a specific disease. These specific factors, called **risk factors**, can be environmental, lifestyle, and psychosocial factors (e.g., sources of exposure, cultural practices, patterns of behaviour, local concerns, direct impact from the service delivery system), or biological factors (e.g., age, sex, or genetic makeup).

When doing **risk assessment**, CHNs identify and target clients who are most likely to contract a particular disease or develop unhealthy behaviours, and assess attributes that affect or potentially affect their health. For example, teens have a higher risk than adults of contracting sexually transmitted infections (STIs) or getting pregnant, as they tend to experiment more with their sexuality; similarly, older adults are more likely to have falls than are younger adults due to the aging process.

## Community Analysis and Nursing Diagnoses

The purpose of data analysis is to identify *actual* and *potential* community strengths and needs that are relevant to the improvement of existing health services. Competent **community analysis** relies on a clear conceptual understanding of how social determinants interact and have an impact on health and on community functions and dynamics. Community data are systematically summarized into categories and compared with other relative community systems for significance; inferences are then made to formulate *community nursing diagnoses*.

Community nursing diagnoses and nursing diagnoses are similar. They differ in that community nursing diagnoses are broad, addressing a community or aggregate, whereas nursing

---

**CASE STUDY**

**What does health mean to people living in a slum area?**

Study the community scene illustrated in Figure 13.3. List and rank what you think the people in this community would say was needed to improve their health. In a group of four to six students, compare the individual rankings and discuss the following questions.

### Discussion Questions

**1.** Who are the experts in identifying the local needs of a community? By priority, rank the areas that you feel would improve the health of this community and relate them to the determinants of health.

**2.** If you were a resident of this community, how would you feel if someone made judgments about your living situation? Why? What do you see as the priority area to improve the health of your community?

**3.** What data sources and data collection methods would you use to establish a community profile as depicted in this figure?

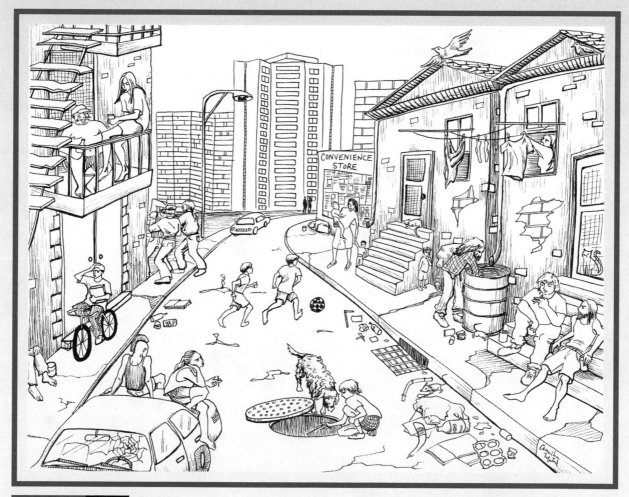

**FIGURE 13.3** Slum Area

*Source:* Slum Area by Camillia F Matuk. Copyright © by Camillia F Matuk. Used by permission of Camillia F Matuk.

diagnoses address individuals or families. All communities have strengths as well as problems. Formulation of community nursing diagnoses must be based on community assessment data collected. **Community nursing diagnoses** may be problem or wellness diagnoses, with statements consisting of the following components:

- specific aggregate or target group;
- actual or potential unhealthy or healthy response/situation that a nurse can change;
- etiology or cause for the unhealthy or healthy response/situation; and
- characteristics (i.e., signs and symptoms) or evidence that describe the response or situation.

Table 13.2 illustrates examples of nursing diagnoses formulation.

**Planning, Implementation, and Evaluation** Once the identified community needs are prioritized, the CHN devises interventions to resolve those needs. The intervention plan should address the *challenges* to achieving health for all: reducing inequalities, increasing prevention, and enhancing

community coping (Epp, 1986). The goals and objectives for intervention are derived from the community nursing diagnoses.

Nursing interventions include primary, secondary, and tertiary preventive services that reflect the five principles of *primary health care*: accessibility, health promotion, intersectoral co-operation, appropriate technology, and public participation (WHO, 1978). Population-focused health promotion strategies include but are not limited to advocacy for healthy public policy, the strengthening of community action, and the creation of supportive environments (CHNC, 2011, revised; Epp, 1986). (See Chapter 8.)

Depending on the role and practice settings, CHNs, such as home health or community-based nurses, focus on direct-care services to individuals and families, whereas public health nurses (PHNs) provide population-focused care. Specific public health nursing interventions include consultation, counselling, health teaching, case management, referral and follow-up, screening, outreach, disease surveillance, policy development and enforcement, social marketing, advocacy, community organizing, coalition building, and collaboration (Canadian Public Health Association [CPHA], 2010). (See Chapters 3

| Table 13.2 | Examples of Community Health Nursing Diagnosis | | |
|---|---|---|---|
| **Focus Population**<br><br>*(Who is your target group or community?)* | **Problem or Wellness Diagnosis**<br><br>*(What is the potential/actual community issue, concern, situation, or response you need to manage or intervene?)* | **Etiology**<br><br>*(Why is there this community issue, concern, situation, or response? Identify the causation factors.)* | **Characteristics**<br><br>*(How did you make this etiologic inference? Give supporting community data/evidence or manifestations, i.e., signs or symptoms.)* |
| 1. Students in high school | Potential for healthy lifestyles | Related to their desire to learn about nutrition and physical activities | As evidenced by integrated school curriculum with an emphasis on healthy lifestyle practices |
| 2. Residents in Kent community | Risk for imbalanced nutrition; more than body requirements | Related to poor optimal lifestyle choices | As evidenced by increased in prevalence of obesity, high consumption rates of fast food, and low physical activity level in the residents |
| 3. West-end community | Optimal waste disposal | Related to effective management of the community recycling system | As evidenced by 98% utilization of the recycling programs, and 25% reduction of rodents in the city area |
| 4. Newcomers | Inadequate income and resources and high family stress level | Related to inadequate language and skilled trades programs to prepare newcomers to be employable | As evidenced by high unemployment rates at 25%, inability to find work because of lack of language skills and Canadian work experience/requirements, high anxiety, and stress expressed by family |

to 5.) Nursing interventions will be successful when the community is fully engaged and empowered throughout the nursing process.

Subjective and objective community data help form the needed indicators for evaluation of any evidence of success. Community planning and interventions will be effective when public policy and supportive environments are addressed and when the community is committed to work on the identified need or issue. (See Chapter 14 for program monitoring and evaluation.) The following section describes common planning and evaluation tools used in community settings.

## Community Participatory Tools for Community Planning

A **community participatory approach** is key to community planning. Through dialogue with stakeholders and community members during the process, the community decides what makes a need become a priority, who is to take the action, what the action will be, and when and how it is to be done. Community participatory tools help quantify and qualify the health issues, needs, or concerns that they identify. Active participation and sharing of experiences can empower people to take responsibility and ownership in health and to effect change.

**Community Needs Matrix Tool** Participants may use the **community needs matrix tool** to discuss, identify, rate, or explain what they perceive to be the most important health problems or the most feasible interventions in their community. The degree of concern about each issue is tallied on a blank chart similar to that in Table 13.3, which shows this community is most concerned about accidents. CHNs facilitate the discussion to learn what the community has to say about their lived experiences. Through mutual planning, the CHNs assist the participants to make informed choices of the needed action and, thus, improved client outcomes (Anuruang et al., 2013).

**Community Mapping** Community mapping is a schematic map of the community indicating the distribution and occurrence of illness, disease, and health; major resources; environmental conditions; and accessibility and barriers to various services. Community members may examine their accessibility and the resources in their environment, and CHNs use the members' expressed perceptions and experiences to mutually formulate the intervention plans. Figure 13.4 illustrates an example of community mapping on the case distribution of spina bifida.

**Present–Future Drawing** CHNs may ask their community clients to draw a **present–future drawing** (see Figure 13.5) to reflect upon their present situation and what resources and constraints contributed to it, and to visualize how the future might appear. This tool allows the nurse and the clients to see where the community wants to go and, hence, to formulate mutual intervention goals and objectives.

## Community Governance and Community Engagement

Community governance and community engagement are pivotal to achieving program sustainability and accountability, building community capacity, and social equity (Nonprofit Quarterly, 2015). **Community governance** refers to management, leadership, and decision making in health organizational matters, which are usually undertaken by a group of community stakeholders, to meet the health needs and priorities of the community through community engagement and empowerment (Totikidis, Armstrong, & Francis, 2005). Effective community governance must encompass three community skills: *engaging citizens, measuring results,* and *getting things done* (Epstein, Coates, Wray, & Swain, 2006).

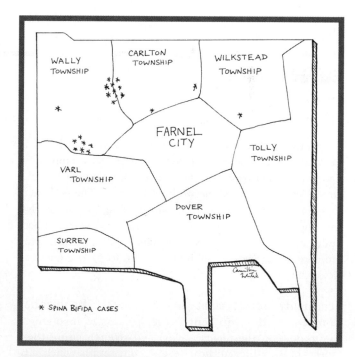

**FIGURE 13.4** Community Map Showing Distribution of Spina Bifida

*Source:* Community Map Showing Distribution of Spina Bifida by Camillia F Matuk. Copyright © by Camillia F Matuk. Used by permission of Camillia F Matuk.

| Table 13.3 | Example of the Results of a Community Needs Matrix Tool | | | |
|---|---|---|---|---|
| Identified Health Need | Not a Concern | Somewhat Concerned | A Concern | Very Concerned |
| Accidents | * | *** | *** | **** |
| Nutrition | * | ** | ** | **** |
| Pneumonia | * | ** | *** | * |
| STIs | * | *** | *** | * |

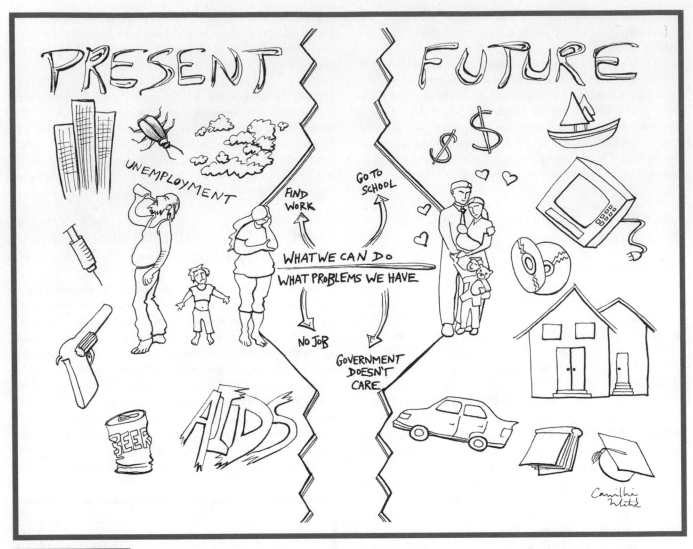

**FIGURE 13.5** Present–Future Drawing

*Source:* Present–future drawing by Camillia F Matuk. Copyright © by Camillia F Matuk. Used by permission of Camillia F Matuk.

**Community engagement** is "a process involving citizens at various levels of participation based on interpersonal communication and trust and a common understanding and purpose" (Ontario Local Health Integrated Network, 2011, p. 4). The purpose of community engagement is "to inform, educate, consult, involve, and empower" stakeholders [and community members] in both health care [and] health service planning and decision-making processes to improve the health care system" (p. 5). (See Canadian Research Box 13.2.)

### Community Development and Community Mobilization

**Community development** is the "process of involving a community in the identification and strengthening those aspects of daily life, culture life, and political life which support health. This might include support for political action to change total environment and strengthen resources for healthy living" (CPHA, 2010, p. 32). Community development begins with a need or a vision for change. The process to bring on the change usually starts with one or a few individuals at a grassroots level, taking collective action to generate solutions to common problems, and it eventually involves the larger community. The process is referred to as **community mobilization**. Community development involves capacity building and community mobilization.

CHNs can engage the community members and work in partnership with their communities as they define their own goals, mobilize resources, and develop action plans for collectively identified issues or problems. Community development focuses on consensus building, improving, strengthening, and sustaining community life and local conditions to enable people, particularly those in disadvantaged situations, and to engage them in decision making to achieve greater control over their circumstances. One example is Terry Fox's Marathon of Hope which started in 1980. As a cancer survivor, Fox had a vision to find a cure for cancer, and he began running across the country to raise funds for cancer research. Since then, his one-person dream has become a world movement. Some examples of community development initiatives related to poverty are community gardens and dragon boat races to raise breast cancer awareness.

**CANADIAN RESEARCH BOX 13.2**

**Does mammography prevent cancer death?**

Miller A. B., Wall, C., Baines, C. J., Sun, P., To, T., & Narod, S. (2014). Twenty-five year follow-up for breast cancer incidence and mortality of the Canadian National Breast Screening Study: Randomized screening trial. *BMJ.* 348:g366. doi:10.1136/bmj.g366

This study, conducted by physicians and statisticians at the University of Toronto, compared the incidence and mortality on a 25-year follow-up in women aged 40–59 who did or did not undergo mammography screening. A total of 89 835 women were randomly assigned to mammography (five annual mammography screens) or control (no mammography) in six provinces (Nova Scotia, Quebec, Ontario, Manitoba, Alberta, and British Columbia) between 1980 and 1985 in 15 screening centres. All women aged 50–59 in both experimental and control groups received annual physical breast examinations. Women aged 40–49 in the experimental group received an annual physical breast examination, and those in the control group received usual care in the community. The comparative analysis on cumulative mortality from breast cancer showed that women aged 40–49 and 50–59 were similar, and there was a residual excess of 106 cancers in the experimental group attributable to over-diagnosis. Overall, 22% (106/484) of mammography screen-detected invasive breast cancers were over-diagnosed, representing one over-diagnosed breast cancer for every 424 women who received mammography screening in the trial. The researchers concluded "annual mammography in women aged 40–59 does not reduce mortality from breast cancer beyond that of physical examination or usual care."

**Discussion Questions**

1. As CHNs, what are some of the questions you should consider with this longitudinal study?
2. When promoting breast health among your target population, what are some of the strategies you could consider?

Community interventions must be evaluated to measure the outcomes, whether the expected results were achieved or not. The steps for **community program evaluation** are (1) determining what needs to be evaluated based on the evaluation criteria; (2) engaging stakeholders throughout the process; (3) determining the appropriate methods of measurement; (4) developing data collection instruments, budget, and timeline for evaluation; (5) collecting and analyzing data; (6) reporting and disseminating the results; and (7) making decisions for action. (See Chapter 14.)

Successes and lessons learned from mistakes or challenges should be shared with the community to benefit other communities. Communities build on successes and work on perfecting problems for future changes and continuous improvement. There are excellent tools described in the Community Tool Box (see http://ctb.ku.edu/en/solveproblem/Troubleshooting_Guide_1.htm). Interventions should be evaluated and documented to support evidence-based practice.

Table 13.4 provides a summary guide that CHNs may use to assess the general health of a community and develop a community intervention plan. The assessment questions should be modified according to the purpose of the assessment.

| Table 13.4 | Guide to Community Health Nursing Process |
| --- | --- |
| **AREAS FOR ASSESSING A COMMUNITY'S GENERAL HEALTH**<br>Modify these general questions to reflect the specific purpose of the community assessment | **DATA/OBSERVATIONS**<br>Gather subjective and objective data and note discrepancies between the CHN and the clients |
| **A. ASSESSMENT**<br><br>**1. Purpose of Community Assessment, Target Group, and Location**<br>– Purpose of assessment (e.g., environmental scan, needs assessment, problem investigation, or resource evaluation)?<br>– Rationale for the assessment?<br>– Who is the target group? What are their characteristics?<br>– Boundaries where target group resides?<br>– Supportive evidence for the health needs of the target group?<br><br>**2. Community Historical and Perception**<br>– Previous history of community actions by local groups or government?<br>– Perceptions of the residents on the community issues, problems, concerns, attitudes, beliefs, felt needs? How are they similar or different from that of the larger community or the nurse? | |

*(continued)*

| **Table 13.4** | **Continued** |
|---|---|

| **AREAS FOR ASSESSING A COMMUNITY'S GENERAL HEALTH**<br>Modify these general questions to reflect the specific purpose of the community assessment | **DATA/OBSERVATIONS**<br>Gather subjective and objective data and note discrepancies between the CHN and the clients |
|---|---|
| **3. Population**<br> – Total composition and characteristics of the population in the community (e.g., age group distribution, gender, marital status, birth rate, and family size)?<br> – Density and rate of population growth, increased or decreased?<br> – Health status<br>  • Mortality and morbidity rates for age-specific diseases or causes, their incidence and prevalence?<br>  • Comparison of mortality and morbidity rates with previous years, with regional, provincial, and national rates?<br>  • Life expectancy and trends?<br>  • Biologic and genetic endowment?<br>  • Health status: indicators and influencing factors related to purpose of assessment (e.g., nutrition; immunization; lifestyles; stress; STIs; unplanned pregnancy; prenatal care; emergency care; primary, secondary, and tertiary care; personal health practices and coping skills (e.g., healthy lifestyle practices, effective or maladaptive coping)?<br><br>**4. Physical Environments**<br> – Location: boundaries, geography, climate, plants, and animals posing threats to health, percentage of urban or rural area?<br> – Housing: type, condition, slum areas, sanitation, adequacy, crowding?<br> – Shopping facilities: types, location, and accessibility?<br> – Safety: crime rates, types, and where? Feeling safe? Police and relationships with the community?<br> – Water supply: quality and adequacy?<br> – Sanitation: sewage and waste disposal?<br><br>**5. Socioeconomic Environments**<br> – Income: income levels, poverty rate, number receiving social assistance?<br> – Social status and mobility<br>  • Percentages for each social class?<br>  • Patterns and impact of mobility on health needs and health service planning?<br> – Employment and working conditions<br>  • Major industries and business establishments?<br>  • Primary occupations? Employment rate? Unemployment or underemployment?<br>  • Occupational hazards?<br>  • Safe and supportive work life?<br> – Social supports and networks: Social isolation? Any support groups and community group involvement?<br> – Social inclusion: embrace diversity and share social experience by gender, sex, sexual orientation, race, ethnicity, and religion?<br> – Recreation: facilities, affordability, accessibility, and appropriateness for all ages?<br><br>**6. Education and Healthy Child Development**<br> – Education: literacy rates, attitudes, and facilities/programs for life skills and technical skills?<br>  • Available and accessible resources, peer support and engagement?<br> – Healthy child development: preconception health, prenatal and parenting class, and daycare?<br>  • Early identification and intervention programs?<br>  • Accessible and affordable resources and services? | |

| Table 13.4 | Continued |
| --- | --- |
| **AREAS FOR ASSESSING A COMMUNITY'S GENERAL HEALTH**<br>Modify these general questions to reflect the specific purpose of the community assessment | **DATA/OBSERVATIONS**<br>Gather subjective and objective data and note discrepancies between the CHN and the clients |

**7. Culture and Religion**
- Ethnic and racial group composition and subcultures, culture, and languages spoken?
- Cultural diversity and tolerance, positive and negative influence on health practices?
- Cultural adaptation, perceptions of health?
- Religious affiliations and spiritual support and influence on health practices?

**8. Health and Social Services**
- Services and community organizations
  - Location, ratios of health workers to rural and urban populations?
  - Number of beds available and type, health service utilization? Wait list? Health budgets priority, amount per capita and spending?
  - Provision of adequate and quality primary, secondary, and tertiary care?
  - Service coordination, gaps, and duplications?
  - Impact of funding on service delivery?
  - Evidence of community engagement and community governance (e.g., inter-sectoral co-operation, health promotion, public participation, and appropriate technology used in service delivery)?
  - Available and adequate social assistance to meet community needs in a timely manner?

**9. Transportation**
- Type, availability, accessibility, affordability, and usage?

**10. Governance and Politics**
- Communications
  - Methods, timing, and locations of verbal and nonverbal communication (e.g., newspapers, radio, television, flyers, Internet, and forums)?
  - Relationships with other organizations, degree of conflict, and collaboration?
  - Evidence of interpersonal relationships, commitment, and partnerships?
- Leadership
  - Who are the formal and informal leaders? What are their visions for the community?
  - Power structure, delegations, politics?
- Decision making: effective and efficient process of decision making (e.g., policy formulation, human resources)?

**B. ANALYSIS**

**1. Wellness Nursing Diagnoses**
- Potential and actual community strengths?

**2. Problem Nursing Diagnoses**
- Potential and actual community needs and gaps?

**C. PLANNED INTERVENTIONS**

- Implementation of primary, secondary, and tertiary preventive care focusing on health promotion challenges such as reducing inequities, increasing prevention, and enhancing coping?
- Evidence of incorporation of primary health care principles, public policy, and supportive environments in nursing care planning?
- Expected outcomes and target dates clearly defined?

**D. EVALUATION**

- Monitoring of progress and gathering of evidence of success based on outcomes objectives?
- Lessons learned, decision for action, and knowledge transfer?

## CONCLUSION

CHNs work in complex social, political, and economic environments as they care for the diverse population. They have the professional and social responsibility to build a healthy community by providing accessible and quality care to meet the needs of individuals, families, aggregates, populations, and their community. CHNs must be competent in using the community health promotion process in which they implement their primary health care roles to address health inequities for the marginalized populations (National Expert Commission, 2012, revised). They engage the community and strategically invest primary, secondary, and tertiary levels of prevention to strengthen individual and community capacity, to identify populations who are at risk, and to provide maintenance, protective care, and palliative care for their clients as needed. Expert CHNs will demonstrate competent leadership in community health promotion and advocate for the importance of population-focused health promotion. They will use various community participatory tools to engage community stakeholders and population groups to address community health needs, to advocate positive change, and to strive to achieve the health for all.

## KEY TERMS

## STUDY QUESTIONS

1. Name four community settings where CHNs work, and describe their role and functions in these settings.

2. What are the characteristics of a healthy community?

3. What nursing process skills will you use to promote the health of the community?

4. What assessment components are used when assessing community health?

5. Define population health, community engagement, community governance, community development, and capacity building.

6. Discuss the benefits of community dialogue between CHNs and Aboriginal communities or any other population groups.

> After working through these questions, go to the MyNursingLab at www.pearsoned.ca/mynursinglab to check your answers.

## INDIVIDUAL CRITICAL-THINKING EXERCISES

1. Why is it important for the nurse to provide care to the community?

2. How does the community health nursing process differ from the individual nursing process?

3. How would you work with your community to identify their health needs and share their community experiences?

4. In developing a health profile for a community, what assessment questions would you ask for each category of the community components? Where and how would you collect the needed data?

5. Why is it important to use participatory tools for community planning?

## GROUP CRITICAL-THINKING EXERCISES

1. Based on the community needs matrix tool (Table 13.3), what are some of the questions you would want to ask the community about their ratings? What would be the next steps?

2. In a group of two to four, spend about an hour visiting and talking to people in your local neighbourhood. Describe your community visit and explain your impression about the felt needs, real needs, and wants of the community. Formulate your nursing diagnoses and propose your actions.

3. Discuss possible ways to engage your community to meet the identified health needs in Question 2.

# REFERENCES

Albert, D., & Herrera, C. (2009, November 20). *Getting lost in the evidence? Part 1: Developing an evidence question and search strategy.* Fireside Chat presentation. Ottawa, ON: University of Ottawa.

Anuruang, S., Hickman, L. D., Jackson, D., Dharmendra, T., Van Balen, J., & Davidson, P. M. (2013). Community-based interventions to promote management for older people: An integrative review. *J Clin Nurs.* doi:10.1111/jocn.12445

Canadian Institute for Health Information. (2013a). *National trauma registry comprehensive data set 2010–2011.* Retrieved from https://secure.cihi.ca/estore/productSeries.htm?pc=PCC46

Canadian Institute for Health Information. (2013b). *Health indicators, 2013.* Retrieved from https://secure.cihi.ca/free_products/HI2013_Jan30_EN.pdf

Canadian Public Health Association. (2010). *Community health–public health nursing in Canada: Preparation and practice* (4th ed.). Ottawa, ON: Author. Copyright © 2010 by Canadian Public Health Association. Used by permission of Canadian Public Health Association.

Clemen-Stone, S., Eigsti, D., & McGuire, S. (2002). *Comprehensive community health nursing* (6th ed.). Toronto, ON: Mosby.

Community Health Nurses of Canada. (2011, revised). *Canadian community health nursing: Professional practice model and standards of practice.* St. John's, NL: Author. Retrieved from http://www.chnc.ca/documents/chnc-standards-eng-book.pdf

Cornelson, K. (2011, December). *Immigrant labour market outcomes in Canada: The benefits of addressing wage and employment gaps.* Retrieved from http://www.hireimmigrants.ca/wp-content/uploads/Immigrant_labour_market_outcomes.pdf

Epp, J. (1986). *Health for all: A framework for health promotion.* Ottawa, ON: Health and Welfare Canada.

Epstein, P. D., Coates, P. M., Wray, L. D., & Swain D. (2006). *Improving communities by engaging citizens, measuring performance and getting things done.* Mississauga, ON: Jossey-Bass (a Wiley imprint).

Kretzmann, J. P., & McKnight, J. L. (1993). *Building communities from the inside out: A path towards finding and mobilising a community's assets.* Chicago, IL: ACTA Publications.

Linsay, S., & McPherson, A. C. (2012). Strategies for improving disability awareness and social inclusion of children and young people with cerebral palsy. *Child Care, Health and Development, 38*(6), 809–816.

McKay, M. (2012). The history of community nursing in Canada. In L. Stamler & L. Yiu. (Eds.), *Community health nursing: A Canadian perspective* (3rd ed., pp. 1–20). Toronto, ON: Pearson Canada.

Minkler, M. (Ed.). (2012). *Community organizing and community building for health* (3rd ed.). New Brunswick, NJ: Rutgers University Press.

Mitic, W., & Rootman, I. (Eds.). (2012). *An inter-sectoral approach to improve health literacy for Canadians: A discussion paper.* Victoria, BC: Public Health Association of BC.

National Expert Commission. (2012, revised). *A nursing call to action.* Ottawa, ON: Canadian Nurses Association. Retrieved from http://www.cna-aiic.ca/~/media/cna/files/en/nec_report_e.pdf

Nonprofit Quarterly. (2015). *Community-engagement governance: Systems-wide governance in action.* Retrieved from https://nonprofitquarterly.org/index.php/governancevoice/12021-community-engagement-governance-systems-wide-governance-in-action

O'Campo, P., & Urquia, M. (2012). Aligning method with theory: A comparison of two approaches to modeling the social determinants of health. *Maternal and Child Health Journal, 16*(9), 1870–1878.

Ontario Local Health Integrated Network. (2011). *LHIN community engagement guidelines and toolkit.* Toronto, ON: Author.

Public Health Agency of Canada. (2002). *Summary table of population health key elements.* Public Health Agency of Canada. Reproduced with permission from the Minister of Health, 2015. © All rights reserved. Retrieved from http://www.phac-aspc.gc.ca/ph-sp/approach-approche/pdf/summary_table.pdf

Public Health Agency of Canada. (2011). *What determines health?* Retrieved from http://www.phac-aspc.gc.ca/ph-sp/determinants

Public Health Agency of Canada. (2012). *What is the population health approach?* Reproduced with permission from the Minister of Health, 2015. © All rights reserved. Retrieved from http://www.phac-aspc.gc.ca/ph-sp/approach-approche/index-eng.php

Public Health Agency of Canada. (2013). *What makes Canadians healthy or unhealthy?* Retrieved from http://www.phac-aspc.gc.ca/ph-sp/determinants/determinants-eng.php

Schofield, R., Valaitis, R., Akhtar-Danesh, N., Baumann, A., Martin-Misener, R., & Underwood, J. (2009). *Phase 2: Strengthening the quality of community health nursing practice: A Pan Canadian survey of community health nurses' continuing education needs study.* Ottawa, ON: CHNC.

Senate of Canada. (2009). *A healthy, productive Canada: A determinant of health approach.* The Standing Senate Committee on Social Affairs, Science and Technology.

Statistics Canada. (2013a). *Canadian community health survey—Annual Component, 2012.* Retrieved from http://www23.statcan.gc.ca/imdb/p2SV.pl?Function=getSurvey&SDDS=3226&lang=en&db=imdb&adm=8&dis=2

Statistics Canada. (2013b). *Health indicators framework.* Retrieved from http://www.statcan.gc.ca/pub/82-221-x/2013001/hifw-eng.htm

Statistics Canada. (2014). *2011 National household survey: Data tables.* Retrieved from http://www12.statcan.gc.ca/nhs-enm/2011/dp-pd/dt-td/Rp-eng.cfm?LANG=E&APATH=3&DETAIL=0&DIM=0&FL=A&FREE=0&GC=0&GID=0&GK=0&GRP=1&PID=105392&PRID=0&PTYPE=105277&S=0&SHOWALL=0&SUB=0&Temporal=2013&THEME=95&VID=0&VNAMEE=&VNAMEF=

Totikidis, V., Armstrong, A., & Francis, R. (2005). The concept of community governance: A preliminary review. Presented at the GovNet Conference, 28–30 Nov, 2005, Melbourne, Australia. (Unpublished).

Traverso-Yepez, M., Maddalena, V., Bavington, W., & Donovan, C. (2012). Community capacity building for health: A critical look at the practical implications of this approach. *Sage Open*. doi:10.1177/2158244012446996

Vollman, A. R., Anderson, E. T., & McFarlane, J. (2012). *Canadian community as partner: Theory and multidisciplinary practice* (Canadian 3rd ed.). New York, NY: Wolters Kluwer/ Lippincott Williams & Wilkins.

World Health Organization. (1978). *Primary health care: Report on the International Conference on Primary Health Care*, Alma Ata, USSR, 6–12, September 1978. Geneva, Switzerland: Author.

World Health Organization, Canadian Public Health Association, & Health and Welfare Canada. (1986). *Ottawa charter of health promotion*. Ottawa, ON: Health and Welfare Canada.

## ABOUT THE AUTHOR

**Lucia Yiu**, RN, BScN, BA (University of Windsor), BSc (University of Toronto), MScN (University of Western Ontario), is an Associate Professor in the Faculty of Nursing at the University of Windsor, and an educational and Training Consultant in community nursing. She has worked overseas and served on various community and social services committees involving local and district health planning. Her practice and research include multicultural health, international health, experiential learning, community development, breast health, and program planning and evaluation. Lucia was the recipient of the 2014 Community Health Nurses of Canada Award of Merit.

# Community Health Planning, Monitoring, and Evaluation

*Nancy C. Edwards, Josephine Etowa, and Wendy E. Peterson*

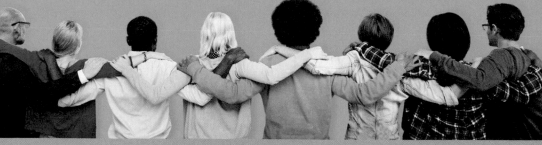
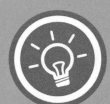
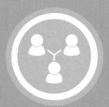
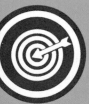
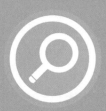
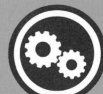

SOLUTION **STRATEGY** PLANNING

GOAL    PROCESS    INSPIRATION    PLANNING    RESEARCH

*Source: Rawpixel/Fotolia*

## LEARNING OUTCOMES

**After studying this chapter, you should be able to:**

1. Describe the importance of program planning, monitoring, and evaluation in the practice of community health nursing.

2. Explain how the socio-structural determinants of health can be reflected in our approach to planning, monitoring, and evaluation.

3. Describe components of the assessment–planning–evaluation cycle and use a logic model to guide the process.

4. Discuss strategies for citizen engagement and involving key stakeholders in the assessment–planning–evaluation cycle.

5. Describe elements of the multiple interventions framework and its application to a complex community health issue.

6. Explain how commonly used evaluation models and the choice of indicators may be structured to address program accountability.

## INTRODUCTION

Planning, monitoring, and evaluating community health programs are fundamental processes used by community health nurses (CHNs) as they work in partnership with the community (Community Health Nurses of Canada [CHNC], 2011, revised). With more scrutiny of how public funds are being expended, increased demands for evidence-based programs, standards of practice, and national and international interest in population health intervention research, these processes have become even more critical (Commission on Social Determinants of

Health, 2008; Senate Subcommittee on Population Health, 2009). The Canadian Community Health Nursing Standards of Practice (CHNC, 2011, revised) describe how nurses are expected to plan new programs, redesign existing services, monitor the implementation of programs, and evaluate their impact. Nurses often make important contributions to these processes with the substantial involvement of community representatives, key stakeholders from a variety of service sectors, and colleagues from multiple disciplines.

There are many tools available to assist CHNs in program planning, but their utility will be diminished if underlying socio-structural determinants of health are ignored, and programs are developed without considering social justice issues. Thus, while research evidence and theory are important, the authentic engagement of the community is also essential in planning, monitoring, and evaluating community health programs.

## PROGRAM PLANNING AND EVALUATION

The planning–evaluation cycle involves several key components. Although various planning frameworks are in common use, all contain similar elements. A classic **planning–implementation–evaluation cycle** (Figure 14.1) involves the following steps:

- conducting a situational analysis or community assessment;
- identifying the problems or issues of concern;
- considering possible solutions or actions to address the problem;
- selecting the best alternative(s);

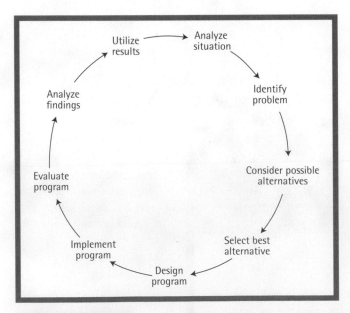

**FIGURE** **14.1** **Planning–Implementation–Evaluation Cycle**

*Source:* Trochim, W. M. K. (2000). *The research methods knowledge base* (2nd ed.). Retrieved from http://www.socialresearchmethods.net/kb/pecycle.php

- designing and implementing the program;
- monitoring and evaluating the program;
- analyzing and interpreting results of the monitoring and evaluation process; and
- using the results to make modifications to the program or to inform decisions about other programs.

The steps in this cycle may need to be repeated as one develops a better understanding of an issue and obtains additional input from partners. It may be necessary to go back to other steps in the planning cycle and try to develop a more complete picture of the factors that are affecting the problem and the potential solutions that need to be considered.

## Selecting a Program Planning and Evaluation Framework

There are many **program planning and evaluation frameworks** available. Frameworks provide a guide for the types of information that need to be assembled and for organizing this information into a coherent plan. Several factors should be considered in selecting a framework for use. First, most community health agencies will have a standard planning framework that is used across departments. Use of a common framework allows for a coherent and consistent approach to planning within an organization. Second, the use of a particular framework may be a requirement of those who fund programs, as this allows them to compare results across funded programs. Third, a framework may be chosen because it helps detail a particular aspect of the planning process that is vexing or challenging. For instance, a framework may be chosen because it is particularly useful in defining the underlying socio-structural determinants of a problem, it guides the choice of theory that will help define program elements, or it is more appropriate for addressing the needs of marginalized populations. Finally, the selection of a framework may be influenced by a set of underlying values or principles such as participatory development or social justice (Edwards & Davison, 2008).

The **program logic model** is used extensively in many public health agencies in Canada, both at regional and municipal levels, and by provincial and federal government agencies (Porteous, Sheldrick, & Stewart, 2002). Logic models provide a coherent structure for complex health programs, help to expose gaps, and yield an overview of programs with appealing visual clarity. As a support to planning, analysis, and program evaluation preparation, the logic model provides means of documenting "what the program is supposed to do, with whom, and why" (Porteous et al., 2002, p. 116).

Wooten et al. (2014) note that the logic model is unique among tools for its simplicity in demonstrating program interrelationships and linkages. Logic models should be developed in collaboration with community and academic partners. In this way, both experiential learning and research findings can inform model development. Joint preparation of a logic model will help build consensus about program priorities among the planning team. In using a logic model, one should avoid positioning it as a rigid guideline, which prevents iterative evolution or lateral exploration of the program under review (see the sample logic model in MyNursingLab).

Development of a logic model consists of two planning stages, referred to as **CAT (components, activities, and target groups)** and **SOLO (short-term outcomes and long-term outcomes)**. For the CAT stage, activities are first clustered thematically into components for the program under review. For example, a suicide prevention program for youth might include the components of risk assessment, crisis intervention, and peer support. Activities are the specific intervention strategies to be used for each component. Using the suicide prevention example, the crisis intervention component may include training youth workers in crisis management, developing community supports for youth in crisis, and establishing better communication among social and health services organizations about youth in crisis. Target groups are the intended recipients of a program. In this example, these might be homeless youth, youth having difficulty in school, and the front-line workers for youth in schools, homeless shelters, and other health and social service organizations.

The purpose of the SOLO stage is to identify program outcomes. **Short-term outcomes** are the immediate and direct results of the program, while **long-term outcomes** reflect the ultimate goals of the program. Building the knowledge and skills of youth workers to identify and support youth in crisis

would be a short-term outcome, while reducing youth suicide rates would be longer-term. Many extraneous factors may influence the achievement of long-term outcomes. Thus, they are more difficult to directly and exclusively attribute to the program.

The **Program Evaluation Tool Kit** (Figure 14.2) incorporates the use of a logic model and identifies which evaluation processes may be used to inform decision making during program planning and implementation (National Collaborating Centre for Methods and Tools, 2010). **Evaluation** is an ongoing, dynamic process that supports further refinement of program activities and helps to identify gaps or flaws in the original program design. It is critical to involve community partners in the evaluation process. They can play key roles in helping with data interpretation and identifying recommendations emerging from program evaluation. (See MyNursingLab, use of Program Evaluation Tool Kit to evaluate H1N1 pandemic planning.)

## Tools and Processes to Support Planning and Evaluation

Many tools and processes may be used in combination with an organizing framework. However, these tools must be used in conjunction with approaches that build relationships and

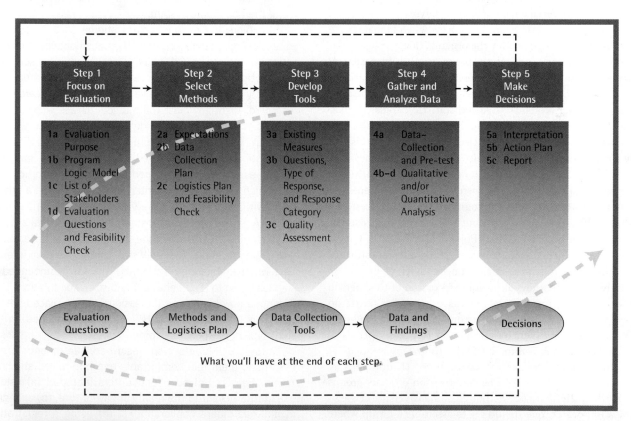

**FIGURE   14.2   PHAC Tool Kit Decision-Oriented Model for Program Evaluation**

*Source:* Public Health Agency of Canada. (2008). *Tool kit decision-oriented model for program evaluation.* Reproduced with permission from the Minister of Health, 2015. © All rights reserved. Retrieved from http://pacificaidsnetwork.org/wp-content/uploads/2012/01/Program-Evaluation-Toolkit1.pdf

create opportunities to hear the voices of disadvantaged groups. Crosby and Noar (2011) suggest that using tools like the **PRECEDE-PROCEED planning model (PPM)** enables the community program developer to think logically about the desired end point and work "backwards" to achieve that goal. The efficient involvement of community partners is important because those working in service delivery sectors have many demands on their time. Involving them in the planning process helps build commitment to the program and aids the design of a program that reflects the dynamic realities and strengths of the community (Angeles, Dolovich, Kaczorowsk, & Thabane, 2013). There are practical tools available to help engage community partners in a planning process. For example, environmental scans can be used to gather information about community needs and priorities. Key informant interviews and focus groups may be conducted (see Chapter 13) or an analysis of strengths, weaknesses, opportunities, and threats (SWOT) may be undertaken.

A **SWOT (strengths, weaknesses, opportunities, and threats) analysis** identifies **internal strengths and weaknesses** of the organization or program, along with **external opportunities and threats**. It may involve **document and policy reviews, community meetings, key informant interviews**, and **focus groups**. It helps those planning a program to customize the fit between an organization (or in this case the program) and its environment (Fraser & Stupak, 2002; Helms & Nixon, 2010). A SWOT may also assist in determining the feasibility of initiating or continuing a program, and may help identify service gaps. SWOT analyses are frequently used as part of a strategic planning process when managers are developing long-term plans for the organization.

**Assessing needs** through the use of **qualitative research strategies** such as individual interviews and focus groups elaborates on those issues and experiences that are not readily understood through quantitative and statistical tools (Pope & Mays, 2013). For example, although quantitative evaluation tools may demonstrate that a particular subpopulation is less likely than others to use community health services, they may not be able to explain why and how. Similarly, quantitative data may not shed light on the perceived appropriateness of community health services and programs. Qualitative research tools not only address these gaps but also can be used to assess the meanings of health and care (Pope & Mays, 2013). Qualitative data can increase the relevance and interpretability of quantitative data generated during a needs assessment.

Individual interviews allow for exploration of first-person experiences and prompt interactive discussions that centre on the perspectives of participants (Patton, 2002). In-depth interviews may yield pertinent examples and rich descriptions of experiences (Rubin & Rubin, 2005). Focus groups are used "to elicit and validate collective testimonies" (Kamberelis & Dimitriadis, 2005, p. 897). The composition of focus groups must be carefully planned. Although some diversity of viewpoints is important, one should try to assemble a group where there is not an underlying power structure among its members that may discourage some participants from openly sharing their viewpoints. For example, it may not be appropriate to have a focus group consisting of both front-line workers and their managers because front-line workers may hesitate to discuss issues concerning organizational leadership or conditions when their managers are present. Focus groups provide opportunities for members to share and validate their individual experiences. The discussion may stimulate participant ownership of the program under development and may prompt participants toward action. Qualitative methods are illustrated in Canadian Research Box 14.1.

## CANADIAN RESEARCH BOX 14.1

**How is stigma experienced by gay male youth living with HIV during healthcare utilization?**

O'Byrne, P., & Watts, J. (2012). Include, differentiate and manage: Gay male youth, stigma and healthcare utilization. *Nursing Inquiry, 21*(1), 20–29. Used by permission of Patrick O'Byrne. doi:10.1111/nin.12014

Stigma has both individual and social dimensions. Although it is experienced by individuals, it is influenced by social, political, institutional, and symbolic contexts. Stigma influences peoples' willingness to access healthcare. Several authors have described the negative impact of stigma on patients' interactions with healthcare providers and the health system as a whole, particularly by marginalized populations. A person who feels judged or perceives that he or she may be stigmatized in the healthcare system may refrain from interacting with health professionals and from using the healthcare system.

To explore the experiences of stigma among gay male youth, this qualitative research study was conducted using a series of semi-structured interviews as the primary source of information. Ethical approval was obtained from the University of Ottawa and Ottawa Public Health Research Ethics Board. Eight gay male youth, aged 20–29, who received services from a local gay-friendly health clinic participated in the study. The average age of study participants was 23 years; 87.3% of them self-identified as homosexual or gay. The highest education level attained by 87% of the participants was a high school diploma. Interviews took place in a private room within this clinic. Interviews were transcribed and coded. A grounded theory constant comparative data analysis process guided this phase of the study. Participants described how stigma related to their HIV status impacted their interactions with healthcare professionals. This was compounded by stigma related to their behaviour and sexual orientation. They described how healthcare professionals often placed greater emphasis on sexuality and HIV transmission based on the stereotype of gay people as promiscuous.

Study participants also described health encounters that made them feel comfortable and minimized stigmatization. Features of such encounters included (a) asking questions relevant to the reality of gay culture, (b) engaging in non-healthcare conversations, (c) using a registration form that provided the clinician with sensitive details prior to patient encounter, and (d) providing STI/HIV counselling related to sex practices, not sexual orientation.

Following analysis, the authors used Hardt and Negri's (2000) three-part theoretical framework to explain participants' narratives and to provide a background for understanding how stigma affects health-seeking behaviour. The study shows how gay male youth experienced stigma and what clinical approaches helped to minimize their experience of stigmatization.

### Discussion Questions

1. How would you assess stigma in a community needs assessment?

2. How can you assess potentially stigmatizing practices among nurses and other health providers?

3. How might you minimize the feeling of being judged among gay male youth who frequently use the health-care services in your local community resource centre?

## Organizing Information and Setting Priorities

The second set of tools help with organizing and understanding data and information, and guide priority-setting (see Chapters 10 and 13 for additional examples). Analyzing and representing qualitative data involves describing, classifying, and connecting the data (Miles, Huberman, & Saldana, 2014). **Content analysis** is frequently used for planning purposes. It is a systematic, replicable technique for compressing large volumes of text data into fewer content categories based on explicit rules of coding. This involves assigning codes or labels to the text data. Data are then grouped into categories to reflect emerging patterns of responses. Systematic counting and recording techniques may also be used to help identify patterns of responses such as the predominant use of certain kinds of phrases by some respondents but not others. Analyzed qualitative data can be packaged in text, matrix, or figure formats. A **text format** involves the use of illustrative quotes. **Matrices** are used to compare major categories of data and highlight differences and similarities among subgroups. For example, a matrix of needs-assessment information may be used to compare responses from homeless men and shelter staff regarding the fairness of the shelter rules or to compare the perspectives of teachers, parents, and students regarding the acceptability and need for school sexual health clinics. **Figures** may be a useful visual tool to reflect emerging relationships among categories of coded data.

Many sources of **quantitative data** may be accessed as you plan a program. These include local and provincial data documenting the magnitude of the problem and contributing factors. These data are often obtained through sources such as special surveys (e.g., school surveys to document patterns of smoking among youth), routinely collected information (e.g., police and ambulance reports, hospital admission data, air pollution records), and surveillance data (e.g., reports of communicable diseases). There are many excellent examples of reporting formats that have been developed to display

quantitative data. A useful starting point is to examine **existing reports** (e.g., health status reports) and to enlist the assistance of someone with epidemiological training. A second use of quantitative data is to estimate program costs and the potential return on investments. Various methods and tools may be of relevance here, including the use of the balanced score card (Woodward, Manuel, & Goel, 2004) and the application of health economics methods (Shiell, Hawe, & Gold, 2008).

Interpreting **systematic reviews** is a third use of quantitative data. Systematic reviews assemble findings from studies with a common research objective (e.g., to examine the effectiveness of exercise and balance programs to reduce the risk of falls among seniors). Those undertaking systematic reviews use a thorough and rigorous set of methods both to identify all potentially relevant studies and to review the methodological quality of these studies. Studies deemed to be relevant and of adequate quality are included in the review. Outcome data are extracted using standard procedures. When possible, the quantitative findings from two or more studies are collapsed into a single estimate of effect. This is done using statistical techniques and the review process is then called a **meta-analysis** (see Chapter 10 for more detail).

Figure 14.3 summarizes the results from 15 studies on the effectiveness of fall prevention interventions. There are three important things to understand in this diagram. First, the **relative risk** is used to indicate whether or not the study group that received the intervention has a lower rate of falls than the study group that did not receive the intervention. If there is no difference between the groups, the relative risk is one. If the intervention group has a lower rate of falls than the control group, the relative risk will be less than one (indicating a protective effect). Fourteen of the 15 studies had a relative risk less than one (range 0.34 to 0.97). Second, if this **intervention effect** is **statistically significant** (indicating that if we repeated the experiment, we are 95% certain that we would again find a difference between groups), then the **confidence interval** around the relative risk will also be less than one. In Figure 14.3, the confidence interval is shown as a horizontal line on the diagram and listed in the right-hand column. We can see that only eight of the 15 studies found statistically significant protective effects of the intervention. Third, results are then pooled across the 15 studies (the meta-analysis part of the exercise). A weighting factor is used in making this calculation so that studies with small sample sizes will contribute less weight to the pooled estimate than studies with large sample sizes. In this example, the pooled relative risk is 0.75 and the result is statistically significant (the test for overall effect yields a $p$ value of 0.000057). Thus, it follows that the recommendation in the abstract for this review concludes that "assessment and multifactorial intervention reduced rate of falls (RR 0.75, 95% CI 0.65 to 0.86)" (Gillespie et al., 2012, p. 1).

## Priority Setting

**Setting priorities** is a vital step in the planning process. An in-depth examination of a problem in the community may leave one overwhelmed at the thought of narrowing down the

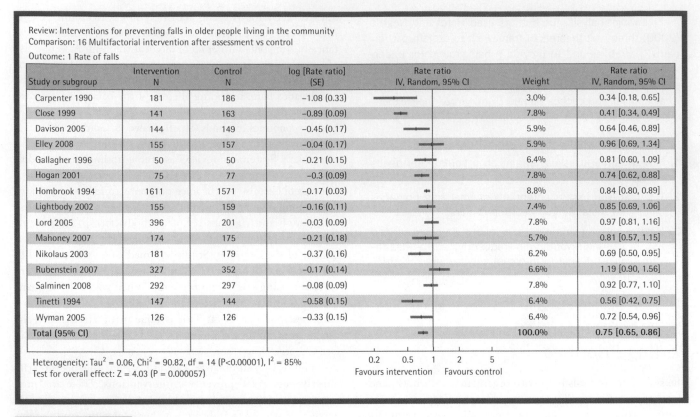

Review: Interventions for preventing falls in older people living in the community
Comparison: 16 Multifactorial intervention after assessment vs control
Outcome: 1 Rate of falls

| Study or subgroup | Intervention N | Control N | log [Rate ratio] (SE) | Rate ratio IV, Random, 95% CI | Weight | Rate ratio IV, Random, 95% CI |
|---|---|---|---|---|---|---|
| Carpenter 1990 | 181 | 186 | −1.08 (0.33) | | 3.0% | 0.34 [0.18, 0.65] |
| Close 1999 | 141 | 163 | −0.89 (0.09) | | 7.8% | 0.41 [0.34, 0.49] |
| Davison 2005 | 144 | 149 | −0.45 (0.17) | | 5.9% | 0.64 [0.46, 0.89] |
| Elley 2008 | 155 | 157 | −0.04 (0.17) | | 5.9% | 0.96 [0.69, 1.34] |
| Gallagher 1996 | 50 | 50 | −0.21 (0.15) | | 6.4% | 0.81 [0.60, 1.09] |
| Hogan 2001 | 75 | 77 | −0.3 (0.09) | | 7.8% | 0.74 [0.62, 0.88] |
| Hombrook 1994 | 1611 | 1571 | −0.17 (0.03) | | 8.8% | 0.84 [0.80, 0.89] |
| Lightbody 2002 | 155 | 159 | −0.16 (0.11) | | 7.4% | 0.85 [0.69, 1.06] |
| Lord 2005 | 396 | 201 | −0.03 (0.09) | | 7.8% | 0.97 [0.81, 1.16] |
| Mahoney 2007 | 174 | 175 | −0.21 (0.18) | | 5.7% | 0.81 [0.57, 1.15] |
| Nikolaus 2003 | 181 | 179 | −0.37 (0.16) | | 6.2% | 0.69 [0.50, 0.95] |
| Rubenstein 2007 | 327 | 352 | −0.17 (0.14) | | 6.6% | 1.19 [0.90, 1.56] |
| Salminen 2008 | 292 | 297 | −0.08 (0.09) | | 7.8% | 0.92 [0.77, 1.10] |
| Tinetti 1994 | 147 | 144 | −0.58 (0.15) | | 6.4% | 0.56 [0.42, 0.75] |
| Wyman 2005 | 126 | 126 | −0.33 (0.15) | | 6.4% | 0.72 [0.54, 0.96] |
| Total (95% CI) | | | | | 100.0% | 0.75 [0.65, 0.86] |

Heterogeneity: $Tau^2 = 0.06$, $Chi^2 = 90.82$, df = 14 (P<0.00001), $I^2 = 85\%$
Test for overall effect: Z = 4.03 (P = 0.000057)

0.2  0.5  1  2  5
Favours intervention   Favours control

**FIGURE 14.3** Assessment Followed by Multi-factorial Interventions versus Control

*Source:* Gillespie, L. D., Robertson, M. C., Gillespie, W. J., Lamb, S. E., Gates, S., Cumming, R. G., & Rowe B. H. (2009). Interventions for preventing falls in older people living in the community. *Cochrane Database of Systematic Reviews,* Issue 2. Art. No.: CD007146. doi:10.1002/14651858.CD007146.pub2

possibilities for action. The guiding principles for priority setting are buy-in, transparency, and communication. Priority setting inevitably means that one can neither address all the identified needs nor operationalize all the proposed interventions. The first principle, **buy-in**, needs to occur early on. Engaging community members and key stakeholders in discussing the problem may initially help with buy-in but runs the risk of backfiring if the priorities selected suggest that their input and ideas were not considered. Thus, it is also important to look at ways to involve the community in the process of setting priorities as one begins to more clearly define program components and activities. While it may not be realistic to involve a community in all phases of a priority-setting process, one can invite input in some critical phases, such as selecting criteria to inform priority setting. Agreement among senior managers on a common priority-setting process for an organization will help ensure managerial support for the priorities identified.

The second principle is **transparency**, whereby the process for selecting priorities is made apparent to those who were not directly involved in the process. In other words, key stakeholders are able to understand how you got from point A (understanding the problem and considering possible intervention strategies) to point B (priority definition of the problem and strategies). Both objective and subjective criteria are important to identifying priority interventions. Objective criteria are measurable facets of a problem and its solutions. For example,

what is the magnitude (prevalence or incidence) of a problem, what are the short- and long-term consequences of the problem (e.g., mortality or morbidity), are there effective strategies to address the problem, and how cost-effective are the strategies relative to other approaches? Subjective criteria require judgment calls that are based on underlying organizational and social values about the issue. For instance, will working on the problem lead to new and stronger partnerships with other community agencies? Is tackling the problem within the mandate of our organization? Is there community readiness and political will to address this problem both in the short and long terms?

The third principle is **communication**. A clear communication strategy needs to accompany efforts to set priorities. Both internal and external communication processes are vital. Internally, the identification of priorities should be directly linked to the approval mechanisms for program funding. Communication and collaborative technologies or tools are increasingly influencing the nature of healthcare interactions and should be used to facilitate internal dialogue. CHNs need to master the use of these tools for a variety of purposes; for example, to instantly debate issues, analyze research, network with peers, use crowd-source information, seek support, and provide advice (van de Belt et al., 2013). Externally, one needs to communicate priorities to partners who have provided input on the program. This will help to ensure more buy-in for program implementation. Social marketing campaigns (see Chapter 8) are one way to facilitate external communication (Gilbert et al., 2013).

| Activities | 2011 | | | | 2012 | | | | | | | | |
|---|---|---|---|---|---|---|---|---|---|---|---|---|---|
| | S | O | N | D | J | F | M | A | M | J | J | A | S |
| Site visit: review of evaluation framework | █ | | | | | | | | | | | | |
| Identify staff & roles for the project | █ | | | | | | | | | | | | |
| Develop project-specific timelines/activities | █ | | | | | | | | | | | | |
| Prepare materials for data collection | | | █ | | | | | | | | | | |
| Prepare for ethical considerations | | | | █ | | | | | | | | | |
| Prepare software/techinical specifications | | | | | █ | | | | | | | | |
| Pilot-test data collection procedures | | | | | █ | | | | | | | | |
| Staff training (if needed) | | | | | | | | | | | | | |
| Collect data; refine measures/procedures | | | | | | | █ | █ | █ | | | | |
| Analyze data | | | | | | | | | | █ | █ | | |
| Share preliminary findings | | | | | | | | | | | █ | | |
| Prepare final report | | | | | | | | | | | | █ | █ |

**FIGURE  14.4**  Example of a Gantt Chart

*Source:* Ontario Centre of Excellence for Child and Youth Mental Health. (2013). *The road to data collection Webinar.* Retrieved from http://www.excellenceforchildandyouth.ca/sites/default/files/docs/webinars/_attach/road_to_data_collection_presentation_02092012.pdf

# Planning, Monitoring, and Evaluating Programs

There are various resources available to assist nurses and other public health professionals to plan, monitor, and evaluate programs (see MyNursingLab, The Online Health Program Planner). **Gantt charts**, depicted in a tabular format, are a commonly used tool to present the sequence and timing of activities that must take place in order to accomplish the specific objectives of the program or project. These charts are particularly helpful when one is planning activities for a complex program with many components. The Gantt chart provides a good starting point for identifying these main components. The timelines for activities that must be undertaken in a particular sequence and details about these activities are then elaborated. For instance, permission must be obtained for the use of space before focus groups with community members can be held, and these focus groups must take place before members of a planning group can convene to consider community input on priority-setting. One example of a Gantt chart is provided in Figure 14.4. Software packages such as Microsoft Project and Excel can also be used to help develop planning and managing timelines with Gantt charts.

## THE SHIFT TO MULTIPLE INTERVENTIONS

Increasingly, community health programs are targeting the complexity and root causes of problems. This requires a socio-ecological examination of the issue of interest and a planning–intervention–evaluation cycle that addresses these underlying determinants. Raphael (2008) defines **social determinants of health** as "the economic and social conditions that influence the health of individuals, communities and jurisdictions as a whole" (p. 1). We use the term "socio-structural determinants" to reinforce the fact that some determinants are embedded in social structures such as legislation, standards, and regulations that generate or perpetuate social and health inequities. Several key features of these **socio-structural determinants** are shaping contemporary community health programs. The determinants do not reside in isolation from each other. Rather, determinants are nested; that is, they are interrelated and as one determinant changes, another may shift. Some determinants are deeply embedded, following from historical inequities such as the oppression that Aboriginal populations have experienced (Smith, Varcoe, & Edwards, 2005) and stigma faced by marginalized groups (Friedman, Cooper, & Osborne, 2009). This notion that health is largely influenced by multiple factors beyond biology, genetics, and the healthcare system provides the foundation for a population health approach. A **population health approach** addresses the health of groups of people and disparities among groups by influencing a range of social, economic, personal, and health-service factors that are well recognized as having an impact on our health (Health Canada, 2001). There have been both national and global calls for a "determinants of health approach" that addresses coherent, multi-level policies in health and other sectors with a specific focus on reducing health disparities (Senate Subcommittee on Population Health, 2009; Commission on Social Determinants, 2008). A **health impact assessment** can be used to examine the potential effects of a policy, including its anticipated impact on health disparities (Taylor & Blair-Stevens, 2002). This socio-structural determinants of health approach recognizes the need to implement population health interventions at multiple levels of the system (individual, community, municipal, provincial, and federal).

The **Multiple Intervention Program (MIP) framework** arises from earlier work by Edwards and Moyer (1999). In Ontario, in the late 1980s, there was a shift away from public health programs that predominantly involved home visits and clinically oriented services in schools and workplaces. As evidence on determinants increased, and as considerations of how best to distribute scarce resources in public health were debated, programs increasingly began to focus on interventions targeting multiple layers of the system. Nurses were being asked to expand their repertoire of interventions to include not only those appropriate for individuals and families (such as home visits and primary care clinics), but also those targeted at community, organizational, and policy levels (such as community action, environment change, and policy strengthening and enforcement). Please re-visit Chapter 3, Nursing Roles, Functions, and Practice Settings for more in-depth discussion about the CHN scope of practice. With the input of front-line public health nurses and managers in Ottawa, a program framework was developed to reflect the integration of self-care capacity and action, collective care capacity and action, and environmental supports (Edwards & Moyer, 1999).

The next generation of this framework was developed 10 years later (Edwards, Mill, & Kothari, 2004). Its evolution arose from the observations and reflections of practitioners and from research. Managers identified the challenges of trying to plan and evaluate MIPs. Research findings were shedding light on a related set of issues. Through the 1990s, results from some well-designed experimental studies of MIPs were yielding unexpected and disappointing findings (Bauman, Suchindran, & Murray, 1999; Merzel & D'Afflitti, 2003; Sorenson, Emmons, Hunt, & Johnston, 1998). For instance, the COMMIT trial (COMMIT Research Group, 1995a) was a four-year multiple intervention study that targeted tobacco cessation and compared 11 matched pairs of communities in the United States and Canada. Eleven communities were in the control group and received no intervention. Eleven communities received a theory-based intervention that aimed to increase cessation rates among heavy smokers. The intervention program that was designed was considered "state-of-the-art-and-science." It included over 50 strategies that were aimed at various levels of the system, including individual behaviour change strategies, community mobilization, and organizational and policy change. However, the goal of reducing smoking rates among heavy smokers was not reached (COMMIT Research Group, 1995b). Authors have attempted to describe reasons why the COMMIT trial and other multiple interventions did not achieve their expected outcomes (Zanna et al., 1994). Common reasons include failing to involve the community in the planning process, the short duration of programs that did not allow enough time for policy change, not planning for long-term sustainability, and inadequate funding (Edwards, MacLean, Estable, & Meyer, 2006; Merzel & D'Afflitti, 2003; Stirman et al., 2012).

Yet, in apparent contradiction to some of the research on MIPs, there have been compelling examples of significant MIP successes in fields such as tobacco control and injury prevention. Prolonged efforts (often over more than a decade) have yielded substantial improvements in health outcomes from multi-strategy, multi-level, and multi-sector interventions. In the case of injury prevention, for example, MIPs have included a combination of strategies aimed at raising awareness (e.g., public media campaigns), supporting behaviour change (e.g., infant car seat clinics), changing social norms (e.g., a generation of children now think that wearing a seat belt is the norm; it is no longer socially acceptable to drink and drive), and developing regulations or passing legislation and setting up enforcement approaches (e.g., traffic calming strategies and police checkpoints for seat belt use and drunk driving).

# THE MULTIPLE INTERVENTION PROGRAM FRAMEWORK

The MIP framework consists of five main elements. Use of the framework involves an iterative cycle whereby emerging lessons from program implementation and new research findings continuously inform program adjustments. Optimal application of the framework should be based on in-depth knowledge of the local community (tacit knowledge), expertise with relevant theories, and up-to-date familiarity with good quality research evidence (both primary studies and systematic and integrative reviews). We describe each element of the framework, using illustrative examples for the problem of preventing falls among seniors. Table 14.1 provides a summary of the types of research studies that are relevant to each element of the model. These are described in more detail below. (See MyNursingLab for MIP examples and interactive exercises.)

## Identification of Community Health Issue

The first element is the identification of a community health issue that is the program focus. It is important to identify **population subgroups** that may be disadvantaged because they bear an unequal or inequitable burden of the health problem.

## Describe Socioecological Features

The second element involves describing the socioecological features of the problem. Here, a socioecological perspective helps to expose the factors that may be contributing to or causing the problem (including socio-structural determinants of health). Similarly, strengths and capacities at different levels of the system may reveal potential solutions to the problem.

Several types of research inform this element of the framework. **Etiological research** examines putative causes of health problems. Both qualitative and quantitative studies may

| Table 14.1 | Assembling the Research Evidence | |
|---|---|---|
| Element of Framework | Description of Relevant Data and Types of Research Studies | Examples from Research on Preventing Falls |
| Burden of illness and inequities | Prevalence and incidence of disease burden<br><br>Age- and gender-specific rates of disease<br><br>Policy coverage for subpopulations | *Burden of Illness:*<br><br>One in three seniors falls each year. Approximately 25% of all falls result in injuries. Falls are the sixth leading cause of death among seniors in Canada.<br>Patterns and risk factors for indoor and outdoor falls differ (Kelsey et al., 2010).<br><br>*Inequities:*<br><br>Although seniors living in publicly subsidized apartment buildings have worse health status than seniors living in privately owned apartment buildings, they are significantly more likely to have universal access to grab bars (Edwards, Birkett, et al., 2006).<br><br>Higher social inequalities (using car availability and home ownership as markers of social class) are associated with an increased risk of falling among women (Syddall, Evancrou, Cooper, & Aihie Sayer, 2009). |
| Socioecological features of the problem | Etiological studies, laboratory studies, integrative reviews, qualitative and quantitative studies provide insights on **micro** (individual, family) and **meso** (community and organizational) factors that are at play, while organizational and policy studies may reveal determinants that operate at a **macro** level | Cumulative findings from individual studies and reviews (Gill, Williams, & Tinetti, 2000; Kearney, Harwood, Gladman, Lincoln, & Masud, 2013; *Letts et al., 2010; Muir, Gopaul, & Montero Odasso, 2012;* O'Loughlin, Robitaille, Boivin, & Suissa, 1993; Rawski, 1998) indicate that major risk factors for falls among community-dwelling seniors are:<br><br>• Use of benzodiazepine sedative hypnotics<br><br>• Polypharmacy (using four or more drugs)<br><br>• Cognitive impairment<br><br>• Problems with balance and peripheral neuromuscular dysfunction<br><br>• Environmental hazards<br><br>Qualitative and quantitative studies describe the perspectives of seniors on risk factors for falls and identify the outcomes that are most important to them (e.g., loss of independence) (Aminzadeh & Edwards, 1998; Grant, Edwards, Sveistrup, Andrews, & Egan, 2010; McInnes, Seers, & Tutton, 2011).<br><br>Laboratory studies identify specific features of the built environment (e.g., configuration of grab bars, height of stairs, dimensions of handrails) that may interact with personal variables (e.g., chronic illness, balance, hand grip strength, cognition) to increase the risk of falls (Guitard, Sveistrup, Lockett, & Edwards, 2011; Maki, Perry, Scovil, Mihailidis, & Fernie, 2006; Sveistrup, Lockett, Edwards, & Aminzadeh, 2006). |

*(continued)*

| Table 14.1 | Continued | |
|---|---|---|
| **Element of Framework** | **Description of Relevant Data and Types of Research Studies** | **Examples from Research on Preventing Falls** |
| | | Policy studies examine policy gaps and the influence of the policy environment on the risk of falls (Edwards, 2008; Grant, Andrews, Edwards, Sveistrup, & Egan, 2011; Perdue, Stone, & Gostin, 2003). |
| Intervention options | Efficacy and effectiveness studies, cost-effectiveness or cost–benefit studies, program evaluation, systematic reviews, best practice guideline documents, and studies that have tested mid-range theories yield evidence to inform intervention options | Cochrane reviews and primary studies provide evidence of the effectiveness and efficiency of strategies to prevent falls and fall-related injuries (Frick, Kung, Parrish, & Narrett, 2010; Gillespie et al., 2003; Gillespie et al., 2012; McClure et al., 2005; Parker, Gillespie, & Gillespie, 2006). |
| | | Best practice guidelines for preventing falls (Registered Nurses' Association of Ontario, 2005; Scott, Dukeshire, Gallagher, & Scanlan, 2001) are informed by effectiveness studies. |
| | | Community health evaluation studies yield promising strategies from fall prevention programs (Gallagher & Scott, 1997). |
| Optimal blend of strategies | Effectiveness studies of multi-strategy and multi-level interventions<br><br>Studies informed by integrated theories and research<br><br>Studies that examine contextual influences on intervention strategies yield data on how intervention strategies may be **synergistic** (working together for positive effect) or **antagonistic** (working against each other for a poor outcome) | Evidence that exercise programs are effective when used in combination with modifications to the built environment (Gillespie et al., 2009). |
| | | Evidence that multi-factor approaches are more effective in reducing falls than single strategies (Gillespie et al., 2012; Tinetti et al., 1994). |
| | | Sociobehavioural factors explain underutilization of efficacious interventions (Edwards, Lockett, Aminzadeh, & Nair, 2003; Fisher, Li, Michael, & Cleveland, 2004; George, Binns, Clayden, & Mulley, 1988; Naik & Gill, 2005). |
| | | Studies examining the application of theory to fall prevention (Sampson & Morenoff, 2000). |
| Monitoring and evaluating process, impact, spin-offs, and sustainability | Identification of potential indicators, ways of assembling data to support decision making | The Ontario Public Health Standards 2008 (Ministry of Health and Long-term Care, 2008) include societal outcomes for injury prevention programs. |

reveal the complex relationships among upstream determinants that perpetuate the problem. **Laboratory studies** may yield insights into biological and environmental issues that are having an impact on the problem, while organizational and policy studies may reveal determinants that operate at a macro level. While individual primary studies may be useful, systematic or integrative reviews that identify causal factors from a synthesis of the best available evidence are more informative. Integrative reviews use findings from both qualitative and quantitative studies (Mays, Pope, & Popay, 2005). The phases of an integrative review process include (a) problem formulation, (b) data collection or literature search, (c) evaluation of data from diverse research designs, (d) data analysis, and (e) interpretation and presentation of results (Whittemore & Knafl, 2005). Integrative reviews may also contribute to the identification of theoretical insights to guide

| Table 14.2 | Socioecological Determinants of Falls among the Elderly |
|---|---|
| **Levels of Socioecological Model** | **Examples and References to Supporting Empirical Literature** |
| Individual | Patterns and type of exercise (Benjamin, Edwards, & Bharti, 2005) |
| | Perceptions of barriers to physical activity (Lockett, Willis, & Edwards, 2005) |
| | Perceptions of risk of falling (McInnes et al., 2011) |
| | Personal barriers to use of hip protectors (Blalock, Demby, McCulloch, & Stevens, 2010) |
| Interpersonal | Buddy systems in apartment buildings where neighbours check on each other to see if anyone has had an injurious fall |
| Community | Coalitions or other organized collectives taking action on preventing falls by raising awareness and addressing policy change (Edwards, 1999) |
| | Promoting safe exercise classes (Hooker & Cirill, 2006) |
| | Skilled volunteers organized in the community to make home modifications such as installing handrails on indoor and outdoor stairs (Edwards, Benjamin, & Lockett, 2006) |
| | Role of community-based organizations in promoting physical activity among seniors (Goodman, Davies, Tai, Dinan, & Iliffe, 2007) |
| Built/Physical Environment | Differences in configuration of bath grab bars and universal access to grab bars in bathrooms (Aminzadeh, Edwards, Lockett, & Nair, 2001; Guitard et al., 2011) |
| | Features of safe stairs (Maki et al., 2006) |
| | Senior-friendly environments (Nova Scotia Seniors' Secretariat, 2005; Ontario Seniors' Secretariat, 2013) |
| Social Environment | Walkable places (Grant et al., 2011) |
| | Accessibility of a esthetically pleasing and safe walking areas near seniors' homes (Giles-Corti & Donovan, 2003; Grant et al., 2010) |
| | Intersection of built and social environment (Hanson, Ashe, McKay, & Winters, 2012) |
| Organizational Policy (e.g., workplace, places of worship, housing) | Organization policies in long-term care settings influencing physical activity (Benjamin, Edwards, Ploeg, & Legault, 2014) |
| Municipal Policy | Policies regarding the marking of cracks in public sidewalks and length of time to fix these cracks (Gallagher & Scott, 1997) |
| Provincial Policy | Provincial building codes for private and public housing (Edwards, Birkett, et al., 2006) |
| National Policy | Recommendations for building codes provided by National Research Council and uptake of empirical evidence in modifications to building codes (Edwards, 2008) |

program strategies. Evidence on determinants is lined up with relevant levels of the socioecological model (see Table 14.2). In consultation with the community, priority levels for action are then selected based on community characteristics and knowledge of the policy context.

The nature or scope of different health issues may render some levels of the model more relevant than others. For instance, in the case of injury prevention, features of the built environment are likely to be a central concern, whereas with tobacco control, the accessibility of tobacco products, addiction, and social norms are particularly important. Furthermore, the level(s) of government (municipal, provincial, federal) to target is determined by who has budgetary and policy jurisdiction over the problem. Community partners will provide much-needed input on the joint action on sociostructural determinants that is required in their setting and opportunities for same.

## Intervention Options

The third element of the framework specifies **intervention options**. Here, one considers strategies that have demonstrated effectiveness and are theoretically sound. This knowledge must be coupled with community input on the feasibility of implementing interventions in their setting and the need to adapt interventions to ensure sociocultural and geographic relevance. For instance, while there is solid evidence of efficacy from laboratory studies (Laing & Robinovitch, 2008) and some evidence of effectiveness from studies with nursing home residents that hip protectors will reduce the risk of a hip fracture when a fall occurs, problems with compliance in using hip protectors have been reported (Gillespie, Gillespie, & Parker, 2010). Reasons for not using these protectors are related to the cost of purchasing them, inconvenience when busy nursing staff in long-term care settings have to help residents with dressing, perceptions of a socially unacceptable appearance if seniors try hip protectors but find them to be bulky under regular clothing, and hygiene problems if seniors who have urge incontinence are more likely to accidentally soil their hip protector garments than regular underwear. These adherence factors reduce the effectiveness of hip protectors as a hip fracture reduction strategy.

A mix of studies is required to inform intervention choices. For example, etiological studies indicate that the use of benzodiazepine sedative hypnotics is consistently a risk factor for falls. This suggests that minimizing use of these medications would be a useful fall prevention strategy. For those planning a program, however, the question that arises is, who is the most effective target, the seniors who use these sedatives or physicians who prescribe the medication? Studies from the field of addictions indicate that it is difficult to wean an individual off this class of drugs following long-term use. However, studies that have targeted changes in prescribing practice suggest that academic detailers (e.g., representatives from pharmaceutical companies who directly market new drugs to physicians) and audit and feedback strategies are effective in modifying physician prescribing (Foy et al., 2002). This combination of evidence indicates that a public health strategy targeting individual counselling for those who are taking benzodiazepines may be less likely to have a population impact than a public health strategy that either targets prescribing patterns among family physicians, discouraging the unnecessary initiation and long-term use of this class of drugs, or targets nurses and nurse practitioners to help elderly clients try new sleep hygiene strategies.

When selecting intervention options, planning teams also need to pay close attention to the reach, dose, and intensity of strategies that are required (Jilcott, Ammerman, Sommers, & Glasgow, 2007) to have their intended effect (see the RE-AIM framework in MyNursingLab). The **reach** of an intervention concerns what proportion and which particular segments of an intended target population receive the interventions. For example, social marketing approaches (Gordon, McDermott, Stead, & Angus, 2006; Luca & Suggs, 2013) such as public service advertisements may be intended for all seniors but will only reach those who are watching television or listening to the radio when the advertisement is run. The **dose** is the amount of intervention required to have an effect. Multiple exposures to a public service announcement are required to change awareness. The **intensity** of the intervention refers to its quality and whether it is tailored to the targeted population subgroup. For instance, a media campaign about the importance of walking regularly may have adequate intensity for seniors who have good functional status but is unlikely to provide suitable messages for very frail seniors who are not independently mobile. A note of caution is important here. If strategies that appear promising are watered down due to funding constraints or other limitations on program delivery capacity, the dose and intensity required for the intervention to make a difference may be diluted and the expected outcome is unlikely to be achieved.

Choosing strategies requires in-depth knowledge of the community characteristics that may influence uptake and effectiveness of the intervention strategies. The readiness and capacity of the community for the intended change is an important consideration that can best be gauged by community partners. The identification of policy windows and policy levers is also important (Kingdon, 1995; Pal, 2006). **Policy windows** are periods of opportunity to get an issue on the policy agenda. Policy windows may open because of a community crisis, mounting concern about a growing problem among the public and substantial press coverage on this issue, or a period of planned change such as the amalgamation of municipalities. These policy windows can create the momentum and public support required for policy change. Identifying **policy levers** requires an understanding of the ways in which different kinds of policies (e.g., community health nursing standards, National Research Council building code recommendations, and legislation) can be introduced or changed. It is important to involve those with expertise in policy change processes such as individuals with political science, public administration, or legal backgrounds in content-specific areas on your planning team.

In addition to evidence on what works and knowledge of the community, theoretical considerations should also drive the planning process. We are often inclined to apply those theories most familiar to us, rather than those theories most pertinent for the problem at hand. Since an MIP approach tackles more than one level of the socioecological system (Edwards & Davison, 2015), a mix of theories is required to guide the program. This involves integrating theories from various disciplines, and involving individuals from different disciplines who know the theories well. Identifying a range of relevant theories may expand the intervention options to be considered. For example, a community-based participatory approach may be used to model respect, reciprocity, and power sharing (Rubin et al., 2012).

## Optimizing Intervention Strategies

The fourth framework element focuses on **optimizing intervention strategies**. That is, how can we increase the likelihood that the combination of interventions works in a well-orchestrated fashion and how can we adapt our interventions to a dynamic context? Sorting this out requires that we attend to the sequence and combination of strategies and to the ways in which the political, social, organizational, and policy environments (contexts) are changing. The integrated theory that guides our program should inform decisions on how to optimize intervention strategies. Since intervention strategies may work together either positively or negatively, questions to consider when discussing how to optimize them include the following:

- What is a particular program trying to achieve and how can we combine intervention strategies to potentiate this?
- Are there ways in which a particular combination of interventions might nullify each other's effects?
- What is going on in the community that might enhance or reduce the impact of the intervention?

Two examples of how selected interventions might be optimized are provided in Table 14.3. The first example, which involves using the media and a risk-counselling approach, illustrates how intervention strategies can be combined to potentiate their effect. The second example shows how a planned intervention strategy can be successfully combined with a contextual influence. Although programs have no direct control over contextual influences, anticipating those that may arise and making program adjustments to reflect contextual influences that do emerge may either optimize the planned intervention strategies or mitigate the negative influences of contextual changes.

## Monitoring and Evaluating Impacts, Spin-Offs, and Sustainability

In the final element, monitoring and evaluating program outputs, outcomes, impacts, spin-offs, and sustainability are the central concern. **Outputs** indicate that a program is being implemented as planned. Identifying **output indicators** involves looking at the critical steps that are required for the program. For instance, initiating partnerships with other community organizations, engaging community members in a coalition, and getting a health issue on a political agenda would be relevant

| Table 14.3 | Optimizing Interventions | |
|---|---|---|
| **Examples of Intervention Strategies and Intended Effect** | **Underlying Theory and Research to Support Plan for Intervention Strategies** | **Optimizing the Intervention** |
| Media campaign to raise awareness about the risk of hazardous stairs, and volunteer program to encourage seniors to take action to improve safety of home stairs. | Social marketing theory (Luca & Suggs, 2013), media communication studies (Van der Belt et al., 2013), and stages of change theory (Prochaska & Velicer, 1997) indicate that a media campaign can shift a segment of the population from precontemplation to contemplation in a short interval (days or weeks). | Media campaign should be timed to coincide with accessible options for action, such as a help line for seniors to call to obtain volunteer assistance to make modifications to stairs (e.g., installation of handrails). van de Belt et al. (2013) define social media as Internet-based applications that build on the ideological and technological foundations of Web 2.0 and that facilitate the development and exchange of user-generated content. These include but are not limited to, YouTube, Facebook, and Twitter. |
| Collective action by a fall prevention coalition may increase community awareness of the importance of bathroom grab bars and can be used in combination with input to technical committees responsible for reviewing building codes. | Collective action, using participatory principles, is an essential component of programs informed by community development theories (Burke et al., 2013). This approach builds on strengths and resources within the community to promote co-learning and action for the mutual benefit of all stakeholders.<br><br>Kingdon's (1995) political science theory on agenda setting indicates that public opinion is a critical influence in the policy change process, both with respect to creating a demand for the change and providing the support necessary for either introducing a new policy or modifying one that already exists.<br><br>Kingdon's (1995) theory also identifies the importance of policy windows, periods of time when a particular policy change is more likely to happen. | Because the process of changing the National Research Council's building code recommendations, and subsequently provincial building code legislation, involves an extended period, coalitions must be ready to mobilize public support for changes to the building codes at several time points.<br><br>Effective and strategic application of Kingdon's (1995) theory by a coalition requires an understanding of how the building code revision process works, how public input on proposed changes is obtained, and whether other key stakeholders such as the home building industry are supporting or opposing proposed changes to the building codes. The action by fall prevention coalitions through this process will require timely interventions to (a) mobilize public awareness and support, (b) work with key stakeholders to mobilize action by them, and (c) network with other coalitions. |

indicators to assess progress toward ultimately achieving policy change. **Outcomes** are medium-term changes that can be attributed to the program. Changes in knowledge, attitudes, and behaviours among the target population would be anticipated at several levels. In the case of fall prevention, these outcomes would be assessed among the elderly, among health professionals (e.g., prescribing practices, assessing patients' risk profile for falls), and among those responsible for policy change (e.g., awareness of existing policies that increase risk for falls). **Impacts** are the longer-term results of a program, often taking some years to achieve. As with outputs and outcomes, impacts may be assessed at various levels of the socioecological model. Thus, one might expect to see impact indicators of individual health status changes, shifts in social norms, changes to the built environment, or policy change, all depending on the original intent of the program.

The selection of **impact indicators** should be guided by what we know about effective interventions and the "dose" of intervention expected to achieve a particular effect. Programs that are overly ambitious may appear ineffective because their resources are spread too thinly. When program managers cannot demonstrate an improvement in program outputs or outcomes, ongoing funding for the program may be threatened. Impact indicators for a multiple intervention program are illustrated in Canadian Research Box 14.2.

**Spin-offs** are unintended effects of a program. They may be positive or negative. One rarely sees formalized plans to assess spin-offs. They may, however, be identified through reflective approaches such as the maintenance of field notes during program implementation or team meeting discussions regarding observed spin-offs, and via mid- or end-of-program interviews with key informants and others who have participated in the program.

**Sustainability** concerns the longer-term viability of the program interventions. Evidence of sustainability at an organizational level may occur when an intervention becomes part of the routine. For instance, the introduction of a new assessment form during a program may become routine when this form becomes part of standard data collection within the agency. Sustainability at a policy level may occur when the policy is established and enforcement strategies are routinely put in place. Sustainability does not necessarily refer to the ongoing funding of a program, nor does it infer that a program will be organized the way it started out or run by the same organization. Rather, the intent of sustainability is to continue addressing the problem and to evolve strategies to match how the problem is changing.

---

### CANADIAN RESEARCH BOX 14.2

**What are the effects of a two-generation preschool program on parenting stress, self-esteem, life skills, risk for child maltreatment, and children's receptive language and global development? Are the identified parent and child effects sustained over time?**

Benzies, K., Mychasiuk, R., Kurilova, J., Tough, S., Edwards, N., & Donnelly, C. (2014). Two-generation preschool programme: Immediate and 7-year-old outcomes for low-income children and their parents. *Child & Family Social Work*, *19*(2), 203–214. doi:10.1111/j.1365-2206.2012.00894.x

Poverty and its sequelae are important determinants of health, and their impact is perhaps most injurious for young children and their families. Lack of school readiness and parenting stress may be associated with poverty, inadequate housing, and unemployment. Early interventions can offset these health effects.

This two-generation program is aimed at the needs of low-income preschool children and their parents. Program interventions included early childhood education (20 hours per week provided by the centre), parenting and life skills education (designed and implemented on-site by program staff), and family support provided by a registered social worker during home visits. This MIP was offered to families at no cost. A single group pretest (program intake) and post-test (at program exit) with follow-up (when children were 7 years old) design was used to evaluate outcomes. Bioecological theory guided the evaluation. In total, 132 children and 79 parents enrolled in the study. At the time of the study's publication, 95 children who had provided both intake and exit data had reached 7 years of age and were eligible to participate in the follow-up portion of the study. Sixty-seven parents (of 79) completed intake and exit data collection and 38 parents provided data at all three time points.

Parents completed a parenting stress index, community life skills scale, self-esteem scale, and a scale measuring attitudes associated with child maltreatment. Measures were self-completed at the outset of their enrolment in the program, following program completion, and when their child was 7 years old. In the portion of the study examining child outcomes, intake and exit data were collected from 109 (of 132) children. Data from all three time points were available for 60 children. A research assistant assessed children's receptive language skills using the Peabody Picture Vocabulary Test, and their global development using the Battelle Developmental Inventory-Screening Test at all three time points. Study participants' results were compared to standardized scores for their age or grade.

Parents reported positive differences in self-esteem, use of community resources, parental distress, and parenting attitudes related to corporal punishment and appropriate parent–child roles. Moreover, at 7 years, parental distress had continued to decrease. The preschool children demonstrated a statistically significant improvement in receptive language skills that was sustained at age 7. Children's global development scores improved during the program and improvements in communication, motor, and personal-social domains were sustained up to age 7 years. Findings suggest that appropriate and timely supports and services for low-income families can reduce the negative impact of their economic pressures.

### Discussion Questions

1. How does poverty affect children living in low-income families?

2. What are the strengths and limitations of the research design used to assess the impact of this program?

3. Were the evaluation measures used examples of output, outcome, or impact indicators?

## CASE STUDY

Rachelle is the public health nurse providing pre- and post-natal visits with pregnant and parenting women at an outreach centre for young single parents. The outreach centre is a "one stop" location where mothers under the age of 25 can access health, educational, and social services. Over the past five years, Rachelle and other staff at the centre have noted an increase in the proportion of young pregnant women attending services at the centre who have been diagnosed with, or exhibit symptoms of, mood disorders (e.g. depression, anxiety) and/or have experienced traumatic childhoods (e.g., violence in the home, parent with addictions, and neglect). Most of the outreach centre's programming focuses on promoting healthy behaviours, prenatal education, and good parenting practices. Rachelle is concerned about the lack of resources to address the mental health of the young mothers currently accessing the centre's services.

### Discussion Questions

1. At what stage in the planning–implementation–evaluation cycle are Rachelle and her colleagues at in their work at the outreach centre?

2. Which community partners should be included in the planning–implementation–evaluation cycle and how can Rachelle engage them?

3. Using a socioecological framework to guide your approach, what sources of literature and community data might help you develop an intervention plan?

## CONCLUSION

Community health nurses are key players in health program delivery, and must also be integral to the dynamic process of program planning and evaluation. Familiarity with the tools and processes described in this chapter will help you contribute fully as a member of a program planning and evaluation team. As our examples have illustrated, community health programs are often aimed at community issues with a complex set of underlying socio-structural determinants. It is not surprising that the planning process needs to be informed by a diverse set of data and evidence. Planning and evaluation should not occur in isolation. Rather, one must pull together an interdisciplinary team with a wide range of experience to help with different facets of this process. By working together, CHNs with program planning experience, academic researchers who are familiar with the theoretical and empirical literature, and community partners who bring important insights and essential experiential learning can substantially strengthen the design and evaluation of MIPs in community health. This in turn will help us meet the complex needs of populations, while demonstrating better accountability for the public funds used when programs are delivered.

## KEY TERMS

antagonistic   p. 276
assessing needs   p. 270
buy-in   p. 272
CAT (components, activities, and target groups)   p. 269
communication   p. 272
community meetings   p. 270
confidence interval   p. 271
content analysis   p. 271
document and policy reviews   p. 270
dose   p. 278
etiological research   p. 274
evaluation   p. 269
existing reports   p. 271
external opportunities and threats   p. 270
figures   p. 271
focus groups   p. 270
Gantt charts   p. 273
health impact assessment   p. 273
impact indicators   p. 280
impacts   p. 280
intensity   p. 278
internal strengths and weaknesses   p. 270
intervention effect   p. 271
intervention options   p. 277
key informant interviews   p. 270
laboratory studies   p. 276
long-term outcomes   p. 269
macro   p. 275
matrices   p. 271
meso   p. 275
meta-analysis   p. 271
micro   p. 275
Multiple Intervention Program (MIP) framework   p. 274
optimizing intervention strategies   p. 278
outcomes   p. 280
output indicators   p. 279
outputs   p. 279
planning–implementation–evaluation cycle   p. 268
policy levers   p. 278
policy windows   p. 278
population health approach   p. 273
population subgroups   p. 274
PRECEDE-PROCEED planning model (PPM)   p. 270
Program Evaluation Tool Kit   p. 269
program logic model   p. 268
program planning and evaluation frameworks   p. 268
qualitative research strategies   p. 270
quantitative data   p. 271
reach   p. 278
relative risk   p. 271
setting priorities   p. 271
short-term outcomes   p. 269
social determinants of health   p. 273
socio-structural determinants   p. 273
SOLO (short-term outcomes and long-term outcomes)   p. 269
spin-offs   p. 280
statistically significant   p. 271
sustainability   p. 280
SWOT (strengths, weaknesses, opportunities, and threats) analysis   p. 270

## STUDY QUESTIONS

1. Are the steps in the planning–implementation–evaluation cycle always followed in a linear fashion? Explain.

2. List four factors that influence the choice of a program planning and evaluation framework.

3. Identify some tools commonly used in planning programs.

4. List three uses of quantitative data in planning and evaluating a program.

5. Identify the three principles of priority setting.

6. List the five main elements of the MIP framework.

> After working through these questions, go to the MyNursingLab at www.pearsoned.ca/mynursinglab to check your answers.

## INDIVIDUAL CRITICAL-THINKING EXERCISES

1. Your healthcare agency is collaborating with a community advocacy group to address escalating substance use among youth aged 12 to 17. What are some of the underlying socio-structural determinants of substance abuse in this age group?

2. Using the substance abuse problem above, what types of evidence would you assemble to support the development of the program plan and why?

3. What are the strengths and weaknesses of each type of evidence you have selected for the substance abuse problem?

4. What are some examples of indicators you can use to assess the impact of the substance abuse program at the individual, organization, community, and policy levels?

5. Identify a community health issue of interest. What are some examples of synergies that might be expected to occur between program strategies and community context?

## GROUP CRITICAL-THINKING EXERCISES

1. You are part of a team evaluating a childhood obesity program delivered through the local schools. What information would you need to develop a logic model for this initiative? Describe to the members of your team why it is important to spend time developing the logic model.

2. Locate a good example of a community health program plan that illustrates the integration of several different theories. Do these theories reflect different levels of a socioecological model?

3. You have been asked to develop a multiple intervention program and evaluation plan to address homelessness among older adults. What community partners would you involve in this process and why? How would you get community partners involved?

## REFERENCES

Aminzadeh, F., & Edwards, N. (1998). Exploring seniors' views on the use of assistive devices in fall prevention. *Public Health Nursing, 15*(4), 297–304.

Aminzadeh, F., Edwards, N., Lockett, D., & Nair, R. C. (2001). Utilization of bathroom safety devices, patterns of bathing and toileting, and bathroom falls in a sample of community living older adults. *Technology and Disability, 13*(2), 95–103.

Angeles, R. M., Dolovich, L., Kaczorowsk, J., & Thabane, L. (2013). Developing a theoretical framework for complex community-based interventions. *Health Promotion Practice 14*(5), 100–108. doi:10.1177/1524839913483469

Bauman, K. E., Suchindran, C. M., & Murray, D. M. (1999). The paucity of effects in community trials: Is secular trend the culprit? *Preventive Medicine, 28*(4), 426–429.

Benjamin, K., Edwards, N., & Bharti, V. (2005). Attitudinal, perceptual, and normative beliefs influencing the exercise decision of community-dwelling physically frail seniors: An application of the theory of planned behaviour. *Journal of Aging and Physical Activity 13*(3), 276–293.

Benjamin, K., Edwards, N., Ploeg, J., & Legault, F. (2014). Barriers to physical activity and restorative care for residents in long-term care homes: A review of the literature. *Journal of Aging and Physical Activity, 22*(1), 154–165.

Blalock, S. J., Demby, K. B., McCulloch, K. L., & Stevens, J. A. (2010). Factors influencing hip protector use among community-dwelling older adults. *Injury Prevention, 16*(4), 235–239.

Burke, J. G., Hess, S., Hoffmann, K., Guizzetti, L., Loy, E., Gielen, A., . . . Yonas, M. (2013). Translating community-based participatory research principles into practice. *Progress in Community Health Partnerships: Research, Education, and Action, 7*(2), 115–122.

Commission on Social Determinants of Health. (2008). *Closing the gap in a generation: Health equity through action on the social determinants of health. Final report of the Commission of Social Determinants on Health.* Geneva, Switzerland: World Health Organization.

COMMIT Research Group. (1995a). Community intervention trial for smoking cessation. (COMMIT). I: Cohort results from a four-year community intervention. *American Journal of Public Health, 85*(2), 183–192.

COMMIT Research Group. (1995b). Community intervention trial for smoking cessation. (COMMIT). II: Changes in adult cigarette smoking prevalence. *American Journal of Public Health, 85*(2), 193–200.

Community Health Nurses of Canada. (2011, revised). *Canadian community health nursing: Professional practice model & standards of practice.* St. John's, NL: Author. Retrieved from https://www.chnc.ca/documents/CHNC-ProfessionalPracticeModel-EN/index.html

Crosby, R., & Noar, S. M. (2011). What is a planning model? An introduction to PRECEDE-PROCEED. *Journal of Public Health Dentistry, 71*(S1), S7–S15. doi:10.1111/j.1752-7325.2011.00235.x

Edwards, N. (1999). Prevention of falls among seniors in the community. In M. Stewart (Ed.), *Community nursing: Promoting Canadians' health* (2nd ed., pp. 296–316). Toronto, ON: W. B. Saunders.

Edwards, N. (2008). Performance-based building codes: A call for injury prevention indicators that bridge health and building sectors. *Injury Prevention, 14*(5), 329–332.

Edwards, N., Benjamin, K., & Lockett, D. (2006, September 25–27). *Environmental hazards and falls prevention: Defining a new research agenda*. Poster presented at the 2006 Australian Public Health Association conference, Sydney, Australia.

Edwards, N., Birkett, N., Nair, R., Murphy, M., Roberge, G., & Lockett, D. (2006). Access to bathtub grab bars: Evidence of a policy gap. *Canadian Journal on Aging, 25*(3), 295–304.

Edwards, N., & Davison, C. (2015). Strengthening communities with a socio-ecological approach: Local and international lessons in whole systems. In L. K. Hallstrom, N. Guehlstorf, & M. Parkes (Eds.), *Ecosystems, society and health: Pathways through diversity, convergence and integration.* Montreal/Kingston: McGill Queen's University Press.

Edwards, N., & Davison, C. (2008). Social justice and core competencies for public health: Improving the fit. *Canadian Journal of Public Health, 99*(2), 130–132.

Edwards, N., Lockett, D., Aminzadeh, F., & Nair, R. (2003). Predictors of bath grab-bar use among community-living older adults. *Canadian Journal on Aging, 22*(2), 217–227.

Edwards, N., MacLean, L., Estable, A., & Meyer, M. (2006). *Multiple intervention program recommendations for Mandatory Health Program and Services Guidelines Technical Review Committees.* Ottawa, ON: Community Health Research Unit, University of Ottawa.

Edwards, N., Mill, J., & Kothari, A. (2004). Multiple intervention research programs in community health. *Canadian Journal of Nursing Research, 36*(1), 40–54.

Edwards, N., & Moyer, A. (1999). Community needs and capacity assessment: Critical component of program planning. In M. Stewart (Ed.), *Community nursing: Promoting Canadians' health* (2nd ed., pp. 420–442). Toronto, ON: W. B. Saunders.

Fisher, K. J., Li, F., Michael, Y., & Cleveland, M. (2004). Neighborhood-level influences on physical activity among older adults: A multilevel analysis. *Journal of Aging and Physical Activity, 12*(1), 45–63.

Foy, R., Penney, G. C., MacLennan, G., Grimshaw, J., Campbell, M., & Grol, R. (2002). Attributes of clinical recommendations that influence change in practice following audit and feedback. *Journal of Clinical Epidemiology, 55*(7), 717–722.

Fraser, D. L., & Stupak, R. J. (2002). A synthesis of the strategic learning planning process with the principles of andragogy: Learning, leading and linking. *International Journal of Public Administration, 25*(9), 1199–1220.

Frick, K. D., Kung, J. Y., Parrish, J. M., & Narrett, M. J. (2010). Evaluating the cost-effectiveness of fall prevention programs that reduce fall-related hip fractures in older adults. *Journal of the American Geriatric Society, 58*(1), 136–141.

Friedman, S. R., Cooper, H. F. L., & Osborne, A. H. (2009). Structural and social contexts of HIV risk among African Americans. *American Journal of Public Health, 99*(6), 1002–1008.

Gallagher, E. M., & Scott, V. J. (1997). The Steps Project: Participatory action research to reduce falls in public places among seniors and persons with disabilities. *Canadian Journal of Public Health, 88*(2), 129–133.

George, J., Binns, V., Clayden, A., & Mulley, G. (1998). Aids and adaptations for the elderly at home: Underprovided, underused, and undermaintained. *British Medical Journal, 296*(6633), 1365–1366.

Gilbert, M., Cook, D., Steinberg, M., Kwag, M., Robert, W., Doupe, G., . . . Rekart, M. (2013). Targeting screening and social marketing to increase detection of acute HIV infection in men who have sex with men in Vancouver, British Columbia. *AIDS, 27*(16), 2649–2654.

Giles-Corti, B., & Donovan, R. J. (2003). Relative influences of individual, social environmental, and physical environmental correlates of walking. *American Journal of Public Health, 93*(9), 1583–1589.

Gill, T., Williams, C., & Tinetti, M. (2000). Environmental hazards and the risk of nonsyncopal falls in the homes of community-living older persons. *Medical Care, 38*(12), 1174–1183.

Gillespie, L. D., Gillespie, W. J., Robertson, M. C., Lamb, S. E., Cumming, R. G., & Rowe, B. H. (2003). Interventions for preventing falls in elderly people. *Cochrane Database System Review, 4,* CD000340.

Gillespie, W. J., Gillespie, L. D., & Parker, M. J. (2010). Hip protectors for preventing hip fractures in older people. *Cochrane Database of Systematic Reviews, 10,* Art. No.: CD001255.

Gillespie, L. D., Robertson, M. C., Gillespie, W. J., Lamb, S. E., Gates, S., Cumming, R. G., & Rowe, B. H. (2009). Interventions for preventing falls in older people living in the community. *Cochrane Database of Systematic Reviews, 2,* Art. No.: CD007146. doi:10.1002/14651858. CD007146.pub2

Gillespie, L. D., Robertson, M. C., Gillespie, W. J., Lamb, S. E., Sherrington, C., Gates, S., . . . Lamb, S. E. (2012). Interventions for preventing falls in older people living in the community. *Cochrane Database of Systematic Reviews,* Issue 9. Copyright © 2012 by John Wiley and Sons. Used by permission of John Wiley and Sons. Art. No.: CD007146. doi:10.1002/14651858. CD007146.pub3

Goodman, C., Davies, S., Tai, S., Dinan, S., & Iliffe, S. (2007). Promoting older people's participation in activity, whose responsibility? A case study of the response of health, local government and voluntary organizations. *Journal of Interprofessional Care, 21*(5), 515–528.

Gordon, R., McDermott, L., Stead, M., & Angus, K. (2006). The effectiveness of social marketing interventions for health improvement: What's the evidence? *Public Health, 120*(12), 1133–1139.

Grant, T., Andrews, C., Edwards, N., Sveistrup, H., & Egan, M. (2011). Creating walkable places: Neighbourhood and municipal level perspectives on the socio-political process in Ottawa, Canada. *Journal of Urbanism, 4*(1), 81–104.

Grant, T., Edwards, N., Sveistrup, H., Andrews, C., & Egan, M. (2010). Neighbourhood walkability: Older people's perspectives from four neighbourhoods in Ottawa, Canada. *Journal of Aging and Physical Activity, 18*(2), 293–312.

Guitard, P., Sveistrup, H., Lockett, D., & Edwards, N. (2011). Use of different bath grab bar configurations following a balance perturbation. *Assistive Technology, 23*(4), 205–215.

Hanson, H. M., Ashe, M. C., McKay, H. A., & Winters, M. (2012). Intersection between the built and social environments and older adults' mobility: An evidence review. Retrieved from http://ncceh.ca/sites/default/files/Built_and_Social_Environments_Older_Adults_Nov_2012.pdf

Hardt, M., & Negri, A. (2000). *Empire*. Cambridge, MA: Harvard University Press.

Health Canada. (2001). *The population health template: Key elements and actions that define a population health approach.* Strategic Policy Directorate of the Population and Public Health Branch, Health Canada. Retrieved from http://www.phac-aspc.gc.ca/ph-sp/pdf/overview_handout_black-eng.pdf

Helms, M. M., & Nixon, J. (2010). Exploring SWOT analysis – where are we now? A review of academic research from the last decade. *Journal of Strategy and Management, 3*(3), 215–251.

Hooker, S. P., & Cirill, L. A. (2006). Evaluation of community coalitions' ability to create safe, effective exercise classes for older adults. *Evaluation and Program Planning, 29*(3), 242–250.

Jilcott, S., Ammerman, A., Sommers, J., & Glasgow, R. E. (2007). Applying the RE-AIM framework to assess the public health impact of policy change. *Annals of Behavioural Medicine, 34*, 105–114.

Kamberelis, G., & Dimitriadis, G. (2005). Focus groups: Strategic articulations of pedagogy, politics and inquiry. In N. K. Denzin & Y. S. Lincoln (Eds.), *The Sage handbook of qualitative research* (3rd ed., pp. 887–907). Thousand Oaks, CA: Sage.

Kearney, F. C., Harwood, R. H., Gladman, J. R., Lincoln, N., & Masud, T. (2013). The relationship between executive function and falls and gait abnormalities in older adults: A systematic review. *Dementia, Geriatric and Cognitive Disorders, 36*(1–2), 20–35.

Kelsey, J. L., Berry, S. D., Proceter-Gray, E., Quach, L., Nguyen, U. S., Li, W., . . . Hannan, M. T. (2010). Indoor and outdoor falls in older adults are different: The maintenance of balanced, independent living, intellect, and zest in the Elderly of Boston Study. *Journal of the American Geriatric Society, 58*(1), 2135–2141.

Kingdon, J. W. (1995). *Agendas, alternatives, and public policies* (2nd ed.). New York, NY: Addison-Wesley.

Laing, A. C., & Robinovitch, S. N. (2008). The force attenuation provided by hip protectors depends on impact velocity, pelvic size and soft tissues stiffness. *Journal of Biomechanical Engineering, 130*(6), 061005. doi:10.1115/1.2979867

Letts, L., Moreland, J., Richardson, J., Coman, L., Edwards, M., Ginis, K. M., . . . Wishart, L. (2010). The physical environment as a fall risk factor in older adults: Systematic review and meta-analysis of cross-sectional and cohort studies. *Australian Occupational Therapy Journal, 57*(1), 51–64.

Lockett, D., Willis, A., & Edwards, N. (2005). Through seniors' eyes: An exploratory qualitative study to identify environmental barriers to and facilitators of walking. *Canadian Journal of Nursing Research, 37*(3), 48–65.

Luca, N. R., & Suggs, L. S. (2013). Theory and model use in social marketing health interventions. *Journal of Health Communication, 18*(1), 20–40.

Maki, B. E., Perry, S. D., Scovil, C. Y., Mihailidis, A., & Fernie, G. R. (2006). Getting a grip on stairs: Research to optimize effectiveness of handrails. In R. N. Pikaar, E. A. P. Koningsveld, & P. J. M. Settels (Eds.), *Proceedings IEA 2006 Congress* (pp. 4669–4674). Amsterdam, The Netherlands: Elsevier.

Mays, N., Pope, C., & Popay, J. (2005). Systematically reviewing qualitative and quantitative evidence to inform management and policy-making in the health field. *Journal of Health Services Research & Policy, 10*(S1), 6–20.

McClure, R., Turner, C., Peel, N., Spinks, A., Eakin, E., & Hughes, K. (2005). Population-based interventions for the prevention of fall-related injuries in older people. *Cochrane Database of Systematic Reviews*, 1, Art. No.: CD004441. doi:10.1002/14651858.CD004441.pub2.

McInnes, E., Seers, K., Tutton, L. J. (2011). Older people's views in relation to risk of falling and need for intervention: A meta-ethnography. *Journal of Advanced Nursing, 67*(12), 2525–2536.

Merzel, D., & D'Afflitti, J. (2003). Reconsidering community-based health promotion: Promise, performance, and potential. *American Journal of Public Health, 93*(4), 557–574.

Miles, M. B., Huberman, A. M., & Saldana, J. (2014). *Qualitative data analysis: A methods sourcebook* (3rd ed.). Thousand Oaks, CA: Sage.

Ministry of Health and Long-Term Care. (2008). *Ontario public health standards 2008.* Retrieved from http://www.health.gov.on.ca/en/pro/programs/publichealth/oph_standards/docs/ophs_2008.pdf

Muir, S. W., Gopaul, K., & Montero Odasso, M. M. (2012). The role of cognitive impairment in fall risk among older adults: A systematic review and meta-analysis. *Age and Ageing, 41*(3), 299–308. doi:10.1093/ageing/afs012

Naik, A. D., & Gill, T. M. (2005). Underutilization of environmental adaptations for bathing in community-living older persons. *Journal of the American Geriatrics Society, 53*(9), 1497–1503.

National Collaborating Centre for Methods and Tools. (2010). *Program evaluation toolkit.* Hamilton, ON: McMaster University. Retrieved from http://www.nccmt.ca/registry/view/eng/68.html

Nova Scotia Seniors' Secretariat. (2005). Strategy for Positive Aging in Nova Scotia. Retrieved from https://www.novascotia.ca/seniors/pub/2005_StrategyPositiveAging.pdf

O'Loughlin, J., Robitaille, Y., Boivin, J. F., & Suissa, S. (1993). Incidence of and risk factors for falls and injurious falls among the community-dwelling elderly. *American Journal of Epidemiology, 137*(3), 342–354.

Ontario Seniors' Secretariat. (2013). Independence, activity, and good health: Ontario's action plan for seniors. Retrieved from http://www.oacao.org/images/ontarioseniorsactionplan-en.pdf

Parker, M. J., Gillespie, W. J., & Gillespie, L. D. (2006). Effectiveness of hip protectors for preventing hip fractures in elderly people: Systematic review. *British Medical Journal, 332*, 571–574.

Pal, L. (2006). *Beyond policy analysis: Public issue management in turbulent times* (3rd ed.). Toronto, ON: Nelson Education.

Patton, M. Q. (2002). *Qualitative research and evaluation methods* (3rd ed.). Thousand Oaks, CA: Sage.

Perdue, W. C., Stone, L. A., & Gostin, L. O. (2003). The built environment and its relation to the public's health: The legal perspective. *American Journal of Public Health, 93*(9), 1390–1394.

Pope, C., & Mays, N. (2013). *Qualitative research in health care.* Toronto, ON: John Wiley & Sons.

Porteous, N., Sheldrick, B., & Stewart, P. (2002). Introducing program teams to logic models: Facilitating the learning process. *The Canadian Journal of Program Evaluation, 17*(3), 113–141.

Prochaska, J. O., & Velicer, W. F. (1997). The transtheoretical model of health behaviour change. *American Journal of Health Promotion, 12*(1), 38–48.

Raphael, D. (Ed.). (2008). *Social determinants of health: Canadian perspectives* (2nd ed.). Toronto, ON: Canadian Scholars' Press.

Rawski, E. (1998). Review of the literature on falls among the elderly. *Journal of Nursing Scholarship, 30*(1), 47–52.

Registered Nurses' Association of Ontario. (2005). *Prevention of falls and fall injuries in the older adult*. (Revised). Toronto, ON: Registered Nurses' Association of Ontario.

Rubin., C. L., Martinez, L. S., Chu, J., Hacker, K., Brugge, D., Pirie, A., . . . Leslie, L. K. (2012). Community-engaged pedagogy: A strengths-based approach to involving diverse stakeholders in research partnerships. *Program Community Health Partnership*. Winter, 6(4), 481–90. doi:10.1353/cpr.2012.0057

Rubin, J. H., & Rubin, I. S. (2005). Listening, hearing and sharing social experiences. In *Qualitative interviewing: The art of hearing data* (pp. 1–18). Thousand Oaks, CA: Sage.

Sampson, R. J., & Morenoff, J. (2000). Listening, hearing and sharing social experiences. In *Qualitative interviewing: The art of hearing data* (2nd ed., pp. 1–18). Toronto, ON: Sage.

Scott, V., Dukeshire, S., Gallagher, E., & Scanlan, A. (2001). *A best practice guide for the prevention of falls among seniors living in the community*. Ottawa, ON: Federal/Provincial/Territorial Ministers of Health and Ministers Responsible for Seniors.

Senate Subcommittee on Population Health. (2009). *A healthy, productive Canada: A determinant of health approach*. The Standing Senate Committee on Social Affairs, Science and Technology. Retrieved from http://www.parl.gc.ca/content/sen/committee/402/popu/rep/rephealth1jun09-e.pdf

Shiell, A., Hawe, P., & Gold, L. (2008). Complex interventions or complex systems? Implications for health economic evaluation. *British Medical Journal, 336*(7656), 1281–1283.

Smith, D., Varcoe, C., & Edwards, N. (2005). Turning around the intergenerational impact of residential schools on Aboriginal people: Implications for health policy and practice. *Canadian Journal of Nursing Research, 37*(4), 38–60.

Sorenson, G., Emmons, K., Hunt, J. K., & Johnston, D. (1998). Implications of the results of community intervention trials. *Annual Review of Public Health, 19*, 379–416.

Stirman, S. W., Kimberly, J., Cook, N., Calloway, A., Castro, F., & Charns, M. (2012). The sustainability of new programs and innovations: A review of the empirical literature and recommendations for future research. *Implementation Science, 7*(17), 1–16.

Sveistrup, H., Lockett, D., Edwards, N., & Aminzadeh, F. (2006). Evaluation of bath grab bar placement for older adults. *Technology and Disability, 18*(2), 45–55.

Syddall, H., Evandrou, M., Cooper, C., Aihie Sayer, A. J. (2009). Social inequalities in grip strength, physical function, and falls among community dwelling older men and women. *Journal of Aging, 21*(6), 913–939.

Taylor, L., & Blair-Stevens, C. (Eds.). (2002). *Introducing health impact assessment (HIA): Informing the decision-making process*. National Health Services Health Development Agency, UK. Retrieved from http://www.apho.org.uk/resource/item.aspx?RID=44263

Tinetti, M. E., Baker, D. I., McAvay, G., Claus, E. B., Garrett, P., Gottschalk, M., & Horwitz, R. I. (1994). A multifactorial intervention to reduce the risk of falling among elderly people living in the community. *The New England Journal of Medicine, 331*(13), 821–827.

van de Belt, T. H., Engelen, L. J., Berben, S. A., Teerenstra, S., Samsom, M., & Schoonhoven, L. (2013). Internet and social media for health-related information and communication in health care: Preferences of the Dutch general population. *Journal of Medical Internet Research, 15*(10), e220.

Whittemore, R., & Knafl, K. (2005). The integrative review: Updated methodology. *Journal of Advanced Nursing, 52*(5), 546–553.

Woodward, G., Manuel, D., & Goel, V. (2004). *Developing a balanced score card for public health*. Institute for Clinical Evaluative Sciences, Toronto, ON. Retrieved from http://www.ices.on.ca/~/media/Files/Atlases-Reports/2004/Developing-a-balanced-scorecard-for-public-health/Full%20report.ashx

Wooten, K. C., Rose, R. M., Ostir, G. V., Calhoun, W. J., Ameredes, B. T., & Braiser, A. R. (2014). Assessing and evaluating multidisciplinary translational teams: A mixed methods approach. *Evaluation & the Health Professions 37*(1), 33–49. doi:10.1177/0163278713504433

Zanna, M., Cameron, R., Goldsmith, C. H., Poland, B., Lindsay, E., & Walker, R. (1994). Critique of the COMMIT study based on the Brantford experience. *Health and Canadian Society, 2*(2), 319–336.

## ABOUT THE AUTHORS

**Nancy Edwards**, RN, PhD, is a Full Professor and distinguished professor at the University of Ottawa, School of Nursing. Nancy's research program examines multiple interventions in community health.

**Josephine Etowa**, RN, PhD, is an Associate Professor and Loyer DaSilva Research Chair in Public Health Nursing at the University of Ottawa, School of Nursing. Her research is in the area of community health, inequity in health, and healthcare.

**Wendy Peterson**, RN, PhD, is an Associate Professor at the University of Ottawa, School of Nursing. Wendy's research focuses on access and utilization of perinatal health services by marginalized women.

The authors would like to acknowledge and thank Margaret Ann Kennedy, RN, PhD, for her important contributions to earlier editions of this chapter.

# CHAPTER 15

# Information Technology

*Linda Ferguson and Tracie Risling*

## LEARNING OUTCOMES

**After studying this chapter, you should be able to:**

1. Explain basic informatics competencies for community health nurses.

2. Discuss the use of the Internet to access health information by various Canadian population groups.

3. Evaluate the quality of a health website.

4. Describe a variety of Internet technology applications with potential to support health promotion, disease prevention, and chronic disease management.

5. Explain ways to increase accessibility to health information on the Internet for the public.

6. Describe emerging technology tools that can support community health nursing practice, professional development, and knowledge exchange in community health nursing.

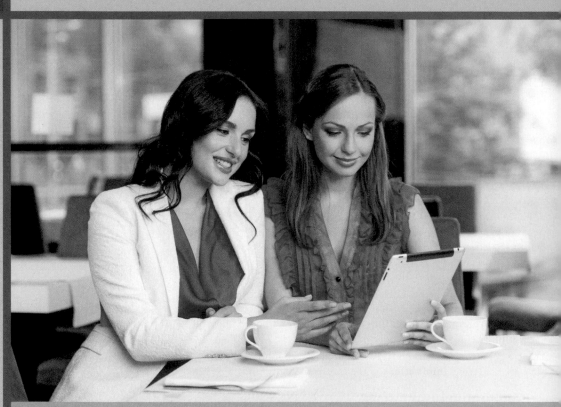

*Source: BlueSkyImages/Fotolia*

## INTRODUCTION

Exponential growth has occurred in the use of Internet-based **information and communication technologies (ICTs)** by health professionals and the public. The term "ICT" represents a variety of computer-based technology systems that support gathering, analyzing, archiving, retrieving, processing, and transmitting information and communication. ICTs can support people to increase control over their health through allowing access to health information, providing social support, facilitating behaviour change, and supporting community mobilization. Primary health care nursing service delivery can be improved through the use of innovative, interactive e-health interventions that are tailored to individual needs. Hebda and Czar (2013) defined **e-health** (also referred to as telehealth) as a "wide range of healthcare activities involving the electronic transfer of health-related information on the Internet" (p. 578). **Telehealth** is defined as "the use of telecommunications technologies and electronic information to exchange healthcare information and to provide and support services such as long distance clinical healthcare to clients" (Hebda & Czar, 2013, p. 505).

**E-nursing** is the integration of ICTs into nursing, as defined by the Canadian Nurses Association's e-Nursing Strategy for Canada (2006). The "e" in *e-nursing* is expected to disappear as the integration of ICTs into nursing becomes part of nursing practice. Community health nurses

(CHNs) can support the effective use of ICTs to promote health, prevent illness; enable consultations; educate clients and families; provide service, therapy, and support; and manage chronic disease using e-health interventions. CHNs are expected to meet the Canadian Community Health Nursing Standards of Practice (Community Health Nurses of Canada [CHNC], 2011, revised), which include specific standards related to nursing informatics (see Appendix A for the full list of standards).

**Nursing informatics** is defined in broad terms as the use of information and computer technology to support all aspects of nursing practice, including direct delivery of care, administration, research, and education (Hebda & Czar, 2013). In 2002, Staggers and Bagley Thompson (2002) had described nursing informatics as facilitating the management and communication of "data, information, and knowledge in nursing practice to support patients, nurses, and other providers in their decision making in all roles and settings" (p. 262).

In this chapter, you will learn about CHN competencies as they relate to nursing informatics and gain an overview of current research on accessing and using the Internet for health information and communication. You will explore innovations in technology that have shown potential to support health promotion, disease prevention, and chronic disease management. Finally, you will be introduced to ICTs that support professional development and knowledge exchange in community health nursing.

## NURSING INFORMATICS COMPETENCIES

Canada Health Infoway (www.infoway-inforoute.ca) is an organization that supports transformation of healthcare in Canada through the appropriate use of information technology and by providing support for clients, healthcare providers, healthcare managers, and organizations. Infoway is a federally supported organization that facilitates the implementation of health information systems needed to manage Canadians' health and healthcare information.

Canada Health Infoway supported the Canadian Association of Schools of Nursing (CASN) in identifying expected information and communication technology competencies of graduates of baccalaureate nursing programs (CASN, 2012) and providing a toolkit to facilitate the teaching of such competencies (CASN, 2013). The overarching competency is the use of ICTs to support information synthesis in accordance with professional and regulatory standards in the delivery of patient or client care. Entry-to-practice competencies of ICT have been highlighted in three distinct areas:

1. uses relevant information and knowledge to support delivery of evidence-informed patient care;
2. uses ICTs in accordance with professional and regulatory standards and workplace policies; and
3. uses ICTs in the delivery of patient/client care.

These informatics competencies build on foundational aspects of existing registered nursing professional standards and expectations, such as these CASN (2014) public health competencies:

1. Applies health literacy when working with clients.
2. Uses social media, community resources, and social marketing techniques appropriately to disseminate health information.
3. Documents population health nursing activities.
4. Uses appropriate communication techniques to influence decision makers.

Because of their importance to the health of nations, national-level nursing informatics competencies are being developed in a number of countries (Borycki, Foster, Sahama, Frisch, & Kushniruk, 2013; U.S. Centers for Disease Control and Prevention and University of Washington's Center for Public Health Informatics, 2009).

**Public health informatics** is defined as "the systematic application of information and computer sciences and technology to public health practice, research and learning" (Hebda & Czar, 2013). This definition reflects a public health perspective on disease surveillance and management, with an emphasis on population health. The Canadian Community Health Nursing Standards of Practice are based on the principles of primary health care that include the appropriate use of technology and resources. Specifically, the standards state that CHNs are expected to use "current evidence and informatics (including information and communication technology) to identify, generate, manage, and process relevant data to support nursing practice" (CHNC, 2011, revised, p. 22). The Canadian Nursing Informatics Association (CNIA) (www. cnia.ca) has also made recommendations concerning basic Internet and computer competencies of nursing graduates (CNIA, 2003). CNIA identified a need to build strong links between nursing informatics and evidence-based practice; increase informatics skills of educators, clinicians, and students; identify how informatics is covered in curricula; build stronger human, material, and financial infrastructure for ICT in clinical and academic settings; and strengthen partnerships with the private sector.

## USE OF THE INTERNET TO ACCESS HEALTH INFORMATION

Rapid growth has occurred in Canadians' use of the Internet to access health information. According to the Internet Use Survey (Figure 15.1), in 2009, 69.9% of individuals searched for medical or health information at home using the Internet (Statistics Canada, 2009). More recent reports indicate 97% of Canadian households have Internet connections (Statistics Canada, 2013a). While 98% of high-income households had high-speed Internet connections, only 58% of low-income households reported the same, a factor that contributes to effective use of the Internet (Statistics Canada, 2013a). In the United States, the Pew Research Internet Survey (2011) also indicated an existing disparity in Internet access, particularly among older citizens and those who do not have Internet connectivity in their homes.

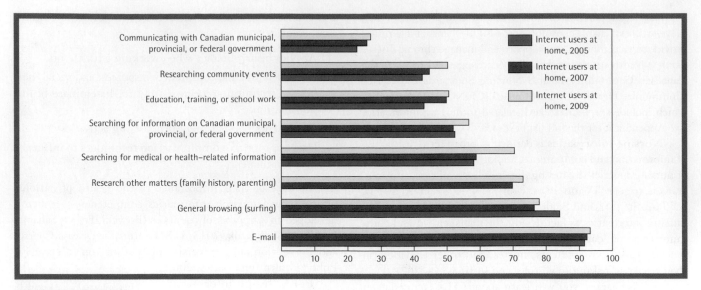

**FIGURE 15.1** Internet Use by Individuals, by Type of Activity, in 2005, 2007, and 2009

*Source:* Statistics Canada. (2010). *Internet use by individuals, by type of activity.* Summary Tables, CANSIM Table 358-0130. Retrieved from http:////www.statcan.gc.ca/tables-tableaux/sum-som/l01/cst01/comm29a-eng.htm

Underhill and McKeown (2008) reported that Internet searches for health information were more likely to be done by women with higher income and education, while young men were least likely to perform this type of search. Health-related Internet searches focused on specific diseases, healthy lifestyle, symptoms, drugs or medications, and alternative therapies.

Rooks, Wiltshire, Elder, BeLue, and Gary (2012) found that racial and ethnic minorities were less likely than Caucasians to seek information online or to use Internet-accessed information in their discussions with physicians. Compared to those who do not seek health information on the Internet, those who frequently use the Internet for health information were also likely to access health services significantly more often (Suziedelyte, 2012). Certain treatment can also prompt Internet use. Half of those who were prescribed contraceptive medications by their physicians, in one recent study, sought additional information on the Internet, suggesting that more health teaching is necessary with these prescriptions (Russo, Parisi, Kukla, & Schwarz, 2013).

Although study participants viewed physicians as the most credible source of health information, 48.6% of respondents reported using the Internet first, while 10.9% reported going to their physicians first (Hesse et al., 2005). In 2012, this number was similar, but over 72% of people discussed the Internet resource with their physicians and found that their relationship with the physician was more positive because of this action (AlGhamdi & Moussa, 2012). Xiao, Sharman, Rao, and Upadhyaya (2014) identified that those individuals who perceive their own health status to be poor, or who have significant anxiety related to their status or lack of diagnosis, use the Internet more frequently, regardless of their relationships with their physicians.

Manafo and Wong (2012) found that the accessibility and availability of online nutrition information enabled some older adults but that the amount of information available online overwhelmed and dis-enabled others. **Health literacy**

is generally defined as an individual's ability to obtain and use health information to make decisions and choices about health behaviours and healthcare, and is related to one's health status, healthcare service use, and self-care behaviours. Age, race, ethnicity, and socioeconomic status can influence health literacy levels (Ownby, Acevedo, Waldrop-Valverde, Jacobs, & Caballera, 2014). These skills are essential to support use of information online (Norman & Skinner, 2006). Xie (2011) has demonstrated that health literacy courses can increase older adults' confidence in the information they access online. Overall, Chaudhuri, Le, White, Thompson, and Demiris (2013) confirmed that older adults preferred sources where they were able to discuss the information. Internet information ranked low in their list of trusted sources, along with newspapers and television.

A random survey of 2038 adults in the Pew Internet Research Project found that although sick or disabled adults were less likely to use the Internet, they did search for online health information more than their healthier counterparts (Goldner, 2006). Another trend is increasing Internet use for personal health maintenance. In Canada in 2009, only 1.4% of Internet users purchased pharmaceuticals online (Statistics Canada, 2010), whereas in 2012, 6% purchased online pharmaceuticals and 15% purchased health or beauty products online (Statistics Canada, 2013b). Approximately 7% communicated with physicians via email—a phenomenon that will have significant management issues for physicians—and 4% participated in online support groups. In addition, incidental online health information acquisition was positively correlated with increased Internet use and seeking online health information for self or others (Tian & Robinson, 2009). Conversely, those persons experiencing a high level of anxiety about their health status searched for online information more frequently and for a longer duration. Significantly, this online search also contributed to an increasing anxiety level for these people (Muse, McManus, Leung, Meghreblain, & Williams, 2012).

Of Internet users, 58% accessed the Internet via a wireless handheld device such as a cellphone or tablet.

Personal empowerment, defined as the development of personal involvement and responsibility, is enhanced by the use of online health resources (Lemire, Sicotte, & Paré, 2008). Through self-report, Internet users identified three aspects of empowerment: compliance with expert advice, self-reliance through individual choice, and social inclusion through the development of collective support. Internet users perceived that all three aspects were enhanced by access to online health information (Lemire, Sicotte, & Paré, 2008). Determinants of use of online health information included its perceived usefulness, concern for personal health, specific health issues experienced, importance given to the opinions of physicians and other healthcare professionals, and trust placed in the online information (Lemire, Paré, Sicotte, & Harvey, 2008).

Khechine, Pascot, and Prémont (2008) demonstrated that people with long-term illnesses were more likely to access websites that were scientific in nature (medical, electronic library, government websites, or foundations). They often accessed online health information at two points in the medical decisional process: identification of possible treatments and treatment follow-up. In this study, only about 25% of respondents frequently used online discussion forums for information, even though Hoffman-Goetz, Donelle, and Thomson (2009) demonstrated that 91% of the advice provided in the forums was congruent with best practice guidelines. See Canadian Research Box 15.1.

Although patients may bring their search results to discuss with their physicians (AlGhamdi & Noussa, 2012), it is worrying that nurses and doctors are rarely asked for advice regarding where to search for health information online (Rice, 2006). This finding highlights an important health education role for CHNs, especially when working with Internet users. Nurses are cautioned that online health information is only one approach to delivering health messages within myriad other communications media.

## Internet Access Issues

Although many populations use the Internet for health information, access to this resource is not equitable, as has previously been noted. Tapscott (1998) first identified the **digital divide** as Internet users, resulting in information "haves" and "have-nots," thus identifying segments of the population that may not use the Internet for health information. Over the past 15 years, this divide has changed. Although youth have been early adopters of the Internet, older adults are now using the Internet in high numbers, and seniors are currently the fastest-growing group of users. Forty-five percent of adults over the age of 65 are using the Internet, and half of those seniors are using the Internet search for health-related information. The number of older seniors using the Internet is lower, about 21% of seniors over the age of 75 (Statistics Canada, 2010); however, this number continues to grow each year. It is older users, however, in the lowest income brackets in Canada who also account for much of the persistent digital divide (Statistics Canada, 2013a). In 2012, only 28% of Canadians aged 65 years and over with the lowest incomes used the Internet in comparison with 95% of those aged 16–24 in similar low-income brackets (Statistics Canada, 2013a).

One of the main limitations to Internet use is the lack of computers and Internet access in the home (Statistics Canada, 2013a). Individuals with low income, limited education, or who are members of minority ethnic groups may have significant limitations to the use of the Internet for health information (Pew Internet Research, 2011). Older adults may also experience limitations in accessing Internet information, or may have concerns about the credibility of the information they have accessed (Chaudhuri et al., 2013).

Despite access limitations and reported low Internet usage, Goldner (2006) encouraged health professionals to provide education to the sick about the quality of online health information to support skill development in the event online health information is sought in the future. Low-income communities, older adults, ethnic groups, and disadvantaged groups have been shown to use and benefit from community-based Internet

---

### CANADIAN RESEARCH BOX 15.1

**Does a website navigation tool facilitate access to health information online?**

Haase, K. R., & Loiselle, C. (2012). Oncology team members' perceptions of a virtual navigation tool for cancer patients. *International Journal of Medical Informatics, 81,* 395–403. Used by permission of Elsevier Science Ltd. doi:10.1016/j.ijmedinf.2011.11.001

Researchers interviewed healthcare providers (HCPs) to determine their perceptions of a virtual navigation tool (Oncology Interactive Navigator [OIN]) in assisting oncology clients to access information on the Internet. All providers offered care or service as part of a multidisciplinary colorectal oncology team at a university-affiliated teaching hospital in Montreal, Quebec. Medicine, nursing, social work, pharmacy, psychology, nutrition, and layperson volunteers were represented in the sample. Through qualitative analysis, researchers demonstrated that HCPs viewed the OIN as a highly accessible repository of high-quality and reliable cancer information, a means of enhancement to HCP–patient communication and trust, and a useful catalyst for patient and family communication and support. A person-centred approach, incorporating a tailored approach to the needs and preferences of cancer patients, was the common thread that linked the perceptions of the participants. Barriers to use were perceived as patient and system specific.

#### Discussion Questions

1. How could you assist clients to use a navigation tool to access credible information relative to their needs?

2. What assessments could nurses make to determine client or family limitations to the use of such a navigation tool?

3. How could nurses support clients who lack computer literacy to use navigation tools to access high-quality oncology information?

access to empower and build healthier neighbourhoods and populations (Chaudhuri et al., 2013; Lober & Flowers, 2011; Valaitis, 2005; Valaitis & O'Mara, 2005). However, the Internet has also been found to be a poor source of health information for some groups, including the Chinese immigrant population of Vancouver, British Columbia, and Seattle, Washington (Woodall et al., 2009). Therefore, nurses should not assume that all clients can, or will, access the Internet for health information.

Youth have been early adopters of technology; therefore, technology has the significant potential to enhance youth's health decision making. Their access issues differ from those of others. Skinner, Biscope, and Poland (2003) studied 210 Ontario youth to explore their perceptions of the Internet for health information and resources. The quality of Internet access was significantly impacted by four factors: privacy, gatekeeping, timeliness, and functionality. Health and education professionals should support interventions to address the "access quality divide" for more vulnerable populations (Skinner et al., 2003). Valaitis (2005) advocated for attention to the factors of privacy, gatekeeping, timeliness, and functionality when designing Internet-based resources for youth.

## Access for Disabled Populations

CHNs often work with disabled populations. The Canadian Council on Social Development (2005) (www.ccsd.ca) reported that more than half a million adult Canadians have some form of vision loss, more than a million have some form of hearing loss, and a number have both. People with disabilities can benefit from using ICTs, since they can reduce social isolation by helping them reach people with similar experiences (Seymour & Lupton, 2004), become better informed, increase communication, and enhance access to health information. The next section will review accessibility standards that guide the design of health information websites, and will provide a basic overview of technology tools to enhance disabled clients' Internet access.

The World Wide Web Consortium (W3C) (www.w3.org) is an international organization that oversees the standardization and operation of the Web. In 1997, to ensure equitable and universal access to information for all populations, including people with disabilities, W3C launched the **Web Accessibility Initiative (WAI)** (W3C, 2014a). Under this initiative, accessibility standards for Web content designers and developers were created. The **Web Content Accessibility Guidelines (WCAG)** document was updated in 2008 (Caldwell, Slatin, & Vanderheiden, 2008), and tutorials are available to support designers in making their websites accessible to those with disabilities (W3C, 2014b). These guidelines define **accessible** as "usable to a wide range of people with disabilities, including blindness and low vision, deafness and hearing loss, learning difficulties, cognitive limitations, limited movement, speech difficulties, photosensitivity, and combinations of these" (W3C, 2014a, para. 1). Standards were grouped into different priority levels. Disability advocates recommend that websites at a minimum meet the Priority Level One standard.

Priority Level One design standards are relatively simple to meet. For example, webpage images need clear text descriptions. Html code should include "alt tags" (alternative text tags) so that when a user rolls over the image, a text description appears. When browser preferences are set for "text only," the option for viewing images is turned off. This option is useful for the visually impaired. Screen readers turn screen text to speech and can read text programmed in the alt tag codes, thereby informing visitors what images are on the page. Another Priority One standard includes the use of contrasting background and text colours. Such standards help to ensure that Web documents are navigable. The Treasury Board of Canada Secretariat has also identified a set of guidelines for all federal government department websites called the "Common Look and Feel for the Internet" (2007). These guidelines incorporate Priority One and Priority Two W3C checkpoints and should be used to ensure accessibility.

Health information websites generally get failing grades with respect to accessibility and usability. Goldberg et al. (2011) indicated that issues of accessibility must be addressed at the onset of development, and that although usability is a quality of the website, it is defined in terms of the people using the site. Hardiker and Grant (2011) explored factors that influence public engagement with e-health, identifying improved access and tailored services as necessary conditions for ease of use. Burns, Jones, Inverson, and Caputi (2013) indicated that there is a lack of current research on the usability of websites that are easily accessible to those with visual and auditory disabilities. In addition, there is also limited access to translation devices to meet the public's needs for accessibility.

Numerous software and hardware devices are available to assist disabled populations. Some commonly used devices for the visually impaired include screen readers, screen magnifiers, Braille displays, voice recognition technologies, data extraction tools that filter content from overly busy webpages, and OCR software to turn a printed page into electronic text for

---

### CASE STUDY

**Testing Website Accessibility**

Identify your favourite health information website or your current clinical placement agency website. Once you have located the website, highlight and copy the URL (universal resource locator—a unique identifier that provides an address for an Internet site). Then proceed to an accessibility checker website. W3C has listed many website accessibility checkers (www.w3.org/WAI/ER/tools/complete). The University of Toronto checker can be found at http://achecker.ca/checker/index.php.

Paste in the URL at the site to obtain a report on how well it complied with W3C Web Content Accessibility Guidelines (Caldwell, Slatin, & Vanderheiden, 2008).

#### Discussion Questions

1. How accessible was your site?
2. Which standards did it fail?

screen reading. Portable note-taking devices can help people with speech communication disorders, and ergonomic adapters, dictation programs, and voice-controlled software can assist the mobility impaired. Simple adjustments can be made with most operating systems to enhance accessibility. For example, explore the "Accessibility Options" folder in the control panel of your own computer to adjust settings for hearing, vision, and mobility.

## QUALITY OF HEALTH INFORMATION ON THE INTERNET

Access to good-quality health information can empower clients to address their health issues; however, increased public access to health information on the Internet has introduced both risks and opportunities. The quality of health information on the Internet is highly variable. The public is challenged to determine the quality and credibility of the health information provided. Health information on the Internet includes health promotion information, screening tests, personal accounts of illness, patient testimonials about treatment effectiveness, patient opinions or perspectives on their illness experiences, product advertisers, treatment providers, patient or client discussion and support groups, peer-reviewed articles, and decision-making aids. A goal for CHNs includes assisting clients to become knowledgeable consumers of information available to them in this medium and that this approach become part of general health management (Anker, Reinhart, & Feeley, 2011; Lemire, Sicotte, & Paré, 2008). Recommendations for nurses, stated in 2006 and true today, are listed in Table 15.1.

Many Internet users have expressed concern about the credibility of Internet-based health information but have an interest in accessing a variety of Internet-based health information resources, including scientific and medical information and patient testimonials about the illness experience (Kivits, 2009). Unfortunately, even though Internet users may indicate they use criteria such as source credibility, language, and transparency to determine the value of online health information, they have tended to disregard these criteria when actually conducting a search. In addition, Internet users often relied only on common sense or personal experience to judge the usefulness of the information (Eysenbach, 2007), and used correspondence with the content of other websites to judge its accuracy (Kivits, 2009). Users have tended to develop a practical knowledge based on their experience to determine what information and sources of knowledge to select (Kivits, 2009). Kitchens, Harle, and Li (2014) found that search techniques and use of search engines were poor, and that users relied heavily on the first few websites or resources identified by the search.

Comfort and familiarity with the Internet does not guarantee the ability to obtain credible online health information. An Internet behaviour and preference study of 60 English-speaking Caribbean immigrant women in New York City revealed that although Internet use was high in this group, many participants did not know the differences among websites with

| Table 15.1 | Recommended Nursing Actions with Respect to Health Information on the Internet |
| --- | --- |

Develop skills in online health information retrieval and evaluation to identify and recommend the best online sites for health information.

Assess clients' Internet access, computer competencies, health literacy, online activity, desired role in decision making, and need for assistive devices to access the Internet.

Identify local community resources for Internet access.

Invite clients to discuss the health information they have found online.

Consider client–provider online communication options (email, bulletin boards, instant messaging), and develop guidelines for email triage in practice settings similar to telephone triage protocols.

When using Internet-based communications with clients, learn about the security of the site and ramifications for client privacy.

Consider gender and culture preferences when developing Web-based health promotion interventions.

Teach clients how to evaluate quality and appropriateness of health information on the Web.

Source: Adapted from Dickerson, S. S. (2006). Women's use of the Internet: What nurses need to know. *Journal of Obstetric, Gynecologic, & Neonatal Nursing, 35*(1), 151–156. doi:10.1111/J.1552-6909.2006.00004.x. Used by permission of Blackwell Publishing, Ltd. (UK).

domain names of .edu, .gov, .com, or .net (Changrani & Gany, 2005). When searching for health information on the Internet, participants used links from the first screen of results displayed by the search engine and rarely refined their search terms or repeated the search. Most searches were concluded within five minutes. If participants repeated a search, they stated it was because they did not trust the source or understand the information. Kivits (2009) reported similar findings.

## Tools Available for Rating Health Information on the Internet

There are many tools available to consumers and healthcare providers that rate the quality of health information on the Internet. Various dimensions of Internet resources can be evaluated, including content, journalistic value, targeted audience, website design, readability and usability, and ethical issues of privacy. These dimensions have changed over time as **Web 2.0** technologies, including collaborative, adaptive, and interactive sites have emerged (Burns et al., 2013). Unfortunately, consumers may have difficulties determining the value of the ratings provided on the health information websites.

Providing clients with clear criteria of credible online information is the best means of enabling them to assess its quality. Using the **HON code** (Health on the Net Foundation, 2009) to examine online information with clients is an

| Table 15.2 | HON Code of Conduct for Medical and Health Websites |
|---|---|
| 1. Authority | Any medical or health advice provided and hosted on this site will only be given by medically trained and qualified health professionals unless a clear statement is made that a piece of advice offered is from a non-medically qualified individual or organization. |
| 2. Complementarity | The information provided on this site is designed to support, not replace, the relationship that exists between a patient/site visitor and his/her existing physician. |
| 3. Privacy | Confidentiality of data relating to individual patients and visitors to a medical/health website, including their identity, is respected by this website. The website owners undertake to honour or exceed the legal requirements of medical/health information privacy that apply in the country and state where the website and mirror sites are located. |
| 4. Attribution | Where appropriate, information contained on this site will be supported by clear references to source data and, where possible, have specific HTML links to that data. The date when a clinical page was last modified will be clearly displayed (e.g. at the bottom of the page). |
| 5. Justifiability | Any claims relating to the benefits/performance of a specific treatment, commercial product, or service will be supported by appropriate balanced evidence in the manner outlined above in Principle 4. |
| 6. Transparency | The designers of this website will seek to provide information in the clearest possible manner and provide contact addresses for visitors that seek further information or support. The webmaster will display his/her email address clearly throughout the website. |
| 7. Financial disclosure | Support for this website will be clearly identified, including the identities of commercial and non-commercial organizations that have contributed funding, services, or material for the site. |
| 8. Honesty in advertising and editorial policy | If advertising is a source of funding, it will be clearly stated. A brief description of the advertising policy adopted by the website owners will be displayed on the site. Advertising and other promotional material will be presented to viewers in a manner and context that facilitates differentiation between it and the original material created by the institution operating the site. |

Source: The HON Code of Conduct for Medical and Health Websites (HON Code). Copyright © 2015 by Health on the Net Foundation. Used by permission of Health on the Net Foundation. Retrieved from http://www.hon.ch/HONcode/Pro/Conduct.html. Reproduced with permission.

effective way of teaching the criteria while simultaneously critiquing the online information. In Table 15.2, eight principles are listed and described.

Although healthcare professionals may be adept at applying HON criteria, most laypersons will not be. Table 15.3 illustrates questions that clients may use in assessing the health information they have accessed on the Internet. Assisting clients to interpret and apply these criteria will empower them to use Internet health information with greater confidence. HON (Health on the Net Foundation, 2009) also supports a service where health information consumers may submit a URL to the "WRAPIN" service (www.wrapin.org) to determine if the site is accredited or trustworthy (WRAPIN, 2014). Sites are searched in various languages. In addition, clients can be encouraged to download the HON code toolbar into their browser, which helps them search for HON-approved sites (www.hon.ch/HONcode/Plugin/Plugins.html).

## Assessment of Health Information Websites

The usability of health information websites may relate to more than the accuracy of the information provided. The Health Information Technology Institute provided another set of criteria that evaluates health information websites on their usability for consumers (Health Summit Working Group, 2010). These criteria include credibility, content, disclosures,

| Table 15.3 | Questions for Clients to Use in Assessing Internet Health Information |
|---|---|

1. Is the health information provided by a qualified medical practitioner or an organization that is committed to the public's health?

2. Does the website encourage you to discuss the health information with your physician or another healthcare professional?

3. Is your identity protected on this website?

4. Does the website indicate sources or references for the information provided? Are these sources credible?

5. Are claims of effectiveness of treatments supported by credible evidence?

6. Is the authorship of this website clear to you? Can you contact the webmaster for more information?

7. Is the sponsorship of the website clearly apparent to you?

8. Are the commercial advertisements clearly separated from the health information presented on the website? Is the advertising policy stated on the website?

9. Is there a link to the homepage of the sponsoring organization from the health information webpages?

10. Does the homepage explain the mission, purpose, and objectives; sources of funding; and governance of the organization?

| Table 15.4 | HITI Criteria for Assessing Health Information Websites |
|---|---|
| 1. Credibility | Source: Sponsoring agency logo and information are displayed, along with relevant personal or financial associations. |
| | Disclosure of sponsorship is clear. |
| | Currency: Includes date of posting and the date of the document on which information is based. |
| | Relevance: Content corresponds to intended purpose of website. |
| | Site evaluation: Editorial/content review process. |
| 2. Content | Accuracy and completeness of content, with source identified. |
| | Disclaimer: Statement that content is general health information and not medical advice. |
| 3. Disclosures | Clear statement of the purpose of the site. |
| | Collection of user information: Indicates any user information collected from site and its intended purpose. |
| 4. Links | Selection: Appropriate links are selected. |
| | Architecture: Ease of navigation to sites and back to original page. |
| | Content of links: Relevant to original website, accurate, external sites clearly identified. |
| 5. Design | Accessibility: For lowest-level browser technology, use by hearing or visually impaired. |
| | Logical organization: Includes design and layout, readability, language, balance of text and graphics. |
| | Navigability: Simple, internally consistent, and easy to use. |
| | Internal search capability: Highly desirable. |
| 6. Interactivity | Feedback mechanisms: Feedback mechanisms and exchange of information among users. |
| 7. Caveats | Clarification of the site's function to market products or services. |

Source: Adapted from the Health on the Net Foundation. (2009). *HON Code of Conduct (HONcode) for medical and health websites.* Health on the Net Foundation. Retrieved from http://www.hon.ch/HONcode/Guidelines/guidelines.html

links, design, interactivity, and caveats (Table 15.4) and relate to the presentation of information and ease of use.

**Readability** of text is an important design aspect of every webpage. Readability is a measure of how easily and comfortably text can be read. People with lower reading skills also use the Internet. For websites intended for laypersons, reading levels should be focused approximately at a Grade 9 level. Reading experts suggest that the majority of the population prefers written materials three grades below the last grade attended at school (Gottlieb & Rogers, 2004). Although this level seems low, it may still be higher than the reading comprehension level of the general population, which is estimated to be on average Grade 5–6 level (Gottlieb & Rogers, 2004). Within the Canadian population, 89% of the population aged 25 to 64 has completed high school and 65% has completed post-secondary education (Statistics Canada, 2014). Nonetheless, 42% of the working-age population scored below the functional level in prose literacy scales and 43% below functional level in document literacy (OECD/Statistics Canada, 2011). The Canadian Literacy and Learning Network (2014) indicates that 42% of Canadian adults between the ages of 16 and 65 have low literacy skills, with 55% of this population possessing inadequate health literacy skills. Eighty-eight percent (88%) of the population over the age of 65 fall into this category. Unfortunately, most websites have much higher reading levels than can be comprehended by a large portion of the general population. Ache and Wallace (2009) found that

Internet-based patient education materials were generally written at the Grade 7 to 12 levels, with a mean of Grade 11, and Lam, Roter, and Cohen (2013) found that 86% of websites for adolescents failed readability standards of less than Grade 8 level.

Health professionals who are recommending or creating websites for clients can assess the readability of written or Internet text using a relatively simple tool, the **SMOG (Simple Measure of Gobbledygook)** Readability Test (McLaughlin, 1969) (see Table 15.5). SMOG reading levels correlate well with grade levels identified by other tests of readability (Gottlieb & Rogers, 2004). Because these tests are based on two variables of reading comprehension, word length and sentence length, the reading level of text materials can be reduced by using simple words and shorter sentences (Table 15.6). The Canadian Public Health Association (CPHA) (1999), in its National Literacy and Health Program, published the Directory of Plain Language Health Information to assist health educators in publishing clear and easily understood written materials. Key points are summarized in Table 15.7. CPHA also offers a plain language service for the assessment and clarification of health resources (CPHA, 2010).

Healthcare professionals may refer clients to well-developed websites specific to their needs. Factors to be considered when judging the utility of online health information include ease of navigation and ease of accessing webpages within the site (Goldberg et al., 2011). Internal links

| Table 15.5 | SMOG Readability Assessment Tool: Document Assessment for Approximate Grade Level of Reading Skills |
|---|---|
| Step 1 Sample selection | Select 30 sentences from the text material: 10 consecutive sentences from each of the start, middle, and end of the material. A sentence is a complete idea with a period, question mark, or exclamation mark, a bulleted point, or both parts of a sentence with a colon included. |
| Step 2 Word count | Count the number of words with more than three syllables (polysyllabic) in the 30-sentence sample. Include all repetitions of a word, proper nouns, the full text of abbreviations, and hyphenated words as one word. |
| Step 3 Short text conversion | For documents of fewer than 30 sentences, multiply the number of polysyllabic words by a factor to simulate a sample of 30 sentences. For example, if the document contained 15 sentences, the factor would be 30 divided by 15 to equal a factor of 2. For documents of 24 sentences, the factor would be 30 divided by 24 to equal 1.25. |
| Step 4 Calculate | Determine the nearest square root of the number of words in the sample. A square root is a number multiplied by itself to equal a perfect square. For example, 8 multiplied by 8 (square root) equals 64 (perfect square). The number that is a square root is usually between 3 and 15. |
| Add the constant "3" to the square root obtained in step 4. | Example: A sample is assessed as having 86 polysyllabic words in 30 sentences. The nearest square root is 9 (9 times 9 equals 81). The constant of 3 is added to give an approximate reading level of 12, or more appropriately described as a reading level requiring the reading skills approximately at the Grade 12 reading level. |

The result is the approximate grade level of reading skills required to read the document. The resultant grade level is correct within 1.5 grades in 68% of cases.

Source: SMOG (Simple Measure of Gobbledygook) Readability Test. Adapted from McLaughlin, G. H. (1969). SMOG-grading: A new readability formula. *Journal of Reading, 12*, 639–646.

for ease of access are beneficial to users. External links should be assessed for their relatedness and ease of return to the original website. Use of graphics to illustrate concepts enhances usability; however, advertising on the website and irritating pop-ups may interfere. Users also find a pleasing appearance and the opportunity for interactivity, such as calculations of body mass index (BMI), daily calorie counters, or self-report progress charts, to be beneficial (Lustria, Cortese, Noar, & Glueckauf, 2009). Ease of usage enhances a user's ability to read and use information contained on a website. Clients can also be referred to government-sponsored health information websites.

| Table 15.6 | Examples of Different Reading Levels |
|---|---|
| Grade 12 reading level* | Include exercise such as walking, biking, swimming, jogging, and active sports, according to your individual preferences. Consider other means of transportation or use stairs instead of elevators. Incorporate physical activities into your interactions with your children.<br><br>The recommended amount of activity per week is 20 minutes of activity daily, on at least five separate occasions per week. Monitor your pulse rate, keeping it within the recommended target level during your activity. To stay physically fit, keep active and have fun. |
| Grade 9 reading level* | Include exercise such as walking, biking, swimming, jogging, and active sports, as you prefer. Consider walking to the store or using the stairs instead of elevators. Be active with your children.<br><br>We recommend 20 minutes of activity daily, at least five times per week. Monitor your pulse rate, keeping it within the target level during your activity. To stay physically fit, keep active and have fun. |
| Grade 6 reading level* | Include walking, biking, swimming, jogging, and active sports in your daily life. Choose other ways of being active. Take the stairs. Walk to the store. Play with your kids.<br><br>We suggest at least 20 minutes of exercise per day, 5 times per week. Include more time as you wish. Learn how to take your own pulse rate. Keep your pulse rate within the target level. Stay fit. Keep active. Have fun. |

Source: SMOG (Simple Measure of Gobbledygook) Readability Test. Adapted from McLaughlin, G. H. (1969). SMOG-grading: A new readability formula. *Journal of Reading, 12*, 639–646.

*Approximate reading levels based on SMOG assessment

| Table 15.7 | Plain Language Strategies |
| --- | --- |

- Use active voice by stating the subject of the action first, for example., "You should eat 5 to 10 fruits and vegetables per day," instead of, "5 to 10 fruits and vegetables should be eaten every day."

- Write directly to the reader, using "you" or implying "you" as the subject of the sentence; for example, "Take this medication once per day," instead of "This medication should be taken once per day."

- Maintain a positive tone, stating actions as positive behaviours rather than avoidance behaviours; for example, "Contact your doctor as soon as you feel sick," instead of "Avoid waiting too long to contact your doctor."

- Use common simple terms rather than technical jargon; e.g., "Medicine will relieve your child's pain," instead of "An analgesic will relieve your child's pain."

- Use short words and short sentences.

- Replace more difficult words with simpler words:
  — *drug* or *medicine* in place of *medication*
  — *heart* in place of *cardiac*
  — *doctor* in place of *physician*
  — *take part in* rather than *participate in*
  — *problems* in place of *difficulties*

- When in doubt, ask your learners what words are most meaningful.

- Do not change verbs into nouns. The action word is a stronger depiction; for example, "Decide when to involve your children in meal planning," instead of "Make decisions about your children's involvement in meal planning."

- List important points separate from the text.
  — Use bullets to highlight important points.
  — Keep bullets short.
  — Use boxes to highlight important information.

- Write instructions in the order that you want them to be carried out.

- List items such as nouns or actions in parallel form.

- Keep your writing in a conversational form.

- Test whatever you write with learners before you formalize it.

Source: Adapted from the Plain Language Service of the Canadian Public Health Association. (1999). http://www.cpha.ca/uploads/portals/h-l/directory_e.pdf

## Targeting Specific Users of Online Health Information

Online health information should be designed for specific users. A combination of health messaging with individual-level participant information permits better targeting. **Targeting** is the development of online resources that allow for personal and direct content presentation based on elements such as preferences, needs, and current health behaviours or behavioural intentions, and that lead to positive outcomes (Lustria et al., 2009). The concept comes from advertising principles that are related to market segmentation.

Although immigrant women use the Internet at the same rate as the general population, only 6% used the Internet for health information, compared to 63% of the general population of Internet users (Changrani & Gany, 2005). Many of these immigrant women indicated a preference for simple navigation sites, simple language, and simple URLs. They preferred soft, soothing colours, images congruent with their culture, "not too much information," and interactive tools such as question-and-answer forums and video and slide show illustrations. They also valued information tailored to their health beliefs and specific needs.

Because scrolling through a website presents challenges for some seniors, website designs that present one paragraph per webpage are a better alternative (Roush, 2006). The U.S. National Institute on Aging maintains a website (www.nihseniorhealth.gov) with common health concerns, where text can be enlarged and a "talking function" can be activated as needed. The site provides links to other credible websites to assist seniors in making decisions about the value of the information they have accessed. Websites with these characteristics will be more useful to seniors.

## Tailoring E-Health Messages

The integration of features that enhance interactivity has long been known to enhance learning (Goldberg et al., 2011; Hardiker & Grant, 2011). **Interactivity** refers to a process where a user is an active participant in using technology and

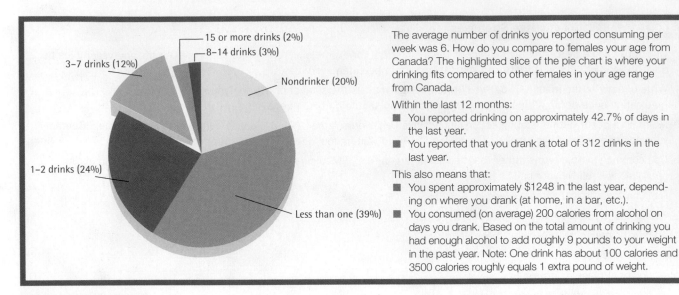

The average number of drinks you reported consuming per week was 6. How do you compare to females your age from Canada? The highlighted slice of the pie chart is where your drinking fits compared to other females in your age range from Canada.

Within the last 12 months:
■ You reported drinking on approximately 42.7% of days in the last year.
■ You reported that you drank a total of 312 drinks in the last year.

This also means that:
■ You spent approximately $1248 in the last year, depending on where you drank (at home, in a bar, etc.).
■ You consumed (on average) 200 calories from alcohol on days you drank. Based on the total amount of drinking you had enough alcohol to add roughly 9 pounds to your weight in the past year. Note: One drink has about 100 calories and 3500 calories roughly equals 1 extra pound of weight.

**FIGURE 15.2** Portion of a Tailored Final Report for a Fictitious Website User Created from Check Your Drinking (CYD)

*Average drinks per week for females aged 35–44 from Canada*

*Source:* From V-AlcoholHelpCentre. Copyright © by Evolution Health Systems Inc. Used by permission of Evolution Health Systems Inc. Retrieved from http://www.alcoholhelpcentre.net/cyd. Reprinted with permission.

information exchange occurs (e.g., chat rooms, calorie calculators, links). For example, computer programs that integrate social cognitive theory to promote behaviour change for management of weight and physical activity have shown positive results (Winett, Tate, Anderson, Wojcik, & Winett, 2005). Features in programs that generate personalized responses can increase positive attitudes and learning about health issues, and have been shown to result in positive health outcomes (Suggs & McIntyre, 2009), as long as anonymity of the user is assured (Hardiker & Grant, 2011). For example, the generation of clear and understandable tailored messages that include the user's name and provide specific information addressing individual health needs is important when designing computer-based health promotion interventions. Compared to the concept of targeting, which focuses on interventions for groups, **tailoring** has been referred to as a "process of creating individualized intervention materials or strategies" (Kreuter & Skinner, 2000, p. 1). Tailored messages are typically "pushed" to the user, as opposed to sites where users "pull" or search for information from fact sheets, booklets, videos, and images. Tailored messages are typically presented with self-comparisons and recommendations based on authoritative research (see Figure 15.2). Suggs and McIntyre (2009) found that only 13 of 497 English-language online health resources were tailored messages, in spite of the identified efficiencies of such websites. However, a study of tailored versus targeted computer-based interventions to promote hearing-protection use among construction workers showed that a targeted intervention was preferred and was more cost effective (Kerr, Savik, Monsen, & Lusk, 2007). Overall, tailoring on individual characteristics (age, gender, readiness) has been shown to outperform static health information (Bennett & Glasgow, 2009).

## TECHNOLOGY TO SUPPORT HEALTH PROMOTION, DISEASE PREVENTION, AND CHRONIC DISEASE MANAGEMENT

The use of ICTs to support e-health promotion interventions has grown. This growth can be attributed to increased Internet use by the public, the low cost of delivery, and public willingness to actively manage their health. It has been argued that e-health promotion interventions can be effective (Hardiker & Grant, 2011). Online interventions for weight management (Bennett & Glasgow, 2009), mental health interventions (Ybarra & Eaton, 2005), cancer care (Becker, Macker, & Kang, 2013), gambling addiction recovery (Mudry & Strong, 2012), smoking-cessation programs (Etter, 2005), asthma care (Letourneau et al., 2012), and hypertension management (Liu et al., 2013), among others, have shown promise. Online counselling interventions can be helpful for people who live in remote areas, value anonymity, belong to a special interest group (Donelle & Hoffman-Goetz, 2008), or have access problems (transportation, scheduling). A systematic review of randomized controlled trials of consumer health informatics interventions (Gibbons et al., 2009) showed that many applications that addressed diet, exercise, physical activity, alcohol abuse, smoking cessation, breast cancer, diabetes, mental health, asthma and chronic obstructive pulmonary disease, and menopause and hormone replacement therapy studies had significant positive impact on at least one intermediate health outcome. No studies identified harm attributed to health informatics interventions. A review of the Internet as a delivery platform for public health interventions showed potential for broad population dissemination of primary and secondary prevention interventions, many of which showed positive results (Bennett & Glasgow, 2009). The authors stressed the importance of intervention designs and components. For example, the most effective weight-loss interventions were highly structured, focused on tailored materials, included a counsellor, and promoted frequent Web logins. Griffiths, Lindenmeyer, Powell, Lowe, and Thorogood (2006) have identified rationales for and drawbacks to delivering health interventions using the Internet.

Web 2.0 technologies and socially oriented sites such as YouTube, Twitter, Facebook, and MySpace have gained popularity, especially among youth. The general use of social media in Canada is on the rise with 67% of Canadians who used the Internet in 2012 reportedly visiting social networking sites such as Facebook or Twitter, an increase from 58% in 2010 (Statistics Canada, 2013a). Research on the use of these technologies to promote health and provide support is also growing (Antheunis, Tates, & Nieboer, 2013; Griffiths et al., 2012; Househ, Borycki, & Kushniruk, 2014). Social media are generally seen as those Internet-based applications that allow the creation and exchange of user-generated content (Antheunis et al., 2013). These tools can afford patients an opportunity to gain access to health information, explore care options, and share health experiences (Househ et al., 2014). "Social media provide online platforms for interactions to occur around various health topics related to patient education, health promotion, public relations, and crisis communication" (Househ et al., 2014, p. 51). Web 2.0 emphasizes the social and participatory nature of Web services, empowering users as well as focusing on content generation and the phenomenon of inclusion. Although these features are well aligned to enhance health promotion and prevention, they have been underutilized for this purpose (Vance, Howe, & Dellavalle, 2009). A Facebook conversation as a health promotion intervention concerning sexual health demonstrated that 93% of the content was generated by users, and 576 users interacted over a five-month period in 2010. However, once advertising for the site discontinued, so did user participation (Syred, Naidoo, Woodhall, & Araitser, 2014). A study reviewing human papillomavirus (HPV) information found on YouTube showed that 146 videoclips on HPV were available on February 8, 2008 (Ache & Wallace, 2008); most clips were sourced from television clips. About 75% portrayed the vaccination in a positive light and one-third generated comments from viewers. In April 2014, a search of the term "human papillomavirus" on YouTube resulted in about 160 000 videoclips, illustrating the growth and potential power of this medium for health information and misinformation. The Canadian Internet Registration Authority (CIRA) reported that in 2011 Canadians watched more online videos than anyone else in the world (CIRA, 2013). Every second video was viewed using YouTube, resulting in a massive reported overall viewing increase in Canada of 170% (CIRA, 2013).

Computer programs that include interactive components have been demonstrated as more effective (Burns et al., 2013; Goldberg et al., 2011; Lustria et al., 2009). Examples of interactive components are calculators that estimate the cost

of smoking, online social support groups where participants communicate with ex-smokers, features that permit posting of personal stories, and email follow-ups before and after quit dates for added support. Such programs can supplement face-to-face programs. It is important for online intervention programs to aim to minimize attrition. Many suffer high attrition over time and the intensity of interventions is also typically low (Bennett & Glasgow, 2009). Newer technologies are also being studied. A Cochrane review of cellphone-based interventions, using text messaging in particular, showed short-term positive effects on smoking cessation, although no long-term effects were found (Whittaker, Borland, & Bullen, 2009).

Tailored messages are particularly appropriate for online screening. Online screening interventions have been implemented with varying degrees of success, including screening for mental health (Farvolden, McBride, Bagby, & Ravitz, 2003),

### CANADIAN RESEARCH BOX 15.2

#### Can social media encourage youth to be tested for sexually transmitted infections (STIs)?

Mann, T. A., Uddin, Z., Hendriks, A. M., Bouchard, C. J., & Etches, V. G. (2013). Get tested, why not? A novel approach to Internet-based chlamydia and gonorrhea testing in Canada. *Canadian Journal of Public Health, 104*(3), e205–e209.

This public-health intervention was focused on a population that traditionally avoids testing for sexually transmitted infections. The target audience was youth between the ages of 15 and 29, the age group most affected by chlamydia and gonorrhea infections (STIs) in Ottawa. Members of the target group were engaged in the development and launch of the website and the communication initiative that used social media and traditional advertising to develop awareness of the campaign. The intervention was a bilingual, youth-friendly website and texting service with the intent of educating youth about the need for testing for STIs. Youth at risk were encouraged to submit urine samples for testing to one of 26 laboratories in Ottawa. The website had more than 13 000 hits, with 104 specimens submitted, most by members of the target group who could download the lab requisition from the website. Ninety-one percent (91%) of the samples were negative. The evaluation demonstrated that the website had a positive effect on knowledge levels and intended behaviours of the target group, and the testing options for youth were acceptable.

#### Discussion Questions

1. What other strategies could be used to direct the target population to the information website?

2. How could youth on the street access such a health information resource?

3. How could you as a community health nurse assure participants of confidentiality in their lab testing and treatment, if necessary?

chlamydia (Gaydos et al., 2006), HIV/AIDS with adolescents (Ybarra, Biringi, Prescott, & Bull, 2012), fruit and vegetable consumption, fitness levels (Kypri & McAnally, 2005), problem gambling (Mudry & Strong, 2012), and alcohol intake (Cunningham, Humphreys, Kypri, & van Mierlo, 2006). U.S. researchers (Saitz et al., 2004) found that screening and management of alcohol problems was a successful Internet health-promotion intervention. Many users were women reporting hazardous amounts of alcohol intake who might not have otherwise looked for help. See Canadian Research Box 15.2.

## Online Social Support Groups

Nine percent of people in the United States who used the Internet for health information used an online social support group (Rice, 2006). In February 2010, Yahoo! listed over 12 000 online groups under the fitness and nutrition topic and Google groups listed over 12 500 English-speaking health groups (Figure 15.3). In particular, online support groups appear useful in supporting those targeted populations who may experience stigma as a result of their conditions (Royer, Fernandez-Lambert, & Moreno, 2013). Internet users have indicated a preference for social interaction on websites (Goldberg et al., 2011; Lustria et al., 2009). A systematic review (Eysenbach, Powell, Englesakis, Rizo, & Stern, 2004) of online support groups found 35 relevant studies. In addition to peer-to-peer support, most studies provided multiple interventions, such as online communication with a professional and psychoeducation programs. Because of this, conclusions about the impact of peer-to-peer social support online as a single intervention cannot be drawn. Studies tended to measure outcomes related to social support and depression, and often reported no effects. Despite this, such groups appear to be growing, and no reported cases of harm were found. Barak, Bonniel-Nissim, and Suler (2008, p. 1867) contend that online support groups foster "well-being, a sense of control, self-confidence, feelings of more independence, social interactions, and improved feelings"—all non-specific but highly important psychological factors.

The growth of online groups for new parents has been rapid. The Internet can provide social support to parents who feel psychologically or geographically isolated, and can meet the needs of parents with unique interests (e.g., adoption, bereavement, multiple births). A review of Internet use by parents showed that many parents turn to the Internet for information and support as a result of weaker supports from family and friends (Plantin & Daneback, 2009; Vennick, Adams, Faber, & Putters, 2014). Problems identified by parents in using online information and supports included usability problems of a technical nature, a lack of confidence in Internet use, large volumes of off-topic chatter, and occasional disagreements in discussion groups. Although some reports of rude or disrespectful communication exist, the opposite has also been reported, possibly related to the application of Internet etiquette or "netiquette" rules.

## Telehealth

Telehealth technologies are used today to provide accessibility to healthcare services that might not be available to clients otherwise, including access to healthcare professionals and specialist services that may be concentrated in urban or high-population areas. In addition, these services may be available to rural, remote, or disadvantaged populations only through telehealth services (see Chapter 24 for examples of telehealth with rural clients). Recently, developments in technology allow healthcare professionals to assess clients, review assessment data, diagnose, treat, and counsel clients at a distance (Godwin et al., 2013). Recent use has involved support of family caregivers in their homes, empowering clients to make decisions about their caregivers and the setting of their care (Stern, Valaitis, Weir, & Jadad, 2012).

## POPULATION HEALTH AND TECHNOLOGY

Many Internet technologies can support population health interventions. Computer and Internet technologies have long been used to support community empowerment and capacity building (Korp, 2006; Valaitis, 2005; Valaitis & O'Mara, 2005). An evaluation of the use of an interactive website to involve local citizens in driving policy related to a smoking bylaw in Calgary was very successful (Grierson, van Dijk, Dozios, & Mascher. 2006). The website sparked public debate about the issue, provided citizens with information about smoking, suggested messages to communicate to city councillors, and updated citizens on how council voted on the issue. Public response was very positive. The website was an effective community capacity-building tool and mobilization strategy that increased citizen participation in building local policy for a healthier community. A similar finding was demonstrated in an Israeli study that engaged stakeholders in consideration of the health impact of a national hazardous industry on nearby land use (Negev, Davidovitch, Garb, & Tal, 2013).

Numerous population-based **surveillance** systems exist within the public health system, which provide valuable data for program planning and evaluation. The Canadian Integrated

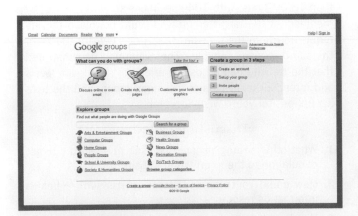

**FIGURE   15.3**  Screen Capture of Google Groups Website

*Source:* Screenshots from Google. Courtesy of Google Corporation.

Public Health Information System (CPHIS), which is being adopted across Canada, combines iPHIS—a client health-reporting surveillance system that supports tracking, follow-up, reporting, and management of cases related to immunization, communicable disease, and population health surveillance—with a laboratory data management system. Panorama, developed by Canada Health Infoway, is being rolled out with tools to support outbreak identification, vaccine inventory management, case management, and notifications (Mowat & Butler-Jones, 2007). CANSIM (Canadian Socioeconomic Information Management System) tables report social trends impacting the lives of Canadians that can be accessed through E-STAT, which also provides access to Canadian census data. It is available at no cost to students and educators through educational institutions (www.statcan.gc.ca/english/Estat/intro.htm). These data are essential for program planners.

## ELECTRONIC DOCUMENTATION FOR COMMUNITY HEALTH NURSING

The use of technology to support electronic documentation systems has been growing across Canada, including in community health organizations (Stonham, Heyes, Owen, & Povey, 2012). Three types of electronic documentation systems that have been developed are the "electronic medical record (EMR)," the "electronic patient record (EPR)," and the "electronic health record (EHR)." Nagle (2007) differentiated these terms with respect to access to information, scope of the information included in the documentation, and custodianship of the record. Typically, EMRs are found in primary health care settings and clinics, whereas EPRs are maintained by healthcare organizations. Access to both of these records is limited to authorized caregivers, and the content typically reflects information that used to be recorded in paper-based systems. The EHR is a more comprehensive record that includes contents from the EPR and EMR. It typically includes most information gathered from encounters with the healthcare system, such as primary care, pharmacies, laboratories, and diagnostic imaging units. The client controls access to his or her record, which is "owned" by the client but is hosted by a jurisdiction (Nagle, 2007, p. 2). The EHR, which provides a longitudinal record of an individual's health history and care, is currently being tested in numerous provinces by Canada Health Infoway.

Nurses in the community are also using point-of-care mobile wireless devices that enable access to health records, documentation, ordering supplies, making appointments, checking inventories, accessing evidence for practice, and reviewing medications. Stonham, Heyes, Owen, and Povey (2012) identified the benefit of being able to document best practice in care and service with clients and Rutten et al. (2014) identified client expectations of the maintenance of an electronic medical record that they could access. For community-based nurses providing care in the home, access to information at the bedside is considered a major advantage (Caligtan, Carroll, Hurley, Gersh-Zaremski, & Dykes, 2012; Luo, Tang, &

Thomas, 2012). A challenge for nurses is the use of mobile devices such as cellphones and tablets at the client's bedside, specifically in terms of contamination of devices (Albrecht et al., 2013; Unstun & Cihangiroglu, 2012), especially for those nurses who access clients in both acute-care and community-based settings. Unstan and Cihangiroglu (2012) demonstrated that virtually all of the cellphones of healthcare workers were contaminated with nosocomial pathogens, 10% with Methicillin-resistant *Staphylococcus aureus* (MRSA), and 11% with E. coli, particularly if the healthcare workers were employed in the intensive care units. Albrecht et al. (2013) demonstrated that tablets used in clinical and nonclinical settings could be disinfected effectively through the use of isopropanol wipes.

## TECHNOLOGIES THAT SUPPORT KNOWLEDGE EXCHANGE AND PROFESSIONAL DEVELOPMENT

ICTs can greatly benefit CHNs through the provision of access to supports for professional development and evidence-based decision making. These technologies include online **communities of practice**, portals, and repositories of evidence-based community health literature. A community of practice refers to groups of people who share common interests, values, and problems about a topic and interact together to deepen their knowledge (Wenger, McDermott, & Snyder, 2002). Canadian nursing researchers investigated networking needs of community health nursing researchers and decision makers (Edwards & Kothari, 2004; Kothari et al., 2005). They identified a need for a formal community health network to assist decision makers, researchers, and practitioners to debate the management of complex community health problems, supported by relevant research. Although face-to-face networks were preferred, there was willingness to try online networks. Findings resulted in an online networking project, CHNET-Works!. Nurses are encouraged to join the asynchronous communication boards and Web-enhanced teleconferences on current community health topics (www.chnet-works.ca).

CHNs can harness the power of social media by creating their own **personal learning network (PLN)**. Gathering online information and resources and organizing these through a PLN can assist with professional development. CHNs unfamiliar with social media should consider adopting one tool, such as Twitter, and begin to explore its use. New users can find how-to resources on the Internet for establishing social media accounts. Once the account is in place, the use of hashtags can assist in creating a dynamic and informative PLN. Hashtags (#) are a means of organizing information in social media platforms. CHNs can explore any of these well-established healthcare hashtags to get a sense of the wealth of information available: #cdnhealth (Canada Healthcare), #CHC (Community Health Centres), #hcsmca (Healthcare Social Media Canada), and #rnchat (Registered Nurses chat).

**NurseONE/INF-Fusion**, developed by the Canadian Nurses Association, is a personalized interactive Web 2.0

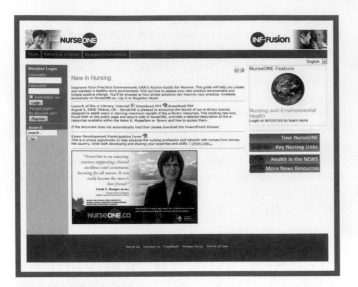

**FIGURE** **15.4** Screen Capture of NurseONE/
INF-Fusion

*Source:* Screenshot from Canadian Nurses Association. Copyright © Canadian Nurses Association. Reprinted with permission. Further reproduction prohibited.

resource designed to assist nurses in Canada to manage their professional development, connect with colleagues, and gain access to current, credible, reliable information resources and tools to support evidence-based nursing practice (www. nurseone.ca; see Figure 15.4). The Public Health Agency of Canada (PHAC) (2006) has developed a portal for knowledge exchange: the Canadian Best Practices Portal for Health Promotion and Chronic Disease Prevention (http://cbpp-pcpe. phac-aspc.gc.ca). It aims to enhance knowledge exchange in best practices and provides a central access point for best practices approaches. PHAC also provides practitioners with online learning modules to enhance skills in public health practice (www.phac-aspc.gc.ca/sehs-acss/index-eng.phpl). Practitioners in public health can register to take the skills enhancement online modules. A reliable source of evidence-based materials relevant to CHNs includes the fully searchable online service Health-Evidence.ca (http://health-evidence.ca). The Effective Public Health Practice Program also provides links to numerous systematic literature reviews and summaries (www.ephpp. ca). The National Collaborating Centre of Methods and Tools (NCCMT) (www.nccmt.ca) provides information and resources about knowledge translation methods and tools relevant for community health students and practitioners. In particular, the NCCMT has collaborated with the Health Communication Unit to develop and disseminate the Online Health Program Planner (www.publichealthontario.ca/en/ServicesAndTools/ ohpp/Pages/default.aspx), which is an interactive, flexible, and intuitive tool to assist with the development of evidence-informed program plans (Ciliska et al., 2009).

## CONCLUSION

ICTs have the potential to provide information, communication, and other supports to empower individuals, groups, and communities. The rapid growth of Internet use by the public to access health information cannot be ignored. CHNs need to incorporate this knowledge into their plan of care and take a leadership role in enabling the public to use this health information resource safely and effectively. CHNs can also help ensure accessibility to quality health information for the populations that they serve. Although research into the use of ICTs to support health promotion, disease prevention, and chronic disease management is relatively new, it shows great promise. ICTs can also foster professional development for CHNs by providing access to communities of practice, online learning modules, and evidence-based materials to support practice.

## KEY TERMS

accessible   p. 290
communities of practice   p. 299
digital divide   p. 289
e-health   p. 286
e-nursing   p. 286
health literacy   p. 288
HON code   p. 291
information and communication technologies (ICTs), p. 286
interactivity   p. 295
NurseONE/INF-Fusion   p. 299
nursing informatics   p. 287
personal learning network (PLN)   p. 299
public health informatics   p. 287
readability   p. 293
SMOG (Simple Measure of Gobbledygook)
  Readability   p. 293
surveillance   p. 298
tailoring   p. 296
targeting   p. 295
telehealth   p. 286
Web 2.0   p. 291
Web Accessibility Initiative (WAI)   p. 290
Web Content Accessibility Guidelines (WCAG)   p. 290

## STUDY QUESTIONS

1. Identify different ways that the "digital divide" has been conceptualized since the term first appeared.

2. Describe three tools that can be used to enhance Internet accessibility for disabled populations.

3. What is the HON code and what is its purpose?

4. Describe three online health promotion interventions that show promise.

5. Where can CHNs get access to evidence-based information on the Web to guide their decision making in practice?

6. What is the nursing role with respect to health information on the Internet?

After working through these questions, go to the MyNursingLab at www.pearsoned.ca/mynursinglab to check your answers.

# INDIVIDUAL CRITICAL-THINKING EXERCISES

1. What criteria would you use to evaluate a health promotion intervention, such as a smoking-cessation website?

2. What would you need to consider when working as a community health nurse with a client who is visually impaired and wants to use the Internet?

3. Discuss the merits and drawbacks of the HON code. Review the editorial and the response to it found in the *Journal of Medical Internet Research* by Eysenbach (2001).

4. What would you need to take into account when designing a Web-based intervention for a senior?

5. How can technology help to empower individuals and communities?

# GROUP CRITICAL-THINKING EXERCISES

1. Discuss the informatics core competencies you think a new graduate working in community health is required to have at a high level of proficiency. Use the Community Health Nurses Standards of Practice (Appendix A) to help you.

2. What trends do you anticipate in the use of the Internet to promote health by youth, senior, new immigrant, and disabled populations? What role could Web 2.0 technologies have in promoting health and preventing disease?

3. Should nurses encourage their clients to join online social support groups? Why or why not?

# REFERENCES

Ache, K., & Wallace, L. (2008). Human papillomavirus vaccination coverage on YouTube. *American Journal of Preventive Medicine, 35*, 389–392. doi:10.1016/jamepre.2008.06.029

Ache, K. A., & Wallace, L. S. (2009). Are end-of-life patient education materials readable? *Palliative Medicine, 23*, 545–548. doi:10.1177/0269216309106313

Albrecht, U. V., von Jan, U., Sedlacek, L., Groos, S., Suerbaum, S., & Vonberg, R. P. (2013). Standardized, app-based disinfection of iPads in a clinical and nonclinical setting: Comparative analysis. *Journal of Medical Internet Research, 15*(8), e176. doi:10.2196/jmir/2643

AlGhamdi, K. M., & Moussa, N. A. (2012). Internet use by the public to search for health-related information. *International Journal of Medical Informatics, 81*, 363–373. doi:10.1016/j.ijmedinf.2011.12.004

Anker, A. E., Reinhart, A. M., & Feeley, T. H. (2011). Health information seeking: A review of measures and methods. *Patient Education and Counselling, 82*, 346–354. doi:10.1016/j.pec/2010.12.008

Antheunis, M. L., Tates, K., & Nieboer, T. E. (2013). Patients' and health professionals' use of social media in health care: Motives, barriers and expectations. *Patient Education and Counselling, 92*, 426–431. doi:10.1016/j.pec.2013.06.020

Barak, A., Boniel-Nissim, M., & Suler, J. (2008) Fostering empowerment in online support groups. *Computers in Human Behavior, 24*(5), 1867–1883. doi:10.1016/j.chb.2008.02.004

Becker, H., Mackert, M., & Kang, S. J. (2013). Using an e-health intervention to promote the health of cancer survivors with preexisting disabling conditions. *Computers, Informatics, Nursing, 31*(3), 107–114. doi:10.1097/nxn.0b013e3182771895

Bennett, G. G., & Glasgow, R. E. (2009). The delivery of public health interventions via the Internet: Actualizing their potential. *Annual review of public health, 30*, 273–292. doi:10.1146/annurev.publhealth.031308.100235

Borycki, E. M., Foster, J., Sahama, T., Frisch, N., & Kushniruk, A. W. (2013). Developing national level nursing informatics competencies for undergraduate nurses: Methodological approaches from Australia and Canada. *Enabling Health and Healthcare through ICT.* IOS Press. doi:10.3233/978-1-61499-203-5-345

Burns, P., Jones, S. C., Inverson, D., & Caputi, P. (2013). Usability testing of AsthmaWise with older adults. *Computers, Informatics, Nursing, 31*(5), 219–226. doi:10.1097/nxn.0b013e31829b0627

Caldwell, B., Slatin, J., & Vanderheiden, G. (2008). Web content accessibility guidelines 2.0. *World Wide Web Consortium W3C.* Retrieved from http://www.w3.org/TR/WCAG20/

Caligtan, C. A., Carroll, D. L., Hurley, A. C., Gersh-Zaremski, R., & Dykes, P. C. (2012). Bedside information technology to support patient-centered care. *International Journal of Medical Information, 81*, 442–451. doi:10.1016.j.ijmedinf.2011.12.005

Canadian Association of Schools of Nursing. (2012). *Nursing Informatics: Entry-to-practice competencies for registered nurses.* Available from http://www.casn.ca/2014/12/nursing-informatics-entry-practice-competencies-registered-nurses-2/

Canadian Association of Schools of Nursing. (2013). *Nursing informatics teaching toolkit: Supporting the integration of the CASN nursing informatics competencies into nursing curricula.* Retrieved from http://casn.ca/wp-content/uploads/2014/12/infowaytoolkit.jpg

Canadian Association of Schools of Nursing. (2014). *Entry-to-Practice Public Health Nursing Competencies for Undergraduate Nursing Education.* Ottawa ON: Author

Canadian Council of Social Development. (2005). *Disability Research Information Sheet #19.* Retrieved from http://www.ccsd.ca/index.php/research/disability-research

Canadian Internet Registration Authority. (2013). *CIRA factbook.* Retrieved from http://www.cira.ca/factbook/2013/index.html

Canadian Literacy and Learning Network. (2014). *Literacy statistics in Canada.* Retrieved from http://www.literacy.ca/

Canadian Nurses Association. (2006). *e-Nursing strategy for Canada.* Retrieved from https://www.cna-aiic.ca/en/download-buy/nursing-informatics

Canadian Nursing Informatics Association. (2003). *Educating tomorrow's nurses: Where's nursing informatics?* (Rep. No. G3-6B-DP1-0054). https://cnia.ca

Canadian Public Health Association. (1999). *Directory of plain language health information.* Retrieved from http://www.cpha.ca/uploads/portals/h-L/directory_e.pdf

Canadian Public Health Association. (2010). *Plain language service.* Canadian Public Health Association. Retrieved from http://www.cpha.ca/en/pls.aspx

Changrani, J., & Gany, F. (2005). Online cancer education and immigrants: Effecting culturally appropriate websites. *Journal of Cancer Education, 20,* 183–186. doi:10.1207/s15430154jce2003_14

Chaudhuri, S., Le, T., White, C., Thompson, H., & Demiris, G. (2013). Examining health information-seeking behaviors of older adults. *Computers, Informatics, Nursing, 32*(11), 547–553. doi:10.1097/01.NCN.0000432131.92020.42

Ciliska, D., Clark, K., Hershfield, L., Jetha, N., Mackintosh, J., & Finkle, D. (2009). *Using an Online Health Program Planner: What's in it for you?* Ottawa, ON: Canadian Public Health Association; 8 pp.

Community Health Nurses of Canada. (2011, revised). *Canadian community health nursing: Professional practice model and standards of practice.* St. Johns, NL: Author.

Cunningham, J. A., Humphreys, K., Kypri, K., & van Mierlo, T. (2006). Formative evaluation and three-month follow-up of an online personalized assessment feedback intervention for problem drinkers. *Journal of Medical Internet Research, 8*(2), e5. doi:10.2196/jmir.8.2.e5

Daneback, K., & Plantin, L. (2008). Research on parenthood and the internet: Themes and trends. *Cyberpsychology: Journal of Psychosocial Research on Cyberspace, 2*(2), article 1. Retrieved from http://cyberpsychology.eu/view.php?cisloclanku=2008110701&article=1

Dickerson, S. S. (2006). Women's use of the internet: What nurses need to know. *Journal of Obstetric Gynecologic and Neonatal Nursing, 35,* 151–156. doi:10.1111/j.1552-6909.2006.00004.x

Donelle, L., & Hoffman-Goetz, L. (2008). An exploratory study of Canadian Aboriginal online health care forums. *Health Communications, 23*(3), 270–281. doi:10.1080/10410230802056388

Edwards, N., & Kothari, A. (2004). CHNET-Works! A networking infrastructure for community health nurse researchers and decision-makers. *Canadian Journal of Nursing Research, 36*(4), 203–207.

Etter, J. F. (2005). Comparing the efficacy of two internet-based, computer-tailored smoking cessation programs: A randomized trial. *Journal of Medical Internet Research, 7,* e2. doi:10.2196/jmir.7.1.e2

Eysenbach, G. (2001). What is e-health? *Journal of Medical Internet Research, 3*(2), e20. doi:10.2196/jmir.3.2.e20

Eysenbach, G. (2007). From intermediation to disintermediation and apomediation: New models for consumers to access and assess the credibility of health information in the age of Web 2.0. *Studies in Health Technology and Informatics, 129*(1), 162–166.

Eysenbach, G., Powell, J., Englesakis, M., Rizo, C., & Stern, A. (2004). Health related virtual communities and electronic support groups: Systematic review of the effects of online peer to peer interactions. *British Medical Journal, 328,* 1166. doi:10.1136/bmj.328.7449.1166

Farvolden, P., McBride, C., Bagby, R. M., & Ravitz, P. (2003). A Web-based screening instrument for depression and anxiety disorders in primary care. *Journal of Medical Internet Research, 5*(3), e23. doi:10.2196/jmir.5.3.e23

Gaydos, M. C., Dwyer, K., Barnes, M., Rizzo-Price, P. A., Wood, B. J., Flemming, T., & Hogan, M. T. (2006). Internet-based screening for Chlamydia trachomatis to reach nonclinic populations with mailed self-administered vaginal swabs. *Sexually Transmitted Diseases, 33*(7), 451–457.

Gibbons, M. C., Wilson, R. F., Samal, L., Lehmann C. U., Dickersin, K., Lehmann, H. P., . . . Bass, E. B. (2009, October). *Impact of consumer health informatics applications* (Evidence Report/Technology Assessment No. 188). (Prepared by Johns Hopkins University Evidence-based Practice Center under contract No. HHSA 290-2007-10061-I.) AHRQ Publication No. 09(10)-E019. Rockville, MD: Agency for Healthcare Research and Quality.

Goldberg, L., Lide, B., Lowry, S., Massett, H. A., O'Connell, T., Preece, J., . . . Shneiderman, B. (2011). Usability and accessibility in consumer health informatics: Current trends and future challenges. *American Journal of Preventative Medicine, 40*(5S2), S187–S197. doi:10.1016/j.amepre.2011.01.009

Goldner, M. (2006). Using the internet and email for health purposes: The impact of health status. *Social Science Quarterly, 87,* 690–710. doi:10.1111/j.1540-6237.2006.00404.x

Godwin, Z. R., Bockhold, J. C., Webster, L., Falwell, S., Bomze, L., & Tran, N. K. (2013). Development of novel smart device based application for serial wound imaging and management. *Burns, 39,* 1395–1402. doi:10.1016/j.burns.2013.03.021

Gottlieb, R., & Rogers, J. L. (2004). Readability of health sites on the internet. *International Electronic Journal of Health Education, 7,* 38–42.

Grierson, T., van Dijk, M. W., Dozois, E., & Mascher, J. (2006). Policy and politics. Using the internet to build community capacity for healthy public policy. *Health Promotion Practice, 7,* 13–22. doi:10.1177/1524839905278590

Griffiths, F., Lindenmeyer, A., Powell, J., Lowe, P., & Thorogood, M. (2006). Why are health care interventions delivered over the internet? A systematic review of the published literature. *Journal of Medical Internet Research, 8,* e10. doi:10.2196/jmir.8.2.e10

Griffiths, F., Cave, J., Boardman, F., Ren, J., Pawlikowska, T., Ball, R., . . . Cohen, A. (2012). Social networks – The future for health care delivery. *Social Science & Medicine, 75,* 2233–2241. doi:10.1016/j.socscimed.2012.08.023

Hardiker, N. R., & Grant, M. J. (2011). Factors that influence public engagement with eHealth: A literature review. *International Journal of Medical Informatics, 80,* 1–12. doi:10.1016/j.ijmedinf.2010.10.017

Health on the Net Foundation. (2009). HON code of conduct (HONcode) for medical and health Web sites. *Health on the Net Foundation.* Retrieved from http://www.hon.ch/HONcode/Guidelines/guidelines.html

Health Summit Working Group. (2010). *Information quality tool. Mitretek Systems.* Retrieved from http://archive.ahrq.gov/research/data/infoqual.html

Hebda, T., & Czar, P. (2013). *Handbook of Informatics for Nurses & Healthcare Professionals* (5th ed.). Boston: Pearson.

Hesse, B. W., Nelson, D. E., Kreps, G. L., Croyle, R. T., Arora, N. K., Rimer, B. K., & Viswanath, K. (2005). Trust and sources of health information. *Archives of Internal Medicine, 165,* 2618–2624. doi:10.1001/archinte.165.22.2618

Hoffman-Goetz, L., Donelle, L., & Thomson, M. D. (2009). Clinical guidelines about diabetes and the accuracy of peer information in an unmoderated online health forum for retired persons. *Informatics for Health and Social Care, 34*(2), 91–99. doi:10.1001/archinte.165.22.2618

Househ, M., Borycki, E., & Kushniruk, A. (2014). Empowering patients through social media: The benefits and challenges. *Health Informatics Journal, 20*(1), 50–58. Published by Sage Publications, Ltd. (UK). doi:10.1177/1460458213476969

Kerr, M., Savik, K., Monsen, K. A., & Lusk, S. L. (2007). Effectiveness of computer-based tailoring versus targeting to promote use of hearing protection. *Canadian Journal of Nursing Research, 39*(1), 80–97.

Khechine, H., Pascot, D., & Prémont, P. (2008). Use of health-related information from the Internet by English-speaking patients. *Health Informatics, 14*, 17–28. doi:10.1177/1460458207086331

Kitchens, B., Harle, C. A., & Li, S. (2014). Quality of health-related search results. *Decision Support Systems, 57*, 454–462.

Kivits, J. (2009). Everyday health and the internet: A mediated health perspective on health information seeking. *Sociology of Health and Illness, 31*(5), 673–687. doi:10.1111/j.1467-9566.2008.01153.x

Korp, P. (2006). Health on the internet: Implications for health promotion. *Health Education Research, 21*, 78–86. doi:10.1093/her/cyh043

Kothari, A., Edwards, N., Brajtman, S., Campbell, B., Hamel, N., Legault, F., . . . Valaitis, R. (2005). Fostering interactions: The networking needs of community health nursing researchers and decision-makers. *Evidence and Policy, 1*, 291–304.

Kreuter, M. W., & Skinner, H. (2000). Tailoring: What's in a name? *Health Education Research, 15*, 4. doi:10.1093/her/15.1.1

Lam, C. G., Roter, D. L., & Cohen, K. J. (2013). Survey of quality, readability, and social reach of websites on osteosarcoma in adolescents. *Patient Education and Counselling, 90*, 82–87. doi:10.1016/j.pec.2012.08.006

Lemire, M., Sicotte, C., & Paré, G. (2008). Internet use and the logics of personal empowerment in health. *Health Policy, 88*, 130–140. doi:10.1016/j.healthpol.2008.03.006

Lemire, M., Paré, G., Sicotte, C., & Harvey, C. (2008). Determinants of Internet use as a preferred source of information on personal health. *International Journal of Medical Informatics, 77*, 723–734. doi:10.1016/j.ijmedinf.1008.03.002

Letourneau, N., Stewart, M., Masuda, J., Anderson, S., Cicutto, L., McGhan, S., & Watt, S. (2012). Impact of online support for youth with asthma and allergies: Pilot study. *Journal of Pediatric Nursing, 27*, 65–73. doi:10.1016/j.pedn.2010.07.007

Liu, S., Dunford, S. D., Leung, Y. W., Brooks, D., Thomas, S. G., Eysenbach, G., & Nolan, R. P. (2013). Reducing blood pressure with Internet-based interventions: A meta-analysis. *Canadian Journal of Cardiology, 29*, 613–621. doi:10.1016/j.cjca.2013.02.007

Lober, W. B., & Flowers, J. L. (2011). Consumer empowerment in health care amid the Internet and social media. *Seminars in Oncology Nursing, 27*(3), 169–182. doi:10.1016/j.soncn.2011.04.002

Lustria, M. L. A., Cortese, J., Noar, S. M., & Glueckauf, R. I. (2009). Computer-tailored health interventions delivered over the web: Review and analysis of key components. *Patient Education and Counselling, 74*, 156–173. doi:10.1016/j.pec.2008.08.023

Luo, G., Tang, C., & Thomas, S. B. (2012). Intelligent personal health record: Experience and open issues. *Journal of Medical Systems, 36*, 2111–2128. doi:10.1007/s10916-011-9674-5

McLaughlin, G. H. (1969). SMOG-grading: A new readability formula. *Journal of Reading, 12*, 639–646.

Manafo, E., & Wong, S. (2012). Exploring older adults' health information seeking behaviors. *Journal of Nutrition and Behavior, 44*(1), 85–89. doi:10.1016/j.jneb.2011.05.018

Mowat, D., & Butler-Jones, D. (2007). Public health in Canada: A difficult history. *Healthcare Papers, 7*, 31–36.

Muse, K., McManus, F., Leung, C., Meghreblian, B., & Williams, J. M. G. (2012). Cyberchondriasis: Fact or fiction? A preliminary examination of the relationship between health anxiety and searching for health information on the Internet. *Journal of Anxiety Disorders, 26*, 189–196. doi:10.1016/j.janxdis.2011.11.005

Mudry, T. E., & Strong, T. (2012). Doing recovery online. *Qualitative Health Research, 23*(3), 313–325. doi:10.1177/1049732312468296

Nagle, L. (2007). Informatics: Emerging concepts and issues. *Nursing Leadership, 20*, 30–32.

National Institute on Aging. (2002). *Making your website senior friendly.* Retrieved from http://www.nlm.nih.gov/pubs/checklist.pdf

Negev, M., Davidovitch, N., Garb, Y., & Tal, A. (2013). Stakeholder participation in health impact assessment: A multicultural approach. *Environmental Impact Assessment Review, 43*, 112–120. doi:10.1016/j.eiar.1013.06.002

Norman, C. D., & Skinner, H. A. (2006). eHealth literacy: Essential skills for consumer health in a networked world. *Journal of Medical Internet Research, 8*(2):e9. doi:10.2196/jmir.8.2.e9

OECD, Statistics Canada. (2011). *Literacy for life: Further results from the adult literacy and life skills survey.* OECD Publishing. doi:9789264091269-en

Ownby, R. L., Acevedo, A., Waldrop-Valverde, D., Jacobs, R. J., & Caballera, J. (2014). Abilities, skills and knowledge in measures of health literacy. *Patient Education and Counselling, 95*, 211–217. doi:10.1016/j.pec/2014.02.002

Pew Research Internet Survey. (2011). *Health information is a popular pursuit online.* Retrieved from http://www5.statcan.gc.ca/subject-sujet/result-resultat.action?pid=2256&id=2256&lang=eng&type=DAILYART

Plantin, L., & Daneback, K. (2009). Parenthood, information and support on the internet. A literature review of research on parents and professionals online. *BMC Family Practice, 10*, 34. doi:10.1186/1471-2296-10-34

Public Health Agency of Canada. (2006). *The Canadian Best Practices Portal for health promotion and chronic disease prevention: About the portal.* Retrieved from http://cbpp-pcpe.phac-aspc.gc.ca

Rice, R. E. (2006). Influences, usage, and outcomes of internet health information searching: Multivariate results from the Pew surveys. *International Journal of Medical Informatics, 75*, 8–28. doi:10.1016/j.ijmedinf.2005.07.032

Rooks, R. N., Wiltshire, J. C., Elder, K., BeLue, R., & Gary, L.C. (2012). Health information seeking and use outside of the medical encounter: Is it associated with race and ethnicity? *Social Science & Medicine, 74*, 176–184. doi:10.1016/j.socscimed.2011.09.040

Roush, K. (2006). Two NIH Web sites on aging: One is for providers and the other is for older adults. *American Journal of Nursing, 106(8),* 17.

Royer, H. R., Fernandez-Lambert, K. M., & Moreno, M. A. (2013). Formative research for the development of an interactive web-based sexually transmitted disease management for young women. *Computers, Informatics, Nursing, 31(9)*, 430–438. doi:10.1097/01.NCN.0000432123.79452.32

Russo, J. A., Parisi, S. M., Kukla, K., & Schwarz, E. B. (2013). Women's information-seeking behavior after receiving contraceptive versus noncontraceptive prescriptions. *Contraception, 87*, 824–829. doi:10.1016/j.contraception.2012.09.028

Rutten, L. J. F., Vieux, S. N., St. Sauver, J. L., Arora, N. K., Moser, R. P., Beckjord, E. B., & Hesse, B. W. (2014). Patient perceptions of electronic medical records use and ratings of care quality. *Patient Related Outcome Measures, 5*, 17–23. doi:10.2147/PROM.S58967

Saitz, R., Helmuth, E. D., Aromaa, S. E., Guard, A., Belanger, M., & Rosenbloom, D. L. (2004). Web-based screening and brief intervention for the spectrum of alcohol problems. *Preventive Medicine, 39(5)*, 969–975. doi:10.1016/j.ypmed.2004.04.011

Seymour, W., & Lupton, D. (2004). Holding the line online: Exploring wired relationships for people with disabilities. *Disability and Society, 19*, 291–305. doi:10.1080/09687590410001689421

Skinner, H., Biscope, S., & Poland, B. (2003). Quality of internet access: Barrier behind internet use statistics. *Social Science and Medicine, 57*, 875–880. doi:10.1016/S0277-9536(02)00455-0

Staggers, N., & Bagley Thompson, C. (2002). The evolution of definitions for nursing informatics: A critical analysis and revised definition. *Journal of the American Medical Informatics Association, 9*, 255–262.

Statistics Canada. (2009). *Internet use by individuals, by type of activity*. Retrieved from http://www40.statcan.gc.ca/l01/cst01/comm29a-eng.htm?sdi=internet

Statistics Canada. (2010). *Online activities of Canadian Boomers and seniors*. Retrieved from http://www.statcan.gc.ca/pub/11-008-x/2009002/article/10910-eng.htm

Statistics Canada. (2011). *Literacy for life: Further results from the adult literacy and life skills survey (Second international ALL report)*. Retrieved from http://www.statcan.gc.ca/pub/89-604-x/89-604-x2011001-eng.pdf

Statistics Canada. (2013a). *Canadian Internet use survey*. Retrieved from http://www5.statcan.gc.ca/subject-sujet/result-resultat.action?pid=2256&id=2256&lang=eng&type=DAILYART

Statistics Canada. (2013b). *Individual Internet usage and e-commerce 2012*. Retrieved from http://www.statcan.gc.ca/daily-quotidien/131028/dq131028a-eng.pdf

Statistics Canada. (2014). Education indicators in Canada: An international perspective. Retrieved from http://www.statcan.gc.ca/daily-quotidien/141215/dq141215b-eng.pdf

Stern, A., Valaitis, R., Weir, R., & Jadad, A. R. (2012). Use of home telehealth in palliative cancer care: A case study. *Journal of Telemedicine and Telecare, 18(5)*, 297–300. doi:10.1258/jtt.2012.111201

Stonham, G., Heyes, B., Owen, A., & Povey, E. (2012). Measuring the nursing contribution using electronic records. *Nursing Management, 19(8)*, 28–32.

Suggs, L. S., & McIntyre, C. (2009). Are we there yet? An examination of online tailored health communication. *Health Education and Behavior, 36*, 278–288. doi:10.1177/1090198107303309

Suziedelyte, A. (2012). How does searching for health information on the Internet affect individuals' demand for health services? *Social Science & Medicine, 75*, 1828–1835. doi:10.1016/j.socscimed.2012.07.022

Syred, J., Naidoo, C., Woodhall, S. C., & Araitser, P. (2014). Would you tell everyone this? Facebook conversations as health promotion interventions. *Journal of Medical Internet Research, 16(4)*, e108. doi:10.2196/jmir.3231

Tapscott, D. (1998). The digital divide. In *Growing up digital: The rise of the net generation* (pp. 255–279). New York, NY: McGraw-Hill.

Tian, Y., & Robinson, J. D. (2009). Incidental health information use on the Internet. *Health Communication, 24*, 41–49. doi:10.1080/10410230802606984

Treasury Board of Canada Secretariat. (2007). Common look and feel standards for the internet (CLF 2.0). *Treasury Board of Canada Secretariat*. Retrieved from http://www.tbs-sct.gc.ca/clf-nsi/index-eng.asp

Unstun, C., & Cihangiroglu, M. (2012). Health care workers' mobile phones: A potential cause for microbial cross-contamination between hospitals and communities. *Journal of Occupational and Environmental Hygiene, 9(9)*, 538–42. doi:10.1080/15459624.2012.697419

U.S. Centers for Disease Control and Prevention and University of Washington's Center for Public Health Informatics. (2009). *Competencies for public health informaticians*. Atlanta, GA: Author.

Vance, K., Howe, W., & Dellavalle, R. P. (2009). Social internet sites as a source of public health information. *Dermatologic Clinics: Epidemiology and Public Health, 27(2)*, 133–36. doi:10.1016/j.det.2008.11.010

Valaitis, R. (2005). Computers and the Internet: Tools for youth empowerment. *Journal of Medical Internet Research, 7(5)*, e51. doi:10.2196/jmir.7.5.e51

Valaitis, R., & O'Mara, L. (2005). Enabling youth participation in school-based computer-supported community development in Canada. *Health Promotion International, 20(3)*, 260–268. doi:10.1093/heapro/dah611

Vennick, F. D., Adams, S. A., Faber, M. J., & Putters, K. (2014). Expert and experiential knowledge in the same place: Patients' experiences with online communities connecting patients and healthcare professionals. *Patient Education and Counselling, 95*, 265–270. doi:10.1016/j.pec.2014.02.003

W3C. (2014a). *Web accessibility initiative (WAI)*. World Wide Web Consortium W3C. Retrieved from http://www.w3.org/TR/2008/REC-WCAG20-20081211

W3C. (2014b). *Web accessibility tutorials*. World Wide Web Consortium W3C. Retrieved from http://www.w3.org/WAI/tutorials

Wenger, E., McDermott, R., & Snyder, W. (2002). *A guide to managing knowledge: Cultivating communities of practice*. Boston, MA: Harvard Business School Press.

Whittaker, R., Borland, R., & Bullen, C. (2009). Mobile phone-based interventions for smoking cessation. *Cochrane Database of Systematic Reviews,* Oct. 7 (4): CD006611.

WRAPIN. (2014). *Worldwide online reliable advice to patients and individuals.* European Project-IST-2001-33260. Retrieved from http://www.wrapin.org

Woodall, J., Taylor, V. M., Chong T., Li, L., Acorda, E., Tu, S., & Hislpo, G. (2009). Sources of health information among Chinese immigrants to the Pacific Northwest. *Journal of Cancer Education, 24*(4), 334–340. doi:10.1080/08858190902854533

Xiao, N., Sharman, R., Rao, H. R., & Upadhyaya, S. (2014). Factors influencing online health information search: An empirical analysis of a national cancer-related survey.

*Decision Support Systems, 57,* 417–427. doi:10.1016/j.dss.2012.10.047

Xie, B. (2012). Improving older adults' e-health literacy through computer training using NIH online resources. *Library & Information Science Research, 34,* 63–71. doi:10.2196/jmir.1880

Ybarra, M. L., & Eaton, W. W. (2005). Internet-based mental health interventions. *Mental Health Services Research, 7*(2), 75–87. doi:10.1007/s11020-005-3779-8

Ybarra, M. L., Biringi, R., Prescott, T., & Bull, S. S. (2012). Usability and navigability of an HIV/AIDS Internet intervention for adolescents in a resource-limited setting. *Computers, Informatics, Nursing, 30*(11), 587–595. doi:10.1097/NSN.0b013e318266cb0e

## ABOUT THE AUTHORS

**Linda Ferguson**, RN, PhD, is a Full Professor in the College of Nursing, University of Saskatchewan. Her undergraduate, master's, and PhD are in the field of nursing, and she has a post-graduate diploma in Continuing Education. She has worked extensively in the field of faculty development within the College of Nursing and the University of Saskatchewan. Linda has taught educational methods courses at the under-graduate (nursing and physical therapy), post-registration, and master's levels for the past 24 years. Her research has focused on the continuing education needs of registered nurses in practice, and of mentoring and precepting nurses, in the areas of teaching excellence, interprofessional education, podcast-ing and nursing education, and the process of developing clinical judgment in nursing practice. She is past director of the Centre for the Advancement of the Study of Nursing Education and Inter-professional Education (CASNIE) within the College of Nursing at the University of Saskatchewan, and was president of the Canadian Association of Schools of Nursing (CASN) (2012–2014).

**Tracie Risling**, RN, PhD, is an Assistant Professor in the College of Nursing at the University of Saskatchewan. Her interests include the use of student response systems, social media, and other collaborative Web-based learning tools in nursing education and patient care. She has explored how the application of technology can improve connectivity and student engagement in both physical and virtual learning environments. She is a member of the Saskatchewan Nurse Peer-to-Peer Network, a group of nurse leaders working to advance the informatics and e-health agenda in the province. The nurse network team is part of a larger provincial health sciences interprofessional group and is connected nationally to other networks sup-ported by Canada Health Infoway.

# CHAPTER 16

# Maternal, Infant, and Child Health

*Deborah Mansell and Aliyah Dosani*

## LEARNING OUTCOMES

**After studying this chapter, you should be able to:**

1. Describe key indicators of maternal, infant, and child health in Canada.

2. Compare and contrast Canada's indicators of maternal, infant, and child health to the global scale.

3. Discuss key challenges of maternal, infant, and child health in Canada.

4. Explore maternal, infant, and child health as it relates to the social determinants of health.

5. Discuss ethical challenges inherent in community health nursing practice with women, infants, and young children, nationally and internationally.

6. Relate community health nursing practice with women, infants, and young children to the Canadian Community Health Nursing Standards of Practice.

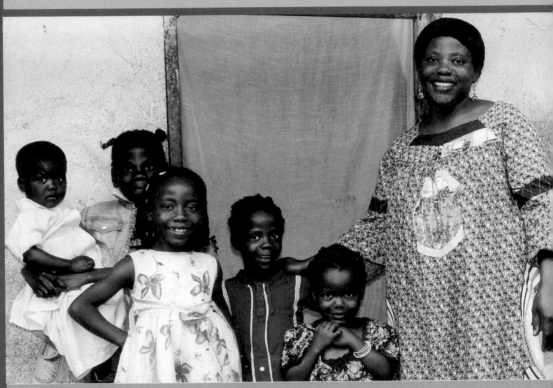

*Source: Sylvie Bouchard/Shutterstock*

## INTRODUCTION

Globally, the health of women and children is considered a key marker for the overall health status of families, communities, and societies, and it is upheld as an indicator for the overall health of people in Canada. In 2010, the Secretary General of the United Nations, Ban Ki Moon, launched the "Every Woman Every Child" initiative to address improving policy and financing related to maternal, infant, and child health. It was hoped that these policy and financing changes would lead to improved services for women, infants, and children around the world (United Nations, 2013). The "Every Woman Every Child" initiative is a sizable intersectoral collaboration that directs the actions of governments, nongovernmental organizations (NGOs), the private sector, and societies to address the substantial health challenges that women, infants, and children face around the world. Each year, more than 280 000 women around the world die in pregnancy or childbirth, as reported by the World Health Organization (WHO) (2013). Approximately 10.9 million children under the age of 5 years die each year from causes that are largely preventable, including undernutrition and diarrhea (WHO, 2013). Women, infants, and children around the world face numerous barriers in achieving an optimal health status. The "Every Woman Every Child" initiative is intended to address and decrease disparities around access to services and health-care providers, decreasing isolation due to remote or rural locations, and increasing access to preventative measures such as immunizations. Recognizing the importance of improving the lives of women and children globally, the Government of Canada, in 2010, launched the "Muskoka Initiative," which directed global effort and actions toward reducing maternal and infant mortality and improving the health of mothers and children around the world (Government of Canada – Foreign Affairs, Trade, and Development Canada, 2014).

Across Canada, the federal, provincial, municipal, and local governments, as well as NGOs, work daily to address the gaps in healthcare that women and children face while creating and implementing health promotion programs. Canada has historically been a leader in promoting the health of women and children across the globe. Yet, even in a country as wealthy as Canada, women and children continue to face barriers to achieving optimal health. Urban and rural women and children in Canada who already face poverty, unemployment, or lower levels of education are at an increased risk of facing disparities in health status, access to healthcare, and health promotion initiatives (Angus et al., 2012). Community health nurses (CHNs), physicians, social workers, youth workers, police, and immigration workers are all playing active roles in identifying and addressing challenges that women and children face in achieving their best health.

## MATERNAL AND CHILD HEALTH AROUND THE WORLD: AN OVERVIEW

Compared to their Canadian counterparts, women and children around the world face barriers in acquiring even the most basic healthcare services. Even though some of the poorest countries in the world have improved maternal health and cut neonatal deaths by half since the mid-1990s, there is a continuing need to improve the health and well-being of women and children around the world (WHO, 2014a). Women and children living in South Asia and in countries in sub-Saharan Africa continue to face the highest rates of maternal, neonatal, and child deaths (see Figure 16.1).

Even though there has been a global decline in maternal mortality rates, it is alarming that in 2013 alone, 289 000 women died in pregnancy or childbirth. The majority of these deaths were preventable if these women had been able to access appropriate healthcare during pregnancy, labour, childbirth, and the postpartum period (WHO, 2014b). In September 2000, 191 United Nations member states signed the Millennium Declaration, which formed the foundation for the eight Millennium Development Goals (MDGs) (WHO, 2014c). The fifth goal of the MDGs, to improve maternal health, set two targets: (a) reduce the **maternal mortality ratio** by 75%, and (b) achieve universal access to reproductive health by 2015. While maternal deaths dropped by 50% between 1990 and 2013 (WHO, 2014d), further progress in reducing maternal mortality in resource-poor countries and providing family planning services continues at a slow rate. Over 10% of all women globally do not have access to, or are not using, an effective method of contraception (WHO, 2014e). The WHO estimates that meeting the need for family planning alone would reduce the number of maternal deaths by almost one-third (2014e). In Table 16.1, 10 facts about maternal health around the world are presented. Table 16.2 provides an overview of key epidemiologic terms related to maternal and infant health.

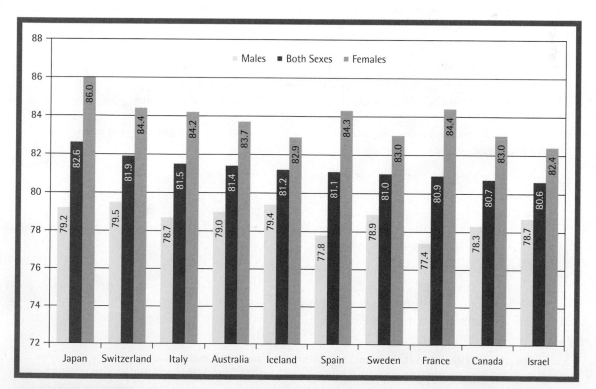

**FIGURE 16.1** Maternal Mortality Ratio (Deaths per 100 000 Live Births) around the World (2013)

*Source:* WHO, UNICEF, UNFPA, The World Bank, and The United Nations Population Division. (2014). *Trends in maternal mortality: 1990–2013.* Retrieved from http://apps.who.int/iris/bitstream/10665/112682/2/9789241507226_eng.pdf?ua=1

| Table 16.1 | 10 Facts about Maternal Health |
| --- | --- |
| Fact 1 | **Almost 800 women die every day due to complications during pregnancy and childbirth.**<br><br>About 289 000 women died worldwide in 2013 due to complications during pregnancy and childbirth. In developing countries, conditions related to pregnancy and childbirth constitute the second leading cause of death (after HIV/AIDS) among women of reproductive age. |
| Fact 2 | **There are four main killers.**<br><br>The four main killers are severe bleeding, infections, unsafe abortions, and hypertensive disorders (pre-eclampsia and eclampsia). Bleeding after delivery can kill even a healthy woman, if unattended, within two hours. Most of these deaths are preventable. |
| Fact 3 | **More than 135 million women give birth per year.**<br><br>About 20 million of these women experience pregnancy-related illness after childbirth. The list of morbidities is long and diverse, and includes fever, anaemia, fistula, incontinence, infertility, and depression. Women who suffer from fistula are often stigmatized and ostracized by their husbands, families, and communities. |
| Fact 4 | **About 16 million girls aged between 15 and 19 give birth each year.**<br><br>They account for more than 10% of all births. In the developing world, about 90% of the births to adolescents occur in marriage. In low- and middle-income countries, complications from pregnancy and childbirth are the leading cause of death among girls aged 15–19. Adolescents face a higher risk of complications and death as a result of pregnancy. |
| Fact 5 | **Maternal health mirrors the gap between the rich and the poor.**<br><br>The majority of maternal deaths (99%) occur in resource-poor countries. Less than 1% of maternal deaths occur in high-income countries. The maternal mortality ratio in developing countries is 230 per 100 000 births versus 16 per 100 000 in developed countries. Also, maternal mortality is higher in rural areas and among poorer and less-educated communities. Of the 800 women who die every day, 500 live in sub-Saharan Africa, 190 in Southern Asia and 6 in high-income countries. |
| Fact 6 | **Most maternal deaths can be prevented.**<br><br>Most of these deaths can be prevented through skilled care at childbirth and access to emergency obstetric care. In sub-Saharan Africa, where maternal mortality ratios are the highest, less than 50% of women are attended by a trained midwife, nurse, or doctor during childbirth. |
| Fact 7 | **Many women do not see a skilled health professional often enough during pregnancy.**<br><br>Although a large proportion of women see skilled health personnel at least once during their pregnancy, only about half receive the recommended minimum of at least four visits during the pregnancy. Women who do not receive the necessary check-ups miss the opportunity to detect problems and receive appropriate care and treatment. This also includes immunization and prevention of mother-to-child transmission of HIV/AIDS. |
| Fact 8 | **About 22 million abortions continue to be performed unsafely each year.**<br><br>Unsafe abortions result in the death of an estimated 47 000 women and more than 5 million complications. Almost every case of death and every case resulting in complications could have been prevented through sexuality education, contraceptive use, and the provision of safe, legal induced abortion and care for complications of abortion. |
| Fact 9 | **Reducing the maternal mortality ratio has been slow.**<br><br>One target of the MDGs is to reduce the maternal mortality ratio by three-quarters between 1990 and 2015. So far, progress has been slow. Since 1990 the global maternal mortality ratio has declined by only 2.6% annually instead of the 5.5% needed to achieve MDG 5, aimed at improving maternal health. |
| Fact 10 | **The lack of skilled care is the main obstacle to better health for mothers.**<br><br>This is aggravated by a global shortage of qualified health workers. |

Source: Adapted from World Health Organization. (2014). *10 Facts on Maternal Health*. Reprinted with permission. Retrieved from http://www.who.int/features/factfiles/maternal_health/maternal_health_facts/en/

| Table 16.2 | Key Epidemiologic Definitions |
|---|---|
| Maternal mortality ratio* | The number of maternal deaths during a given period per 100 000 live births during that same period. |
| Maternal mortality rate* | The number of maternal deaths in a given period per 100 000 women of reproductive age during the same time period. |
| Maternal death+ | "The death of a woman while pregnant or within 42 days of termination of pregnancy, irrespective of the duration and the site of pregnancy, from any cause related to or aggravated by the pregnancy or its management but not from accidental or incidental causes." Maternal mortality is usually expressed per 100 000 deliveries. |
| Preterm birth** | An infant born with less than 37 weeks of gestation completed. |
| Small-for-gestational-age birth** | An infant who falls in the less-than-10th percentile at birth, based on the Canadian Fetal Growth Standard. |
| Low birth weight** | An infant who weighs less than 2500 grams at birth. |
| High birth weight** | An infant who weighs more than 4000 grams at birth. |
| Large-for-gestational-age birth** | An infant who falls in the greater-than-90th percentile at birth, based on the Canadian Fetal Growth Standard. |
| Neonatal death** | An infant who dies 0–27 days after birth. |
| Post-neonatal death** | An infant who dies 28–364 days after birth. |
| Total infant death** | An infant who dies 0–364 days after birth. |

Sources: *World Health Organization. (2012). Trends in maternal mortality: 1990 to 2010, WHO, UNICEF, UNFPA, and The World Bank estimates. Retrieved from http://www.unfpa.org/sites/default/files/pub-pdf/9789241507226_eng.pdf; +International statistical classification of diseases 10th revision (ICD-10).

** Luo, Z. C., Wilkins, R., Heaman, M., Martens, P., Smylie, J., Hart, L., Simonet, F., . . . Fraser, W. D. (2010). Birth outcomes and infant mortality by the degree of rural isolation among First Nations and non-First Nations, in Manitoba, Canada. *Journal of Rural Health, 26*(2), 175–181.

In 2013, 6.3 million children under five years of age died—nearly 17 000 every day (WHO, 2014f). Internationally, infants and young children also face higher morbidity and mortality rates compared to their Canadian counterparts (Table 16.3). In many low-income countries, the probability of a child dying before age five grows exponentially, despite global efforts to reduce childhood mortality (see Figure 16.2). Internationally, the first 28 days of life, known as the neonatal period, is when infants are at the highest risk of dying. According to the WHO (2013), approximately 44% of all childhood deaths under the age of five years occur during the neonatal period. Three-quarters of all newborn deaths occur within the

| Table 16.3 | Trends in Estimates of Maternal Mortality Ratio (Maternal Deaths per 100 000 Live Births), 1990–2013, by WHO Region | | | | | | | |
|---|---|---|---|---|---|---|---|---|
| Region | MMRa | | | | | | % change in MMR between 1990 and 2013b | Average annual % change in MMR between 1990 and 2013b |
| | 1990 | 1995 | 2000 | 2005 | 2010 | 2013 | | |
| Africa | 960 | 920 | 820 | 670 | 550 | 500 | −49 | −2.8 |
| Americas | 110 | 92 | 81 | 71 | 70 | 68 | −37 | −2 |
| Eastern Mediterranean | 340 | 330 | 300 | 240 | 190 | 170 | −50 | −3 |
| Europe | 42 | 36 | 29 | 22 | 20 | 17 | −59 | −3.8 |
| South-East Asia | 520 | 430 | 340 | 260 | 210 | 190 | −64 | −4.4 |
| Western Pacific | 110 | 93 | 78 | 63 | 49 | 45 | −60 | −3.9 |
| World | 380 | 360 | 330 | 270 | 230 | 210 | −45 | −2.6 |

Source: World Health Organization. (2014). Trends in maternal mortality: 1990 to 2013, WHO, UNICEF, UNFPA, and The World Bank estimates. Reprinted with permission. Retrieved from http://www.unfpa.org/sites/default/files/pub-pdf/9789241507226_eng.pdf

a MMR estimates have been rounded according to the following scheme: <100, no rounding; 100–999, rounded to nearest 10; and >1000, rounded to nearest 100. b Negative values indicate a decreasing MMR from 1990 to 2013, while positive values indicate an increasing MMR. Percentages have been calculated using unrounded estimates. The average annual per cent change is estimated by: For countries with MMR ≥100 in 1990, they are categorized as 'on track' if MMR has had 5.5% or more average annual decline; 'making progress' if MMR has had 2% to 5.5% average annual decline; 'insufficient progress' if MMR has had less than 2% average annual decline; and 'no progress' if MMR has had an average annual increase. Countries with MMR <100 in 1990 are not categorized.

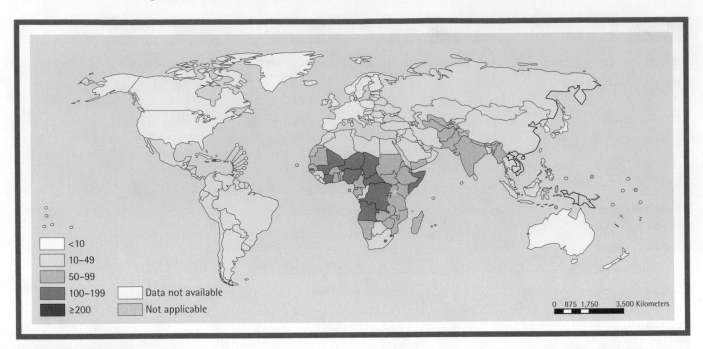

**FIGURE 16.2** Under-Five Childhood Mortality Rates around the World (the Probability of Dying by Age Five per 1000 Live Births), WHO (2013)

*Source:* WHO, UNICEF, UNFPA, The World Bank, and The United Nations Population Division (2014). Reprinted with permission from World Health Organization from Global Health Observatory Map Gallery. Retrieved from http://gamapserver.who.int/mapLibrary/app/searchResults.aspx

first week of life (WHO, 2012). Preterm birth (birth before 37 weeks gestation), birth asphyxia (a lack of breathing at birth), and infections are the main reasons for the majority of neonatal deaths globally (see Figure 16.2). However, from the

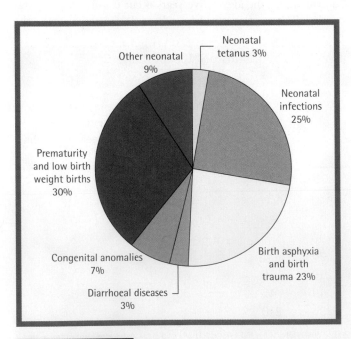

**FIGURE 16.3** Causes of Neonatal Death

*Source:* WHO. (2008). The global burden of disease. 2004 update. Reprinted with permission from World Health Organization. Retrieved from http://www.who.int/mediacentre/factsheets/20090804_figure1.jpg?ua=1

end of the neonatal period through to the first five years of life, the primary causes of death for this population are pneumonia, diarrhea, and malaria (see Figure 16.3). Malnutrition is also a major contributing factor in about 45% of all child deaths, as malnutrition makes infants and children more susceptible to severe diseases. Malnutrition also makes prevention and treatment more challenging. Access to health promotion activities such as vaccinations and exclusive breastfeeding, and access to basic necessities such as clean water and antibiotics have all been shown to reduce neonate, infant, and child mortality (WHO, 2013). Yet in many developing or resource-poor countries, access to health promotion and illness prevention programs can be limited and there may be varying levels of implementation and accessibility.

# HEALTH OF WOMEN AND CHILDREN IN CANADA: AN OVERVIEW

Canada is known internationally as having a healthcare system that is accessible to all its citizens regardless of socioeconomic status, gender, or age. Fortunately, many women in Canada receive high-quality pre-conception, prenatal, and postpartum care, which inevitably leads to increased health and wellness for both mother and child. However, even within a wealthy country with a publicly funded healthcare system, there are women and children who face barriers and inequities that can prevent or limit achieving the best possible health outcomes.

| Table 16.4 | Maternal Mortality Rates in Canada from 1997 to 2011 | |
| --- | --- | --- |
| **Fiscal Years** | **Number of Maternal Deaths** | **Maternal Deaths per 100 000 Hospital Deliveries (95% CI)** |
| 1997–1998 to 1998–1999 | 42 | 8.3 (6.0–11.2) |
| 1999–2000 to 2000–2001 | 42 | 8.5 (6.2–11.6) |
| 2001–2002 to 2002–2003 | 58 | 11.9 (9.1–15.4) |
| 2003–2004 to 2004–2005 | 42 | 8.2 (5.9–11.1) |
| 2005–2006 to 2006–2007 | 48 | 8.9 (6.6–11.8) |
| 2007–2008 to 2008–2009 | 50 | 8.8 (6.5–11.6) |
| 2009–2010 to 2010–2011 | 35 | 6.1 (4.3–8.6) |

Source: Public Health Agency of Canada. (2013). *Perinatal health indicators for Canada 2013: A report from the Canadian perinatal surveillance system*. Ottawa, ON: Author. Adapted and reproduced with permission from the Minister of Health, 2015. Retrieved from http://publications.gc.ca/collections/collection_2014/aspc-phac/HP7-1-2013-eng.pdf. CI – Confidence interval

# Maternal Health in Canada— Statistical Trends

Overall, Canada is a leader in achieving quality outcomes for women of childbearing age (i.e., 15–49 years of age) (WHO, 2014g). The concept of **maternal healthcare**, in Canada, includes family planning, prenatal care, and postnatal care. Maternal mortality rates in Canada remain some of the lowest in world. According to Statistics Canada, approximately 97% of mothers with children ages 0 to 11 months received prenatal care, but it is not known exactly what physical, emotional, or pregnancy-related care and/or information was provided at each of these prenatal visits (Canadian Institute for Health Information, 2006). Despite the void related to information provided to mothers during pregnancy, Canada has seen decreases in known harms to both mothers and fetuses (see Canadian Research Box 16.1). For example, maternal smoking

in pregnancy has steadily decreased from a high of approximately 30% to a rate of 12.3%. Furthermore, alcohol consumption during pregnancy decreased from 15.5% in 2001–2004 to 10.7% between 2005 and 2008, as reported by the Public Health Agency of Canada (PHAC) (2013).

The **maternal mortality rate** in Canada has dropped from 11.9 deaths per 100 000 deliveries in 1997–1998 to 6.1 deaths per 100 000 deliveries in 2010–2011 (PHAC, 2013). In Table 16.4 we can see that over the past decade the maternal mortality rate of hospital deliveries has decreased by almost 50%. It is clear that many of the factors relating to maternal deaths in various parts of the world are related to the accessibility of healthcare services and are preventable. In Table 16.5, the main causes of maternal mortality in Canada are presented. While Canada fares well with respect to maternal mortality on the global scale, it is clear that there are some parts of Canada, mainly eastern Canada

| Table 16.5 | Causes of Maternal Mortality in Canada | |
| --- | --- | --- |
| **Diagnosis** | **Number of Maternal Deaths** | **Maternal Deaths per 100 000 Hospital Deliveries (95% CI)** |
| Diseases of the circulatory system | 76 | 3.1 (2.5–3.9) |
| Other indirect causes | 59 | 2.4 (1.9–3.1) |
| Postpartum hemorrhage | 39 | 1.6 (1.1–2.2) |
| Hypertension complicating pregnancy, childbirth, and the puerperium | 34 | 1.4 (1.0–1.9) |
| Obstetric embolism | 34 | 1.4 (1.0–1.9) |
| Major puerperal infection | 22 | 0.9 (0.6–1.3) |
| Ectopic and molar pregnancy/abortive outcome | 21 | 0.9 (0.5–1.3) |
| Antepartum hemorrhage, abruptio placentae, and placenta previa | 15 | 0.6 (0.3–1.0) |

Source: Public Health Agency of Canada. (2013). *Perinatal health indicators for Canada 2013: A report from the Canadian perinatal surveillance system*. Ottawa, ON: Author. Adapted and reproduced with permission from the Minister of Health, 2015. Retrieved from http://publications.gc.ca/collections/collection_2014/aspc-phac/HP7-1-2013-eng.pdf. CI – Confidence interval

| Table 16.6 | Maternal Mortality by Provinces in Canada | |
|---|---|---|
| **Province/Territory** | **Number of Maternal Deaths** | **Maternal Deaths per 100 000 Hospital Deliveries (95% CI)** |
| Newfoundland and Labrador | 12 | 16.7 (8.7–29.3) |
| Prince Edward Island | ** | 19.0 (5.2–48.6) |
| Nova Scotia | 8 | 5.9 (2.6–11.7) |
| New Brunswick | 6 | 5.4 (2.0–11.7) |
| Ontario | 195 | 9.6 (8.2–11.0) |
| Manitoba | 6 | 5.6 (2.1–12.3) |
| Saskatchewan | 13 | 6.8 (3.7–11.7) |
| Alberta | 49 | 7.9 (5.8–10.4) |
| British Columbia | 52 | 8.4 (6.3–11.0) |
| Yukon | ** | 18.8 (0.5–104.4) |
| Northwest Territories | 0 | 0.0 (0.0–37.5) |
| Nunavut | 0 | 0.0 (0.0–54.7) |
| CANADA | 346 | 8.8 (7.9–9.8) |

Source: Public Health Agency of Canada. (2013). *Perinatal health indicators for Canada 2013: A report from the Canadian perinatal surveillance system*. Ottawa, ON: Author. Adapted and reproduced with permission from the Minister of Health, 2015. Retrieved from http://publications.gc.ca/collections/collection_2014/aspc-phac/HP7-1-2013-eng.pdf. ** Number suppressed for privacy reasons (cell size between 1 and 5) CI – Confidence interval

and the Yukon Territory, that appear to have significantly higher rates of maternal mortality than the rest of Canada (see Table 16.6).

## MATERNAL HEALTH PROMOTION IN CANADA

**Maternal health** and maternal healthcare generally refer to the health and services provided to women who are of childbearing age (after menses) and include pre-conception care, pregnancy, childbirth, and the postpartum period (PHAC, 2013). Sometimes, this period of time just before conception, during pregnancy, and after labour and delivery may also be referred to as the **perinatal period**. One of the main goals for the United Nations MDGs is for all women globally to have universal access to safe and reliable reproductive health services and education by 2015 (United Nations, 2013). "**Reproductive health**" is understood to address the reproductive processes and functions, and the bodily systems impacted throughout all stages of life. The term "reproductive health" implies that every individual has the ability to reproduce and the right to decide when, if, and how this occurs (WHO, 2014a). This means that both men and women must therefore have access to healthcare services and knowledgeable healthcare providers who can safely support women and their families through pregnancy, labour and delivery, and in the postpartum period. Furthermore, it is of utmost importance that women be able to make

decisions about their reproductive health free from coercion and/or discrimination.

**Reproductive rights** are a series of legal rights that were established at the United Nations 1968 International Conference on Human Rights and have been taken up in varying degrees by countries around the world since then. In 1994, reproductive rights were clarified and endorsed internationally in the Cairo Consensus that emerged from the International Conference on Population and Development (United Nations Population Fund, 2012). The rights that were reaffirmed at that time included:

- reproductive health as a component of overall health, throughout the life cycle, for both men and women;
- reproductive decision making, including voluntary choice in marriage, family formation and determination of the number, timing and spacing of one's children and the right to have access to the information and means needed to exercise voluntary choice;
- equality and equity for men and women, to enable individuals to make free and informed choices in all spheres of life, free from discrimination based on gender; and
- sexual and reproductive security, including freedom from sexual violence and coercion, and the right to privacy (United Nations Population Fund, 2012, para. 3).

**Reproductive justice** is a term that was developed to connect the right of reproductive health with the concept of social justice. Reproductive justice acknowledges that, while every woman may have reproductive rights, there are barriers that women face every day in accessing those rights, including lower socioeconomic status and lack of political influence and advocacy.

> Reproductive justice is the complete physical, mental, spiritual, political, economic, and social well-being of women and girls, and will be achieved when women and girls have the economic, social, and political power and resources to make healthy decisions about our bodies, sexuality, and reproduction for ourselves, our families, and our communities in all areas of our lives. (Asian Communities for Reproductive Justice, 2005, p. 1)

Experts around the world agree that until issues that women face, including economic disparities, racial discrimination, and inequalities in power, are addressed, women will never have full control over their reproductive lives and decisions.

When CHNs work with women, men, children, adolescents, and families within the context of promoting sexual health and/or providing access to education or healthcare services, they may face ethical issues that either impact themselves or their clients. Discussing sexual health, sexual health education, and supporting sexual decision making may bring CHNs into environments where their own personal ethics or those of their clients may be challenged. The Community Health Nurses of Canada practice guidelines offer that CHNs should be able to "make decisions using ethical standards and principles, taking into consideration one individual's rights over the rights of another, individual or societal good, allocation of scarce resources, and quantity versus quality of life" (2011, revised, p. 22). CHNs may assess their values, attitudes, beliefs, and assumptions about reproductive health in order to determine when or if ethical tensions may impact their nursing practice. In addition, using critical reflection, seeking help and support, using current evidence, knowing who the experts are in your community, and referring your clients to the other professionals working in the area of reproductive health are all supportive ways in which CHNs can negotiate the ethical tensions that they or their clients may experience.

## Mothering: A Kaleidoscope of Ideologies

Mothering . . .
. . . is fundamental to all beings.
. . . involves nurturing and raising children.
. . . extends far beyond biology and bodies.
. . . is the act and practice of love and the passing on of knowledge.
. . . occurs across multiple times and spaces.
. . . is political.
. . . is life.

(National Collaborating Centre for Aboriginal Health, 2012)

In Western societies such as Canada, becoming a mother is often exalted and envisioned as a beautiful state that all women should embrace. The reality is that for many women in Canada, mothering can be profoundly different from this. The discussions that societies, communities, families, and individuals have about mothering can both help and hinder the health of women and their families. For example, a positive message of the importance of mothering in Canadian society is the public health policy of a

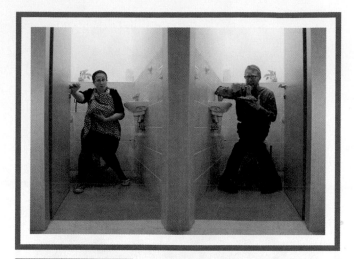

**PHOTO 16.1** If you are not willing to eat your lunch in the bathroom, then don't expect me to feed my kid there!

*Source: Tamar Shugert Photography*

paid 50-week maternity and parental benefit that enables many women to stay home with their child during the first year after birth (Service Canada, 2014). Many families benefit from the paid leave as childcare costs can be reduced and children can benefit from time with a parent over their first year of life. However, there are contradictory messages about mothering, which can isolate women and setup unrealistic or unfair disconnects. Breastfeeding, for example, is widely accepted as the best nutrition a mother can offer her baby. Yet, when mothers across Canada have attempted to breastfeed in public, they have faced discrimination. For example, some mothers have been asked to stop feeding their infant or to continue to feed in a "private" area such as a public bathroom (Photo 16.1). Breastfeeding campaigns across North America are moving to bring this issue to light in order to promote social justice for mothers and babies and to change the culture of how breastfeeding is viewed.

Over the past 150 years, Canadian mothers have faced the medicalization of pregnancy and birth, where the biomedical model of being cared for by a physician, often in a tertiary care centre or doctors' office, has been considered the "gold standard" of care for women and their children. For mothers who require close medical supervision, physicians, obstetricians, and tertiary care centres are the best choice. In Canada, the majority of women received their prenatal care from an obstetrician and gynecologist (58%) or a family physician (34%). Approximately 7% of women received their prenatal care from a midwife or nurse/nurse practitioner (PHAC, 2009a). Midwives provide a holistic model of care, which promotes normal birth, enables women and their families to make informed choices, and provides continuity of care and support throughout the childbearing experience at births in hospitals, birth centres, and at home. However, in 2009 nearly all births (97.9%) occurred in hospitals or clinics, with only 2% taking place in a private home or in a birthing centre (PHAC, 2009a). Midwives support traditional birthing practices—such as water births and the natural delivery of the placenta, for example—which had been lost within the modern medical system (Canadian Association of

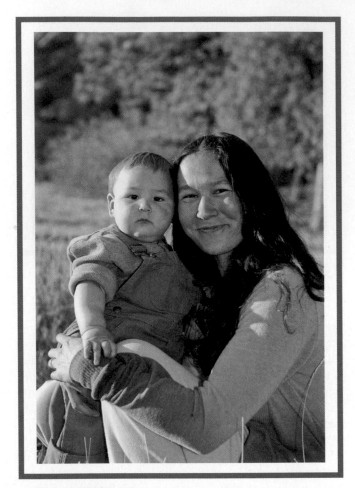

Midwives, 2014). Receiving medicalized prenatal/birth care and information about fundamentals of childcare, such as breastfeeding, from medical professionals can send the message to mothers that, even though mothering should be a very natural and safe process, it must be monitored by healthcare professionals.

The concept of mothering and how to become a mother is not a uniformly held belief across Canada. Aboriginal, First Nation, Inuit, and Métis cultures all hold traditional beliefs about how women become mothers, what is expected of mothers, and how families and communities work together to raise children and support families. Traditionally, in many Aboriginal, First Nation, Inuit, and Métis communities, pregnant women and mothers are supported by the entire community, provided with healthy foods, supported to be physically active, and cared for spiritually through prayers and traditional ceremonies that have been passed down through the millennia.

"A Saulteaux Elder describes how in the past, the whole community celebrated pregnancy: Everybody knew about it. Everybody wanted to be part and parcel of that child within that womb. [The child] had to have a sense of belonging through the mother, and the woman had to have a sense of pride because she was

contributing to the life of the community. She was bringing in new life, and she was treated special." (Excerpt from Until Our Hearts Are On The Ground: Aboriginal Mothering, Oppression, Resistance And Rebirth by D.M. Lavell-Harvard and J. Corbiere Lavell in Journal of Comparative Family Studies, Vol. 39, No. 2. Published by Journal of Comparative Family Studies, © 2013.)

Colonization and the dominance of the biomedical model have resulted in many Aboriginal, First Nation, Inuit, and Métis women receiving prenatal care and giving birth in non-traditional settings that do not support sacred and traditional practices. Many First Nation communities are isolated, requiring women and families to travel great distances to receive prenatal care or to give birth, and traditional, community-based midwives were eliminated due to the imposed belief that giving birth in a hospital and being attended by a physician is safer (Browne, McDonald, & Elliott, 2009). As a result, Aboriginal, First Nation, Inuit, and Métis traditional practices surrounding pregnancy, mothering, and giving birth have been lost from many tertiary care centres in Canada. However, many communities across Canada are taking up grassroots initiatives and political advocacy to bring social justice to women of childbearing age within Aboriginal, Frist Nation, Inuit, and Métis communities. From the education of a new generation of midwives from within First Nations communities to the creation of birthing centres in large urban cities in Canada that enable urban First Nation women to deliver in a home-like setting, attended by an Aboriginal midwife, health-promotion activities are recognizing the importance of supporting a positive, culturally sensitive, and safe transition to motherhood. (See Photo 16.2). Think about how such initiatives align with the seven CHNC (2011, revised) Standards of Practice.

## CANADIAN RESEARCH BOX 16.1

### Does disaster-related stress during pregnancy impact the motor function of the child?

Cao, X., Laplante, D., Brunet, A., Ciampi, A., & King, S. (2012). Prenatal maternal stress affects motor function in 5½-year-old children: Project ice storm. *Developmental Psychology, 56,* 117–125. doi:10.1002/dev.21085

The impact of maternal stress on the fetal development of children has been studied over the past several decades. Both animal and human research has shown that maternal stress may have an impact on the cognitive development of infants and children. However, there has been little work on connecting the impact of maternal stress to the motor function of infants and children. Since 1980 in Canada, there have been 81 events that have been classified as natural disasters, including wildfires, floods, storms, and extreme temperatures. Yet this statistic does not represent the local disasters that mothers and their families may face, such as localized building or home fires, nor does it take into account events that may impact a smaller number of women in a very local area. In 1998, the province of Quebec faced an ice storm of a large magnitude, resulting in a natural disaster that had never been seen before in the province's history. At the same time as the Quebec ice storm, there were a relatively large number of pregnant women living within the affected areas of the province. Since the ice storm had precise parameters—for example, the exact dates of the storm were known, along with the areas of power outages—the authors were able to identify the exact week(s) of exposure of higher levels of stress and link this data directly back to a week in the pregnancy of the mothers in their study. Ultimately, the authors' goal was to "determine the exact extent to which disaster-related objective and/or subjective maternal stress predicted motor functioning in the . . . cohort of children at 5½ years . . ." (p. 118). The study participants included 87 children (42 boys and 47 girls) whose mothers were in the first, second, or third trimester of their pregnancy on January 9, 1998, the height of the worst conditions of the ice storm.

The authors discovered that high levels of both subjective (perceived) and objective (measurable) maternal stress while pregnant were associated with lower motor scores on two-thirds of the motor assessment tests of the preschool children. The results indicated that both subjective and objective maternal stresses may have impacted the children's motor functioning. However, it appears from the research data that it may be the subjective stress of mothers that has a greater impact on the overall motor function of their children. The authors also concluded that female fetuses may experience a higher risk of being impacted by increased levels of maternal cortisol (stress hormone) than the male fetuses.

This research study highlights the complexity of fetal development and its relationship to maternal stress. While the effect of a higher socioeconomic status had been shown to be positively correlated to better overall motor function of children (Venetsanou & Kambas, 2010), there continues to be a knowledge gap among practitioners about the direct or indirect impact of maternal stress in disaster situations or in situations where mothers subjectively perceive their situation as extremely stressful. CHNs need to be aware of the impact that adverse events can have on maternal stress levels, and recognize that intervening to reduce maternal stress may be necessary in order to ensure optimal motor development of the unborn child.

### Discussion Questions

1. Aside from natural disasters, what other situations can you identify that may increase stress levels during pregnancy?

2. How do the social determinants of health impact a pregnant woman's stress level?

3. If you were going to set up a stress reduction program for pregnant women in your community, what areas would you want to focus on for the women you care for? What unique strengths and challenges does your community have that a CHN could address?

# INDICATORS OF MATERNAL HEALTH IN CANADA

There are many indicators of the status of maternal health in Canada. This section briefly examines only two of the commonly found indicators used to examine maternal health in Canada. For a complete list, along with supporting statistics and discussion, please access the "Perinatal Health Indicators Report" (PHAC, 2013).

## Breastfeeding

**Breastfeeding** is considered the normal and best method of infant feeding, and the WHO (2014g) recommends that all infants be exclusively breastfed for the first six months (180 days) of life. There are numerous benefits, both long and short term, for the mother and her infant. The benefits of breastfeeding for mothers include a measure of protection against breast cancer and ovarian cancer, protection against weak bones later in life, cost effectiveness, and portability, allowing breastfeeding to be done anywhere and supporting mothers to be active as their children grow (PHAC, 2009b). The long-term disadvantages of not breastfeeding are becoming increasingly recognized as significant. Yet, there are women who either do not initiate breastfeeding or who are not able to continue breastfeeding through to the recommended age of six months. Breastfeeding initiation rates in Canada, in 2009–2010, ranged from 61.5% in Newfoundland and Labrador to 97.2% in the Yukon. The rates of breastfeeding initiation are lower in the east and steadily increase as you move west across Canada (PHAC, 2013). The rates of exclusive breastfeeding for at least six months after birth in Canada increased from 20.3% in 2005 to 25.9% in 2009–2010 (PHAC, 2013). As shown in Figure 16.4,

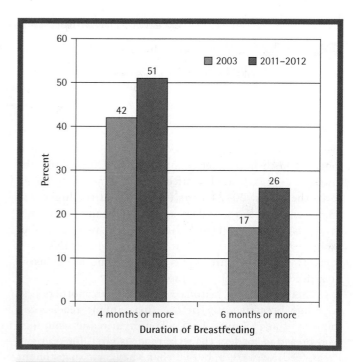

**FIGURE  16.4**  Rates of Exclusive Breastfeeding for Four Months or More and Six Months or More in Canada 2003, 2011–2012

*Source:* Statistics Canada. (2003; 2011–2012). *Canadian Community Health Survey. Breastfeeding Trends in Canada.* Retrieved from http://www.statcan.gc.ca/pub/82-624-x/2013001/article/11879-eng.htm

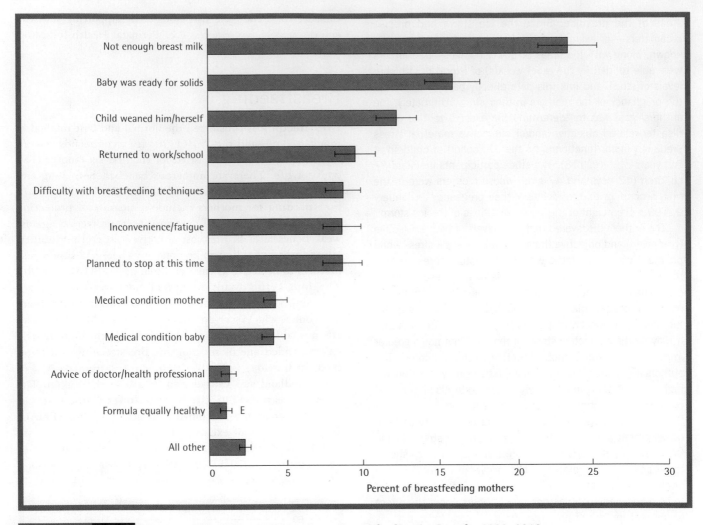

**FIGURE 16.5** Reasons Why Women Discontinue Breastfeeding in Canada, 2009–2010

*Source:* Statistics Canada. (2012). *Canadian Community Health Survey, 2009–2010.* Adapted and reproduced with permission from the Minister of Health, 2015. Retrieved from http://www.hc-sc.gc.ca/fn-an/surveill/nutrition/commun/prenatal/exclusive-exclusif-eng.php

over the past decade, older mothers exclusively breastfed longer than their younger counterparts. In 2009–2010, the lowest rates of exclusive breastfeeding at six months belonged to mothers aged 20–24 years (13.8%), and the highest at 33.3% and 28.4% to mothers aged 35–39 and 40 years and over, respectively (PHAC, 2013). These percentages of exclusive breastfeeding are less than ideal and CHNs must actively support initiatives that promote exclusive breastfeeding for the first six months of life.

There are many reasons why Canadian mothers discontinue breastfeeding before their infant reaches six months of age (Figure 16.5). The main reasons mothers who breastfed for less than six months cited for quitting breastfeeding were a belief that they had insufficient breast milk (44%) and difficulties with their breastfeeding technique (18%) (Gionet, 2012). Additionally, babies who consume other liquids and solids before the recommended initiation at six months tend to breastfeed less. In 2011–2012, 76% of mothers who breastfed exclusively for six months (or more) had post-secondary education,

compared with the mothers who breastfed less than six months (partially or exclusively) or those mothers who did not breastfeed at all (Gionet, 2012). Furthermore, mothers who are older and have higher education levels are more likely to initiate and continue with breastfeeding. CHNs are in an ideal position to use the information about why mothers may choose not to initiate breastfeeding (or the reasons for discontinuing breastfeeding) to implement various interventions that promote breastfeeding-friendly environments.

## Smoking in Pregnancy

It is well researched that smoking is harmful to the health of individuals and their family members. Smoking in pregnancy not only impacts the mother, but it directly impacts the fetus. When mothers smoke during their pregnancy, their fetus is exposed to dangerous chemicals like nicotine, carbon monoxide, and tar, which can result in the fetus receiving less oxygen and directly impacting growth and development (March of Dimes, 2014). Women who smoke in pregnancy are more likely to be younger, to be of lower socioeconomic status, and not to have attended a post-secondary educational institution (PHAC, 2009a). It is important for CHNs to identify women who are ready to quit smoking and provide relevant information about how to access smoking cessation programs. Maternal smoking while breastfeeding has been linked to early weaning, lowered milk production, and inhibition of the milk ejection ("let-down") reflex (La Leche League International, 2013). However, the risks of not breastfeeding even though mother smokes outweigh the risks (to mother and infant) of not breastfeeding at all. It is important to convey the following illness prevention information related to smoking:

- a smoke-free home environment should be encouraged for pregnant and breastfeeding women in order to avoid exposure to second-hand smoke. During pregnancy and breastfeeding, behavioural and cognitive therapies are recommended as first-line treatment for smoking cessation;
- partners, friends, and family members should also be offered smoking cessation interventions;
- nicotine levels in breast milk are halved about 97 minutes after a cigarette. The longer the time between smoking a cigarette and breastfeeding, the less nicotine the baby will be exposed to through breast milk; and
- do not smoke in the house or in the car. Keep the area around baby as smoke free as possible. Do not allow anyone else to smoke near your infant (Australian Breastfeeding Association, 2012).

# HEALTH PROMOTION AND DISEASE PREVENTION: TEENAGE MOTHERHOOD

## Teenage Pregnancy: An Introduction

Trends in teenage pregnancy over time are a significant marker of young women's sexual and reproductive health as well as overall well-being (McKay, 2013). According to the WHO (2014h), approximately 16 million females, aged 15–19 years, give birth each year constituting approximately 11% of all births worldwide. Ninety-five percent of these births take place in both low- and middle-income countries. Overall, the average adolescent birth rate in middle-income countries is almost 100% higher than high-income countries, with the birth rate among teenaged girls in low-income countries being five times higher when compared to high-income countries (WHO, 2014g). Although the majority of teenage pregnancies occur in low-income countries, there are approximately one million babies born annually to teenage mothers in high-income countries (Shrim et al., 2011). In Canada, 40 000 teenaged girls become pregnant every year with 20 000 of them terminating their pregnancies, and roughly 20 000 give birth (see Table 16.7). Teenagers, in Canada, may be more likely to become pregnant if they are of a lower socioeconomic status, are from an Aboriginal background, are the children of teen mothers, or if they experience barriers to accessing education and birth control services (Luong, 2014). Pregnant adolescents often experience unique challenges during pregnancy and after childbirth. Pregnant teenagers are at higher risk of obstetric complications, including anemia, toxemia, eclampsia, and hypertension (Al-Sahab, Heifetz, Tamim, Bohr, & Connolly, 2012). Furthermore, infants of adolescent mothers are at two times higher risk of being of low birth weight or born premature.

| Table 16.7 | Number and Percent of Live Births in Teenagers by Year across Canada (Excluding Ontario) | | | | | | |
|---|---|---|---|---|---|---|---|
| | 10–14 years | | 15–17 years | | 18–19 years | | |
| Year | Number of Live births | Percent of Total Live Births | Number of Live Births | Percent of Total Live Births | Number of Live Births | Percent of Total Live Births | Total Number of Live Births** |
| 2001 | 90 | 0.04 | 3443 | 1.7 | 7942 | 3.9 | 202 020 |
| 2002 | 100 | 0.05 | 3089 | 1.5 | 7569 | 3.8 | 200 263 |
| 2003 | 82 | 0.04 | 2900 | 1.4 | 7242 | 3.5 | 204 265 |
| 2004 | 90 | 0.04 | 2879 | 1.4 | 6875 | 3.4 | 204 500 |
| 2005 | 95 | 0.05 | 2784 | 1.3 | 6774 | 3.3 | 208 399 |
| 2006 | 99 | 0.05 | 2943 | 1.3 | 7030 | 3.2 | 218 993 |
| 2007 | 94 | 0.04 | 3147 | 1.4 | 7378 | 3.2 | 229 401 |
| 2008 | 110 | 0.05 | 3173 | 1.3 | 7599 | 3.2 | 237 049 |
| 2009 | 80 | 0.03 | 3237 | 1.3 | 7636 | 3.2 | 240 408 |
| 2010 | 75 | 0.03 | 2933 | 1.2 | 7107 | 3.0 | 237 538 |

** Excludes live births to mothers ≥50 years and those with unknown maternal age.
Source: Public Health Agency of Canada. (2013). *Perinatal health indicators for Canada 2013: A report from the Canadian perinatal surveillance system*. Ottawa, ON: Author. Adapted and reproduced with permission from the Minister of Health, 2015. Retrieved from http://publications.gc.ca/collections/collection_2014/aspc-phac/HP7-1-2013-eng.pdf

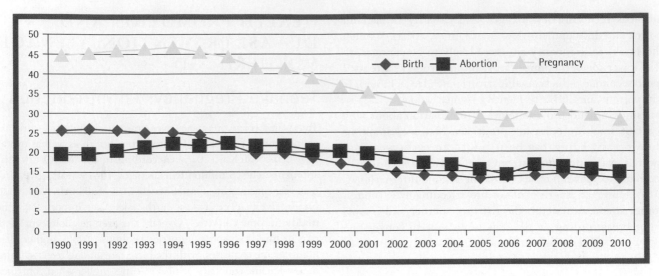

**FIGURE   16.6**   Birth/Abortion/Pregnancy Rates per 1000, Canada, Ages 15–19, 1990–2010

*Source:* Community Health Nursing, 4e. Copyright © 2010 by Sex Information and Education Council of Canada. *The Canadian Journal of Human Sexuality.* Used by permission of Sex Information and Education Council of Canada.

While childbearing is often initiated at an earlier age in various parts of the world, rates of teenage pregnancy in Canada have decreased steadily from 2001 to 2010 (see Table 16.7). Figure 16.6 represents the long-term trends of teenage pregnancy, abortion, and birth rates in Canada from 1990 to 2010 in girls aged 15–19 years. At a basic level, collecting and monitoring trends in teenage pregnancy rates can provide an indication of changing levels of effective contraceptive use among sexually active young women and their partners (McKay, 2013). Levels of effective contraceptive use among adolescents are determined by factors such as access to effective and affordable contraception, reproductive health services, and high-quality sexual health education. At a broader level, monitoring trends in teenage pregnancy rates can also reveal changes in population demographics and community sociocultural, norms, values, attitudes, and beliefs related to adolescent sexuality and teenage childbearing.

## Teenage Motherhood and the Social Determinants of Health

There are a variety of ways in which the social determinants of health impact teen parenthood. This section is meant to provide you with a general discussion about some of these ways. With respect to income and social status, Al-Sahab et al. (2012) examined the prevalence and characteristics of adolescent pregnancy in Canada. The authors of this study found that when compared to average-aged mothers, adolescent childbearing is more common in teenagers who are of lower socioeconomic status; come from non-immigrant families; have no partner; come from Saskatchewan, Manitoba, and Alberta; and have experienced physical or sexual abuse, or both. In addition, teenage mothers are less likely to complete high school or post-secondary education (Luong, 2014). Lastly, children of teen mothers have higher rates of becoming teen parents themselves, perpetuating the cycle of teen pregnancy (Ontario Ministry of Health & Long-Term Care, 2012).

While it is important to note that teenage mothers are twice as likely to experience postpartum depression as adult mothers are, teen mothers also report having more social support during and after pregnancy than adult mothers (Kim, Connolly, & Tamim, 2014). However, it is well known that children born to adolescent mothers are more likely to engage in juvenile delinquency, to be less successful in school, and to be at greater risk of violence and neglect (Sen & Ariizumi, 2014). Not surprisingly, Sen and Ariizumi (2014) have discovered a positive correlation between increasing minimum wage and teen pregnancy rates. The higher minimum wage may be associated with greater increases in average earnings in male teens, relative to females, leading to family formation. Sen and Ariizumi also found that higher minimum wage may result in a higher birth rate for married, versus unmarried, teenagers. Adolescent mothers are more likely to be smokers either before they get pregnant, while they are pregnant, or after they give birth (PHAC, 2009a). Tackling teenage smoking as a community health nurse requires that the CHN examine the broad social determinants of health and social influences that surround teenage mothers (see box titled "Tobacco and Alcohol Use of Teenage Girls during Pregnancy and Postpartum Period in Canada"). In summary, there are a variety of ways in which the social determinants of health impact adolescent parents and their children. If this area is of interest to you, we invite you to conduct a review of the literature to help you understand how the social determinants of health impact teenage parents and their offspring.

## Teenage Women and Smoking: Health Promotion and Prevention

While smoking among teenagers in Canada has been on the decline over the past decade, it is interesting to note that a higher proportion of female adolescents smoke (24.4%) when compared to their male counterparts (22.2%) (Bottorff et al.,

2014). Smoking rates are often found to be significantly higher within specific vulnerable populations. For example, 46% of Aboriginal women aged 13 to 18 years reported smoking (Bottorff et al., 2014). Internationally, we see that rural adolescent women who are pregnant have higher rates of smoking than their non-pregnant counterparts, and that smoking may increase in the first and third trimesters.

The federal, provincial, and municipal governments in Canada have taken an active role in implementing smoking prevention programs targeting adolescents and young adults. Multifaceted primary prevention programs include media campaigns and in-school education programs. Additionally, there are active efforts to create the new normal of a tobacco-free lifestyle by preventing the promotion of tobacco at venues and events that appeal to young people, such as organized sports (Canadian Partnership Against Cancer, 2014). In 2009, policy makers in Ontario introduced legislation that prohibits smoking in a motor vehicle when a child is present. Under this law, any driver or passenger smoking in a motor vehicle while someone under the age of 16 is present is committing an offence and can be fined $125 (Ontario Ministry of Health & Long-Term Care, 2013). The use of modern media tools like Facebook has enabled campaigns such as "Quit the Denial," which compares social smoking at parties to activities such as social farting (www.youtube.com/watch?v=w8762zEOkSo). Opening space to promote an anti-smoking social marketing campaign in

### CASE STUDY

You are a CHN working to provide postpartum care services to new mothers and their families. You are visiting the home of a family who has just arrived in Canada from Southeast Asia. While the mother is friendly and keen to interact with you, you notice that there are language barriers. While it appears that the mother understands what you are saying, you are unsure if she fully understands the messages you are trying to convey. She tells you that while she has one cousin in the city it takes over an hour to commute to his house by public transportation. In addition, many of her immediate family members do not live in Canada. While she receives some support over the phone, she indicates that she feels alone much of the time. When you arrive back at your community health centre, in discussions with a few colleagues you realize that this is a pattern that you are seeing in one quadrant of the city.

#### Discussion Questions

1. Which of the determinants of health would you want to consider in your community health nursing interventions?
2. Based on your responses to Question 1 above, what CHN interventions might you consider implementing?
3. Based on the perceived language barriers, how might you ensure that the messages you are trying to convey are received as intended?

### TOBACCO AND ALCOHOL USE OF TEENAGE GIRLS DURING PREGNANCY AND POSTPARTUM PERIOD IN CANADA

- Teenage girls are more likely than women of older ages to smoke, drink alcohol, and binge drink during pregnancy.
- There are important health-related consequences of smoking and/or drinking on maternal, fetal, and infant health.
- Teenage girls who smoke cigarettes pre-pregnancy are more likely to relapse during the postpartum period and becoming life-long smokers.
- There are few examples of gender-informed prevention and treatment programs to prevent and reduce alcohol and tobacco use among teenage girls, despite this being strongly encouraged.
- There is a clear need for effective and integrated approaches to prevent and reduce alcohol and tobacco use among teenage girls pre-pregnancy, during pregnancy, and postpartum.
- Approaches must consider the influence of partner and friends on cigarette smoking and alcohol consumption in a sensitive and culturally safe manner.

*Source:* Bottorff et al. (2014). Tobacco and alcohol use in the context of adolescent pregnancy and postpartum: A scoping review of the literature. *Health and Social Care in the Community,* 2(6), 561–574. Copyright © 2014 by U.S. National Library of Medicine.

places that are frequented by Canadian youth is intended to prevent young people from taking up smoking in the first place. Various programs are available that are aimed at smoking prevention, reduction, and cessation among teenagers and teenage mothers. CHNs play a pivotal role in identifying, supporting, and connecting teenage women and mothers to the most appropriate primary, secondary, or tertiary smoking cessation programs in each case.

## INFANT AND EARLY CHILD HEALTH IN CANADA

Infancy and early childhood (up to four years of age) is a critical period of time for healthy growth and development. While infants, toddlers, and preschool children in Canada generally have better health than their counterparts in various other countries around the world, the health of Canada's children when compared with other developed countries "is mediocre at best" (Raphael, 2014, p. 220). The health of Canada's children is closely linked to their social determinants of health, which are of generally lower quality than those of other developed countries (Raphael, 2014). It is important for children to be healthy and have access to health-promotion strategies, as this sets the foundation for the rest of their lives (Beaglehole et al., 2014). Currently there is no central Canadian agency responsible for tracking the health of children; independent researchers have taken up this challenge (Raphael, 2012), a situation that makes it difficult to identify trends (or changes in trends) of infant and early childhood health in Canada.

One important key indicator of child health is the **infant mortality rate**. It is worrisome that Canada's infant mortality rate ranked 10th among 24 OECD (Organisation for Economic Co-operation and Development) countries in 1980 (Robert Wood Johnson Foundation, 2008), and dropped even further down the list to 27th of 36 countries in 2010, a span of just three decades (Organisation for Economic Co-operation and Development, 2011). Clearly, our challenges in Canada are unique, and the social determinants of child health must be taken into account. In Table 16.8, indicators of **child well-being** are presented. In this section, an overview of current health status indicators for infants, toddlers, and preschool children is presented. We will also discuss current health challenges of infants, toddlers, and preschool children with respect to sudden infant death syndrome, breastfeeding, nutrition, obesity, and intended and unintended injuries. While the topic of immunizations is also relevant to this discussion, Chapter 12, Communicable Diseases, presents an in-depth discussion of immunizations.

The term "infants" is used to describe babies who are in the 0–12 months age range. The Canadian Perinatal Surveillance System (CPSS) is used to capture current information on major maternal, fetal, and infant health determinants and outcomes in Canada. Please refer to Table 16.2 to compare and contrast specific terms that are often used in discussions about infant health. In Figure 16.7, the infant, neonatal, and post-neonatal mortality rates are presented by province or territory. The main causes of infant deaths are immaturity (29.4%), congenital anomalies (22%), asphyxia (10.4%), infection (6.5%), and sudden infant death syndrome (SIDS) (6.4%). The remainder of infant deaths (25.3%) are unexplained (PHAC, 2013). Lower socioeconomic status and lower levels of neighbourhood income have been found to be associated with a higher risk of adverse perinatal health outcomes, particularly infant mortality (de Graff, 2013). Aboriginal populations have historically had poor health outcomes relative to non-Aboriginal peoples. A similar trend has been observed in infant health. Luo et al. (2010) have observed that in urban areas, First Nations infants fare more poorly than non-Aboriginal populations. In contrast, rural residence, regardless of degree of isolation, appears to be a protective factor against preterm birth, small for gestational age, and low birth weight for both Aboriginal and non-Aboriginal populations.

| Table 16.8 | How We Measure Child Well-Being | |
|---|---|---|
| **Dimensions** | **Components** | **Indicators** |
| Dimension 1: Material well-being | Monetary deprivation | Relative child poverty rate |
| | | Relative child poverty gap |
| | Material deprivation | Child deprivation rate |
| | | Low family affluence rate |
| Dimension 2: Health and safety | Health at birth | Infant mortality rate |
| | | Low birthweight rate |
| | Preventive health services | Overall immunization rate |
| | Childhood mortality | Child death rate, age 1 to 19 |
| Dimension 3: Education | Participation | Participation rate: early childhood education |
| | | Participation rate: further education, age 15–19 |
| | | NEET rate (% age 15–19 not in education, employment or training) |
| | Achievement | Average PISA scores in reading, maths and science |
| Dimension 4: Behaviours and risks | Health behaviours | Being overweight |
| | | Eating breakfast |
| | | Eating fruit |
| | | Taking exercise |
| | Risk behaviours | Teenage fertility rate |
| | | Smoking |
| | | Alcohol |
| | | Cannabis |
| | Exposure to violence | Fighting |
| | | Being bullied |
| Dimension 5: Housing and environment | Housing | Rooms per person |
| | | Multiple housing problems |
| | Environmental safety | Homicide rate |
| | | Air pollution |

Sources: From Raphael, D. (2014). Social determinants of children's health in Canada: Analysis and implications. *International Journal of Child, Youth and Family Studies*, 5(2), 220–239; Innocenti Research Centre (2013). Child well-being in rich countries: A comparative overview, Box 1, p. 5. Florence: Innocenti Research Centre.

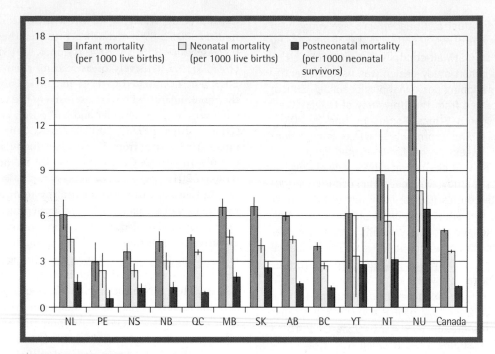

**FIGURE 16.7** Rate of Infant, Neonatal, and Post-Neonatal Mortality by Province or Territory, Canada (Excluding Ontario), 2005–2009

*Source:* Public Health Agency of Canada. (2013). *Perinatal health indicators for Canada 2013: A report from the Canadian perinatal surveillance system.* Ottawa, ON: Author. Adapted and reproduced with permission from the Minister of Health, 2015. Retrieved from http://publications.gc.ca/collections/collection_2014/aspc-phac/HP7-1-2013-eng.pdf

## Sudden Infant Death Syndrome (SIDS)

In 1992, the American Academy of Pediatrics released a statement recommending that all healthy infants be placed to sleep on their backs (American Academy of Pediatrics Task Force on Infant Positioning and SIDS, 1992). Canada followed suit in February 1999, when the Canadian Foundation for the Study of Infant Deaths, the Canadian Paediatric Society, and the Canadian Institute for Child Health released a joint statement entitled "Reducing the Risk of Sudden Infant Death Syndrome (SIDS) in Canada." The current version of the statement recommends that all healthy infants be placed to sleep on their backs (in the supine position) (Government of Canada, Canadian Paediatric Society, Canadian Institute of Child Health, & Canadian Foundation for the Study of Infant Deaths, 2011). There is compelling evidence indicating that the **SIDS** rate has decreased with the introduction of the "Back to Sleep" campaign. SIDS mortality in Canada decreased from 144 deaths (26% of all post-neonatal deaths) in 1999 to 76 deaths (18% of all post-neonatal deaths) in 2004 (Smylie & Sauvé, 2009). While the benefit of supine sleeping is reduced infant mortality, it is not without consequences. In the last decade, the supine sleep position has been thought to contribute to an increase in **positional plagiocephaly** across Canada (Dubé & Flake, 2003; Neufeld & Birkett, 2000). The first population-based incidence study of positional plagiocephaly was conducted in Calgary, Alberta, where the incidence of positional plagiocephaly was estimated at 46.6% (Mawji, Robinson Vollman, Hatfield, McNeil, & Sauvé, 2013) (see

Canadian Research Box 16.2). Although infant mortality related to SIDS has decreased overall, Gilbert, Auger, Wilkins, & Kramer (2013) have found higher rates of neonatal deaths, post-neonatal deaths, and SIDS deaths in lower-income neighbourhoods across Canada. While Canada has experienced significant gains in infant health over the past decade, inequalities in infant health continue to persist across the country.

---

**CANADIAN RESEARCH BOX 16.2**

**What are the risk factors for developing positional plagiocephaly in infants aged 7–12 weeks?**

Mawji, A., Robinson Vollman, A., Fung, T., Hatfield, J., McNeil, D. A., & Sauvé, R. (2014). Risk factors for positional plagiocephaly and appropriate timeframes for prevention messaging. *Paediatrics and Child Health, 19*(8), 423–427.

Plagiocephaly is defined as a deformation of the skull producing the appearance of a lopsided head. If this condition is not identified and treated early, the associated changes in skull shape and facial features can be permanent. Minimal literature exists on what the risk factors are for developing positional plagiocephaly. We also know that risk factors vary by infant age. When this idea for a research project was being developed, there were two published studies that addressed the risk factors for developing positional plageiocephaly in infants aged 6–7 weeks. The objective of this study was to identify risk factors for developing positional plagiocephaly in infants 7–12 weeks of age in Calgary, Alberta, Canada. This age range was selected because it is during this time that they are seen by a public health nurse at well-child immunization clinics.

A prospective cohort study design was used to identify risk factors for developing positional plagiocephaly. Ethical approval was received from the University of Calgary Conjoint Health Research Ethics Board on June 3, 2010. Healthy full-term infants (born at ≥37 weeks of gestation) ranging from 7–12 weeks of age that presented for immunization at two-month well-child clinics in the city of Calgary, were included in the study. Data collection occurred in four community health centres (CHCs) from July to September 2010. Each CHC was situated in one quadrant of the city, increasing the likelihood that the results would be representative of the larger population in Calgary. The incidence of positional plagiocephaly was estimated to be 46.6%. The following risk factors were identified using multiple logistic regression: right-sided head positional preference (OR 4.66 [95% CI 2.85 to 7.58]; $P < 0.001$), left-sided head positional preference (OR 4.21 [95% CI 2.45 to 7.25]; $P < 0.001$), supine sleep position (OR 2.67 [95% CI 1.58 to 4.51]; $P < 0.001$), vacuum/forceps assisted delivery (OR 1.88 [95% CI 1.02 to 3.49]; $P = 0.04$), M and male sex (OR 1.55 [95% CI 1.00 to 2.38]; $P = 0.05$).

### Discussion Questions

1. Based on the risk factors that were identified in this study, what prevention messaging could you provide?

2. Since the incidence of positional plagiocephaly was found to be 46.6% in infants attending the two-month well-child immunization appointments, when would be an ideal time for parents or guardians to hear messaging about how to prevent positional plagiocephaly?

3. Which of the seven CHNC (2011, revised) Standards of Practice would prevention messaging align with and why?

## Infant–Toddler Nutrition

"Breast milk is custom made by each mother for her own baby, and contains the perfect amount of protein, carbohydrate, fat, vitamins and minerals" (PHAC, 2009b, p. 3). As the infant grows, breast milk also changes in order to meet the infant's nutritional needs. Breast milk is known to have both short-term and long-term benefits for infants and children. Short-term benefits include protection against various infectious diseases in infancy, including acute otitis media, gastroenteritis and diarrhea, severe lower respiratory infections, and SIDS (Rennick Salone, Vann, & Dee, 2013). Long-term benefits include protection against obesity (Rennick Salone et al., 2013) and enhanced cognitive development (Quigley et al., 2012). Furthermore, breast milk is easier to digest than formula (Gionet, 2013).

Although the infant benefits of breastfeeding are widely documented, the rates of exclusive breastfeeding at four to six months are sub-optimal in many countries, including

Canada (Cai, Wardlaw, & Brown, 2012; PHAC, 2009c). In 2011–2012, 89% of mothers breastfed their infant, a slight increase from 85% in 2003 (Gionet, 2013). More mothers (26%) were exclusively breastfeeding their infant in 2011–2012 when compared to 17% in 2003 (Gionet, 2013). Furthermore, infants who were exclusively breastfed had mothers who were 30 years or older and had post-secondary education (Gionet, 2013; PHAC, 2009c). Across Canada, breastfeeding rates varied widely from 57% in Newfoundland and Labrador to 96% in British Columbia and the Yukon in 2011–2012 (Gionet, 2013).

In Canada, **nutrition** for healthy term infants (up to six months of age) is organized around seven principles (Table 16.9), which may be classified as primary prevention initiatives. While exclusive breastfeeding from birth through six months is recommended, there may be instances due to personal, medical, or social reasons when the decision is made to use breast milk substitutes. The CHN must provide additional support so that parents and caregivers may make the best nutritional decisions for their infant(s). It is interesting to note that among formula-fed infants, introduction of solid foods before four months was associated with a six-fold increase in odds of obesity at age 3 years (Huh, Rifas-Shiman, Taveras, Oken, & Gillman, 2011). For example, formula-fed babies may be at a higher risk of being obese later in life (Oddy, 2012). Due to various instances in which the use of breast milk substitutes have caused infants harm, the International Code of Marketing of Breast-Milk Substitutes was developed by the WHO in 1981. This code protects and promotes breastfeeding by ensuring that marketing of breast milk substitutes is conducted in an ethical manner. The main points of this code are as follows:

- formula, bottles, artificial nipples, and pacifiers may not be advertised to the public;
- free samples of formula, bottles, artificial nipples, and pacifiers may not be offered to mothers directly from companies producing such products;
- healthcare facilities may not promote artificial feeding products, including the distribution of free or low-cost supplies;
- individuals working for companies producing artificial feeding products may not advise mothers about infant nutrition;
- individuals working for companies producing artificial feeding products may not offer gifts or personal samples to health workers;
- individuals working for companies producing artificial feeding products may not use words or pictures that idealize artificial feeding (including pictures of infants on the labels of products);
- all information coming from companies producing artificial feeding products should be scientific and factual;
- all information on artificial infant feeding, including labels, should explain the benefits of breastfeeding and the cost and hazards associated with artificial feeding;
- unsuitable products, such as sweetened condensed milk, should not be promoted for infants; and

| Table 16.9 | The Seven Principles and Recommendations of Nutrition for Healthy Term Infants' (0–6 Months) Nutrition | |
|---|---|---|
| **Number** | **Principle** | **Recommendations** |
| 1 | Breastfeeding is the normal and unequalled method of feeding infants. | Exclusive breastfeeding for the first 6 months is recommended. |
| 2 | Breastfeeding initiation and duration rates increase with active protection, support, and promotion. | Implement the policies and practices of the Baby-Friendly Initiative for hospitals and community health services. |
| 3 | Supplemental vitamin D is recommended for breastfed infants. | Recommend a daily vitamin D supplement of 10 µg (400 IU) for breastfed infants. |
| 4 | First complementary foods should be iron-rich. | Recommend meat, meat alternatives, and iron-fortified cereals as infant's first complementary foods. |
| 5 | Routine growth monitoring is important to assess infant's health and nutrition. | Use WHO growth charts for Canada for optimal monitoring of infant growth. |
| 6 | Feeding changes are unnecessary for most common health conditions in infancy. | Explain that feeding changes do little to manage infantile colic; educate about the wide variation in normal bowel function, noting that true constipation is rare; reassure that reflux or regurgitation is common and rarely needs treatment; manage mild to moderate dehydration from acute gastroenteritis with continued breastfeeding and oral rehydration therapy. |
| 7 | Breastfeeding is rarely contraindicated. | Recommend an acceptable alternative to breastfeeding for mothers who are HIV infected; advise that most medications are compatible with breastfeeding; take a case-by-case approach when a mother is using medications or drugs. |

Source: Critch, J. N., Canadian Pediatric Society Nutrition and Gastroenterology Committee. (2013). *Nutrition for healthy term infants, birth to 6 months: An overview*. Adapted and reproduced with permission from the Minister of Health, 2015. Retrieved from http://www.hc-sc.gc.ca/fn-an/nutrition/infant-nourisson/recom/index-eng.php

- all products marketed should be of high quality and take into account the climatic and storage conditions of the country where they are marketed (Breastfeeding Committee for Canada, 2012; WHO, 1981).

According to Health Canada (2014), cow milk–based infant formula is currently used as the standard formula for healthy term infants who are not exclusively breastfed. An assortment of cow milk–based formulas are found on the market, with different types of proteins (hydrolyzed or non-hydrolyzed), varying levels of iron, and even lactose-free formulas. Furthermore, infant formulas may also contain nucleotides, amino acids, and live micro-organisms. Infant formula selections also include soy-based formula and formulas manufactured for different medical purposes. It is important to note that animal milks, including cow and goat milk, are not suitable substitutes to breast milk for young infants (WHO, 2014i).

## Nutrition in Children Aged 6–24 Months

Breastfeeding that is continued for up to two years or longer, with appropriate complementary feeding, is important for the nutrition, immunologic protection, growth, and development of infants and toddlers (Health Canada, 2014). By about six months of age, infants are developmentally ready for other foods. The signs of this readiness include:

- improved head control;
- the capacity to sit up and lean forward;
- the ability to let the parent or caregiver know when they are full (e.g., turns head away); and
- the ability to pick up food and try to put it in their mouth.

From six to 12 months, older infants are able to meet their nutrition requirements with a combination of breast milk and complementary foods (Sanders & Schor, 2014). In 2011–2012, 26% of mothers in Canada breastfed exclusively for six months (or more), up from 17% in 2003 (Gionet, 2012). About 77% of mothers who breastfed exclusively for six months (or more) were aged 30 years and older and had completed post-secondary education (Gionet, 2012). From 12 to 24 months, an estimated one-third of a young child's energy can come from breastfeeding and the remaining two-thirds from complementary foods. At this stage, infants should be offered nutrient-dense and safe complementary foods, along with continued breastfeeding (Health Canada, Canadian Paediatric Society, Dietitians of Canada, & Breastfeeding Committee for Canada, 2014). The first foods introduced should be rich in iron. Unpasteurized cow or goat milk (raw milk) should never be offered to infants and young children due to the risk of food-borne illness from pathogens such *as salmonella, escherichia coli, campylobacter,* and *listeria monocytogenes* (Moore, Canadian Paediatric Society, & Infectious Diseases and Immunization Committee, 2008).

## Nutrition in Pre-School-Aged Children

Pre-school-aged children should be following Canada's Food Guide. Health Canada has since developed a publication specifically for Aboriginal peoples titled "Eating Well with Canada's Food Guide—First Nations, Inuit and Métis." This document considers food items that are culturally appropriate for our Aboriginal populations, including bannock and wild game (Langlois, Findlay, & Kohen, 2013). Very little information is available on the nutrition of pre-school children. Often this type of information for younger children is grouped together with that for school-aged children. For instance, one in five children aged one to eight years in Canada have a calorie intake that exceeds their daily calorie expenditure (Health Canada, 2012). Surprisingly, a significant portion of children aged one to three years old do not have the recommended fat intake, and there appears to be a general concern that children are not getting enough potassium or fibre (Health Canada, 2012).

The health of Canada's children is closely tied to the health of their parents. One's personal identity or **social location**—for example, gender, race, class, Aboriginal, immigrant, or disability status—influences our ability to access healthcare services (Anderson, 2011, as cited in Raphael, 2014). Where one is socially located is related to if, how, or when one may leverage power and influence in order to affect the distribution of economic and social resources that are significant to achieving health (Raphael, 2011). Raphael (2014) views the distribution of economic and social resources as the **social determinants of child health**. Children who come from poorer households are more likely to experience food insecurity. Childhood hunger is an extreme consequence of food insecurity and leads to inadequate dietary intake, resulting in poor health. Some factors that are related to child hunger include older child age, lone-parent households, large household size, low household income, and poor family dynamics (McIntyre, Bartoo, & Potestio, 2012). It is clear that health promotion programs that are related to childhood nutrition in Canada must focus on the broader determinants of health in order to greatly improve the nutrition, and thus health, of our preschool-aged children.

## Physical Activity

The early years represent a critical period for **child development** in terms of growth. It is during this time that active living habits, including healthy eating and physical activity, are established. Physical activity during the preschool years is associated with improved motor skill development as well as improved psychosocial health, cardiac health, and measures of adiposity (LeBlanc et al., 2012; Timmons et al., 2012).

Conversely, high levels of sedentary behaviour, including high levels of screen time, is associated with increased adiposity and lower measures of psychosocial and cognitive development. According to a recent study conducted by Colley et al. (2013), 84% of three- and four-year-olds across Canada met the current physical activity guidelines (defined as being active at any intensity for at least 180 minutes every day). However, only 18% of children aged three and four years met the screen-time recommendation within the sedentary behaviour guidelines, which states that children of this age should accumulate less than one hour of screen time per day. Interestingly, Colley et al. (2013) observed the opposite trend in five-year-old children, with 14% meeting their age-specific physical activity guideline and the majority (81%) meeting their screen-time recommendation.

## Injuries

**Childhood injuries** represent a significant public health problem in Canada (Soubhi, Raina, & Kohen, 2004). Injuries related to physical activity are the main reasons children present in emergency departments across the country (Molcho & Picket, 2011). There is currently a lack of documented evidence about statistical trends in injuries sustained in the zero to four years age group. However, evidence does exist regarding the causes of the injuries. For both males and females aged zero to four years, Kang, Emery, Senger, and Meeuwisse (2013) found that injuries were caused by playground equipment, bicycling, trampolines, swimming, and tobogganing. Consumer product–related injuries in young children include hazards associated with bunk beds (risks of falls and strangulation), magnets, baby walkers (falling while in a baby walker), and other household products. Injuries from household products were associated with trampolines, bath seats, dangling blind or curtain cords, furniture, appliances, and televisions (PHAC, 2012).

**Injury prevention**, an example of primary prevention, must entail a surveillance system (Kang et al., 2013). The Canadian Hospitals Injury Reporting and Prevention Program (CHIRPP) is a surveillance system that is currently in place in emergency departments of 16 hospitals in Canada. Surveillance systems give rise to epidemiologic information, which then can quantify the magnitude of injuries across various age groups. This information than may be used to develop and tailor various health promotion and injury prevention programs for specific regions, cities, and communities.

## CONCLUSION

The health of mothers and children is a priority for governments and healthcare providers globally. CHNs have the opportunity to play an integral role in promoting the health of some of the most vulnerable people. CHNs who care for mothers and children in Canada can advocate for evidence-informed healthcare strategies that promote health versus just mitigating or preventing illness or injury. CHNs are uniquely positioned to care for women and children within the community, enabling them to assess this population with an understanding of the socio-environmental influences that overtly and subtly shape health. CHNs also have an *ethical* responsibility to advocate for improved access to services that are culturally safe. CHNs across Canada can play an active role in advocating for the health and well-being of mothers and children globally. Women and children around the world deserve the same quality and timely care that their counterparts in Western countries receive.

## KEY TERMS

breastfeeding   p. 315
child development   p. 324
child well-being   p. 320
childhood injuries   p. 324
infant mortality rate   p. 320
injury prevention   p. 324
maternal health   p. 312
maternal healthcare   p. 311
maternal mortality rate   p. 311
maternal mortality ratio   p. 307
nutrition   p. 322
perinatal period   p. 312
positional plagiocephaly   p. 321
reproductive health   p. 312
reproductive justice   p. 312
reproductive rights   p. 312
SIDS   p. 321
social determinants of child health   p. 324
social location   p. 324

## STUDY QUESTIONS

1. Describe key indicators that influence maternal health.
2. Name one strategy that has been implemented to improve the health of women around the world.
3. Define the difference between reproductive rights and reproductive justice.
4. Name a few benefits of breastfeeding.
5. What are the seven principles and recommendations of nutrition for healthy term infants zero to six months of age?
6. By about six months of age, infants are developmentally ready for other foods. What are the signs of this readiness?

After working through these questions, go to the MyNursingLab at www.pearsoned.ca/mynursinglab to check your answers.

## INDIVIDUAL CRITICAL-THINKING EXERCISES

1. Visit the Public Health Agency of Canada Healthy Pregnancy Guidelines (www.phac-aspc.gc.ca/hp-gs/guide/index-eng.php) and compare the recommended guidelines to the resources that are being offered in your local area. Are there differences or similarities? Are there policies or programs in your area that offer unique guidelines based on the population that program/policy is trying to serve?

2. What is positional plagiocephaly and why is it important that we discuss this potential health issue with respect to infant health?
3. What is reproductive justice? What are the resources in your community that would support a client to have access to reproductive justice? What gaps in services exist in your community and how could a CHN help to fill that void?

## GROUP CRITICAL-THINKING EXERCISES

1. Assume your group is a team of CHNs that have been asked to develop a health promotion drop-in program aimed at pregnant teens in your community. What four main topic areas would your group propose as essential for pregnant teens to know about? What may be three barriers that your program could face in engaging this population?
2. Consider Table 16.8. Do you agree with the indicators that are being used to measure child well-being? Why do you think these indicators are being used? Discuss with your group any indicators you think should be added or removed and why.
3. Consider the concept of mothering. What responsibilities do CHNs have to ensure that women have a positive self-image as mothers? What cultural influences in your communities shape the idea of a "good mother"? What barriers do women face in getting support for positive mothering education and support?

## REFERENCES

Al-Sahab, B., Heifetz, M., Hamim, H., Bohr, Y., & Connolly, J. (2012). Prevalence and characteristics of teen motherhood in Canada. *Maternal and Child Health Journal, 16*(1), 228–234. doi:10.1007/s10995-011-0750-8

American Academy of Pediatrics Task Force on Infant Positioning and SIDS. (1992). Positioning and SIDS. *Pediatrics. 89*(6), 1120–1126.

Angus, J. E., Lombardo, A. P., Lowndes, R. H., Cechetto, N., Ahmad, F., & Bierman, F. (2012). Beyond barriers in studying disparities in women's access to health services in Ontario, Canada: A qualitative metasynthesis. *Qualitative Health Research, 23*(4), 476–494. doi:10.1177/1049732312469464

Asian Communities for Reproductive Justice. (2005). *A new vision for advancing our movement for reproductive rights, reproductive health, and reproductive justice.* Retrieved from http://strongfamiliesmovement.org/assets/docs/ACRJ-A-New-Vision.pdf

Australian Breastfeeding Association. (2012). Breastfeeding and smoking. Retrieved from https://www.breastfeeding.asn.au/bfinfo/breastfeeding-and-smoking

Beaglehole, R., Bonita, R., Ezzati, M., Alleyne, G., Dain, K., Kishore, S. P., & Horton, R. (2014). NCD countdown 2025: Accountability for the 25 × 25 NCD mortality reduction target. *Lancet, 384*(9938), 105–107. doi:10.1016/S0140-6736(14)61091-6

Breastfeeding Committee for Canada. (2012). Breastfeeding committee for Canada baby-friendly initiative. Retrieved from http://www.breastfeedingcanada.ca/documents/2012-05-14_BCC_BFI_Ten_Steps_Integrated_Indicators.pdf

Browne, A. J., McDonald, H., & Elliott, D. (2009). First Nations urban Aboriginal health research discussion paper: A report for the First Nations Centre, National Aboriginal Health Organization. Ottawa, ON: National Aboriginal Health Organization. Retrieved from http://www.naho.ca/documents/fnc/english/UrbanFirstNationsHealthResearchDiscussionPaper.pdf

Bottorff, J. L., Poole, N., Kelly, M. T., Greaves, L., Marcellus, L., & Jung, M. (2014). Tobacco and alcohol use in the context of adolescent pregnancy and postpartum: A scoping review of the literature. *Health and Social Care in the Community, 22*(6), 561–574. doi:10.1111/hsc.12091

Cai, X., Wardlaw, T., & Brown, D. W. (2012). Global trends in exclusive breastfeeding. *International Breastfeeding Journal, 7*, 12. Retrieved from http://www.internationalbreastfeedingjournal.com/content/7/1/12

Canadian Association of Midwives. (2014). *What is a Canadian midwife?* Retrieved from http://www.canadianmidwives.org/what-is-a-midwife.html

Canadian Institute of Health Information (2006). *Giving birth in Canada: The costs.* Ottawa, ON: Author. Retrieved from https://secure.cihi.ca/free_products/Costs_Report_06_Eng.pdf

Canadian Partnership against Cancer. (2014). *What we do.* Retrieved from http://www.partnershipagainstcancer.ca/what-we-do

Community Health Nurses of Canada. (2011, revised). *Canadian community health nursing: Professional practice model & standards of practice.* St. John's, NL: Author. Retrieved from https://www.chnc.ca/documents/CHNC-ProfessionalPracticeModel-EN/index.html

Centre for Addiction and Mental Health. (2011). *Smoking cessation knowledge exchange network & clinical practice guidelines.* Retrieved from https://www.nicotinedependenceclinic.com/English/CANADAPTT/Pages/Home.aspx

Colley, R. C., Garriguet, D., Adamo, K. B., Carson, V., Janssen, I., Timmons, B.W., & Tremblay, M. S. (2013). Physical activity and sedentary behaviour during the early years in Canada. *International Journal of Behavioral Nutrition and Physical Activity, 10*, 54. Retrieved from http://www.ijbnpa.org/content/10/1/54

de Graaf, J. P. (2013). Living in deprived urban districts increases perinatal health inequalities. *Journal of Maternal-Fetal and Neonatal Medicine, 26*(5), 473–481. doi:10.3109/14767058.2012.735722

Dubé, K., & Flake, M. L. (2003). Early prevention: Occipital flattening of positional origin. *Canadian Nurse, 99*(1), 16–21.

Gilbert, N. L., Auger, N., Wilkins, R., & Kramer, M. S. (2013). Neighbourhood income and neonatal, postneonatal, and sudden infant death syndrome (SIDS) mortality in Canada, 1991–2005. *Canadian Journal of Public Health, 104*(3), e187–e192.

Gionet, L. (2012). Statistics Canada: Breastfeeding trends in Canada. Retrieved from http://www.statcan.gc.ca/pub/82-624-x/2013001/article/11879-eng.htm

Gionet, L. (2013). Breastfeeding trends in Canada. *Health at a Glance.* November. Statistics Canada Catalogue no. 82-624-X.

Government of Canada–Foreign Affairs, Trade, and Development Canada. (2014). *Muskoka Initiative Partnership program.* Retrieved from http://www.pm.gc.ca/eng/news/2011/09/20/projects-under-muskoka-initiative-partnership-program

Government of Canada, Canadian Paediatric Society, Canadian Institute of Child Health, & Canadian Foundation for the Study of Infant Deaths. (2011). *Joint statement on safe sleep: Preventing sudden infant deaths in Canada.* Retrieved from

http://www.phac-aspc.gc.ca/hp-ps/dca-dea/stages-etapes/childhood-enfance_0-2/sids/pdf/jsss-ecss2011-eng.pdf

Health Canada. (2012). *Do Canadian children meet their nutrient requirement through food intake alone?* Ottawa, ON: Author. Retrieved from http://www.hc-sc.gc.ca/fn-an/alt_formats/pdf/surveill/nutrition/commun/art-nutr-child-enf-eng.pdf

Health Canada. (2014). *Nutrition for healthy term infants: Recommendations from birth to 6 months.* Ottawa, ON: Author. Retrieved from http://www.hc-sc.gc.ca/fn-an/nutrition/infant-nourisson/recom/index-eng.php#a5.4

Health Canada, Canadian Paediatric Society, Dietitians of Canada, & Breastfeeding Committee for Canada. (2014). *Nutrition for healthy term infants: Recommendations from 6–24 months.* Ottawa, ON: Author. Retrieved from http://www.hc-sc.gc.ca/fn-an/nutrition/infant-nourisson/recom/recom-6-24-months-6-24-mois-eng.php

Huh, S. Y., Rifas-Shiman, S. L., Taveras, E. M., Oken, E., & Gillman, M. W. (2011). Timing of solid food introduction and risk of obesity in preschool-aged children. *Pediatrics, 127*(3), e544-e551. doi:10.1542/peds.2010-0740

Kang, J., Emery, C. A., Senger, T., & Meeuwisse, W. (2013). Assessing the representativeness of Canadian Hospitals Injury Reporting and Prevention Programme (CHIRPP) sport and recreational injury data in Calgary, Canada. *International Journal of Injury Control and Safety Promotion, 20*(1), 19–26. doi:http://dx.doi.org/10.1080/17457300.2012.656315

Kim, T. H. M., Connolly, J., & Tamim, H. (2014). The effect of social support around pregnancy on postpartum depression among Canadian teen mothers and adult mothers in the Canadian Maternity Experiences Survey. *BioMed Central Pregnancy and Childbirth, 14*, 162. Retrieved from http://www.biomedcentral.com/1471-2393/14/162

La Leche League International. (2013). Breastfeeding and lifestyle choices. Retrieved from http://www.lalecheleague.org/nb/nblifestyle.html

Langlois, K. A., Findlay, L. C., & Kohen, D. E. (2013). *Dietary habits of Aboriginal children.* Statistics Canada Catalogue No. 82-003-X.

LeBlanc, A. G., Spence, J. C., Carson, V., Connor Grober, S., Dillman, C., Janssen, I., & Trembley, M. S. (2012). Systematic review of sedentary behavior and health indicators in the early years (aged 0–4 years). *Applied Physiology, Nutrition, and Metabolism Journal of Public Health, 37*, 753–772. doi:10.1139/H2012-063

Luo, Z. C., Wilkins, R., Heaman, M., Martens, P., Smylie, J., Hart, L., . . . . Fraser, W. D. (2010). Birth outcomes and infant mortality by the degree of rural isolation among First Nations and non-First Nations, in Manitoba, Canada. *Journal of Rural Health, 26*(2), 175–181.

Luong, M. (2014). Statistics Canada. *Life after teenage motherhood.* Retrieved from http://www.statcan.gc.ca/pub/75-001-x/2008105/article/10577-eng.htm

March of Dimes. (2014). Smoking, drugs, and alcohol. Retrieved from http://www.marchofdimes.com/pregnancy/smoking-during-pregnancy.aspx?gclid=CIWf-fm2wr4CFZ-KCfgodiYUATA

Mawji, A., Robinson Vollman, A., Hatfield, J., Mcneil, D., & Sauve, R. (2013, August 1). The incidence of positional plagiocephaly: A cohort study. *Pediatrics, 132*(2), 298–304. doi:10.1542/peds.2012-3438

McKay, A. (2013). Trends in Canadian national and provincial/territorial teen pregnancy rates: 2001–2010. *The Canadian Journal of Human Sexuality, 21*(3–4), 161–175.

McIntyre, L., Bartoo, A. C., & Potestio, M. L. (2012). Coping with child hunger in Canada: Have household strategies changed over a decade? *Canadian Journal of Public Health, 103*(6), e428–e432.

Molcho, M., & Pickett, W. (2011). Some thoughts about "acceptable" and "non-acceptable" childhood injuries. *Injury Prevention, 17*(3), 147–148. doi:10.1136/ip.2010.030023

Moore, D. L., Canadian Paediatric Society, and the Infectious Diseases and Immunization Committee. (2008). Food borne infections. *Paediatrics and Child Health, 13*(9), 779–782.

National Collaborating Centre for Aboriginal Health. (2012). *The sacred space of womanhood across the generations: A national showcase on First Nations, Inuit, and Métis women and mothering.* Ottawa, ON: Public Health Agency of Canada. Excerpt from Until Our Hearts Are On The Ground: Aboriginal Mothering, Oppression, Resistance And Rebirth by D.M. Lavell-Harvard and J. Corbiere Lavell in Journal of Comparative Family Studies, Vol. 39, No. 2. Published by Journal of Comparative Family Studies, © 2013.

Neufeld, S., & Birkett, S. (2000). What to do about flat heads: Preventing and treating positional occipital flattening. *AXON, 22*(2), 29–31.

Oddy, W. H. (2012). Infant feeding and obesity risk in the child. *Breastfeeding Review: Professional Publication of the Nursing Mothers' Association of Australia, 20*(2), 7.

Ontario Ministry of Health and Long-Term Care. (2012). Teenage pregnancy. Retrieved from http://www.health.gov.on.ca/en/public/publications/pubhealth/init_report/tp.html

Ontario Ministry of Health and Long-Term Care (2009). Smoke free Ontario Act. Retrieved from http://www.e-laws.gov.on.ca/html/statutes/english/elaws_statutes_94t10_e.htm

Organisation for Economic Co-operation and Development. (2011). OECD health data 2011 – Frequently requested data. Paris: Author. Retrieved from http://www.oecd.org

Porta, M. (Ed.). (2008). *A dictionary of epidemiology* (5th ed.). New York, NY: Oxford University Press.

Public Health Agency of Canada. (2009a). *What mothers say: The Canadian maternity experiences Survey.* Ottawa, ON: Author.

Public Health Agency of Canada. (2009b). *10 great reasons to breastfeed your baby.* Ottawa, ON: Author. Retrieved from http://www.phac-aspc.gc.ca/hp-ps/dca-dea/stages-etapes/childhood-enfance_0-2/nutrition/reasons-raisons-eng.php

Public Health Agency of Canada. (2009c). *What mothers say: The Canadian maternity experiences survey.* Ottawa, ON: Author.

Public Health Agency of Canada. (2012). *Consumer product related injuries.* Ottawa, ON: Author. Retrieved from http://www.phac-aspc.gc.ca/publicat/cyi-bej/2009/index-eng.php

Public Health Agency of Canada. (2013). *Perinatal health indicators for Canada 2013: A report from the Canadian perinatal surveillance system.* Ottawa, ON: Author.

Quigley, M. A., Hockley, C., Carson, C., Kelly, Y., Renfrew, M. J., & Sacker, A. (2012). Breastfeeding is associated with improved child cognitive development: A population-based cohort study. *Journal of Pediatrics, 160*(1), 25–32. doi:10.1016/j.jpeds.2011.06.035

Raphael, D. (2011). Who is poor in Canada? In D. Raphael (Ed.), *Poverty in Canada: Implications for health and quality of life* (2nd ed., pp. 62–89). Toronto: Canadian Scholars' Press.

Raphael, D. (2012). Canadian experiences. In D. Raphael (Ed.), *Tackling health inequalities: Lessons from international experiences.* Toronto: Canadian Scholars' Press.

Raphael, D. (2014). Social determinants of children's health in Canada: Analysis and implications. *International Journal of Child, Youth and Family Studies, 5*(2), 220–239.

Rennick Salone, L., Vann, W. F., & Dee, D. L. (2013). Breastfeeding: An overview of oral and general health benefits. *The Journal of the American Dental Association, 144*(2), 143–151. doi:10.14219/jada.archive.2013.0093

Robert Woods Johnson Foundation. (2008). *Overcoming obstacles to health: Stories, facts and findings.* Princeton: Robert Woods Johnson Foundation.

Sanders, K. M., & Schor, J. (2014). Introducing baby to solid foods. The Townsend Letter Group.

Sen, A., & Ariizumi, H. (2014). Teen families, welfare transfers, and the minimum wage: Evidence from Canada. *Canadian Journal of Economics, 46*(1), 338–360.

Service Canada. (2014). Employment insurance, maternity, and parental benefits. Retrieved from http://www.servicecanada.gc.ca/eng/sc/ei/benefits/maternityparental.shtml

Shrim, A., Ates, S., Mallozzi, A., Brown, R., Ponette, V., Levin, I., . . . Almod, B. (2011). Is young maternal age really a risk factor for adverse pregnancy outcome in a Canadian tertiary referral hospital? *Journal of Pediatric and Adolescent Gynecology, 24*, 218–222. doi:10.1016/j.jpag.2011.02.008

Smylie, J., & Sauvé, R. (2009). Chapter 37: Infant sleep position. *What mothers say: the Canadian maternity experiences survey.* Ottawa, ON: Public Health Agency of Canada.

Soubhi, H., Raina, P., & Kohen, D. (2004). Neighbourhood, family, and child predictors of childhood injury in Canada. *American Journal of Health Behavior, 28*(5), 397–409.

Timmons, B.W., Leblanc, A. G., Carson, V., Connor Gorber, S., Dillman, C., Janssen, I., Tremblay, M. S. (2012). Systematic review of physical activity and health in the early years (aged 0–4 years). *Applied Physiology, Nutrition, and Metabolism Journal of Public Health, 37*, 773–792. doi:10.1139/H2012-070

United Nations. (2013). *Millennial development goals and beyond 2015: Improve maternal health.* Retrieved from http://www.un.org/millenniumgoals/pdf/Goal_5_fs.pdf

United Nations Population Fund. (2012). *Supporting the constellation of reproductive rights.* Retrieved from http://www.unfpa.org/rights/rights.htm

Venetsanou, F., & Kambas, A. (2010). Environmental factors affecting preschoolers' motor development. *Early Childhood Education Journal, 37*(4), 319–327.

World Health Organization. (1981). *International code of marketing breast-milk substitutes.* Geneva, Switzerland: Author. Retrieved from http://www.who.int/nutrition/publications/code_english.pdf

World Health Organization. (2012). *Newborns: Reducing mortality.* Geneva, Switzerland: Author. Retrieved from http://www.who.int/mediacentre/factsheets/fs333/en

World Health Organization. (2013). *Children: Reducing mortality.* Fact sheet N. 178. Geneva, Switzerland: Author. Retrieved from http://www.who.int/mediacentre/factsheets/fs178/en

World Health Organization. (2014a). *Reproductive health*. Geneva, Switzerland: Author. Retrieved from http://www.who.int/topics/reproductive_health/en

World Health Organization. (2014b). *10 facts on maternal health*. Geneva, Switzerland: Author. Retrieved from http://www.who.int/features/factfiles/maternal_health/en

World Health Organization. (2014c). *Millennium development goals (MDGs)*. Geneva, Switzerland: Author. Retrieved from http://www.who.int/topics/millennium_development_goals/en

World Health Organization. (2014d). *Maternal mortality. Fact Sheet N348*. Geneva, Switzerland: Author. Retrieved from http://www.who.int/mediacentre/factsheets/fs348/en

World Health Organization. (2014e). *MDG 5: Improve maternal health*. Retrieved from http://www.who.int/topics/millennium_development_goals/maternal_health/en

World Health Organization. (2014f). *Under five mortality*. Geneva, Switzerland: Author. Retrieved from http://www.who.int/gho/child_health/mortality/mortality_under_five_text/en

World Health Organization. (**2014g**). *Maternal, newborn, child and adolescent health: Adolescent pregnancy*. Geneva, Switzerland: Author. Retrieved from http://www.who.int/maternal_child_adolescent/topics/maternal/adolescent_pregnancy/en

World Health Organization. (2014h). *10 facts on breastfeeding*. Geneva, Switzerland: Author. Retrieved from http://www.who.int/features/factfiles/breastfeeding/en

World Health Organization. (2014i). *Infant and young child feeding. Fact Sheet N. 342*. Geneva, Switzerland: Author. Retrieved from http://www.who.int/mediacentre/factsheets/fs342/en

## ABOUT THE AUTHORS

**Deborah Mansell**, RN, MN, is an Assistant Professor in the School of Nursing and Midwifery, Faculty of Health, Community and Education at Mount Royal University. Her nursing practice includes community health and public health nursing, caring for childbearing/childrearing families, breastfeeding, parenting programs, legal issues in nursing, and teaching nursing students in Bachelor of Nursing programs. Deborah's research and research interests include caring for and promoting the health of diverse populations, maternal and child health, and community-based programs and interventions.

**Aliyah Dosani**, RN, BN, MPH, PhD, is an Associate Professor in the School of Nursing and Midwifery, Faculty of Health, Community Education Studies at Mount Royal University in Calgary Alberta. She holds a PhD from the University of Calgary with a specialization in population/public health. Her nursing practice includes instructing students in the Bachelor of Nursing Program, population and public health, community health nursing, and legal issues in nursing. Her work focuses on maternal, newborn, and child health. Her research interests include working with vulnerable populations through community-based programs and interventions. She also shares a passion for global health issues.

# School Health

*Yvette Laforêt-Fliesser,
Carol MacDougall, and Cheryl MacLeod*

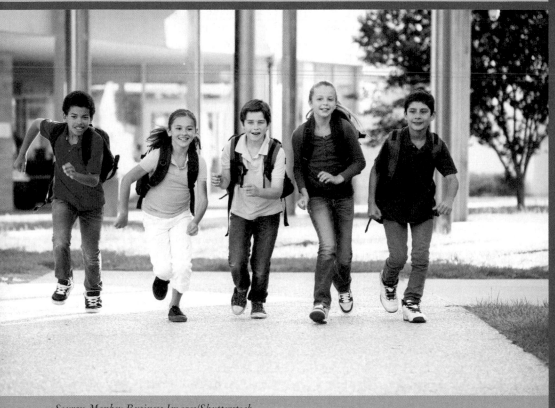

*Source: Monkey Business Images/Shutterstock*

## LEARNING OUTCOMES

**After studying this chapter, you should be able to:**

1. Explain the importance of the school as a setting for child and youth health promotion.

2. Identify common health and developmental challenges encountered in the school-aged population.

3. Discuss the importance of mental health promotion in schools.

4. Discuss how concepts and strategies from population health, comprehensive school health, and primary health care are relevant to school-based health promotion.

5. Examine the roles and functions of the public health nurse within a comprehensive school health approach.

6. Discuss the challenges and opportunities for maximizing the contribution of public health nursing in school settings.

## INTRODUCTION

School-aged children and youth need a supportive, healthful environment to achieve optimal development and educational milestones. The academic success and health and well-being of school-aged children and youth will ultimately determine Canada's place in the world (Health Council of Canada, 2006). Today, just over five million Canadian children and adolescents attend school every day (Statistics Canada, 2014). While many factors influence the physical, social, and emotional well-being of children and youth, research has shown that school settings have a positive impact on most of the health behaviours and outcomes of this population (Boyce, King, & Roche, 2008; Joint Consortium for School Health, 2014a).

For over a century, schools have been an important setting where public health nurses (PHNs) provide health promotion services and programs. They are settings where children and youth learn, play, and love; where adults work; and where families and neighbourhoods gather to engage in various educational and community activities. With the integration of children with complex health needs into publicly funded schools during the 1980s, many jurisdictions developed special nursing services within their home care program or community and social services to provide treatments in the school setting and consultation on health issues related to individual students (see Chapter 5). While these nursing services play a valuable role in supporting students with special health needs, PHNs focus on promoting the overall health of the whole school population. In some communities, especially in rural Canada, the PHN may be the only health professional providing service on an ongoing basis in schools. PHNs work within a primary health care and population health approach by offering a broad spectrum of services to promote and protect the health of individuals, families, groups, and aggregates within the school community (see Chapter 4).

This chapter presents a brief overview of growth and development in school-aged children and youth, and a discussion of some of the important health determinants and outcomes in this population. Current socio-environmental frameworks for comprehensive health promotion in schools will be presented, followed by a brief historical perspective on the role of the PHN in promoting school health. Finally, the diverse roles and activities of school-based PHNs in promoting the health of students, staff, families, and school communities will be discussed.

## THE IMPORTANCE OF SCHOOL YEARS

Over a period of 12 to 15 years, the school-aged population experiences dramatic physical, cognitive, emotional, and social transformations that can create uncertainty and anxiety for some children and youth (DeBell, Buttigieg, Sherwin, & Lowe, 2007). How children and adolescents manage the transitions from early to middle childhood and from adolescence to adulthood are important indicators of how healthy and well they will be as adults. **Middle childhood** extends from age 6 to the onset of puberty at 10 to 12 years, when children shift from seeing themselves as the centre of the world to realizing that the world is a complex environment in which they must find a place (Davies, 2011). The transition to middle childhood is marked by entry into the formal education system, when children begin to move from home and their family into wider social contexts that strongly influence their development. **School-aged children** seek opportunities to master and demonstrate new skills, make independent decisions, control their own behaviour, and form positive relationships with peers and adults outside the family (Mah & Ford-Jones, 2012). Nearing the end of this period, children who have successfully mastered these developmental tasks and not yet entered puberty are likely to appear confident, competent, reasonable, and composed. They are capable of reasoning, looking at situations from multiple perspectives, and using many adaptive strategies of self-regulation (Davies, 2011).

**Adolescence** begins with puberty and ends with the beginning of adulthood. The transition to this life stage involves a balance of school, extracurricular activities, and engagement in the workforce. The developmental tasks associated with adolescence include achieving independence, adjusting to sexual maturation, establishing co-operative relationships with peers, preparing for meaningful work or a career, establishing intimate relationships, and developing a core set of values (Registered Nurses Association of Ontario, 2010). Adolescents begin to develop greater autonomy and a stronger sense of who they are and who they want to become, and the sequencing, timing, and success of youth transitions into adulthood vary. Completing post-secondary education, entering the full-time labour force, leaving home, and entering into marriage or co-habitation are being delayed compared to previous generations (Ontario Ministry of Children and Youth Services, 2012; Public Health Agency of Canada [PHAC], 2011a).

A child's family and home environment are the most important and influential settings during the school-age years. The school provides the second most important social and physical environment where the child will experience nurturing and caring outside the family. During these formative years, the school and home interact with each other as determinants of child and youth health (DeBell et al., 2007).

## HEALTH DETERMINANTS AND OUTCOMES

Child and youth development and health status are shaped by multiple determinants of health (DeBell et al., 2007). Contexts and environments where young people learn, live, and play can have a significant impact on health status. Social exclusion and poorer socioeconomic circumstances can increase the likelihood of adopting risky behaviours (Davison et al., 2013; PHAC, 2011a). Approximately 20% of Canadian children live in small towns or rural areas that have limited access to public transportation, specialist services, and recreational facilities, which can significantly impact their health (Government of Canada, 2011).

About 1.3 million (19%) of Canadian children and youth under 18 live in poverty, with the plight being even worse for indigenous youth where 50% live in poverty (Campaign 2000, 2014). Child poverty rates are also very high for new immigrants, visible minorities, and children with disabilities. In 2014, of the more than 841 000 Canadians who used food banks, 37% of food bank clients were children less than 18 years of age (Food Banks Canada, 2014). Children and youth living in poverty are disadvantaged in almost every way and the health effects last a lifetime. They are more likely to live in unsafe neighbourhoods where exposure to violent and illegal activity occurs. These same conditions also create fewer opportunities for them to be physically and socially active and increase their chances of being overweight or obese compared to children living in higher socioeconomic groups. More importantly, inadequate nutrition impacts a child's ability to learn and to develop physically (Gupta, de Wit, & McKeown, 2007).

While most Canadian children and youth are in good health, risk-taking behaviours normally increase as they experience the social, biological, and psychological changes during these formative years (Davison et al., 2013; Freeman, King, & Pickett, 2011). Health concerns commonly addressed in school settings include unintentional injuries, communicable diseases, unhealthy weights, mental health issues, and **risky behaviours**. These are briefly discussed below.

## Unintentional Injuries

Unintentional injuries due to motor vehicle collisions (67%) and drowning (6%) are the leading cause of death for children and youth aged 10–19 years old (Statistics Canada, 2011). Sports and recreational activities such as running, biking, and skating are the leading causes of non-fatal injury (Pickett, 2011). For Aboriginal children and youth, the unintentional injury rate is three to four times higher than the rate for other children in Canada (Banerji, 2012). Youth who reside in rural areas experience more injuries per capita than their urban counterparts. Rural boys are also more likely to drive a motor vehicle while drinking alcohol or using drugs and rural girls are more likely to drive while impaired compared to youth in large urban centres (Davisonet et al., 2013).

## Communicable Diseases

Just 100 years ago, infectious diseases were the leading cause of death around the world. Immunization against vaccine-preventable communicable diseases is one of the most cost-effective public health interventions. Public health units are mandated by provincial health legislation to collect and review immunization information on students related to measles, mumps, rubella, tetanus, diphtheria, pertussis, polio, and varicella, and, in some jurisdictions, to hepatitis B, human papilloma virus, and meningitis, as well as annual influenza immunization. Routine childhood immunization without cost to the child is, for the most part, accepted as standard practice in Canada, as reported by the Public Health Agency of Canada (PHAC, 2013). Low immunization coverage rates are related to low socioeconomic status, urban dwelling, impoverished neighbourhoods, single-parent families, transient populations, and minority cultural status (Lemstra et al., 2007).

## Unhealthy Weights

The prevalence of overweightness and obesity among Canadian children remains unchanged in the last decade. Approximately one-third (31.5%) of 5- to 17-year-olds are overweight or obese; the percentage of boys who are obese (19.5%) is three times greater than the percentage of girls (6.3%) (PHAC, 2011b). For Aboriginal children, the numbers are of great concern, with 55% of on-reserve children and 41% of off-reserve children being either overweight or obese (Roberts, Shields, de Groh, Aziz, & Gilbert, 2012). Overweight children are more likely to develop type 2 diabetes, high blood pressure, heart disease, and arthritis (Ontario Ministry of Health and Long-term Care, 2013). While many of these conditions may not appear until adulthood, social and emotional problems can start during childhood. Overweight and obese young people, particularly young girls, are more likely to have mental health problems than young people with a healthy weight, and they often suffer from low self-esteem, social isolation, and depression (Freeman et al., 2011).

Overweightness and obesity are complex health factors that are linked to a number of determinants of health that have been proven to be difficult to manage. Reduced access to healthy foods and low levels of physical activity, education, and income can increase the risk of obesity (PHAC, 2011a, 2011b). Today, only one in three Canadian youth use active methods such as walking and biking to get to school, with the majority getting there by car or bus. Physically active children tend to perform better in school, manage stress and anxiety better, and have high levels of self-esteem (Freeman et al., 2011; Government of Canada, 2011).

## Risky Behaviours

While risk taking is an expected behaviour in adolescence, in some cases it can be a symptom of deeper underlying issues. Risky behaviours can include alcohol and drug use, smoking, and unprotected sexual activity. Alcohol and cannabis are the most common substances used by students in Grades 7 to 12 in Canada. In 2011, 45% of youth reported drinking alcohol, down significantly from the 53% reported in 2008–09. Binge drinking (i.e., five or more drinks for males and four or more drinks for females) has also decreased, with 33% of students reporting this activity compared to 39% in 2011. Tobacco smoking among youth 15 to 19 years declined to 11% in 2013 from 15% in 2008, with more boys (13%) reporting smoking than girls (8%). Six percent (6%) of youth, or 126 000 youth aged 15 to 19, and 10% of young adults (233 000) aged 20 to 24 reported having ever tried smokeless tobacco (Health Canada, 2013). The prevalence of smokers in Grades 6 to 9 significantly decreased between 2008 (3%) and 2011 (2%). The use of cannabis among students in Grades 7 to 12 has continued to decrease significantly between 2009 (27%) and 2011 (21%), with more boys (23%) than girls (19%) using this drug. There is concern that many Canadian adolescents, especially in Grades 9 and 10, perceive that smoking cannabis is less risky than smoking cigarettes (Freeman et al., 2011; Health Canada, 2013).

In 2010, 30% of youth ages 15 to 17 reported having had sex compared to 68% of 18- to 19-year-olds; these figures were not significantly different than those reported in 2003 (Rotermann, 2012). While these trends are encouraging, 35% of youth reported having multiple partners and 20% of 15- to 17-year-olds and 26% of 18- to 19-year-olds reported having sex without a condom. These patterns of sexual activity have contributed significantly to the increasing number of chlamydia and gonorrhea cases among young people, particularly women. When compared to other age groups, Canadian youth have the highest reported rates of sexually transmitted infections (PHAC, 2011a).

From 1990 to 2010, the teen pregnancy rate in Canada declined 20.3% from 35.4 per 1000 to 28.2 per 1000. However, during the period of 2006–2010, the national rate did increase 1.1%, with New Brunswick, Newfoundland, Nova Scotia, and Manitoba seeing a 15% increase in their teen pregnancy rates (McKay, 2013). Declining rates may reflect increasing use of contraceptives, exposure to reliable sexual health education, and better access to reproductive health services.

The risky behaviours just discussed are mostly responsible for the morbidity and mortality in adolescence. There is strong evidence that teens who engage in one "risky behaviour" tend to engage in several other risk behaviours (Alamian & Paradis, 2009). Many of the behaviours that begin during this time can continue into adulthood, with negative long-term health consequences (PHAC, 2011a). Positive relationships with families, peers in schools, and community members may lessen the potential harm of these high-risk behaviours and encourage more health-enhancing behaviours (Weare, 2010). Individual capacity and coping skills, such as personal competence and a sense of control over one's life, also play an important role in supporting mental and physical health (Boyce et al., 2008; Government of Canada, 2011).

## Mental Health

The mental health of children and youth has emerged as an urgent matter in Canada and around the world (WHO, 2013). An estimated 1.2 million young Canadians (15%) live with anxiety, attention deficit, depression, addiction, and other disorders (Mental Health Commission of Canada, 2006, 2012). Mental health problems among children and youth are expected to increase 50% by the year 2020 (Canadian Paediatric Society, 2009). Many mental health issues are gender specific, and the gender gap continues to increase. In Canada, 22% of boys in Grade 6 and 24% of boys in Grade 10 reported that they felt low or depressed at least weekly in the previous six months, as compared to 28% and 38% of girls in Grades 6 and 10, respectively (Freeman et al., 2011).

In 2011, there were 227 suicides among young Canadians (152 males and 75 females), accounting for 22% of all deaths for people aged 10 to 19 years, and compared with 1.5% deaths by suicide among the entire population. It is the second leading cause of death, behind unintentional injury, for Canadian youth between ages 15 and 24 (Statistics Canada, 2014). Suicide rates among female children and adolescents are increasing, whereas those among male children and adolescents are decreasing (Skinner & McFaull, 2012). The suicide rate for Aboriginal young people is three to five times higher than that for non-Aboriginal youth (PHAC, 2011a).

The mental health strategy for Canada recognizes that greater attention to prevention of mental illness and promotion of mental health for the whole population is essential. The first strategic direction, "to promote mental health across the lifespan in homes, schools, and work-places, and prevent mental illness and suicide wherever possible" (Mental Health Commission of Canada, 2012, p. 11), lends support to comprehensive school health approaches that promote the mental health of all students and provide targeted prevention efforts for those at risk. With early detection and intervention, most children can experience improvement in mental health conditions. Programs and services are more effective when they are part of a comprehensive approach for nurturing all children (Weare, 2010).

## SCHOOL-BASED HEALTH PROMOTION MODELS

The term "comprehensive school health" (CSH) was coined in the 1980s to describe a socioecological approach to school-based health promotion in Canada and in the United States. In essence, this comprehensive approach was undertaken when it became evident that an educational approach alone was inadequate for changing student behaviours. Students require a social environment, physical environment, and school policies that reinforce educational messages. They also require school partnerships to improve access to programs and services supporting the messages. CSH and the "health-promoting schools" approaches integrate the principles of primary health care and the strategies of the Ottawa Charter for Health Promotion. CSH is a health-promotion approach that empowers individuals and school communities to take action for health.

The **comprehensive school health approach** involves mobilizing an action group of students, parents, school staff, and community partners, including PHNs, forming a *planning structure*. This group then undertakes a *planning process,* where it

- creates a shared vision of the school as a "healthy school,"
- assesses existing strengths and needs,
- prioritizes an issue,
- develops a comprehensive plan addressing the four pillars in the diagram that follows (see Figure 17.1),
- implements the plan,
- monitors/evaluates, and
- celebrates and communicates successes (Alberta Healthy Schools Wellness Fund, 2011; Ontario Ministry of Health Promotion, 2010).

In Canada, CSH gained momentum following a national conference in 1990 that produced a consensus statement on CSH subsequently endorsed by more than 20 national organizations. In 2007, the consensus statement was revised to reflect a unifying vision for educators, health professionals, policy makers, parents, and youth (Canadian Association for School Health, 2007). Health Canada, Canadian Association for School Health (CASH), Public Health Agency of Canada (PHAC), and Physical and Health Education (PHE) Canada have played important roles in promoting CSH through research, education, project development, and networking activities. An increasing emphasis on school improvement and school effectiveness has resulted in schools linking student health and academic success. Since its establishment in 2005, the Pan-Canadian Joint Consortium for School Health (JCSH) has facilitated federal–provincial or territorial co-operation and inter-ministerial coordination to promote the wellness and achievement of children and youth in the school setting. The consortium serves to

- strengthen co-operation among ministries, agencies, departments and others in support of healthy schools;
- build the capacity of the health and education sectors to work together more effectively and efficiently; and
- promote understanding of, and support for, the concept and benefits of comprehensive school health initiatives (JCSH, 2014a, pp. 8–9).

According to the JCSH, comprehensive school health encompasses the *whole* school environment that supports students in becoming healthy and productive members of society, through actions illustrated in four distinct but interrelated pillars (see Figure 17.1): social and physical environment, teaching and learning, healthy school policy, and partnerships and services. Internationally and within Canada, the pillars and terminology may vary but the essence of the models (e.g., Health Promoting Schools, Coordinated School Health Program, Healthy Schools, and Healthy School Communities) is the same. For clarity, we will use the term "comprehensive school health" (CSH) in the remainder of this chapter. Table 17.1 outlines the key components of CSH.

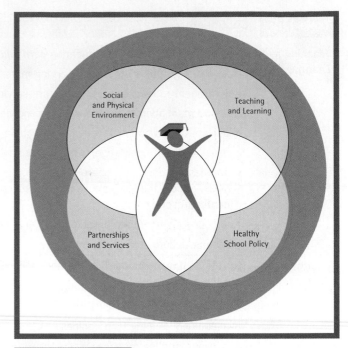

**FIGURE 17.1** The Pan-Canadian Joint Consortium for School Health Model for Comprehensive School Health

*Source:* Pan-Canadian Joint Consortium for School Health (JCSH). (2014). *Annual Report.* Used by permission of Joint Consortium for School Health. *Retrieved from* http://www.jcsh-cces.ca/upload/JCSH_AnnualReport_Eng_Sept14.pdf, p. 7.

| TABLE 17.1 | Components of a Comprehensive School Health/Health Promoting Schools Approach |
|---|---|
| **Supportive Social and Physical Environment** | Welcoming and positive environment |
| | Supportive relationships |
| | Clear expectations and limits |
| | Inclusive environment that celebrates diversity and ensures *equity* |
| | Collaborative, partnership approach with input from students, parents, administration, teachers, and local community agencies |
| | Establishment of *sustainable structures* and processes (e.g., school health committee/team) to identify and address health issues and *measure success* |
| | *Democracy*/involving students in decision making/active student participation (e.g., in setting classroom rules, on a school health committee, on a student council, in peer leadership) |
| | High degree of staff participation |
| | Encouragement of staff and student autonomy |
| | Role-modelling by parents, teachers, peers |
| | Mentoring programs |
| | Promotion of social-emotional learning and positive mental health |
| | Clean and hygienic *environment* |
| | Acceptable air quality and ventilation |
| | Safe water |
| | Adequate lighting |
| | Low-allergen environment |
| | Safe playground equipment and injury prevention measures in the school |
| | Universal, non-stigmatizing student nutrition/food programs |
| | Media reinforcing healthy behaviours |

*(continued)*

| Table 17.1 | Continued |
|---|---|
| **Teaching and Learning** | K–12 Health and Physical Education *curriculum*<br><br>Relevant, high-quality teaching/learning materials<br><br>Commitment to *teacher preparation*: pre-service and in-service training<br><br>*Empowerment* approaches that consider individual and social contexts, promote *action competence,* and:<br><br>• use active and cooperative learning techniques<br><br>• develop health knowledge, attitudes, and behaviours<br><br>• emphasize generic skill development (e.g., information seeking, decision making, problem solving, refusal skills, critical thinking, media awareness, coping, personal goal setting, social skills, building relationships, conflict resolution)<br><br>• encourage students to participate in local *community action*<br><br>Cross-curriculum support for health |
| **Healthy School Policy** | Government, school board, and school policies/guidelines supporting health<br><br>Funding and agreements facilitating access to services, including partnership policies<br><br>Smoke-free policy enforcement<br><br>Availability of healthy food choices<br><br>Safe food-handling practices<br><br>Daily physical activity policies<br><br>Injury prevention policies<br><br>Sun safety policies<br><br>Mental health and well-being policies<br><br>Safe and healthy school policies/guidelines (e.g., prohibiting harassment) |
| **Partnerships and Services** | Health services (e.g., physical, mental, public health)<br><br>Guidance and career education<br><br>Social work<br><br>Psychology<br><br>Child protection<br><br>Police services<br><br>Early identification, assessment, referral, treatment, and follow-up<br><br>Parks and recreation/Boys' and Girls' Clubs/YMCAs and YWCAs<br><br>Access to community-based services<br><br>"Healthy School" coordinators (provincial level, school board level, and local school level) |

Note: The words in bold italics refer to the 10 key principles of the Health Promoting School concept as identified at the First Conference of the European Network of Health Promoting Schools in Greece, 1997: 1. Democracy, 2. Equity, 3. Empowerment and Action Competence, 4. School Environment, 5. Curriculum, 6. Teacher Training, 7. Measuring Success, 8. Collaboration, 9. Communities, 10. Sustainability. Source: WHO. (1997). First Conference of the European Network of Health Promoting Schools Conference Report. Retrieved from http://www.euro.who.int/__data/assets/pdf_file/0013/120307/E72971.pdf

## HISTORICAL PERSPECTIVES ON SCHOOL NURSING IN CANADA

PHNs in Canada have a long history of working in school communities. With the emergence of public health nursing at the turn of the 20th century, schools became one of the initial settings for the provision of health education and preventive programs (see Chapter 1). Medical inspection programs were initiated in most schools to counteract absenteeism of children due to communicable disease. Public health officials proposed that poor health inhibited a child's academic performance and could potentially have harmful effects on that child's future economic and social well-being.

In several Canadian cities, boards of education initially established school health programs in which the PHNs moved between school and home providing preventive health teaching, screening, and counselling, in addition to their primary role in communicable disease control. A nurse's ability to move between home and school was seen as key to improving the health of children and young families (McKay, 2012).

For most of the 20th century, PHNs in school settings primarily focused on individual and family counselling, classroom health teaching, screening, case-finding programs, immunization programs, and advising school staff about student health problems (see Chapters 1 and 4). Interventions were based on a biomedical model where the emphasis was on the prevention and control of disease. Schools were one of the settings in a district or neighbourhood that received the services of the generalist PHN. **District nursing** created opportunities for the nurse to really know the community, where regular communication and collaboration with local family physicians, pharmacists, businesses, and other health professionals occurred. School children and their families were often known to the nurse through home visiting or clinic work in the district. With the emergence of health promotion in the mid-1970s, PHNs addressed lifestyle issues through health education, health communication campaigns, and individual or group counselling, in addition to the traditional screening and immunization programs. The 1986 Ottawa Charter introduced a new way of thinking about health promotion, and PHNs incorporated its principles of equity, participation, empowerment, and collaboration in their practices (see Chapter 1).

In the 1990s, the shift to population health and program-based delivery of public health programs led to the reduction or elimination of PHNs in schools. Such constraints took place at a time when CSH was being introduced in many jurisdictions, and resulted in erosion of the relationships that PHNs had built with principals, teachers, and students and their families, and diminished their overall visibility in the community (Cohen & McKay, 2010; Crouch & Chalmers, 2010).

Despite these challenges, the nursing profession in Canada has continued to advocate for school-based PHNs working to their full scope of practice within a comprehensive school health approach (Canadian Nurses Association, 2012; Community Health Nurses Initiatives Group, 2015; Ordre des infirmières et infirmiers du Québec, 2015). Internationally, there is a growing call for expanding the role of school nurses to include a multi-dimensional and multi-sectoral approach to the health promotion and health protection of school-aged children (Brooks, Kendall, Bunn, Bindler, & Bruya, 2007; Crouch & Chalmers, 2010; Department of Health, 2012). (See Canadian Research Box 17.1.)

---

**CANADIAN RESEARCH BOX 17.1**

**What are the barriers in providing school-based health services?**

Seigart, D., Dietsch, E., & Parent, M. (2013). Barriers to providing school-based health care: International case comparisons. *Collegian, 20,* 43–50. Used by permission of Elsevier Inc. – Health Sciences Division. http://dx.doi.org/10.1016/j.colegn.2012.03.003

This research used a case-study approach to gather data from in-depth interviews with key stakeholders, on-site observations, agency reports, and the literature. Forty school nurses or community health nurses who worked in schools were interviewed and additional interviews were conducted with 33 parents, teachers, administrators, nursing faculty, and other community leaders in two states or provinces in Australia, Canada, and the U.S. Grounded theory approaches such as analysis of interview transcripts, field notes, and records of observations for emerging themes were used in the data analysis.

Common concerns expressed in all three countries included high student-to-nurse ratios especially in Australia

and Canada; limited knowledge of the roles and benefits of school nurses and school-based healthcare; and a lack of timely access to primary care services. Canadian and Australian community health nurses (CHNs) tended not to engage in hands-on care, but to focus on surveillance, health education, infection control, vaccinations, and staff education. U.S. school nurses provided more primary care services, such as medication administration, health education and promotion, staff education, counselling, referrals, and networking with other health professionals. Another difference observed in Canada and Australia was the lack of school nurse practitioners and school-based health centres as compared to the U.S., where both are more common. In all three countries, funding was the most common barrier mentioned to expanding school health services. Australia and Canada also reported an increase in teacher stress due to taking on responsibilities for monitoring the health of children.

### Discussion Questions

1. What are some of the unique features about providing health services in schools?

2. From the above findings, what might explain the differences or similarities among the three jurisdictions in this study?

3. How might provincial and national nursing leadership help PHNs in Canada to practise within the scope of practice identified in Table 17.2?

---

# ROLES OF THE SCHOOL-BASED PUBLIC HEALTH NURSE

In Canada, PHN practice is guided by the Community Health Nurses of Canada (CHNC, 2011, revised), Professional Practice Model and Standards of Practice, the Public Health Nursing Discipline Specific Competencies (CHNC, 2009), and the roles and activities described by the CPHA (2010) (see Chapter 4). A recent discussion paper by the Community Health Nurses' Initiatives Group (CHNIG) on the role of PHNs in Ontario schools proposes that

> The practice of school-based PHNs is situated within a primary health care and population health approach that emphasizes the importance of addressing determinants of health. Social justice and equity are foundational to the work of school-based PHNs and are derived from the core principle of caring, made visible as compassion, sensitivity to diversity, and respect for all people. These core values ground their interventions, so these are timely, responsive, targeted to community priorities and needs, and based on best available evidence. Knowledge and skills in community development, comprehensive health promotion, illness and injury prevention, primary health care, and community participation underpin this collaborative way of nursing. (CHNIG, 2015, p. 12)

Within schools, PHNs simultaneously plan and deliver care at multiple levels: individual students or staff, families, groups, classrooms, the entire school population, the community, or the whole school board or jurisdiction. One-on-one work with individuals, whether counselling or providing clinical services, can evolve into identifying a need for small-group or psycho-educational interventions. Individually focused or small-group-focused strategies may also uncover specific health trends within the school community requiring a whole-school intervention using a CSH approach. Table 17.2 summarizes a recommended scope of practice for school PHNs in Ontario (cited in CHNIG, 2015, pp. 41–42).

| TABLE 17.2 | Recommended Scope of Practice for School-Based Public Health Nurses |
|---|---|

**Goal:** To enable all children and youth to attain and sustain optimal health and development, and learning potential ["health" refers to physical, mental/emotional, and social health]

**Philosophy:** Strengths based/solution focused

**Clients:** Students and families/school staff/school board/community

**Promoting Health with Individuals**

– Assessment, supportive counselling, and referral of students to needed services
– Health education and skill development with students, families, school staff
– Provision of some clinical services per locally identified need
– School-based health or wellness clinics or youth health centres in secondary schools
– Consultation and coordination with school staff
– Participation in case conferences
– Communication and coordination with families via school visits, home visits, phone calls
– Coordination with other service or care providers

**Promoting Health with Small Groups or Classrooms**

– Small group programming with students in areas of identified need (e.g., healthy relationships, self-esteem, communication, social skills, anger management)
– Staff education on health and development issues and on youth engagement
– Parenting education
– Training of groups of peer leaders in various topic areas (e.g., playground activity leaders, nutrition, mental health leaders, healthy school committees)
– Providing or recommending curriculum materials to teachers
– Classroom education sessions on health topics

**School-Wide Health Promotion**

– Assessment, surveillance, and data analysis to identify strengths and priority needs in school populations
– Ensuring a group to address school health or school improvement issues is established, and that it includes significant student participation and leadership
– Supporting the group in creating comprehensive action plans (i.e., the plans should include the components of teaching and learning; partnerships and services; social and physical environment; healthy school policies)
– Encouraging youth across the school to become involved in health action
– Working with school staff, students, and communities to develop and implement healthy school policies and to create supportive school environments
– Ensuring equitable access to health and social services for the school population

**Board- or District-Wide and Community-Level Health Promotion**

– Contributing to health policy development on school board working groups
– Participating on board/inter-agency committees related to school services or coordination of care to ensure equitable access
– Engaging young people in the development and implementation of health-related communications/campaigns (including ensuring connection with appropriate health unit staff and maintaining website information)
– Acknowledging school successes at board or community events
– Collecting statistics to identify trends and prevailing issues
– Conducting evaluations as indicated

Source: Community Health Nurses Initiatives Group. (2013). *Healthy schools, healthy children: Maximizing the contribution of public health nursing in school settings. Version 2.0*, Appendix B: pp. 41–42. "Used with the permission of CHNIG and Carol MacDougall" with "Used by permission of Community Health Nurses Initiatives Group."

## Working with Individuals

Today, PHNs provide clinical services that may include immunization, sexual health services, vision and hearing screening, and health counselling and referral. The counselling role of PHNs in schools, especially high schools, contributes to successful adolescent health programs, along with personal skill training in learning life and social skills and dealing with peer pressure and peer influences (Brooks et al., 2007). PHNs provide this initial assessment, support, and referral as they practise from a solution-focused, strengths-based approach that optimizes the problem-solving and coping abilities of young people and families. PHNs communicate and coordinate care with a student's family and school staff, and serve as a consultation resource for school staff. For some children, a one-to-one approach may be the most appropriate approach to address sensitive issues such as bullying, sexual health, or obesity (Crouch & Chalmers, 2010).

In Canada and other countries, there is great variability within mandated public health services regarding the provision of individual counselling to students. (See Canadian Research Box 17.1.) Even in jurisdictions supportive of this role, most PHNs are on-site only a few hours per week, so it is important that additional counselling services be provided by other professionals such as social workers, guidance counsellors, and psychologists. Collaborative partnerships among public health, school boards/districts, and community agencies can share responsibility for funding these types of support services in schools. Delivery of this type of school-based counselling service by PHNs yields a high degree of satisfaction among staff, students, and parents (Moynagh & Singleton, 2011; Saewyc, Roy, & Foster, 2014; Trim, 2011).

The school-based health clinic (e.g., teen health clinic) is another model that is gaining acceptance and, therefore, being used in many areas of the country. Health services offered in a school setting that integrate clinical care with public health interventions and environmental change strategies offer an opportunity to address multiple determinants of health (Clayton, Chin, Blackburn, & Echeverria, 2009; Saewyc, Roy, & Foster, 2014). Students often have limited access to community services or they have to take time out from classes to attend off-site medical appointments. Public health agencies can work with a number of community partners, including school police officers, physicians, and alcohol and drug service workers, to provide school-based comprehensive health services to high school youth. In Nova Scotia, the Youth Health Centre (YHC) model operates within high schools, where youth access comprehensive, confidential, and non-judgmental programs and services, including health education, health assessment and intervention, referral, support, and follow-up by PHNs and other health providers (Nova Scotia Department of Health Promotion and Protection, 2009). Additionally, the YHC coordinators support student action teams, provide health curriculum support through classroom presentations, and coordinate immunization clinics in the school. The Nova Scotia model integrates individual-focused services as well as opportunities for group work and peer-led student action teams that address whole-school issues.

## Working with Small Groups

Group learning or group discussion is an effective approach to actively engage children and youth in creating peer support and formal or informal learning. Topics may include smoking cessation, healthy relationships, sexual health and sexuality, parenting, anger management, self-esteem, decision making, birth control methods, or puberty. It can involve the training of peer leaders to lead a variety of activities during lunch, at recess, or after school. Such group learning is particularly valuable because it enables a peer group as a whole to experience a shift in social norms and collectively increase its awareness, knowledge, and critical-thinking skills in a caring, supportive, and non-judgmental environment. (See Canadian Research Box 17.2.)

---

**CANADIAN RESEARCH BOX 17.2**

**What is the long-term impact of the Teen Esteem program on pre-teen girls?**

Brown, K. (2013). *Teen Esteem impact evaluation: The voices of young women in Perth County.* Stratford, ON: Perth District Health Unit. Used by permission of Perth District Health Unit. Retrieved from http://www.pdhu.on.ca/wp-content/uploads/2015/04/Teen-Esteem-Evaluation-Report-2014.pdf

Teen Esteem is a school-based program designed to improve girls' self-esteem and has been offered for the past 10 years to Grades 7 and 8 girls in Perth County schools with self-identified need and interest. It consists of seven weekly lunch-hour sessions coordinated by a public health nurse, and women from the community volunteer to lead discussions with small groups of four to eight girls. The main areas of focus are self-esteem, body image, communication, conflict management, dating relationships, stress management, and goal setting. Of the 658 past participants from 2006 to 2012, 454 were located and 75 completed the survey (16% response rate). The findings revealed that Teen Esteem had a positive influence across the seven areas of focus. The greatest influences were on the girls' knowledge that there was not one ideal body shape (76%), on their ability to distinguish between healthy versus unhealthy relationships (83%), on how to access help for handling unhealthy relationships (77%) and stress (69%), and on their ability to make decisions based on their own values as opposed to their friends' decisions (65%). Respondents suggested expanding content in the areas of mental health, stress management, mental illness, handling difficult friendship issues, and what to expect at high school. They also suggested a similar program in high school, expanding on the existing topics and adding mental health, motivation, sex, drugs, and alcohol.

## Working with Whole Schools, Boards or Districts, and Communities

Some health concerns that arise during individual or small-group work may benefit from further school-wide health promotion. PHNs can facilitate the implementation of a structure and process to address health in schools. They can raise awareness among principals, teachers, students, and parents about "the possibility of addressing school health issues in a partnership structure" through school health committees or action teams (MacDougall, 2004a, p. 48) (see Photo 17.1). It is critical to involve a diverse group of representatives so they can share their concerns about various aspects of school life that need to be improved. Ideally, the chairperson should come from the school community itself to encourage local ownership of the health committee from the outset. Engagement of a critical mass of students is essential for the success of healthy school initiatives (MacDougall & Laforêt-Fliesser, 2009). When youth are engaged in decisions concerning their health and their school, they feel more connected to their school and are better able to build relationships with peers and other adults. Meaningful youth participation on a school health committee or action team provides an opportunity to share ideas, be involved with planning and implementing new programs or policies, and to learn new skills in consensus building, project planning, and communication (JCSH, 2014b).

The CSH process is, in essence, the nursing process applied in collaboration with a school community. Integral to this process is the development of effective working relationships with the groups and populations. The core nursing skills of mutual respect, caring, listening, assessing, enabling, and empowering are critical to the PHN's work with school communities and school boards. A PHN's practice in school can be complex and challenging because relationships with school staff, parents, students, superintendents, or community partners occur within a complex, changing, and often ambiguous environment that may present conflicting circumstances for the PHN (Athwal et al., 2014). In addition to meeting the needs of individuals, families, or groups, a PHN uses a macroscopic approach in assessing and planning interventions that address the broader determinants of health within a community. The use of community development principles is particularly relevant when building capacity in school communities.

In facilitating CSH, it is important to determine the school community's level of readiness, its strengths or assets, and its areas of interest or concern. Some school communities may have a health champion who can easily facilitate the school's participation in health-promotion activities. Other school communities may be immersed in their academic focus and the PHN has a role in assisting them to see the link between health and learning before any action is possible. The PHN can support the health action team in using the CSH framework to examine how health promoting the school is overall. A PHN can engage a school in reflecting on the following questions:

- How effective is the health, physical education, and other curriculum delivery?
- Is the school aware of and able to access support services from the board and local community to support the health of students, staff, and families in the school community?
- Does the school have a democratic and supportive social environment with shared decision making?
- Is the physical environment supportive of the health curriculum being taught in the classroom?
- Does the school implement and enforce health-supporting policies? (MacDougall, 2004b).

The PHN can also support the health action team in using the CSH framework to comprehensively address a specific issue. The JCSH (2010) provides a Healthy School Planner, an online tool that helps Canadian schools assess the state of their environment and surveys students on specific health issues such as healthy eating, physical activity, or tobacco. Several jurisdictions have developed their own assessment tools that foster discussion about the school's strengths and health issues and what it can do about them. Potential activities, services, and programs within the four components of the CSH approach are also illustrated in Table 17.1.

Health promotion programs in schools frequently focus on increasing students' awareness about healthy eating, active living, safety issues, avoiding substance use, and developing healthy relationships, including sexual health and violence

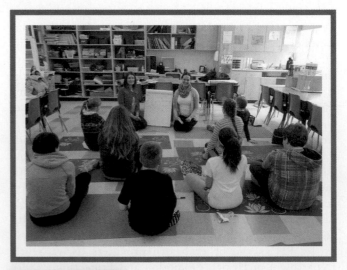

**PHOTO 17.1** A public health nurse and public health promoter co-facilitating a Healthy School Committee at an elementary school

*Source: Photo courtesy of Carol Arnott, for the Perth District Health Unit.*

prevention. The "school health committee" or "action team" creates a place to discuss and build upon a school's strengths or assets while addressing health concerns and planning appropriate action. When formulating a plan to address an identified health issue, the PHN can support the action team in identifying strategies or activities within each of the four component areas to achieve a degree of comprehensiveness that is more likely to have a meaningful impact on the school community. For example, if student nutrition is the priority concern of the school, then the components of the plan might look like this:

1. Supportive social and physical environment—Assist students to run a healthy tuck shop; engage youth in finding solutions for healthier high school cafeteria menus; encourage parents to reinforce healthy eating in the purchases they make for lunches and home meals.
2. Teaching and learning—Ensure the provision of in-service for teachers so they are better prepared to deliver the nutrition curriculum.
3. Healthy school policies—Establish universal student nutrition programs, such as breakfast, snack, or lunch programs; establish healthy school nutrition policies that address foods offered at school events and for fundraising.
4. Partnerships and services—Consult with a public health nutritionist, dietitian, or nurse to explore the many ways student nutrition could be addressed throughout the school, and suggest community agencies that could assist students who may have significant nutritional issues, such as eating disorders or unhealthy weights.

PHNs can also support school board or district-wide and community-wide health promotion. The formation of strong partnerships between boards or districts of education and public health agencies at the local level enables sustainable implementation of CSH. Examples of effective partnerships include joint committees for curriculum and policy development, which support the health of students and the school environment (MacDougall & Laforêt-Fliesser, 2009). (See Case Study.) Joint development of a local CSH initiative or adoption of a provincial initiative greatly increases the commitment of principals and school staff, as their participation becomes part of expected school improvement efforts and is actively recognized by school board leaders (Ontario Ministry of Health Promotion, 2010). Participation of PHNs on interagency community planning tables enables coordination of efforts to address youth health trends; for example, self-harm and suicide.

## Promoting Positive Mental Health

Recent research supports the importance of moving beyond a problem-focused approach to embrace a positive mental health view, where there is recognition that the assets within individuals and their social settings can contribute to healthy growth and development (Morrison & Peterson, 2013). The PHAC describes **positive mental health** as "the capacity of

### CASE STUDY

Personnel in one Calgary high school approached their school PHN and shared their concerns about the increasing number of students coming to school hungry. Despite instituting a school breakfast program and purchasing foods for a mobile food cart, the magnitude of the issue exceeded the school's capacity to respond effectively. The PHN brought together school personnel, parents, and students to discuss their perspective on this concern. She shared her community assessment that described the characteristics, assets, and potential needs of the school. Additionally, she facilitated a meeting to create a greater awareness of the issue with a view to mobilizing community action. Community agencies that supported food security were also invited to the meeting to explore options for collaboration. By bringing together key agencies, the PHN enabled conversations among all the stakeholders, resulting in the development of new partnerships and collaborative strategies for food security within the school and eventually throughout the school jurisdiction/board. For example, the local Meals-on-Wheels program expanded its service delivery model to include youth in need at the school. Secondly, the school established a partnership with the food bank that allowed school staff to pick up food on a weekly basis for distribution at the school.

### Discussion Questions

1. When creating an interest in working together, it is important to recognize what the focus of action will be and how others perceive it. How can the PHN be sure that there is support for this collaborative action from the community, other organizations, and the individuals who are to benefit most by it?
2. What actions can the PHN take to assist the group in articulating its goal and planning appropriate action?
3. Community capacity influences readiness for community action. Define community capacity in the context of this case study.

each and all of us to feel, think, and act in ways that enhance our ability to enjoy life and deal with the challenges we face. It is a positive sense of emotional and spiritual well-being that respects the importance of culture, equity, social justice, interconnections and personal dignity" (PHAC, 2006). The key concepts that describe the nature of positive mental health approaches include social-emotional learning, positive youth development, resiliency, protective factors, diversity, acceptance and understanding of student mental health needs, connectedness, strength-based perspectives, mental fitness, and self-efficacy (JCSH, 2014a). These approaches create supportive environments that promote and sustain positive mental health for all individuals. The development of mental health skills are especially important during the school-aged years as they can help youth cope with the challenges of growing up (Weare, 2010).

Promoting positive mental health through schools provides another opportunity for PHNs to use their clinical knowledge and expertise in prevention and health promotion. Comprehensive mental health promotion programs, when delivered for over a year or more, can reduce risky behaviours (Stewart-Brown, 2006). The characteristics of effective *mental health promotion programs* in schools include the following:

1. providing a backdrop of universal, multi-dimensional, coherent programs and services that promote the mental health of all and then effectively targeting those with special needs;
2. creating supportive climates that promote warmth, empathy, positive expectations, and clear boundaries;

3. tackling mental health problems early when they first manifest themselves and then taking a long-term approach that considers the child's development over time;
4. identifying and targeting vulnerable and at-risk groups and helping people acquire the skills and competencies that underlie mental health; and
5. involving end users and their families in ways that encourage a feeling of ownership and participation, and providing effective training for those who run the programs, including helping them to promote their own mental health (Morrison & Peterson, 2013; Weare, 2010).

Table 17.3 summarizes components of a comprehensive approach to mental health promotion.

| TABLE 17.3 | A Comprehensive Approach to Mental Health Promotion: The PHN's Contribution |
|---|---|
| Supportive Social and Physical Environment | – Build trusting and positive relationships with school principal, staff, students, and parents |
| | – Use strengths-based and solution-focused approaches in creating positive interactions with students, staff, and parents |
| | – Foster student participation and opportunities for leadership on school health committee and/or planning committee for health-awareness campaigns |
| | – Provide formal recognition of student/staff/parental contributions to health initiatives in the school |
| | – Incorporate student performances—music, art, and media skills—in health-promotion events |
| | – Provide posters and other media that promote positive health messaging |
| | – Ensure that students are seen by the PHN in a designated physical space so that student concerns can be shared in a respectful and confidential manner |
| | – Participate in school-based events that bring the school, family, and community together |
| Teaching and Learning | – Identify health-related curriculum resources that build skills and strategies to enhance student confidence, coping, and problem solving |
| | – Collaborate with teachers in designing and implementing resources related to self-care |
| | – Co-facilitate group sessions to build skills and/or change behaviour; for example, smoking cessation, anger management, and self-esteem |
| | – Show how positive mental health practices can be embedded within curriculum in order to avoid being seen as an "add on" |
| | – Provide educational opportunities for parents and school staff related to positive mental health |
| Partnerships and Services | – Promote the services and programs available through public health that may assist the school staff in addressing needs in their school |
| | – Share health status reports and/or community assessment data to assist the school in addressing health and social issues |
| | – Ensure engagement and participation of parents and students in healthy school initiatives |
| | – Offer opportunities for parent participation in learning activities or health-awareness events; for example, health fairs, workshops for students, board- or district-wide events |
| | – Participate in joint meetings to develop coordinated approaches to address mental health concerns in the school |
| | – Engage students in peer leader training opportunities; for example, playground leaders and mental health coaches |

| Table 17.3 | Continued |
|---|---|
| Healthy School Policies | – Act as a champion for school-wide adoption of policies that support school connectedness and student inclusion<br><br>– Participate in processes that develop policies to promote healthy lifestyle behaviour; for example, smoke-free policies, safe parties, sun safety, and bullying prevention<br><br>– Advocate for coordinated and responsive services to address emerging needs in children and youth<br><br>– Respect, and be aware of, the crisis or emergency routines in the school following traumatic events in the school or community<br><br>– Advocate for policies that assist pregnant teens and justice-involved students to complete their education<br><br>– Ensure protocols for referral of students and families to partnership agencies when additional support is required |

Source: Adapted from Morrison, P., & Peterson, W. (2013). *Schools as a setting for promoting positive mental health: Better practices and perspectives* (2nd ed.). Retrieved from http://www.jcsh-cces.ca/upload/JCSH%20Best%20Practice_Eng_Jan21.pdf

## CONCLUSION

This chapter describes the importance of the school years and the role of PHNs in promoting the healthy growth and development of children and youth in the school setting. It describes CSH and the role of PHNs in building committee structures and processes within schools. CSH offers PHNs the opportunity to work within a broad scope of practice that incorporates one-on-one, small group, and school-, board-, and community-wide health-promotion strategies. Schools are unique settings in which PHNs can work collaboratively to optimize the health of school-aged children and youth, their families, and school personnel. By virtue of their presence in schools, PHNs work within the cultures of education and health and bring unique insight that combines both an individual and population perspective (CHNIG, 2015). The significant health concerns in this population identified at the beginning of this chapter reinforce the need for an expanded health-promotion role for the PHN in schools.

While CSH has gained momentum in this country, PHNs struggle to work within a broad scope of practice that is consistent with socio-environmental and population health approaches. The Canadian Nurses Association (2014) asserts that PHNs are well positioned to significantly influence the health and education outcomes of Canada's school-age population. Efforts are mounting to develop a national strategy that clearly defines the roles and contributions of PHNs within a CSH approach.

## KEY TERMS

adolescence   p. 330
comprehensive school health approach   p. 332
district nursing   p. 335
middle childhood   p. 330
positive mental health   p. 339
risky behaviours   p. 331
school-aged children   p. 330

## STUDY QUESTIONS

1. Compare and contrast health promotion work with individuals versus school communities.
2. Discuss the challenges for PHNs working in school settings.
3. Research the various comprehensive school-based health-promotion models and describe the commonalities amongst them; for example, comprehensive school health, health-promoting schools, coordinated school health program.
4. List the potential partners on a school health committee/action team.
5. Identify some key principles of effective youth or student engagement and discuss the importance of using these in a PHN's daily practice.
6. List common health concerns or problems found in school settings.
7. List the 10 key ingredients for effective child and youth health programs.

> After working through these questions, go to the MyNursingLab at www.pearsoned.ca/mynursinglab to check your answers.

## INDIVIDUAL CRITICAL-THINKING EXERCISES

1. What are the main assumptions underlying comprehensive school health work, in particular work with school health committees?
2. Think of a school you attended in your past, and identify an issue that you believe would have benefitted from a comprehensive school health approach. Devise a comprehensive action plan.
3. How might a PHN in a school promote the health of families who have children in the school?
4. Considering the growth and development of children and youth, what potential health issues are likely to arise and how would you use the CSH framework to address them?
5. What are the benefits of a CSH approach for students, teachers, and the entire school community?
6. Analyze your level of comfort, knowledge, and skill base in facilitating a CSH approach. What would increase your comfort, knowledge, and skill with the structure and process?

# GROUP CRITICAL-THINKING EXERCISES

1. Imagine a high school has a sudden increase in the number of teens becoming pregnant. (or, imagine an elementary school is experiencing a high incidence of bullying.) Describe how you would work with the school community to assist it to address this issue.

2. Review current provincial or territorial legislation to determine what health services are provided in schools.

3. In developing a health profile for a school community, what assessment questions would you ask for each component of CSH? What methods might you use for various stakeholders: students, parents, teachers, administration, and community members?

4. A high school administrator wants to find ways to prevent substance use and abuse among the school's students. Identify five or six points that you would want to address with school staff, students, and parents.

5. Discuss the meaning of a "strengths-based approach" and how a PHN could operationalize this in working with students and schools.

# REFERENCES

Alamian, A., & Paradis, G. (2009). Clustering of chronic disease behavioural risk factors in Canadian children and adolescents. *Preventive Medicine, 48*, 493–499. Retrieved from http://www.sciencedirect.com/science/article/pii/S0091743509001133

Alberta Healthy Schools Wellness Fund. (2011). *Developing healthy school communities handbook.* Retrieved from http://www.wellnessfund.ualberta.ca/en/~/media/abhealthy-schools/Wellness_Fund_Handbook_2015-English.pdf

Athwal, L., Marchuk, B., Laforêt-Fliesser, Y., Castanza, J., Davis, L., & LaSalle, M. (2014). Adaptation of a best practice guideline to strengthen client-centred care in public health. *Public Health Nursing, 31*(2), 134–143. doi:10.1111/phn.12059

Banerji, A. (2012). Preventing unintentional injuries in indigenous children and youth. *Paediatric Child Health, 17*(7), 393. Retrieved from http://www.cps.ca/documents/position/unintentional-injuries-indigenous-children-youth

Boyce, W. F., King, M. A., & Roche, J. (2008). *Healthy settings for young people in Canada.* Ottawa, ON: Public Health Agency of Canada. Retrieved from http://publications.gc.ca/collections/collection_2008/phac-aspc/HP35-6-2007E.pdf

Brooks, F., Kendall, S., Bunn, F., Bindler, R., & Bruya, M. (2007). The school nurse as navigator of the school health journey: Developing the theory and evidence for policy. *Primary Health Care Research and Development, 8*, 226–234.

Campaign 2000. (2014). *Child poverty, 25 years later: We can fix this.* Retrieved from http://campaign2000.ca/anniversaryreport/CanadaRC2014EN.pdf

Canadian Association for School Health. (2007). *Comprehensive school health: Canadian consensus statement* (revised). Retrieved from http://www.albertahealthservices.ca/SchoolsTeachers/if-sch-csh-canadian-consensus-statement-on-comprehensive-school-health.pdf

Canadian Nurses Association. (2012). *Resolution 13: The role of public health nurses in schools.* Retrieved from http://www.cna-aiic.ca/~/media/cna/page-content/pdf-fr/report_on_resolutions_2012_e.pdf?la=en

Canadian Nurses Association. (2014). *CNA decision support policy synthesis: Public health nursing in schools.* Ottawa, ON: Author.

Canadian Paediatric Society. (2009). *Are we doing enough? A status report on Canadian public policy and child and youth health.* Ottawa: Author. Retrieved from http://rightsofchildren.ca/wp-content/uploads/are-we-doing-enough-cps-report.pdf

Canadian Public Health Association. (2010). *Public health–community health nursing practice in Canada: Roles and activities.* Ottawa, ON: Author. Retrieved from http://www.cpha.ca/uploads/pubs/3-1bk04214.pdf

Clayton, S., Chin, T., Blackburn, S., & Echeverria, C. (2010). Different setting, different care: Integrating prevention and clinical care in school-based health centers. *American Journal of Public Health, 100*, 1592–1596. doi:10.2105/AJPH.2009.186668

Cohen, B. E., & McKay, M. (2010). The role of public health agencies in addressing child and family poverty: Public health nurses' perspectives. *The Open Journal, 4*, 60–71.

Community Health Nurses of Canada. (2009). *Public health nursing discipline specific competencies Version 1.0.* St. John's, NL: Author. Retrieved from http://www.chnc.ca/documents/competencies_june_2009_english.pdf

Community Health Nurses of Canada. (2011, revised). *Canadian community health nursing: Professional practice model & standards of practice.* St. John's, NL: Author. Retrieved from http://www.chnc.ca/documents/chnc-standards-eng-book.pdf

Community Health Nurses Initiatives Group. (2015). *Healthy schools, healthy children: Maximizing the contribution of public health nursing in school settings Version 2.0.* Toronto, ON: Author. Retrieved from http://draftohsc.files.word-press.com/2014/05/policy-paper-school-health-pdf.pdf

Crouch, V., & Chalmers, H. (2010). The role of the school nurse. In P. Aggleton, C., Dennison, & I. Warwick (Eds.), *Promoting health and well-being through schools* (pp. 147–161). New York, NY: Routledge.

Davies, D. (2011). *Child development: A practitioner's guide* (3rd ed.). New York, NY: Guilford Press.

Davison, C. M., Russell, K., Piedts, S., Pike, I., Pickett, W., & the CIHR team in Child and Youth Injury Prevention. (2013). *Injury among young Canadians: A national study of contextual determinants.* Vancouver, BC: CIHR team in Child and Youth Injury Prevention.

DeBell, D., Buttigieg, M., Sherwin, S., & Lowe, K. (2007). The school as location for health promotion. In D. DeBell (Ed.), *Public health practice and the school-age population* (pp. 93–130). London, UK: Edward Arnold Publishers Inc.

Department of Health. (2012). *Getting it right for children, young people and families: Maximizing the contribution of the school nursing team: Vision and Call to Action.* Retrieved from https://www.gov.uk/government/uploads/system/uploads/attachment_data/file/216464/dh_133352.pdf

Food Banks Canada. (2014). *Hunger count 2014.* Retrieved from http://www.foodbankscanada.ca/getmedia/76907192-263c-4022-8561-73a16c06dd2f/HungerCount_2014_EN_HR.pdf.aspx

Freeman, J. G., King, M., & Pickett, W. (2011). *The health of Canada's young people: A mental health focus.* Retrieved from http://www.phac-aspc.gc.ca/hp-ps/dca-dea/publications/health-young-people-sante-jeunes-canadiens/assets/pdf/health-young-people-sante-jeunes-canadiens-eng.pdf

Government of Canada. (2011). *The well-being of Canada's young children*. Ottawa, ON: Author. Retrieved from http://www.dpe-agje-ecd-elcc.ca/eng/ecd/well-being/sp_1027_04_12_eng.pdf

Gupta, R., de Wit, M. L., & McKeown, D. (2007). The impact of poverty on the current and future health status of children. *Paediatric Child Health, 12*(8), 667–672.

Health Canada. (2013). *Summary of results: Canadian tobacco, alcohol and drugs survey (CTADS)*. Retrieved from http://healthycanadians.gc.ca/science-research-sciences-recherches/data-donnees/ctads-ectad/summary-sommaire-2013-eng.php

Health Canada. (2014). *Tobacco use in Canada: Patterns and trends 2014 edition*. Retrieved from http://www.mantrainc.ca/assets/tobaccouseincanada_2014.pdf

Health Council of Canada. (2006). *Their future is now: Healthy choices for Canada's children and youth*. Retrieved from http://www.healthcouncilcanada.ca/rpt_det.php?id=147

Joint Consortium for School Health. (2010). *The healthy school planner*. Retrieved from http://www.healthyschoolplanner.uwaterloo.ca

Joint Consortium for School Health. (2014a). *Annual report*. Retrieved from http://www.jcsh-cces.ca/upload/JCSH_AnnualReport_Eng_Sept14.pdf

Joint Consortium for School Health. (2014b). *Youth engagement toolkit*. Retrieved from http://www.jcsh-cces.ca/ye-book

Lemstra, M., Neudorf, C., Opondo, J., Toye, J., Kurji, A., Kunst, A., & Tournier, C. (2007). Disparity in childhood immunizations. *Paediatric Child Health, 12*(10), 847–852.

MacDougall, C. A. (2004a). *School health committees: Perceptions of public health staff*. ProQuest Digital Dissertations database Publication No. AAT MQ91427. Toronto, ON: Ontario Institute for Studies in Education University of Toronto.

MacDougall, C. A. (2004b). School health committees: Making "healthy schools" happen. *Canadian Association for Health Physical Education Recreation and Dance Journal, 70*(2), 27–29.

MacDougall, C. A., & Laforêt-Fliesser, Y. (2009). Canada: The evolution of healthy schools in Ontario, Canada: Top-down and bottom-up. In C. Vince Whitman & C. Aldinger (Eds.), *Case studies in global school health promotion: From research to practice* (pp. 143–157). New York, NY: Springer.

Mah, V. H., & Ford-Jones, E. L. (2012). Spotlight on middle childhood: Rejuvenating the "forgotten years." *Paediatrics and Child Health, 17*(2), 81–83.

McKay, A. (2013). Trends in Canadian national and provincial/territorial teen pregnancy rates: 2001–2010. *The Canadian Journal of Human Sexuality, 21*(3&4), 161–175.

McKay, M. (2012). The history of community health nursing in Canada. In L. L. Stamler & L.Yiu (Eds.), *Community health nursing: A Canadian perspective* (3rd ed., pp. 1–20). Toronto, ON: Pearson Canada.

Mental Health Commission of Canada. (2006). *Out of the shadows at last: Transforming mental health, mental illness and addiction services in Canada*. Retrieved from http://publications.gc.ca/collections/collection_2011/sen/yc17-0/YC17-0-391-2-1-eng.pdf

Mental Health Commission of Canada. (2012). *Changing directions, changing lives: The mental health strategy for Canada*.

Calgary, AB: Author. Retrieved from http://strategy.mentalhealthcommission.ca/pdf/strategy-images-en.pdf

Morrison, P., & Peterson, W. (2013). *Schools as a setting for promoting positive mental health: Better practices and perspectives* (2nd ed.). Ottawa, ON: Joint Consortium for School Health. Retrieved from http://www.jcsh-cces.ca/upload/JCSH%20Best%20Practice_Eng_Jan21.pdf

Moynagh, K., & Singleton, M. (2011). *Mental health liaison program evaluation: Client outcomes and satisfaction with services*. Halton, ON: Halton Region Health Department. Retrieved from http://www.halton.ca/living_in_halton/public_health/halton_health_statistics/mental_health/mental_health_liaison_program_evaluation__client_o

Nova Scotia Department of Health Promotion and Protection. (2009). *An evaluation of youth health centres in Nova Scotia: Executive summary*. Retrieved from http://novascotia.ca/dhw/healthy-development/documents/Youth-Health-Centres-in-Nova-Scotia-An-Evaluation.pdf

Ontario Ministry of Children and Youth Services. (2012). *Stepping stones: A resource on youth development*. Toronto, ON: Author. Retrieved from http://www.children.gov.on.ca/htdocs/English/documents/topics/youthopportunities/steppingstones/SteppingStones.pdf

Ontario Ministry of Health and Long-Term Care. (2013). *No time to wait: The healthy kids strategy*. Toronto, ON: Author. Retrieved from http://www.health.gov.on.ca/en/common/ministry/publications/reports/healthy_kids/healthy_kids.pdf

Ontario Ministry of Health Promotion. (2010). *School health guidance document*. Retrieved from http://www.health.gov.on.ca/en/pro/programs/publichealth/oph_standards/docs/guidance/SchoolHealth.pdf

Ordre des infirmières et infirmiers du Québec. (2015). *Standards de pratique pour l'infirmière en santé scolaire* (2nd ed.). Montreal, QC: Author. Retrieved from https://www.oiiq.org/sites/default/files/SanteScolaire-Abrege-Final%20Web.pdf

Pickett, W. (2011). Injuries. In J. G. Freeman, M. King, & W. Pickett (Eds.), *The health of Canada's young people: A mental health focus*. Retrieved from http://www.phac-aspc.gc.ca/hp-ps/dca-dea/publications/health-young-people-sante-jeunes-canadiens/assets/pdf/health-young-people-sante-jeunes-canadiens-eng.pdf

Public Health Agency of Canada. (2006). *The human face of mental health and mental illness in Canada*. Ottawa, ON: PHAC.

Public Health Agency of Canada. (2011a). *The chief public health officer's report on the state of public health in Canada: Youth and young adults—Life in transition*. Retrieved from http://www.phac-aspc.gc.ca/cphorsphc-respcacsp/2011/index-eng.php

Public Health Agency of Canada. (2011b). *Our health our future: A national dialogue on healthy weights dialogue report*. Ottawa, ON: Ascentum. Retrieved from http://www.phac-aspc.gc.ca/hp-ps/hl-mvs/ohof-nsna/index-eng.php?utm_source=VanityURL&utm_medium=URL&utm_campaign=ourhealthourfuture.gc.ca

Public Health Agency of Canada. (2013). *The chief public health officer's report on the state of public health in Canada: Infectious disease—The never-ending threat*. Retrieved from http://www.phac-aspc.gc.ca/cphorsphc-respcacsp/2013/index-eng.php

Registered Nurses Association of Ontario. (2010). *Nursing best practice guideline: Enhancing healthy adolescent development.* Toronto, ON: Author.

Roberts, K. C., Shields, M., de Groh, M., Aziz, A., & Gilbert, J. (2012). Overweight and obesity in children and adolescents: Results from the 2009 to 2011 Canadian health measures survey. *Health Reports 23*(3). Statistics Canada, Catalogue no. 82-003-XPE.

Rotermann, M. (2012). Sexual behaviour and condom use of 15- to 24-year-olds in 2003 and 2009/2010. *Health Reports, 23*(1). Statistics Canada, Catalogue no. 82-003-XPE.

Saewyc, E., Roy, J., & Foster, S. (2014). *An evaluation of North Shore public health nurses' child and youth school-linked practice.* Vancouver, BC: Vancouver Coastal Health. Retrieved from http://www.saravyc.ubc.ca/files/2014/11/NorthShore-PHN-Evaluation.pdf

Skinner, R., & McFaull, S. (2012). Suicide among children and adolescents in Canada: Trends and sex differences, 1980–2008. *Canadian Medical Association Journal, 184,* 1029–34. doi:10.1503/cmaj.111867

Statistics Canada. (2014). Table 1: Headcount enrolments in public elementary and secondary schools, Canada, provinces and territories, 2008/2009 to 2012/2013. *The Daily,* November 21, 1–2.

Statistics Canada. (2011). *Table 102-0551: Deaths and mortality rate by selected group causes, age group and sex, Canada, annual.* CANSIM database. Retrieved from http://www5.statcan.gc.ca/cansim/a26?lang=eng&retrLang=eng&id=1020551

Stewart-Brown, S. (2006). *What is the evidence on school health promotion in improving health or preventing disease and, specifically, what is the effectiveness of the health promoting schools approach?* Copenhagen: WHO Regional Office for Europe. Retrieved from http://www.euro.who.int/__data/assets/pdf_file/0007/74653/E88185.pdf

Trim, K. (2011). *Perth District Health Unit and Avon Maitland District School Board: 2006–2010 School-based public health nurse program evaluation.* Retrieved from http://www.pdhu.on.ca/wp-content/uploads/2015/04/PDHU-and-AMDSB-2006-2010-School-Based-PHN-Program-Evaluation.pdf

Weare, K. (2010). Promoting mental health through schools. In P. Aggleton, C. Dennison, & I. Warwick (Eds.), *Promoting health and well-being through schools* (pp. 24–41). New York, NY: Routledge.

World Health Organization. (2013). *Investing in mental health: evidence for action.* Geneva, Switzerland: Author. Retrieved from http://apps.who.int/iris/bitstream/10665/87232/1/9789241564618_eng.pdf

## ABOUT THE AUTHORS

**Yvette Laforêt-Fliesser**, RN, BScN, MScN (Western University), CCHN(C), is an independent Consultant in community and public health with 40 years of progressive experience in public health and community nursing, academia, and management. As a volunteer, she has served on a number of boards and committees including the Community Health Nurses of Canada, the CNA CHN Certification Exam Committee, and the Ontario Healthy Schools Coalition and is currently on the board of the London Intercommunity Health Centre. Yvette is an adjunct associate professor at Western University and is a recipient of the CHNIG Award of Excellence in Community Health Nursing and an Honorary Lifetime Membership in CHNC for her contributions to advancing community health nursing in Canada.

**Carol MacDougall**, RN, BScN (McGill University), MA (Ontario Institute for Studies in Education, Department of Curriculum, Teaching and Learning, University of Toronto), has worked for 12 years as a public health nurse in Toronto schools, five years as the school health consultant in planning and policy with Toronto Public Health, and since 2006, as the public health manager, School and Sexual Health, at the Perth District Health Unit in Stratford, Ontario. She has been involved in provincial advocacy for comprehensive school health since 1990, and is co-chair of the Ontario Healthy Schools Coalition.

**Cheryl MacLeod**, RN, BScN (University of Saskatchewan), MEd (University of Calgary), CCHN(C), is the area Manager for the East Calgary Health Centre and Sheldon M. Chumir Health Centre. Prior to this, she was the lead for public health nursing practice for school and well-child nursing services with Alberta Health Services, Calgary Zone. Over her 30-plus year nursing career, she has provided direction, leadership, support, and development for public health nursing. Cheryl is chair of the Alberta Coalition for Healthy School Communities. Since 2008, she has volunteered as a mentor with the UNITAR (United Nations Institute for Training and Research) Fellowship for Afghanistan, building leadership and management skills of Afghan professionals.

# Family Health

*Lucia Yiu, Marilyn Sutton, and Candace Martin Ryan*

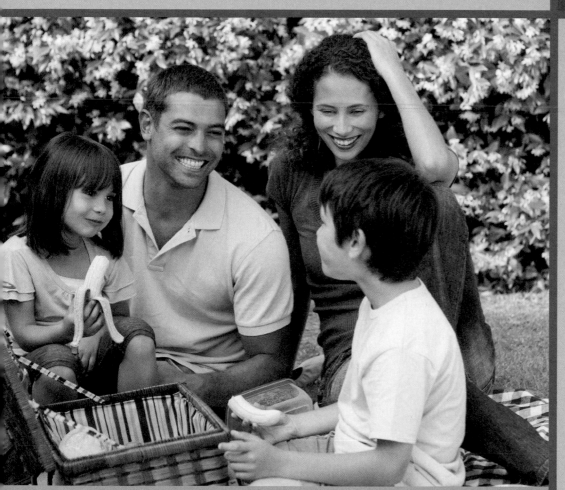

*Source: Wavebreakmedia/Shutterstock*

## LEARNING OUTCOMES

**After studying this chapter, you should be able to:**

1. Define family and its basic purposes.

2. Describe the theoretical frameworks of family health-care nursing.

3. Discuss the components and basic characteristics of family assessment.

4. Relate family home visits to the Canadian Community Health Nursing Standards.

5. Discuss case management in relation to family-centred care.

6. Discuss future research and challenges for community family health nurses.

## INTRODUCTION

Families are the basic units of the society and a major source of functional, emotional, psychological, and informational support for members of the family unit. We all begin life as daughters or sons to our biological or adopted parents. We become sisters or brothers, grandchildren, nieces or nephews, and cousins within the traditional view of the family. For many, friends and pets are also treated as family members. We all play many different roles within our family units and in the lives of our significant others.

Community health nurses (CHNs) practising family nursing find personal rewards when they can make a difference in promoting health or reducing suffering in the lives of their family clients. This chapter describes the social and cultural context of the family and a brief overview of theoretical frameworks that guide family nursing practice, family case management, and family-centred care. Opportunities and challenges for CHNs will also be discussed.

# WHY STUDY FAMILY NURSING?

Because we all came from a family unit, many individuals, including nurses, tend to believe that they are experts in the family based on their personal experiences. Some of these personal experiences may present a romantic view of a nuclear family where there may be two loving heterosexual parents and two well-accomplished children living in a middle-class neighbourhood; the children have good grades in school, the parents have successful careers, and the family attends religious services and has a wide network of social support. In contrast, some other personal experiences may result in a stigmatized view of a chaotic, dysfunctional family, where there may be multiple problems, such as poverty, substance abuse, and violence; where the family members "bring on" their problems as a result of poor decisions and lifestyles; and where multiproblem families are regarded as a burden to society. Thus, CHNs must be aware of the impact of their own values and beliefs about family and how these may shape their approach to providing family nursing care.

Family nursing practice is guided by the Community Health Nurses of Canada (CHNC) (2011, revised) and the Canadian Nurses Association (CNA) (2013), both of which state that CHNs care for families as clients in their practice, and that nurses must act on ways to improve social determinants of health to promote family health. Some of these social determinants of health can impact the health of individuals, families, and populations, and result in inequity in the health status of populations. Social determinants of health can affect the conditions in which people live, play, learn, and work; they determine the extent to which people attain the physical, social, and personal resources to meet their family needs and cope with ongoing problems in these areas: food security, income, job security, housing, physical and social environments, access to education, early childhood development, transportation, safety, and social inclusion (Public Health Agency of Canada, 2013) (see Chapter 8).

CHNs also recognize the need to study family nursing for these reasons: (1) health behaviours are learned in the family, (2) the health of one family member affects the health of the rest of the family, and (3) family plays a key healthcare function role, from health promotion and maintenance to palliative care (Rowe Kaakinen, Padgett Coehlo, Steele, Tabacco, & Harmon Hanson, 2014).

# FAMILY NURSING

Family nursing has evolved considerably since early 1980s and is now a specialty practice in nursing (Wright & Leahey, 2013). **Family nursing** is a provision of care where the nurse uses nursing processes to assist the family and its members in achieving their highest potential health through coping and adapting to various health and illness situations. **Family health** is the changing, relative state of well-being that includes wellness in the biological, psychological, sociological, cultural, and spiritual aspects of the family system (Stanhope & Lancaster, 2014).

Hunt (2013) stressed that when working with families, besides developing a therapeutic relationship with the family, the nurse needs to view the family as a system, functioning to achieve a state of equilibrium or optimal health at all times. Any changes introduced to any parts of the family will cause changes in other parts of the family system. CHNs strive to provide competent family nursing care that promotes family health by understanding the trends of today's families and their health challenges as they move through various life events.

# TRENDS IN CANADIAN FAMILIES

According to Statistics Canada (2012a), currently married couples comprise the predominant family structure (67%), followed by common-law couples (16.7%), and then lone-parent families (16.3%). Figure 18.1 illustrates that common-law families are the fastest-growing family structure, followed by lone-parent families, while the proportion of married couples has decreased. Despite the legalization and growing number of same-sex marriages since 2005, same-sex couples (married and common-law) account for only 0.6% of all Canadian families. One significant change impacting family composition is the large cohort of aging *baby boomers* (born between 1946 and 1964) now entering their senior years. Many of these older adults now are living with their adult children, forming **multigenerational households** that typically consist of children less than 14 years of age, their parents, and at least one grandparent. (See Photo 18.1.)

The *baby busters*, born between 1965 and 1976, following the baby boom when the birthrate dropped dramatically, contributed to the increasing numbers of couples without children (Bushnik, Cook, Hughes, & Tough, 2012). As Canadian families became smaller over the past 50 years, the fertility rate dropped to 1.61 in 2011 (Statistics Canada, 2013a), the average number of children per Canadian family

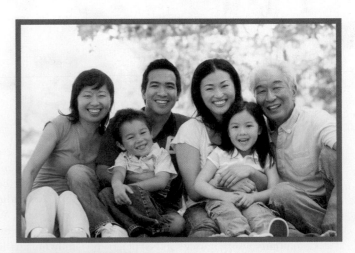

**PHOTO 18.1** Three-generation households are becoming increasingly common in Canada.

*Source: Monkey Business Images/Shutterstock*

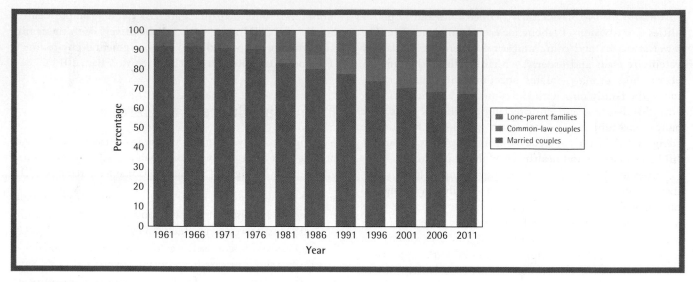

**FIGURE** **18.1** Distribution (in percentage) of Census Families by Family Structure, Canada, 1961 to 2011

*Source:* Statistics Canada. (n. d.). *Fifty years of families in Canada: 1961 to 2011.* (98-312-X2011003). Retrieved from http://www12 .statcan.gc.ca/census-recensement/2011/as-sa/98-312-x/98-312-x2011003_1-eng.pdf

also decreased from 2.7 in 1961 to 1.9 in 2011, and the average number of people per family declined from 3.9 in 1961 to 2.9 in 2011 (Statistics Canada, 2012a).

Despite the shrinking family size, the number of Canadian households has increased. This phenomenon was largely due to the aging population and the higher rates of separation and divorce leading to a growing number of non-traditional families. CHNs should note that the current low fertility rate is below the expected population replacement rate; there will be fewer children sharing the caregiving responsibilities for aging parents. Both trends will have economic and healthcare impacts on society.

## WHAT IS FAMILY?

The definition of family has changed significantly over the last five decades. Traditional definitions of family have used the legal concepts of relationships, such as genetic ties, adoption, guardianship, or marriage (Stanhope & Lancaster, 2014). Today, the definitions of family are more encompassing. The Vanier Institute of the Family (2010) defines the **family** as "any combination of two or more persons who are bound together over time by ties of mutual consent, birth and/or adoption or placement" (p. xii). Wright and Leahey (2013) also state that "the family is who they say they are" (p. 55). Some families, especially the elderly who live alone, consider their pet a valued family member. Nurses therefore should ask families who they consider to be members of their family and include them in healthcare planning (Hunt, 2013).

**Family forms** refer to how the family is structured or composed, as families can take various forms: nuclear, extended, lone parent, blended, and homosexual families. In Canada, same-sex marriages have been legalized since July 2005 with the enactment of the Civil Marriage Act (Government of Canada, 2015).

**Family structure** refers to the characteristics and demographics (i.e., gender, age, and number) of individual members who make up the family unit. The structure of a family defines the roles and positions of family members (Stanhope & Lancaster, 2014). Friedman, Bowden, and Jones (2003) examine how the family is organized, and they stress four structural dimensions: family power and decision making, roles, values, and communication. For example, a father unilaterally decides where the family will go on vacation. He communicates this decision to his wife with the expectation that she will inform the children. Here we see a *patriarchal family* where power and decision making reside with the father who has indirect communication patterns with his children.

**Family functions** are defined as "behaviours or activities performed to maintain the integrity of the family unit and to meet the family's needs, individual members' needs, and society's expectations" (Stanhope & Lancaster, 2014). How well the family fulfills its functions or attains its goals is related to family structure. Thus, these two concepts are intimately connected (Freistadt & Strohschein, 2012).

The Vanier Institute of the Family (2010) described the following functions or responsibilities characterized by **healthy families:**

- physical maintenance and care of group members;
- addition of new members through procreation or adoption;
- socialization of children;
- social control of members;
- production, consumption, and distribution of goods and services; and
- affective nurturance—love (p. xii).

*Healthy families* have clearly defined roles and responsibilities and division of labour for each family member. The power structure and communication system for the family system are clear and orderly, which enhances the family's relationships, problem-solving or coping skills, and socialization of the family unit with the community. When working with childbearing and childrearing families, CHNs have many opportunities to work with beginning families to strengthen the family system by promoting healthy parent–child relationships and healthy child development.

All families experience many developmental and situational crises throughout their various family developmental stages (see Table 18.1). Healthy families cope with these crises as they acquire new skills and confidence to cope with other developmental tasks. **Dysfunctional families** often lack problem-solving skills and resources to deal with these crises, which result in the buildup of problems. A **multiproblem family** is one with "needs in several areas simultaneously, difficulty achieving developmental tasks, illness or loss, inadequate resources and support, or environmental stressors" (Smith, 2013a, p. 374). An example of a multiproblem family would be a single, unemployed mother with limited support who has just given birth to a baby with Down syndrome. The intensity and multiplicity of stressors associated with life events can put these families at increased risk and vulnerability (Smith, 2013a).

To effectively work with multiproblem families, CHNs must consider three key factors. First, the CHN must understand that external factors such as poverty, unemployment, isolation, and lack of support system can shape the family biologically, psychologically, and interpersonally. Second, the CHN must help the family anticipate risks and subsequently mobilize resources to mitigate risks and promote health. Finally, the CHN must work collaboratively with the family in a trusting, respectful, and non-judgmental environment (Browne, Doane, Reimer, MacLeod, & McLellan, 2011).

## Family as Context of Care

Viewing the family as context of care is the traditional focus of nursing. There are five ways of viewing the family (Friedman et al., 2003) (see Figure 18.2 and Canadian Research Box 18.1):

- The *first level* is to view the family as context to the client. The CHN focuses nursing care on the individual, with the family as a secondary focus. For example, the CHN might provide counselling for a depressed teenager in clinic settings or care for hospitalized clients.
- In the *second level*, the family is viewed as the sum of its individual family members or parts. The focus of care is on the individual family member, and members are seen as separate entities rather than interacting units. For example, the CHN might provide counselling to each member of a family facing divorce.
- In the *third level* of family nursing practice, family dyads, triads, and other family subsystems are the focus of care. For example, a CHN might focus on the care of the new mother and her baby during a home visit.
- Viewing the family as client is the *fourth level* of family nursing practice. It is the most unique type of family nursing. Here the entire family is the unit of care. The nurse provides care for both the individual and the whole family and society simultaneously, and provides healthcare for all family members. The focus is placed on internal family dynamics, relationships, family structure, and functions. The CHN assesses the interactions among the family subsystems within its own family system and with their external environment. An example is the nurse caring for a family with a family member experiencing cancer or a chronic or acute illness.
- A *fifth level* of family nursing conceptualizes family as a component of society. The family is seen as one of society's basic institutions. An example would be clients living in long-term care facilities.

## Theoretical Frameworks of Family Health Nursing

Theories help us to "make sense" of our world and they guide our nursing practice. Family social science theories, family therapy theories, and nursing models and theories all contribute to the emerging field of family nursing theories. No one theory or conceptual model, however, is sufficient for describing the multifaceted nature of family processes and relationships (Rowe Kaakinen et al., 2014). CHNs will need to be competent in knowledge and skills to integrate multiple theories in order to fully understand the perspectives on families,

| TABLE 18.1 | Family Life Cycle Stages and Tasks |
|---|---|
| **Stages** | **Task** |
| Launching of the single young adult | Differentiation from family of origin |
| | Financial independence |
| Marriage: The joining of families | Commitment to and establishing a new family |
| Families with young children | Adjustment to parenthood and new family members |
| | Meeting age-appropriate developmental needs of children |
| | Maintaining supportive relationships with children and across generations |
| Families with adolescents | Adjustment to needs of young adults leaving and/or re-entering the family |
| Launching children and moving on | Adjusting to changes in the partner relationship |
| Families in later life | Adjustments to retirement, end of life |

Source: Adapted from Wright, L. M., & Leahey, M. M. (2012). *Nurses and families: A guide to family assessment and intervention* (6th ed.). Philadelphia, PA: F. A. Davis. (pp. 95–110).

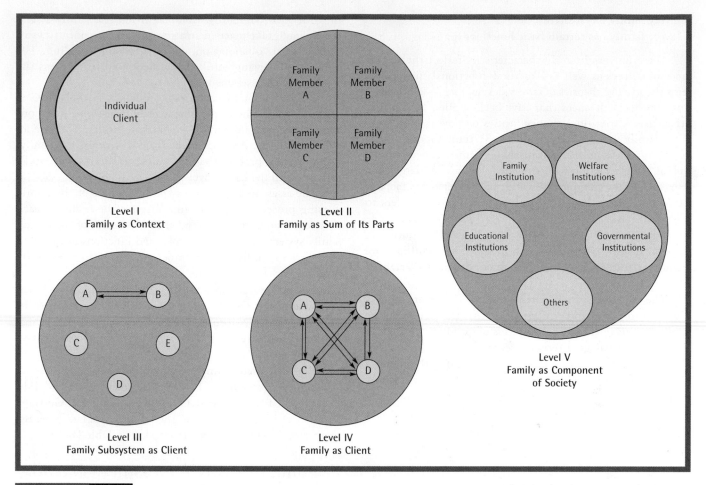

**FIGURE 18.2** Five Ways of Viewing the Family

*Source:* Reproduced with permission from Friedman, M. M., Bowden, V. R., & Jones, E. G. (Eds.). (2003). *Family nursing: Research, theory, and practice* (5th ed.). Upper Saddle River, NJ: Prentice Hall, p. 37. © Reprinted by permission of Pearson Education, Inc. Upper Saddle River, NJ.

---

### CANADIAN RESEARCH BOX 18.1

#### How to improve the quality of care for hospitalized older adults?

Parke, B. I., Hunter, K. F., Bostrom, A. M., Chambers, T., & Manraj, C. (2014). Identifying modifiable factors to improve quality for older adults in hospital: A scoping review. *International Journal of Older People Nursing, 9*(1), 8–24. doi:10.1111/opn.12007

Nurses have been attending to the social climate; physical design; care systems; and processes, policies, and procedures when providing age-friendly hospital care. Yet, modifiable factors that may contribute to hospitalized elderly clients' disability were often ignored. This exploratory scoping review of primary research evaluated a total of 66 studies for modifiable factors related to the healthcare systems and processes among hospitalized community-dwelling older adults. Four theoretical dimensions were identified: models of care, assessment of potential geriatric issues, targeting care to specific clinical or health issues, and supporting client's transition to home. The researchers stressed that to provide competent gerontological nursing for hospitalized older adults, nurses must have further understanding of the older adult and family as a unit of care in the hospital environment, and design competent nursing interventions based on the modifiable factors.

#### Discussion Questions

1. Discuss your thoughts on the level of family nursing addressed in this study.
2. What might the nurse do to provide family-focused care for hospitalized clients?

---

then to design effective nursing interventions within the contexts of health promotion and the social determinants of health.

Although every family is unique, all families share some universal characteristics. Drake (2014) lists five most important *characteristics of a family*:

- every family is a small social system;
- every family moves through stages in its life cycle;
- every family has its own cultural values and rules;

- every family has structure; and
- every family has certain basic functions (p. 571).

These universal family characteristics reflect the importance of culture as well as structural–functional theory, systems theory, and theories of family development—all theories from the social sciences that have been applied to families. **Structural–functional theory** focuses on how the structure of the family affects family functions. **Systems theory** focuses on the interactions within and among family subsystems as well as the interaction with extended families and larger systems such as the community, world, and universe (Stanhope & Lancaster, 2014). **Family developmental theory** refers to stages and tasks as presented in Table 18.1. This family life cycle approach refers to the generally predictable sequence of stages that most North American middle-class families move through despite their cultural or ethnic variations (Wright & Leahey, 2013).

The theories, frameworks, and assessment models discussed in this chapter all recognize that the CHN and the family are engaged in a social process of exploration, negotiation, and mutual goal setting, centred within the family–nurse relationship. Interventions are grounded in the contexts of family structure and function, family development, family support and environment, health work and potential health promotion, education and advocacy, the social determinants of health, and the principles of primary health care.

## FAMILY ASSESSMENT

The purpose of **family assessment** is to determine family roles, communication, division of labour, decision making, power structure, boundaries, styles of problem solving, coping abilities, and health promotion practices (Friedman et al., 2003; Wright & Leahey, 2013). During the assessment process, the nurse facilitates the family in discovering and articulating the often unexamined assumptions, context, and expectations underlying its perception of reality. The family assessment process takes time, sensitivity, and flexibility and requires the CHN to have effective interviewing skills. The nurse conducts the assessment starting from the perspective of the family at the time when the nurse begins

to work with the family. Competent holistic family assessment should take place in an atmosphere of openness, awareness, mutual collaboration, and relationship building. The nurse uses relevant family assessment tools to address the purpose of the assessment.

Regardless of the concepts, models, and tools used, a comprehensive family assessment uses open-ended questions and is detailed and inclusive. Nursing assessments are an ongoing process. An assessment is not "done to" the family; rather, it is a process that the nurse facilitates and works through with the family over time.

The assessment process is the first phase of the family nursing process. The nurse first assesses the health of each individual family member and then the health of the overall family system in terms of its roles and functions in fulfilling the needs of individual members. Such collective family assessment data provide the foundation for planning, interventions, and evaluation of nursing care. Both family strengths and weaknesses will be identified during the assessment. However, the CHN focuses on how to assist the family to recognize its own strengths and use various resources to achieve its family goals.

The Friedman Family Assessment Model (Friedman et al., 2003), the Calgary Family Assessment Model (Wright & Leahey, 2013), and the McGill Model (Gottlieb & Gottlieb, 2007; Gottlieb & Rowat, 1987) are examples of family assessment models which will be discussed. (See Table 18.2.)

## Friedman Family Assessment Model

The **Friedman Family Assessment Model** has six broad categories (Friedman et al., 2003). *Identifying data* include family composition, cultural background, religious identification, social class status, and recreational activities. The *developmental stage* is assessed along with the family's history and the history of both parents' family of origin. *Environmental data* include characteristics of the home, neighbourhood, and community; the family's geographic mobility; associations with the community and use of community resources; and the family's social support system. *Family structure* looks at communication patterns, power structure, role structure, and family values. *Affective, socialization, and healthcare functions* are assessed in the family functions category. The sixth category, *family*

| TABLE 18.2 | Components of Family Assessment Models | | |
|---|---|---|---|
| **Friedman Family Assessment Model** | **Calgary Family Assessment Model** | **McGill Model** | |
| Identifying data | Developmental stage and history of family | The family as the subsystem | |
| Developmental stage and history of family | Structural | Health as the focus of work | |
| Environmental data | Developmental | Learning as the process through which health behaviours are acquired | |
| Family structure | Functional | Family collaborates with the nurse in the learning process | |
| Family functions | | | |
| Family coping | | | |

Source: Adapted from Registered Nurses' Association of Ontario. (2006). *Supporting and strengthening families through expected and unexpected life events* (rev. suppl.). Toronto, ON: Registered Nurses' Association of Ontario.

*stress and coping*, includes assessment of stressors and strengths along with coping strategies. Each category has many subcategories. The nurse and the family decide which areas need in-depth exploration based on the focus for nursing intervention.

## Calgary Family Assessment Model

Wright and Leahey (2013) first developed the **Calgary Family Assessment Model (CFAM)** in 1983 at the University of Calgary in Canada. The CFAM has been conceptualized as a branching model with three major categories: structural, developmental, and functional (see Figure 18.3). The nurse decides which subcategories should be explored and to what extent, and assesses each family accordingly. The nurse and the family move back and forth across the branches to integrate all relevant data and build a holistic picture of the family's strengths, problems, and current situation.

Interventions conceptualized in the **Calgary Family Intervention Model (CFIM)** provide a framework for family functions in three domains: cognitive, affective, and behavioural, and these interventions focus on promoting, improving, and sustaining effective family functioning. Interventions that affect changes in family's beliefs and values (cognition domain) provide the most significant and lasting changes. A change in cognition can, in turn, influence the affective and behavioural domains (Wright & Leahey, 2013).

## McGill Model

The **McGill Model** has been developed and refined over time by faculty and students at the McGill University School of Nursing (Gottlieb & Gottlieb, 2007; Gottlieb & Rowat, 1987). This model emphasizes family, health, collaboration,

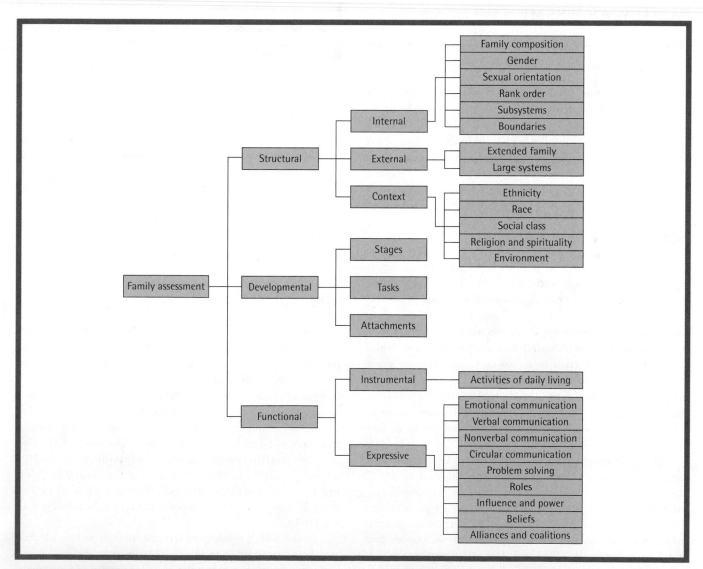

**FIGURE 18.3** Branching Diagram of Calgary Family Assessment Model

*Source:* Wright, M. L., & Leahey, M. M. (2012). *Nurses and families: A guide to family assessment and intervention* (6th ed.). Philadelphia, PA: F. A. Davis, p. 52. Used by permission of F. A. Davis & Company.

and learning; and health consists of processes that are dynamic and multi-dimensional, especially the processes of coping and development. The family is an active participant throughout the healthcare process. In this model, one of the nursing goals is to help families use the strengths of the individual family members and of the family as unit, as well as resources external to the family system, to cope, achieve their goals, and develop.

The assessment phase of the McGill Model requires the nurse to explore and create a supportive environment so that the family's perceptions and strengths can emerge. Learning needs are identified and the initiative for planning can be with the nurse or the family (Gottlieb & Rowat, 1987). During the implementation phase, the family becomes an active learner in collaboration with the nurse. The nurse, as an empowering partner, fosters the families to reach a potential for positive growth.

## FAMILY ASSESSMENT TOOLS

There are various family assessment tools to assist the nurse in collecting and organizing family data. So how does the CHN decide on an assessment tool that will then guide interventions? It is not a case of "one size fits all" or of designing the "perfect" model. Rather, it is having the openness, knowledge, and skill to evaluate existing theories, models, and tools in light of what would be most appropriate and effective for the client, and integrating and adapting as necessary. Two valuable tools for all assessments are the genogram and ecomap.

## Genogram

**Genograms** are a visual sketch providing a picture of family structure, relationships, and boundaries. Usually, the nurse constructs a three-generational genogram (or more, as needed) to examine the patterns and relationships of family events. Effective family assessment skills specific to communication and interviewing are essential to constructing meaningful genograms. A genogram is a tool that can help the nurse uncover the roots of significant family problems related to intergenerational health and social problems (e.g., alcoholism, diabetes, heart problems, cancer, hereditary diseases, and critical family events such as births, divorces, twin births, miscarriages, etc.). (See Figure 18.4.)

The genogram illustrated in Figure 18.4 shows the family of Mr. and Mrs. W., who were married in 1990. Mrs. W. is 52 years of age and lives with her 53-year-old husband and their two children, who are 9 and 13 years of age. The oldest daughter is in Grade 8 and the younger daughter is in Grade 4 at the local elementary school. Mr. W.'s father died of stomach cancer in 2000 and Mrs. W.'s mother died of pancreatitis in 1962. Mrs. W. did not know her father. Mrs. W. was diagnosed with locally advanced breast cancer in 2008. Mrs. W. works as a researcher and Mr. W. works as an administrator. The W. family is used as a case study later in the chapter.

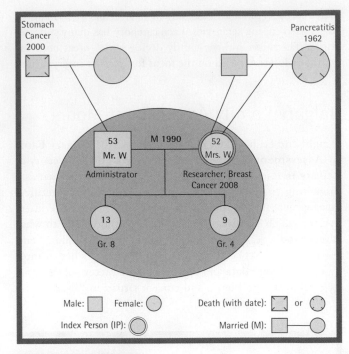

**FIGURE 18.4** Genogram

## Ecomap

An **ecomap** is a visual representation of a family's connections and the nature and degree of its relationships with the larger community, such as schools, friends, workplace, social and health workers or agencies, etc. The nurse constructs a family ecomap to assess the family strengths, such as available resources and support systems, including strains or conflicting relationships experienced by the family (Wright & Leahey, 2013) (see Figure 18.5).

## The ABCX Model

All families encounter stressful events. While some families can overcome these stressful events and maintain family cohesion and function, other families cannot. The **ABCX model**, developed by Rueben Hill (1958), is used to explain "the crisis-proneness and freedom from crisis among families" (p. 143). Also known as the stress model, Hill's ABCX model focuses on the interaction of four common factors faced by families in any crisis state: A (a crisis or precipitating *event/stressor*) interacting with B (the *resources* available to the family during the crisis), interacting with C (family's *perception* of the event/stressor) to produce X (the *crisis* state experienced by the family) (see Figure 18.6).

In the ABCX model, the stressor encountered by a family may be a life event or transition that impacts the family system, thereby affecting the roles and functions of various members in the family system. **Stressors** may be normative changes experienced along the life cycle, unpredictable challenges, or catastrophic events. A positive stressor might be a job promotion or winning a lottery, whereas a negative stressor might be

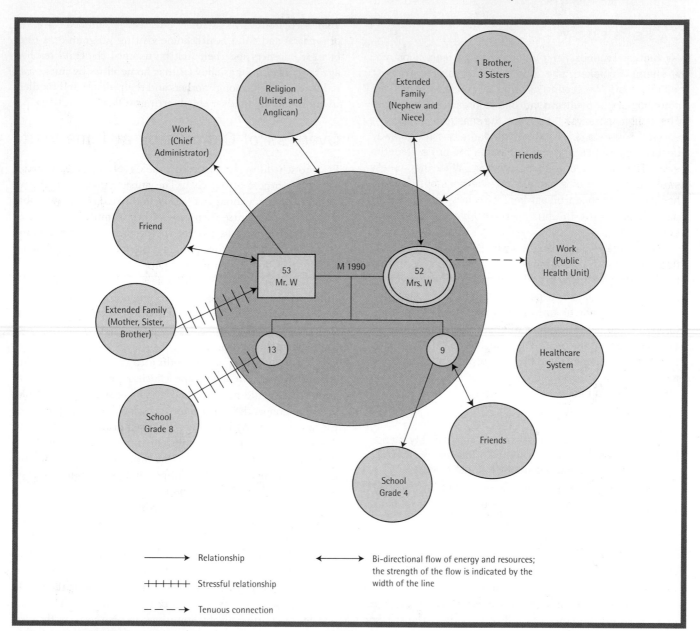

**FIGURE** **18.5** Ecomap

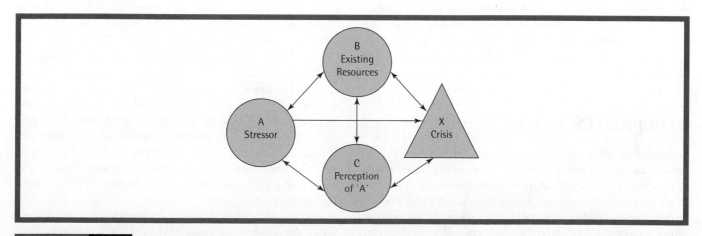

**FIGURE** **18.6** ABCX Model

*Source:* Adapted from McCubbin, H. I., & Patterson, J. M. (1983). Family transitions: Adaptation to stress. In H. I. McCubbin & C. R. Figley (Eds.), *Stress and the family, Volume I: Coping with normative transitions* (pp. 5–25). New York, NY: Brunner/Mazel. (p. 12). Used with permission of Psychology Press.

**A**mother touches her right breast and feels a painful lump. Panicked, she tells herself it is probably just another cyst. The feeling of relief is wonderful when the mammogram and ultrasound of the breast are negative. The radiologist says, "It's from the mastitis you experienced 13 years ago." However, the lump doesn't go away despite antibiotics and anti-inflammatory drugs. Months pass. The lump seems to be growing. When her breast swells to the size of a cantaloupe, she finds out that she has locally advanced breast cancer. Now what? She wonders if she will live to Christmas and what she is going to tell her girls.

Rose, the younger daughter who is 9 years old, is terrified. Her best friend's mother has just died of a brain tumour; Rose wonders if her mom is next. Rose begins to have stomach pains and headaches, and is not sleeping. She does not want to go to school and leave her mother. Charlotte, the older daughter who is 13 years old, focuses all of her attention on school and has difficulty talking about what is happening to her mother. John, her husband, must leave for a week-long conference. He wonders if he should leave his family.

### Discussion Questions

1. Describe how you would assess the family's ability to cope with the cancer diagnosis and help this family "survive" this unexpected and potentially traumatic event.

2. What family nursing interventions could you employ, and how would you assess the effectiveness of those interventions?

an illness in a family member (e.g., spouse, child, or grandparent) or a job loss. **Strains** are additional demands and hardships placed on the family as a direct result of the stressor. Families with good problem-solving and coping skills will learn to adapt and accept life stressors or events in a positive way by using available resources to overcome changes or hardships, thereby avoiding the crisis. Families who view their life events negatively are likely to be reluctant to seek help and will live in crisis or dysfunctional mode (McCubbin & McCubbin, 1993). (See Case Study.)

## THE FAMILY HOME VISIT

Historically, CHNs cared for the sick and the poor and visited families in their homes (see Chapter 1); thus, the family home visit is seen as the "root" of community health nursing practice. Family home visits allow the nurse to observe and interact with a family in their natural environment. It also allows nurses to better understand the needs of the collective family in addition to the individual family members (Wright & Leahey, 2013). The key benefit of the home visit is supported by a recent randomized clinical trial conducted in Memphis,

Tennessee, from 1990 to 2011. This study examined the effect of prenatal and child health home visiting program on a total of 1238 mothers and their first-borns until the child reached age two. The findings showed that home visits by nurses can reduce mortality among mothers and their infants and toddlers living in highly disadvantaged settings (Olds et al., 2014).

## Overview of Conducting a Home Visit

Prior to scheduling a home visit, the CHN must clearly articulate the purpose of the visit. The nurse collects and reviews all pertinent data about the family, and based on the available family data, the nurse then proceeds to formulate hypotheses and tentative plans as part of the preparation for the home visit. This is done before phoning the family to schedule an appointment for the home visit. Drop-in visits are not encouraged and would be seen as unprofessional, and would not be time and cost effective if the family is not home; however, it may be done depending on the situation, such as if the client is well-known to the nurse, has no phone connection, or agrees to the nurse doing drop-in visits.

Active listening and attending to the family's needs are crucial throughout the home-visiting process. The initial home visit should be scheduled by phone as soon as possible. Over the phone, the nurse begins to establish the rapport with the family client by introducing himself or herself and stating the reason and anticipated length of home visit. The visit usually is no more than an hour. This first contact to the family, usually by phone, is of prime importance as the nurse enters a working relationship with the family. The nurse conducts a skilful assessment of the family needs during the phone interview, hypothesizes what the nursing diagnoses might be, and plans for the visit to meet the client needs accordingly.

At the first home visit, the nurse uses the first few minutes of the home visit to gain rapport and put the family at ease. The nurse clarifies his or her role and informs the family of the agency policies, including confidentiality. The nurse restates the purpose of the home visit to set a focus of the visit or to ensure that the family situation has not changed since the last phone contact or scheduled home visit. The family interview usually is carried out either in the living room or kitchen, usually as determined by the client.

When the family assessment begins, priority is given to the important needs as identified by the family. Ideally, the whole family should be present at the home visit. If not possible, and at times not all family members need to be present at the family interview, the nurse would interview the decision maker of the family or the person who needs to be visited by the nurse. Each family member is given an opportunity to provide input where appropriate. Families have the right to terminate the nursing visit anytime. CHNs must use effective interviewing skills, including active listening, when conducting a home visit.

Nurses plan for mutually set goals with the family according to the desires and needs of the family. Developing contracts concerning the plan of care and frequency of visits is a way to clearly identify roles and expectations. If the situation arises, it is important for the CHNs to discuss with the family their professional and legal responsibility to report to authorities such as Children's Aid Society or the police (Stanhope & Lancaster, 2014; Wright & Leahey, 2013).

When the visit comes to a close, it is important for the nurse to summarize what was discussed or accomplished at the visit, to review mutually agreed-upon roles and actions, to discuss referrals if needed, and to schedule the next visit or terminate the visits where appropriate. Over the course of the working relationship with the family, the nurse works on assisting the family to develop needed knowledge and skills, and acquire resources to sustain the progress made. The nurse acts as a helper and not as a rescuer (Stanhope & Lancaster, 2014; Wright & Leahey, 2013). When the goals are achieved, the nurse plans for termination of the visits. If achieving the goals is beyond the nurse's ability or scope of practice, referrals must be made for continuity of care for the family.

Clinical notes should be documented after each visit to record the assessment data, the plan of care, the implementation of the interventions, as well as an evaluation of any progress toward the goals. When the care for the family is beyond the CHNs' scope of practice or ability to care, the nurse will initiate a referral to ensure that the family will receive the right care by the right personnel in a timely fashion. Professional nursing home visits must be purposeful and goal oriented.

CHNs must pay particular attention to their personal safety. When home visiting, CHNs are most likely going into unknown environments. This is one of the reasons for nurses to be knowledgeable about their neighbourhoods in the community. Nurses could attend to their personal safety by sharing their visiting schedules with the agency, including the location of the visits. A plan of action should be in place in case of emergencies. Once in the home, nurses can quickly determine an exit route and sit in a barrier-free location near the door. If nurses feel uncomfortable or encounter a dangerous situation, they leave at once and notify their supervisor (Stanhope & Lancaster, 2014). CHNs use their judgment and follow the College of Nurses' guidelines when accepting gifts from their family clients.

## CHNC STANDARDS

The CHNC standards clearly outline the specific roles and function of CHNs when they care for community clients. The following describes how family nurses adhere to these standards as they care for their family clients.

## Professional Relationships, Responsibility, and Accountability

Nurse–client interaction begins with relationship building (Porr, 2013). Successful family home visits require the nurse to establish mutuality, respect, and trust with the family. This is especially necessary if the family feels vulnerable or fears that family members will be judged or reported to a social welfare authority. When the nurse can establish a collaborative, respectful relationship with the family, she or he can facilitate an assessment of family strengths; gain an understanding of the family fears, issues, and concerns; and identify opportunities to collaboratively plan, intervene, and evaluate the desired goals.

**Family Interview** Each family member's perceptions of an event or a situation need to be validated through active listening and patience. CHNs need to skilfully ask meaningful questions to elicit the family's current level of knowledge on the health issues, its past history of approaches to resolve issues, and its desired approaches toward change prior to providing advice (Eddy & Doutrich, 2014; Eggenberger & Regan, 2010; Rowe Kaakinen et al., 2014).

Examples of family interview questions are listed in Table 18.3. These interview questions serve to promote family healing through reflection. For example, the question "What worries you the most in the family?" can provide the family an opportunity to identify its fears and concerns. Other questions

**TABLE 18.3  Family Interview Questions**

1. How can I be most helpful to you and your family (or friends) during your care? (Clarifies expectations and increases collaboration.)
2. What has been most and least helpful to you and your family in past healthcare experiences? (Identifies past strengths, problems to avoid, and successes to repeat.)
3. What is the greatest challenge facing your family right now? (Identifies actual or potential suffering, roles, and beliefs.)
4. With which of your family members or friends would you like us to share information? With which ones would you like us not to share information? (Indicates alliances, resources, and possible conflictual relationships.)
5. What do you need to best prepare you or your family for _____? (Identifies appropriate community resources.)
6. Who do you believe is suffering the most in your family right now? (Identifies the family member who has the greatest need for support and intervention.)
7. What is the one question you would like to have answered during our meeting right now? I may not be able to answer this question at the moment, but I will do my best or will try to find the answer for you. (Identifies most pressing issue or concern.)
8. How have I been most helpful to you today? How could we improve? (Shows a willingness to learn from families and to work collaboratively.)

Source: Adapted from Wright, L. M., & Leahey, M. M. (2012). *Nurses and families: A guide to family assessment and intervention* (6th ed.). Philadelphia, PA: F. A. Davis. (p. 271). Used by permission of F. A. Davis & Company.

will allow the family to name its strengths and reinforce coping mechanisms that assisted them in managing past complex situations. CHNs can purposively use silence while asking questions to allow the family time to reflect on its experiences.

The decision to end the family visits should be mutual. The CHN reviews and summarizes the family's strengths and lists the strategies used for health promotion, healing, and building capacity at the termination of the visits.

Wright and Leahey (2013) identified three common errors when working with families: (1) failure to establish the context for change, (2) taking sides, and (3) giving too much advice prematurely. CHNs can avoid making these errors by ensuring that they obtain a clear understanding of the family's most pressing concern while validating each family member's perspective. Each family member needs equal time to acknowledge the suffering in the family and the sufferer. CHNs need to remain engaged, not take sides, and seek mutual understanding of the situation.

CHNs should not offer advice or guidance until a thorough assessment has been completed and after they have established that the advice "fits" with the family's perspective of a possible solution. CHNs should always be aware of their own personal experiences and biases. Finally, the intervention needs to be evaluated from the family's perspective and adapted according to the family's response.

## Health Promotion, Prevention, and Health Protection; and Capacity Building

CHNs promote family health by addressing a family's physical, psychological, spiritual, and sociocultural needs. In promoting family health, CHNs may address the social determinants of health on *healthy child development* by providing education on preconception health in schools or provide prenatal and parenting information to parents in classes or in their homes. For *health and social services*, CHNs can act as a resource person and help families navigate the health system to obtain the needed support and preventive services or care, such as cancer and sexually transmitted infection (STI) screenings or geriatric assessment. Through these nursing activities, families are empowered by having the needed knowledge, skills, and resources to protect the health of their own family members.

**Family Caregiving** When a family member is struck with an acute illness or other debilitating or chronic condition, CHNs also play a key role to help the family acquire the needed resources or capacity for the care it needs. (See Chapter 5 for the role of the home health nurse.) While the ill family member is the focus of care, the caregivers often are the forgotten clients. In 2012, 8.1 million or 28% of Canadians 15 years or older provided care for a family member or a friend with a chronic health condition, disability, or aging need (Statistics Canada, 2013b). The majority of caregivers tended to be women, often mothers (Paulson & Lichtenberg, 2011; Statistics Canada, 2012b).

The term **caregiver** refers to an individual "who provides a broad range of financially uncompensated care to . . . family members in need due to physical, cognitive or mental health condition" (Duxbury, Higgins, & Smart, 2011, p. 30). A family caregiver may be an elderly adult caring for her or his spouse, an adult child caring for her or his aging parent, or a parent caring for a child with a chronic illness. When a chronic illness or dependency arises, the family unit as a whole is impacted and each member must adapt to new demands and a redistribution of roles and functions (Wright & Leahey, 2013).

The emotional, physical, and financial health of family caregivers and the family may be negatively impacted by the numerous, ongoing responsibilities of caregiving. Prolonged caregiving may result in caregivers experiencing overall poor health and limited opportunity to employ measures to prevent their own illness (Duxbury et al., 2011). For example, adult children caring for an aging parent may experience role reversal and grieve over the deterioration of their parent's health. Caring tasks may significantly reduce caregivers' social interactions and leisure time while increasing disruptions of personal schedules, leading to feelings of guilt, social isolation, stress, depression, or anger (MacNeil et al., 2010; Paulson & Lichtenberg, 2011). Financial strain may result from numerous

---

### CANADIAN RESEARCH BOX 18.2

#### What are the safety risks of caregivers?

Macdonald, M., & Lang, A. (2014). Applying risk society theory to findings of a scoping review on caregiver safety. *Health & Social Care in Community, 22*(2), 124–133. Retrieved from http://onlinelibrary.wiley.com/doi/10.1111/hsc.12056/pdf

With the rise of chronic illness, individuals living with chronic illness at home are mainly cared for by family caregivers. The authors conducted a scoping review of the home care literature (2004–2013) on unpaid caregivers across the lifespan from Canada, the United States, England, Australia, Sweden, Denmark, Norway, the United Kingdom, and Israel. Findings revealed four key safety-related concerns among the caregivers: caregivers are conscripted to the role, economic hardship, risk for being abused and abusing, and becoming the "hidden" patients themselves. The authors used their findings to develop their Risk Society Theory to construct a macro-level view of the risk in society and healthcare. They asserted the need to support home care programs and recognize the valuable contribution of caregivers. They also called for a recommitment to sustainable programs that support the aging population to improve the quality of life and safety for caregivers.

#### Discussion Questions

1. Explain why should CHNs be concerned about the health and safety needs of the caregivers.
2. How should the CHN work with the caregiver and the ill family member to promote optimal family health?

out-of-pocket medical expenses not covered by insurance. The many issues described above can also ultimately lead to caregiver burnout or strain (Stanhope & Lancaster, 2014). (See Canadian Research Box 18.2.)

CHNs can also build capacity by promoting family resilience among families experiencing stressors. **Family resilience** is the ability of a family to withstand and rebound from disruptive life challenges, emerging strengthened and more resourceful (Walsh, 2013). CHNs foster family resilience by helping families to view themselves in terms of (1) their existing and potential strengths, and (2) their seeing problems as challenges to be overcome to enhance family coping (Walsh, 2013). CHNs help families to reflect and build on their strengths and available resources and empower them to develop a positive outlook regarding their circumstances (Wright & Leahey, 2013).

## Access, Equity, Health Maintenance, Restoration, and Palliation

In Canada, health system restructuring during the 1990s and early discharge from hospital resulted in challenges faced by clients requiring home care. Cost containment further impacted the provision of quality services to clients and their families. The deterioration in home care and fragmentation in community services have had detrimental impacts on clients and their families. Scarce resources and supportive care were being redirected away from those needing care (e.g., the frail and elderly, chronically ill, or those with disabilities), and the shortage for long-term care beds keeps mounting (see Chapter 2). Increasingly, families are forced to assume complex care for their ill family members. CHNs are in the ideal position to act as a liaison between acute and community care settings, and to facilitate and coordinate the care needed by their clients and families.

**Case management** is a collaborative approach used by CHNs to coordinate and facilitate the delivery of healthcare services. A CHN case manager works with individuals, families, and other healthcare providers to facilitate all necessary services for care provided in community settings during times of illness, or for other healthcare conditions requiring nursing intervention. Often these clients are marginalized, powerless, and vulnerable, and they lack experience in navigating the healthcare system. CHNs, acting as case managers, identify and assess clients' needs, plan care, provide or delegate care, and follow up with an evaluation of care. The goal of case management is to arrive at quality, cost-effective client outcomes (Smith, 2013b).

Just gathering a team of healthcare providers to provide care will not yield quality health outcomes (Creemers et al., 2014). CHNs need to ensure that their clients will receive the *right care* by the *right people* and at the *right time* to yield optimal health outcomes. Case management supports the client's right to achieve their self-determined goals for optimal health, maximum self-care, and independence. It is a collaborative process in which the client (or substitute decision maker) provides informed consent and input for all aspects of planned care. It is a purposeful process addressing the specific needs of the client. Case management involves accountability and facilitating the coordinated and timely delivery of appropriate planned services, while monitoring and responding to changes in the client's needs and abilities. It must also ensure provision of care that reflects cultural safety, respect, problem-solving strategies, spiritual, and religious considerations (National Case Management Network, 2012).

## FUTURE RESEARCH DIRECTIONS AND CHALLENGES

Progress in family nursing research has been made over the years. The First International Family Nursing Conference was hosted in May 1988 by the University of Calgary's Faculty of Nursing under the leadership of Dr. Lorraine M. Wright (Bell, 2014). The Canadian Family Practice Nurses Association (2014) was established by a group of seven dynamic nurses in 2008. Both the conference and association brought nursing researchers, educators, practitioners, and nursing students together to share their vision, experiences, and new knowledge in family nursing practice.

On the international scene, the International Family Nursing Association (2014) disseminates a collection of family research studies in areas such as conceptual and methodological issues, underpinnings of family research, nature and purpose of research, intervention search, family dyadic studies, and synthesis research. The association has been instrumental in advancing family nursing research and noted the future directions for family nursing research are in new analytical strategies, evidence-based interventions, determinations of critical dimensions for tailoring family interventions, and establishment of links between family system characteristics and individual outcomes.

The need for family nursing as a specialty has never been greater with the movement toward increased levels of community-based care (Rowe Kaakinen et al., 2014). CHNs target their interventions with family members in the cognitive, affective, and behavioural domains as they promote and improve the effectiveness of family functioning (Wright & Leahey, 2013). To do so, nursing educators must be familiar with the specialty practice of family and community nursing. They need to select meaningful and quality family nursing clinical placements to prepare their students to provide competent family nursing care. Family nurse practitioners must support vulnerable or priority families in need through empowerment, capacity building, and advocacy. Family nursing researchers must advance family nursing research and foster knowledge utilization of their findings. Finally, family nurse leaders must play a key role in promoting the allocation of resources available for family nursing development. They also play an advocacy role in health policy and health legislation to improve the care of families.

# CONCLUSION

This chapter is an overview of family nursing care in community settings. It is not all encompassing, but it provides a glimpse into this nursing specialty. The changing demographics of the family and the key conceptual frameworks for family assessment have been presented. How CHNs could adhere to the CHNC standards when providing family nursing care has been outlined, as well as the importance of case management and the challenges and future directions for family nursing. With this understanding, CHNs will provide family care with more confidence and will continue to advance their skills in promoting family health.

## KEY TERMS

ABCX Model    p. 352
Calgary Family Assessment Model
   (CFAM)    p. 351
Calgary Family Intervention Model
   (CFIM)    p. 351
caregiver    p. 356
case management    p. 357
dysfunctional families    p. 348
ecomap    p. 352
family    p. 347
family assessment    p. 350
family developmental theory    p. 350
family forms    p. 347
family functions    p. 347
family health    p. 346
family nursing    p. 346
family resilience    p. 357
family structure    p. 347
Friedman Family Assessment Model    p. 350
genogram    p. 352
healthy families    p. 347
McGill Model    p. 351
multigenerational households    p. 346
multiproblem family    p. 348
strains    p. 354
stressors    p. 352
structural–functional theory    p. 350
systems theory    p. 350

## STUDY QUESTIONS

1. Define the concept of family and identify some common family functions.
2. Describe the demographic shifts that are changing the composition of Canadian families.
3. What are the levels of conceptualizing the family in family nursing theory?
4. Describe the key differences between a genogram and an ecomap.
5. Identify the components of a family home visit.
6. Define case management and its role in family-centred care.

After working through these questions, go to the MyNursingLab at www.pearsoned.ca/mynursinglab to check your answers.

## INDIVIDUAL CRITICAL-THINKING EXERCISES

1. Draw your family genogram and ecomap. Describe the roles of family members, the quality of the intra-family relationships, and the strengths of your family.
2. Identify some factors that make a family vulnerable.
3. Describe a crisis experience in your family and the family resilience factors that assisted your family to cope with the crisis.
4. Compare your beliefs about your family with those of a romanticized or a stigmatized family.
5. What impact could your values and beliefs about family have on your nurse–family relationships?

## GROUP CRITICAL-THINKING EXERCISES

1. Differentiate between viewing the family as client and the family as context. Drawing on your experiences, provide an example to illustrate each concept (family as client and family as context).
2. Describe an approach to the assessment of a family for each of the CCHN standards: promoting health, building capacity, building relationships, facilitating access and equity, and demonstrating professional responsibility and accountability. Provide concrete examples to illustrate the application of each standard in family nursing.
3. Role play a family–nurse situation. Practise the family interview questions listed in Table 18.3.

## REFERENCES

Bell, J. M. (2014). *The history of the International Family Nursing Conferences*. Retrieved from http://janicembell.com/2009/09/history-of-the-international-family-nursing-conferences

Browne, A. J., Doane, G. H., Reimer, J., MacLeod, M. L., & McLellan, E. (2011). Public health nursing practice with "high priority" families: The significance of contextualizing "risk." *Nursing Inquiry, 17*(1), 26–37.

Bushnik, T., Cook, J., Hughes, & Tough, S. (2012). Seeking medical help to conceive. *Health Reports, 23*(4). Statistics Canada Catalogue no. 82-003-XPE. pp. 1–9. Retrieved from http://www.statcan.gc.ca/pub/82-003-x/2012004/article/11719-eng.pdf

Canadian Family Practice Nurse Association. (2014). *History*. Retrieved from http://www.cfpna.ca/history.cfm

Community Health Nurses Association of Canada. (2011, revised). *Canadian community health nursing standards of practice*. St. John's, NL: Author. Retrieved from http://www.chnc.ca/documents/chnc-standards-eng-book.pdf

Canadian Nurses Association. (2013). *Social determinants of health*. Retrieved from http://www.cna-aiic.ca/PositionStatement

Creemers, H., Veldink, J. H., Grupstra, H., Nollet, F., Beelen, A., & van den Berg, L. H. (2014). Cluster RCT of case management on patients' quality of life and caregiver strain in ALS. *Neurology, 82*(1), pp. 23–31. doi:10.1212/01.wnl.0000438227.48470.62

Drake, M. A. (2014). Theoretical bases for promoting family health. In J. A. Allender, C. Rector, & K. Warner (Eds.), *Community health nursing: Promoting and protecting the public's health* (8th ed., pp. 568–583). Philadelphia, PA: Wolters Kluwer/Lippincott, Williams & Wilkins.

Duxbury, L., Higgins, C., & Smart, R. (2011). Elder care and the impact of caregiver strain on the health of employed caregivers. *Work, 40,* 29–40. Published by IOS Press, © 1989.

Eddy, L. L., & Doutrich, D. (2014). Families and communities/public health nursing. In J. Rowe Kaakinen, V. Gedaly-Duff, D. P. Coehlo, & S. M. Harmon Hanson (Eds.), *Family health care nursing: Theory, practice and research* (5th ed., pp. 470–489). Philadelphia, PA: F. A. Davis.

Eggenberger, S. K., & Regan, M. (2010). Expanding simulation to teach family nursing. *Journal of Nursing Education, 49*(10), 550–558.

Friedman, M. M., Bowden, V. R., & Jones, E. G. (Eds.). (2003). *Family nursing: Research, theory, and practice* (5th ed.). Upper Saddle River, NJ: Prentice Hall.

Freistadt, J., & Strohschein, L. (2012). Family structure differences in family functions: Interactive effects of social capital and family structure. *Journal of Family Issues, 34*(7), 952–974.

Gottlieb, L. N., & Gottlieb, B. (2007). The developmental/health framework within the McGill Model of Nursing: "Laws of nature" guiding whole person care. *Advances in Nursing Science, 30*(1), E43–E57. PMID: 17299275.

Gottlieb, L., & Rowat, K. (1987). The McGill model of nursing: A practice-derived model. *Advances in Nursing Science, 9*(4), 51–61.

Government of Canada. (2015). *Civil Marriage Act*. Retrieved from http://laws-lois.justice.gc.ca/eng/acts/c-31.5/page-1.html

Hill, R. (1958). Generic features of families under stress. *Social Casework, 49,* 139–150.

Hunt, R. (2013). Family care. In R. Hunt (Ed.), *Introduction to community-based nursing* (5th ed., pp. 77–118). Philadelphia, PA: Lippincott.

International Family Nursing Association. (2014). *Research, bibliography/seminal works*. Retrieved from http://internationalfamilynursing.org/resources-for-family-nursing/research/research-bibliography

McCubbin, H. I., & McCubbin M. A. (1993). Families coping with illness: The resiliency model of family stress, adjustment, and adaptation. In C. B. Danielson, B. Hamel-Bissel, & P. Winsted-Fry (Eds.), *Families, health and illness: Perspectives on coping and intervention* (pp. 21–63). St. Louis, MO: Mosby.

MacNeil, G., Kosberg, J. I., Durkin, D. W., Dooley, W. K., Decoster, J., & Williamson, G. M. (2010). Caregiver mental health and potentially harmful caregiving behaviour: The central role of caregiver anger. *The Gerontologist, 50,* 76–86.

National Case Management Network. (2012). Canadian core competency profile for case management providers. Retrieved from http://www.ncmn.ca/Resources/Documents/NCMN%20VALIDATION%20DRAFT%20July%202012.pdf

Olds, D. L., Kitzman, H., Knudtson, M. D., Anson, E., Smith, J. A., & Cole, R. (2014). Effect of home visiting by nurses on maternal and child mortality: Results of a 2-decade follow-up of a randomized clinical trial. *JAMA Pediatr, 68*(9), 800–806. doi:10.1001/jamapediatrics.2014.472. (Original) PMID: 25003802

Paulson, D., & Lichtenberg, P. A. (2011). Effect of caregiver family status on care recipient symptom severity and caregiver stress at nursing home intake. *Clinical Gerontologist, 34,* 132–143.

Porr, C. J. (2013). Important interactional strategies for everyday public health nursing practice. *Public Health Nursing*. doi:10.1111/phn.12097

Public Health Agency of Canada. (2013). *What makes Canadians healthy or unhealthy?* Retrieved from http://www.phac-aspc.gc.ca/ph-sp/determinants/determinants-eng.php

Rowe Kaakinen, J., Padgett Coehlo, D., Steele, R., Tabacco, A., & Harmon Hanson, S. M. (2014). *Family health care nursing: Theory, practice, and research* (5th ed.). Philadelphia, PA: F. A. Davis Company.

Smith, C. M. (2013a). Multiproblem families. In F. A. Maurer & C. M. Smith (Eds.), *Community/public health nursing practice* (5th ed., pp. 372–391). St. Louis, MO: Saunders.

Smith, C. M. (2013b). Family case management. In F. A. Maurer & C. M. Smith (Eds.), *Community/public health nursing practice* (5th ed., pp. 340–371). St. Louis, MO: Saunders.

Stanhope, M., & Lancaster, J. (2014). *Foundations of nursing in the community: Community-oriented practice* (4th ed.). St. Louis, MO: Mosby Elsevier.

Statistics Canada. (2012a). *Fifty years of families in Canada: 1961 to 2011*. Statistics Canada Catalogue no. 98-312-X2011003. Retrieved from http://webcache.googleusercontent.com/search?q=cache:http://www12.statcan.gc.ca/census-recensement/2011/as-sa/98-312-x/98-312-x2011003_1-eng.pdf&gws_rd=cr&ei=PnVqVYK7CpGcyASr64L4Ag

Statistics Canada. (2012b). *Portrait of caregivers, 2012*. Statistics Canada Catalogue no. 89-652-X2011003. Retrieved from http://www.statcan.gc.ca/pub/89-652-x/89-652-x2013001-eng.pdf

Statistics Canada. (2013a). Births and total fertility rate, by province and territory (Fertility rate). Retrieved from http://www.statcan.gc.ca/tables-tableaux/sum-som/l01/cst01/hlth85b-eng.htm

Statistics Canada. (2013b). Study: Caregivers in Canada 2012. *The Daily*, September 10. Retrieved from http://www.statcan.gc.ca/daily-quotidien/130910/dq130910a-eng.pdf

Vanier Institute of the Family. (2010). *Families count: Profiling Canada's families IV*. Ottawa, ON: Author.

Walsh, F. (2012). Successful aging and family resilience. *Annual Review of Gerontology & Geriatrics, 32,* 153–172.

Wright, L. M., & Leahey, M. M. (2012). *Nurses and families: A guide to family assessment and intervention* (6th ed.). Philadelphia, PA: F. A. Davis.

## ABOUT THE AUTHORS

**Lucia Yiu**, RN, BScN, BA (University of Windsor), BSc (University of Toronto), MScN (University of Western Ontario), is an Associate Professor in the Faculty of Nursing at the University of Windsor, and an educational and training consultant in community nursing. She has worked overseas and served on various community and social services committees involving local and district health planning. Her practice and research include multicultural health, international health, experiential learning, community development, breast health, and program planning and evaluation. Lucia is the recipient of the 2014 Community Health Nurses of Canada Award of Merit.

**Marilyn A. Sutton**, RN, BScN (University of Windsor), MA (University of Windsor), currently teaches Community Health Clinical Nursing Experience at the University of Windsor. Marilyn has previously taught family health nursing, both theory and clinical nursing experience. Interests include community nursing, critical reasoning, and ethics.

**Candace Martin Ryan**, RN, BSc (University of Toronto), BScN (University of Windsor), MSc (University of Windsor), has experience in family nursing in both the community and hospital settings. She has taught community health nursing courses at the University of Windsor. She currently works in a Neonatal Intensive Care Unit. Interests include family nursing, family integrated care, and infection control.

# Gender and Community Health

*Aliyah Dosani and Deborah Mansell*

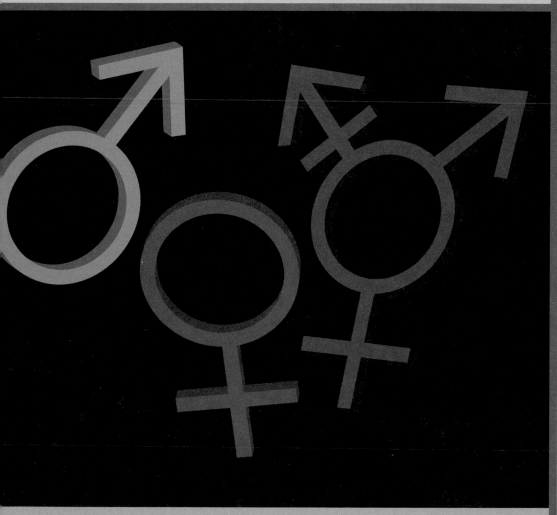

*Source: Paw/Fotolia*

## INTRODUCTION

"Gender equality is more than a goal in itself. It is a precondition of meeting the challenge of reducing poverty, promoting sustainable development, and building good governance" (Kofi Annan, as cited in Unicef, 2006). Yet, over the last several decades, gender is a concept that is often taken for granted, with a one-size-fits-all approach that is limited to men and women only. We design health programs and interventions without asking whether they are well suited to the needs of men, women, or those individuals who consider themselves transgendered. Before reading further, think about the ways your own gender influences your life. Consider the ways it influences how you dress, what you talk about, with whom you are friends, when and where you may feel unsafe, and to whom you go for help. While we often think about gender as something that is not within our control, gender is a concept that we as individuals cultivate, develop, and understand based on what society reinforces through social relations and institutional norms. This can mean that in our society men and women are thought of, live their lives, and are treated as different kinds of people with different bodies and different roles, responsibilities, and opportunities (Jackson, Pederson, & Boscoe, 2009). When we really begin to think about gender, we realize that it influences, overtly and subtly, many aspects of our lives. Indeed, it has been recognized as a key social determinant of health (World Health Organization, 2008).

The **social determinants of health** are mostly responsible for health inequities—the unfair and preventable differences in health status seen within and between countries. Responding to increasing concern about these persisting and widening inequities, the World Health Organization (WHO) established the Commission on Social Determinants of Health (CSDH) in 2005 to provide advice on how to reduce them (WHO, 2008). One of the chapters in this report focuses on gender equity and health. The authors of this report argue that gender inequities damage the health of women and girls throughout the world, particularly in low- and middle-income countries. As a result, girls and women have less power, privilege, and access to resources than do men. In some countries girls are valued less, receive less education, are fed less, and are restricted in what they can do. In many areas of the world, transgender people may be forced to live on the edges of mainstream society, leaving them isolated, facing discrimination and bullying (WHO, 2010). The topic of gender and health is now widely recognized and continues to be discussed at the global level. This difference in how gender is taken up by societies inevitably influences their health outcomes. Is the same true in Canada, where it is often assumed that women and men have equal opportunities, or that people who do not "fit" as either male or female have equal access to healthcare and employment opportunities? This chapter will focus on gender, its influence on health, and various roles that community health nurses (CHNs) can play to promote health equity between men and women, boys and girls.

## HEALTH OUTCOMES OF CANADIAN MEN AND WOMEN: STATISTICS AND TRENDS

As demonstrated in Table 19.1, women live longer than men in all developed countries and nearly all developing countries (WHO, 2013a). The disparity in life expectancy between males and females varies by country, although Canada's life expectancy ranks among the top 10 in the world (Figure 19.1). Women in Canada tend to live longer than men, on average, and have done so for nearly a century (Nagunar, 2011). In Canada, women are expected to live an average of

| Table 19.1 | Life Expectancy at Birth (Years) for Males and Females, Selected Countries, 1990 and 2012 | | | |
|---|---|---|---|---|
| Country | Men | | Women | |
| | 1990 | 2012 | 1990 | 2012 |
| Afghanistan | 48 | 58 | 50 | 61 |
| Australia | 74 | 81 | 80 | 85 |
| Austria | 72 | 80 | 79 | 83 |
| Canada | 74 | 80 | 81 | 84 |
| China | 67 | 74 | 71 | 77 |
| Costa Rica | 75 | 77 | 78 | 81 |
| Cuba | 73 | 76 | 76 | 81 |
| Czech Republic | 68 | 75 | 75 | 81 |
| Egypt | 63 | 69 | 67 | 74 |
| Ethiopia | 42 | 62 | 48 | 65 |
| France | 73 | 79 | 82 | 85 |
| Ghana | 55 | 61 | 58 | 64 |
| Haiti | 52 | 61 | 56 | 64 |
| India | 57 | 64 | 58 | 68 |
| Iraq | 67 | 66 | 71 | 74 |
| Ireland | 72 | 79 | 78 | 83 |
| Japan | 76 | 80 | 82 | 87 |
| Kenya | 58 | 59 | 62 | 62 |
| Saudi Arabia | 67 | 74 | 71 | 78 |
| Sierra Leone | 38 | 45 | 38 | 46 |
| Singapore | 73 | 80 | 78 | 85 |
| Sudan | 54 | 61 | 57 | 65 |
| Switzerland | 74 | 81 | 81 | 85 |
| Uganda | 44 | 56 | 49 | 58 |
| United Kingdom | 73 | 79 | 79 | 83 |
| United Republic of Tanzania | 49 | 59 | 52 | 63 |
| United States of America | 72 | 76 | 79 | 81 |
| Vietnam | 66 | 71 | 75 | 80 |
| Zambia | 40 | 45 | 47 | 58 |

Source: Based on WHO. (2014). Life expectancy and mortality. World Health Statistics 2014. Reprinted with permission. Retrieved from http://www.who.int/gho/publications/world_health_statistics/EN_WHS2014_Part3.pdf?ua=1

4.7 years longer than men (Greenberg & Normandin, 2011). The discrepancy in life expectancy between males and females varies across Canada, from 3.2 years to 7.5 years (Greenberg & Normandin, 2011). The gap is generally smaller among regions with higher life expectancy and greater among regions with lower life expectancy (Greenberg &

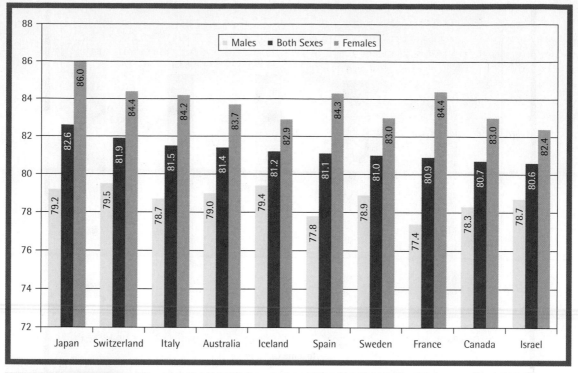

**FIGURE  19.1**  Life Expectancy at Birth, Top 10 OECD Countries

*Source:* Statistics Canada. *Life expectancy at birth, top 10 OECD countries.* Retrieved from http://www.statcan.gc.ca/pub/82-624-x/2011001/article/chart/11427-01-chart1-eng.htm. Last modified: 2013-05-13.

Normandin, 2011). These regional figures also reveal important differences with respect to the social determinants of health within Canada. Parts of the country facing the lowest life expectancy also hold some of the highest rates of smoking, obesity, and heavy drinking (Greenberg & Normandin, 2011). These regions have high long-term unemployment rates, lower levels of education, small immigrant populations, relatively large Aboriginal populations, and are situated in rural or remote locations (Greenberg & Normandin, 2011). In addition, higher neighbourhood income is also associated with longer life expectancy (Figure 19.2).

The basis of this degree of difference in life expectancy between men and women is clearly complex. It is important to recognize that men and women are not monolithic categories but groups of individuals with multiple and intersecting identities connected to all of the social determinants of health. Even as Canadians enjoy a publicly funded health system and generally good health, access to and utilization of healthcare services are not equal across the board. And while Canada ranks well internationally in terms of life expectancy and quality of life for its citizens, not every Canadian's health reflects this. It is important to note that differing social locations impact Canadians' health in important ways. Assessing differences and disparities in health status, health behaviours, and utilization of healthcare services based on sex and gender is one step toward ensuring that all Canadians benefit equally from Canada's public health system.

## CONCEPTUAL DEFINITIONS

The differences between the concepts of sex and gender are often misunderstood. Although these terms are related, they are *not* synonymous. CHNs must be mindful of the implications of both "sex" and "gender" as programs and interventions are planned, delivered, and evaluated.

**Sex** refers to the biological and physiological characteristics that define men and women (WHO, 2013b, para. 2). Sex differences result from the classification of organisms based on genetic constitution at the cellular level as well as the anatomy and physiology of reproductive organs (Jenkins, Kemnitz, & Tortora, 2010). Obvious examples of sex-specific diseases are cervical cancer and prostate cancer. However, there has been increasing evidence that cells beyond those involved in reproduction have sex differences and that these sex differences can create distinctive patterns of morbidity and mortality in men and women. Indeed, some researchers contend "every organ in the body, not just those related to reproduction, has the capacity to respond differently on the basis of sex" (Gesensway, 2001, p. 935). There is a growing body of research that suggests there are differences in the incidence, symptoms, natural history, and outcome of many other conditions, and those differences are shaped by genetic, hormonal, and metabolic effects (Senie, 2014). For instance, Ghandi et al. (2002) found that women have lower levels of human immunodeficiency virus (HIV) RNA than do men at similar stages of HIV

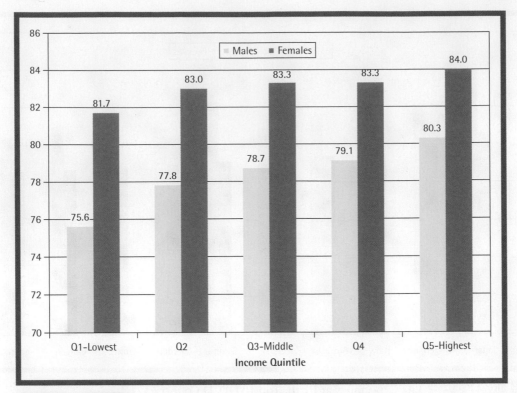

**FIGURE 19.2** Life Expectancy at Birth, by Sex, Neighbourhood Income Quintiles, 2005–2007

*Source:* Statistics Canada. *Life expectancy at birth, by sex, neighbourhood income quintiles, 2005–2007.* Special Tabulation. Retrieved from http://www.statcan.gc.ca/pub/82-624-x/2011001/article/chart/11427-06-chart5-eng.htm. Last modified: 2013-05-13.

infection. This finding is significant because viral loads are often used to guide the initiation and adjustment of antiretroviral therapy. Furthermore, Soldin, Chung, and Mattison (2011) found that males and females might differ in drug pharmacokinetics and pharmacodynamics. Therefore, it is imperative that we understand such sex differences in order for interventions to be safe and effective. It is imperative that healthcare providers be aware of the sex differences of various conditions, regardless of the settings in which they work.

**Gender** "refers to the socially constructed roles, behaviours, activities, and attributes that a given society considers appropriate for men and women . . ." (WHO, 2013b, para. 3). Gender is often expressed in terms of masculinity and femininity and is rooted in culture and history. For example, women in Canada are allowed to drive while women in Saudi Arabia are not; and more men in Vietnam smoke, as it is customary for men but not women (WHO, 2013a).

**Transgendered** refers to "persons whose gender identity, gender expression, or behaviour does not conform to that typically associated with the sex to which they were assigned at birth" (American Psychological Association, 2011, p. 1). It is important to note that the term "transgendered" does not relate directly to sexuality. People who are transgendered may categorize themselves as straight, gay, lesbian, bisexual, or

with any other label or term that non-transgendered people use to define themselves.

**Gender identity** describes how we see ourselves as women, men, neither, or both, and this affects our feelings and behaviours. Women and men develop their gender identity in the face of strong societal messages about the "correct" gendered role for their presenting sex. Gender identities are actively constructed over time and within cultures (Greco, 2013). "Gender identity is linked to an individual's intrinsic sense of self and, particularly, the sense of being male or female. Gender identity may or may not conform to a person's birth assigned sex" (Edmonds, 2012, p. 2).

Often closely tied to gender identity are the concepts of **masculinity** and **femininity**. Masculinity theories suggest that men's performance, perceptions, and practices around health and illness may be informed and influenced by gender norms (Tyler, 2012). For example, traditionally, men have been viewed as reluctant to seek professional help for depression because the illness and their actions in seeking help suggest weakness, and illness and seeking help are decidedly non-masculine. As a result, masculine ideals including self-reliance, stoicism, and emotional control can be lost and negatively impact many men's self-perceptions about their masculinity (Oliffe & Phillips, 2008). Likewise, traditional femininity can be thought of as the gender norms that are ascribed to women. In the context of health, women often subscribe to feminine ideals about being competent in self-care, as well as being the primary health provider to the men and children in their lives (Lee & Owens, 2002).

Despite many societies and organizations entrenching the idea of gender being either male or female, the concept of gender as being *only* either a man or a woman is being challenged in some societies. For example, the Harvard University application process enables students to choose male, female, or enter in the words that best describe their gender (or nothing at all). The University of Victoria in British Columbia has renovated several washroom facilities throughout the campus to be gender neutral, enabling those who do not identify themselves as male or female to use bathrooms that they feel safe to access. Native American and First Nations cultures have long recognized that gender is a much more fluid notion than just being a man or a woman. The term "Two Spirit," which was recognized at the Third Annual Spiritual Gathering of Gay and Lesbian Native People in 2001, refers to Native Americans who were born with masculine and feminine spirits in one body (Sheppard & Mayo, 2013). CHNs must be aware of the debate and dialogue that is happening around the changing notions of the concept of gender in order to best serve the diverse members of the communities with which they work.

**Gender roles** are defined as the social *and* cultural expectations that different societies assign to men and women (WHO, 2013a). Gender roles of men and women have changed over time and place as they engage in different activities than they did traditionally. Furthermore, gender is relational and refers not simply to women or men, but also to the relationship that exists between them (WHO, 2013b). In all societies, gender impacts opportunities to access resources and societal benefits, thus impacting health.

Gender roles are expressed and enacted in a range of ways, from how we dress or talk, to what we may aspire to do as a career, to what we feel are valuable contributions to make as a woman or a man. In some cultures, these roles are sharply defined and differentiated, allowing and disallowing women (and men) from certain tasks, jobs, opportunities, and spaces. Gender roles often categorize and control individuals within institutions such as the family, community, labour force, and educational systems. For example, a woman may not receive required healthcare because norms in her community expect that she be accompanied when travelling (WHO, 2013c). In addition, in many cultures men are ascribed the "breadwinner" role in the family, while women are expected to fulfill more nurturing and caretaking roles that include domestic chores, childcare, and the emotional work of relationships (Figure 19.3). Societies continue to discuss women in "non-traditional jobs," thereby giving recognition to the fact that there is a pattern in which certain forms of paid employment are seen as men's jobs and others women's. These differences in gender roles are associated with social status: in almost every society, higher power and prestige is conferred on individuals occupying masculine gender roles (WHO, 2013a).

**Gender relations** refer to how we interact with or are treated by people in the world around us, based on our ascribed gender. They affect us at all levels of society and can restrict or make available various opportunities.

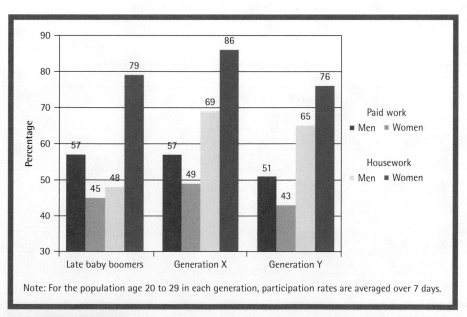

**FIGURE  19.3**  Paid and Unpaid Work over Three Generations

*Source:* Marshall, K. (2012). Paid and unpaid work over three generations. *Perspectives on Labour and Income.* Component of Statistics Canada Catalogue no. 75-001-X. Retrieved from http://www.statcan.gc.ca/pub/75-001-x/2012001/article/11612-eng.pdf. Last modified: 2013-15-03.

Gender relations interact with our race, ethnicity, class, and other identities. In most societies, gender relations reflect differential power between women and men and often disadvantage women (WHO, 2013b). Gender affects not only our personal relationships with others, but also guides our interactions within larger social units, including family and the workplace. For example, the gendered relationships between men and women have been found to influence the interpersonal dynamics related to tobacco reduction in pregnant and postpartum women (Bottorff et al., 2006). Likewise, prostate cancer is often referred to as a couples' disease because the illness and many treatments directly impact gender relations (Bottorff et al., 2008). Furthermore, in many societies around the world married women are at risk for contracting HIV because societal standards encourage her husband's promiscuity while simultaneously preventing her from negotiating condom use (WHO, 2013d).

**Institutionalized gender** reflects the distribution of power between the genders in the political, educational, religious, media, medical, and social institutions in any society. These powerful institutions shape the social norms that define, reproduce, and often justify different expectations and opportunities for women and men and girls and boys. This may translate into job segregation, job limitations, dress codes, health practices, and different access to resources such as money, food, or political power. Institutions in society often impose social controls through the ways in which they organize, regulate, and uphold differential values for men and women. While pay equity is viewed as a fundamental human right, and is outlined clearly in section 11 of the Canadian Human Rights Act (Government of Canada, 2013a), it is important to acknowledge how employers often enforce these roles and power differentials by providing higher rates of pay to men for performing similar jobs as women. The Conference Board of Canada (2014) estimates that while most Canadians believe that men and women are earning an equal salary for equal work, there is, in fact, an approximately 19% gap in income between men and women. Women face deficits in pay ranging from 6% to as high as 53% (Figure 19.4). In 2011, on average, women in Canada earned a mere 72% of what men were paid for the same work (see Photo 19.1). The pay equity gap is even wider for women who are older, Aboriginal, belong to visible minority groups, and living with disabilities (Canadian Labour Congress, 2009).

As demonstrated in this discussion around gender roles, gender relations, and institutionalized gender, gender norms and values, and resulting behaviours, may adversely impact health. In fact, how gender is valued, understood, and translated into behaviours in any given time, place, and space can be one of the most significant barriers standing between improving overall health and well-being of men and women. Nevertheless, it is also important to acknowledge that gender norms and values are not static. They evolve over time, differ considerably from place to place, and are subject to change. Thus, the poor health consequences resulting from gender differences and gender inequalities are not fixed either. They can be modified and transformed (WHO, 2013d).

| Relative Earnings of Women and Men by Occupation, Canada (Ratio of Female to Male Earnings) | 1986 | 2010 |
|---|---|---|
| Natural and applied sciences | 0.63 | 0.94 |
| Art, culture, recreation, and sport | 0.54 | 0.88 |
| Management | 0.59 | 0.71 |
| Social science, education, government service, and religion | 0.57 | 0.70 |
| Processing, manufacturing, and utilities | 0.52 | 0.65 |
| Business, finance, and administrative | 0.58 | 0.60 |
| Trades, transport, and equipment | 0.50 | 0.59 |
| Sales and service | 0.48 | 0.57 |
| Primary industry | 0.46 | 0.49 |
| Health | 0.48 | 0.47 |

Source: Statistics Canada, *Income in Canada 2010.*

**FIGURE 19.4** Relative Earnings of Men and Women by Occupation, Canada, 1986–2010

*Source:* Conference Board of Canada. *Gender income gap.* Used by permission of The Conference Board of Canada. Retrieved from http://www.conferenceboard.ca/hcp/details/society/gender-income-gap.aspx. Last modified: 2014.

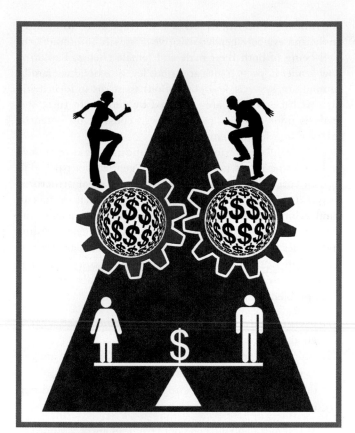

**PHOTO 19.1** It often appears that men and women have equal opportunities for salary and advancement in the workplace, yet the evidence demonstrates that women face barriers in achieving workplace equality.

*Source: Sangoiri/Fotolia*

### CANADIAN RESEARCH BOX 19.1

**How do heteronormative discourses affect sexually transmitted infection testing?**

Knight, R., Shoveller, J. A., Oliffe, J. L., Gilbert, M., & Goldenberg, S. (2012). Heteronormativity hurts everyone: Experiences of young men and clinicians with STI testing. *Journal of Men's Health, 7*(5), 441–459. doi:10.1177/1363459312464071

Heteronormativity can be defined as the world view that endorses heterosexuality as the "normal" or preferred sexual orientation (Oxford Dictionary, 2013). The terms "heterosexual" and "homosexual" often bring about a society's belief that men who are either heterosexual or homosexual should behave, or do behave, in particular ways. This belief about *how* a man should act or behave quietly infiltrates modern societies, where heterosexual men may be identified as strong and stoic. In contrast, homosexual men may be identified as bright, bubbly, and outgoing. While Canada may appear to be a pluralistic society, where people are free to live as they desire, the overall view of Canadian society in terms of the **gender norms** that are associated with heterosexually or homosexuality can be detrimental to the experience of men attempting to access sexually transmitted infection (STI) testing and information. How men are

*expected* to behave impacts the care they receive from healthcare professionals such as registered nurses.

A team of Canadian researchers in British Columbia examined the influence of how society believes heterosexual men versus homosexual men behave to better understand the influence of gender norms on the experiences of young men seeking STI testing. The researchers conducted in-depth qualitative interviews with 45 men (15–24 years old) and 25 clinicians. The researchers discovered that the risk assessment questions related to STIs for the young men were described as "interrogative" (Knight et al., 2010, p. 301). Furthermore, the questions and comments from healthcare practitioners positioned the behaviours of gay men as being risky and "other" in a society that believes heterosexual behaviours are the norm and valued by Canadian society. In the STI clinics, "heterosexual men's concern for STI exposure was often alleviated by virtue of their sexual identity. Clinicians affirmed their relative safety, rather than the sexual practices in which they engaged. This in turn frequently resulted in closing down discussions around men's sexual health needs and promotion" (Knight et al., 2010, p. 302). The clinicians working in the STI clinics stated that some had implemented "gender neutral services" (Knight et al., 2010, p. 302); however, their practice with young men continued to be influenced by the broader set of social norms and opinions about how men should behave. This includes what is considered "normal" for each gender, and both the men and clinicians were influenced by these societal views in their lives every day. These beliefs shaped how the clinicians interacted with the young men, and often shut conversations down about the men's sexual health promotion needs and illness prevention. This was particularly true of heterosexual men, who were expected to behave a certain way and, therefore, were not engaging in risky sexual behaviours.

This research study illuminates the complexity Canadian men face through the very nature of being male and the gender role expectations that follow them. Entering into the STI clinic, the men may have faced gender-based bias in accessing both testing and informational support—perhaps not getting the information they needed or wanted because of the beliefs about how men behave. The clinicians more closely associated those behaviours that were viewed as risky in acquiring STIs with gay men than straight men, even though the men who are heterosexual may have actually wanted to discuss those risky behaviours. Clinicians unintentionally may reinforce what it is to "be a man," and therefore may close down the collaborative conversations that promote health and prevent illness.

### Discussion Questions

1. In your view, what beliefs does Canadian society have about how both heterosexual and homosexual men should act?

2. If you were going to set up a health clinic in the community, how might you create an environment that respects the fluid nature of gender and gender roles?

3. What is the responsibility of a CHN in creating healthcare spaces that respect all people?

# GENDER AND EQUITY

Increasingly, governments and other agencies are using **gender-based analyses** to ensure that the programs and policies they develop are equitable. For example, Health Canada's (2000) "Gender Based Analysis Policy" (Figure 19.5) is an important driver in encouraging policy makers to account for gender in their work (Tudiver, 2009). The Government of Canada (2013b) suggests the following factors be considered when examining policies and programs through a gender-based analysis process:

1. Access: The ability for all people to have equal access to policy, program, and legislative activities.
2. Inclusion: Representation of diverse groups of men and women throughout the policy or program process.
3. Benefits: The intended advantages of any program or policy are equally available to both men and women of diverse cultures, socioeconomic status, and at various levels of identity.
4. Equity: Ensuring that Government of Canada programs and health promotion strategies identify the unique elements, opportunities, and challenges that men, women, and transgendered people face.

The Government of Canada (2013b) suggests that the following model can be used to visualize and guide healthcare practitioners can identify how gender-based analysis (GBA) should be included when planning community health–based interventions or strategies.

CHNs can engage in this type of analysis when considering how notions of gender impact services, programs, interventions, and policies. Perceiving gender as a modifiable determinant of health, CHNs will be empowered to identify, apply, and evaluate gender-sensitive strategies to promote the well-being of both their male and female clients. Exploring how gender impacts health at various levels (individual, family, community, systems, and population) assists us in identifying how health outcomes are impacted by gender. In turn, this analysis informs CHN practice when considering potential interventions for implementation.

The valuation of men and masculine ideals over women and feminine ideals is one way that "gender is a part of all human interactions" and "is a 'stable' form of structured inequality" (Ettorre, 2004, p. 329). These experiences and cultural values may constrain our everyday life decisions, and thereby affect decisions about income, employment, housing, and childcare. **Gender inequity** occurs when men and women are not provided the same opportunities in society. **Gender bias** is the root of gender inequities and generally arises from three problems:

1. overgeneralization—when it is assumed that what is good for men is good for women;
2. gender and sex insensitivity—ignoring gender and sex as important variables; and
3. double standards—assessing the same situation differently on the basis of gender.

When men's and women's opportunities are constrained by gender, this creates inequities that affect health. To combat gender inequity in our practices, as CHNs we need have a strong understanding of sex and gender in order to identify mechanisms by which sex and gender issues translate into inequitable health outcomes. We must then plan, implement, and evaluate our community health nursing interventions accordingly.

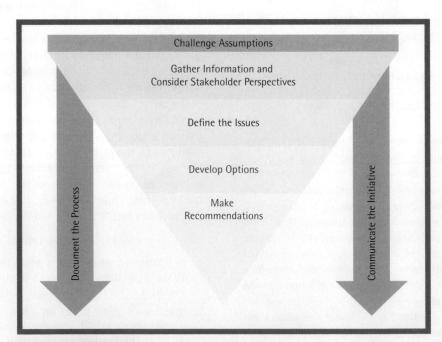

**FIGURE 19.5** Gender-Based Analysis Policy

*Source:* Government of Canada. (n. d.). *Gender-based analysis, status of women.* Retrieved from http://www.swc-cfc.gc.ca/gba-acs/course-cours/eng/mod06/mod06_03_01.php

## GENDER, SEX, AND HEALTH OUTCOMES

Sex and gender are powerful determinants that influence the health of individuals, families, communities, systems, and populations. *This is because every cell in our body is sexed and every person is gendered.* This means that biologically men and women differ in terms of the diseases they develop, the symptoms they experience, and the ways in which they respond to medicines and other treatments. Likewise, women's and men's varying alignments to gender ideals mediate their experiences and expressions about health and illness. While women generally live longer than men, women commonly experience poorer health than men (WHO, 2013a). Women have higher levels of depression, psychiatric disorders, distress, and a variety of chronic illnesses than men. Men have more life-threatening health conditions (WHO, 2013c). However, it is important to note that the direction and magnitude of gender differences in health may vary according to the symptom, condition, and/or phase of life cycle (Denton, Prus, & Walters, 2003).

The effects of sex and gender sometimes combine and lead to particular health outcomes. For example, research has found that women are more likely to experience depression because of both their sex characteristics and gender roles. Hormones, the activity of the hypothalamic–pituitary–adrenal (HPA) axis in response to stress, and reduced thyroid function have all been posited as important biological factors that make women more likely than men to suffer from depression (Senie, 2014). Gender is also associated with different rates of depression among men and women. Factors such as poverty, low level of education, social isolation, and lack of power can increase the risk for depression, and are often unequally distributed among men and women. Additionally, women's multiple roles within work and family settings can result in work overload, and can adversely affect women's mental health (Senie, 2014).

Although men and women develop and experience diseases differently, they share the 10 leading causes of death (Table 19.2). A limitation in many of the studies examining gender differences in health is the use of only a dichotomous classification of diseases (i.e., fatal and non-fatal). A clearer depiction of gender differences in health may require a more complex paradigm in order to gain a stronger understanding of the interplay between sex and gender and their respective contributions to morbidity and mortality. This may be further compounded by the fact that little is known about the health outcomes of those people who identify themselves as transgendered, two sex, or intersex (Health Canada, 2001). And while those who identify themselves as transgendered, two sex, or intersex may not experience different disease processes, the institutional nature of recognizing male or female requires consideration "to avoid the potential for isolation and inequities in service" (Health Canada, 2007, para. 42).

## THE GENDER LENS AND COMMUNITY HEALTH NURSING PRACTICE

The use of a **gender lens** is another way to ensure that policies, programs, services, and interventions are appropriate for men and women boys and girls. Using a gender lens to examine a context helps to purposefully illuminate the unique constraints and opportunities men and women face. You can liken the use of a gender lens to putting on a pair of eyeglasses. Through one lens of the glasses, you see the participation, needs, and realities of women and transgendered people. Through the other lens, you see the participation, needs, and

| Table 19.2 | The Ten Leading Causes of Death among Canadian Men and Women, 2011 | | | |
|---|---|---|---|---|
| **Leading Causes of Death, Both Sexes** | | **Rank** | **Number** | **Percent** |
| All causes of death | | | 242 074 | 100 |
| Total, ten causes of death | | . . . | 181 625 | 75.0 |
| Malignant neoplasms (cancer) | | 1 | 72 476 | 29.9 |
| Diseases of heart (heart disease) | | 2 | 47 627 | 19.7 |
| Cerebrovascular diseases (stroke) | | 3 | 13 283 | 5.5 |
| Chronic lower respiratory diseases | | 4 | 11 184 | 4.6 |
| Accidents (unintentional injuries) | | 5 | 10 716 | 4.4 |
| Diabetes mellitus (diabetes) | | 6 | 7 194 | 3.0 |
| Alzheimer's disease | | 7 | 6 356 | 2.6 |
| Influenza and pneumonia | | 8 | 5 767 | 2.4 |
| Intentional self-harm (suicide) | | 9 | 3 728 | 1.5 |
| Nephritis, nephrotic syndrome, and nephrosis (kidney disease) | | 10 | 3 294 | 1.4 |

Source: Statistics Canada. (2014). *Leading causes of death by sex.* CANSIM Table 102-0561 and Catalogue no. 84-215-X. Retrieved from http://www.statcan.gc.ca/pub/82-625-x/2014001/article/11896-eng.htm

| Table 19.3 | Gender Lens Tool | | | | | | |
|---|---|---|---|---|---|---|---|
| | | **What Factors Might Contribute to These Differences?** | | | | | |
| | **Biological** | **Psychosocial** | | | | | |
| **Are There Gender Differences in:** | | **Social** | **Cultural** | **Economic** | **Political** | **Educational** | |
| Incidence/Prevalence | Yes  No | | | | | | |
| Diagnosis/Investigation | Yes  No | | | | | | |
| Risk Factors | Yes  No | | | | | | |
| Natural History | Yes  No | | | | | | |
| Treatment | Yes  No | | | | | | |
| Response | Yes  No | | | | | | |

Source: Adapted from A. Day, University of Toronto. (2009). *Using the gender lens tool.* Retrieved from http://www.genderandhealth.ca/en/modules/lens/gender-lens-identifying-gaps-02.jsp

realities of men and transgendered people. Your sight or vision is the combination of what each eye sees. Table 19.3 represents a gender lens tool that you may use in your community health nursing practice.

Using a gender lens enables CHNs to examine the impact of biological sex, gender, and gender bias to uncover where men, women, and transgendered people are facing barriers in accessing programs and services to promote their health (see Canadian Research Box 19.1). However, caution must be exercised when planning gender-appropriate community health interventions. We do not want to inadvertently enforce gendered stereotypes or gender dominance. For example, youth-directed anti-tobacco campaigns seeking to counter the "gendered cool" of smoking present in tobacco advertising can also run the risk of reinforcing gender biases by focusing on young women who take smoking up to fit in or be popular versus boys who may have it reinforced that smoking makes them look tough and independent (Government of Canada, 2013b). While tending to structures that design and deliver community health policy and programs, it is important to consider their potential for reinforcing or disrupting gender ideals. By delivering and evaluating gender-appropriate community health nursing programs, we will better engage end-users to advance the well-being of all Canadians. In addition, CHNs will develop their collective expertise for how gender can most effectively be integrated to future community health programs, services, and interventions.

### CANADIAN RESEARCH BOX 19.2

**What are young men's grief experiences and how do they express a masculine identity after the death of a friend?**

Creighton, G., Oliffe, J. L., Butterwick, S., & Saewyc, E. (2013). After the death of a friend: Young men's grief and masculine identities. *Social Science & Medicine, 84,* 35–43. http://dx.doi.org/10.1016/j.socscimed.2013.02.022

One of the most powerful experiences for human beings is the experience of grief. While researchers have paid close attention to the impacts of grief on the health and wellness of individuals, families, and communities, there has been little analysis on the impact of gender on the experience of grief. Particularly absent from the literature is the experience of young men and the influence of society's construction of what grief for young men "should look like." To begin to address this gap, Creighton, Oliffe, Butterwick, and Saewyc (2013) used qualitative interviews with 25 men aged 19–25 who had experienced the sudden death of a friend from various causes, including motor vehicle accidents, fights, and drug overdose. The purpose of this study was to explore the influence of gender on the expression of grief.

Through their work, Creighton et al. (2013) discovered that the men who experienced grief did so in particular ways. Three main models or masculine identities were identified in relation to the young men's grief processes: *the adventurer* (journeying out into the unknown), *the father figure* (focusing on caring for family and friends), and *the lamplighter* (overcoming similar hardships that their friend may have passed away from, such as drug addiction). The results of the study indicated that the men were influenced by the socially acceptable ideals of how men should grieve in public. Ideals such as being stoic and angry were perceived as being acceptable for them to show while grieving in public. Crying, however, was perceived by study participants as "a feminine activity that would be seen as unacceptable or signifying weakness to their friends" (p. 42).

### Discussion Questions

1. In your view, what beliefs does Canadian society have about how men should act after the loss of a friend or family member?

2. Think about some of the stereotypes you've seen in movies and television. How do the media influence the perception of how men should act while grieving?

3. Are there areas within your own developing nursing practice where you have witnessed men being expected to behave in a certain way, just because they are men?

The research evidence suggests that while many women quit smoking during pregnancy, many relapse in the postpartum period. One of the major factors associated with relapse is having a partner who smokes. Women smoke for a variety of reasons. In addition to struggling with addiction, they may smoke as a coping strategy to manage stress, difficult emotions, or to get a much needed time-out from their hectic schedules.

### Discussion Questions

1. In what ways is tobacco use a women's health issue?
2. How might gender relations affect women's tobacco use?
3. What might a women-centred approach to smoking cessation programming involve?

## CARDIOVASCULAR DISEASE, SEX, GENDER, AND COMMUNITY HEALTH NURSING INTERVENTIONS

The healthcare of Canadians can be examined through the application of a gender lens. The impact of gender on the health of individuals, families, communities, sectors, and populations can be very subtle and hard to see if you are not directly looking for it (see Canadian Research Box 19.2). Using cardiovascular health as the vehicle, the impact of sex and gender will be explored to show how these concepts can impact individuals, families, communities, and populations.

## Cardiovascular Disease and Sex

Although cardiovascular disease is the second leading cause of death for both sexes (Table 19.2), research has demonstrated widespread differences between men and women in terms of clinical profiles, presentation, and outcomes. In their study, Dey et al. (2009) discovered that women were more likely to have adverse outcomes such as death, myocardial infarction, stroke, and re-admittance to the hospital at six months when compared to men. Other symptoms of acute coronary syndrome specific to women include fatigue, difficulty breathing, shortness of breath, neck and jaw pain, heart palpitations, cough, nausea and vomiting, and indigestion (Norris, Dasgupta, & Kirkland, 2007). Sex differences in anatomic, physiologic, and biologic characteristics may explain differences in symptoms of acute coronary syndrome.

> Women have smaller coronary artery lumens and less collateral circulation than men, which may lead to an increase in ischemia, particularly during exertion or stress. Sex hormones may partly account for symptom differences. For example, diminishing estrogen levels in premenopausal and menopausal women may affect lipid metabolism and the activation of the coagulation cascade and vasoactive mediators. (Norris et al., 2007, p. S22)

Women are more likely to be diagnosed with unstable angina whereas men are more likely to have an acute myocardial infarction (Norris et al., 2007). Hochman et al. (1999) also found that women had more complications than men during hospitalization. Differences in base-line characteristics could not account for these differences and could reflect pathophysiologic and anatomical distinctions between men and women. Rieves, Wright, Gupta, and Shacter (2000) were able to determine that men die earlier than women do after acute myocardial infarction. Hence, it is imperative that CHNs to understand sex differences in the clinical profile, presentation, and outcomes of specific disease processes.

## CARDIOVASCULAR DISEASE, GENDER, AND THE LEVELS OF PREVENTION

## Secondary and Tertiary Prevention with Families

It is important to note that women are socialized to stress and how to cope with stress in distinctive ways. This is evident in a variety of circumstances, and cardiovascular disease is no exception. For example, women have been known to delay seeking treatment after the onset of symptoms of a myocardial infarction and to minimize the impact of cardiovascular disease (Bjarnason-Wehrens, Grand, Loewel, Voller, & Mittag, 2007). Women have also been known to be reluctant in involving family members in lifestyle changes required by their health problems (Bjarnason-Wehrens et al., 2007). Conversely, men often place responsibility for necessary lifestyle changes on their spouses. This may be related to women's role as the primary caregiver in the home, which often means that women sacrifice their own health and personal preventative health practices to improve those of other family members. For instance, women are less likely to engage in regular physical exercise, a health-promotion activity known to decrease risk of cardiovascular disease (Kristofferzon, Lofmark, & Carlsson, 2003).

With respect to gender roles and gender relations, research points to distinct differences in the social support of men and women within families. Although it has been shown that women have more confidants and are more likely to utilize emotional social support resources (Davidson, Trudeau, van Roosmalen, Stewart, & Kirkland, 2006), they often do not want to burden family members with their health problems (Kristofferzon et al., 2003). With respect to lifestyle changes, women reported that they received less support from their partners, in spite of having expressed a greater need for support (Kristofferzon et al., 2003). Men reported having more support from their spouses than women did, and men are more likely to involve their spouses in the recovery process. Although women reported that engaging in household activities was important to them and aided in their recovery, they received less assistance with household duties from others (Kristofferzon et al., 2003). Women also reported having less social support one year after a myocardial infarction when compared to men. It is important for CHNs to understand the ways in which gender roles and gender relations impact the health and well-being of men and women differently.

CHNs are in an ideal position to intervene with health-promotion messaging when working with families who are living through cardiovascular disease. In fact, one of the roles of CHNs working at the family level is to assist families to take responsibility for establishing, maintaining, or improving their health. This can be accomplished by adding to family members' knowledge of the determinants of health. (Canadian Public Health Association, 2010). This, in turn, could empower family members' ability to influence modifiable factors to the benefit of their loved one who is ill. Using the population health-promotion model (Flynn, 1999), nurses can create supportive environments within families by involving family members in discussions with the women experiencing cardiovascular disease. Care planning should include family members and significant others so that they can support and encourage women to cope with issues that may arise as a result of their illness (Wright & Leahey, 2013). For example, family members can be encouraged to engage in physical activity together, as a form of secondary or tertiary prevention. Framing physical activity as a family activity may increase the chance that women will participate. Part of the cardiac rehabilitation process includes working with families to explore how unpaid work, including household duties and family responsibilities, may impact recovery from a myocardial infarction. CHNs can also create supportive environments by encouraging the sharing of domestic responsibilities (Artazcoz, Borrell, & Benach, 2001). Furthermore, family members can be taught the signs and symptoms of myocardial infarction and the importance of seeking prompt treatment if a second episode occurs. Thus, exploring gender roles, gender identities, and gender relations within the family context may influence the recovery of women who have experienced a myocardial infarction.

## Tertiary Prevention with Communities

CHNs have a responsibility to work with other colleagues in the healthcare community to promote and protect health (Canadian Public Health Association, 2010). Working with communities of various health professionals opens up opportunities to develop capacity around how gender impacts cardiovascular health. This is important, since recent evidence suggests that women receive less information about their cardiovascular illness than men, women receive different treatments for their cardiac symptoms, women are more likely to experience delayed diagnosis and treatment when compared to men, and women receive less information about rehabilitation options and support groups (Genesway, 2001; Kristofferzon et al., 2003; Norris et al., 2007). These differences may be the result of institutionalized gender. Using the population health-promotion model (Flynn, 1999), a CHN can strengthen community action by bringing together a community of healthcare professionals involved in cardiovascular health in

order to explore if these differences exist across the continuum of the healthcare system, particularly in the community setting. CHNs can work with communities of healthcare professionals to explore potential solutions in order to reduce such gender differences, when and where they exist.

# TOWARD GENDER-APPROPRIATE COMMUNITY HEALTH NURSING PRACTICE

## Community Health Nursing Practice and Gender Advocacy—A Form of Primary Prevention

As demonstrated in this chapter, CHNs have wide-ranging and far-reaching roles and responsibilities. One function of CHNs is to link the health and illness experiences of individuals, families, and communities to advocacy and the development of health public policy. Indeed, CHNs are known for their role in activism for specific population groups. CHNs show a strong commitment to equity and social justice and speak out for equity in population health through policy-making activities (Canadian Public Health Association, 2010).

It is well known that the caregiving burden is a major societal cost that women often bear to the detriment of their health (Davidson et al., 2006). How the caregiving burden affects the health of women at the individual, family, and community levels are detailed in earlier sections. In order to address this, CHNs can use the population health-promotion model (Flynn, 1999) to engage in the policy cycle to assist in building healthy public policy. One area of policy focus could be the issue of the caregiving burden on a larger scale. CHNs are in an ideal position to advocate for a change in how governments, employers, and Canadians think about unpaid caregiver work. CHNs can serve as activists in this cause related to gender inequity by advocating for public policies around family care. This may result in reduced gender health inequities that are attributable to the unequal distribution of caregiving expectations. Engaging in discussions that frame healthy public policy is a fundamental role of CHNs in Canada (Canadian Public Health Association, 2010).

There are numerous ways in which the labour market contributes to gender inequities. According to the Global Employment Trends for Women 2012 report (International Labor Organization, 2012), there are key gaps between women and men (also known as gender differentials) that clearly disadvantage women. CHNs may serve as activists to decrease such gender inequities in the following:

■ work on various initiatives to reduce the burden of housework. Depending on the level of development in any given country, this may range from advocating for the availability of electricity and safe drinking water to sanitation, roads, and transportation infrastructure;

- balancing the gender division of paid and unpaid work;
- changing the costs and benefits of gender specialization; ensuring that taxes and transfers do not create disincentives for dual-earner families;
- compensating for unequal employment opportunities based on gender. This may include initiatives to eliminate the adverse impact of career breaks through well-paid leave and the right of return to post; and
- engaging in public social marketing campaigns to challenge gender stereotypes and to ensure the proper implementation of legislation against discrimination (International Labor Organization, 2012).

Gender considerations are relevant to *all* community health nursing practice. By applying a gender lens, we can start to consider the ways in which policies, programs, services, and interventions can better meet the needs of men, women, and people who identify themselves as transgender. CHNs adhere to standards of practice that guide their professional responsibilities (Canadian Nurses Association & Community Health Nurses of Canada, 2010, CHNC, 2011, revised). Within those standards are areas of advocacy that CHNs should be attending to in their practice. This includes ensuring that gender does not interfere with access to health resources and advocacy for healthy public policies that are influenced by gender (Canadian Nurses Association & Community Health Nurses of Canada, 2010).

## CONCLUSION

It is clear that "one size does not fit all" when it comes to community health. Nursing strategies in community health need to be gender appropriate. We cannot assume that the approaches commonly used with women will be effective with men and vice versa. CHNs must also acknowledge that gender is a fluid concept. **Gender-appropriate community health nursing interventions** are tailored approaches that ensure that the unique needs of men, women, and transgendered people are met. Assessing differences and disparities in health status, health behaviours, and utilization of healthcare services based on gender is an important step in ensuring that all Canadians benefit equally from Canada's healthcare system.

In this chapter, we have highlighted the differences between the concepts of sex and gender and have demonstrated how these concepts are relevant to community health practice. Applying a gender lens to one's practice can help to shed light on the unique health needs that men, women, and transgendered people have, and can help CHNs to appropriately tailor their approaches.

## KEY TERMS

femininity   p. 364
gender   p. 364
gender bias   p. 368
gender identity   p. 364
gender inequity   p. 368
gender lens   p. 369
gender norms   p. 367
gender relations   p. 365

gender roles   p. 365
gender-appropriate community health nursing interventions   p. 373
gender-based analyses   p. 368
institutionalized gender   p. 366
masculinity   p. 364
sex   p. 363
social determinants of health   p. 362
transgendered   p. 364

## STUDY QUESTIONS

1. What distinguishes sex from gender?
2. What is a gender lens and how is it used?
3. How do Canadian men's and women's life expectancy and causes of death differ?
4. When should gender considerations be made in community health nursing?
5. Why is it important to consider gender as part of community health nursing practice?
6. What is institutionalized gender?

> After working through these questions, go to the MyNursingLab at www.pearsoned.ca/mynursinglab to check your answers.

## INDIVIDUAL CRITICAL-THINKING EXERCISES

1. Imagine a world without gender—what would the world be like?
2. Are there countries that are trying to reduce gender disparities? Do an Internet search and see how gender disparities are being reduced around the world. Do you believe that any of the strategies that you have discovered could be applied in Canada?
3. How do I as a community health nurse improve the health of my clients from a gender-based perspective? In what ways are my expectations different for men and women in my practice?
4. In your practice experiences, who is more likely to engage in health-promoting behaviour—men or women?
5. What barriers do CHNs face within the institutions that they work in to create spaces where gender role diversity can flourish?

## GROUP CRITICAL-THINKING EXERCISES

1. Stand up and position yourself on a continuum from one side of the room to another. On one side of the room is feminine; on the other side of the room is the most masculine. After placing yourself on the continuum, look around and see where everyone else is. Discuss why you placed yourself where you did. How do your observations inform our understanding of gender?

2. Now place yourself on a continuum of how men and women typically engage in health promotion activities. What notions of gender informed your positioning?

3. Consider the labour market and its effects on gender. What are some specific ways in which CHNs can serve as activists to decrease the inequities related to gender in the workplace?

# REFERENCES

American Psychological Association. (2011). What does transgender mean? In *Answers to your questions about transgendered people, gendered identity, and gender expression.* Retrieved from http://www.apa.org/topics/sexuality/transgender.aspx

Artazcoz, L., Borrell, C., & Benach, J. (2001). Gender inequalities in health among workers: The relation with family demands. *Journal of Epidemiology and Community Health, 55*(9), 639–647.

Bottorff, J. L., Kalaw, C., Johnson, J. L., Stewart, M., Greaves, L., & Carey, J. (2006). Couple dynamics during women's tobacco reduction in pregnancy and postpartum. *Nicotine and Tobacco Research, 8*(4), 499–509. doi:10.1080/14622200600789551

Bottorff, J. L., Oliffe, J. L., Halpin, M., Phillips, M., McLean, G., & Mroz, L. (2008). Women and prostate cancer support groups: The gender connect? *Social Sciences and Medicine, 66*(5), 1217–1227. doi:10.1016/j.socscimed.2007.11.018

Bjarnason-Wehrens, B., Grand, G., Loewel, H., Voller, H., & Mittag, O. (2007). Gender-specific issues in cardiac rehabilitation: Do women with ischaemic heart disease need specially tailored programmes? *European Journal of Cardiovascular Prevention and Rehabilitation, 14*(2), 163–171. doi:10.1097/HJR.0b013e3280128bce

Canadian Labour Congress. (2009). Closing the gender pay gap. Retrieved from http://canadianlabour.ca/issues-research/closing-gender-pay-gap

Canadian Nurses Association and Community Health Nurses of Canada (2010). Assessment of current CHNC programs, policies, and products using the CAN social justice gauge. Retrieved from http://www.chnc.ca/documents/SocialJusticeGaugeAssessmentofCommunityHealthNursesofCanadaCHNCMarch312010.pdf

Canadian Public Health Association. (2010). *Public health–community health nursing practice in Canada: Roles and activities.* (4th ed.). Ottawa, ON: Author.

Community Health Nurses of Canada. (2011, revised). *Canadian community health nursing: Professional practice model & standards of practice.* St. John's, NL: Author. Retrieved from https://www.chnc.ca/documents/CHNC-ProfessionalPracticeModel-EN/index.html

Conference Board of Canada. (2014). Gender income gap. Retrieved from http://www.conferenceboard.ca/hcp/details/society/gender-income-gap.aspx

Davidson, K. W., Trudeau, K. J., van Roosmalen, E., Stewart, M., & Kirkland, S. (2006). Gender as a health determinant and implications for health education. *Health Education & Behavior, 33*(6), 731–743. doi:10.1177/1090198106288043

Denton, M., Prus, S., & Walters, V. (2003). Gender differences in health: A Canadian study of the psychosocial, structural and behavioural determinants of health. *Social Science &*

*Medicine, 58*(2004), 2585–2600. doi:10.1016/j.socscimed.2003.09.008

Dey, S., Flather, M. D., Devlin, G., Brieger, D., Gurfinkel, E. P., Steg, P. G., . . . Eagle, K. A. (2009). Sex-related differences in the presentation, treatment and outcomes among patients with acute coronary syndromes: The global registry of acute coronary events. *Heart, 95*(1), 20–26. doi:10.1136/hrt.2007.138537

Edmonds, R. (2012). *Ontario's human rights code amendments: Deconstructing "gender identity" and "gender expression." Sexual Orientation and Gender Identity Section.* Retrieved from http://www.oba.org/en/pdf/sec_news_sog_dec12_gen_edm.pdf

Ettorre, E. (2004). Revisioning women and drug use: Gender sensitivity, embodiment, and reducing harm. *International Journal of Drug Policy, 15*(5), 327–335. doi:10.1016/j.drugpo.2004.06.009

Flynn, L. (1999). *Population health promotion model.* Revised from original model developed by N. Hamilton and T. Bhatti, Health Promotion Development Division, Health Canada, 1996. Winnipeg, MB: Health Canada, Manitoba/Saskatchewan Region.

Gesensway, D. (2001). Reasons for sex-specific and gender-specific study of health topics. *Annals of Internal Medicine, 135*(10), 935–938.

Ghandi, M., Bacchetti, P., Miotti, P., Quinn, T. C., Veronese, F., & Greenblatt, R. M. (2002). Does patient sex affect human immunodeficiency virus levels? *Clinical Infectious Disease, 35*(3), 313–322.

Government of Canada. (2013a). *Introduction to pay equity.* Retrieved from http://www.labour.gc.ca/eng/standards_equity/eq/pay/intro.shtml#links

Government of Canada. (2013b). *GBA+.* Ottawa, ON: Status of Women Canada. Retrieved from http://www.swc-cfc.gc.ca/gba-acs/overview-apercu-en.html

Greco, J. (2013). Gender: A social construction. *Sociological Imagination: Western's Undergraduate Sociology Student Journal, 2*(2). Retrieved from http://ir.lib.uwo.ca/si/vol2/iss2/8

Greenberg, L., & Normandin, C. (2011). *Health at a glance: Disparities in life expectancy at birth.* Retrieved from http://www.statcan.gc.ca/pub/82-624-x/2011001/article/11427-eng.htm#a3

Health Canada (2001). *"Certain circumstances": Issues in equity and responsiveness in access to health care in Canada.* Ottawa, ON: Author. Retrieved from http://www.hc-sc.gc.ca/hcs-sss/pubs/acces/2001-certain-equit-acces/index-eng.php

Health Canada (2007). *Chronic disease prevention and management.* Ottawa, ON: Author. Retrieved from http://www.hc-sc.gc.ca/hcs-sss/pubs/prim/2006-synth-chronic-chroniques/index-eng.php

Heteronormative (2013). In Oxford Dictionary online. Retrieved from http://www.oxforddictionaries.com/definition/english/heteronormative

Hochman, J. S., Tamis, J. E., Thompson, T. D., Weaver, W. D., White, H. D., Van de Werf, F., . . . Califf, R. M. for the Global Use of Strategies to Open Occluded Coronary Arteries in Acute Coronary Syndromes IIb Investigators. (1999). Sex, clinical presentation, and outcome in patients with acute coronary syndromes. *The New England Journal of Medicine, 341*(4), 226–232.

International Labor Organization. (2012). Global employment trends for women. Geneva: Author. Retrieved from http://www.ilo.org/global/research/global-reports/global-employment-trends/WCMS_195447/lang--en/index.htm

Jackson, B. E., Pederson, A., & Boscoe, M. (2009). Waiting to wait: Improving wait times evidence though gender-based analysis. In P. Armstrong & J. Deadman (Eds.), *Women's health: Intersections of policy research and practice* (pp. 35–52). Toronto, ON: Women's Press.

Jenkins, G. W., Kemnitz, C. P., & Tortora, G. J. (2010). *Anatomy and Physiology: From science to life.* (2nd ed.). Hoboken, NJ: John Wiley & Sons, Inc.

Kristofferzon, M. L., Lofmark, R., & Carlsson, M. (2003). Myocardial infarction: Gender differences in coping and social support. *Journal of Advanced Nursing, 44,* 360–374.

Lee, C., & Owens, R. (2002). *The psychology of men's health.* Philadelphia, PA: Open University Press.

Nagunar, D. (2011). Longevity and historical life tables (for 1920–1922 through 1980–1982); Statistics Canada Catalogue no. 84–537, Life Tables (for 1985–1987 and 1990–1992); Statistics Canada, Vital Statistics, CANSIM Table 102–0512, Life expectancy (for 1995–1997 through 2005–2007). Retrieved from http://www.statcan.gc.ca/pub/82-624-x/2011001/article/chart/11427-02-chart2-eng.htm

Norris, C. Dasgupta, K., & Kirkland, S. (2007). Differences in cardiovascular presentation in women and men. *Canadian Medical Association Journal, 176*(6), S22–S23. Published by Canadian Nurses Association.

Oliffe, J. L., & Phillips, M. (2008). Depression, men and masculinities: A review and recommendations. *Journal of Men's Health, 5*(3), 194–202. doi:10.1016/j.jomh.2008.03.016

Rieves, D., Wright, G., Gupta, G., & Shacter, E. (2000). Clinical trial (GUSTO-1 and INJECT) evidence of earlier death for men than women after acute myocardial infarction. *American Journal of Cardiology, 85,* 147–153. doi:10.1016/S0002-9149(99)00652-9

Senie, R. T. (2014). *Epidemiology of women's health.* Burlington, MD: Jones and Bartlett.

Sheppard, M., & Mayo, J. B. (2013). The social construction of gender and sexuality: Learning from two spirit traditions. *The Social Studies, 104*(6), 259–270.

Soldin, O. P., Chung, S. H., & Mattison, D. R. (2011). Sex differences in drug disposition. *Journal of Biomedicine and Biotechnology.* 2011. doi:10.1155/2011/187103

Tudiver, S. (2009). Integrating women's health and gender analysis in a government context: Reflections on a work in progress. In P. Armstrong & J. Deadman (Eds.), *Women's health: Intersections of policy research and practice* (pp. 21–34). Toronto, ON: Women's Press.

Tyler, R. E. (2012). Adolescent and young adult male health: A review. *Pediatrics, 132,* 535–546.

Unicef (2006). Statement on International Women's Day. Retrieved from http://www.unicef.org/media/media_35134.html

Wright, L., & Leahey, M. (2013). *Nurses and families: A guide to family assessment and intervention* (6th ed.). Philadelphia, PA: F. A. Davis Company.

World Health Organization. (2008). *Closing the gap in a generation: Health equity through action on the social determinants of health.* Geneva, Switzerland: Author. Retrieved from http://www.who.int/social_determinants/thecommission/finalreport/en/index.html

World Health Organization. (2010). *Gender, women and primary health care renewal.* Discussion Paper. Geneva, Switzerland: Author.

World Health Organization. (2013a). *Trade, foreign policy, diplomacy, and health: Gender.* Geneva, Switzerland: Author. Retrieved from http://www.who.int/trade/glossary/story032/en

World Health Organization. (2013b). What do we mean by gender and sex? *Gender, women, and health.* Geneva, Switzerland: Author. Retrieved from http://www.who.int/gender/whatisgender/en

World Health Organization. (2013c). *Gender and women's mental health.* Geneva, Switzerland: Author. Retrieved from http://www.who.int/mental_health/prevention/genderwomen/en

World Health Organization. (2013d). *Why gender and health?* Geneva, Switzerland: Author. Retrieved from http://www.who.int/gender/genderandhealth/en

## ABOUT THE AUTHORS

**Aliyah Dosani**, RN, BN, MPH, PhD, is an Associate Professor in the School of Nursing and Midwifery, Faculty of Health, Community and Education at Mount Royal University in Calgary, Alberta. She holds a PhD from the University of Calgary with a specialization in population/public health. Her nursing practice includes instructing students in the Bachelor of Nursing Program, population/public health, community health nursing, and legal issues in nursing. Her work focuses on maternal, newborn, and child health. Her research interests include working with vulnerable populations through community-based programs and interventions. She also shares a passion for global health issues.

**Deborah Mansell**, RN, MN, is an Assistant Professor in the School of Nursing and Midwifery, Faculty of Health, Community and Education at Mount Royal University. Her nursing practice includes community health/public health nursing, caring for childbearing/childrearing families, breastfeeding, parenting programs, legal issues in nursing, and teaching nursing students in Bachelor of Nursing programs. Deborah's research and research interests include caring for and promoting the health of diverse populations, maternal/child health, and community-based programs and interventions.

# Lesbian, Gay, Bisexual, Transgender, and Queer Clients

*Elizabeth M. Saewyc*

LEARNING OUTCOMES

**After studying this chapter, you should be able to:**

1. Describe the developmental processes and dimensions that are part of sexual orientation and of gender identity.

2. Recognize different sexual orientations and gender identities generally found within Canadian communities.

3. Understand the societal attitudes and health risks that may be experienced by lesbian, gay, bisexual, transgender, and queer or questioning (LGBTQ) clients in communities and healthcare settings.

4. Explore the challenges and potential consequences of disclosing sexual orientation to family, peers, and healthcare providers.

5. Reflect on and identify your own assumptions, values, beliefs, and judgments related to LGBTQ people, and on how these influence your approach to community health nursing with LGBTQ populations.

6. Identify community health nursing interventions for promoting the health of LGBTQ people.

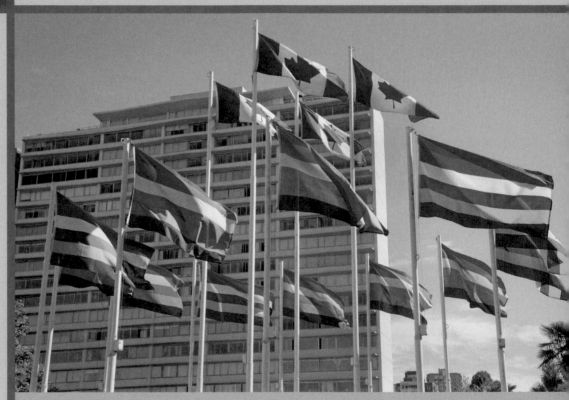

*Source: Maxdigi/Fotolia*

## INTRODUCTION

Sexual orientation and gender identity are two major characteristics that develop during childhood and adolescence. Sexual orientation can be defined as romantic and sexual attractions toward people of one or more genders (Saewyc, 2011). Other dimensions of sexual orientation include sexual relations with people of one or more genders as well as self-labelling as heterosexual, gay, lesbian, bisexual, and queer or "questioning." **Homosexuality** refers to romantic and sexual attractions toward persons of the same gender, and people with this orientation are commonly referred to in Canada as gay men and lesbian women (Photo 20.1). **Heterosexuality** refers to romantic and/or sexual attractions to another gender, such as men attracted solely to women or women attracted solely to men. People with this orientation are called heterosexual men or women. **Bisexuality** refers to romantic and/or sexual attractions to more than one gender, and people with this orientation are commonly called bisexual men or bisexual women. Some sexual minority people prefer the term **queer** as a label to indicate a non-heterosexual orientation. However, this term used to carry strongly negative connotations, and older lesbian, gay, or bisexual people may be offended by its use, so it should generally only be used when someone has self-identified using that term. Some people may be unsure of their orientation, especially adolescents, and so may prefer to identify as "questioning" their orientation. Since society tends to assume a "default" orientation of heterosexual for most people (see "heterosexism" discussed later in this chapter), when lesbian, gay, bisexual, or queer people disclose their orientation publicly to others, it is termed **coming out**.

**Gender identity** is a complex development of one's sense of self as a gendered person, with the attributes and social traits assigned in one's culture to a particular gender role. This most commonly means identifying as a man or woman, as masculine or feminine. But the traits, appearance, and behaviours associated with various genders may differ across cultures and social groups. Gender identity is not the same as **physiological sex**, which is based on chromosomes and phenotypic expression in the body that is commonly labelled as either male or female, even though physical bodies do not always fit neatly into these two categories; there are chromosomal variations and some congenital conditions that lead to variations in physiological development. Most of the time, gender identity aligns with physiological sex, also identified by the term "cisgender" (see below).

**Transgender** or **gender diverse** people may feel their core gender identity does not match what others think it is or should be (e.g., their gender assigned at birth might have been male, but they identify as a woman) or that their gender does not fit within a binary model of man or woman (e.g., they might identify as gender queer, gender fluid, or another unlabelled gender). They might feel as though their physical bodies do not accurately reflect their internal gender identity. Transgender or gender diverse persons may see their gender as being more fluid. These individuals may want to dress and act according to their gender identity rather than according to others' expectations of how they should behave based on their assigned birth gender. They may also choose to take hormones or undergo surgery to help align their external body and appearance with their gender identity. In the same way the term "heterosexual" is an acknowledgement that everyone has an orientation, not just sexual minority people, the term **cisgender** has emerged in some health and social circles as somewhat of an equivalent in gender identity, referring to the majority of people whose internal gender identity matches their external body appearance and gender performance (Schilt & Westbrook, 2009). Aboriginal or First Nations people may prefer the term **Two Spirit**, or two-spirited, as a culturally specific term referring to gender identity or sexual orientation or a combination of both (Balsam, Huang, Fieland, Simoni, & Walters, 2004).

According to the 2009 Canadian Community Health Survey (CCHS), about 1% of adults aged 18 to 59 identify as gay or lesbian, and another 1% identify as bisexual (Statistics Canada, 2011). Studies of adolescents and adults that include more measures of orientation than just self-labelling suggest that a larger percentage of people report same-gender or both-gender attractions—as many as 4% to 7%. Among adolescents, those reporting bisexual attractions outnumber exclusively same-gender attractions by three to one or more. Same-gender or both-gender sexual behaviour is less common than attractions among adolescents, in part because most Canadian adolescents are not sexually active until the later

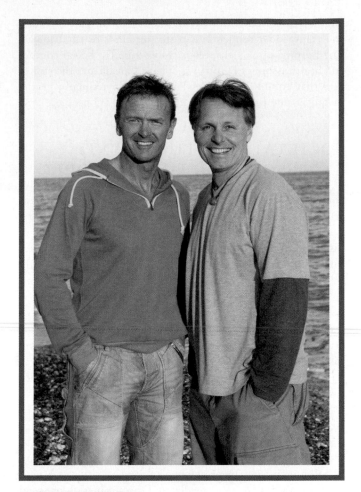

**PHOTO 20.1** Cisgender and transgender men in relationships with each other may identify as gay or as bisexual.

*Source: Andrew Lever/Fotolia*

teen years or young adulthood (Saewyc, Poon, Homma, & Skay, 2008). Among adults, however, self-identifying as lesbian, gay, or bisexual is less common than attractions or behaviour, so the estimates from the CCHS are likely an undercount of the population of **LGBTQ** people in Canada.

There are various theories about the nature of sexual orientation and development of gender identity, but most scientific evidence at present seems to lean toward a genetic basis for sexual attraction, potentially influenced in part by environment, with identity and behaviour influenced more strongly by culture and societal attitudes (Mustanski, Chivers, & Bailey, 2002). Family studies as well as studies of monozygotic and dizygotic twins have found enough concordance in sexual orientation to suggest there is some genetic basis for orientation, but specific genes have not been identified. As well, the variety of cultural meanings and practices around sexual orientation and gender identity across the world suggests that people's expression of their romantic attractions and their gender performance are influenced by culture.

Most nurses can expect to encounter at least some lesbian, gay, bisexual, and, less commonly, transgender clients in all age groups, from adolescents to older adults. The numbers will reflect regional variation and type of health service, with large metropolitan cities having more lesbian, gay, bisexual, and transgender residents than smaller cities or rural towns. The purpose of this chapter is to describe the social context and health issues of LGBTQ people in Canada and the strategies that community health nurses use in reducing health inequities and promoting the health of LGBTQ people.

## SOCIETAL ATTITUDES AND STRESSORS FOR LGBTQ PEOPLE

Some LGBTQ clients choose to not disclose their sexual orientation or gender identity, or to limit disclosure to people they trust. This reluctance to disclose or fear of the consequences of disclosure relates to several essential concepts: homophobia, biphobia, transphobia, and heterosexism. **Homophobia** describes a fear or hatred, often irrational, of gay men and lesbian women (Oxford Dictionary, 1993). This prejudice is not usually based on experience or knowledge of actual gay or lesbian people but rather on myths and assumptions. It is often demonstrated through derogatory language, jokes, and discriminatory treatment of individuals perceived or known to be gay or lesbian. Similarly, **biphobia** is an extreme prejudice toward bisexual people (Eliason, 1997), and **transphobia** is a fear of or hatred toward transgender people (Norton, 1997). At its worst, these prejudices can involve extreme violence (gay bashing or trans bashing) toward those perceived to be lesbian, gay, bisexual, or transgender. More often it shows up as bullying or harassment in schools and social situations, negative comments on social media, and discrimination or social exclusion of people thought to be LGBTQ.

Being surrounded by negative or rejecting messages or open hostility and discrimination can create significant stress in LGBTQ people's lives. This type of stress can contribute to challenges with coping and long-term, stress-related health issues. Some LGBTQ individuals may subconsciously accept negative societal views about sexual minority or gender diverse people and, thus, experience a loss of self-worth and a lack of self-acceptance (Herek, Cogan, Gillis, & Glunt, 1998); this is termed **internalized homophobia** (or biphobia or transphobia). It can show up as low self-esteem and reduced self-care, and may lead to adopting health-compromising activities, such as substance abuse and unprotected or high-risk sexual activities, as a way to cope with distress.

**Heterosexism**, on the other hand, refers to the assumption that heterosexuality is the norm and a lack of awareness or acknowledgement that other orientations or genders exist along the spectrum of "normal." This is acted out constantly in everyday society through behaviours or practices that assume everyone is heterosexual, or should be. Examples of heterosexism in healthcare systems include asking clients about their marital status or sexual relationships using gendered terms, such as asking a man, "and do you have a wife?" This emphasizes that you expect a man would only have a female spouse even though in Canada it is legal for a man to marry another man. Likewise, asking all women what type of contraception they use without first assessing whether they are sexually active and if their sexual partners are women, men, or

another gender assumes that every woman has male sexual partners and needs some form of contraception. Heterosexism alienates LGBTQ people, and while it is not as overtly threatening as homophobia, it can cause people to avoid or delay access to needed healthcare. In addition to heterosexism, cissexism privileges cisgender identities and bodies over trans identities and trans bodies. Cissexism may be apparent in the health, social service, and justice sectors. For example, on most medical forms there is an option for male or female, but rarely for other genders. Another example is gender-segregated spaces, such as public washrooms, change rooms, sports leagues, shelters, and prisons, which can become inaccessible to trans people due to fear of transphobia and violence.

## HEALTH INEQUITIES AMONG LGBTQ PEOPLE

Because of the relatively smaller size of the population of LGBTQ people in our society, their health issues and healthcare needs are not readily apparent. Up until the mid-1970s, homosexuality was classified as a mental illness, and attention was focused on "curing" LGBTQ people (Brotman, Ryan, Jalbert, & Rowe, 2002). This usually involved intensive psychiatric therapy, including classical aversion therapy using electric shock. Today, this type of "conversion" or "reparative therapy" is considered unethical by most professional health organizations, as there is no credible evidence of its effectiveness. There is significant evidence that indicates conversion or reparative therapy is harmful, especially for adolescents when parents force them into therapy to try to change their orientation. This practice has been condemned by the World Health Organization (WHO), which has called on governments to ban reparative therapy (Pan American Health Organization/World Health Organization, 2012).

LGBTQ people face a variety of health inequities in Canada, and while the causes of these higher risks are complex, a key component is the health-related effects of societal stigma and discrimination. Although laws in Canada are changing, attitudes tend to be slower to shift. Population-based studies have shown LGBTQ youth in school still face high levels of discrimination and harassment (Taylor & Peter, 2011), as well as higher rates of physical and sexual abuse (Friedman et al., 2011). LGBTQ adults may also face hate crimes and assault in the community, harassment or discrimination in the workplace, and rejection within their families.

The stress that LGBTQ experience as a result of stigma, prejudice, and discrimination has been termed "minority stress" (Meyer, 2003), and it contributes to the higher risk for health problems and poorer self-rated health (Saewyc, 2011; Steele, Ross, Dobinson, Veldhuizen, & Tinmouth, 2009). LGBTQ people may face widespread negative attitudes within some communities, as well as witnessing or even personally experiencing hostility and violence. These types of negative experiences foster an expectation of personal rejection, the need to hide or conceal relationships and identity, and the need for coping mechanisms to handle distress from unsafe environments and lack of social support.

As mentioned, LGBTQ people face significant health inequities. Population-based research in Canada has documented higher rates of mental health issues, including depressive symptoms and anxiety, self-harm, suicidal thoughts, and suicide attempts among both adolescents and adults (Brennan, Ross, Dobinson, Veldhuizen, & Steele, 2010; Saewyc, 2011; Steele et al., 2009; Rotondi Khobzi et al., 2011a; Rotondi Khobzi et al., 2011b). These studies and others also document higher rates of tobacco use, alcohol use (including binge drinking), and substance use and abuse among LGBTQ youth, and to a lesser extent, among adults. Researchers have found that lesbian and bisexual adolescent girls have higher overweight and obese levels of body-mass index (BMI) when compared to heterosexual peers (Saewyc, Homma, Hitchcock, & Prior, 2012). Gay and bisexual boys and men have been demonstrated to have lower BMI and increased risk of eating-disordered behaviours when compared to their heterosexual peers (Brennan et al., 2010; Saewyc et al., 2007).

Sexual health is another important area of health inequities among LGBTQ people. Although most healthcare providers are aware of the higher risk for HIV/AIDS among men who have sex with men, lesbian and bisexual women in Canada have also reported higher prevalence of STIs (Steele et al., 2009). Similarly, lesbian, gay, and bisexual adolescents in western Canada have reported higher levels of sexual risk-taking behaviours than heterosexual students. Such high-risk behaviours include engaging in sexual intercourse before age 14, having a higher number of sexual partners, participating in unprotected sexual intercourse, and sex while intoxicated (Saewyc et al., 2006). These high-risk behaviours may be explained, in part, by higher rates of sexual abuse history (Saewyc et al., 2006). As a result, LGBTQ youth are also more likely to become pregnant or cause a pregnancy during adolescence (Saewyc et al., 2008). Pregnancy may be used as a way to deflect discrimination and heterosexism (Travers, Newton, & Munro, 2011). Pregnancy among lesbian and bisexual women is also increasingly common (see Photo 20.2), whether as a result of opposite-sex relationships or through assisted reproductive technologies, and many fertility clinics in Canada provide services for lesbian and bisexual women (Corbett, Frecker, Shapiro, & Yudin, 2013).

LGBTQ people from racialized ethnocultural backgrounds, such as Aboriginal or South Asian heritage, and those with visible or invisible disabilities face additional challenges. They may experience rejection and stigma both from larger society and within the wider LGBTQ community (Balsam et al., 2004; Parks, Hughes, & Matthews, 2004). The intersection of sexual orientation, gender, and ethnocultural background creates varying levels of health inequity as it can lead to multiple levels of discrimination (Poon, Saewyc, & Chen, 2011; Steele et al., 2009; Veenstra, 2011).

# COMING OUT, OR DISCLOSURE OF LGBTQ IDENTITY

Disclosure of a non-heterosexual sexual orientation or transgender identity can be difficult no matter when it occurs in the lifespan. The amount of difficulty relates to the nature of the relationship (e.g., telling a parent), the age of the individual

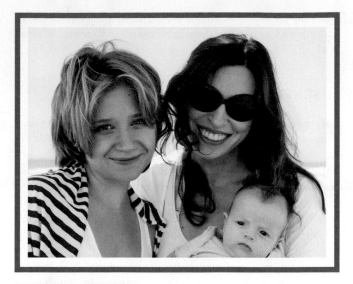

**PHOTO  20.2** Lesbian and bisexual women may have children together through assisted reproductive technologies.

*Source: Dubova/Fotolia*

(e.g., adolescent versus adult), and the value placed on the relationship (e.g., friend or relative versus stranger). Hiding one's sexual orientation or gender identity can be stressful and lead to poor health outcomes and health-compromising behaviours. LGBTQ adolescents' increased risk for depression and suicidal ideation may be highest just before disclosure within important relationships, such as to parents (Igartua, Gill, & Montoro, 2003). The response to that disclosure can also be an important predictor of suicidal ideation and attempt, as well as of long-term coping responses (Ryan, Huebner, Diaz, & Sanchez, 2009). Parents' negative responses can include violence or forcing the young person out of home; a disproportionate number of homeless and street-involved youth are LGBTQ (Frederick, Ross, Bruno, & Erickson, 2011). Even parents' less-severe negative or neutral responses are often interpreted by youth as rejection and are still linked with suicide attempts, problem substance use, and other challenges into young adulthood. In contrast, parents' supportive responses, such as continuing to state their love and acceptance of their child, can improve self-esteem and help buffer the stress of other negative reactions in school or among peers (Ryan, Russell, Huebner, Diaz, & Sanchez, 2010).

Transgender youth are especially vulnerable as society is particularly blind to the existence of individuals who do not fit into traditional masculine or feminine gender presentations. Gender diverse behaviour is less accepted among school-age children and adolescents than among young children, and trans and gender diverse youth experience significant adversity within school, their family, and the wider community. They may run away or be kicked out, become street-involved or homeless, and may need to engage in survival sex (exchanging sex for food, shelter, money, or drugs), all of which put them at significant risk for adverse health outcomes (Grossman & D'Augelli, 2006). When youth present and dress either gender ambiguously or in their felt gender they frequently experience ridicule, harassment, and sometimes violence. Fear of the consequences of disclosing transgender identity is a major factor in mental health and affects their personal safety in many social as well as family situations (Rotondi Khobzi et al., 2011a; Rotondi Khobzi et al., 2011b).

## Disclosing to Healthcare Providers

Coming out or disclosing sexual orientation or transgender identity can support good health and appropriate healthcare for LGBTQ people. However, in healthcare and community settings it can be a constant process—with each new care provider encountered the process must be repeated, and the same fears and concerns about the provider's reaction are experienced over again (Brotman et al., 2002). Not disclosing (being "closeted") is associated with shame and hiding and can lead to physical and psychological health challenges. LGBTQ people may be in the position of having to educate their healthcare providers, who may lack knowledge or comfort in providing appropriate care. Or they may actually experience unethical and unprofessional treatment by healthcare providers who have homophobic, biphobic, or transphobic attitudes as well as misinformation and prejudiced assumptions (for an example, see Canadian Research Box 20.1).

Many healthcare providers describe themselves as being "neutral" in their practice related to the sexual orientation or gender identity of their clients. This is based on the belief that healthcare should be accessible to all and not based on the particular needs of any one group or population (Brotman et al., 2002). This may result in healthcare providers not asking about sexual orientation when meeting a new client, or ignoring disclosure in an attempt to appear accepting. It is more appropriate to acknowledge the disclosure and reflect acceptance and caring, which will further encourage the client to share sensitive information that may influence care (Williams-Barnard, Mendoza, & Shippee-Rice, 2001). Acting in a "neutral" or unresponsive manner may in fact be read as a rejecting or negative response (Boehmer & Case, 2004).

## RESPONSES THAT PROMOTE HEALTH OR CONTRIBUTE TO HARM FOR LGBTQ PEOPLE

How can nurses provide safe and inclusive care for LGBTQ people? The first step is to address our own assumptions, beliefs, values, and attitudes about sexual orientation and gender diversity. These are likely to be reflective of the attitudes we absorbed growing up in our own families. Many of us may not ever have explored our attitudes about homosexuality, bisexuality, or gender diversity and may not be aware of how heterosexist we are. Think about what you believe about sexual orientation and gender identity, and where those beliefs came from. Have they changed over the years or are they the same as they were when you were growing up? How many different people do you know who are lesbian, gay, bisexual, or transgender? Can you recall caring for a self-identified

---

### CANADIAN RESEARCH BOX 20.1

**What are the experiences of transgender people in the Canadian healthcare system?**

Bauer, G. R., Scheim, A. I., Deutsch, M. B., & Cassarella, C. (2014). Reported emergency department avoidance, use, and experiences of transgender persons in Ontario, Canada: Results from a respondent-driven sampling survey. *Annals of Emergency Medicine, 63*(6), 713–720. http://dx.doi.org/10.1016/j.annemergmed.2013.09.027

This study involved the Trans PULSE survey of transgender people in Ontario, which involved 433 trans people ages 16 to 65. The study used a respondent-driven sampling design, a public health method for the accessing relatively hidden populations and using complex statistical adjustments to calculate estimates for entire population. Although one in three transgender Ontarians described needing emergency department (ED) care in the past year, only 71% of those who needed care were actually able to get care. Half of those who accessed ED care reported negative experiences, including hurtful and insulting language (32%), being told the provider does not know enough to provide care (31%), being told they thought gender on the ID bracelet was a mistake (27%), being belittled or ridiculed (24%), refusal to discuss trans-related concerns (18%), being told they were not really trans (13%), refusal to examine parts of body (12%), and actually refused or ended care (10%). As a result of these negative experiences, one in five trans people in the survey said they had avoided ED care, even when they needed it.

Implications of this research are significant. This is important information for health policy makers, clinical educators, and community health nurses who advocate for access to care. Emergency department staff may need further training, and EDs may need improved protocols for ensuring safe and supportive care for trans people accessing the ED. This training and improved protocols may help to meet the needs of this population in the future. It is equally important to note that healthcare providers should facilitate access to trans-friendly preventive and primary health care services in order to reduce the need for emergency services.

#### Discussion Questions

1. Why do you think ED clinical staff treat transgender people presenting for care in the ways this study reported?

2. What are the potential consequences, both to individuals and to society, when people with emergency health needs avoid the ED?

3. If you were providing community health nursing care to a transgender person who disclosed being treated badly in the ED, what are some ways you could respond to the issue in terms of your response to your individual client and for the wider population of trans people in your community?

LGBTQ client and what that was like? Did you recognize any assumptions or attitudes that got in the way of providing non-judgmental care?

Reflect whether you regularly use inclusive language when taking a history from a new client. Do you ask if the client has a partner and if that partner is a man, woman, or other gender? Most heterosexual clients will readily tell you that their partner is a man (or woman), and even if LGBTQ clients do not disclose to you at that point, or say they are not partnered at the present time, you have shown by your choice of language that you know that more than just heterosexual relationships exist. This may allow the LGBTQ client to be more open at this or a future appointment. If a client does identify as being lesbian, gay, bisexual, or transgender, do not ignore the comment, but rather thank them for sharing the information and indicate how knowing this can be important to providing the right care. Another way of dealing with this question is to ask whether the client is sexually active, and if so, whether their partners are men, women, trans, or some combination. This removes the assumption that sex is only something that happens in the context of a relationship and also shows you recognize the diversity of possibilities in people's relationships. Directly asking if the client is gay, lesbian, or bisexual can be a problem because social stigma or previous negative experiences by healthcare providers may make the client reluctant to disclose. As well, the client may not self-identify by those labels but still be having sexual relations with people of the same gender or more than one gender.

Consider the forms that we ask clients to complete. Is the language contained in these forms inclusive or exclusive? Think about advocating for a change in the options for gender identity, beyond just male and female. Consider whether the section usually marked as "marital status" is really necessary for healthcare, and if so, is it is as appropriate as asking about "relationship status" and having a space for "name of partner" if the answer is yes, rather than the usual "single, married, separated/divorced, or widowed." Since same-gender relationships can also be legal or common-law marriages in Canada, just having a box to check the usual single, married, separated, or widowed options are relevant but it may send the implicit message of heterosexual relationships only.

It is also important to be clear about the level of confidentiality that is possible in the clinical and public health agency charting. As with most people, LGBTQ clients, especially adolescents, are very concerned about this. Though complete confidentiality is an important standard in healthcare and usually a requirement within Canadian privacy laws and provincial health system policies, there are some circumstances where it is not possible, usually related to imminent safety concerns. Clients need to know what information about them may be accessible to others, and when you might be required to break confidentiality (e.g., when a minor discloses abuse or suicidal intent), and to tailor their disclosure and health-related information accordingly.

Think about the educational material you give to clients, and look to see if there are any images of same-gender couples or gender diverse people used as illustrations. The same goes for posters displayed on the walls of clinics and hospitals. These seemingly minor details can speak volumes to LGBTQ clients attending the clinic or hospital about their safety in disclosing sexual orientation. Familiarize yourself with resources in the community that are LGBTQ friendly; know the names and contact information of supportive counsellors and other healthcare providers. Have information on hand to give out to clients, including websites and other resources that provide information for LGBTQ individuals.

# ROLES FOR COMMUNITY HEALTH NURSES IN PROMOTING THE HEALTH OF LGBTQ POPULATIONS

Community health nurses have a vital role to play in both modelling and encouraging respect and support in all aspects of daily life, and especially in the various arenas where they work with members of the community. Nurses who work in schools have a particularly important role to play in affecting the health and physical and mental safety of lesbian, gay, bisexual, or transgender youth. It is vitally important that the needs of this vulnerable and invisible population are identified and addressed, both on an individual and a school-based level. There is much work to be done in sensitizing teachers, coaches, aides, and other youth to the challenges facing these youth every day in our schools and on playgrounds. This needs to occur within the context of the community's cultural and religious affiliations. Where cultural norms or religious beliefs have problems with sexual minority orientations, there may be resistance, misinformation, or heightened concern about creating safer, more supportive environments. There may be significant challenges for the individual who wants to come out but also wants to maintain ties with family and members of the community.

Though it is important to consider our own attitudes, values, beliefs, and practices, it is also important to challenge these same attitudes and actions among fellow students, coworkers, and colleagues. While you may be LGBTQ positive, other people you encounter in class, in clinics, and in the community may not be, and in their opportunities to interact with LGBTQ clients they may potentially cause harm through their words or actions. Including fellow students in an exploration of attitudes, knowledge, values, and beliefs will give you a good idea of how easy or difficult it may be to change homophobic or heterosexist attitudes and practices.

Community health nursing interventions for working with LGBTQ people do not end with advocacy to reduce stigma and foster respect. Since many of their health issues are also those of the general population, nurses will also use primary prevention approaches, secondary prevention (e.g., screening), and tertiary prevention interventions to help reduce health inequities in this group. The interventions may need to be adapted to be appropriate to the unique perspectives of LGBTQ groups, and to pay attention to culture and gender as well. In designing or adapting health-promotion

## CANADIAN RESEARCH BOX 20.2

**What interventions can school nurses promote to reduce discrimination and suicide attempts among lesbian, gay, and bisexual adolescents?**

Saewyc, E., Konishi, C., Rose, H., & Homma, Y. (2014). School-based strategies to reduce suicidal ideation and attempts among lesbian, gay, and bisexual, as well as heterosexual adolescents in western Canada. *International Journal of Child, Youth and Family Studies, 5*(1), 89–112.

This study used data from the B.C. Adolescent Health Survey, a province-wide survey of students in Grades 8–12 that is conducted in classrooms every five years by public health nurses. Information is collected from students and school districts on whether their schools had explicit anti-homophobia policies or gay-straight alliances (GSAs—social justice and social support clubs). More than one in four lesbian, gay, and bisexual students had attempted suicide in the past year, compared to fewer than 5% of heterosexual students. Where GSAs and school policies had been in schools for at least three years, LGB boys and girls had lower odds of sexual-orientation discrimination and suicidal thoughts. Similarly, for girls, suicide attempts were reduced by more than half compared to no GSAs. When there had been a policy in place for at least three years, the odds of overall suicide attempts were more than two-thirds lower than in schools with no policy. Even heterosexual students in schools with GSAs and policies that had been in place for three years or more benefitted; the odds of suicidal thoughts for girls and suicide attempts for boys were cut significantly compared to students in schools without policies or GSAs.

This research suggests that policies and programs take time to have an effect on the entire school environment. However, when programs and policies are put into place to reduce homophobia and foster school belonging, suicidal ideation and attempts are reduced for sexual minority youth. Such initiatives may also benefit heterosexual students. School nurses can use this research to counter concerns from parents and school staff that LGBTQ-friendly policies and programs would harm heterosexual students.

### Discussion Questions

1. Why might policies or programs focused on preventing homophobic bullying and fostering inclusion for LGBTQ students also improve the health of heterosexual students?

2. The schools in this study were public schools in western Canada. Do you think a study like this in Quebec, or Ontario, or Nova Scotia would have similar results? Why or why not?

3. What further questions does this research raise for you? What additional research do you think would be useful to augment this study?

interventions for LGBTQ people, as with all groups, community health nurses should engage with community members regularly and listen closely in order to ensure their views and needs are considered in population health approaches.

Primary prevention interventions around healthy living and stress management are salient for all people. Creating groups or classes for LGBTQ people to learn stress coping techniques, or healthy nutrition and physical activity, could be useful strategies for helping them deal with the distress caused by stigma and discrimination. Primary prevention approaches to prevent health problems might also aim even further upstream, toward preventing harassment and violence, and so focus on the structural environments of laws and policies. Community health nurses can recommend policies in workplaces, schools, and healthcare environments that foster community inclusion and connectedness for LGBTQ people and address bullying or harassment. Primary prevention might also include home visits for lesbian and bisexual first-time mothers as part of a community's maternal home visiting program, or parenting classes for gay and bisexual fathers advertised through the LGBTQ community newspapers and community groups. LGBTQ-inclusive sexual health education among secondary school students, as well as for young adults, may help prevent unintended pregnancy and STIs. (For an example, see the Canadian Research Box 20.2.)

At the secondary prevention level, community health nurses might screen for hypertension among older LGBTQ people at a local LGBTQ community centre, or provide counselling and testing for sexually transmitted infections, including HIV, for men, women, and trans people. Given the concerns about stigmatizing healthcare that transgender people have expressed, they may not get regular screening for health issues. Community health nurses could engage in outreach to the transgender community with information about mammograms and pap smears or testicular and prostate exams, using trans-sensitive language, and offer referrals to trans-friendly service providers. Smoking cessation programs for LGBTQ youth and young adults may help prevent cardiovascular problems or cancers later in life. Screening for family violence or intimate partner violence, for suicidal ideation, or for substance use and abuse can be incorporated into any confidential healthcare interactions, although it would be important to have a list of referrals for LGBTQ-welcoming services for these issues.

Tertiary prevention approaches can include interventions to help HIV-positive LGBTQ people with medication adherence, as well as referrals to appropriate healthcare services to manage the side effects from some HIV medication regimens. Locating LGBTQ-specific substance abuse treatment programs that attend to societal stigma and unaddressed trauma may be needed for effective support. If the community does not have such services, community health nurses may need to advocate for the development of appropriate programs. Many of the tertiary prevention interventions for chronic health conditions—such as supporting effective self-care among people with diabetes, or strategies for managing depression, or exercise programs for people with arthritis or after cardiac bypass surgery—would all be

## CASE STUDY

**Y**ou are a CHN in a child and youth health service, and for part of your time you are assigned as a school nurse in a local high school. During a school health committee meeting (part of your school's comprehensive school health initiative) the vice-principal says he has been approached by some students who want to start a gay-straight alliance. They want to make the school climate safer for LGBTQ students, and they need a staff sponsor for their club. The health committee thinks you would be the best professional to support the GSA, and the principal agrees. However, the committee's parent representative voices a concern about opposition to a GSA from some parents, especially some who believe this would cause distress for heterosexual students. The principal, vice-principal, and other committee members look to you expectantly.

### Discussion Questions

1. What support or assistance might you want to request from the school health committee, or the vice-principal and principal, in taking on this role?

2. What kinds of health information and skills-building support do you think the students who start the GSA will want or need?

3. How would you suggest engaging with parents before a GSA becomes a controversy? Or after there is opposition?

relevant for older members of the LGBTQ community. However, outreach for services may need to take place within LGBTQ venues. By offering services to targeted groups, community health nurses (CHNs) may encourage access to health information and care that otherwise may be missed due to stigma.

Ultimately, the diverse population of LGBTQ people in Canada experiences an array of health inequities that may be addressed with improved outreach and LGBTQ-inclusive approaches. Culturally safe care that respects and acknowledges sexual orientation and gender diversity, and is sensitive to clients' prior experiences of stigma within the healthcare system, can promote the health of LGBTQ people across the lifespan.

## CONCLUSION

This chapter has described some of the challenges and health inequities that lesbian, gay, bisexual, and transgender people face in our society as a whole and in our healthcare systems in particular. The importance of CHNs' consideration of their own attitudes, values, beliefs, and assumptions about LGBTQ clients is highlighted. Examples of community health nursing interventions in terms of primary, secondary, and tertiary prevention are proposed. It is imperative that CHNs engage with LGBTQ populations in a culturally safe way in order to not only reduce inequities in health status but to actively work to promote the health of this population.

## KEY TERMS

biphobia   p. 378
bisexuality   p. 376
cisgender   p. 377
coming out   p. 377
gender diverse   p. 377
gender identity   p. 377
heterosexism   p. 378
heterosexuality   p. 376
homophobia   p. 378
homosexuality   p. 376
internalized homophobia   p. 378
LGBTQ   p. 377
physiological sex   p. 377
queer   p. 376
transgender   p. 377
transphobia   p. 378
Two Spirit   p. 377

## STUDY QUESTIONS

1. How is homophobia, biphobia, or transphobia usually enacted?

2. What are some of the risks of being neutral about homosexuality as a nurse or other healthcare provider?

3. Why is internalized homophobia a threat to general well-being?

4. What are some of the special health inequities experienced by LGBTQ adolescents?

5. When is the time of highest risk of suicide for LGBTQ youth?

6. What are some of the health issues of LGBTQ adults?

7. How can we make healthcare settings safer and more supportive for their gay, lesbian, bisexual, and transgender clients?

8. How can nurses work within their communities to support LGBTQ populations?

9. What can you as a school nurse contribute to the health and well-being of LGBTQ youth?

10. What are issues for LGBTQ youth of colour or of minority social groups?

> After working through these questions, go to the MyNursingLab at www.pearsoned.ca/mynursinglab to check your answers.

## INDIVIDUAL CRITICAL-THINKING EXERCISES

1. What is your belief about sexual orientation? Do you think it is genetic or a learned phenomenon (i.e., nature or nurture)? What factors in your life may have influenced your thinking?

2. A client discloses to you that she is a lesbian. Do you enter this into her chart or tell other members of the health team about this? Why or why not?

3. How would you address a transgender client who has male genitalia but dresses as a woman?

4. What are your feelings regarding caring for a patient with HIV/AIDS? What are your ethical responsibilities regarding caring for such a patient? You may find it helpful to draw upon the CNA Code of Ethics when thinking about these questions.

5. What, if any, ethical issues can arise from refusing to care for a patient with HIV/AIDS?

6. Do you think that LGBTQ people should have access to specialized clinics for their healthcare? Why or why not?

## GROUP CRITICAL-THINKING EXERCISES

1. Identify homophobic, biphobic, transphobic, or heterosexist attitudes that you have witnessed as a student at the university and during your clinical experiences. How did you deal with these?

2. Do you think that a gay, lesbian, bisexual, or transgender nurse should be "out" in the workplace? Why or why not?

3. A client expresses discomfort with being cared for by one of your colleagues who is LGBTQ. How do you think you and/or the clinical setting should respond? Would your response be different if the patient had expressed discomfort with being cared for by a nurse of colour? Or a nurse who is Jewish, Muslim, or Sikh?

## REFERENCES

Balsam, K., Huang, B., Fieland, K., Simoni, J., & Walters, K. (2004). Culture, trauma, and wellness: A comparison of heterosexual and lesbian, gay, bisexual, and two-spirit Native Americans. *Cultural Diversity and Ethnic Minority Psychology, 10*(3), 287–301.

Boehmer, U., & Case, P. (2004). Physicians don't ask, sometimes patients tell: Disclosure of sexual orientation among women with breast carcinoma. *Cancer, 101*(8), 1882–1889.

Brennan, D. J., Ross, L. E., Dobinson, C., Veldhuizen, S., & Steele, L. S. (2010). Men's sexual orientation and health in Canada. *Canadian Journal of Public Health, 101*(3), 255–258.

Brotman, S., Ryan, B., Jalbert, Y., & Rowe, B. (2002). The impact of coming out on health and health care access: The experiences of gay, lesbian, bisexual and two-spirit people. *Journal of Health and Social Policy, 15*(1), 1–29.

Corbett, S. L., Frecker, H. M., Shapiro, H. M., & Yudin, M. H. (2013). Access to fertility services for lesbian women in Canada. *Fertility and Sterility, 100*(4), 1077–1080.

Eliason, M. J. (1997). The prevalence and nature of biphobia in heterosexual undergraduate students. *Archives of Sexual Behavior 26*(3), 317–326.

Frederick, T. J., Ross, L. E., Bruno, T. L., & Erickson, T. G. (2011). Exploring gender and sexual minority status among street-involved youth. *Vulnerable Children and Youth Studies, 6*(2), 166–183.

Friedman, M. S., Marshal, M. P., Guadamuz, T. E., Wei, C., Saewyc, E., Wong, C. F., & Stall, R. (2011). A meta-analysis to examine disparities in childhood sexual abuse, parental physical abuse, and peer victimization among sexual minority and non-sexual minority individuals. *American Journal of Public Health, 101*(81), 1481–1494. doi:10.2105/AJPH.2009.190009

Grossman, A., & D'Augelli, A. (2006). Transgender youth: Invisible and vulnerable. *Journal of Homosexuality, 51*(1), 111–128.

Herek, G. M., Cogan, J. C., Gillis, J. R, & Glunt, E. K. (1998). Correlates of internalized homophobia in a community sample of lesbians and gay men. *Journal of the Gay and Lesbian Medical Association, 2*(1), 17–26.

Igartua, K., Gill, K., & Montoro, R. (2003). Internalized homophobia: A factor in depression, anxiety, and suicide in the gay and lesbian population. *Canadian Journal of Community Mental Health, 22*(2), 15–30.

Meyer, I. (2003). Prejudice, social stress, and mental health in lesbian, gay, and bisexual populations: Conceptual issues and research evidence. *Psychological Bulletin, 129*(5), 674–697.

Mustanski, B. S., Chivers, M. L., & Bailey, J. M. (2002). A critical review of recent biological research on human sexual orientation. *Annual Review of Sex Research, 13,* 89–140.

Norton, J. (1997). "Brain says you're a girl, but I think you're a sissy boy": Cultural origins of transphobia. *Journal of Gay, Lesbian and Bisexual Identity, 2*(2), 139–164.

Oxford English Dictionary, 2nd Edition. (1993). Oxford University Press.

Pan American Health Organization/World Health Organization. (2012). "Cures" for an illness that does not exist. Purported therapies aimed at changing sexual orientation lack medical justification and are ethically unacceptable. Retrieved from http://www.paho.org/hq/index.php?option=com_content&view=article&id=6803&Itemid=1926

Parks, C., Hughes, T., & Matthews, A. (2004). Race/ethnicity and sexual orientation: Intersecting identities. *Cultural Diversity and Ethnic Minority Psychology, 10*(3), 241–254.

Poon, C., Saewyc, E., & Chen, W. (2011). Enacted stigma, problem substance use, and protective factors among Asian sexual minority youth in British Columbia. *Canadian Journal of Community Mental Health, 30*(2), 47–64.

Rotondi Khobzi, N., Bauer, G. R., Travers, R., Travers, A., Scanlon, K., & Kaay, M. (2011a). Depression in male-to-female transgender Ontarians: Results from the Trans PULSE Project. *Canadian Journal of Community Mental Health, 30*(2), 113–133.

Rotondi Khobzi, N., Bauer, G. R., Scanlon, K., Kaay, M., Travers, R., & Travers, A. (2011b). Prevalence of and risk and protective factors for depression in female-to-male transgender Ontarians: Trans PULSE Project. *Canadian Journal of Community Mental Health, 30*(2), 135–155.

Ryan, C., Huebner, D., Diaz, R. M., & Sanchez, J. (2009). Family rejection as a predictor of negative health outcomes in white and Latino lesbian, gay, and bisexual young adults. *Pediatrics, 123*(1), 346–352.

Ryan, C., Russell, S. T., Huebner, D., Diaz, R. M., & Sanchez, J. (2010). Family acceptance in adolescence and the health of young adults. *Journal of Child and Adolescent Psychiatric Nursing, 23*(4), 205–213. doi:10.1111/j.1744-6171.2010.00246.x

Saewyc, E. M. (2011). Research on adolescent sexual orientation: Development, health disparities, stigma and resilience. *Journal of Research on Adolescence, 21*(1), 256–272.

Saewyc, E., Homma, Y., Hitchcock, C., & Prior, J. (2012). Sexual orientation, stigma, and menarche among adolescent girls in Canada. *Journal of Adolescent Health, 50*(2), S28.

Saewyc, E. M., Poon, C., Homma, Y., & Skay, C. L. (2008). Stigma management? The links between enacted stigma and teen pregnancy trends among gay, lesbian and bisexual students in British Columbia. *Canadian Journal of Human Sexuality, 17*(3), 123–131. PMC2655734

Saewyc, E., Poon, C., Wang, N., Homma, Y., Smith, A., & the McCreary Centre Society. (2007). *Not yet equal: The health of lesbian, gay, & bisexual youth in BC.* Vancouver, BC: McCreary Centre Society. Retrieved from www.mcs.bc.ca

Saewyc, E., Richens, K., Skay, C. L., Reis, E., Poon, C., & Murphy, A. (2006). Sexual orientation, sexual abuse, and HIV-risk behaviours among adolescents in the Pacific Northwest. *American Journal of Public Health, 96*(6), 1104–1110. doi:10.2105/AJPH.2005.065870

Schilt, K., & Westbrook, L. (2009). Doing gender, doing heteronormativity: "Gender normals," transgender people, and the social maintenance of heterosexuality. *Gender & Society, 23,* 440–464.

Statistics Canada. (2011). *Gay pride by the numbers.* Ottawa, ON: Author. Retrieved from http://www42.statcan.gc.ca/smr08/2011/smr08_158_2011-eng.htm

Steele, L. S., Ross, L. E., Dobinson, C., Veldhuizen, S., & Tinmouth, J. M. (2009). Women's sexual orientation and health: Results from a Canadian population-based study. *Women & Health, 49*(5), 353–367. doi:10.1080/03630240903238685

Taylor, C., & Peter, T. (2011). "We are not aliens, we're people, and we have rights." Canadian human rights discourse and high school climate for LGBTQ students. *Canadian Review of Sociology, 48*(3), 275–312.

Travers, R., Newton, H., & Munro, L. (2011). "Because it was expected": Heterosexism as a determinant of adolescent pregnancy among sexually diverse youth. *Canadian Journal of Community Mental Health, 30*(2), 65–79.

Veenstra, G. (2011). Race, gender, class, and sexual orientation: Intersecting axes of inequality and self-rated health in Canada. *International Journal of Health Equity, 10*(3), 1–11. doi:10.1186/1475-9276-10-3

Williams-Barnard, C., Mendoza, D., & Shippee-Rice, R. (2001). The lived experience of college student lesbians' encounters with health care providers. *Journal of Holistic Nursing, 19*(2), 127–142.

## ABOUT THE AUTHOR

**Elizabeth M. Saewyc**, RN, PhD, PHN(Minn.), FSAHM, FCAHS, is a Professor of nursing and adolescent medicine at the University of British Columbia, Vancouver, Canada. She held a Canadian Institutes of Health Research/Public Health Agency of Canada national Chair in Applied Public Health Research, focused on youth health. She has worked as a public health nurse in both the United States (in Seattle and Minnesota) and Canada, and has taught community health nursing for more than 15 years. She heads the Stigma and Resilience among Vulnerable Youth Centre at the UBC School of Nursing. Dr. Saewyc conducts research about the health issues of vulnerable populations, including gay, lesbian, bisexual, and transgender youth, and she has been consulted about school nursing and public health nursing roles provincially, nationally, and internationally, including most recently with the World Health Organization.

# Older Adult Health

*Suzanne Dupuis-Blanchard*

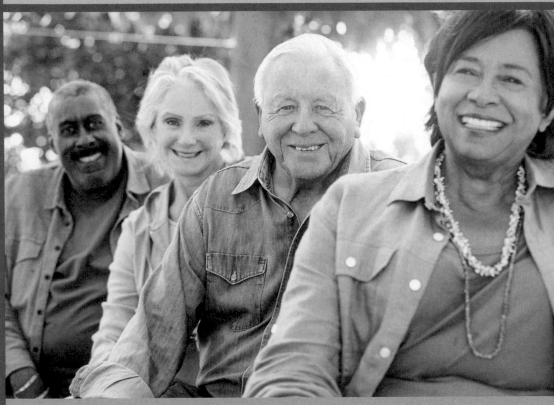

*Source: Monkey Business Images/Shutterstock*

## INTRODUCTION

Community health nurses (CHNs) interact with older adults in various community settings; this includes at-home visits, outpatient clinics, health fairs, and seniors' centres. As many of these older adults seek health information to make informed decisions about their health, CHNs use various opportunities for health promotion and disease-prevention information dissemination. It is never too late to strive toward disease prevention or to promote healthy lifestyles among older adults. This chapter will examine demographic trends, present key health-promotion and disease-prevention needs for older adults, and describe the role of CHNs and their challenges when working with this population group. In this chapter, the terms "seniors" and "older adults" will be used interchangeably.

## PORTRAIT OF SENIORS

As a result of longer life expectancy and lower fertility rates, population aging is a global trend, as reported by the World Health Organization (WHO) (World Health Organization, 2013). It is estimated that by the year 2015, 22% of the world population will be over the

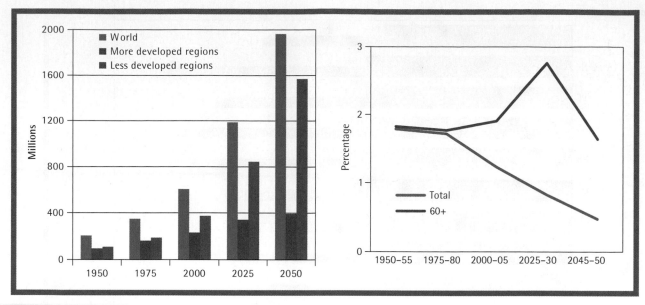

**FIGURE 21.1** World Aging Population

*Source:* United Nations. (2002). *World population ageing 1950–2050.* New York, NY: Author. Copyright © 2001 by United Nations. Used by permission of United Nations. Retrieved from http://globalag.igc.org/ruralaging/world/ageingo.htm

age of 60 years. More people will live well into their 80s and 90s, and countries such as Brazil and China will experience the most rapid demographic change (Figure 21.1). Although many older adults have at least one chronic disease, many rate their own health as good or excellent (WHO, 2013). Worldwide, even in poorer countries, many seniors die prematurely of cardiovascular disease, cancer, and diabetes. Health promotion, disease prevention, and early detection are key public health interventions in order for older adults to remain independent and in good health.

The first cohort of **baby boomers**, those individuals born between 1945 and 1965, entered the senior years in 2011. Typically, **seniors** or **older adults** are defined as those aged 65 years and older; however, many community agencies consider 55 years and older as defining the senior years. It is estimated that by the year 2036, 10.4 million Canadians will be over the age of 65; one in four citizens will be a senior, and older adults will outnumber youths in Canada (Statistics Canada, 2013, 2014). As shown in Figure 21.2, the provinces of New Brunswick and Nova Scotia have the highest percentage of seniors at 18.3% of the population compared to 11.4% in Alberta. In general, the Maritime provinces have a more rapidly aging population than the rest of Canada (Statistics Canada, 2014).

## SOCIETAL ATTITUDE ON AGING

Canadian society has embraced positive and active aging in the last few years; and positive aging movements have become prominent in our society as means of primary prevention toward ageism (see "Seniors are Cool" video, www.gov.mb.ca/shas/seniors_are_cool/seniors_are_cool.html). There are many aspects to active and positive aging, such as self-determination,

actively contributing to the community, good physical and mental health, supportive social relationships, and financial security (National Seniors Council, 2011). For older adults, an active lifestyle will contribute to prolonged independence, prevention of disease, promotion of health, and delay of memory loss.

Although older adults make significant contributions to our communities, negative attitudes toward older adults still prevail in society. Often referred to as **ageism**, it is based on the assumption that everyone is young, therefore stereotyping those that are dependent, frail, and older (Ontario Human Rights Commission, 2013). This results in a societal belief that older adults are a burden to society, especially on healthcare resources. Although spending per capita on seniors is more than that of non-senior adults, the rate of spending growth for seniors has actually decreased over the past 10 years (Canadian Institute of Health Information, 2011a). In reality, other factors such as technology, medical tests, and medication contribute to the high cost of healthcare in Canada (Canadian Foundation for Healthcare Improvement, 2011) and population aging does not hold sole responsibility.

Disappointingly, negative attitudes toward older adults are not limited to the general population. Studies conducted with physicians and nurses reveal that working with older adults is not often a domain of interest based on the misconception that their conditions are untreatable, therefore influencing quality of care (Eymard & Douglas, 2012; Meisner, 2011). Some nursing students also believe that they will lose their technical skills, assuming that care for older adults is uncomplicated and unspecialized and that geriatrics is for nurses who are toward the end of their career (Gould, MacLennan, & Dupuis-Blanchard, 2012; Holroyd, Dahlke, Fehr, Jung, & Hunter, 2009; Liu, Norman, & While, 2013).

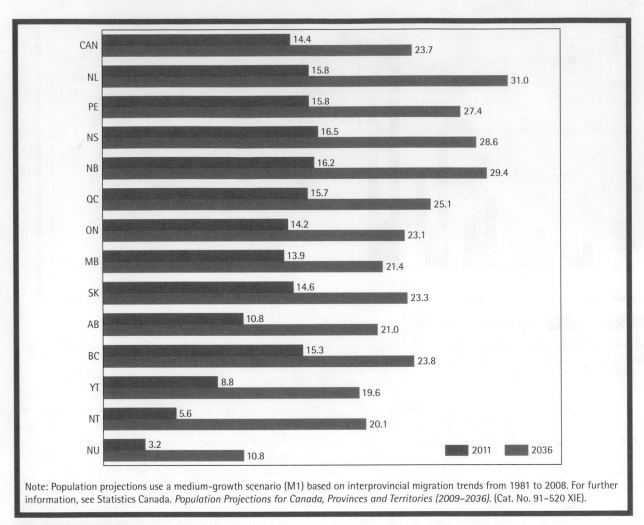

Note: Population projections use a medium-growth scenario (M1) based on interprovincial migration trends from 1981 to 2008. For further information, see Statistics Canada. *Population Projections for Canada, Provinces and Territories (2009–2036).* (Cat. No. 91–520 XIE).

**FIGURE 21.2** Population Aging by Canadian Provinces

*Source:* Statistics Canada. (2013). *Canadians in context—Population aging.* Ottawa, ON: Author. Retrieved from http://www4. hrsdc.gc.ca/.3ndic.1t.4r@-eng.jsp?iid=33

# COMMUNITY GERONTOLOGICAL PRACTICE

Gerontological nursing is a complex specialty of nursing care. Nurses working with older adults must have advanced knowledge of how chronic illness and acute conditions affect the everyday lives of older adults and their families. CHNs working with older adults in the community setting must value the *competencies* required for practice but also embrace the different approaches congruent with community and population health approaches. Older adults have a right to dignity and privacy and to make informed choices. Family and friends play a central role, and CHNs must collaborate with them when caring for older adults. The Canadian Gerontological Nursing Association's (CGNA) framework for care of older client states,

> Gerontological nursing is a dynamic interaction between the client and nurse to achieve health and well-being. The client and the nurse both contribute to the interaction. Clients bring their unique experiences, personal knowledge and expertise

about themselves whereas nurses bring their specific body of knowledge of gerontology and geriatrics, their skills and the art and science of nursing. The historical and current social and cultural climates, political influence and values of the community and society also influence the interaction. (CGNA, 2010, p. 7)

Most importantly, CHNs must collaborate with older adults to achieve health goals. Collaboration implies that nurses and seniors work together to realize shared outcomes and that CHNs intervene to empower individuals by acknowledging past experiences, recognizing strengths, respecting limitations, and providing necessary information and education for well-being. Within the context of the social determinants of health, CHNs must address physiological health issues, optimize functional health, respond to communication challenges, address educational needs, support advanced care planning, provide relationship care, advocate for proper care and services, and assess environmental hazards while empowering older adults and their families. A *population health approach* guided by the "Ottawa Charter for Health Promotion" allows CHNs and older adults to focus on broader issues, such as creating supportive environments for vulnerable seniors who may be in need of appropriate housing, building healthy public policy to improve access to appropriate services and care, and developing the personal skills of seniors who may have a low level of education or literacy difficulties.

## DETERMINANTS OF ACTIVE AGING

**Active aging** is a process with a vision to keep older adults healthy, active, and secure (WHO, 2002). It has become an important component for many community organizations because it applies to both the community and the individual. Active aging is not limited to physical activity but includes participation in social, economic, cultural, and civic affairs. Maintaining autonomy and quality of life is essential for active aging.

A number of factors are important for active aging (National Seniors Council, 2011):

■ active participation in all aspects of community life;
■ self-determination;
■ recognition as an active and contributing member of society;
■ a positive outlook about self and the future;
■ good health;
■ mutually supportive social relationships;
■ financial security;
■ safe and supportive community; and
■ availability of services and support.

Active aging can prolong independence, help manage chronic disease, prevent poor health, and slow memory loss, as well as contribute to an extended participation in the labour force. *Older workers* play an important role in the economy through employment and consumption of goods. Finding employment after age 50 can be challenging due to lack of opportunities when competing for jobs with the younger workforce. Low skill levels, lack of job search skills, low self-esteem or self-confidence, inability to relocate due to family responsibilities, and age discrimination also are challenges (National Seniors Council, 2013). Seniors also make significant contributions to society through volunteer work and support for family and friends. The notions of active aging are consistent with the concept of age-friendly communities.

## AGE-FRIENDLY COMMUNITIES

In 2006, the WHO launched a project with interested cities around the world who were concerned with supporting healthy aging. An **age-friendly community** recognizes that seniors have skills and abilities, respects the decisions and lifestyle choices of seniors, protects those that are most vulnerable, and recognizes the importance of including seniors in all aspects of community life (WHO, 2007). A total of four

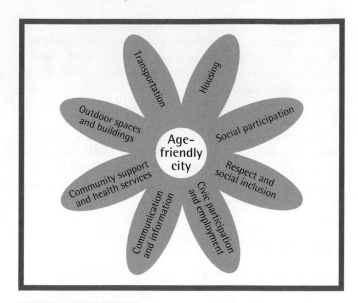

**FIGURE 21.3** Eight Domains of Age-Friendly Communities

*Source:* World Health Organization. (2007). *Global age-friendly cities: A guide.* Geneva, CH: Author. Reprinted with permission of World Health Organization. Retrieved from http://www.who.int/ageing/age_friendly_cities_guide/en/index.html

Canadian cities took part in the Global Age-Friendly Cities Project that gathered information to help identify eight key domains of community life important to an aging population (Figure 21.3).

Many Canadian communities in urban and rural settings realize the importance of policies, services, and structures that relate to the eight domains of age-friendly communities. These communities recognize the important contribution seniors make and understand that needs change with age. CHNs can collaborate with municipalities and seniors' groups to ensure that communities in which older adults reside are age friendly and conducive to well-being.

Age-friendly communities facilitate **aging-in-place** for older adults by providing an environment that supports seniors' independence and optimal health or quality of life. Only 8% of older adults live in institutions; therefore, the majority of seniors reside in the community (Statistics Canada, 2012). To remain independent, some older adults seek home care and home services. For many, home maintenance services are their greatest needs and include help with household chores such as cleaning, mowing the lawn, snow shovelling, filling out forms, and providing transportation (Dupuis-Blanchard, Simard, Gould, & Villalon, 2013). Although many seniors will not ask for help, when offered it they are more than likely to accept. CHNs need to inform older adults of services available to help them remain independent and aging at home. CHNs must assess reasons for refusing services as well as evaluate the specific individual needs of seniors.

*Transportation* is one of older adults' greatest community-based needs. In both rural and urban communities, seniors who want to remain in their home and be active in their community need a mode of transportation to access various services and activities. Many seniors are able to drive for many years after retirement; it is their health limitations and not advanced age that increase the risk of motor vehicle accidents (Turcotte, 2012). Seniors who do not drive can use alternative methods of transportation such as public transportation, family members or friends, and neighbours. To promote well-being and independence and prevent social isolation, CHNs must assess transportation needs and assist seniors who have difficulties accessing transportation as this can have an impact on seniors' lives, for errands such as grocery shopping, attending social functions, and visits to the doctor or hospital.

## POPULATION GROUPS

Although aging is often discussed as a global occurrence for those over the age of 65 years, older adults are not a homogenous group but individuals with different experiences. CHNs must respect individuality by considering the defining factors of culture and the wide range of experiences and care contexts in which seniors and CHNs interact.

## Official Language Minority

French-speaking seniors living outside of the province of Quebec and English-speaking older adults residing in Quebec are considered citizens living in "official language minority communities." Living in these communities implies that many seniors experience difficulties accessing services and support services in their own language, thereby augmenting the risk of social isolation (Dupuis-Blanchard et al., 2013; Office of the Commissioner of Official Languages, 2013). As a result, older adults may forgo home services and health consultations and wait too long to access services. Health coordinators and CHNs need to recognize the importance of language for seniors' health. Seniors fear not being able to express themselves correctly during times of healthcare needs, especially when they are faced with language and cultural barriers. (See Chapter 9.)

## Rural

Twenty-two percent of Canadian seniors reside in rural communities. **Rural aging** is complex and sometimes challenging; it is "an area of scholarship focusing on issues affecting quality of life for older persons living in areas of low population density" (Ritzer, 2007). Older adults living in rural areas often have less education and fewer financial resources, and habits such as smoking and obesity result in higher rates of mortality (DesMeules, Luo, Wang, & Pong, 2007). An advantage of living in rural communities is the sense of belonging, which has a direct influence on health; however, difficulties accessing health services, dependency on family members for help, isolation, and the lack of public transportation are important challenges that impact health promotion, illness prevention, and medical consultations.

## Aboriginal

Statistics Canada (2013) notes that the Aboriginal population is younger than the rest of the Canadian population, but First Nations seniors face more challenges staying healthy and Aboriginal life expectancy is 10 years less than that of the rest of the population. First Nations, Inuit, and Métis seniors live on lower incomes, in less-than-adequate housing, and in poorer health with multiple chronic conditions and disabilities than their non-Aboriginal counterparts (Health Council of Canada, 2013). Figure 21.4 provides an overview of innovative practices in Aboriginal seniors' healthcare although few initiatives are developed specifically for the Aboriginal population. Obesity, diabetes, and heart disease are prevalent, as are mental health issues. Chronic conditions are often not detected because of lack of access to healthcare services such as prevention, screening, treatment, and rehabilitation. There is currently a lack of palliative care and rehabilitation services in Aboriginal communities (Beatty & Berdhal, 2011). (See Chapter 22.)

## Immigrants

According to Statistics Canada (2010), older immigrants to Canada also face certain challenges related to health. Fifty percent of new immigrant seniors in the years 2001 to 2009 were unable to speak English or French. Often, they have had a different life course, including poor socioeconomic conditions and life histories involving difficulties such as trauma or torture (Durst, 2005; Edmonston, 2013), that differs from older non-immigrants and that can result in poorer health. Some issues are higher rates of hypertension, nutritional deficiencies, and cataracts; however, they may also present with less arthritis and with better psychological health. Although recent immigrant seniors need more help with daily activities of living, they are less likely than non-immigrants to receive home care or home support services. Because immigrant seniors have lower income and education levels, it is likely more difficult for them to access healthcare services. In addition, many immigrant seniors have no private insurance, making it challenging to fill prescriptions for medications and access certain home support services. Accessing income support such as pensions and benefits may also prove challenging for older immigrants. To benefit from Old Age Security, a person must meet the legal status and residency requirements of the federal government, which means that they must be a Canadian citizen and have evidence of living in Canada for at least 10 years. Given the importance of income on health, CHNs need to provide appropriate information on how to apply for income supplements and how to access appropriate healthcare services.

## Older Offender

In Canada, almost one in five federally incarcerated offenders is over the age of 50 years. The aging process is accelerated by 10 years for older offenders in custodial settings, exacerbated by substance abuse, poor diet, and unhealthy lifestyle (Office of the Correctional Investigator, 2013). Issues of concern for older offenders include access to health and social programs, healthcare, the conditions of confinement, and post-release supervision (Correctional Services, 2013). CHNs need to attend to older offenders needs, such as difficulties maintaining everyday routine, palliative care, and being a victim of intimidation by society. The older offender may also present with reduced mobility and chronic conditions such as diabetes, hepatitis, and cardiovascular disease. (See Chapter 26.)

# HEALTH PROMOTION, DISEASE PREVENTION, AND CHRONIC ILLNESS

Healthcare for older adults in the community must be viewed on a continuum of care. At one end, health promotion and prevention are provided to healthy seniors, and at the other end, home care and home support services are available for those still living at home or in assisted living communities. This vision incorporates the principles of primary health care, such as

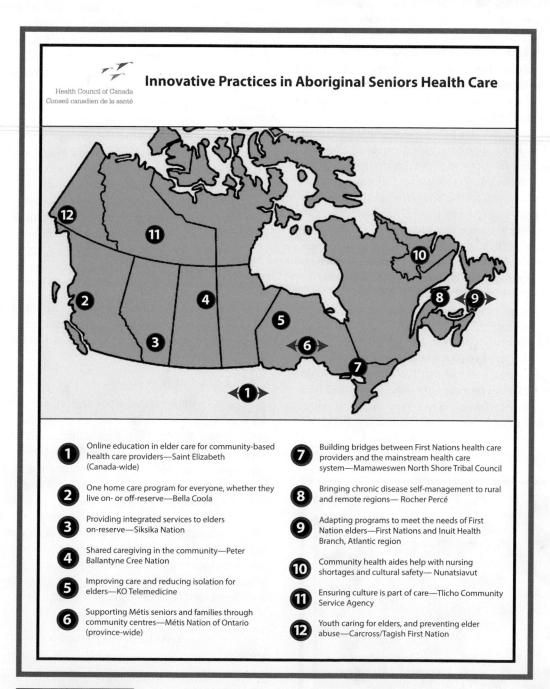

**FIGURE 21.4** Aboriginal Seniors Health

*Source:* Health Council of Canada. *Innovative practices in Aboriginal seniors health care.* Copyright © 2013 by Health Council of Canada. Used by permission of Health Council of Canada. Retrieved from http://www. healthcouncilcanada.ca/content_ab.php?mnu=2&mnu1=48&mnu2=30&mnu3=55

public participation, health promotion, and accessibility, while considering the influences of the social determinants of health.

## Physical Activity and Fall Prevention

Self-reported health in seniors is often based on levels of mobility. **Mobility** is influenced by eyesight, balance, strength, reaction time, coordination, chronic illness such as arthritis, and is reported by 17% of older adults over the age of 65 years (Employment and Social Development Canada, 2013a). Foot problems, difficulty climbing stairs, and having less flexibility can also cause mobility challenges. In fact, mobility is a direct result of being physically active. Very few older Canadians meet the physical activity guidelines of 10 000 steps per day or 150 minutes of activity per week despite the known benefits of reduced risk of illness. Being physically active can also decrease the risk of premature death and help maintain functional independence, bone health, and an overall feeling of well-being. (See Photo 21.1.)

CHNs must promote active aging and physical activity in older adults by providing appropriate information on the benefits of exercise, and facilitate supportive environments to encourage seniors to be physically active. Through understanding and collaboration, CHNs and their aging clients can develop activity goals and identify likeable activities that can be achieved on a weekly basis either alone or in the company of others. Activities such as walking the dog at a moderately brisk pace around the block or following an exercise video on television or computer can be achieved alone. Others may be more motivated to join an exercise group for older adults, a mall walking group, or an afternoon line dancing session at a local seniors' community group, all of which serve as social support for older adults. CHNs must be knowledgeable regarding various community physical activity programs and act as resource persons for older adults. For example, it would be beneficial for CHNs to be aware of when, where, and how to access mall walking programs, classes for dancing, singing, Tai Chi classes, and aqua fitness in the community. In certain situations, CHNs may collaborate with other health professionals, such as physiotherapists, and community organizations, such as municipal offices, to develop supportive environments for active living for older adults.

A major benefit of physical activity in seniors is fall prevention. Falls are the most common injury in older adults, and one in three seniors have one or more falls during a one-year period; these are the cause of high morbidity and mortality rates in older adults (Public Health Agency of Canada, 2014a). The consequences of falls can be devastating to the health and well-being of older adults. Best practices for prevention of falls address falls risk assessment and multi-factorial falls risk management programs. Assessment should include a history of falls, medication, balance and mobility evaluation, and a medical history. Falls prevention programs must include the proper use of assistive devices, clinical disease management, education, environmental modifications, exercise programs, medication review, nutritional assessment, and vision correction. CHNs can educate older adults about the risk factors for falls as part of a physical activity program. Modifiable risk factors for falls include a review of medications, handrails on stairs and grab bars in the washroom, proper lighting, and control of hazards such as unattached carpets and pets. CHNs can perform a home evaluation for falls risk and safety issues, and make recommendations to older adults (Edwards, 2011). Such recommendations can include information on obtaining a personal safety device system that can be used to call for help in an emergency. CHNs must also advocate for accessible and safe housing for older adults (see Case Study).

## Healthy Eating

Although many older adults are aware of Canada's Food Guide, food choices are related to health status and functional ability (Payette & Shatenstein, 2005). Low vision, altered taste, poor

### CASE STUDY

Mrs. Myers lives alone in her apartment. She relocated to this seniors-designated apartment building when her husband died two years ago. Since moving, she has developed good relationships with a few of her neighbours. Three weeks ago, Mrs. Myers fell while going to the bathroom at night. She was able to get up and get back into bed. She did not want to tell anyone but decided to confide in a neighbour, who also revealed that she had fallen many times in her apartment in the last year. Both verbalized to the activity director in their apartment building that they were reluctant to go out and were thinking of not attending group exercises in the social room. The concerned activity director called the local health clinic and a CHN was asked to visit the apartment building.

#### Discussion Questions

1. What are the key issues in this case?
2. What assessments should the CHN complete to address falls in this building?
3. How can the CHN best facilitate tenants' feelings of empowerment?

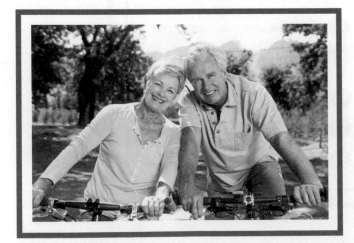

**PHOTO 21.1** Active aging

*Source: Monkey Business/Fotolia*

dentition, widowhood, and loneliness contribute to inappropriate food choices. Although portions may become smaller, vitamins and nutrient intake remain important. During home visits, CHNs must question older adults' nutrition by asking specific questions about what they ate within the last three days, what they will consume during the current day, and what meals may be planned for the coming days. CHNs must discuss with older adults the challenges of healthy eating, such as transportation to the grocery store, financial worries, meal planning, and cooking for one or two people. Information about community resources should be provided to seniors, such as referral to a dietitian if needed, home delivery of meals or groceries, availability of group meals at a local seniors club, locations of food banks, and other community services that can facilitate healthy eating. CHNs can also collaborate with community groups to offer opportunities for group meals or with grocery stores to create awareness around the grocery shopping needs of older adults. An often neglected aspect of seniors' health is oral health, which can alter older adults' food intake. CHNs need to ask questions about dental health, specifically inquiring about the last visit to the dentist, ill-fitting dental prostheses, or tooth sensitivity that can impact proper nutrition (Canadian Dental Association, 2009).

## Medication Compliance

Almost all seniors in institutions and over three-quarters of those living in the community consume at least one type of medication (McPherson, Ji, Hunt, Ranger, & Gula, 2012). In fact, 62% of seniors consume five or more types of medications (Canadian Institute of Health Information, 2010), also known as **polypharmacy**. Polypharmacy increases the risk of medication compliance, and failure to follow the proper medication regimen can result in adverse drug effects, drug interactions, frequent visits to a primary care provider, and hospitalization. During home visits, CHNs need to inquire about the sort of medication being consumed and have a conversation about how the individual is taking the medication. Questions about the time of day a medication is taken, what is done about a missed dose, fear of addiction, adverse effects, and cost can be discussed in a non-threatening manner. CHNs can also organize individual or group sessions to provide information on safe medication use, suggesting blister packs or medication organizers, discussing the importance of discarding unused medications, emphasizing maintenance of an accurate list of medications, and offering referral to the community pharmacist, as needed.

## Immunizations

CHNs advise older adults on the importance of routine immunizations against vaccine-preventable diseases. Many older adults and healthcare professionals neglect the need for immunizations in advanced age. The Public Health Agency of Canada (2014b) recommends that older adults be immunized against diphtheria and tetanus every 10 years, against herpes zoster (shingles) for those over 50 as well as pneumococcal infections once after age 65, and have the influenza vaccination yearly. If older adults travel outside Canada, they may require additional immunizations, such as for hepatitis A and hepatitis B.

## Sexuality

Sexual activity is a normal part of healthy aging; it includes sexual intercourse but also touching, hugging, holding hands, and emotional intimacy. Many older adults say they enjoy sexual activity more than when they were younger because of feelings of closeness, privacy, and less stress in life (Health Canada, 2012).

Common underlying health problems such as diabetes, hypertension, incontinence, arthritis, and the use of certain medications can alter sexual desire and performance. Sexual orientation can also be difficult for seniors to disclose in fear of discrimination (see Chapter 31). Increasing numbers of cases of sexually transmitted infections (STIs) are being reported in older adults (Public Health Agency of Canada, 2014c). Cases of chlamydia and gonorrhea have the highest relative rate increase among women aged 60 years and over. Also, STIs can have long-term impacts while some, like HIV, are becoming chronic conditions. It is important for CHNs to remember that STIs do not respect age and older adults need to be informed about preventing and detecting chlamydia, gonorrhea, HIV, and genital herpes. Seniors often lack information about prevention methods and transmission modes (Canadian AIDS Society, 2013). Although mixed perceptions exist about older adults' sexuality, it is important for CHNs to provide sexual education similar to younger age groups (Ross, Humble, & Blum, 2013) (see Canadian Research Box 21.1).

## Cognitive Decline

Cognitive decline affects individuals differently. There are many reasons for cognitive decline: chronic inflammation (such as in certain forms of arthritis), hormonal imbalance (e.g., thyroid disease), cerebrovascular health, diabetes, obesity, anxiety, stress, delirium, dementia, and depression. It is especially important to differentiate among delirium, dementia, and depression as proper treatment can alleviate cognitive decline. Often referred to as the 3Ds, all three can manifest with cognitive symptoms. In Canada, 10% of older adults in the community have had an episode of delirium. **Delirium** is characterized by a disturbance in consciousness, a change in cognition, or perceptual disturbance with acute onset, while **dementia** has a gradual onset and continuous cognitive decline. **Depression** affects the person's thoughts and emotions and is present in 15–20% of older adults in the community. Thus, recognizing the cause of cognitive impairment is complex.

According to the Alzheimer Society of Canada (2010), our country and the world are facing a dementia epidemic within the next 20 years. In Canada, 15% of older adults have developed Alzheimer's disease. The number of Canadians with Alzheimer's disease or other types of dementia will double, and so will the time to be devoted by caregivers, and the costs attributed to dementia care will reach $153 billion. It is

**CANADIAN RESEARCH BOX 21.1**

**What knowledge do women who are 50 years old and older have in regard to sexuality and HIV/AIDS?**

Ross, P., Humble, A., & Blum, I. (2013). Sexuality and HIV/AIDS: An exploration of older heterosexual women's knowledge level. *Journal of Women & Aging, 25,* 165–182. doi: 10.1080/08952841.2013.760366. Reproduced by permission of Taylor & Francis LLC (http://www.tandfonline.com).

A survey was distributed to heterosexual women 50 years of age and older in the province of Nova Scotia. A total of 202 questionnaires were returned for a return rate of 40%. HIV/AIDS knowledge was measured using the HIV/AIDS Knowledge Scale, a Likert scale survey format. Sexual knowledge was measured with the Aging Sexual Knowledge and Attitudes Scale, comprised of 35 questions answered by Likert scale. Participants were mostly married (71%), Roman Catholic (37%), and retired (58%). Of the respondents, 70% had a current sex partner and only 20% were sexually inactive in the last month. Women had moderate levels of knowledge in regards to general sexual health. The majority knew that prescription medication can alter sex drive and 88% correctly answered that sexual activity is not harmful to health for older adults. HIV/AIDS knowledge scores varied widely. Only one in five participants correctly answered that it is not possible to get the AIDS virus from eating in a restaurant where the cook has AIDS, and half of the participants believed AIDS could be contracted by shaking hands. Overall, participants knew AIDS could be obtained from sexual activity, but they also believed many myths about the disease.

Although the majority had knowledge about sexual health and HIV/AIDS, the study concluded that women have limited understanding of how the aging process affects older adults' sexual health.

### Discussion Questions

1. What implications do the study results have for health promotion education?

2. Describe the best ways to disseminate sexual health information to this population.

3. What additional information could the CHN ask for during a sexual health assessment?

imperative that CHNs be prepared to care for older adults with dementia and provide family members with the information and support needed for care. CHNs should assess older adults for health conditions making them susceptible to increased risks of cognitive decline, and refer them to family health practitioners for testing. Disclosure of diagnosis to friends and family can be difficult, and CHNs should also be aware that seniors experiencing cognitive decline may need to change certain habits, such as driving, and require assistance with medication management, legal affairs, and safety issues. CHNs can also provide prevention information pertaining to cognitive decline, such as proper nutrition (Shatenstein et al., 2012),

physical activity (Bherer, Erickson, & Liu-Ambrose, 2013), and brain exercises (Nagamatsu, Handy, Hsu, Voss, & Liu-Ambrose, 2012).

## Isolation

Social isolation is a significant problem among older adults living in the community and can impact health, quality of life, and well-being. Isolation can lead to depression, loneliness, falls, and hospitalization in about 20% of older adults (Miedema, 2014). The causes of isolation can vary from vision and hearing loss, cognitive impairment, incontinence, to life events such as widowhood (Nicholson, 2012). Despite the negative effects of social isolation on health, few CHNs assess for isolation in seniors. Many instruments exist to evaluate social isolation but CHNs can also ask older adults about visits from friends and family, feelings of loneliness or isolation, and activities outside the home. Assessment and prevention of social isolation should be the goal of the CHN as isolation is often part of a cascade of complex psychosocial factors. Linking older adults to community resources, to local social activities for seniors, and to small regular group meetings with a focus on health education can alleviate feelings of isolation and provide self-confidence to older adults. (See Chapter 23.) Other means by which CHNs can help alleviate isolation in older adults include the use of a computer as a form of social support. In fact, half of all older adults are online (Zickuhr & Madden, 2012) and 43% of social media users are adults over the age of 65 years (Zickuhr, 2014). CHNs may want to assess older adults' interest and ability to join online communities such as social media or specific topic groups, or in emailing friends and family (see Chapter 15).

## Elder Abuse

**Elder abuse** affects up to 10% of older adults in Canada but very few incidents are reported due to fear of retribution (Registered Nurses' Association of Ontario, 2014). Forms of elder abuse can be physical, sexual, financial, emotional, and neglect, which can have an impact on health (Government of Canada, 2013) and quality of life (Registered Nurses' Association of Ontario). CHNs must recognize the signs of abuse, such as changes in behaviour or appearance, depression, physical injuries or deterioration, and changes in financial resources. Abusers often have power or control over the older adult and can be a partner, family member, friend, or care provider. CHNs have a responsibility to report any suspicions or confirmed cases of elder abuse to the local police. High-risk seniors often include frail, isolated, and dependent persons (Perel-Levin, 2008). (See Chapter 28.)

## Emergency Preparedness

Disasters or emergencies can happen any time and seniors who are frail and live alone are especially vulnerable in situations such as the flood in Calgary in June 2014 and the December 2013 ice storms in parts of Toronto and New Brunswick, both of which resulted in power outages for several days. Help may not be available, electricity may be out, and pharmacies, grocery stores, and hospitals may be inaccessible. CHNs have a vital role in the preparedness and planning for emergency situations. Seniors must be educated on how to prepare to stay in their home or how to access shelter or follow evacuation procedures, or how to determine their safety priorities. CHNs should help older adults determine a communication strategy and identify local emergency and evacuation information. It is important for seniors to stock up on bottled water, non-perishable foods, and at least a two-week supply of medications, and to have an emergency kit ready that contains water, blankets, a change of clothes, and cash (Public Safety Canada, 2012). (See Chapter 32.)

## Informal Caregivers

**Caregivers** are people that provide care and support to family members and friends because of age, health dependency, or injury. In 2012, 28% of the Canadian population over the age of 15 years identified themselves as a caregiver (Turcotte, 2013). The majority of caregivers are daughters caring for an older parent for an average of four hours per week while still having children at home and working full time. Thus, 20% of caregivers to older adults identify experiencing financial difficulties as well as feelings of depression. There are benefits to caregiving, including the feeling of satisfaction in making a difference by allowing a loved one to remain as independent as possible. However, there can also be negative consequences and strain in caring for a loved one. CHNs must recognize the impact of caregiving on the caregiver's employment, physical and mental health, reduced time for other activities, feelings of stress and being overwhelmed, as well as sleeping difficulties. Caregivers must receive appropriate support through community services, their employers, and other family members. Caregivers also need information about available financial support, such as the caregiver amount available on the income tax return, and how to navigate the various health and social services in their community. Caregivers play a fundamental role as more and more seniors want to age at home. CHNs need to offer education, information, and resources to support caregivers in providing care for a family member or friend. (See Chapter 25 and Canadian Research Box 21.2.)

## Chronic Illness

For many years, infectious disease was the principal cause of death. At present, chronic diseases such as cardiovascular disease, cancer, respiratory illnesses, and diabetes are prevalent and the primary causes of 60% of mortality. Arthritis affects one in six Canadians, and is the most common chronic disease in Canada (Canadian Institute of Health Information, 2011b). It is also one of the most debilitating conditions due to pain and swelling. CHNs must recognize the impact of chronic illness on older adults, such as loss of independence, disengagement, social isolation, immobility, depression, and poor self-esteem. Furthermore, if more than one chronic condition is present or combined with an acute illness, the older adult may become vulnerable to reduced quality of life. CHNs need to support older adults and their families in

---

### CANADIAN RESEARCH BOX 21.2

**What is the experience of spouse caregivers in early-onset dementia?**

Ducharme, F., Kergoat, M. J., Antoine, P., Pasquier, F., & Coulombe, R. (2013). The unique experience of spouses in early onset dementia. *American Journal of Alzheimer's Disease and Other Dementias, 28*(6), 634–641. doi:10.1177/1533317513494443

Early-onset dementia affects people after age 50 but before 65 years. This qualitative phenomenology study identified the experience of spouse caregivers with a goal of developing professional support for their specified needs. Twelve spouse caregivers, eight women and four men, were recruited via a memory clinic and interviewed individually. Broad, open-ended questions were posed to cover different topics related to the caregiving experience, the first symptoms, the diagnosis, and the difficulties encountered. On average, the spouses were 55 years old and had been caregivers for 6.5 years, providing 102 hours a week of support and care. Findings revealed six themes in relation to caregiver's experience: difficulty managing behavioural and psychological symptoms; a long quest for diagnosis; non-disclosure to others and denial of diagnosis; grief for loss of spouse, married life, and family projects; difficulty juggling unexpected roles and responsibilities; and difficulty planning for the future. Many of these experiences are similar to those of caregivers for older individuals. With the growing number of dementia diagnoses, the role of CHNs in providing support and encouragement is paramount. This study is important as younger seniors are being diagnosed with early-onset dementia.

#### Discussion Questions

1. What implications do the study results have for the health education that a CHN would provide to a caregiver of early-onset dementia?
2. How could a CHN support the caregiver in accepting the diagnosis?
3. Discuss the specific strategies that a CHN would use in such a scenario.

---

finding appropriate care and services in order to restore optimal health. Education about healthy lifestyle such as smoking cessation, increased physical activity, limited alcohol consumption, and improved diet can enhance the quality of life for seniors with one or many chronic conditions. (See Chapter 25.)

## FAVOURABLE CONDITIONS FOR HEALTH AND WELLNESS

The present cohort of older adults and the baby-boomer generation have realized the importance of staying active during advanced age. Therefore, personal habits such as proper nutrition, exercise, and stress reduction are critical to optimal health. In addition to considering healthy lifestyles, CHNs must also consider factors such as income, education, housing, social relationships, and other social determinants of health that have an impact on older adults' health and well-being. Other factors such as empowerment, research, and public policy also influence health and wellness.

## Empowerment

Healthy aging can only be achieved if older adults, their families, the community, CHNs, and other healthcare professionals work in partnership. Shifting the balance of power can empower individuals and communities to take charge and build capacity for an aging population. **Empowerment** is a process by which capacity and competence are built and it is an essential component of health promotion and disease prevention programs. The Community Health Nurses Association of Canada (2008) defined empowerment as "an active involved process where people, groups and communities move towards increased individual and community control, political efficacy, improved quality of community life and social justice" (p. 7).

Older adults need the proper knowledge, skills, and attitude to feel empowered and CHNs play an essential role in providing educational opportunities and leadership. To achieve optimal health, older adults need to be actively involved in all aspects of their lives. CHNs can motivate and support older adults to engage at different levels (individual, small groups, or community) and to contribute to society. To assist seniors in getting involved, CHNs must first understand the needs of this population, then facilitate goal development, identify opportunities for engagement, and provide sufficient information and skills development. This can be achieved in small group sessions where information is provided and participants can share experiences among themselves or at home with family members. CHNs are privileged members of the healthcare team as they get to interact with older adults in different community settings, including where they live and socialize and one-on-one or in groups. Any information provided must be accessible; that is, expressed in simple language and with appropriate adaptations for the visually impaired or those with auditory needs. CHNs must also respect the principles of primary health care when developing or renewing services to older adults. (See Chapter 8.)

## Research

Research on aging issues is vital to older adults' quality of life and wellness. In Canada, there are approximately 15 research centres on aging as well as the national Canadian Institutes of Health Research (CIHR)–Institute of Aging (IA), which sets research priorities on aging (CIHR, 2013). The 2013 to 2018 CIHR–IA's research plan includes cognitive impairments, caregivers' health, end-of-life issues, lifestyle improvement, and social and environmental conditions. Also, the Canadian Longitudinal Study on Aging (CLSA) is currently researching ways to improve the health of aging individuals. The CLSA is a long-term project that will recruit 50 000 participants over a 20-year period and all aspects of aging will be studied. CHNs can actively participate in research by collaborating with research team members, by being identified as an expert, and by disseminating research results with colleagues and clients. The Canadian Gerontological Nurses Association (CGNA) and the Canadian Association on Gerontology (CAG) provide opportunities for disseminating results of recent research and networking with other professionals working with older adults. (See Chapter 10.)

## Public Policy

The Government of Canada (Echenberg, Gauthier, & Leonard, 2011) has identified three *public policy priorities* related to aging: public pensions, healthcare, and caregiving. Other priorities include community planning, such as age-friendly communities; reframing the labour market for an aging workforce; and affordable medications (Elgersma, Simeone, Roy-César, & Theckedath, 2012; Martin-Matthews, Tamblyn, Keefe, & Gillis, 2009). Public policies on aging are essential as they protect and benefit older adults. CHNs must voice their opinions and get involved in public policy development. In fact, the Canadian Public Health Association (CPHA) (2010) identifies policy development as an activity of CHNs for health promotion. (See Chapter 2.)

## ROLE OF THE COMMUNITY HEALTH NURSE

Community health nurses collaborate with older adults and communities toward optimal health and well-being by integrating complex knowledge sources such as the social determinants of health, the Population Health Promotion Model, the Canadian Community Health Nursing Standards of Practice, and the principles of primary health care as well as knowledge-based practice (see Chapters 3 and 7). Such practice is defined as specialized with a focus on promoting population and community health. CHNs may provide home visits with older clients, support family members, or focus on a community's health. Regardless of the clientele, CHNs aim to promote health and prevent illness as well as protect and restore health.

A wide range of social and personal factors determine seniors' health, and CHNs need to pay special attention to the influence of the social determinants of health. Income, education, social support networks, and social and physical environments are identified as determinants of healthy aging (British Columbia Ministry of Health, 2005). The population health-promotion model can guide CHNs' strategies for healthy aging by focusing on educational programs for health promotion and disease prevention, personal skills development, and working with government collaborators to develop or strengthen healthy public policy for seniors. Key issues that CHNs can address for an aging population are healthy eating, physical activity, smoking cessation, injury prevention, and social connectedness. And, while addressing these key issues and planning appropriate strategies, CHNs should support the principles of primary health care, especially geographical or financial accessibility, and the active participation of older adults in identifying priorities for health promotion and disease prevention.

CHNs incorporate primary and secondary prevention in their practice and support tertiary prevention mostly through education of individuals and groups. They collaborate with community groups and other health professionals to maximize opportunities for health promotion and disease prevention. Such primary and secondary prevention activities include raising awareness among older adults about the importance of mammography, prostate exams, PAP tests, regular eyesight exams and dental visits, and cardiovascular risks. Tertiary prevention includes disease management to avoid complications from chronic conditions such as arthritis, osteoporosis, diabetes, and vascular disease. CHNs are often the first line of contact for seniors and their families, and they are well positioned to mobilize resources and the community (College and Association of Registered Nurses of Alberta, 2011) by identifying the strengths of individual seniors, groups, or communities.

## FUTURE CHALLENGES AND OPPORTUNITIES

Population aging creates many challenges and opportunities. The organization of the healthcare system is a significant challenge for an aging population as it remains uncoordinated and in silos among acute, chronic, long term, and home care (International Federation on Ageing, 2012). In Canada, home care is absent from the Canada Health Act; therefore, provinces and territories have the responsibility of allocating resources to this sector, resulting in different types of home care programs across the country.

The rise in chronic illnesses combined with acute conditions creates situations of complex care. Seniors living in the community need CHNs who are well trained and informed in gerontological nursing care and the availability of local community resources. As a significant number of older adults with dementia age at home, many of them will be vulnerable to isolation and abuse. CHNs must collaborate with community organizations to help develop or improve existing services for older adults to include social care and prevention of abuse. For many seniors, staying in the community is possible because of the support they receive from family members. Support to caregivers is essential, and although a six-week leave program is available with the Employment Insurance Compassionate Care Benefits, more strategies are needed to assist families. Other important challenges to seniors' health include falls prevention, emergency response and preparedness, housing, and older workers (Employment and Social Development Canada, 2013b). These situations will necessitate multifaceted coordination between health professionals, service providers, family, friends, neighbours, and the community.

Health-conscious baby boomers will seek health-promotion and disease-prevention programs in the community, and CHNs will have a central role in assessing seniors' needs and developing interventions. Aging-in-place is likely to remain popular but

may necessitate a shift to include other types of housing, such as apartment living in a senior-designated building. CHNs will be involved in transitional psychosocial care, an issue which, at present, is believed to be part of the normal aging process. Communities will also have important responsibilities in leading positive change for an aging population. Home care and long-term care facilities will also need to open their doors to cater to seniors aging at home through program and service offerings.

## CONCLUSION

This chapter presented the health promotion and disease prevention needs of older adults in Canada while addressing the roles of CHNs. Population aging will force the healthcare system to transition from institutional care to community care, and CHNs need to be knowledgeable of seniors' health needs. Older adults contribute greatly to society and CHNs must seize opportunities in which seniors and the community can collaborate for health-promotion and disease-prevention programming.

## KEY TERMS

active aging   p. 389
age-friendly community   p. 389
ageism   p. 387
aging-in-place   p. 389
baby boomers   p. 387
caregivers   p. 395
delirium   p. 393
dementia   p. 393
depression   p. 393
elder abuse   p. 397
empowerment   p. 396
mobility   p. 392
older adults   p. 387
polypharmacy   p. 393
rural aging   p. 390
seniors   p. 387

## STUDY QUESTIONS

1. Describe socio-demographic trends in Canada and the world related to aging.

2. Explain the components of age-friendly communities.

3. Name the challenges faced by the different population groups featured in this chapter.

4. Describe the importance of mobility and physical activity for older adults.

5. Outline the health-promotion and illness-prevention roles of the CHN.

6. List three future challenges or opportunities related to population aging.

After working through these questions, go to the MyNursingLab at www.pearsoned.ca/mynursinglab to check your answers.

# INDIVIDUAL CRITICAL-THINKING EXERCISES

1. Arrange a visit with an older adult and have a conversation about the healthcare system of the past and how the system has changed with the years. Does the person have any advice for you as a future nurse?

2. In your surroundings, observe how older adults are portrayed. Is ageism present? How? Why?

3. You are an older adult seeking information on exercise (general information and locating an exercise group). What process is involved in finding this information and how long did it take to find an exercise group?

4. In your community, investigate the availability and cost of transportation for seniors who rely on public transportation. Verify schedules and calculate a minimum of two outings per week, one to the grocery store and the other to a community centre, for one month. Are there direct routes from your home to these locations? How long will the bus trip last? Is the bus stop close? How much will it cost?

5. Visit the Alzheimer's Society of Canada website (www .alzheimer.ca/en) and identify what information would be useful to a CHN preparing to meet with a group of caregivers. Did you find all the information that you wanted? Would a caregiver be satisfied with the content of the website? What would you modify?

# GROUP CRITICAL-THINKING EXERCISES

1. With other students, discuss your findings from the Individual Critical-Thinking Exercises.

2. Find out about your province's policy regarding older drivers. Discuss if the policy is appropriate and how it is enforced. What are the implications of losing one's driver's licence?

3. Call a public health office or home care agency in your community and ask to speak with a CHN who works with older adults. Plan to meet in person or talk on the telephone to discuss the following questions: How are health promotion and illness prevention integrated in the CHN's daily actions with older clients? How does the CHN describe her roles? What is the most important health issue for older adults as described by the CHN? Explain. After the meeting, as a group, discuss the CHN's answers. Are they what you expected? Why or why not?

# REFERENCES

Alzheimer Society of Canada. (2010). *Rising tide: The impact of dementia on Canadian society.* Toronto, ON: Author. Retrieved from http://www.alzheimer.ca/~/media/Files/national/Advocacy/ASC_Rising_Tide_Full_Report_e.ashx

Beatty, B. B., & Berdahl, L. (2011). Health care and Aboriginal seniors in urban Canada: Helping a neglected class. *The International Indigenous Policy Journal, 2*(1), 1–18.

Bherer, L., Erickson, K. I., & Liu-Ambrose, T. (2013). A review of the effects of physical activity and exercise on cognitive and brain function in older adults. *Journal of Aging Research*, article ID 657508, 8 pages. Retrieved from http://www.hindawi.com/journals/jar/2013/657508

British Columbia Ministry of Health. (2005). *Healthy aging through healthy living.* Retrieved from http://www.health.gov.bc.ca/library/publications/year/2005/healthy_aging.pdf

Canadian AIDS Society. (2013). *HIV and aging in Canada: Prevention.* Toronto, ON: Author.

Canadian Dental Association. (2009). *Optimal health for frail older adults: Best practices along the continuum of care.* Ottawa, ON: Author. Retrieved from http://www.cda-adc.ca/_files/becoming/practising/best_practices_seniors/optimal_oral_health_older_adults_2009.pdf

Canadian Foundation for Healthcare Improvement. (2011). *Myth busters: The aging population is to blame for uncontrollable healthcare costs.* Retrieved from http://www.cfhi-fcass.ca/sf-docs/default-source/mythbusters/Myth_AgingPopulation_EN_FINAL.pdf?sfvrsn=0

Canadian Gerontological Nursing Association. (2010). *Gerontological nursing competencies and standards of practice 2010.* Vancouver, BC: Author. Used by permission of Canadian Gerontological Nursing Association.

Canadian Institute for Health Information. (2010). *Drug use among seniors on public drug programs in Canada.* Ottawa, ON: Author. Retrieved from https://secure.cihi.ca/free_products/drug_use_in_seniors_2002–2008_e.pdf

Canadian Institute for Health Information. (2011a). *Health care in Canada: A focus on seniors and aging.* Ottawa, ON: Author. Retrieved from https://secure.cihi.ca/free_products/HCIC_2011_seniors_report_en.pdf

Canadian Institute for Health Information. (2011b). *Seniors and the health care system: What is the impact of multiple chronic conditions?* Ottawa, ON: Author. Retrieved from https://secure.cihi.ca/free_products/air-chronic_disease_aib_en.pdf

Canadian Institute of Health Research. (2013). *IA Strategic plan 2013–2018: Living longer, living better.* Retrieved from http://www.cihr-irsc.gc.ca/e/47179.html

Canadian Public Health Association. (2010). *Public health–community health nursing practice in Canada: Roles and activities.* Ottawa, ON: Author. Retrieved from http://www.cpha.ca/uploads/pubs/3-1bk04214.pdf

College and Association of Registered Nurses of Alberta. (2011). *Seniors and healthy aging: A position statement.* Edmonton, AB: Author. Retrieved from http://www.nurses.ab.ca/content/dam/carna/pdfs/DocumentList/PositionStatements/SeniorsHealthyAging_Jan2011.pdf

Community Health Nurses Association of Canada. (2008). *Canadian community health nursing: Standards of practice.* St. John's, NL: Author.

Correctional Services. (2013). *Summary of issues and challenges facing older and aging offenders in federal custody.* Ottawa, ON: Government of Canada. Retrieved from http://www.oci-bec.gc.ca/cnt/comm/presentations/presentationsAR-RA0911 Info-eng.aspx

DesMeules, M., Luo, W., Wang, F., & Pong, R. (2007). Lieux ruraux: Disparités de santé. *Bulletin de recherche sur les politiques de santé, 14*, 19–22.

Dupuis-Blanchard, S., Simard, M., Gould, O., & Villalon, L. (2013). La perception des aînés francophones en situation minoritaire face aux défis et aux enjeux liés au maintien à domicile en milieu urbain néo-brunswickois. *Canadian Journal of Public Health, 104*(6), S71–S74.

Durst, D. (2005). Aging amongst immigrants in Canada: Population drift. *Canadian Studies in Population, 32*(2), 257–270.

Echenberg, H., Gauthier, J., & Leonard, A. (2011). *Some public policy implications of an aging population.* Ottawa, ON: Parliament of Canada. Retrieved from http://www.parl.gc.ca/content/lop/researchpublications/cei-07-e.htm

Edmonston, R. (2013). Life course perspectives on immigration. *Canadian Studies in Population, 40*(1–2), 1–8.

Edwards, N. (2011). Preventing falls among seniors: The way forward. *Journal of Safety Research, 42,* 537–541.

Elgersma, S., Simeone, T., Roy-César, E., & Theckedath, D. (2012). *Canada's aging population and public policy.* Ottawa, ON: Parliament of Canada. Retrieved from http://www.parl.gc.ca/content/lop/researchpublications/2012-07-e.pdf

Employment and Social Development Canada. (2013a). *Defining seniors with disabilities.* Ottawa, ON: Government of Canada. Retrieved from http://www.esdc.gc.ca/eng/disability/arc/federal_report2011/section1.shtml

Employment and Social Development Canada. (2013b). *Addressing the challenges and opportunities of ageing in Canada.* Ottawa, ON: Government of Canada. Retrieved from http://www.esdc.gc.ca/eng/seniors/reports/aging.shtml

Eymard, A. S., & Douglas, D. H. (2012). Ageism among health care providers and interventions to improve their attitudes toward older adults. *Journal of Gerontological Nursing, 38*(5), 26–35. doi:10.3928/00989134-20120307-09

Gould, O., MacLennan, A., & Dupuis-Blanchard, S. (2012). Career preferences of nursing students. *Canadian Journal on Aging, 31*(4), 471–482. doi:http://dx.doi.org/10.1017/S0714980812000359

Government of Canada. (2013). *Elder abuse: It's time to face the reality.* Ottawa, ON: Author. Retrieved from http://www.seniors.gc.ca/eng/pie/eaa/elderabuse.shtml#b

Health Canada. (2012). *Seniors and aging – sexual activity.* Ottawa, ON: Government of Canada.

Health Council of Canada. (2013). *Canada's most vulnerable: Improving health care for First Nations, Inuit and Métis seniors.* Ottawa, ON: Author. Retrieved from http://healthcouncilcanada.ca/content_ab.php?mnu=2&mnu1=48&mnu2=30&mnu3=55

Holroyd, A., Dahlke, S., Fehr, C., Jung, P., & Hunter, A. (2009). Attitudes toward aging: Implications for a caring profession. *The Journal of Nursing Education, 48*(7), 374–380.

International Federation on Ageing. (2012). *Current and emerging issues facing older Canadians.* Toronto, ON: Author. Retrieved from http://www.ifa-fiv.org/wpcontent/uploads/2012/12/current-and-emerging-issues-facing-older-canadiansfinal-report-30-march-2012.pdf

Liu, Y., Norman, I. J., & While, A. E. (2013). Nurses' attitude towards older people: A systematic review. *International Journal of Nursing Studies, 50*(9), 1271–1282.

Martin-Matthews, A., Tamblyn, R., Keefe, J., & Gillis, M. (2009). Bridging policy and research on aging in Canada: Recognizing an anniversary, realizing an opportunity. *Canadian Journal on Aging, 28*(2), 185–193. doi:10.1017/S0714980809090217

McPherson, M., Ji, H., Hunt, J., Ranger, R., & Gula, C. (2012). Medication use among Canadian seniors.

*Healthcare Quarterly, 15*(4), 15–18. doi:10.12927/hcq.2012.23192

Meisner, B. (2011). Physicians' attitudes toward aging, the aged and the provision of geriatric care: A systematic narrative review. *Critical Public Health, 22*(1), 61–72.

Miedema, D. (2014). Among Canadian seniors, a social isolation epidemic. *eReview, 14*(7), 1–2.

Nagamatsu, L., Handy, T. C., Hsu, L., Voss, M., & Liu-Ambrose, T. (2012). Resistance training promotes cognitive and functional brain plasticity in seniors with probable mild cognitive impairment. *Archives of Internal Medicine, 172*(8), 666–668. doi:10.1001/archinternmed.2012.379

National Seniors Council. (2011). *Report of the National Seniors Council on volunteering among seniors and positive and active aging.* Ottawa, ON: Author. Retrieved from http://www.seniorscouncil.gc.ca/eng/research_publications/volunteering.pdf

National Seniors Council. (2013). *Older workers at risk of withdrawing from the labour force or becoming unemployed: Employers' views on how to retain and attract older workers.* Ottawa, ON: Author. Retrieved from http://www.seniorscouncil.gc.ca/eng/research_publications/older_workers/page0.shtml

Nicholson, N. (2012). A review of social isolation: An important but underassessed condition in older adults. *Journal of Primary Prevention, 33,* 137–152. doi:10.1007/s10935-012-0271-2

Office of the Commissioner of Official Languages. (2013). *Enjoying your senior years in your own language, culture and community.* Ottawa, ON: Minister of PublicWorks and Government Services Canada. Retrieved from http://www.ocol-clo.gc.ca/sites/default/files/stu_etu_112013_e.pdf

Office of the Correctional Investigator. (2013). *Summary of issues and challenges facing older and aging offenders in federal custody.* Ottawa, ON: Government of Canada.

Ontario Human Rights Commission. (2013). *Ageism and age discrimination.* Toronto, ON: Author. Retrieved from http://www.ohrc.on.ca/en/time-action-advancing-human-rights-older-ontarians/ageism

Payette, H., & Shatenstein, B. (2005). Determinants of healthy eating in community dwelling elderly people. *Canadian Journal of Public Health, 96*(3), S2731.

Perel-Levin, S. (2008). *Discussing screening for elder abuse at primary health care levels.* Geneva, CH: WHO. Retrieved from http://whqlibdoc.who.int/publications/2008/9789241594530_eng.pdf

Public Health Agency of Canada. (2014a). *Seniors' falls in Canada: Second report.* Ottawa: ON: Author. Retrieved from http://www.phac-aspc.gc.ca/seniors-aines/publications/public/injury-blessure/seniors_falls-chutes_aines/assets/pdf/seniors_falls-chutes_aines-eng.pdf

Public Health Agency of Canada. (2014b). *Canadian immunization guide.* Ottawa, ON: Author. Retrieved from http://www.phac-aspc.gc.ca/publicat/cig-gci/

Public Health Agency of Canada. (2014c). *Reporting on sexually transmitted infections in Canada: 2011.* Ottawa, ON: Author. Retrieved from http://www.positivelivingbc.org/files/64-02-14-1200-sti-report-2011_en-final.pdf

Public Safety Canada. (2012). *Your emergency preparedness guide.* Ottawa, ON: Author. Retrieved from http://www.getprepared.gc.ca/cnt/rsrcs/pblctns/yprprdnssgd/yprprdnssgd-eng.pdf

Registered Nurses' Association of Ontario. (2014). *Preventing and addressing abuse and neglect in older adults*. Toronto, ON: Author. Retrieved from http://rnao.ca/bpg/guidelines/abuse-and-neglect-older-adults

Ritzer, G. (Ed). (2007). *Blackwell encyclopedia of sociology*. Blackwell Reference Online: Blackwell Publishing Inc. Retrieved from http://www.blackwellreference.com/public/tocnode?id=g9781405124331_yr2012_chunk_g978140512433124_ss1-83

Ross, P., Humble, A. M., & Blum, I. (2013). Sexuality and HIV/AIDS: An exploration of older heterosexual women's knowledge levels. *Journal of Women & Aging, 25*(2), 165–182.

Shatenstein, B., Ferland, G., Belleville, S., Gray-Donald, K., Kergoat, M. J., Morais, J., . . . Greenwood, C. (2012). Diet quality and cognition among older adults from the NuAge study. *Experiential Gerontology, 47*(5), 353–360. doi:10.1016/j.exger.2012.02.002

Statistics Canada. (2010). *A portrait of seniors in Canada: Immigrant seniors*. Ottawa, ON: Author. Retrieved from http://www.statcan.gc.ca/pub/89-519-x/2006001/4122094-eng.htm

Statistics Canada. (2012). *Population and dwelling counts*. Ottawa, ON: Author. Retrieved from https://www12.statcan.gc.ca/census-recensement/2011/dp-pd/hlt-fst/pd-pl/index-eng.cfm

Statistics Canada. (2013). *The Canadian population 2011*. Ottawa, ON: Author. Retrieved from http://www12.statcan.ca/census-recensement/2011/as-sa/98-310-x/98-310-x2011001-eng.cfm

Statistics Canada. (2014). *Canada's population estimates: Age and sex, 2014*. Ottawa, ON: Author. Retrieved from http://www.statcan.gc.ca/daily-quotidien/140926/dq140926b-eng.htm

Turcotte, M. (2012). *Profile of seniors' transportation habits*. Ottawa, ON: Statistics Canada. Retrieved from http://www.statcan.gc.ca/pub/11-008-x/2012001/article/11619-eng.pdf

Turcotte, M. (2013). *Family caregiving: What are the consequences?* Ottawa, ON: Statistics Canada. Retrieved from http://www.statcan.gc.ca/pub/75-006-x/2013001/article/11858-eng.htm

World Health Organization. (2002). *Active ageing: A policy framework*. Geneva, Switzerland: Author. Retrieved from http://whqlibdoc.who.int/hq/2002/WHO_NMH_NPH_02.8.pdf

World Health Organization. (2007). *Global age-friendly cities: A guide*. Geneva, Switzerland: Author. Retrieved from http://www.who.int/ageing/publications/Global_age_friendly_cities_Guide_English.pdf

World Health Organization. (2013). *Ageing*. Geneva, Switzerland: Author. Retrieved from http://www.who.int/topics/ageing/en

Zickuhr, K. (2014). *Older adults and technology*. New York, NY: Pew Research Center.

Zickuhr, K., & Madden, M. (2012). *Older adults and internet use*. Pew Research Centers. Washington, DC: Author. Retrieved from http://www.pewinternet.org/files/oldmedia/Files/Reports/2012/PIP_Older_adults_and_internet_use.pdf

## ABOUT THE AUTHOR

**Suzanne Dupuis-Blanchard**, RN, PhD, is research chair in Population Aging CNFS-Université de Moncton in New Brunswick, Associate Professor at the School of Nursing, and director of the Centre for Aging Research at Université de Moncton. She began her nursing career as a public health nurse in the older adult directorate of the Ottawa-Carleton Health Department, followed by different academic positions. Her program of research focuses on aging-in-place, health resources for aged care, and access to healthcare services of French-speaking older adults living in official language minority communities. She teaches in the undergraduate and graduate nursing programs. Suzanne is the current president of the Canadian Association on Gerontology and is a board member of the Atlantic Institute on Aging. She is past member of the executive for the New Brunswick Gerontological Nursing Association (NBGNA).

# Aboriginal Health

*Rose Alene Roberts*

# CHAPTER 22

*Source: Courtesy of Rose Roberts*

## LEARNING OUTCOMES

**After studying this chapter, you should be able to:**

1. Identify culturally appropriate nursing practice for Aboriginal communities.

2. Describe historical impacts that relate to the current health status of Aboriginal peoples in Canada.

3. Describe Aboriginal peoples' healthcare delivery systems, including funding implications.

4. Identify healthcare issues that are important in Aboriginal communities.

5. Discuss how culture can impact policy on the health of Aboriginal communities.

6. Apply concepts of the medicine wheel in understanding the holistic world views of Aboriginal peoples.

## INTRODUCTION

This chapter provides a general overview of the health status of the Canadian Aboriginal population, with specific focus on the historical, sociocultural, geographic, and economic impacts on health status. Terminology and how one is named are important considerations when it comes to Aboriginal people. The term **Aboriginal** is one that has been created by the federal government as an umbrella term for all First Nations, Métis, and Inuit peoples. Waldram, Herring, and Young (2006) state, "Currently, the Indian, Inuit, and Métis peoples are recognized as 'Aboriginal peoples' under Section 35 of the Constitution, and their 'existing Aboriginal and treaty rights [are] recognized and affirmed.' While the courts and politicians continue to wrangle about the legal implication of this section, clearly the Constitution establishes the Aboriginal peoples as unique, with special status within Canada" (p. 12). As part of the decolonizing process, Indian organizations are more commonly referring to themselves as **First Nations**; the Inuit and Métis have already decolonized their names. First Nations, Métis, and Inuit peoples are often recognized as being **vulnerable populations**, meaning they are more likely than other populations to have adverse health outcomes (Flaskerud & Winslow, 1998). This has occurred not only through colonization, but also by the overwhelming poverty found within many of the communities. Community health nurses (CHNs) need to adapt knowledge and skills to provide meaningful community health nursing care in Aboriginal communities. Nurses who choose to practise in Aboriginal communities must come prepared to deal with complex issues in health and nursing.

In this chapter, the history of Aboriginal people is outlined from **pre-European contact** (prior to exploration and settlement by Europeans) to contemporary times. The historical context is important in order to provide culturally appropriate community healthcare to Aboriginal populations. Healthcare services are delivered to First Nations and Inuit by a distinctly different system, whereas healthcare is delivered to the Métis in typically the same method as to non-Aboriginals. Included is the description of the funding of First Nations and Inuit healthcare systems. Finally, culture, policy, and health issues important to the Aboriginal people of Canada in the modern context are discussed. The CHN can influence changes to improve the health of the descendants of Canada's First Peoples.

# FIRST NATIONS HISTORY

## Pre-European Contact

North America's Aboriginal peoples have maintained that they are the original inhabitants of the Americas. That fact is not questioned; however, the date and path of the arrival of humans on this continent are still being debated (Dickason, 2002a). Most tribes have a version of a creation story of being the original inhabitants of North America. Unearthed artifacts prove that humans arrived and resided in the Americas during the later Ice Ages. The first inhabitants of the Americas arrived with the necessary skills to survive in harsh environments (Ricciuti, 1990). Despite the hardships, cultures developed and adapted to the locale (Ballantine & Ballantine, 1993). However, the lives of Aboriginal people were profoundly altered by colonization. Mann (2005) presents somewhat controversial theories, based on research, of the possibility that the Americas may have been more densely populated as many as 20 or 30 thousand years earlier than history accepts.

Before the arrival of the Europeans on this continent, an estimated 18 million inhabitants and more than 2 200 languages flourished. First Nations peoples of Canada had an oral history (Dickason, 2002a). Aboriginal languages evolved into dialects spoken in different areas of a region, leading to the following linguistic and cultural groupings: Arctic, Western Subarctic, Eastern Subarctic, Northeastern Woodlands, Plains, Plateau, and Northwest Coast (Waldram et al., 2006). These cultures were based on the resources of the area that the people inhabited. For example, the Plains people were hunter-gatherers who provisioned their bands or tribes by hunting and harvesting the fauna and flora of the prairies, including

following the bison herds (Schultz, 1962). The Haudenosaunee (Six Nations) in the Ontario regions grew up to 80% of their food requirements, while the tribes along the Northwest Coast met their needs from the abundance in the oceans (Dickason, 2002a). Thus, cultural and historical diversity of Aboriginal peoples in Canada clearly existed before the arrival of the colonizers.

Childcare and education were the responsibility of the extended family (Sherman, 1996). The adults provided for themselves and the community. Methods of food preservation were devised to store food for less plentiful seasons. Housing materials included animal hides or the trees of the woodlands. Any less fortunate members of the band were provided sustenance by the whole group. Sharing of resources among the group was expected and ensured the survival of the community; for example, among the Northwest Coast tribes, the potlatch was a method of redistributing resources. Transgression by anyone was dealt with according to custom law. The culture of the group included spirituality; one facet involved connection with all living and non-living things—this was a belief shared by most Aboriginal people. Life, if not ideal, was valued, and individuals knew their roles and purpose (Fleet, 1997).

Aboriginal communities had traditional beliefs about health. Shamans and herbalists held the knowledge of curing illness. Mothers or grandmothers practised folk medicine to care for their families, using medicines that were common to their geographical area. The medicine wheel philosophy, which encompassed all nature, was extensively used by numerous tribes, with regional variability.

## European Contact

Initial contact with Europeans was on Canada's east coast and extended into the Hudson Bay area over a significant period of time. Explorers and fur traders from England and France began to explore and harvest the plentiful animals for the fur trade. Missionaries made their way westward to bring Christian doctrine. The newcomers brought diseases such as smallpox, tuberculosis, and measles, which decimated the population by the thousands. For example, Mann (2005) cites research that the initial Aboriginal population's small homogeneous gene pool made them more susceptible to European diseases. Biochemistry research of measles vaccine responses of an Aboriginal group concluded that "virgin-soil Indians" were more susceptible to European diseases, while "virgin-soil Europeans" had acquired immunity. The result was the devastation and fragmenting of Aboriginal cultures. Furthermore, resources that had supplied Aboriginal livelihoods, such as the buffalo and the beaver, became scarce, thus increasing susceptibility to depopulating epidemics.

The establishment of Canada as a country brought settlers from Europe into virtually all areas of the country. The process of establishing colonies and settlements in Canada required treaty negotiations with the original inhabitants and the subsequent establishment of reserves, which created further problems, including malnutrition, starvation, and death. At the time of European contact, Canada was estimated to have 50 to 60 languages. Many of those languages became extinct, and the rest continued to dwindle over time (Waldram et al., 2006), further contributing to the decimation of Aboriginal culture (Chrisjohn, Young, & Maraun, 1994).

## Post-European Contact

Even though there were about 500 distinct tribes in the early 1600s, the land was legally considered empty and therefore claimable (Fleet, 1997). Britain developed the **treaty** method with the Indians to claim land that the Aboriginal people occupied. The **British North America (BNA) Act** of 1867 gave Canada its birth as a country, but the Royal Proclamation specified that only the British government could buy Indian lands or negotiate treaties. In contrast, the Aboriginal people entered the treaties with the understanding that it was land sharing, not land cession (Office of the Treaty Commissioner, 2013). Private individuals or other nations (including Canada) could not go into Indian communities to buy land directly (Dickason, 2002b). The **Indian Act** of 1876 was passed to ensure that the terms of the treaties were observed.

As a result of the treaties, First Nations peoples were relegated to living on **reserves**. Those who came from agrarian cultures had lived their entire lives in villages; however, hunter-gatherers were a nomadic society whose territories were reduced to small plots of land, some as small as a few acres, and in many cases the land was of no economic value. The Indian reserves were governed by the federal government under the Indian Act (Venne, 2002). Individuals called **Indian agents**, hired and paid by the federal government, were assigned to carry out the terms of the Indian Act and often lived on the reserve or in very close proximity. Once accustomed to having freedom, First Nations people found that they now required written permission from the Indian agents to leave the reserve and became dependent on the agents for all aspects of their sustenance. First Nations reserves are located in all of Canada's provinces and territories, with the exception of Nunavut (Aboriginal Affairs and Northern Development Canada, 2013a). Some reserves are adjacent to or located within urban centres. The reserves located in the south are easily accessible. Farther north, most reserves are remote and isolated unless they are located near an urban centre. Most reserves are governed by an elected Chief and council for two- to four-year terms of office. **Aboriginal Affairs and Northern Development Canada (AANDC)** is one of the federal government departments responsible for meeting the Government of Canada's obligations and commitments to First Nations, Inuit, and Métis and for fulfilling the federal government's constitutional responsibilities in the North (Aboriginal Affairs and Northern Development Canada, 2013a).

## The Residential School Legacy

**Residential schools** were first established by the missionaries in the late 1800s in various locations of Canada. The federal government took over the administration of some residential schools as a response to the treaty right to education. Leaders of First Nations communities wanted schools built on the reserves. However, the federal government decided that residential schools would be cheaper; furthermore, a similar system in the United States was showing promise in assimilating the American Indian children into the white society. Approximately 135 residential schools were operated through an agreement between the federal government and the Roman Catholic Church, the Church of England, the Methodist Church, and the Presbyterian Church between 1892 and 1969 (Aboriginal Healing Foundation, 1999). After the withdrawal of the federal government, some residential schools continued to operate into the 1970s, 1980s, and 1990s. The vast majority of residential schools were in the western provinces. The number of children sent to residential schools has been estimated to be more than 150 000, and in 1991 the Assembly of First Nations estimated that approximately 105 000 to 107 000 survivors were still alive; that figure has dropped to about 80 000 today (Legacy of Hope Foundation, 2013). The Métis population was living in very similar conditions to the First Nations at the turn of the century and, despite the federal government's resistance, approximately 9% of residential school students identified themselves as Métis (Aboriginal Healing Foundation, 2006).

The premise of the residential schools was to **assimilate** the children into the general population through a process of education, religious and otherwise, as well as cultural degradation—teaching the children to be ashamed of their heritage in order to facilitate the assimilation process. Parents were legally required to send their children; failure to do so meant incarceration, at which point the children became wards of the state and would be sent to residential schools anyway. Physical, emotional, and sexual abuse were rampant in the schools, and little was done to stop it or to punish the abusers. Living conditions were often far below acceptable levels in modern society's terms. Children often went hungry; children report their parents bringing them food on their weekend visits to supplement their substandard diet (Aboriginal Healing Foundation, 1999). Some children report being forced to steal food from the kitchens. The education they received was also substandard. As late as the 1950s, more than 40% of the teaching staff at the schools had no professional training (Aboriginal Healing Foundation, 1999). Cultural degradation practices included physical and emotional abuse for speaking a traditional language, cutting of hair (hair has strong cultural and spiritual implications), imposing foreign religious practices, and intentional separation from visiting parents. The residential school experiences of Aboriginal peoples continue to have a detrimental impact on Aboriginal communities. Generational and intergenerational issues such as high rates of suicide, addictions, violence, and abuse plague Aboriginal communities. The intergenerational impact of loss of parenting skills has now been felt by three generations and is starting to be felt by a fourth generation.

The **Aboriginal Healing Foundation (AHF)** was established in 1998 as a response to the findings of the 1996 Royal Commission on Aboriginal Peoples regarding residential school survivors (AHF, 2007). The AHF was provided with a one-time $350 million fund to assist communities in healing from the residential school trauma (AHF, 2007). The AHF received an additional $40 million in 2005 and $125 million in 2007 (AHF, 2013). There were 1 345 community-based healing initiatives funded through the AHF that have helped the healing process in some communities. The AHF operated for 11 years until March 31, 2009 (AHF, 2013).

In 2005, the federal government signed the Indian Residential Schools Settlement Agreement, which was intended to acknowledge every survivor's experience. There are three sections of the agreement: Common Experience Payment for every survivor—$10 000 for ever having attended and $3 000 for each year of attendance; an Independent Assessment Process (IAP) for students who suffered sexual abuse, serious physical abuse, and other wrongful acts; and a commemorative section including more funding for the AHF (Aboriginal Affairs and Northern Development Canada, 2013b). Compensation for survivors began following the legal ratification of the agreement on September 17, 2007, until September 19, 2012 (Aboriginal Affairs and Northern Development Canada, 2013b). There were 105 510 applicants under the Common Experience Payment clause, and the average amount paid out was $19 412 for a total payout of $1 613 419 106 (Aboriginal Affairs and Northern Development Canada, 2013b). The Independent Assessment Process (IAP) had the same application deadline of September 19, 2012; each claim required a hearing by an adjudicator (Aboriginal Affairs and Northern Development Canada, 2013c); therefore, the final statistics are not available at the time of writing. The commemorative section of the agreement is being carried out by the federally mandated Truth and Reconciliation Commission of Canada (TRC). The TRC's mandate is to inform all Canadians about what happened in Indian residential schools through documentation of the truth of survivors, families, and communities (Truth and Reconciliation Commission of Canada, 2013). The TRC has a five-year lifespan and committed to national and regional gatherings to collect and document survivors' stories. Over 6200 stories have been collected, mostly through video and audio recordings (Truth and Reconciliation Commission of Canada, 2013). The University of Manitoba has recently been selected by the TRC to house the documentation of the residential school legacy in its newly established National Research Centre on Residential Schools (University of Manitoba, 2013).

## Treaty Status

An understanding of how treaty status is acquired and defined is indispensable to understanding the healthcare of Aboriginal people. The status of being a treaty Indian in Canada is not only acquired by birth but also legislated by the Indian Act. A **registered or status Indian** is recognized under the Indian Act and has a unique registration number called a treaty number. **Non-status Indians** are culturally Indians, but because their tribe did not sign a treaty or their treaty status was lost through the Indian Act policies, they are not recognized as status Indians by the federal government. One of the main goals of the Indian Act was assimilation. There were several ways one could lose treaty status, otherwise known as enfranchisement, such as by entering the armed forces; obtaining a university education; becoming a Christian minister, doctor, or lawyer; gaining access to vote; or, for a woman, marrying a non-status man (Furi & Wherrett, 2003).

Prior to 1985, the definition of an Indian was any male person of Indian blood belonging to a recognized band, any child of such a person, and any woman legally married to such a person (Furi & Wherrett, 2003). There was an amendment to the Indian Act in 1985. Many of the issues relating to loss of treaty status were intended to be resolved through the passing of **Bill C-31**. For example, a status woman who marries a non-status man no longer loses her treaty status and neither do her children. Furthermore, an individual who had lost his or her status could apply for its return. However, the assimilative intent of the Indian Act remains in Bill C-31, because there are limitations on how far treaty status can be passed on generationally. In two generations of intermarriage, whether the non-status spouse is male or female, the children lose their treaty status. There have been several court challenges to this aspect of Bill C-31; however, no definitive changes or decisions have been made since it was enacted in 1985 (Furi & Wherrett, 2003). The **Inuit** are in a separate category, because no treaties were signed in the Far North, but they are treated in the same manner as registered Indians by the federal government (Waldram et al., 2006). The isolation, cold, and inhospitable environment are the likeliest reasons treaties were not signed in the Far North; that is, settlers were unlikely to have wanted the land. The **Métis**, who were the mixed-blood children born of Aboriginal and non-Aboriginal parents, are legally considered the same as non-status Indians. The Métis are considered Aboriginal peoples of Canada under the Constitution and are acquiring rights, such as hunting rights. Métis acquire services through the Office of the Interlocutor at the federal government level.

## CONTEMPORARY ABORIGINALS

A White Paper was written in 1969 (First Nations and Inuit Health Branch, 2007) for the purpose of abolishing the treaties and the Indian Act and disassembling the government departments responsible for reserves and treaty Indians. Generally, a White Paper is a government report on an investigation into a given topic. Often, a White Paper offers recommendations that become policy or law. However, this White Paper never became policy or legislation (Department of Indian and Northern Affairs, 1997) because of an unprecedented show of force and unity among Aboriginal communities. Though the White Paper did not succeed in terminating the First Nations and Inuit relationship with the federal government, its very attempt to do so appears to have created a resurgence in the culture of Canada's Aboriginal people (Schouls, 2002). Today, there is increasing interest in speaking the languages of the remaining 11 language families: Algonquian, Athapaskan,

Eskimo–Aleut, Haida, Tlingit, Siouan, Tsimshian, Wakashan, Salishan, Kutenai, and Iroquoian.

Canada's Aboriginal peoples' rights were given recognition in the Canadian Constitution. Several attempts have been made to define the treaty rights. The federal government attempted to clarify governance issues through its First Nations Governance Act (FNGA). The FNGA would allow effective self-governance for Aboriginal people (Department of Indian and Northern Affairs, 2002). However, once again, Aboriginal communities, political bodies, and community groups acted in unity to prevent this act being passed by parliament into law. Another federal initiative spearheaded by then-Prime Minister Paul Martin was intended to improve the lives of Aboriginal people, with a $5 million dollar budget over a 10-year period (Patterson, 2006). This agreement was signed by the federal government, all provincial and territorial governments, as well as Aboriginal organizations in November 2005. However, due to the change in government, the principles of the agreement were never formally adopted at the federal government level (Patterson, 2006).

## First Nations, Métis, and Inuit Health Disparities

The deplorable health status of First Nations, Métis, and Inuit populations has been a controversial issue within Canadian society for decades. Applying the health determinants to the Aboriginal population shows disparities in virtually all areas. It is often easier to access statistical data on First Nations due to the unique identifying number on their health cards; finding data about Métis and Inuit populations is more difficult. Information presented here is as current and comprehensive as possible; however, the reader is encouraged to keep in mind the limitations inherent in missing or unavailable data.

According to the 2011 National Household Survey, the population of Aboriginal peoples in Canada was 1 400 685 (4.3% of total population) (Employment and Social Development Canada, 2013). First Nations make up 61%, Métis 32%, Inuit 4%, and a category of "multiple & other" Aboriginals make up the remaining 3% (Employment and Social Development Canada, 2013). Aboriginal people are dispersed throughout Canada, with Ontario and the four western provinces having the highest total numbers. The highest proportion to the total population are found in Nunavut (86.3%), Northwest Territories (51.9%), and the Yukon (23.1%) (Employment and Social Development Canada, 2013). There are 614 First Nations communities, otherwise known as reserves, in Canada (Aboriginal Affairs and Northern Development Canada, 2011), and 49.3% of the First Nations population live on these reserves (Statistics Canada, 2013). There are also Métis settlements, and most are found in the western prairie provinces; however, only in Alberta are they recognized as legal land bases (Government of Alberta, 2013). Statistics Canada reports that 25% of the Métis population live in the metropolitan areas of Winnipeg, Edmonton, Vancouver, and Calgary (Statistics Canada, 2013). The majority of the Inuit population continues to live in settlements throughout the Far North, with 73.1% found within Inuit Nunangat (Statistics Canada, 2013). The population of Aboriginal peoples continues to grow (20.1% Aboriginal growth versus 5.2% general population growth), with the highest growth rate found among First Nations people at 22.9% (Employment and Social Development Canada, 2013). A higher fertility rate indicates a younger population; the median age among Aboriginal peoples is 27.7 compared to 40.6 in the non-Aboriginal population (Employment and Social Development Canada, 2013). The youngest age category of 0–14 years has the highest rate among Aboriginal people at 28%, whereas non-Aboriginal people have the highest rate in the 45–54 age group (16.2%) (Employment and Social Development Canada, 2013).

Low socioeconomic status can be found in all Aboriginal populations, regardless of rural, urban, or remote location; the median total income of the Aboriginal population aged 25 to 54 in 2005 was just over $22 000, compared to over $33 000 for the non-Aboriginal population in the same age group (Statistics Canada 2010a), and more than 50% of Aboriginal children live in poverty (Chansonneuve, 2005). Métis have the highest median income at $28 000, followed by Inuit at $25 000, First Nations living off-reserve at $22 500, and First Nations living on-reserve bringing up the rear at $14 000 (Statistics Canada 2010a). To help put these figures into perspective, the low-income cut-off (LICO) for 2010 was $29 623 (Statistics Canada, 2011) (see Chapter 29).

Education, as one of the health determinants, is often seen as a marker for the ability to earn sufficient income. While there continue to be effects of the residential school legacy on education levels, with 33% of the Aboriginal population having less than high school education compared to 13% in the non-Aboriginal population (Statistics Canada, 2010b), there is improvement in other areas. The rate of post-secondary school graduates is estimated at 44%: 14% with trade credentials, 19% with a college diploma, and 8% with a university degree (Statistics Canada, 2008). This is an increase from 38% in 2001 and 33% in 1996 (Statistics Canada, 2008). Looking at the figures from the three categories of Aboriginal peoples, 51% of Inuit aged 25–64 do not have a high school education, however 36% had a post-secondary certificate (Statistics Canada, 2008). Among the Métis, 50% had a post-secondary education, while 26% had a less than high school education level (Statistics Canada, 2008). Within the First Nations populations, 42% indicated post-secondary education as the highest level attained, compared to 38% with less than high school (Statistics Canada, 2008). First Nations communities have been reclaiming their own educational institutions, including curriculum and the training of Aboriginal teachers, and this is becoming evident in the statistics. A teaching degree was the most common university degree obtained by First Nations (27%) and Inuit at 39% (Statistics Canada, 2008).

Employment indicators are closely related to education levels and socioeconomic status; therefore, it is not surprising that employment rates among Aboriginal peoples continue to be below the non-Aboriginal population rates. Overall, the employment rate of Aboriginal people was 65.8% in the

2006 census (First Nations, 60.4%; Métis, 74.5%; Inuit, 61.1%), compared to 81.6% in the non-Aboriginal population (Statistics Canada, 2010c). As previously stated, many reserves are located in remote or rural areas and the job opportunities are often scarce. First Nations living on-reserve have employment rates of 51.8%, slightly lower than for those First Nations who live off-reserve, at 66.3% (Statistics Canada, 2010c). There is improvement in the labour participation rates and the employment rates of Aboriginal peoples; the employment rate gap decreased from 19.1% in 2001 to 15.8% in 2006. The employment gap decrease was seen within the Métis and First Nations populations; however, it remained unchanged between the Inuit and non-Aboriginal population (Statistics Canada, 2010c).

Health determinants cite physical environment as one of the factors that determine the health of individuals in a community. On-reserve housing is often subpar by Canadian standards, and 29% of First Nations 2006 census participants lived in homes that were in need of major repairs, an increase from 26% in 1996 (Statistics Canada, 2010d). First Nations living on-reserve had higher rates, at 45% (Statistics Canada, 2010d). Houses that needed major repairs among those that reported Métis ancestry decreased (17% to 14%), and the highest increase was among Inuit homes (28% from 19%) (Statistics Canada, 2010d). Utilities that are considered essential in urban homes, such as electricity, heating, and indoor plumbing, are not always available to First Nations community homes. Furthermore, urban-dwelling Aboriginal peoples are often found in the poorer areas of town, such as the inner city, which is often rampant with substandard rental housing. First Nations people living off-reserve reported 17% living in houses that needed major repairs (Statistics Canada, 2010d).

Risk factors inherent with unsafe physical environments affect health. This is demonstrated in the high rates of mortality and morbidity from injury and trauma, chronic illness, depression, and family violence (Sebastian, 2000). Illnesses such as TB and respiratory diseases, transmission of which are exacerbated by crowded housing, continue to be a health threat. For example, the rate of TB in the Aboriginal population is six times higher than the non-Aboriginal population, with the highest rate found within the Inuit population at 38 times the national average (Canadian Public Health Agency, 2013). Respiratory diseases among Aboriginal children are among the leading causes of hospitalization and death (Smylie & Adomako, 2009). Burns caused by fires are another area of concern. First Nations and Inuit Health (2009) reports that nearly half of the Aboriginal communities under its jurisdiction lack adequate fire protection services. The nurse must be an advocate for clients and the community to improve housing standards and safety for Aboriginal communities.

Trauma and injury, whether accidental or intentional, are also related to physical environments and are high on the list of health issues besetting Aboriginal populations. Communities that practise a hunting and gathering culture may be prone to injuries related to their particular lifestyle, such as from firearms, boats, ATVs, snowmobiles, or other hunting equipment. Alcohol is often a contributing factor to injuries

and death caused by injuries, both accidental and intentional. (See Chapter 30.)

In the area of personal health practices and coping skills, lifestyle illnesses caused by drug and alcohol abuse, such as organ damage and FASD, continue to be overrepresented among Aboriginal populations. Smoking rates continue to be very high—59% among First Nations living on-reserve and 58% of Inuit in the North. The majority started smoking between the ages of 13 and 16 (Health Canada, 2011). Obesity, which has recently become classified as a disease by the American Medical Association, has higher rates among the Aboriginal population than the non-Aboriginal population. The obesity rates are similar for Inuit, Métis, and off-reserve First Nations populations (23.9%, 26.4%, and 26.1%, respectively) (Canadian Public Health Agency, 2011a). Obesity among children and youth (ages 6–14) is also high, ranging from 16.9% among the Métis, to 20.0% among off-reserve First Nations, to 25.6% among the Inuit (Canadian Public Health Agency, 2011a). Therefore, it is not surprising that diabetes, for which being overweight is a common risk factor, has reached epidemic proportions in Aboriginal communities. First Nations living on-reserve have the highest prevalence of diabetes at 17.2%. First Nations living off-reserve have a prevalence of 10.3%, and Métis are at 7.3%. The prevalence rate for the general population is 5.0% (Canadian Public Health Agency, 2011b). Mortality rates from diabetes for Aboriginal women living in First Nations communities are five times higher than the national average. Diabetes is also being diagnosed at a younger age and with increasing rates among youth and children (Canadian Public Health Agency, 2011b). (See Canadian Research Box 22.1.) Rates of amputation, blindness, and kidney failure are also higher among Aboriginal populations. Nurses must understand the health promotion and health education needed to influence change in the lifestyle of those affected by diabetes (McMurray, 1999). Cancer, which has been relatively uncommon in Aboriginal populations, has steadily been increasing and there are certain issues that are common in relation to cancer screening, diagnosis, and treatment. Screening programs have generally received a low uptake, diagnosis is often at advanced stages, and remote locations hamper cancer treatment, which typically takes place in larger urban centres (Shahid & Thompson, 2009).

Healthy child development is an important health indicator for Aboriginal populations, because the birth rate is almost twice that of the general Canadian population. Furthermore, the overall Aboriginal population is younger, with 28% of the population in the 0–14 years age category, compared to 16.5% for the non-Aboriginal population (Employment and Social Development Canada, 2013). Lack of childcare, lack of food security (see Chapter 29), and low immunization rates for children are serious concerns for Aboriginal communities, both on- and off-reserve.

Aboriginal peoples are moving to urban communities in increasing numbers, often to seek a better life for their children. However, the same problems that plague reserve and remote communities can be apparent for urban dwellers. Those problems present themselves as unemployment, inadequate housing, social exclusion, lack of childcare, food insecurity, lack of transportation, and intermittent access to healthcare.

Even considering all of these issues, it is important to remember that the picture is not all bleak. Aboriginal people are adapting to Western society and are represented in all occupations, including education, health, justice, business, and the trades. Some individuals receive a Western-based education and return to work and live in their communities, while others elect to remain in urban settings. The National Aboriginal Achievement Awards showcase the talent in the Canadian Aboriginal community. It is important to become aware of the positive aspects of being Aboriginal. It counteracts the negative stereotyping of Aboriginal people.

The national profile of First Nations communities and their health status highlights the dire need for change. The relatively new health determinants have emphasized the health needs of the Canadian Aboriginal peoples. Changes have to be made to the social determinants of health, such as income, physical environments, and employment, to overcome the poverty and third-world conditions present in too many First Nations communities.

## First Nations Healthcare

Working with First Nations communities requires knowing the larger healthcare system that enacts the policy which establishes the practice and standards for First Nations healthcare systems. Healthcare provision is considered a treaty right by First Nations and Inuit; however, government policy states that healthcare provided to First Nations is benevolence by the federal government. Deagle (1999) contends that Canada's healthcare system operates under a three-tier system, with the Aboriginal populations in the lowest position. The federal government, through its health minister and department and the **First Nations and Inuit Health Branch (FNIHB)**, provides the health services and support for First Nations and Inuit living on reserves. The FNIHB is based in Ottawa, where policy is planned. The First Nations and Inuit health policy is administered by the regional branches in each province, each headed by a regional director. First Nations are increasingly assuming local control through the transfer of health services (see Appendix 2A at the end of Chapter 2). Health services for the Métis are provided by the provincial healthcare systems. Furthermore, First Nations and Inuit living off-reserve have their healthcare services provided within the provincial healthcare system, and then the province asks for reimbursement from the federal government. The territories assume responsibility for their Aboriginal populations through their agreements with Ottawa.

Part of the politics of First Nations, Métis, and Inuit are the national organizations that represent their interests in Ottawa. For example, the Assembly of First Nations elects a Grand Chief, who negotiates with federal officials for program funding of First Nations healthcare. The Inuit Tapiriit Kanatami represents the Inuit, and the Métis National Council represents the Métis.

Why do CHNs need to know about government and its functions? The answer is because it affects how healthcare is delivered to First Nations on a daily basis. It is advantageous to know and understand policies, thereby increasing the effectiveness of healthcare practitioners. When the governing party changes, often the agreements that have been in place are altered, deleted, or replaced by new legislation.

For acute-care services, First Nations healthcare systems interface with the greater Canadian healthcare system, primarily because hospitals are a provincial responsibility. The degree of interfacing required with the surrounding communities depends on the type and scope of health services that exist on the reserves. The more remote and isolated the reserve, the more likely it is that the healthcare services include comprehensive care, including short-term acute-care services. The federal government operated Indian hospitals but has been divesting itself of this responsibility. Rather, it has entered into tripartite agreements with the provinces and the First Nations government to fund hospitals, such as the Fort Qu'Appelle All Nations Healing Hospital in Saskatchewan.

The process for community-based health services is different. The governance for health services is derived from the Chief and council, the governing authority for First Nations. Once the band council resolution is signed, a health committee or health board can be formed to begin the process of exploring community-based health services for its membership. First Nations health authorities were established to prepare for the transfer of control of health services to First Nations. Various types of funding arrangements are available to First Nations groups seeking to administer their own health programs (see Appendix A). The most recent funding arrangement has been the complete transfer of all First Nations health services from both the federal and provincial governments in British Columbia. The tripartite agreement has been signed, and the newly established First Nations Health Authority is currently in the process of staffing its respective units (First Nations Health Authority, 2013). Other regional offices of FNIHB now serve primarily a financial accountability role.

### CANADIAN RESEARCH BOX 22.1

#### How are sleep and screen time affecting weight among First Nations youth?

Gates, M., Hanning, R. M., Martin, I. D., Gates, A., & Tsuji, L. J. S. (2013). Body mass index of First Nations youth in Ontario, Canada: Influence of sleep and screen time. *Rural and Remote Health, 13,* 2498.

This study was an observational, population-based study of cross-sectional design attempting to connect physical activity, screen time, and sleep time to the high rates of overweight and obese youth being reported among First Nations populations. A group of 348 youth, 10–18 years of age, from five remote northern First Nations communities and one southern First Nations community in Ontario participated in the study. The measurement tool was a

Web-based survey questionnaire administered through the school system. The research team measured the height and weight of the participants, entered the data into the survey, and body mass index was then electronically calculated. Screen time was divided into time spent watching television and time spent on the Internet and playing video games. Sleep time was determined by questions that asked the time one normally went to bed and number of hours of sleep per night.

Significant findings of the study are as follows:

1. There was a positive correlation between time spent using the Internet or playing video games and BMI for boys only: 56.7% of boys who reported two or more hours of screen time were obese.
2. There was a negative correlation between time spent outside and BMI, again for boys only, where only 9.5% of obese boys reported that they spent "most of the time" outside.
3. Although not statistically significant, a higher-than-expected number of obese youth had a television in their bedroom.

Consistent with patterns seen in the general population, youth in the current study demonstrated low levels of after-school physical activity and excess screen time relative to national guidelines. One possible cause offered in this study is the loss of traditional lifestyles. Implications for policy and practice indicate that local knowledge systems need to be incorporated in health-promotion and prevention programs.

### Discussion Questions

1. As a CHN, how might you use the findings in your program planning for working with school-age youth and the teachers?
2. In the Western education system, physical activity programming does not often include traditional lifestyle activities such as snowshoeing, canoeing, kayaking, or walking to check snares or traps. How could you facilitate ways of incorporating traditional lifestyle components into the school system?

## Cultural Issues in Community Health Nursing in Aboriginal Communities

First Nations' healthcare systems are varied in scope and practice. The nurse may practise in a large healthcare system that utilizes nursing skills in a limited scope. In contrast, the nurse may arrive in a remote northern community where the expectation is that all nursing roles will be met by one individual (Cradduck, 1995). Giger and Davidhizar's (1998) conceptual framework states that there are six key phenomena in all cultures: communication, space, time, social organization, environmental control, and biological variations. The Giger and Davidhizar transcultural assessment model is one tool that can be utilized in assessing Aboriginal populations with the goal of developing culturally appropriate community health nursing care.

Development of competent, culturally appropriate nursing care (Andrews & Boyle, 1999) for Aboriginal clients requires the CHN to keep in mind the historical, cultural, and changing clinical healthcare delivery system. As noted earlier, the traditional lifestyles of Canada's Aboriginal peoples profoundly changed because of colonization. Reserves effectively excluded First Nations from participating in mainstream Canadian society (McMurray, 1999).

Aboriginal populations continue to remain a distinct cultural segment of Canadian society. Traditional holistic health beliefs, traditional medicine, and herbal medicine are deemed acceptable alternatives to Western medicine by some Aboriginal people. First Nations communities are societies in themselves. Based on a culture continuum, the society may have different members who are traditionalists, traditionalists/modernists, or modernists. Each group's strengths and challenges present for interesting nurse practice. The CHN must learn protocol for communicating with the traditionalists, who may possess cultural manners, diet, and health beliefs contrary to nursing knowledge and skills (Holland & Hogg, 2001). For example, some individuals believe that bear grease is the best treatment for abrasions and wounds. The CHN must respect the client's health beliefs while attempting to maintain sterile wound care. The outcome is establishing sufficient trust with the client so that the wound heals without infection and the client continues to seek the required healthcare.

Rumbold (1999) states that ethics provide a framework for dealing with issues, problems, and dilemmas. An understanding of ethical or moral theories helps a person decide on an appropriate line of action, although it may not necessarily provide the answer. Nurses need to study ethics because they often have to deal with moral or ethical problems, and they also need to examine their own beliefs and values. Rumbold makes the case that nurses who move from one culture to another need to be informed of the values and norms of the society to which they are moving. It does not mean that they should abandon their own ethical values (Rumbold, 1999). Aboriginal communities can present dilemmas for which it is crucial that CHNs make wise choices. Dilemmas may be related to childcare, family violence, or geriatric abuse (Dumont-Smith, 2001). Aboriginal nurses working with First Nations communities may find different challenges, such as a personal tension between cultural practices and their knowledge of health science. Clients may assume a belief system (e.g., traditional medicine) that is not included in the nurse's practice. The Aboriginal Nurses Association of Canada (ANAC) provides support to Aboriginal and non-Aboriginal nurses practising in First Nations communities and can be accessed on their website (www.anac.on.ca). One of their projects concerns cultural competency and cultural safety in nursing education (Aboriginal Nurses Association of Canada, 2013). (See Chapter 9.)

Nurses contemplating employment with FNIHB or a First Nations health authority should prepare by doing research on the tribe's culture, language, geographic location, education, economy, and healthcare system. CHNs require excellent skills for assessment, planning, implementing, and evaluating community health programs (see Chapters 13 and 14). Knowing your client, whether it is the individual, family, or community, facilitates evidence-based decision making.

## CANADIAN RESEARCH BOX 22.2

### Are influenza pandemic plans effective in remote and isolated First Nations communities?

Charania, N. A., & Tsuji L. J. S. (2013). Assessing the effectiveness of implementing mitigation measures for an influenza pandemic in remote and isolated First Nations communities: A qualitative community-based participatory research approach. *Rural and Remote Health, 13,* 2566. Retrieved from http://www.rrh.org.au

In this study, researchers used a community-based participatory approach to assess the effectiveness of 41 interventions (identified from a literature review) to mitigate the 2009 H1N1 influenza pandemic. The participants were nine health professionals working in three remote and isolated communities in northern Ontario during the outbreak. Effectiveness was measured through constructs of feasibility, cost, logistics, operational and infrastructure constraints, and acceptability.

The results indicate that 30 of the 41 interventions were used during the outbreak, that all measures used were considered to be effective, and that additional measures which would be more appropriate for the community were suggested. Promoting the use of traditional medicine as a treatment option worked well for the communities, and point-of-care testing would have been beneficial as remote location hampers time for sending samples out. Three measures were considered to be not effective: travel restrictions or advisories on all arriving and departing passengers, because there were not enough healthcare staff; workplace closures, because all businesses in the small communities were considered essential; and quarantine, because of a lack of infrastructure to use as a quarantine base, and homes were not viable due to overcrowding. Increased education of community members would likely have increased adherence to travel restrictions.

### Discussion Questions

1. The non-pharmaceutical interventions were seen to be more effective in the communities. How would the CHN be able to use this information for future pandemic planning?

2. Historically, influenza outbreaks have had depopulating effects in First Nations communities but traditional medicine was used. How might the CHN access this knowledge in the respective communities and incorporate it into the pandemic plan?

3. Educating community members was suggested as a possibility in future pandemic planning. What are several educational avenues that a CHN could pursue that would be culturally appropriate?

The nurses should be genuinely interested in the health of the Aboriginal clients requiring community health nursing. Required skill sets include the ability to remain objective and to resist stereotyping the community and its residents despite frequent negative media attention. Health personnel are continually being recruited, and nurses often must relocate to remote or isolated First Nations communities (Tarlier, Johnson, & Whyte, 2003). Retention of health personnel for only short lengths of time can result in some communities becoming distrustful of new nurses. This can provide another challenge to the nurse's communication skills (Sundeen, Stuart, Rankin, & Cohen, 1998).

Formal and informal leadership in First Nations communities can be difficult to grasp. CHNs require the skills to assess the community and outline the health priorities and health issues of the population. They have to decide on the course of action in consultation with the community. Historically, First Nations people made decisions on a consensus basis; some communities continue to make decisions in this way (Cookfair, 1991). CHNs have to find roles that can be filled by a non-member health professional, perhaps as a consultant who provides information the community can use to make its best decision. Alternatively, the nurse may be seen as the individual who makes the decisions. The nurse must rely on community development knowledge and allow the community to make its own decisions over time. It is easy to assume control of the decision making if you are seen as the individual with the best health knowledge. However, it is important to consult and work with the community in all phases of health program development (Smylie, 2000). (See Canadian Research Box 22.2.) Elders are traditionally seen as the knowledge keepers of communities, and as such, they can be important allies and sources of knowledge.

## POLICY ISSUES AFFECTING COMMUNITY HEALTH NURSING IN ABORIGINAL COMMUNITIES

Unlike public health nursing in urban communities, First Nations and Inuit healthcare systems vary in size and services offered. Nurses who seek employment in an Aboriginal community must establish a network of colleagues who can assist with information when required. Health professionals establish liaisons with other service agencies or professional organizations, such as the ANAC, to promote the population health approach.

CHNs must also be aware of competing policies and jurisdictions. For instance, the federal government is responsible for the healthcare of Aboriginal people on-reserve; thus, nursing services are provided for home care clients by FNIHB. However, Aboriginal Affairs and Northern Development Canada is responsible for funding personal-care and home-support services as well as infrastructure, such as housing and water treatment plants. The nurse must be innovative in coordinating the home-care services for clients from two service agencies, and that may also include the provincial healthcare system if the client is being transferred from the hospital. In addition, the CHN may be requested to supervise staff responsible for personal care, homemaking, and transportation.

Health education and promotion are part of the everyday contact with communities and groups. CHNs need to make the effort to make these activities culturally appropriate (see Chapter 9). The medicine wheel framework is an excellent teaching tool and, because of its diversity, can be adapted to virtually any health issue. Medicine wheels made of stone and small boulders set in various circular patterns are found in the United States and southern Canada, mostly in Alberta and Saskatchewan. However, their origins and meaning have been lost in time. Some say they are for navigation using the stars, or to mark events such as the solstice. Whatever significance they had for the original inhabitants of North America, they still influence the thinking and lives of Canadian Aboriginal peoples today. Not unlike other Aboriginal cultures in the world, Canadian Aboriginal peoples have a holistic belief about life.

Traditional world views of Aboriginal peoples emphasize the interconnectedness of all things, and this concept is the basis of the medicine wheel framework. Most First Nations in Canada maintain holistic beliefs, yet not all believe in the medicine wheel philosophy. The present significance of the medicine wheel is that it provides a framework for the holistic beliefs of the descendants of those original inhabitants of Canada.

The medicine wheel usually represents four quadrants of emotional, physical, mental, and spiritual aspects of health and wellness (see Figure 22.1). It is said that a balance has to be maintained in the four aspects for an individual to maintain optimal health. On first glance, the medicine wheel model can seem simple; however, the concepts it represents are complex. The four directions are represented, just as the races of humankind are represented. The different teachings of how one can lead a purposeful life are also represented. The four life stages of infancy, childhood, adulthood, and the elder are also represented. The four components of our humanness are the physical, the intellectual, the spiritual, and the emotional. Colours, animals, and characteristics such as strength, humility, and illumination are also assigned to their respective quadrants. Today, the medicine wheel philosophy is being taught by elders to the youth in Aboriginal populations across North America. Examples can be found online, where communities have adapted the medicine wheel to issues including HIV/AIDS, diabetes, family violence, and addictions.

An alternative framework can be found in the First Nations cultural framework of the national First Nations and Inuit Regional Longitudinal Health Survey (First Nations Information Governance Centre, 2012). The two models are similar but cannot be deemed to be the same. Another model, one that is similar to the WHO Determinants of Health model, has been put forward by the Four Worlds International Institute. This model has a list of 14 health determinants (Four Worlds International Institute, 2011) that are more focused on Aboriginal world views and ways of being. These are displayed in Table 22.1.

Part of the community health nursing practice in Aboriginal communities is the evaluation component of health programs. Nurses should recognize that nursing standards of practice can be maintained through continuous quality improvement. First Nations health organizations are becoming members of the Canadian Council on Health Services Accreditation.

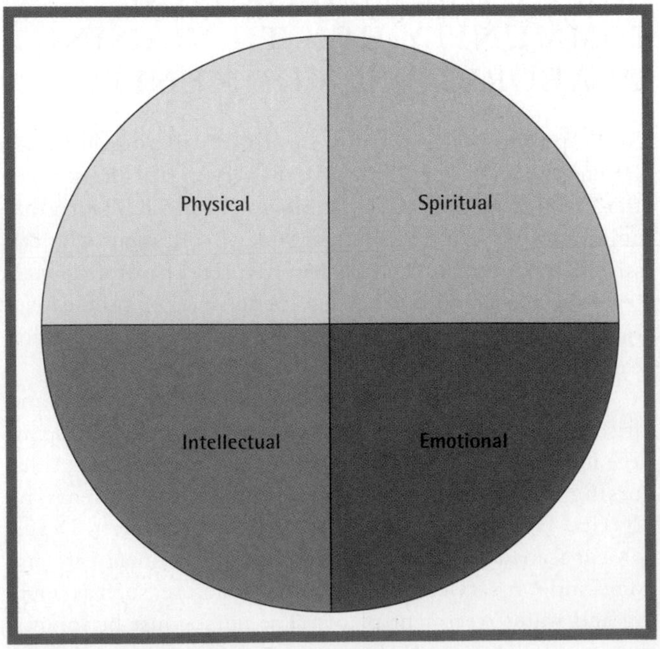

FIGURE 22.1 A medicine wheel

| Table 22.1 | **Four Worlds Institute Determinants of Well-Being and Health** |
| --- | --- |

1. Basic physical needs
2. Spirituality and a sense of purpose
3. Life-sustaining values, morals, and ethics
4. Safety and security
5. Adequate income and sustainable economies
6. Adequate power
7. Social justice and equity
8. Cultural integrity and identity
9. Community solidarity and social support
10. Strong families and healthy child development
11. Healthy eco-system and a sustainable relationship between human beings and the natural world
12. Critical learning opportunities
13. Adequate human services and social safety net
14. Meaningful work and service to others

Source: Four Worlds International Institute. (2011). *Identifying determinants of well-being and health.* Used by permission of Four Worlds International Inc. Retrieved from Four Worlds International Institute at http://www.4worlds.org/4w/visionsanddeterminants/fuldeter.htm

## CASE STUDY

A First Nations community has a total population of 3 200. Two thousand members live on the reserve and 1 200 members live off-reserve. The community is located near a mid-sized city. The unemployment level is consistently at 70%. Most families rely on social services for their subsistence. Sixty percent of the population is 18 years of age or less. The education level ranges from Grade 8 to Grade 12. The community is governed by an elected Chief and eight Councillors.

Most homes are 25 to 35 years old and have indoor plumbing, central heating, and electricity. However, potable water is delivered by water trucks. Sewage disposal is done by the community sewage system, but rural homes have a septic tank sewage disposal system. The region's climate is temperate, with cold winters and dry summers.

The community-controlled school system goes from Kindergarten to Grade 8, and eight of the 10 teachers are Aboriginal. Very few community members practise the traditional lifestyle, and fewer than 5% of the school children speak their language. High school students are bused 40 minutes each way to attend school in the nearby city. Most families end up being single-parent households.

The economy is based on school transportation and employment with the band administration, the band-controlled school, the health centre, and two privately owned gas stations/convenience stores. The school principal has initiated a good recreation program for the students, and Aboriginal teacher assistants keep the students interested in being physically active. Parents participate in the school activities. However, once the students are bused to attend school in the city, parents no longer display much interest in school activities. Most of the adults attended a residential school located in the city, where they completed middle school.

The health centre is readily accessed by the population for all community health programs. The First Nations band received transfer of their health funding five years ago. The health centre employs a health director, who is from the community, three primary care nurses, one home care nurse, two community health representatives, one addictions counsellor, one medical taxi driver, and you are the newly hired community health nurse. Immunization levels are at 33% for all ages. Chronic disease rates for diabetes, arthritis, and circulatory diseases have not been assessed since prior to the health program transfer. The First Nations and Inuit Health Branch continues to provide support for the CHN, primarily through federally approved programs and materials. During your orientation at the regional FNIHB office, the zone nurse manager informs you that one of the priorities is the immunization program because the Canada Disease Weekly has reported pertussis in the area. There have been disturbing developments in the community in the last several years. On weekends, parents leave the community to shop in the nearby city. However, with the opening of the First Nations casino, they are now spending their money gambling and drinking. Children are often left in the care of elderly grandparents or alone at home to fend for themselves until their parents return. Family violence, child neglect, and an increased number of motor vehicle accidents and house fires are causing concern for the various community agencies. In the last five months, five teenagers have attempted suicide.

As the new nurse, you are greeted by the health director when you arrive and given a tour of their new health centre. At the staff meeting you meet the other staff members, including the community health representatives, who seem to know the community very well. The other three nurses have been there between one and seven years, two are First Nations and from the community, one was born there, and one married into the community. They tell you their day is non-stop primary care and they don't have time for community health. The addictions counsellor is very eager to assist in any way he can.

### Discussion Questions

1. How would you, as the CHN, use the nursing process to begin planning your community health program?

2. Whom would you ask to help you familiarize yourself with the community?

3. List the resiliency factors of the community.

4. What factors make this First Nations community a vulnerable community?

5. Describe how you will begin to work on the immunization program.

## CONCLUSION

The chapter outlined the historical and current health issues affecting Aboriginal populations in Canada. Nurses working in Aboriginal communities must understand the distinction between First Nations, status and non-status; Métis; and Inuit because it affects nursing services delivery. The employers of nurses working in Aboriginal communities can be the federal, provincial, or local health authorities, each with its own organizational complexities.

Aboriginal populations have immense health challenges that nurses must assess in order to plan health services. Nurses may be responsible for the implementation of health services and programs, and should have the skills to evaluate the efficacy of health programs for Aboriginal communities. In addition, nurses must have the communication skills to allow effective interaction with Aboriginal leadership and other service agency personnel. Advance preparation for working with First Nations and Inuit should be a priority for nurses contemplating employment in First Nations and Inuit communities to lessen the possible effects of culture shock. Nurses working with Canadian Aboriginal peoples often face complex challenges in what is often a rewarding practice setting.

## KEY TERMS

## STUDY QUESTIONS

1. What is the difference between a status and a non-status Indian?

2. Why are Aboriginal persons more likely to be diagnosed with diabetes at a younger age?

3. Is healthcare a treaty right for First Nations people in Canada?

4. What did the 1969 White Paper unintentionally create?

5. Describe five effects of the residential school legacy that can still be seen in Aboriginal communities today.

6. Bill C-31 created a spike among which sectors of the Aboriginal population in Canada?

After working through these questions, go to the MyNursingLab at www.pearsoned.ca/mynursinglab to check your answers.

## INDIVIDUAL CRITICAL-THINKING EXERCISES

1. The Chief of the First Nations community that employs you has just asked to see the chart of one of the clients in your care. How would you handle the situation? How do you maintain security for client records?

2. An Elder in the community believes cancer is spread through personal contact. How would you go about ameliorating this knowledge deficit?

3. A mother brings in her child for immunization and you notice the mother has several large bruises on her face and arms. What course of action do you take?

4. There is an increase in dental caries among the school-age children, which corresponds with the installation of a pop machine in school. The proceeds from the pop machine are to be used to build a skating rink. What are your options?

5. An intoxicated female client comes into the clinic with lacerations on her arms and face. During your treatment of her, she starts swearing at you and attempting to hit you. What are your professional and personal responsibilities in this situation?

## GROUP CRITICAL-THINKING EXERCISES

1. The routine water sample of the First Nations community indicates heavy growth of E. coli. As the nurse manager, how would you deal with this threat to public health? Whom would you contact?

2. There is an unexpected increase in the school-age children's responses to the yearly tuberculin Mantoux test. As the community health nurse, what would you do, in addition to instituting a preventive medication regime for the children? Whom could you contact for assistance?

3. The community you work in believes that children are a gift from the Creator; therefore, there doesn't seem to be any incentive to prevent teen pregnancy. You know the health risks to teen moms and their babies. What are some ways you could approach this issue from a community health promotion perspective?

## REFERENCES

Aboriginal Affairs and Northern Development Canada. (2011, April 18). *First Nations People of Canada*. Retrieved from Information Sheets: http://www.aadnc-aandc.gc.ca/eng/1303134042666/1303134337338

Aboriginal Affairs and Northern Development Canada. (2013a, November 11). *First Nations in Canada map*. Retrieved from http://www.aadnc-aandc.gc.ca/DAM/DAM-INTER-HQ-AI/STAGING/texte-text/ai_mprm_fnc_wal_pdf_1344968972421_eng.pdf

Aboriginal Affairs and Northern Development Canada. (2013b). *Statistics on the implementation of the Indian Residential Schools Settlement Agreement*. Retrieved from http://www.aadnc-aandc.gc.ca/eng/1315320539682/1315320692192

Aboriginal Affairs and Northern Development Canada. (2013c). *Independent assessment process*. Retrieved from http://www.aadnc-aandc.gc.ca/eng/1100100015632/1100100015633

Aboriginal Healing Foundation. (1999). *Annual report 1999*. Retrieved from http://www.ahf.ca/about-us/annual-reports

Aboriginal Healing Foundation. (2006). *Métis history and experience and residential schools in Canada*. Retrieved from http://www.ahf.ca/downloads/metiseweb.pdf

Aboriginal Healing Foundation. (2007). *Lump sum compensation payments research project: The circle rechecks itself*. Ottawa: Aboriginal Healing Foundation.

Aboriginal Healing Foundation. (2013). *FAQs*. Retrieved from http://www.ahf.ca/faqs

Aboriginal Nurses Association of Canada. (2013, March 31). *ANAC Summary of AHHRI funded Making It Happen Projects.*

Retrieved from http://www.anac.on.ca/Documents/ANAC%20 Summary%20of%20AHHRI%20funded_Making%20It%20 Happen%20Projects_March%20312013.pdf

Andrews, M. M., & Boyle, J. S. (1999). *Transcultural concepts in nursing* (3rd ed.). Philadelphia, PA: Lippincott.

Ballantine, B., & Ballantine, I. (1993). *Native Americans: An illustrated history*. Atlanta, GA: Time.

Canadian Public Health Agency. (2011a, June 23). *Prevalence among Aboriginal Peoples*. Retrieved from Obesity in Canada: http://www.phac-aspc.gc.ca/hp-ps/hl-mvs/oic-oac/abo-aut-eng.php

Canadian Public Health Agency. (2011b, December 15). *Chapter 6 – Diabetes among First Nations, Inuit, and Métis populations*. Retrieved from Diabetes in Canada: Facts and figures from a public health perspective: http://www. phac-aspc.gc.ca/cd-mc/publications/diabetes-diabete/ facts-figures-faits-chiffres-2011/chap6-eng.php

Canadian Public Health Agency. (2013). *TB and Aboriginal People*. Retrieved from Control of Infectious Diseases: http:// www.cpha.ca/en/programs/history/achievements/02-id/tb-aboriginal.aspx

Chansonneuve, D. (2005). *Reclaiming connections: Understanding residential school trauma among Aboriginal people*. Ottawa, ON: Aboriginal Healing Foundation.

Chrisjohn, R. D., Young, S. L., & Maraun, M. (1994). *The circle game: Shadows and substance in the residential school experience in Canada: A report to the Royal Commission on Aboriginal Peoples*. Penticton, BC: Theytus.

Cookfair, J. M. (1991). *Nursing process and practice in the community*. Toronto, ON: Mosby.

Cradduck, G. R. (1995). Primary practice. In M. J. Stewart, *Community nursing: Promoting Canadians' health* (pp. 454–471). Toronto, ON: Saunders.

Deagle, G. (1999). The three-tier system [Editorial]. *Canadian Family Physician*, 247–249.

Department of Indian and Northern Affairs. (1997). *First Nations in Canada*. Ottawa, ON: Government of Canada.

Department of Indian and Northern Affairs. (2002). *A summary of the First Nations Governance Act*. Ottawa, ON: Government of Canada.

Dickason, O. (2002a). Reclaiming stolen land. In J. Bird, L. Land, & M. Macadam, *Nation to nation: Aboriginal sovereignty and the future of Canada* (pp. 34–42). Toronto, ON: Irwin.

Dickason, O. P. (2002b). *Canada's First Nations: A history of founding peoples from earliest times* (3rd ed.). Don Mills, ON: Oxford.

Dumont-Smith, C. (2001). *Exposure to violence in the home: Effects on Aboriginal children*. Ottawa, ON: Aboriginal Nurses Association of Canada.

Employment and Social Development Canada. (2013, December 30). *Canadians in Context – Aboriginal Population*. Retrieved from Indicators of Well-being in Canada: http://www4.hrsdc.gc.ca/.3ndic.1t.4r@-eng.jsp?iid=36

First Nations and Inuit Health. (2009, February). *A statistical profile on the health of First Nations in Canada: Determinants of health, 1999 to 2003*. Retrieved from http://www.hc-sc. gc.ca/fniah-spnia/pubs/aborig-autoch/2009-stats-profil/ index-eng.php

First Nations and Inuit Health Branch. (2007, July 25). *Indian Health Policy 1979*. Retrieved from http://www.hc-sc.gc.ca/ ahc-asc/branch-dirgen/fnihb-dgspni/poli_1979-eng.php

First Nations Health Authority. (2013). *Governance and accountability*. Retrieved from http://www.fnha.ca/about/ governance-and-accountability

First Nations Information Governance Centre. (2012). First Nations regional health survey (RHS) Phase 2 (2008/10). *National report on adults, youth and children living in First Nations communities*. Ottawa, ON: First Nations Information Governance Centre.

Flaskerud, J., & Winslow, B. (1998). Conceptualizing vulnerable populations health-related research. *Nursing Research*, 69–78.

Fleet, C. (1997). *First Nations firsthand: A history of five hundred years of encounter, war, and peace inspired by the eyewitnesses*. Edison, NJ: Chartwell.

Four Worlds International Institute. (2011). *Identifying determinants of well-being and health*. Retrieved from http:// www.4worlds.org/4w/visionsanddeterminants/fuldeter.htm

Furi, M., & Wherrett, J. (2003, February). *Indian status and band membership issues*. Retrieved from http://www.parl.gc.ca/ content/lop/researchpublications/bp410-e.htm#a registrationtx

Giger, J. N., & Davidhizar, R. E. (1998). *Canadian transcultural nursing assessment and intervention*. Toronto, ON: Mosby.

Government of Alberta. (2013). *Métis settlements*. Retrieved from http://www.aboriginal.alberta.ca/965.cfm

Health Canada. (2011, July 19). *Tobacco*. Retrieved from http://www.hc-sc.gc.ca/fniah-spnia/substan/tobac-tabac/ index-eng.php

Holland, K., & Hogg, C. (2001). *Cultural awareness in nursing and health care: An introductory text*. New York, NY: Oxford University Press.

Legacy of Hope Foundation. (2013). *About residential schools*. Retrieved from http://www.legacyofhope.ca/about-residential-schools

Mann, C. C. (2005). *1491: New revelations of the Americas before Columbus*. New York, NY: Vintage Books.

McMurray, A. (1999). *Community health and wellness: A sociological approach*. Toronto, ON: Mosby.

Office of the Treaty Commissioner. (2013). *Aboriginal rights and title*. Retrieved from http://www.otc.ca/pdfs/aboriginal_ rights.pdf

Patterson, L. L. (2006, May 4). *Aboriginal roundtable to Kelowna Accord: Aboriginal policy negotiations, 2004-2005*. Retrieved from http://www.parl.gc.ca/Content/LOP/researchpublications/ prb0604-e.pdf

Ricciuti, E. (1990). *The natural history of North America*. New York, NY: Gallery.

Rumbold, G. (1999). *Ethics in nursing practice* (3rd ed.). Toronto, ON: Bailliere Tindall.

Schouls, T. (2002). The basic dilemma: Sovereignty or assimilation. In J. Bird, L. Land, & M. Macadam, *Nation to nation: Aboriginal sovereignty and the future of Canada* (pp. 34–42). Toronto, ON: Irwin.

Schultz, J. W. (1962). *Blackfeet and buffalo: Memories of life among the Indians*. Norman, OK: University of Oklahoma Press.

Sebastian, J. G. (2000). Vulnerability and vulnerable populations: An overview. In M. Stanhope, & J. Lancaster, *Community and public health nursing* (pp. 638–661). Toronto, ON: Mosby.

Shahid, S., & Thompson, S. C. (2009). An overview of cancer and beliefs about the disease in Indigenous people of

Australia, Canada, New Zealand and the US. *Australian and New Zealand Journal of Public Health*, 109–118. doi: 10.1111/j.1753-6405.2009.0035.x.

Sherman, J. (1996). *Indian tribes of North America*. New York, NY: Todri Productions.

Smylie, J. (2000). A guide for health professionals working with Aboriginal people. *Journal of the Society of Obstetricians and Gynecologists of Canada*, 1056–1061.

Smylie, J., & Adomako, P. (2009). *Indigenous children's health report: Health assessment in action*. Retrieved from http://www.stmichaelshospital.com/pdf/crich/ichr_report.pdf

Statistics Canada. (2008, March). *Educational portrait of Canada, 2006*. Retrieved from http://www12.statcan.ca/census-recensement/2006/as-sa/97-560/pdf/97-560-XIE2006001.pdf

Statistics Canada. (2010a, June 21). *Income*. Retrieved from http://www.statcan.gc.ca/pub/89-645-x/2010001/income-revenu-eng.htm

Statistics Canada. (2010b, June 21). *Education*. Retrieved from http://www.statcan.gc.ca/pub/89-645-x/2010001/education-eng.htm

Statistics Canada. (2010c, June 21). *Aboriginal statistics at a glance*. Retrieved from http://www.statcan.gc.ca/pub/89-645-x/89-645-x2010001-eng.htm?fpv=10000

Statistics Canada. (2010d, June 21). *Housing conditions*. Retrieved from http://www.statcan.gc.ca/pub/89-645-x/2010001/housing-logement-eng.htm

Statistics Canada. (2011, August 23). *Low income cut-offs*. Retrieved from http://www.statcan.gc.ca/pub/75f0002m/2011002/lico-sfr-eng.htm

Statistics Canada. (2013, July 11). *Aboriginal Peoples in Canada: First Nations People, Métis and Inuit*. Retrieved from http://www12.statcan.gc.ca/nhs-enm/2011/as-sa/99-011-x/99-011-x2011001-eng.cfm#a4

Sundeen, S. J., Stuart, G. W., Rankin, A. D., & Cohen, S. A. (1998). *Nurse-client interaction: Implementing the nursing process* (6th ed.). Toronto, ON: Mosby.

Tarlier, D. S., Johnson, J. L., & Whyte, N. B. (2003). Voices from the wilderness: An interpretive study describing the role and practice of outpost nurses. *Canadian Journal of Public Health*, 180–184.

Truth and Reconciliation Commission of Canada. (2013). *FAQs*. Retrieved from http://www.trc.ca/websites/trcinstitution/index.php?p=10

University of Manitoba. (2013). *Learning from the past*. Retrieved from http://www.umanitoba.ca/about/trc.html

Venne, S. (2002). Treaty-making with the crown. In J. Bird, L. Land, & M. Macadam, *Nation to nation: Aboriginal sovereignty and the future of Canada* (pp. 45–52). Toronto, ON: Irwin.

Waldram, J. B., Herring, D. A., & Young, T. K. (2006). *Aboriginal health in Canada: Historical, cultural and epidemiological perspectives*. Toronto, ON: University of Toronto Press.

## ABOUT THE AUTHOR

**Dr. Rose A. Roberts,** RN, PhD, is a member of the Lac La Ronge Indian Band and is originally from the community of Stanley Mission, Saskatchewan. She has an undergraduate degree in nursing, and master's and doctoral degrees in community health and epidemiology, all from the University of Saskatchewan. Dr. Roberts has held faculty positions in the College of Nursing and the School of Public Health, University of Saskatchewan, and was the CEO of the Northern Inter-Tribal Health Authority. She is a Fulbright Scholar in Residence recipient and spent a year teaching at the Northwest Indian College in Bellingham, WA. Her research interests include cancer in Aboriginal populations, alternative healing modalities, residential school survivorship, and traditional indigenous knowledge systems as a mode of healing.

# Mental Health

*Elaine Mordoch*

Source: Courtesy of David C. Stacey

LEARNING OUTCOMES

**After studying this chapter, you should be able to:**

1. Describe the historical context and current challenges surrounding mental health and illness in Canadian society.

2. Discuss the effects, impact, and risk factors for mental illness and how they affect the vulnerable populations.

3. Examine the causes of suicide, the at-risk groups, and the related assessment, intervention, and prevention strategies.

4. Explain mental health legislation that dictates the provision of services for people with mental illness.

5. Analyze the organization of services in the mental health system and selected models of care.

6. Consider nursing roles in community mental health and future directions for practice.

## INTRODUCTION

Mental illness (MI) affects the life trajectory of individuals, disrupts family processes, and impacts communities and society with lost productivity and costly treatment. Stigma and discrimination influence the identification and treatment of people with MI and their families. Services are often neither timely nor adequate to facilitate recovery from MI. Realizing that community services must incorporate mental health promotion, prevention, treatment, and rehabilitation of MI, community mental health nurses (CMHNs) must strive to establish best practices when working with this population. Mental health impacts the ability of all people to enjoy life and deal with its challenges. This chapter discusses challenges facing persons with MI, available services, and strategies to promote mental health within Canadian society.

## HISTORICAL CONTEXT AND CHALLENGES

Historically, mental healthcare in Canada has taken place within a context of culture, gender, and sociopolitical attitudes. Formal management of people with MI (PMI) began in poorhouses and jails that provided little but containment. In the mid-19th century, large institutional hospitals or asylums were built to provide more humane care. Hospitals were first built in Quebec, New Brunswick, Nova Scotia, Manitoba, British Columbia, and Prince Edward Island, followed by Saskatchewan and Alberta. Although physically isolated from their homes and families, PMI were believed to be in safe healing environments where they followed structured therapeutic routines (Sussman, 1998).

Efforts to define psychiatry (which was introduced in 1846) and to find a cure for mental illnesses prevailed. When expectations that patients would return to the community proved unrealistic, the asylums became overcrowded and understaffed, deteriorating to warehouses for PMI (Nolan, 1993). The resultant inhumane care evoked public outcry, demanding humane treatment and educated caregivers.

In the 1960s, a philosophical shift proposed that humane treatment would be best achieved in the community. Concurrently, the discovery of the psychotropic medications chlorpromazine and lithium, and cost-containment measures associated with large institutions, contributed to deinstitutionalization. Long-stay institutions were depopulated and people with major mental illnesses were placed in community hospitals and other community facilities. Deinstitutionalization resulted in a decrease in bed capacity in provincial mental hospitals from 47 633 beds in 1960 to 15 011 beds in 1976, and a rise in general hospital psychiatric beds from 844 to 5836 (Goering, Wasylenki, & Durbin, 2000). The resources that former residents needed to live in the community were underestimated. People discharged from the institutions were marginalized and vulnerable, with families lacking adequate resources to assist them (Davis, 2006).

## CURRENT DEVELOPMENTS IN CANADA

Today, several important trends influence psychiatric and mental health services: the consumer and family movements, the rehabilitative recovery model, the Kirby report, and more recently, the national mental health strategies developed by the Mental Health Commission of Canada (MHCC) (2012). Through effective lobbying, consumer and family movements advanced health promotion strategies and rehabilitative resources for patients (Davis, 2006). Concurrently, the **recovery model of rehabilitation** identified life beyond symptom management; it is based upon a collaborative, consumer-driven process that challenges previous conceptions of intervention goals (Anthony, 2000). Consumers expect active collaboration with care providers rather than passive participation in dictated treatment. These trends are influencing changes within the Mental Health Act, service delivery, research, policy development, and the relationship between service providers, PMI, and their families. "Out of the Shadows at Last: Transforming Mental Health, Mental Illness and Addictions Services in Canada," also known as the Kirby report, was Canada's first national report that addressed deficiencies and inequities of mental health services in the Canadian healthcare system (Kirby, 2008; Kirby & Keon, 2006).

Based on the recommendations presented in the Kirby report, the federal government initiated the MHCC in 2007. Its mandate is to reform mental health policies and improve service delivery, facilitate a national approach to mental health issues, diminish stigma and discrimination, and disseminate evidence-based research to governments, stakeholders, and the public. The Commission had developed five strategic initiatives: (1) a 10-year anti-stigma campaign to change public attitudes toward mental illness; (2) development of a national strategy to address mental illness in collaboration with all members of the mental health community; (3) the homelessness research demonstration projects; (4) the Partners for Mental Health Program; and (5) the development of a Knowledge Exchange Centre to facilitate access to evidence-based information and encourage collaboration across Canada (Kirby, 2008). In 2012, a national mental health strategy for Canada was developed. This strategy aims to improve both the mental health outcomes for all Canadians and to rectify inadequacies within the current mental health system (MHCC, 2012).

While most PMI receive services within their communities, poor integration of services and alienation among psychiatric hospitals, community mental health programs, and private practitioners continue to fragment service delivery. Rural and remote areas lack access to appropriate and timely mental health services (Ryan-Nicholls & Haggarty, 2007). Comprehensive services that address socioeconomic factors such as housing, income, and supportive resources to facilitate living in the community are required to assist PMI and their families in their daily lives (Kirby & Keon, 2006). Recognition of the impact of social health determinants, the need for consumer involvement within policy development, the value of self-help groups and peer consultations, and the importance of policy based on a recovery model will assist PMI to live more satisfying, hopeful, and productive lives.

## STIGMA AND DISCRIMINATION

The 10-year anti-stigma campaign "Opening Minds," initiated by the MHCC, addresses the fact that stigma and discrimination are a reality facing PMI. Cultural beliefs, superstitions, and poor understanding of MI contribute to fear, stereotyping, and avoidance of PMI. Stigma affects health determinants such as housing, where discrimination limits consumers' ability to secure safe and affordable housing. People with co-morbid MI and physical disabilities are doubly jeopardized by stigma from society and healthcare professionals. Stigma causes people to conceal their illness and delay or refuse treatment and follow-up care. One in seven Canadians reported feelings of being discriminated against in the past five years. This perception is linked to increased vulnerability and poor physical and mental health outcomes (MHCC, 2015). Youth with mental illness identified stigma as the major barrier to their reintegration to society and experienced feelings of exclusion related to their perceived loss of social status once the diagnosis became known (Leave, 2015). Also, some people with depression tend not to seek treatment for their depression, they believe that the most effective way is to self-manage on their own (Griffiths, Crisp, Jorm, & Christensen, 2011).

Efforts to reduce stigma toward MI in Canadian society include the following target groups:

- youth—most mental illnesses began before age 18; early intervention would make an important difference in the quality of life;
- healthcare providers—people with lived mental health experiences perceived stigma from the providers;
- media—it plays an important role in shaping public opinion; and

| Table 23.1 | Anti-Stigma Initiatives | | |
|---|---|---|---|
| **YOUTH** | **HEALTHCARE PROVIDERS** | **MEDIA** | **WORKPLACE** |
| Iris the Dragon series, *He Shoots He Scores!* One of a series of books addressing children's mental health challenges; used with school children in Perth, Ontario.<br><br>Durham, Talking About Mental Illness (TAMI).<br><br>Five-class teaching curriculum for Grades 7–12, with professional development workshop.<br><br>Stigma Summit – Mind your Mind Youth website provides information, personal stories, coping tools; used in London, Ontario. | Practice Support Program for physicians<br><br>Central Local Health Integrated Network (LHIN) for hospital and support workers with stories from people with mental illness; DVD for discussion points.<br><br>University programs with specific curriculum content: Occupational therapy, Alberta; Psychiatric nurses, Brandon, Manitoba; Pharmacy, Dalhousie, Memorial, and Saskatchewan; Mind Course, Medicine Calgary. | Mindset: Reporting on Mental Health: Contract with Canadian Journalism Forum on Violence and Trauma to develop a media resource guide; Canadian Broadcasting Corporation is a partner.<br><br>Media monitoring project on mental illness issues (McGill University). | Programs for government employees: Mental Health Works (MHW) is a national program created by the Canadian Mental Health Association; Mind Matters, a program for business leaders developed by Mood Disorders Ontario, creates healthy work-places.<br><br>Department of National Defence: Road to Mind Readiness aims to increase resiliency and mental health in soldiers and civilians.<br><br>Economic analysis of the impact of mental illness in the workplace. |

Source: Mental Health Commission of Canada. (2013a). *Interim report on opening minds*. Retrieved from http://www.mentalhealthcommission.ca/English/system/files/private/document/opening_minds_interim_report.pdf

- workforce—employees avoid treatment for fear of stigma and discrimination from their employers and coworkers (MHCC, 2013a) (see Table 23.1).

Many community efforts are in place to promote community awareness. Public education campaigns such as Bell's "Let's Talk" and the National Hockey League of Canada's "Hockey Talks" programs use champion spokespersons to raise awareness and funds for community mental health promotion programs (http://letstalk.bell.ca/en/).

Language is embedded with underlying biases and requires careful consideration in its use. Nurses must be sensitive to terminology that they use and respect the language that PMI prefer. Currently, the term *people with lived experience* is often used. This term is generally acceptable to most people; however, the nurse is responsible to appropriately address the person as he or she wishes to be addressed.

## CANADIAN MENTAL HEALTH ORGANIZATIONS

In Canada, it is the provincial governments' responsibility to provide community mental health services (see Chapter 2). In most provinces, mental health services are governed by regional health authorities without an overriding national strategy (Kirby, 2008). Many community organizations exist that have arisen from the consumer, recovery, and family movements. Community mental health programs such as the Canadian Mental Health Association operate under the provincial mental health division. The **Canadian Mental Health Association (CMHA)** is an umbrella organization founded in 1918 to prevent MI and promote the mental health of people living in their own communities. The CMHA has

a national office, provincial divisions, and local community-based branches. Local branches provide resources, mental health programs, and other human services to individuals, families, and groups. This is accomplished through self-help, community resources, and the support of family, friends, and neighbours. Services such as housing, income, education, leisure opportunities, employment, peer and social supports, and self-esteem are based on factors that determine health and wellness.

## MENTAL ILLNESS AND ITS EFFECTS

**Mental illness (MI)** refers to a group of diagnosable diseases or disabilities of the mind described as some combination of altered thinking, mood, behaviour, or will that can be linked with distress or impaired functioning (Mental Health Act, 1990, amended 2010). **Mental health** is the capacity to think, feel, and act in ways that enhance the enjoyment of life and ability to face life's challenges. "It is a positive sense of emotional and spiritual well-being that respects the importance of culture, equity, social justice, interconnections, and personal dignity" (Government of Canada, 2006, p. 2).

By the year 2041, the number of Canadians living with mental illness is estimated at over one million people and is expected to increase by 30%. Children and adolescents between the ages of 9 and 19 years are expected to number over 1.2 million (Smetanin et al., 2011). One in four Canadian seniors over the age of 65 years has a mental illness such as depression, anxiety, or dementia; and it is likely that a considerable additional number do not get diagnosed. (See Figure 23.1.) In Canada, the *Diagnostic and Statistical Manual* (DSM), recently updated to the DSM-5, is used to diagnose MI. It has been criticized for gender bias, cultural insensitivity, and reliance on non-empirical evidence. Attempts to address some of these biases are apparent in the DSM-5. For example, chronic trauma experiences, such as childhood sexual abuse, have not been adequately explained by post-traumatic stress disorder. The terms "complex post-traumatic stress disorder" and "disorders of extreme stress" have been suggested in order to capture the experience of chronic traumatization and better understanding of the issues that people may face in their life circumstances (McGibbon, 2012). (See Figure 23.2.)

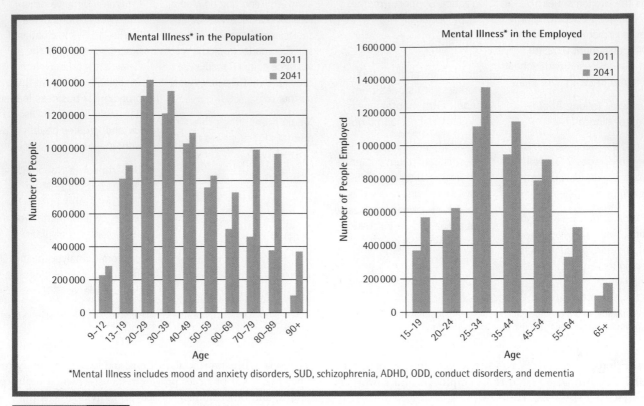

**FIGURE 23.1** Estimated Number of People with Mental Illness in the Canadian Population and Employed Population

*Source:* Smetanin, P., Stiff, D., Briante, C., Adair, C. E., Ahmad, S., & Khan, M. (2011). *The life and economic impact of major mental illnesses in Canada 2011–2041.* Risk Analytica, on behalf of the Mental Health Commission of Canada 2011, p. 7. Used by permission of the Mental Health Commission of Canada.

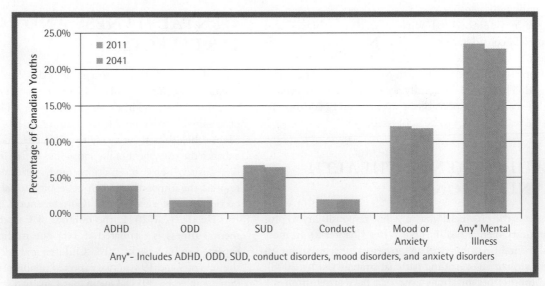

**FIGURE 23.2** Estimated Percentage of Canadian Youth with Mental Illness in 2011–2041 (Ages 9–19 Years)

*Source:* Smetanin, P., Stiff, D., Briante, C., Adair, C. E., Ahmad, S., & Khan, M. (2011). *The life and economic impact of major mental illnesses in Canada 2011–2041.* Risk Analytica, on behalf of the Mental Health Commission of Canada 2011, p. 8. Used by permission of the Mental Health Commission of Canada.

# THE IMPACT OF MENTAL ILLNESS

The global burden of disease attributable to mental and substance use disorder has increased by 37% since 1990; and the largest proportion of the population affected is between the ages of 10 and 29 years, representing a significant loss of productivity and potential. One in five Canadians will experience a mental illness or mental health problem with a cost to the Canadian economy of $50 billion per year (MHCC, 2012). This represents a significant amount of lost potential, disruption to personal and family lifestyles, and costs of medical treatment. Population mental health promotion strategies are urgently needed to address the growing problem of mental illness (Degenhardt et al., 2013).

# RISK FACTORS

The etiology of MI is not fully understood, and the links between specific brain dysfunction and disorders remain unclear. Psychiatric illness is best explained as a combination of complex interactions between genetics, environment, biology, and personality.

**Genetic and Hereditary Influences** Regions of chromosomes have been identified as linking with five major psychiatric disorders: depression, schizophrenia, autism, attention deficit disorder, and bipolar disorder. These genome studies are providing more evidence for the neurological underpinnings of mental illness (McGibbon, 2012). Future research focusing on neurobiology will undoubtedly discover important links to risk and causation.

Alternatively, the root causes of mental illness can be considered through a systemic lens which identifies that people who live with chronic oppression embedded within a social system will develop both physical and mental illnesses. McGibbon (2012) raises the issue of how mental illness must be viewed beyond the biomedical model and that the societal and systemic issues that impact mental illness must converge to the understanding and treating of mental illnesses. McGibbon shows research evidence of physiological needs (such as food, shelter, and safety) and mental illnesses that develop from living in chronic poverty and oppression, which limit one's ability to influence positive changes. Many women and children in Canada also experience domestic violence, which can lead to accumulative complex trauma situations, some of which may be a response to intergenerational trauma related to the colonization of Aboriginal peoples in Canada. Racism, ageism, classism, and heterosexism are identified as factors that contribute to both the poor mental health of populations and debilitating living conditions, such as chronic poverty and lack of opportunities. In addition to broad social changes, community development models require a shift from their central focus of pathology to incorporate individual and collectives strengths of a community.

Schissel (2011) discusses in this report, "About Canada Children and Youth," the state of child and youth mental health in Canada. One in seven children and youth has a mental illness; these children experience anxiety, mood disorders leading to suicidal thoughts and actions, conduct disorder, attention deficit disorder, developmental delays, substance abuse, and eating disorders. Only one in seven of these children and youth received treatment. Causative factors for MI in this population group include genetic and hereditary influences, traumatic and abusive experiences, social pressures, and low self-esteem.

Youth suicide is concerning, with a high incidence in some First Nations and Inuit communities. Current estimates suggest that a significant number (15.6%) of Canadian children are exposed to parental MI, which puts them at risk for psychopathology and behavioural and emotional problems, especially when services for these children are not well integrated into the mental health system (Bassani, Padoin, & Veldhuzein, 2008). A significant number of Canadian college students (6.6%) reported self-harm behaviours, indicative of emotional distress and increased potential for suicide, within the past 12 months (MHCC, 2015). Post-secondary students from 34 Canadian universities represent a population with significant mental health challenges, particularly stress, anxiety, and depression. They struggle with negative feelings and may require significant supports to manage transitions in their lives (see Table 23.2).

The lack of professionals specializing in children's mental health, the stigma related to MI, and the difficulty of diagnosing children's behaviour over their growth and developmental lifespans all contribute to untimely diagnosis and inadequate treatments. Canada urgently requires a multifaceted approach to children's mental health concerns inclusive of assessment, treatment, and universal mental health promotion for all children (see Table 23.3). To respond to this concern, the Canadian Institutes of Health Research's strategic plan for 2013–2017 has targeted integration and improved accessibility of mental health services as a research priority. However, prevention programs remain a low priority in Canadian health policy. Researchers are working toward informing policy makers

| Table 23.2 | Percentage of Canadian Post-Secondary School Students with Mental Health Indicators in the Past Twelve Months |
|---|---|

| Mental Health Indicators | % |
|---|---|
| Exhausted | 89.9% |
| Overwhelmed | 89% |
| Hopeless | 54% |
| Anxiety | 56% |
| Seriously considered suicide in the past 12 months | 10% |

Source: American College Health Assessment. (2013). *National College Association of Health Assessment 11. Canadian Reference Group Data Report, Spring.* Hanover, MD: American College Health Association.

| Table 23.3 | Signs of Mental Illness in Children and Youth |
|---|---|

**Changes in behaviour:** an active child becomes quiet and withdrawn; a good student starts getting poor grades, avoiding places

**Changes in feelings:** feeling unhappy, worried, guilty, angry, fearful, hopeless, or rejected

**Physical symptoms:** frequent headaches, stomach or backaches, problems eating or sleeping, decreased energy

**Changes in thoughts:** saying things that indicate low self-esteem, self-blame, or **suicidal thoughts**, **repetitive thoughts**

**Abuse** of alcohol and/or drugs

**Difficulty coping** with regular activities and everyday problems

**Little regard** for the rights of others: thefts, vandalism

**Odd or repetitive movements** beyond regular play, such as spinning, hand flapping, or head banging

**Deliberate self-harm or talk of suicide**

Source: Adapted from Could my child have mental disorders? *Mental Health in Children and Youth*. Retrieved from http://www.heretohelp.bc.ca/factsheet/mental-illnesses-in-children-and-youth

about evidence-based programs that may be replicated in Canada (Waddell, Hua, Garland, Peters, & McEwan, 2007). (See Canadian Research Box 23.1.)

## Refugees and Immigrants

The 2011 National Household Survey indicated that one in five people living in Canada is a visible minority, with 20.6% of the Canadian population being foreign born. The largest group of immigrants is Asian, including Middle Eastern people (Statistics Canada, 2011). Current high-priority conditions in recently arriving immigrants and refugees, mainly from Africa, include domestic violence, abuse, anxiety, adjustment disorders, depression, torture, and post-traumatic stress disorder (Swinkels, Pottie, Tugwell, Rashid, & Naraslah, 2011). Most clients present with physical symptoms that, if not recognized and investigated as potential mental health problems, may go untreated. Often, clients are uncomfortable with discussing these concerns with healthcare professionals. The use of cultural brokers and interpreters may be helpful, as well as research into patterns of symptom presentation (Kirmayer et al., 2011).

Accessing mental health services is often problematic due to cultural and language barriers. Immigrant and refugee Iranian and Sri Lankan Tamil women who experienced current and pre-immigration abuse from domestic partners reported their experiences as physical symptoms and were silent on mental health symptoms. If practitioners inquire only about physical health symptoms, there is a danger that mental health

### CANADIAN RESEARCH BOX 23.1

**Caregiver Satisfaction with Mental Health Services**

Perreault, M., Provencher, H., Roberts, S., & Milton, D. (2012). Predictors of caregiver satisfaction with mental health services. *Journal of Community Mental Health, 48*, 232–237.

This multidisciplinary team study aimed to determine what factors impact caregivers' satisfaction with services for a family member with mental illness. The sample consisted of 174 family caregivers who spent five hours a day with their family member, were between 18 and 74 years of age, and spent the most time with their family member. The mental health patient had to have a diagnosed mental illness and be between the ages of 18 and 65. Telephone interviews were conducted with family members and scales for Opinion of Outpatient Services, Mental Health Resources, and a service continuity questionnaire were administered. Logistic regression was used in data analysis. Caregivers reported a lack of rehabilitation services, more dissatisfaction with access and organization of services, and increased satisfaction when collaboration was high between professionals and themselves. Caregivers require better access to services and more rehabilitation services.

#### Discussion Questions

1. As a community mental health nurse, what measures can you employ to ensure that family caregivers' needs for rehabilitation services are met?

2. What is the role of the community mental health nurse to advocate and support the caregiver?

issues will not be revealed (Guruge, Roche, & Catallo, 2012) (see Chapter 9, and Canadian Research Box 23.2). Refugees who have experienced collective violence prior to emigration may find it difficult to seek help for the aftermath of these experiences. Nurses need to be aware that females are more willing to discuss trauma experiences, while males may remain silent about their trauma. Mental health services to address these issues must be built in partnership with community engagement (Mabaya & Ray, 2014).

## Prison Inmates

Mental health services in prisons are inadequate. According to the "Annual Report of the Correctional Investigator 2013–2014" (Government of Canada, 2014), there are increasing numbers of federal prisoners who are both mentally ill and addicted, with mental health issues being two to three times more prevalent in prisons than in the general population. Suicide rates for these inmates with co-morbid illnesses are elevated. Due to overcrowding, disease, and violence, the prison environment in Canada is not conducive to

## CANADIAN RESEARCH BOX 23.2

### Mental health and tuberculosis in immigrants

Bender, A., Guruge, S., Hyman, I., & Janjua, M. (2012). Tuberculosis and common mental disorders: International lessons for Canadian immigrant health. *Canadian Journal of Nursing Research, 44*(4), 56–57.

Tuberculosis (TB) is a global concern that often is present in immigrants to Canada. The authors of this study reported on the connections between tuberculosis, mental disorders (anxiety and depression), and underlying social conditions influencing the prevalence of the disease. The article summarized 13 studies in a table that outlines their purpose and immigration focus. Results from the analysis indicate that a high percentage of patients with TB also have co-morbidities of depression and anxiety, as well as social factors of stigma and poverty. Specific implications for Canada are as follows: (a) further exploration of depression, TB, and resettlement stress, (b) research to fully understand the complexity of the experience of TB beyond the medical model, (c) awareness that healthcare providers can inadvertently stigmatize patients by rushing education strategies, and (d) research the racialization of TB to examine why certain populations are prone to this disease. Global research can inform Canadian issues and should be considered. Nurses need to build trust and culturally sensitive care into their helping relationships with new immigrants who have TB.

### Discussion Questions

1. Scoping reviews are one form of nursing research. They are a type of literature review that provides an overview of the type, extent, and quantity of research available on a given topic and can be done prior to a more detailed literature reviews. How can this type of nursing research help people with conditions like TB and co-morbid depression or anxiety?

2. In developing a helping relationship with a new immigrant from Africa who has tested positively for TB, what steps would you take to gain the trust of your client?

the management of mood, behaviour, and disability problems. Often, mentally ill inmates are dealt with by force, solitary confinement, and pepper spray, and yet they do not respond well to punitive measures. A disproportionate number of Aboriginal people are in prisons with a significant number of Aboriginal youth being involved in gang activities. (See Chapter 26.)

Canada's penal system has been criticized for overcrowding, use of solitary confinement for people with serious mental illness, and lack of treatment for mental illness (Canadian Medical Association, 2013). The 2007 death of Ashley Smith, a 19-year-old youth with severe mental illness who died in prison while guards watched her complete a suicide, highlighted the extreme punitive practices of solitary confinement and misguided treatment of a person with a mental illness.

Her death has been ruled a homicide and is now used as a case study to demonstrate the failure of both the healthcare and correctional systems (CBC News, 2013).

## Aboriginal People

Aboriginal people have a suicide rate twice the national average. Societal changes, socioeconomic conditions, and interpersonal problems are risk factors influencing the high mental health needs of Aboriginal people. These risk factors include historical oppression, post-colonization, and the lack of appropriate mental health therapies honouring their cultural perspectives. The legacy of colonization contributes to elevated rates of alcoholism, substance abuse, suicide, domestic violence, overcrowding, poverty, and community demoralization, in addition to the social structural problems experienced in many communities (Bell, 2013; Elias et al., 2012; Kirmayer, Tait, & Simpson, 2009) (see Chapter 22).

The overall suicide rate varies among Aboriginal communities, showing little change since 1979. However, suicide rates for Inuit youth are among the highest in the world, at 11 times the national average rate of suicide in Canada (Health Canada, 2015). High suicide rates, particularly among Inuit youth younger than 25 years, are attributed to the intergenerational effects of historical trauma and its legacy of addictions, depression, and abuse (Chavchamovich & Tomlinson, 2013). Currently, Canada is leading an international study on ways to prevent youth suicide within eight countries with indigenous Arctic populations (Nunavut Bureau of Statistics, 2015; Weber, 2014).

The high incidence of youth suicide in many communities represents a significant loss of potential years of life for the nation. Addictions and depression, both factors in increasing the risk of suicide, are disproportionately represented in the First Nations population. For many First Nation youth, home is not a haven but may be a place where youth are exposed to violence, intergenerational trauma, and multi-systemic problems.

Suicide prevention efforts need to be coordinated and holistic in their approach (Health Canada, 2013). Despite a high proportion of mental health problems, services are underused by Aboriginal people. This is likely due to the fact that most mental health services do not incorporate an Aboriginal understanding of mental health, illness, and healing, and the effects of historical oppression. In the treatment of individual mental health problems, CMHNs must consider the impact of the collective identity and political situations of Aboriginal people and its importance in healing.

## Serious and Persistent Mental Illness

**Serious and persistent mental illness (SPMI)**, formerly described as chronic mental illness, is a term used to describe a non-specific diagnosis, usually schizophrenia, bipolar disorder, substance abuse, personality disorder, or severe depression, resulting in social and functional disability, a prolonged illness, and long-term treatment inclusive of social interventions. Pervasive stigma and fragmented services impede healthcare delivery for this marginalized population (Lawrence & Kisley, 2010).

People with SPMI are disproportionately represented in the Canadian homeless population, with estimates that one-third of homeless people have an SPMI (Forchuk et al., 2008). People who become homeless may develop MI as a result of their circumstances. Poverty, lack of affordable housing, and inadequate discharge planning from hospitals to shelters or the street exacerbate this societal problem. (See Chapter 29.) The recent national multi-site Home/Chez/Soi Housing First project has demonstrated that supportive housing based on recovery principles can decrease prison and psychiatric hospital costs and increase quality of life for people with mental illness (MHCC, 2013b).

## SUICIDE IN CANADA

Suicide is a public health concern affecting all ages and socio-economic classes. In 2011, the prevalence of suicide in Canada was 10.85% per 100 000, with men (16.3%) completing suicides at a significantly higher rate than the rate of 5.4% for women (MHCC, 2015). For every completed suicide, it is estimated that there are 20 suicide attempts. Suicide is one of the leading causes of death in Canadian youth, and is highest in the age group 40 to 59 years with an increased trend in late life for men (MHCC, 2015; Navanneelan, 2012). Deaths by suicide are likely underestimated, as deaths may be labelled as undetermined or accidental. Stigma surrounding suicide prevents populations at risk and their families from seeking help and discussing suicide. Survivors of suicide often feel isolated and experience complex emotions. Survivors of suicide need encouragement to attend self-help groups where they may benefit from discussion with other group members who have experienced suicide deaths. The Public Health Agency of Canada (2013) is working on developing a national strategy on suicide prevention in Canada.

## Contributing Factors to Suicide

**Suicidal behaviours** are classified as suicidal ideation, suicide attempt, and completed suicide. **Suicidal ideation** refers to thoughts about suicide; 13.4% of people have seriously thought about suicide during their lifetime. As suicide attempts are not always reported, their incidence is likely under reported. Statistics indicate that 3.1% of the population over 5 years of age has attempted suicide, with women attempting more than men. Hospitalization rates are higher for women, peaking between the ages of 15 and 19 years and again in mid-life. Mortality due to completed suicides is four times higher among men. Men have historically chosen more fatal methods and been reluctant to seek help. This trend is

changing with some women choosing more lethal suicide methods. A significant proportion of people with suicidal ideation and attempts do not perceive a need for or do not access mental healthcare prior to the event. Community outreach and educational programs for suicide prevention may help decrease this trend.

Developmental crisis, impulsivity, and lack of life experiences make youth particularly vulnerable to suicidal thoughts and attempts. Aboriginal youth aged 15 to 24 years are at increased risk, with suicide and self-inflicted injuries being the leading cause of death for youth and adults under the age of 45. Inuit youth have one of the highest suicide rates in the world (MHCC, 2012). Seniors also face multiple losses of friends and family, health problems, and diminished capacity, and in facing their own mortality may choose to end life (see Chapter 21).

Due to the stigma associated with their sexual identity, lesbian, gay, bisexual, and transgender (LGBT) youth are also at increased risk for suicide. People who "come out" may face increased harassment, while not "coming out" may lead to extreme isolation. LGBT youth require sensitive assessment to determine their suicide risk. Recent trends in Canada include recognition of bisexual, lesbian, gay, queer, and transgendered youth as at risk for suicide with few resources to assist them with mental health issues; teen suicides as a result of cyber bullying; and suicide among armed forces veterans (Dyck, 2013) (see Chapter 20).

A prompt and accurate assessment of suicide lethality is crucial to ensuring the safety of the individual. CMHNs must be comfortable asking directly about suicidal ideation, the suicide plan, the means, and if the person has access to the means. Ropes, firearms, and medications should be removed until the person has received treatment and is safe. Acutely suicidal people require suicide observation in a safe environment. Survivors of suicide often feel isolated and emotionally overwhelmed. They require specific resources to manage their grief and to restore their mental health. Suicide prevention efforts at the provincial, territorial, and national levels must be population-wide and target at-risk populations. Efforts to reduce stigma, increase public awareness of suicidal behaviours, restrict access to lethal means (guns, access to bridges, quantities of over-the-counter medications), and incorporate universal and culturally sensitive mental health promotion in public policy are needed to address the problem of suicide in Canada (Government of Canada, 2006).

## CARING FOR MENTAL HEALTH CLIENTS IN THE COMMUNITY

CMHNs work with individuals, families, aggregates, and populations affected by the major mental illnesses; personality, eating, and trauma-related disorders; and mental health issues across the lifespan. They contribute to population-wide interventions and have a unique opportunity to advocate on issues that impact the mental well-being of Canadians and mental healthcare for people with MI.

## Community Mental Health Service Delivery

The **Mental Health Act** (2010) is a legal document that provides humane and just care to people with MI, while protecting society and individuals with MI from harm. It is evoked when acute treatment services are needed on an involuntarily basis. PMI and family members often have diverse opinions when an involuntary admission is enacted, with PMIs feeling that their rights are violated and family members expressing concerns that their loved ones require treatment. While the Mental Health Act covers multiple details on the rights of PMI, this discussion focuses on two central issues: committal and compulsory treatment orders.

**Committal** Mental Health Acts across Canada vary in their wording and focus on the criteria for curtailing an individual's freedom. There is general consensus that harm to others or self-harm are key deciding factors, with some provinces adding the criteria of potential physical and mental deterioration. Manitoba, Alberta, and British Columbia include potential physical and mental deterioration, while Ontario has specified this may be a criterion only when there is evidence of past successful psychiatric treatment (Davis, 2006). CMHNs need to be familiar with the Mental Health Act in their province and issues related to the diverse perspectives of PMI, their families, and the public.

**Compulsory Treatment Orders** Compulsory treatment orders (CTOs) decree that PMIs must be compliant with treatment or they must return to the hospital. The laws on CTOs vary among provinces, with Saskatchewan, Ontario, and British Columbia having statutes for CTOs. Manitoba has a statue on Leave Certificates. There is a trend toward this type of legislation (Davis, 2006).

## SERVICE ORIENTATION

Discussion regarding resource allocation for an adequate balance of mental health services in the institutional and community sectors continues. Service reorganization has not yet provided comprehensive supports to enable recovery from MI, nor has it implemented a national, population-based mental health promotion strategy. Practising CMHNs will be aware of the need for improvement in mental health services.

Three main problems affect service orientation. First, while the move from institutions to intersectoral community services is expected to ultimately reduce costs, currently both systems must be operated with continued community services investment. An institutional bias requiring public funding of physician and hospital services disadvantages people with limited incomes when trying to obtain alternative services. In remote and rural regions, adequate mental health services are lacking. Second, comprehensive services must be intersectoral and address the basic determinants of health to enable recovery. Housing remains a major problem, with 27% of people with MI unable to find and afford adequate housing (Kirby & Keon, 2006). Third, stigma and discrimination are formidable barriers preventing people from accessing services. The principles of recovery, which challenge society's assumptions regarding MI, are beginning to be implemented into policy and services.

Mental health resources are organized around primary, secondary, and tertiary services. Primary intervention's goal is to prevent new cases and reduce the rate of development of mental disorder in the community. It occurs through mental health promotion. Key strategies involve promoting healthy growth and development of individuals and resourcefulness of the family and the community. Secondary intervention focuses on the early screening and diagnosis of PMI, healing strategies, and the health promotion of individuals, families, and communities. The goal is to reduce episodes of acute distress and the prevalence of MI in the community. Tertiary intervention focuses on treatment and case management of people with MI, with emphasis on rehabilitation and recovery through tangible resources, psycho-education, and rehabilitative strategies. The goal of tertiary intervention is to reduce the severity of the illness and associated disability and to assist people in recovery from MI.

## Organization of Services in the Mental Health System

**Emergency Services** Emergency services, consisting of admissions to hospital and crisis stabilization units, are initiated through general hospitals' emergency wards, where services are organized for medical emergencies, not psychiatric emergencies. General or psychiatric hospitals provide services for serious acute illness, while **crisis stabilization units** provide services to less-acutely ill people, generally judged by indicators of self-harm or homicide. Additional services include 24-hour mobile crisis response teams and professional and peer support telephone crisis lines.

Outpatient clinics and specialized programs, for example, as well as eating disorder programs and child and adolescent treatment clinics may be offered as follow-up services in the form of day hospitals, day treatment, and daycare settings. Community mental health workers follow people with MI in the community but often carry large caseloads that leave little time for consistent intervention.

**Case Management** Case management is a best-practice model providing assistance to PMIs and families to negotiate the mental health system. Case managers coordinate long-term care, providing and negotiating services for holistic needs related to physical health, leisure, education, and housing. Case management fosters continuity and coordination of care.

**Assertive Community Treatment** **Assertive community treatment (ACT)** is a comprehensive, long-term intensive case management approach to treating persons who have an SMI, a functional impairment, and are intensive users of the healthcare system. **Functional impairment** refers to an inability to look after hygiene, nutritional needs, and finances, and inability to develop or sustain support systems. Outreach services decrease hospitalizations by addressing compliance issues and improving the quality of community life. Programs exist in many areas of Canada and are noted in best-practice documents as vital to the coordination of services for this difficult-to-serve population.

**Primary Health Care Services** **Primary health care services** include a wide range of services, and the first contact is often a general practitioner with little time and limited expertise in mental illness. This can result in over-prescribing of medications and fewer people being assessed by mental health specialists. Integrating mental health practitioners with primary health care providers is a goal of the collaborative care movement. This shared care could involve telephone access to psychiatrists or on-site psychiatrists at clinics.

**Early Intervention Programs** **Early intervention programs** arose in response to treatment delays. These programs attempt to intervene prior to a full-blown episode of MI to mitigate the illness's effects. The **early psychosis intervention (EPI) program** addresses the stigma and demoralization associated with MI, supports family, and actively seeks timely treatment and follow-up (Thomas & Nandrha, 2009).

**Co-occurring Disorder Programs** **Co-occurring disorders** refer to the existence of a psychiatric diagnosis and an additional diagnosis of substance abuse. Currently, programs exist that address both MI and addiction. People with anxiety disorders and depression have higher rates of substance dependence than the general population. Acceptance of both addictions and MIs as conditions requiring treatment that may be long term, inclusive of relapse, is crucial (Davis, 2006).

**Self-Help and Peer Support** These programs are an integral part of services for PMI and their families and allow them to share their lived experiences with one another. Recommendations to fund these programs from public funding attest to their value. Current discussion suggests increasing the number of paid peer support helpers and peer counsellors. Research in this area is new but shows promise for innovation (Kirby & Keon, 2006).

**Mental Health Promotion** **Mental health promotion** emphasizes positive mental health and recognizes the personal, social, economic, and environmental factors that contribute to mental health. Mental health promotion is becoming increasingly prominent in the mental health and public health systems. Recommendations to include mental health promotion

in a "Pan-Canadian Healthy Living Strategy" and the development of a "Canadian Mental Health Guide" demonstrate the growing trend to incorporate mental health promotion at a policy level. Suicide prevention efforts inclusive of a national policy to decrease suicidal behaviour and completed suicides in Canada are under discussion.

# Mental Health Service Delivery Models

**The Recovery Model** The **recovery model** arose from the writings of PMIs who challenged the need for professional attitudes and suggested that MI irrevocably led to deterioration and diminished lives (Anthony, 2000). In consultation with the Boston University Center for Psychiatric Rehabilitation, the recovery model has been implemented in parts of the mental health system. The assumptions of recovery challenge the status quo to re-examine psychiatric mental health service delivery. Essential services are crisis intervention, case management, rehabilitation, enrichment, rights protection, basic support, self-help, wellness, and prevention. The Canadian Mental Health Association, Ontario (2014) describes recovery as a personal process where some people may live with mental illness symptoms in recovery and others look to being symptom free, but both experience more control and optimism about their diagnoses. (See Table 23.4.)

**Collaborative Mental Healthcare Model** The Canadian Collaborative Mental Health Initiative has created a body of evidence-based research papers and toolkits (available from www.ccmhi.ca). The initiative has proposed collaboration among primary health care services, consumers and families, and interdisciplinary healthcare providers to provide optimal mental healthcare for all Canadians. A **collaborative mental healthcare model** consists of consumers, family and caregivers, and multidisciplinary healthcare providers from mental health and primary care services to provide more

| Table 23.4 | Recovery Principles |
|---|---|

Recovery is unique. There is no one path.

Recovery occurs even though symptoms reoccur. Recovery occurs within MI.

Recovery increases control, meaning, and purpose while living with a mental illness.

Recovery orientation to services emphasizes the person is central to planning care.

WRAP—Wellness Recovery Action Plans help people self-manage their illness, connect with helpers, and become empowered and optimistic.

Source: Adapted from http://ontario.cmha.ca/mental-health/mental-health-conditions/recovery. Canadian Mental Health Association, Ontario.

coordinated and effective service. This model delivers mental health promotion, prevention, detection, and treatment of mental illness, rehabilitation, and recovery support.

## Nursing Role in Case Finding and Referral

Early identification and treatment of MI reduces its severity and promotes quicker recovery. For example, timely referral can decrease secondary problems of substance abuse and depression commonly associated with anxiety disorders. CMHNs providing mental health promotion programs will have opportunities to assess people at risk or who are not receiving appropriate services. CMHNs play an important role in screening for physical health problems and adherence to medical treatment in the SMI population who are at risk for physical disorders and non-adherence to treatment plans. Within family nursing, CMHNs can assess children living with a parent with MI and ensure that the children's needs are met. CMHNs may also refer parents to parenting programs to assist them with parenting skills.

Advocacy is needed to negotiate the mental health system (Kirby & Keon, 2006). Finding services when one is stressed is difficult. CMHNs ease this tension for PMI and their families, ensuring their concerns are represented and their rights are protected, and accessing appropriate services. CMHNs advocate for funding for new community programs based on needs and best-practice evidence, serve on advisory boards, and lobby to influence healthy public policy. They play a significant advocacy role in reducing social inequities that impede mental health and recovery from MI.

## Nursing Role in Education and Counselling

CMHNs provide education to the general public, to targeted groups, and to individuals and families. The recovery and collaborative care models provide a framework for developing therapeutic relationships with consumers, families, and communities. Within therapeutic relationships, CMHNs promote self-care, develop coping abilities, and foster social support networks. In crises, these nurses work with PMI and families to find appropriate resources. Individual and group educational counselling promotes discussion of the signs of MI, medication, treatment options, and the recovery model. CMHNs support peer and self-help recovery-based programs; facilitate cognitive behavioural therapy groups; and organize educational programs for the general public to promote mental health and reduce risk factors associated with mental illness, including programs to inform schools and children of ways to help protect children and to reduce the risk of abuse, which is a precursor to mental health problems. Such programs can offer information on specific illnesses, stigma, and suicide prevention. CMHNs can create educational programs to increase public awareness of the issues surrounding MI and mental health.

# FUTURE DIRECTIONS AND IMPLICATIONS FOR NURSING

Reports on mental health services in Canada demonstrate the need for continued support for PMI and their families and have called for integrated comprehensive services from diverse sectors, such as income and housing (Davis, 2006; Goering et al., 2014). Increased recognition of peer support programs, family contributions to care, self-help, and the principles of recovery are beginning to change service delivery. CMHNs will face challenges to address the needs of specific populations at risk for mental health problems, contribute to innovative programs for mental health promotion targeted at the Canadian population, and support policy changes at the national level and commit to the anti–mental health stigma campaign.

Changes in the community mental health system call for comprehensive funding to address societal barriers that impede PMI. Vulnerable target populations such as children, adolescents, First Nations people, inmates, people with co-occurring disorders, and SMI will require specific nursing intervention and health promotion strategies. CMHNs have the opportunity to be part of the changes that are occurring. They can prepare themselves to address gaps in mental health services. CMHNs play a key role in facilitating peer programs, self-help groups, and family advocacy and support groups. The recovery model outlines approaches to working with

## CASE STUDY

You are a community health nurse working with inner-city youth whose daily lives include challenges with poverty, racism, substance abuse, and trauma. For the past six months you have been conducting weekly "Ask the Nurse" health clinics at Youth Power, an organization that assists youth to return to school and find housing, counselling, and educational supports. You have frequently worked with Gary, a 24-year-old young man who is a well-liked peer counsellor who encourages youth to return to school and live healthy lifestyles. Gary has had many personal challenges related to substance abuse, poverty, and homelessness. He is a role model for youth who come to the program. On Monday, you arrive at Youth Power and the program director tells you that Gary has died by suicide on the weekend after learning that the apartment he planned on renting would not be available. You feel an overwhelming sense of sadness and discouragement.

### Discussion Questions

1. What resources can help you to process your feelings in order to practise self-care and continue to work with the youth?

2. How will you assist the youth to understand why Gary died by suicide and process their emotions?

3. How can CHNs support peer youth workers who may still be struggling with their personal circumstances?

people with MI while acknowledging the support structures that people require to live successfully in the community. Future directions require focused nursing efforts to affect policy and health determinants and to work collaboratively in new ways and relationships.

CMHNs have the capacity to encourage and support clients and families to become actively involved in the work of the Mental Health Commission. CMHNs' grounding in the realities that clients, families, and communities face propels them to advocate for services and to work collaboratively with their family and community partners. CMHNs will provide valuable input in knowledge exchange and translation by engaging in pertinent research and facilitating dissemination of research findings (Mental Health Commission of Canada, 2012).

## CONCLUSION

When working with PMI, their families, and their communities, nurses are practising in a system that is undergoing change. New models propose reconfigurations of care that honour personal narratives of PMI and families and change the nurse–person relationship. These changes will challenge nursing to examine practice and nursing's openness to innovations. Population data sets will assist nurses to identify vulnerable groups and direct healthcare and promotion efforts toward them. As colonialism's effects on mental health are recognized and traditional Aboriginal wisdom is incorporated into therapies for Aboriginal peoples, nurses are also challenged to understand the effects of historical oppression on health and incorporate new ways to promote healing. As cultural diversity increases within Canadian society, nurses will consider alternative ways of understanding MI. Perhaps, most importantly, the recovery model and the integration of a collaborative model of mental healthcare will help nurses to focus on consumers' abilities to build meaningful lives and will strengthen nurses' resolve to change the inequities that influence the mental well-being of people living with MI.

## KEY TERMS

assertive community treatment (ACT)   p. 424
Canadian Mental Health Association (CMHA)   p. 417
case management   p. 423
collaborative mental healthcare model   p. 424
co-occurring disorders   p. 424
crisis stabilization units   p. 423
early intervention programs   p. 424
early psychosis intervention (EPI) program   p. 424
emergency services   p. 423
functional impairment   p. 424
Mental Health Act   p. 423
mental health promotion   p. 424
mental health   p. 417
mental illness (MI)   p. 417
primary health care services   p. 424
recovery model of rehabilitation   p. 416
recovery model   p. 424
serious and persistent mental illness (SPMI)   p. 421

suicidal behaviours   p. 422
suicidal ideation   p. 422

## STUDY QUESTIONS

1. Knowing the history of the mental health system in Canada can help nurses understand current issues. From what you have read about the process of deinstitutionalization, how do you think this may have impacted the current problems in the mental health system?

2. Suicide continues to be a troubling problem in Canadian society. Identify groups who are at risk for suicide. Explain four strategies you might use in your community nursing practice to decrease suicide in these groups.

3. Define mental health promotion and consider how you would implement strategies to promote mental health in the frail elderly living in the community, new immigrant mothers, and suburban high school students.

4. Consider the risk factors for mental illness. How can community mental health nurses reduce risk factors within their practice communities?

5. Recently there has been a national report on the state of mental health services in Canada. Identify and discuss four recommendations from this report.

After working through these questions, go to the MyNursingLab at www.pearsoned.ca/mynursinglab to check your answers.

## INDIVIDUAL CRITICAL-THINKING EXERCISES

1. What strategies might a community mental health nurse use to promote the mental health of elementary school age children?

2. How would a community mental health nurse implement the recovery model with a depressed client and their family?

3. Why do you think "people first" language (i.e., a person with schizophrenia rather than schizophrenic) is important?

4. What issues are important to consider in designing mental health services for diverse cultural groups?

5. What are the unique challenges that face First Aboriginal people in restoring mental health and healing to their communities?

## GROUP CRITICAL-THINKING EXERCISES

1. How might CMHNs ensure that the physical and mental health needs of people with MI are met within a primary health care clinic?

2. How might CMHNs influence and develop a national suicide prevention strategy?

3. How can the principles of recovery be implemented and researched within the mental health system?

# REFERENCES

Anthony, W. A. (2000). A recovery service system: Setting some systems level standards. *Psychiatric Rehabilitation Journal, 24*(2), 160–166.

Bassani, D. G., Padoin, C. V., Phillip, D., & Veldhuzein, S. (2008). Estimating the number of children exposed to parental psychiatric disorders through a national health survey. *Child and Adolescent Psychiatry and Mental Health, 3*(1), (6). doi:10.1186/1753-2000-3-6

Bell, J. (2013, June 6) *Suicide in Nunavut: Child abuse, pot smoking, mental disorders the biggest factors.* Retrieved from http://www.nunatsiaqonline.ca/stories/article/65674suicide_in_nunavut_child_abuse_pot_smoking_mental_disorders_the_bigges/

CBC News. (2013). *Ashley Smith's coroner's jury rules prison death a homicide.* Retrieved from http://www.cbc.ca/news/canada/new-brunswick/ashley-smith-coroner-s-jury-rules-prison-death-a.-homicide-1.2469527

Canadian Institute of Health Research. (2012). *The first decade.* Institute of Human Development, Child and Youth Health. Retrieved from http://www.cihr-irsc.gc.ca/e/45247.html#a1

Canadian Medical Association. (2013). Imprisoning the mentally ill. *Canadian Medical Association Journal, 19, 185*(3), 201–202.

Canadian Mental Health Association, Ontario. (2014). *Recovery.* Retrieved from http://ontario.cmha.ca/mental-health/mental-health-conditions/recovery

Chachamovich, E., & Tomlinson, M. (2013). Nunavut suicide follow-back study: Identifying the risk factors for Inuit suicide in Nunavut. *Learning from lives that have been lived.* Retrieved from https://torontodistresscentre.com/sites/torontodistresscentre.com/files/Learning%20from%20lives%20that%20have%20been%20lived.pdf

Davis, S. (2006). *Community mental health in Canada: Policy, theory, and practice.* Vancouver, BC: UBC Press.

Degenhardt, L., Whitford, H. A., Ferrari, A. J., Baxter, A. J., Charlson, F. J., Hall, W. D., & Vos, T. (2013). Global burden of disease attributable to illicit drug use and dependence: Findings from the Global Burden of Disease Study 2010. *The Lancet, 382*(9904), 1564–1574. doi:10.1016/S0140-6736(13)61530-5

Dyck, D. R. (2013). *Report on outcomes and recommendations: LBGTQ youth suicide prevention summit.* Egale Canada Human Rights Trust. Retrieved from http://egale.ca/wp-content/uploads/2013/02/YSPS-Report-online.pdf

Elias, B., Mignone, J., Hall, M., Hong, S., Hart, L., & Sareen, J. (2012). Trauma and suicide behaviour histories among a Canadian indigenous population: An empirical exploration of the potential role of Canada's residential school system. *Social Science and Medicine, 74*(10), 1560–1569.

Forchuk, C., MacClure, S. K., Van Beers, M., Smith, C., Csternik, R., Hoch, J., & Jensen, E. (2008). Developing and testing an intervention to prevent homelessness among individuals discharged from psychiatric wards to shelters and "no fixed address." *Journal of Psychiatric and Mental Health Nursing, 15*, 569–575.

Goering, P., Veldhuizen, S., Watson, A., Adair, C., Kopp, B., Latimer, E., Nelson, G., MacNaughton, E., Streiner, D., & Aubry, T. (2014). National At Home/Chez Soi Final Report. Calgary, AB: Mental Health Commission of Canada. Retrieved from: http://www.mentalhealthcommission.ca

Goering, P., Wasylenki, D., & Durbin, J. (2000). Canada's mental health system. *International Journal of Law and Psychiatry, 23*(3–4), 345–359.

Government of Canada. (2006). *The human face of mental health and mental illness in Canada 2006* (Cat. no. HP5-19/2006E). Ottawa, ON: Minister of Public Works and Government Services. Retrieved from http://www.phac-aspc.gc.ca/publicat/human-humain06/pdf/human_face_e.pdf

Government of Canada. (2014). *Annual report of the office of the correctional investigator 2013–14.* Office of the correctional investigator. Retrieved from http://www.oci-bec.gc.ca/cnt/rpt/annrpt/annrpt20132014-eng.aspx

Griffiths, K. M., Crisp, D. A., Jorm, A. F., & Christensen, H. (2011). Does stigma predict a belief in dealing with depression alone? *Journal of Affective Disorders, 132*, 413–417.

Guruge, S., Roche, B., & Catallo, C. (2012). Violence against women: An exploration of the physical and mental health trends among immigrant and refugee women in Canada. *Nursing Research and Practice, 434*–592. doi:10.1155/2012/434592

Health Canada, First Nations and Inuit Health. (2015). *Mental health and wellness.* Ottawa, ON: Government of Canada. Retrieved from http://www.hc-sc.gc.ca/fniah-spnia/promotion/mental/index-eng.php

Kirby, M. J. (2008). Mental health in Canada: Out of the shadows forever. *Canadian Medical Association Journal, 178*(10), 1320–1322.

Kirby, M. J., & Keon, W. J. (2006). *Out of the shadows at last: Transforming mental health, mental illness and addictions services in Canada.* Ottawa, ON: Standing Senate Committee on Social Affairs, Science and Technology.

Kirkmayer, L. J., Tait, C., & Simpson, C. (2009). The mental health of Aboriginal peoples in Canada: Transformations of identity and community. In L. J. Kirkmayer & G. Guthrie Valaskakis (Eds.), *Healing traditions. The mental health of Aboriginal peoples in Canada.* (pp. 3–35). Vancouver: UBC Press.

Kirmayer, L. J., Narashlah, L., Munoz, M., Rashid, M., Ryder, A., Guzder, . . . Pottie, K. (2011). Common mental health problems in immigrants and refugees: General approach in primary care. *Canadian Medical Association Journal, 183*(12), 959–967.

Lawrence, D., & Kisley, S. (2010). Inequities in healthcare provision for people with severe mental illness. *Journal of Psychopharmacology, 24*(4 Suppl), 61–68. Retrieved from http://www.ncbi.nlm.nih.gov/pmc/articles/PMC2951586

Leavey, J. E. (2015). *Living recovery: Youth speak out on "owning" mental illness.* Waterloo: Wilfred Laurier University Press.

Mabaya, G., & Ray, S. L. (2014). The meaning of health and help-seeking behaviours among refugees who have experienced collective violence prior to emigration: A Canadian perspective. *Canadian Journal of Community Mental Health, 33*(3), 71–85.

McGibbon, E. (2012). *Oppression: A social determinant of health.* Winnipeg, MB: Fernwood.

Mental Health Commission of Canada. (2012). *Changing directions, changing lives. The mental health strategy for Canada, Summary.* Calgary, AB: Author.

Mental Health Commission of Canada. (2013a). *Opening minds interim report.* Used by permission of the Mental Health Commission of Canada. Retrieved from http://www.mentalhealthcommission.ca/English/system/files/private/document/opening_minds_interim_report.pdf

Mental Health Commission of Canada. (2013b). *Housing and homelessness*. Retrieved from http://www.mentalhealthcommission.ca/English/issues/housing-and-homelessness

Mental Health Commission of Canada. (2015). *Informing the future: Mental health indicators for Canada*. Retrieved from http://www.mentalhealthcommission.ca/English/system/files/private/document/MHCC_MentalHealthIndicators_Jan2015_ENG.pdf

Navanneelan, N. (2012). *Suicide rates: An overview*. Cat. no. 82-624 X. Ottawa: Health Canada. Retrieved from http://www.statcan.gc.ca/pub/82-624-x/2012001/article/11696-eng.pdf

Nolan, P. W. (1993). A history of the training of asylum nurses. *Journal of Advanced Nursing, 18*(8), 1193–1201.

Nunavut Bureau of Statistics. (2015, June 3). Nunavut suicides by region, sex, age group and ethnicity, 1999 to 2014. Retrieved from http://www.stats.gov.nu.ca/Publications/Historical/Deaths/Nunavut%20Suicides%20by%20Region,%20Sex,%20Age%20Group%20and%20Ethnicity,%201999%20to%202014.xlsx

Public Health Agency of Canada. (2013). *Consultations on the development of a federal framework for suicide prevention*. Retrieved from http://www.phac-aspc.gc.ca/mh-sm/mhp-psm/new-nouv-eng.php

Ryan-Nicholls, K. D., & Haggarty, J. M. (2007). Collaborative mental health care in rural and isolated Canada: Stakeholder feedback. *Journal of Psychosocial Nursing, 45*(12), 37–45.

Schissel, B. (2011). *About Canada: Children and youth*. Black Point, NS: Fernwood Publishing.

Smetanin, P., Stiff, D., Briante, C., Adair, C. E., Ahmad, S., & Khan, M. (2011). The life and economic impact of major mental illnesses in Canada, 2011–2041.

Risk Analytica, on behalf of the Mental Health Commission of Canada 2011.

Statistics Canada. (2003, updated 2004, 2007). *Canadian community health survey: Mental health and well-being*. Retrieved from http://www.statcan.ca/bsolc/english/bsolc?catno=82-617-X&CHROPG=1

Statistics Canada. (2011). *National Household Survey: Immigration, place of birth, citizenship, ethnic origin, visible minorities, language and religion*. Retrieved from http://www.statcan.gc.ca/daily-quotidien/130508/dq130508b-eng.htm?WT.mc_id=twtB3796

Sussman, S. (1998). The first asylums in Canada: A response to neglectful community care and current trends. *Canadian Journal of Psychiatry, 43*, 260–264.

Swinkels, H., Pottie, K., Tugwell, P., Rashid, M., & Naraslah, L. (2011). Development of guidelines for recently arrived immigrants and refugees to Canada: Delphi consensus on selecting preventable and treatable conditions. *Canadian Medical Association Journal, 183*(12), 928–932.

Thomas, S. P., & Nandrha, H. S. (2009). Early intervention in psychosis: A retrospective analysis of clinical and social factors influencing duration of untreated psychosis. *Primary Care Companion Journal of Clinical Psychiatry, 11*(5), 212–214.

Waddell, C., Hua, J., Garland, O., Dev Peters, R., & McEwan, K. (2007). Preventing mental disorders in children: A systematic review to inform policy-making. *Canadian Journal of Public Health, 98*(3), 166–173.

Weber, B. (2014, November 12). Canada leading global effort to curb high Inuit suicide rate. Retrieved from http://www.theglobeandmail.com/news/national/canada-leading-global-effort-to-curb-high-rate-of-inuit-suicide/article21419168

## ABOUT THE AUTHOR

**Elaine Mordoch**, RN, PhD, is an Associate Professor in the College of Nursing, Faculty of Health Science at the University of Manitoba. She has practised as a primary nurse in acute psychiatry, and facilitated community groups for the well elderly living with depression and for women identifying abuse in their relationships. She has developed and managed COPE (Care of Psychiatric Emergencies) for a tertiary hospital general emergency unit with a focus on family care and intermediate follow-up services. Her research interest focuses on children and families living with parental mental illness. She is particularly interested in children's perceptions of their lives and ways to strengthen families. She is also interested in the long-term effects of childhood trauma on adult survivors. Currently she conducts research on mental health topics, teaches psychiatric/mental health nursing, qualitative research methods, and counselling skills in Nursing and in the Aboriginal Focus Programs at the University of Manitoba.

# Rural Health

*Judith Kulig, Martha MacLeod, Norma Stewart,
Mary Ellen Andrews, Erin Wilson, and Kelley Kilpatrick*

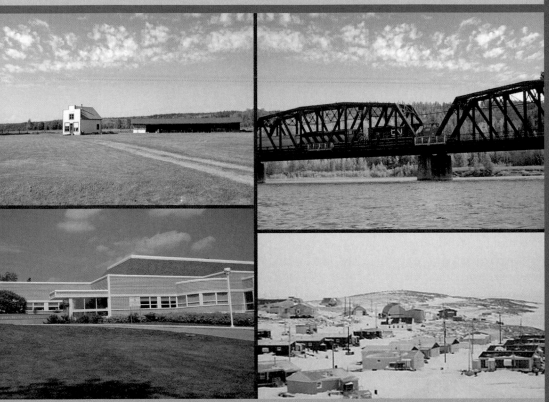

Sources: *Courtesy of Mary Ellen Andrews/University of Saskatchewan; Erin Wilson/University of Northern British Columbia; Erin Wilson/University of Northern British Columbia; Martha MacLeod/University of Northern British Columbia*

## LEARNING OUTCOMES

**After studying this chapter, you should be able to:**

1. Describe the meaning of rural in a Canadian context.

2. Analyze the impact of rural contexts on the health status and access to care of rural residents.

3. Recognize challenges and rewards associated with being a rural resident in Canada.

4. Explain the context of rural nursing practice and its interrelationship with the care of clients in rural areas.

5. Identify barriers to, and facilitators of, the development of a nursing role in a rural community and identify evidence-informed strategies that support role development.

6. Apply the intervention levels of prevention (primary, secondary, and tertiary) in relation to rural nursing practice.

7. Formulate an example of how a rural nurse can implement evidence-informed practice when providing care to rural residents.

8. Identify how the Canadian Community Health Nursing Standards for Practice can be utilized to work with unique populations within rural communities.

## INTRODUCTION

This chapter introduces concepts relevant to caring for clients in rural areas. The character of rural and remote Canada is delineated, with an emphasis on diversity. This discussion provides a contextual understanding of clients who live in these areas and some of the practice characteristics of rural nurses. We refer to nursing practice in both rural and remote sites as "rural." The reason for this decision is that the definitions of rural and remote given by registered nurses (RNs) in a national survey (Kulig et al., 2008) fit within the same overarching themes. These include community characteristics; geographical location; health, human, and technical resources; and nursing practice characteristics. In addition, some rurality indexes include "remote" but there is no consensus in the literature about the definition of this term, which is often context dependent. In the chapter, key features of rural nursing practice are identified and explained in depth. Critical-thinking questions enable opportunities for discussion and application of the materials presented.

# THE CHARACTERISTICS OF RURAL AND REMOTE CANADA

## Definitions

Approximately 95% of Canada's land mass, or 9.5 million square kilometres, can be considered rural and remote (Public Health Agency of Canada, 2005). However, longstanding debate exists about the definitions of key terms, including "rural," "remote," "northern," and "isolated." Pitblado (2005) has noted two main ways to define rural: technical and social.

**Technical approaches** to the definition of rural include locators or geographic regions, like the location of hospitals, roads, or specific political areas (i.e., provinces, counties). Statistics Canada (du Plessis, Beshiri, & Bollman, 2001) has examined six possible ways to define rural, with each emphasizing different criteria, such as population size, population density, and settlement or labour market contexts. One example is the definition of "census rural," which refers to "individuals living in the countryside outside centres of 1 000 or more population" (du Plessis et al., 2001, p. 6). The Canadian Institute for Health Information (CIHI) adds the notion of distance to, and relationship with, urban areas (CIHI, 2013). The First Nations and Inuit Health Branch (FNIHB) within Health Canada (2005) defines the degrees of rurality as follows:

1. *non-isolated community* includes communities with road access of less than 90 kilometres to physician services;
2. *semi-isolated community* includes communities with road access greater than 90 kilometres to physician services;
3. *isolated community* refers to communities with good telephone service, scheduled air transportation flights, but no road access; and
4. *remote, isolated community* means the communities have no scheduled air flights, minimal telephone or radio access, and no road access.

The FNIHB designations highlight the importance of access to services and the types of locally available health services while considering transportation and communication limitations as important factors in their differentiation. (See Photo 24.1 for illustration of alternate transportation.) A wide variety of indices of rurality exist, such as the Canadian General Practice Rurality Index (Leduc, 1997) or the Rurality Index of Ontario (Kralj, 2001). Many of these indices of rurality are only of theoretical value as they have never been put into operation. And almost all of them have been designed with physicians—not nurses—in mind. In the analysis of the perceptions of rurality by rural RNs, Kulig et al. (2008) concluded that there was no benefit in developing a national numerical index of rurality based on distance to services because of the variability of absolute distance (ranging from 20 to 1000 kilometres). In addition, most rurality models focus on deficits rather than the strengths of rural communities.

**Social approaches** to defining rural refer to the nature of the rural community, including such features as specific services that are normally associated with larger population sizes (e.g.,

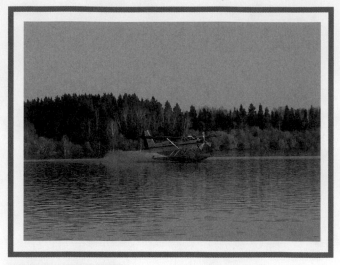

**PHOTO 24.1** Float plane landing on Lac La Ronge, adjacent to La Ronge, Saskatchewan

*Source: Courtesy of Judith C. Kulig/University of Lethbridge*

specific types of stores or restaurants) (Pitblado, 2005). Although the social nature of place in defining rural is relevant to health-care service delivery, particularly the recruitment and retention of health professionals, including registered nurses (RNs), there has been limited work done on examination of its specific meaning or application. The definition offered by Statistics Canada identifies "rural and small town" as "individuals in towns or municipalities outside the commuting zone of larger urban centres" (du Plessis et al., 2001, p. 6). Using this definition, in 2011, 6 041 723 or 18% of Canadians lived in communities with populations of less than 10 000 people (CIHI, 2013). This is the definition of rural employed in this chapter. It is selected because of its growing use in studies of rural issues in Canada, including the determinants of health and the delivery of healthcare.

## Diversity of Rural

Rural Canada is not homogeneous. Rural economies vary by the specific geographic features of the land itself. Traditionally, rural economies have been dependent on the natural resources reflective of the geographic landscape, such as oil and gas extraction, forestry, fishing, and agriculture. It is incumbent on nurses to understand the socioeconomic context in the community where they work, given its influence on the determinants on health.

The resource base of the community will influence the health status of those who live in it. In rural, remote, and isolated communities where there is a heavy reliance on industries such as oil and gas, logging, mining, fishing, and agriculture, there are interrelated injuries and illnesses that impact the affected individual as well as the community at large. For example, in 2011 there were 293 925 farm operators across Canada (Statistics Canada, 2011). Operators on medium-sized farms had the highest incidence of injury because they worked the longest hours without reliance on hired help in comparison to those on the largest farms (Maltais, 2010). Farm operators are also aging, possibly contributing to the higher incidences of injury in an industry that continues to have one of the highest fatality rates (Maltais, 2007). According to statistics from the Association of Workers' Compensation Boards of Canada (AWCB), in 2011, there were 3 083 accepted time-loss injuries (i.e., "an injury where a worker is compensated for a loss of wages following a work-related injury") and 18 fatalities in the agriculture and related service industry across Canada. The Canadian Agricultural Injury Reporting (CAIR) system found that between 1990 and 2008 there were 104 annual average number of deaths, with 70% being machine related and 92% of the fatalities being male (CAIR, 2012).

Other natural resource industries also employ a significant number of individuals and impact rural areas; for example, the oil and gas sector employs 230 000 individuals (Electric Canadian, n. d.). Individuals who work within the oil and gas, logging, and mining industries may experience personal health issues, such as respiratory problems from environmental exposure to reduced air and water quality as well as the potential for accidents while on the job (Fraser Basin Council, 2012). For instance, those in the logging industry and specifically individuals who work in sawmills are exposed to wood dust, which can lead to acute and chronic upper and lower respiratory health conditions (Demers, 2011). In 2011, there were 1 391 accepted time-loss injuries and 15 deaths in the logging and forestry industry, and 2 814 accepted time-loss injuries and 75 deaths in the mining, quarrying, and oil well industries across Canada (AWCB, 2011). Events such as explosions (e.g., the Burns Lake Sawmill in 2012), oil spills, and mining accidents all have the potential to affect not just those who are directly impacted by the event but also family and friends who must deal with death or long-term health impacts of community members, as well as the potential for the loss of employment and the ultimately negative long-term changes in the community. Finally, the fishing industry has its own associated issues, as noted in the 2011 statistics: 477 accepted time-loss injuries in the fishing and trapping industry and five fatalities (AWCB, 2011).

In some natural-resource-dependent areas, industrial camps are set up for varying periods of time. The local health regions may be responsible for enforcing environmental and public health regulations for the camp as well as helping to address health issues that may arise (Northern Health, 2012). Specific health issues that may arise involve impacts of shift work, which might include obesity, emotional distress, and domestic issues, all of which may be interrelated with substance abuse (Northern Health, 2012). Another issue that community health nurses (CHNs) will need to address is the perception among workers that cancer can be attributed to working in the oil and gas industry (Fraser Basin Council, 2012); this has implications for individual and community health assessments in identifying trends among such diseases.

The socioeconomic status of rural communities is not static. For example, in areas where these resources are depleted, or when global pricing and demand decreases, communities often seek alternate economic ventures, such as tourism, to sustain their economic and social viability. As the populations change, so do the health needs of the communities. The village of Queen Charlotte, illustrated by the hospital pictured in Photo 24.2, is a place where tourism is valued.

## Being Rural

Emphasizing such notions as a "type" of rural person can lead to generalizations and inaccurate descriptions of the variety of people who live in rural settings. Rural areas reported higher proportions of people with low income and less than a secondary education level. At the same time, a greater proportion of rural residents reported a strong sense of community belonging than did their urban counterparts (DesMeules et al., 2006). Instead of resorting to stereotypes of rural residents, it is more useful for nursing practice to discuss the intersection between rural living and the meanings of health and health status.

Rural residents have been the focus of studies examining the meaning of health. Research that focused on the health beliefs of rural Canadians in two western provinces found that being healthy was defined as having a holistic relationship among mental, social, physical, and spiritual aspects. The participants defined sickness as being a curable and short-term condition, whereas illness was perceived as chronic and life-threatening (Thomlinson, McDonagh, Baird, Crooks, & Lees, 2004). Rural domestic violence in general and elder abuse in particular are of special concern. Rural communities often lack the resources to address these issues from legal and social standpoints (Spencer, 2000) or from social services perspectives (Dimah & Dimah, 2013). In addition, rural elderly who experience abuse are often women who are reluctant to come forward (Cornes, Manthorpe, & Haselden, 2010) and to alter their identity as good wives who protect their husbands (Harbison, 2008). One study found that service delivery for those who experience elder abuse in rural communities is under threat through the centralization of such services, including the removal of clergy, police, and care providers (Harbison, Coughlan, Karabanow, & VanderPlaat, 2005). Finally, in general, rural issues are often seen to be of marginal concern to those responsible for policy making, which further compounds the lack of assistance for the rural elderly who experience abuse (Cornes et al., 2010).

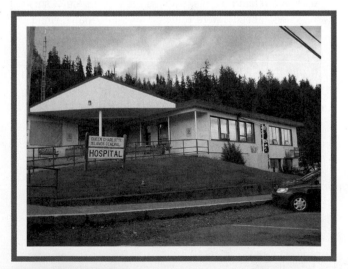

PHOTO    24.2  **Queen Charlotte Islands General Hospital, Queen Charlotte City, British Columbia**

*Source: Courtesy of Martha MacLeod/University of Northern British Columbia*

Other research with rural residents focuses specifically on their health status—examining differences in disease patterns and occurrences. For example, one study found that a lower proportion of those living in small town regions, rural regions, and northern regions rated their health as excellent. Specific conditions such as arthritis are higher than the national average among rural regions, and those in northern regions had a higher prevalence of hypertension (Mitura & Bollman, 2003). An important Canadian study (DesMeules et al., 2006) that examined health status and health determinants among the rural population found that there are variations of prevalence, incidence, and being at risk for specific diseases in different rural settings, and also among rural compared to urban residents, as noted in the box titled "Health Variations in Rural Settings."

Rural health status and rural-specific determinants of health point to the importance of disease prevention and health promotion through public health initiatives in order to address these issues in rural settings. However, what is less clear is whether conventional strategies, mostly developed by urban program planners for urban residents, are equally effective in rural settings. In addressing rural health concerns, RNs can apply the three levels of prevention: primary (reducing risks for a potential problem), secondary (providing screening and early detection and treatment), and tertiary (maintaining health). For instance, primary prevention would include providing health education for individuals in rural communities to maintain the lower incidence rates of cause-specific cancers, secondary prevention activities would include developing and implementing diabetes screening programs for rural women who are at risk for death from diabetes, and tertiary prevention would include monitoring the effectiveness of treatment for circulatory and respiratory diseases.

---

### HEALTH VARIATIONS IN RURAL SETTINGS

■ Rural areas reported higher proportions of people with low income and less than secondary education level.

■ Health-related factors, such as the prevalence of smoking and obesity, were elevated in rural Canada, while other health influences, such as dietary practices and leisure-time physical activity, were lower in rural areas.

■ Life expectancy at birth was significantly higher in urban areas.

■ Higher overall mortality risks among rural communities appear to be driven by higher death rates from such causes as circulatory diseases, injuries, and suicide; residents of the most-rural areas are often at highest risk.

■ Incidence rates of most cause-specific cancers were lower in rural areas.

■ Respiratory disease mortality risks were, for the most part, significantly higher among rural residents.

■ Women living in the most-rural areas had higher risks of dying from diabetes.

*Source:* Health variations in rural settings. From *How healthy are rural Canadians? An assessment of their health status and health determinants.* Copyright © 2006 by Canadian Institute for Health Information. Used by permission of Canadian Institute for Health Information.

## Unique Groups of People in Rural Areas

**Demographic Variations in Rural Areas** In addition to unique geographic features that affect the livelihood and everyday life cycle of rural residents, a number of **unique groups** of people live in rural areas. For many of these groups, there are challenges in being diverse and living in a rural environment. Thus, some may feel excluded from rural community life, whereas others, who want to live apart, prefer rural living where they can co-exist with other groups but not be expected to interact with others. It is part of the role for nurses to assess the rural community within which they live to determine its diversity and the strengths or needs that arise from such diversity. The changing face of immigration, which includes the influx of temporary foreign workers in some rural communities, adds to the **diversity of rural** community people. See Canadian Research Box 24.1.

Many groups could be included for further discussion in this chapter. Predominant among them are Aboriginal peoples, who are the focus of Chapter 22. General principles in relation to assessing and caring for multicultural clients are identified in Chapter 9 and for those with alternative sexual orientations are discussed in Chapter 20. The complexity of such individual situations is beyond the scope of this chapter but needs to be considered by rural nurses who may encounter such individuals in their practice. Identifying unique groups in rural areas is important for the development and implementation of appropriate nursing care that also incorporates the social determinants of health. For example, in some rural areas of Canada there are unique religious groups, such as the Amish, Hutterites, Mennonites, and Conservative Dutch, which may mean that some health behaviours such as immunization (Vandenberg, 2013) are not commonly accessed. These examples highlight that it is important for the rural CHNs to conduct community assessments that acknowledge the religious, socio-historical, and policy contexts within which individuals, families, and groups are located. Rather than focus on describing specific groups and practices, the principle of cultural safety that is a reflective process based on cultural awareness, sensitivity, and competence is the appropriate focus. The five principles of cultural safety are protocols (i.e., respect for cultural forms of engagement), personal knowledge (i.e., understanding one's own cultural identity), process (i.e., engaging in mutual learning), positive purpose (i.e., ensuring the process yields the right outcome for the client), and partnerships (i.e., promoting collaborative practice) (Polaschek, 1998; Smye & Browne, 2002).

## The Challenges Experienced by Rural Communities

Numerous challenges are faced by residents of rural Canadian communities. While the challenge of out-migration from distant rural areas to more-urban areas is recognized (Rothwell, Bollman, Tremblay, & Marshall, 2002), particularly for youth (Tremblay, 2001), the population is actually increasing for rural communities within commuting distance of urban areas (du Plessis et al., 2001). This, however, presents its own concerns when rural residents engage in work and leisure activities outside the rural community in the nearby urban centre. Rural communities by nature have less infrastructure and services, such as retail businesses or healthcare delivery options. Boom-and-bust cycles affect economic opportunity and availability of employment for rural residents, and rural poverty is a significant issue. Rural poverty is largely "invisible" to urban dwellers. The rural poor are also disadvantaged because they have to travel longer distances for services and pay more for services and resources in their home communities (Fairbairn & Gustafson, 2008). Rural poverty is exacerbated by the declining population and the subsequent declining resources in rural communities.

All of these challenges have impacts on health status in general and on healthcare delivery in particular. For example, the loss of youth and economic opportunities in rural communities leads to fewer individuals available to provide care to elderly parents and other relatives. In communities that are dependent on oil and gas extraction, there may be many single men or young families with few supports. Therefore, nursing practice needs to be designed to specifically address the particular situation in each rural community. For example, in some rural communities, there is access to technologies such as telehealth. This virtual environment allows for health education, such as prenatal teaching or online support programs for individuals with chronic illnesses. Rural-based CHNs need to become familiar with e-health initiatives and their use in order to positively impact their clients' health (Wathen & Harris, 2007).

# THE REALITIES OF RURAL NURSING PRACTICE

Although all graduates of nursing programs in Canada are prepared for generalist practice, working in rural communities stretches the meaning of being a generalist nurse. Nurses experience a wide range of practice demands in small communities.

## Who Are the Rural Registered Nurses?

Analyses (Pitblado et al., 2013) of the Nurses Database (NDB) reveal that there were 28 799 RNs working in rural Canada in 2010. Of those rural RNs, 6 595, or 22.9%, worked in community settings. Nurse-to-population ratios vary by rural region, but on average there were 477 nurses per 100 000 people in rural Canada compared to 871 per 100 000 in urban Canada. There is also an east-to-west trend, with higher nurse-to-population ratios in eastern Canada. The majority of rural RNs were female (88.2%), with 53.6% working full time. Although rural RNs have a lower level of education at entry to practice than their urban counterparts, there has been a

significant positive change in the percentage of rural RNs with a baccalaureate degree. In 2010, 32.5% of rural RNs had achieved a baccalaureate degree as their highest level of education compared to 18.5% in 2003 (Pitblado et al., 2013). Despite this improvement, limited access to nursing education remains a concern for rural RNs.

---

### CANADIAN RESEARCH BOX 24.1

**What is the role of rural nurses in wildfire disasters?**

Kulig, J., Edge, D., & Smolenski, S. (2014). Wildfire disasters: Implications for rural nurses. *Australasian Emergency Nursing Journal, 17*(3), 126–134. Copyright © 2014 by Elsevier Ltd. Used by permission of Elsevier Ltd. doi:10.1016:j.aenj.2014.04.003

There has been a notable increase in disasters around the globe, highlighting the role of rural nurses in disaster mitigation, response, and recovery. This article discusses a research program that focused on the human impacts of four wild fires, using community resiliency as a theoretical framework. The findings are placed within the World Health Organization/International Council of Nurses framework of disaster nursing competencies.

The findings across the four study sites were discussed within each of the WHO/ICN competencies in order to emphasize their relevance for rural settings as the following examples indicate. The care of vulnerable persons during and after the wildfire is particularly important in rural settings, where there may be limited capacity to address the needs of seniors and other vulnerable people. Sustained support is needed for rural communities during their recovery phase while ensuring that the community does not become overwhelmed with the response to assist them. Clear communication is needed in all phases of disaster mitigation, response, and recovery. The underlying strength of the community is an important variable to consider post-wildfire; that is, communities that are strong before a disaster will be stronger afterwards and, hence, it is important to help all rural communities become stronger in preparation for disasters. Divisions among groups within communities may occur and tax recovery of the rural community.

Rural nurses' intimate knowledge of their communities makes them ideal members of disaster planning teams as well as advocates for their rural communities during all phases of the disaster. Preparation of nursing students to act in this role and ongoing training for rural nurses are essential.

#### Discussion Questions

1. What initiatives can nursing organizations take to support nurses who work in rural settings?

2. What is the responsibility of health regions in preparing rural nurses to address disasters?

3. Given the geographic isolation of many rural nurses, what is the best way to ensure ongoing training in disaster preparation and recovery?

# A DAY IN THE LIFE

The generalist practice of a rural nurse differs by setting and across regions in Canada. The following instances of "a day in the life" of nurses in various settings are meant to illustrate the diversity in nursing practice in rural, remote, and isolated communities. The descriptions that follow here combine elements of practice and do not represent a particular nurse in a rural location.

## Rural

Sandra lives on a farm in rural British Columbia. She is married, with two school-age children. Her husband manages their mixed-farming operation year round while Sandra leaves home each day and commutes 50 kilometres to the next community where she is employed full time as a home care nurse. For Sandra, and the other two nurses described below, the only typical part of their day is leaving home and travelling to work. The commute for Sandra to begin her workday changes depending on weather and road conditions. The first 20 kilometres are a gravel road that leads to the highway, which makes driving a challenge on stormy winter mornings.

Sandra's workday begins at her office, planning her day and route to client homes within and outside of the small town. Like her urban colleagues, Sandra provides wound-care and chronic-care services to her clients. Unlike her urban colleagues, she knows most of her clients and their families outside the context of her job, even though they are in the next community, as this is where her family also does their shopping and her children go to school. Sandra finds that knowing her clients well is sometimes positive. It helps her to focus quickly on what might be affecting their pain. It also might be negative when they withhold information because they are concerned about potential breaches of confidentiality due to Sandra's dual role as nurse and neighbour.

## Remote and Isolated

Nurses in remote and isolated communities often practise in clinics, but the distance from other services may shape their practice differently. Daniel, a nurse working in a northern Ontario nursing station, begins his day walking down the hall from his apartment to the attached clinic. The close proximity of work and home can be a benefit to clients, as they know Daniel is there and feel free to come to the clinic at any time of day for treatment. But it can be a challenge for nurses, as there is little separation between work and home life. Daniel also finds that it can be difficult living in accommodations attached to his workplace, as he lives and works with his coworkers over a long period of time.

The typical day for Daniel as a nurse in a remote community includes a number of primary-care and health-promotion activities. On this typical day, Daniel finds himself applying primary prevention through immunizing infants, children, and adults. Secondary prevention occurs through collecting, ordering, and reviewing client laboratory results; assessing and treating common medical conditions; and monitoring and referring chronic care and prenatal clients. Tertiary prevention occurs through caring for wounds and suturing lacerations. In remote communities, a nurse like Daniel might also provide care to clients in emergency situations, such as status epilepticus or trauma from a motor vehicle collision.

Carol works in the Far North. Her practice is much the same as Daniel's in her remote setting. Carol may have more technologies available to her that help to bridge the gap between her location and the urban health centre that she accesses in an emergency or for client consultations. Canadian communities that might be considered more isolated include small Arctic and other communities, such as in northern Newfoundland, where road access is not available and planes arrive infrequently.

A typical day for Carol may involve taking a picture of a wound and emailing the picture to a dermatologist in the south for assessment and treatment advice. She offers a chronic care clinic in the afternoon that includes connecting via telehealth to a specialist for client follow-up appointments. In the evening when a client comes in with a severe traumatic injury, Carol connects with ER physicians over telehealth. They support Carol, in real time, with assessment and treatment prior to air ambulance personnel arriving and transporting the client to a larger facility.

Although nursing practice in the above descriptions use the word "typical," most nurses practising in these settings will suggest that while there are common elements in their day, little is typical. All nurses in these settings experience a high demand for ongoing flexibility and openness to changes in routine (Tarlier, Johnson, & Whyte, 2003). The attraction to rural practice for nurses like Sandra, Daniel, and Carol includes the challenging nature of the work and the chance to live and work in a rural community setting that is or becomes their home.

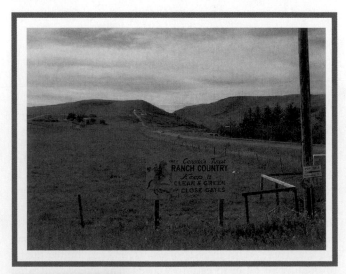

**PHOTO    24.3** Ranch country, near Nanton, Alberta

*Source: Courtesy of Judith C. Kulig/University of Lethbridge*

# KEY FEATURES OF RURAL NURSING

Regardless of practice setting, all rural nurses are faced with addressing issues in clinical practice, leadership, and the work environment. Rural nursing practice is shaped by the context of rural communities, with their limited transportation, communications, and other resources. (See Photo 24.3 for an example if a part of the country where population is more sparse.) Within small communities, rural nurses provide care to clients, who also may be friends and neighbours, with a wide range of conditions. Rural nurses experience practice as being multifaceted and complex, with considerable decision-making challenges, few resources, and little backup (MacLeod et al., 2008). It demands considerable knowledge and skills to be responsive to community needs (CARRN, 2008). For example, CHNs in northern British Columbia found they could be more responsive to high-risk and vulnerable families when they focused on creating working relationships with families instead of on "home visiting" protocols, because their services to families happened in many locations in the community, including the grocery store (Moules, MacLeod, Hanlon, & Thirsk, 2009).

# REGISTERED NURSES PROVIDING PRIMARY CARE IN RURAL AND REMOTE COMMUNITIES

As a cornerstone of Canada's healthcare system, primary health care is the focus of intensive renewal efforts (Kates et al., 2012). In rural and remote communities, RNs provide **primary care services** or work as part of a team providing primary health care to rural populations. The roles and responsibilities of nurses in primary health care vary based on the needs and services of the community (MacLeod et al., 2008) as well as the complexity of the rural setting.

Rural communities are diverse in characteristics and context, yet many face similar issues and challenges in healthcare service delivery (Mitton, Dionne, Masucci, Wong, & Law, 2011). It is important to be aware of successful examples of rural healthcare innovation (Wakerman & Humphreys, 2011). For example, recognition that rural and remote stakeholder collaboration could support the spread of rural innovation represents a step forward in improving the health of rural populations (Canadian Foundation for Healthcare Improvement, 2013). Innovations that reflect changes to rural nursing roles, settings, and modes of practice are of particular interest as health systems transition toward a primary health care model of service provision and delivery (Banner, MacLeod, & Johnston, 2010).

RNs in rural primary health care settings may practise in a particular setting, such as mental health or occupational health. Alternatively, the CHN role that is often identified with nursing practice in northern rural and remote communities blends specialized knowledge for performing activities related to public health, home care, emergency care, palliative care, and management of episodic and chronic conditions. CHNs frequently work in an expanded practice role (Mitton et al., 2011) that initially developed in the context of widespread physician shortages (Martin-Misener et al., 2010).

While numerous initiatives and innovative models have evolved to attract and retain healthcare providers in rural communities (Mitton et al., 2011; Wakerman et al., 2008), nurses remain instrumental to optimizing primary health care services and delivery in rural and remote communities. Rural nurses have the capacity to effectively collaborate and lead interprofessional teams to improve health outcomes for rural populations (Canadian Health Services Research Foundation, 2012), and in so doing will contribute to the health and sustainability of rural populations and lifestyles.

Nursing practice, as part of an interprofessional primary health care team, may appear very different from the practice of urban-based teams. A rural team may include only one or two RNs and a community health worker (Mills et al., 2010) collaborating with a physician or other healthcare professionals via telephone, telehealth, or itinerant specialist visits to the community (e.g., dentists, pediatricians). In urban settings, all team members typically can interact daily in a face-to-face manner. As such, the scope, autonomy, and breadth of practice of a rural nurse may go beyond that of his or her urban colleague, depending on the focus of the team and client's health concerns.

The vast physical distances that can separate team members necessitate deliberate consideration for professional and collegial communication in order to ensure a degree of interprofessional collaboration (Bainbridge, Nasmith, Orchard, & Wood, 2010) and to provide high quality comprehensive primary health care services. Telehealth is one technology that has been successfully implemented in some locations and is used to complement primary health care services. In Takla Landing, a remote Aboriginal community in northern British Columbia, the nurses who work in the community lead most of the care and are able to use telehealth to consult with off-site healthcare providers (Mah, 2013). In this community, nurses assist patients to optimize management of acute and chronic health conditions without leaving their community. This reduces the stress experienced by patients and their families while also saving the patients and the healthcare system money. The telehealth initiative currently offers several medical specialties to Takla Landing, including general surgery, infectious disease, dermatology, and addictions, among others. Nurses manage and support the patient onsite while patients receive the same specialist care as their urban counterparts. Nursing practice in settings such as this requires excellent assessment skills and clinical reasoning to make decisions about when and who to consult for patient care.

Technologies such as telehealth are increasingly considered as a resource to improve access and comprehensiveness of care for rural populations (Gibson et al., 2011; Taylor, Stone, & Huijbregts, 2012), but it is not yet the norm for rural and remote communities. See Canadian Research Box 24.2. Rural nurses often work in settings of chronic resource shortages in the form of equipment, other providers, and services (Forbes & Edge, 2009; Kulig et al., 2008). Given that nurses are front-line providers working at significant distances from tertiary care settings, rural nursing practice requires a broad knowledge base (Jackman, Myrick, & Yonge, 2012; Kulig et al., 2008) and advanced educational preparation (Cant, Birks, Porter, Jacob, & Cooper, 2011; MacLeod et al., 2008). In an analysis of responses from a national nursing survey (MacLeod, Kulig, Stewart, & Pitblado, 2004), the most common reason nurses reported intent to leave their position within the next year was to undertake further nursing education (Stewart et al., 2011).

Rural nurses working in primary health care assume multiple roles that may not be captured by a formal job description (Mitton et al., 2011). Program planning and evaluation, such as well-woman clinics and immunization clinics, quality assurance initiatives such as practice audits, and extended periods of time on call are all activities that a rural nurse may be expected to perform in addition to being competent in direct patient care, illness prevention, health promotion, and emergency care. A rural nurse in primary health care may conduct a group medical visit for chronic disease management one morning, attend the local school to provide immunizations in the afternoon, and medevac a patient with appendicitis in the evening.

The demands of providing primary health care in rural communities are challenging, and turnover rates can be high in some circumstances (Tarlier, Johnson, Browne, & Sheps, 2013; Vukic & Keddy, 2002). A rural nurse's intent to leave a position is influenced by interrelated individual, workplace, and community factors (Stewart et al., 2011). Increasingly, and particularly in northern, remote communities, primary health care is provided by relief nurses who stay only short periods of time in the communities (Minore et al., 2005). When primary health care service provision is fragmented, continuity of care and health outcomes may worsen for populations already enduring significant health disparities (Tarlier et al., 2013).

Rural and remote nurses are resourceful and innovative. Rural healthcare environments may be open to trying things differently (CFHI, 2013), and nurses can enjoy and take pride in accepting the challenge of providing best practices in rural and remote communities. Rural nurses providing primary health care services must be adaptable, perseverant, critical thinkers who are willing to listen and learn (Martin-Misener et al., 2008).

**Leadership** In the first study of rural and remote nursing practice in Canada, almost all nurses talked about issues related to **nursing leadership** (Bish, Kenny, & Nay, 2012; MacLeod, Martin-Misener, et al., 2008; Martin-Misener et al., 2008; Ulrich & MacLeod, 2005). Issues included finding ways of working through conflicting priorities, coping with having leaders at a distance, and creating support networks. Leadership was more effective when leaders set up possibilities for quality practice, even in situations of few resources. When leaders planned for the realities of rural practice, nurses felt supported. For nursing leaders, providing the appropriate support at a distance was a challenge; for nurses, seeking and accepting that support was equally challenging. Both nursing managers and nurses needed to work creatively within organizations that did not always understand the realities of their practice.

---

## CANADIAN RESEARCH BOX 24.2

### Does telehealth offer an alternative to in-person group support for caregivers of a spouse with atypical dementia?

O'Connell, M. E., Crossley, M., Cammer, A., Morgan, D., Allingham, W., Cheavins, B., . . . Morgan, E. (2013). Development and evaluation of a telehealth videoconferenced support group for rural spouses of individuals diagnosed with atypical early-onset dementias. *Dementia: The International Journal of Social Research and Practice, 13*(3). Reproduced by permission of SAGE Publications Ltd., London, Los Angeles, New Delhi, Singapore and Washington DC. Copyright © SAGE Publications Ltd., 2013. doi:10.1177/1471301212474143

The purpose of this research was to describe the development and evaluation of a novel use of telehealth videoconferencing to provide a support group for rural caregivers of spouses with atypical and early-onset dementia, such as frontotemporal dementia (FTD). Individuals with FTD tend to present with behavioural problems such as disinhibition, impulsiveness, socially inappropriate behaviour, and aggression. Caregivers of family members with FTD report high levels of distress due to behaviour changes and the unique social and financial issues resulting from dementia onset in midlife. Rural residence adds another stressor for families who may become isolated and lack formal services for support.

In this study, all participants were family members referred with their spouse to a Rural and Remote Memory Clinic (RRMC) at the University of Saskatchewan for dementia diagnosis and follow-up. The intervention was a monthly 90-minute videoconferenced support group, co-facilitated by two members of the neuropsychology team at the urban centre of the RRMC.

Qualitative data were collected after 18 months at an in-person retreat of nine group members to evaluate the group effectiveness. The findings included key aspects of the group that contributed to success, as well as challenges. The group effectively provided access to support across a large geographic area. Strengths included the open group structure, the lack of preplanned agenda, and learning what worked for others in their caregiving relationships. While members experienced much support from the group, they also reported a sense of distance that differed from in-person meetings. Technology had some challenges but it reduced travel for group members (distances to rural telehealth sites versus to the urban site) by 262 to 532 kilometres per session, demonstrating the feasibility of this group intervention for rural caregivers.

### Discussion Questions

1. In what ways are telehealth strategies currently used to address health issues in rural and remote settings?

2. What other groups of individuals with chronic diseases who are dependent upon caregivers would benefit from the telehealth strategy discussed in this example?

3. What is the responsibility of educational institutions in the preparation of CHNs to use telehealth in rural and remote settings?

**Quality Work Environments** Creating quality work environments in rural practice settings is particularly challenging. A central challenge is that many nurses in rural settings work alone much of the time (Andrews et al., 2005) or with few colleagues during much of their everyday work. Orientations that include discussion about working alone and safety issues when entering homes or travelling on isolated roads can help. A strategy for developing a **quality work environment** in rural or remote practice includes developing consistent expectations and approaches among managers and nurses to address practice issues at the site level. This includes relevant rural practice standards; policies and practices that support rural nurses' scope of practice; practice-driven, rural-focused nursing education programs; rural reality-based preceptorship and mentorship programs; and the development of sustained processes for direct rural nursing involvement in local and regional planning (Ulrich & MacLeod, 2005).

### CASE STUDY

The Gibbons family lives on their family farm 90 kilometres east of a small city (population 68 000). After completing high school at the local community school, Nancy and John were married in the Anglican church. Nancy is now 45 and John is 46. Nancy has been an active mother, raising their three sons while also volunteering in the community. John and his son Peter work on the farm together, which has been in the family for two generations. The two older sons, Jack and Ian, live and work in cities that are three hours and five hours, respectively, from the family farm. Both Jack and Ian are married and have children. Their jobs, family life, and other responsibilities mean that they are not able to visit the farm very often.

Nancy has had an uneventful health history; she had regular physical examinations and three normal pregnancies. A few years ago she had a hysterectomy, and from a health perspective was expecting to enjoy retirement with her husband and their sons, daughters-in-law, and grandchildren. About a year ago, Nancy began to feel "unwell." She was tired, shaky, and having difficulties sleeping. Four months ago, tests revealed that she had amyotrophic lateral sclerosis (ALS), a terminal condition for which there is no cure.

She was referred to home care for assessment, but John refused to have them in the home and instead has provided all care to Nancy. The ALS Society was notified by home care about Nancy's diagnosis and has called and offered to visit and assist in any way possible. John would agree only after Peter convinced his mother and father that it could be helpful. While the ALS Society was at the home, John expressed his frustration at his wife's deteriorating condition and related he was unsure if he could continue providing care by himself. Nancy is now dependent upon John to bathe her, assist her with feeding, and transfer her to the toilet. She is also frequently in pain, and due to the muscle weakness, is at risk for falls. Depression has set in and Nancy has said that "life is not worth living." At the same time, she wants to die peacefully at the farm and does not want to be moved into the city hospital. John is increasingly upset about his wife's condition and appears overwhelmed and bewildered; he realizes that he needs support to continue to care for Nancy in their home.

It takes some time but John finally agrees to have a home care nurse return, do another assessment, and set up equipment resources such as oxygen and personal care aides on a routine basis. The home care nurse also refers the family to the palliative care nurse. Peter calls his brothers and asks that they come home to visit their mother as soon as possible.

### Discussion Questions

1. Describe the roles and responsibilities of a home care and palliative care nurse in this case study.

2. Identify three factors related to living in a rural setting that provide challenges in the delivery of nursing care for Nancy Gibbons. Identify how a home care nurse could address these factors.

3. Identify three rural community factors that could provide assistance to the Gibbons family. Identify how a home care nurse could incorporate these factors into a care plan for Nancy.

*Source:* This case study is a modified version from the Nursing Education in Southern Alberta (NESA) curriculum used by the collaborative partners, the University of Lethbridge and Lethbridge College.

**Policy Issues in Rural and Remote Environments** Most policies in Canada, with health policies being no exception, are based upon an urban perspective with little consideration of their applicability in rural environments. In order for this situation to be changed, the following key issues need to be addressed.

- Having a specific individual champion in Canada who focuses on the importance of addressing the unique situation experienced by rural residents would be beneficial.
- Few RNs are educationally prepared for work in the policy arena (Kulig, Nahachewsky, Thomlinson, MacLeod, & Curran, 2004), and although nurse educators have been encouraged to include information about the policy cycle and its application in their curriculum (Murphy, 1999), it will be some time before any change is realized.
- Relevant information about the nature of rural communities, including the number and location of rural residents and their health issues, is not readily available. Some organizations have lobbied to have this altered (e.g., Canadian Rural Health Research Society, 2008).
- The perspectives of rural residents and their involvement in setting the policy agenda, even at their local level, need to be acknowledged and respected as a key component of rural development (Morton, Glasgow, & Johnson, 2004). Rural RNs have a key role in helping this to transpire (Kulig et al., 2004).

# CONCLUSION

This chapter has focused on the unique nature of caring for clients in rural areas. Precise definitions of "rural" are lacking and need to include both technical and social characteristics. Rural residents experience challenges, including depopulation, distance to services, and the need to develop local initiatives. Nurses who practise in rural areas would benefit from educational supports, including continuing education by distance delivery methods and the development of appropriate work expectations, given the nature of the rural settings in which they work. Many diverse groups within rural Canada offer opportunities for a rewarding nursing practice.

## KEY TERMS

diversity of rural    p. 432
nursing leadership    p. 436
primary care services    p. 435
quality work environment    p. 437
social approaches    p. 430
technical approaches    p. 430
unique groups    p. 432

## STUDY QUESTIONS

1. Identify what public health nurses can do to generate information about the communities they work within.

2. Identify four concepts that would be discussed in a rural nursing course for nursing students.

3. Identify four challenges to working as a nurse in a northern community.

4. A group of undergraduate nursing students is developing a health-promotion project for a farming community. What level of prevention is this an example of? In order to be successful, what do they need to take into consideration?

5. Maria is a 35-year-old Low German Mennonite woman who has just had her fifth child. She was diagnosed with gestational diabetes and requires follow-up to more closely monitor her health. How would you apply the principles of cultural safety in the care of Maria?

6. Timothy has been working as a public health nurse in an Aboriginal community for the past four years. Over a year ago the community experienced the loss of several family members in a house fire. Identify the levels of prevention and specific strategies that Timothy can address in collaboration with community members to deal with the loss and prevent such tragedies in the future.

After working through these questions, go to the MyNursingLab at www.pearsoned.ca/mynursinglab to check your answers.

## INDIVIDUAL CRITICAL-THINKING EXERCISES

1. Examine the provincial or territorial nursing standards related to professional boundaries and identify three challenges in the provision of care within rural communities. As a professional registered nurse, how would you address the challenges without jeopardizing ethical standards and professional boundaries?

2. A new work camp for the oil industry has been set up 50 kilometres north of the rural community where you reside and work. The health authority is responsible for the health of the workers. There are unsubstantiated reports of high stress levels among the workers. What health issues are associated with high stress levels? Identify the appropriate levels of prevention. What are examples of relevant strategies to reduce stress within this work camp?

3. The community care office you work within as a home care nurse will be moving to a primary care model in the next year. Identify how you can describe this change to your home care clients and what it means to the care that they will receive. What does it mean for you as a nurse? How might it affect your practice?

4. You work in a public health office within a large agriculture area that includes established farm families and feedlot operators. Over the past few years there has been an increase in migrant farm workers from Mexico that has added to the diverse mix of the area, which includes conservative religious groups who also work in the agricultural industry. Locating and communicating with all of these groups has become increasingly challenging, and ensuring routine public health programs such as immunizations has become even more difficult due to their beliefs and practices. What are three barriers that need to be addressed? Who can you turn to in order to receive some guidance and support? What actions on your part might facilitate collaboration? What are short- and long-term goals in this situation?

5. You work in collaboration with a long-term care facility that has just developed a support group for rural families caring for a relative with dementia, which is most commonly caused by Alzheimer's disease. After the first six months of the service, only three family members have attended the group, even though you are sure that many others could benefit from the support. What issues could make families reluctant to participate in this service? In what ways can technology (e.g., Skype, telehealth) be used to facilitate participation?

## GROUP CRITICAL-THINKING EXERCISES

1. You work part time as a CHN in a two-nurse office in a rural community. The other nurse works full time. You are both responsible for implementing the full range of public health programs. Because of the difficulty in finding casual replacements over the last two months, you deferred your vacation and have worked more than full time. You have just received a call that the full-time nurse has gone on sick

leave. As your manager, who works 200 kilometres away, tells you this, she adds that the medical health officer has identified two TB cases in your community. Your manager asks you to work overtime again and you are debating what your answer should be. As a group, identify the following:

a. personal and professional concerns you would face in this situation
b. dilemmas being faced by the public health administration
c. potential impacts on client and community safety
d. strategies, including ones that reflect interprofessional practice, to address the above concerns

2. You are the new community nurse in an outpost setting on a community-based Aboriginal reserve. Two other nurses are stationed at the centre but they are from the community and live with their spouses away from the station. You are the only nurse who works at the outpost accommodation. This particular community (population of 545) is fly-in only with interruptions of flight service due to inclement weather. As a group, identify the following:

a. priorities you would engage in as the new nurse
b. the process you would use to assess the community
c. how you would develop a relationship with the other nurses and community residents

3. You are part of a group of CHNs who receive the latest statistics that discuss the health status of Canadian residents. The report lacks sufficient detail about rural Canadians and their health status. In order to address this scenario, identify and discuss the following:

a. the shortfalls of using inappropriate data in your work as CHNs
b. agencies that collect information about rural residents and their health status
c. a process to work with your program managers to address the limitations of the data
d. a process to work with your program managers to contact the relevant agencies about the limitations of the data

4. You are a CHN in a logging/ranching community of 1 500 residents. There is only one physician in town and a limited health centre facility. In the community, when the logging and ranching slows down over winter, some individuals are able to go south for a vacation. This year, when one couple returns, the husband develops symptoms indicative of a new flu strain. A few days later it is confirmed that the man has the new flu strain. Within a week, several other people have similar symptoms and are also confirmed to have the new flu strain.

a. Identify the key individuals you would need to work with in this circumstance; include a list of their roles in addressing the situation.
b. Identify the main elements of a pandemic plan, including the levels of prevention to curtail the spread of the new flu strain.
c. Identify the process that you would use to work with community members in implementing a pandemic strategy.
d. Discuss the ramifications to your regular workload and the impact on your personal life.

5. You have been a home care nurse working in several eastern coastal communities for the last five years. It is a job that you love mostly because of the people you care for and the diversity within your everyday work. You are currently mentoring an undergraduate nursing student from an urban-based university nursing program. The student has made it clear that it was not her choice to come to a rural area or to do home care. As a group, identify how you will address the student's issues in a productive manner. Identify ways in which you can encourage the student to see the benefits of her education experience in a rural area.

## REFERENCES

Andrews, M. E., Stewart, N. J., Pitblado, J. R., Morgan, D. G., Forbes, D., & D'Arcy, C. (2005). Registered nurses working alone in rural and remote Canada. *Canadian Journal of Nursing Research, 37*(1), 14–33.

Association of Workers' Compensation Boards of Canada. (n. d.). *National work injury statistics program: Number of accepted time-loss injuries, by industry and jurisdiction.* Toronto, ON: Author. Retrieved from http://awcbc.org/en/statistics.asp

Bainbridge, L., Nasmith, L., Orchard, C., & Wood, V. (2010). Competencies for interprofessional collaboration. *Journal of Physical Therapy Education, 24*(1), 6–11.

Banner, D., MacLeod, M. L. P., & Johnston, S. (2010). Role transition in rural and remote primary health care nursing: A scoping literature review. *Canadian Journal of Nursing Research, 42*(4), 40–57.

Bish, M., Kenny, A., & Nay, R. (2012). A scoping review identifying contemporary issues in rural nursing leadership. *Journal of Nursing Scholarship, 44*(4), 411–417. doi:10.1111/j.1547-5069.2012.01471.x

Canadian Agricultural Injury Reporting. (2012). Agricultural fatalities in Canada 1990–2008. Retrieved from http://www.cair-sbac.ca

Canadian Association of Rural and Remote Nurses. (2008). *Rural and remote nursing practice parameters: Discussion document.* Unpublished document: Author.

Canadian Foundation for Healthcare Improvement. (2013). *Northern, rural and remote pan-provincial collaboration.* Ottawa, ON: Author. Retrieved from http://www.cfhi-fcass.ca/WhatWeDo/Collaborations/NorthernRuralRemote.aspx

Canadian Health Services Research Foundation. (2012). *Evidence synthesis for the effectiveness of interprofessional teams in primary care.* Ottawa, ON: Author.

Canadian Institute for Health Information. (2013). *Hospital births in Canada: A focus on women living in rural and remote areas.* Ottawa, ON: Author.

Canadian Rural Health Research Society. (n.d.). *About us.* Retrieved from http://crhrs-scrsr.usask.ca

Cant, R., Birks, M., Porter, J., Jacob, E., & Cooper, S. (2011). Developing advanced rural nursing practice: A whole new scope of responsibility. *Collegian: Journal of the Royal College of Nursing Australia, 18*(4), 177–182. doi:10.1016/j.colegn.2011.08.001

Cornes, M., Manthorpe, J., & Haselden, N. (2010). Rural dimensions of elder abuse: Contributions to the No Secrets review from rural older people. *The Journal of Adult Protection, 12*(3), 20–29.

Demers, P. (2011). Disease and injury patterns: Lumber industry. In P. Demers & K. Teschke, (Eds.), *Encyclopedia of Occupational Health and Safety*. Geneva, CH: International Labor Organization.

DesMeules, M., Pong, R., Lagacé, C., Heng, D., Manuel, D., Pitblado, R. J., & Koren, I. (2006). *How healthy are rural Canadians? An assessment of their health status and health determinants*. Ottawa, ON: Canadian Population Initiative, Canadian Institute for Health Information.

Dimah, K., & Dimah, A. (2013). Elder abuse and neglect among rural and urban women. *Journal of Elder Abuse and Neglect, 15*(1), 75–93. doi: 10.1300/J084v15n01_06

du Plessis, V., Beshiri, R., & Bollman, R. (2001). Definitions of rural. *Rural and Small Town Analysis Bulletin, 3*(3), 1–17. #21-006-XIE. Ottawa, ON: Statistics Canada. Available at statcan.gc.ca

Electric Canadian. (n.d.) Retrieved from http://www.electriccanadian.com/transport/oilgas/index.htm

Fairbairn, J., & Gustafson, L. (2008). Beyond freefall: Halting rural poverty. Final report of the Standing Committee on Agriculture and Forestry. Ottawa, ON: Government of Canada.

Forbes, D. A., & Edge, D. S. (2009). Canadian home care policy and practice in rural and remote settings: Challenges and solutions. *Journal of Agromedicine, 14*(2), 119–124. doi:10.1080/10599240902724135

Fraser Basin Council. (2012). Identifying health concerns relating to oil and gas development in northeastern BC. Victoria, BC: BC Ministry of Health.

Gibson, K., Coulson, H., Miles, R., Kakekakekung, C., Daniels, E., & O'Donnell, S. (2011). Conversations on tele-mental health: Listening to remote and rural First Nations communities. *Rural and Remote Health, 11*. Retrieved from http://www.rrh.org.au/publishedarticles/article_print_1656.pdf

Harbison, J. (2008). Stoic heroines or collaborators: Ageism, feminism and the provision of assistance to abused old women. *Journal of Social Work Practice, 22*(2), 221–234. doi:10.1080/02650530802099890

Harbison, J., Coughlan, S., Karabanow, J., & VanderPlaat, M. (2005). A clash of cultures: Rural values and service delivery to mistreated and neglected older people in Eastern Canada. *Practice: Social Work in Action, 17*(4), 229–246. doi:10.1080/09503150500425091

Health Canada. (2005). *Ten years of health transfer First Nation and Inuit control*. First Nations and Inuit Health Branch. Adapted and reproduced with permission from the Minister of Health, 2015. Retrieved from http://www.hc-sc.gc.ca/fniah-spnia/pubs/finance/_agree-accord/10_years_ans_trans/index-eng.php

Jackman, D., Myrick, F., & Yonge, O. J. (2010). Rural nursing in Canada: A voice unheard. *Online Journal of Rural Nursing and Health Care, 10*(1), 60–69.

Kates, N., Hutchison, B., O'Brien, P., Fraser, B., Wheeler, S., & Chapman, C. (2012). Framework for advancing improvement in primary care. *Healthcare Papers, 12*(2), 8–21.

Kralj, B. (2001). Measuring "rurality" for purposes of health-care planning: An empirical measure for Ontario. *Ontario Medical Review, 67*(9), 33–52.

Kulig, J., Andrews, M. E., Stewart, N., Pitblado, R., MacLeod, M., Bentham, D., & Smith, B. (2008). How do registered nurses define rurality? *Australian Journal of Rural Health, 16*(1), 28–32. doi:10.1111/j.1440-1584.2007.00947.x

Kulig, J., Nahachewsky, D., Thomlinson, E., MacLeod, M., & Curran, F. (2004). Maximizing the involvement of rural nurses in policy. *Nursing Leadership, 17*(1), 88–96.

MacLeod, M. L. P., Martin-Misener, R., Banks, C., Morton, M., Vogt, C., & Bentham, D. (2008). "I'm a different kind of nurse": Advice from nurses in rural and remote Canada. *Canadian Journal of Nursing Leadership, 21*(3), 24–37.

MacLeod, M., Kulig, J., Stewart, N., & Pitblado, R. (2004). *Nursing practice in rural and remote Canada*. Canadian Health Services Research Foundation. Retrieved from http://www.chsrf.ca

Mah, S. (2013). Telehealth in northern B.C. *Canadian Health Care Technology, 18*(7), 4.

Maltais, V. (2007). *Risk factors associated with farm injuries in Canada*. Ottawa, ON: Statistics Canada.

Maltais, V. (2010). *Risk factors associated with farm injuries in Canada*. 2010 catalogue #21-601-MWE. From the Agriculture and Rural Working Paper Series. Retrieved from http://www.statcan.gc.ca/bsolc/olc-cel/olc-cel?catno=21-601-MWE&lang=eng

Martin-Misener, R., MacLeod, M. L. P., Vogt, C., Morton, M., Banks, C., & Bentham, D., (2008). "There's rural and then there's rural": Advice from nurses providig health care in northern remote communities. *Canadian Journal of Nursing Leadership, 30*(7), 785–800.

Mills, J. E., Francis, K., Birks, M., Coyle, M., Henderson, S., & Jones, J. (2010). Registered nurses as members of interprofessional primary health care teams in remote or isolated areas of Queensland: Collaboration, communication and partnerships in practice. *Journal of Interprofessional Care, 24*(5), 587–596. doi:10.3109/13561821003624630

Minore, B., Boone, M., Katt, M., Kinch, P., Birch, S., & Mushquash, C. (2005). The effects of nursing turnover on continuity of care in isolated First Nation communities. *Canadian Journal of Nursing Research, 37*(1), 87–100.

Mitton, C., Dionne, F., Masucci, L., Wong, S., & Law, S. (2011). Innovations in health service organization and delivery in northern and rural and remote regions: A review of the literature. *International Journal of Circumpolar Health, 70*(5), 460–472. doi:http://dx.doi.org/10.3402/ijch.v70i5.17859

Mitura, V., & Bollman, R. (2003). The health of rural Canadians: A rural–urban comparison of health indicators. *Rural and Small Town Analysis Bulletin, 4*(6), 1–23. #21-006-XIE. Ottawa: Statistics Canada. Retrieved from http://www.statcan.gc.ca

Morton, L., Glasgow, N., & Johnson, N. (2004). Reaching the goal: Less disparity, better rural health. In N. Glasgow, L. Morton, & N. Johnson (Eds.), *Critical Issues in Rural Health* (pp. 283–291). Ames, IA: Blackwell.

Moules, N. J., MacLeod, M. L. P., Hanlon, N., & Thirsk, L. (2009). "And then you'll see her in the grocery store": The working relationships of community health nurses and high priority families in rural and northern Canadian communities. *Journal of Pediatric Nursing, 25*(5), 327–334. doi:10.1016/j.pedn.2008.12.003

Murphy, N. (1999). A survey of health policy content in Canadian graduate programs in nursing. *Journal of Nursing Education, 38*(2), 88–91.

Northern Health. (2012). *Understanding the state of industrial camps in northern BC*. Prince George, BC: Northern Health.

Pitblado, R., Koren, I., MacLeod, M., Place, J., Kulig, J., & Stewart, N. (2013). *Characteristics and distribution of the regulated nursing workforce in rural and small town Canada, 2003 and 2010*. Prince George, BC: Author.

Pitblado, J. R. (2005). So, what do we mean by "rural," "remote," and "northern"? *Canadian Journal of Nursing Research, 37*(1), 163–168.

Polaschek, N. R. (1998). Cultural safety: A new concept in nursing people of different ethnicities. *Journal of Advanced Nursing, 27*, 452–457. doi:10.1046/j.1365-2648 .1998.00547.x

Public Health Agency of Canada (2005). *The rural think tank 2005—Understanding issues families face living in rural and remote communities*. Retrieved from http://www.phac-aspc .gc.ca/hp-ps/dca-dea/publications/rtt-grr-2005/2-eng.php

Rothwell, N., Bollman, R., Tremblay, J., & Marshall, J. (2002). Migration to and from rural and small town Canada. *Rural and Small Town Analysis Bulletin, 3*(6), 2–22. #21-006-XIE. Ottawa, ON: Statistics Canada. Retrieved from http://www.statcan.gc.ca

Smye, V., & Browne, A. J. (2002). "Cultural safety" and the analysis of health policy affecting aboriginal people. *Nurse Researcher, 9*(3), 42–56. Retrieved from http://dx.doi.org/ 10.7748/nr2002.04.9.3.42.c6188

Spencer, C. (2000). Abuse and neglect of older adults in rural communities. *Gerontology Research News, 19*(1), 7–10.

Statistics Canada. (2011). *Farm and operator data*. Retrieved from http://www.statcan.gc.ca/daily-quotidien/141117/ dq141117b-eng.htm

Stewart, N. J., D'Arcy, C., Kosteniuk, J., Andrews, M. E., Morgan, D., Forbes, D., . . . Pitblado, J.R. (2011). Moving on: Predictors of intention to leave among rural and remote RNs in Canada. *Journal of Rural Health, 27*(1), 103–113.

Tarlier, D. S., Johnson, J. L., Browne, A. J., & Sheps, S. (2013). Maternal-infant health outcomes and nursing practice in a remote First Nations community in northern Canada. *Canadian Journal of Nursing Research, 45*(2), 76–100.

Tarlier, D., Johnson, J. L., & Whyte, N. B. (2003). Voices from the wilderness: An interpretive study describing the role

and practice of outpost nurses. *Canadian Journal of Public Health, 94*(3), 180–184.

Taylor, D., Stone, S., & Huijbregts, M. (2012). Remote participants' experiences with a group-based stroke self-management program using videoconference technology. *Rural and Remote Health, 12,* 1947. Retrieved from http://www.rrh.org.au

Thomlinson, E., McDonagh, M., Baird Crooks, K., & Lees, M. (2004). Health beliefs of rural Canadians: Implications for rural practice. *Australian Journal of Rural Health, 12*, 258–263. doi:10.1111/j.1440-1854. 2004.00627.x

Tremblay, J. (2001). Rural youth migration between 1971 and 1996. *Rural and Small Town Analysis Bulletin, 2*(3), 1–10. #21-006-XIE. Ottawa, ON: Statistics Canada. Retrieved from http://www.statcan.gc.ca

Ulrich, C., & MacLeod, M. (2005). *Overcoming distance and accommodating diversity: Creating a practical northern nursing strategy*. Proceedings of the National Nursing Leadership Conference, Ottawa, ON, February 13–15, 2005.

Vandenberg, S., (2013). *Saying no to childhood immunization: Perceptions of mothers and health care professionals in southern Alberta*. Lethbridge, AB: University of Lethbridge.

Vukic, A., & Keddy, B. (2002). Northern nursing practice in a primary health care setting. *Journal of Advanced Nursing, 40*(5), 542–548. doi:10.1046/j.1365-2648. 2002.02411.x

Wakerman, J., & Humphreys, J. S. (2011). Sustainable primary health care services in rural and remote areas: Innovation and evidence. *Australian Journal of Rural Health, 19*(3), 118–124. doi: 10.1111/j.1440-1584.2010. 01180.x

Wakerman, J., Humphreys, J. S., Wells, R., Kuipers, P., Entwistle, P., & Jones, J. (2008). Primary health care delivery models in rural and remote Australia: A systematic review. *BMC Health Services Research, 8*, 276. doi:10. 1186/1472-6963-8-276

Wathen, C. N., & Harris, R. (2007). "I try to take care of myself": How rural women search for health information. *Qualitative Health Research, 17*, 639–651. doi:10.1177/ 1049732307301236

## ABOUT THE AUTHORS

**Judith Kulig**, RN, PhD (University of California, San Francisco), is a Professor within the Faculty of Health Sciences at the University of Lethbridge, Lethbridge, Alberta. Her research program focuses on rural health, including resiliency of rural communities (e.g., communities that have experienced wildfires), unique populations in rural communities (e.g., Low German–speaking Mennonites), and rural nursing practice. She is a co-principal investigator for the current study "The Nature of Nursing Practice in Rural and Remote Canada, II." In all her research, she has worked closely with community members and health and social service personnel and managers to ensure that the research meets local needs. The principle of integrated knowledge translation is also noteworthy in her research program. Judith is widely published and is senior co-editor of *Health in Rural Canada*, the only comprehensive book of its kind in Canada that examines rural health issues in our country. She is a member of the study.

**Martha L. P. MacLeod**, RN, PhD (University of Edinburgh), is a Professor in the Schools of Nursing and Health Sciences at the University of Northern British Columbia. She comes from a background in nursing management and continuing education, and teaches in the areas of leadership, qualitative research, knowledge development, and moving evidence into practice. Her research takes a qualitative approach to examining health services and health human resources, particularly in rural and northern settings. She has published and presented widely on rural and northern nursing issues, nursing education, knowledge translation, and network development. Currently, Martha is undertaking a national study on the nature of rural and remote nursing practice, "The Nature of Nursing Practice in Rural and Remote Canada, II." She has a long-standing partnered research program with B.C.'s Northern Health Authority and is currently investigating the processes of system transformation in primary health care. Martha continues to be active in developing national and regional multidisciplinary research and knowledge translation networks.

**Norma J. Stewart**, RN, PhD (University of British Columbia), is a Professor in the College of Nursing at the University of Saskatchewan. Her research interests are in rural dementia care and rural health services. She is a co-principal investigator of the national study "The Nature of Nursing Practice in Rural and Remote Canada, II." Norma has worked extensively with graduate students in the health sciences through her career and she has had administrative roles related to graduate studies and research.

**Mary Ellen Andrews**, RN(NP), PhD (University of Saskatchewan), is an Assistant Professor in the College of Nursing, University of Saskatchewan, and director of the Nurse Practitioner programs. She refers to her nursing experiences as "my adventures in nursing." Her background in nursing includes working in rural and urban acute care settings and in northern outpost and mining settings in Manitoba, Saskatchewan, Alberta, NWT, and Nunavut. Mary Ellen's tour of nursing practice settings also included employment in Addictions Services, Community Health, Sexual Health, and as a clinical nurse specialist in LTC. Research interests include rural and remote nursing, and the delivery of primary

health care that addresses the unique determinants of health for a population. She is a member of the study "The Nature of Nursing Practice in Rural and Remote Canada, II."

**Erin Wilson**, RN(NP[F]), MSN, PhD(c) (University of British Columbia), is a Family Nurse Practitioner and Assistant Professor in Prince George, British Columbia. She has lived and worked in rural regions of four provinces and one territory. She completed her undergraduate degree in nursing at the University of Manitoba, her master's at the University of British Columbia, and is currently a doctoral student at the University of Northern British Columbia. She teaches in the Rural Nursing Certificate Program and the Family Nurse Practitioner Program at UNBC and practises as a nurse practitioner two days per week. She is passionate about rural health and rural nursing practice, and is a member of the study "The Nature of Nursing Practice in Rural and Remote Canada, II."

**Kelley Kilpatrick**, RN, PhD (McGill University), is an Assistant Professor with the Faculty of Nursing at the Université de Montréal, a researcher with the Maisonneuve-Rosemont Hospital Research Centre, and an affiliate faculty member with the Canadian Centre for Advanced Practice Nursing Research. She completed a postdoctoral fellowship at McMaster University (2011). She also received a junior researcher award from the Fonds de recherche du Québec-Santé (2013–2017). Kelley's research interests include nurse practitioner and clinical nurse specialist roles, boundary work activities, perceptions of team effectiveness, acute and primary care, and the effects of healthcare service delivery on patients and families. She is a member of the study "The Nature of Nursing Practice in Rural and Remote Canada, II." Kelley has used different approaches, including mixed methods, case study, surveys, systematic reviews, and qualitative description to answer her research questions.

# Chronic Care, Long-Term Care, and Palliative Care

*Lorraine Holtslander and Shelley Peacock*

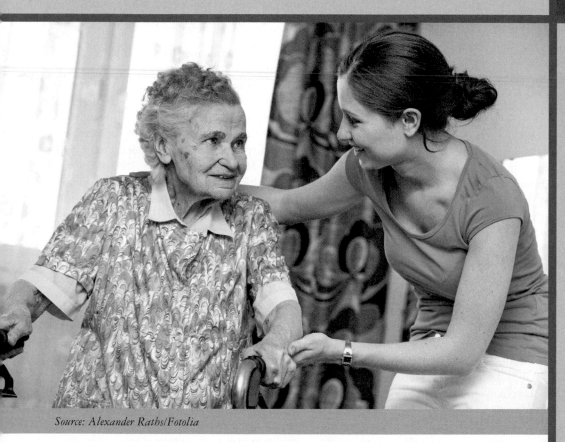

*Source: Alexander Raths/Fotolia*

## INTRODUCTION

The number of Canadians living with and dying from chronic diseases is steadily increasing due to an aging population. Often negatively described as a "tsunami" of aging, this global phenomenon is expected to occur over the next 20 to 30 years. The role of the community health nurse (CHN) to promote health and strive for positive outcomes at all levels, including palliation, will be greatly impacted. More than 68% of all deaths in Canada are due to a chronic disease such as cancer (30%), heart disease and stroke (26%), and dementia (3%) (Statistics Canada, 2013). The overall goal of this chapter is to introduce the learner to important considerations for the role of the CHN as they relate to providing excellent care for people living and dying with chronic conditions. An emphasis on supporting the essential role of the family caregiver in these settings is mandated by international and national guidelines within a continuum of care.

Chronic care, long-term care, and palliative care are interrelated, interconnected, and overlapping concepts, a relationship that is difficult to explain and becoming even more linked within our current healthcare systems. Although palliative care models and programs have historically focused on the cancer-care trajectory, current trends in the numbers of aging adults, living longer with serious chronic illnesses and other life-limiting conditions have made it imperative that a new approach is sought. The concept of a "palliative approach," advocated by the Canadian Hospice Palliative Care Association (CHPCA) (CHPCA, 2012), integrates palliative care principles into any setting of care (Stajduhar, 2011). There is an emphasis on impeccable symptom management, pain control, quality of life, and open discussions with patients and families on the goals of care in order to meet their needs in a holistic and integrated way. Access and support for this approach across all healthcare sectors require an even greater need for coordination, accessibility, and continuing care focused on prevention and health promotion.

# CHRONIC CARE: DEFINITION AND MODELS OF CARE

Many Canadians live with one or more chronic diseases or conditions that can lead to ill health, impaired functioning, and being unable to live independently (Hollander, Liu, & Chappell, 2009). It is challenging to define what is meant by chronic disease, and limiting classification of chronic health to individual diseases is inadequate, as indicated by the Canadian Academy of Health Sciences (CAHS) (CAHS, 2010). For our purposes, **chronic conditions** may be broadly defined as persistent conditions that require ongoing medical management over many years (Goodman, Posner, Huang, Parekh, & Koh, 2013). Common chronic conditions include arthritis, diabetes, cardiovascular disease, dementia, and chronic obstructive pulmonary disease, as well as infectious diseases such as HIV/AIDS or hepatitis. Each condition imposes different physical and psychological needs on patients and, as such, requires different healthcare and informal services. For example, 2.4 million Canadians over the age of 20 years have diabetes (Public Health Agency of Canada, 2011), while 747 000 Canadians live with some form of dementia (Alzheimer Society of Canada, 2011). Patients with chronic conditions require and should have access to comprehensive, coordinated healthcare services from knowledgeable healthcare professionals; this is known as **chronic care**.

Advances in medicine and an aging population have resulted in an increase in the prevalence of chronic conditions. Many Canadians lead normal lives despite having a chronic condition, while others have considerable disruption in their lives due to more complex or multiple conditions that at times are manageable and at other times may be acute. Although chronic conditions exist across all stages of life, the majority of these conditions occur in adults older than 65 years of age. It is important to note that, even though there is a perception that as a person ages his or her health declines, as many as 50% of older adults up to the age of 85 years indicate they are in good health (Statistics Canada, 2011). Patients living with chronic conditions have diverse experiences, and all require care and support from healthcare and informal systems (Canadian Academy of Health Sciences, 2010; Goodman et al., 2013). Chronic care must address how chronic conditions are managed in the community so as to improve patient outcomes and quality of life (Coleman, Austin, Brach, & Wagner, 2009).

All over the world, countries are recognizing the need for a comprehensive approach to the provision of appropriate care for patients with chronic conditions (CAHS, 2010). This is challenging because, in general, healthcare is attuned toward curing and managing of acute care illnesses. To manage chronic conditions or illnesses requires a shift in perspective to emphasize *care*, particularly with the needs and perspective of the patient at the forefront, rather than the disease being the focus. This means a move away from an ambulatory visit to an individual family physician who assesses and evaluates the needs of a passive patient and toward a **comprehensive care model** made up of an interprofessional team that engages with an informed, activated patient to arrive at appropriate clinical outcomes marked by patient satisfaction (Bowen et al., 2010).

Integrated comprehensive care models that have their foundation in a population-oriented primary care approach are becoming established internationally (CAHS, 2010). The best-known comprehensive model to address chronic care needs of patients is the **Chronic Care Model** (CCM); it is a primary care-based framework aimed at supporting the complex needs of patients in the community living with one or more chronic conditions (Tsai, Morton, Mangione, & Keeler, 2005; Wagner, 1998). The CCM is a multicomponent intervention that includes "self-management support, decision support, delivery system design, clinical information systems, healthcare organization, and community resources" (Coleman et al., 2009, p. 76). Having informed, activated patients working with a proactive team of healthcare professionals is essential to the successes of the CCM.

The **Expanded Chronic Care Model** (ECCM) was developed in Canada to broaden the clinical focus of the CCM to include elements of population health promotion with the aim to improve prevention of illness and enhance community participation (Barr et al., 2003). The ECCM acknowledges the association between healthcare and communities (see Figure 25.1). As a result, individual functional and clinical outcomes are enhanced, with the addition of measures for population health outcomes. The major aim of the ECCM is to combine population health promotion with improved treatment of conditions to provide the best option for improved healthcare outcomes in the long run. As an example, Alberta Health has successfully incorporated the ECCM in the province's approach to chronic disease management (Delon & MacKinnon, 2009).

In recent decades, management and treatment of chronic conditions has advanced, yet deficiencies continue to exist; this is cause for concern, owing to the increasing prevalence of chronic conditions globally (Tsai et al., 2005; World Health Organization, 2002a). There must be a continued effort to develop effective strategies to promote health and prevent and manage chronic conditions. As illustrated in the Canadian Research Box 25.1, challenges and opportunities remain in implementing best practices for the management of type 2 diabetes in the community. With the support of an effective chronic care model, many patients can and do manage their chronic conditions. When this is no longer the case there is often a shift to long-term care, where chronic care is further aligned with essential support from family or other often unpaid caregivers.

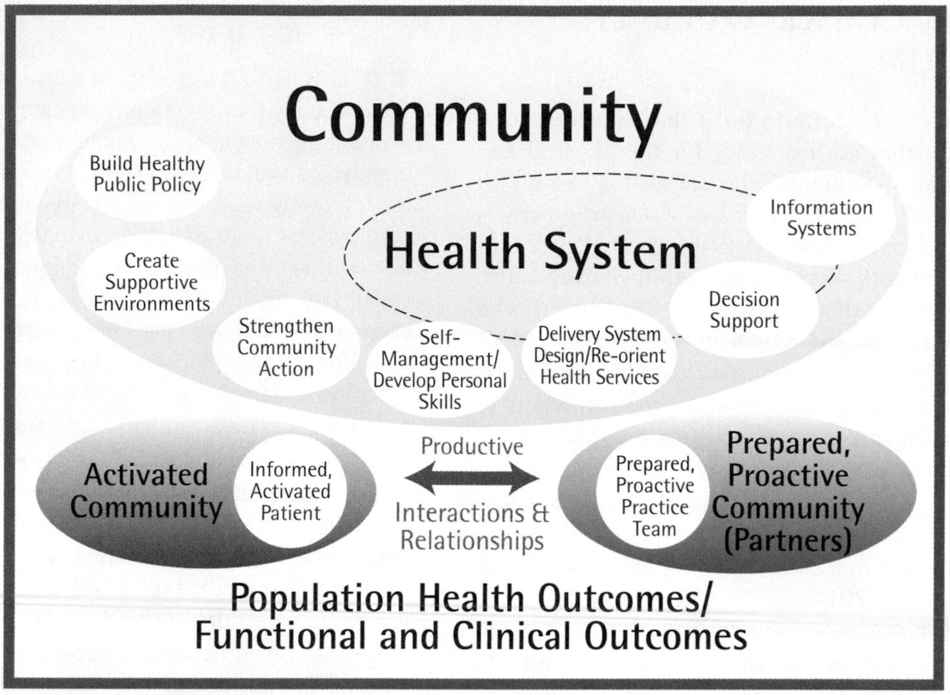

**FIGURE** **25.1** The Expanded Chronic Care Model

*Source:* Created by V. Barr, S. Robinson, B. Marin-Link, L. Underhill, A. Dotts, and D. Ravensdale. (2002). Adapted from Glasgow, R., Orleans, C., Wagner, E., Curry, S., & Solberg, L. (2001). Does the Chronic Care Model also serve as a template for improving prevention? *The Milbank Quarterly, 79*(4), and World Health Organization, Health and Welfare Canada, and Canadian Public Health Association. (1986). Ottawa Charter of Health Promotion.

### CANADIAN RESEARCH BOX 25.1

**Do diabetes clinical care best practice guidelines address the chronic care needs of Canadians with type 2 diabetes?**

Baillot, A., Pelletier, C., Dunbar, P., Geiss, L., Johnson, J., Leiter, L., & Langlois, M. (2014). Profile of adults with type 2 diabetes and uptake of clinical care best practices: Results from the 2011 survey on living with chronic diseases in Canada – diabetes component. *Diabetes Research and Clinical Practice, 103*, 11–19. Used by permission of Elsevier Science Ireland Ltd. doi:10.1016/j.diabetes.2013.11.22

This study described the profile of Canadian adults with type 2 diabetes and examined the uptake of the Canadian Diabetes Association's (CDA) Clinical Practice Guidelines (CPGs). Diabetes is reaching epidemic levels in Canada, and considerable resources are directed to its treatment, management, and care. This study utilized data from the 2011 "Survey on Living with Chronic Diseases in Canada" and the CDA CPGs as indicators of optimum care. The clinical care best practices specifically assessed in this study included six clinical monitoring indicators (e.g., HbA1c tests, eye screening, or weight measurement, etc.), as well as recommendations by healthcare providers regarding self-monitoring (e.g., assessing blood glucose) and lifestyle management (e.g., changing type/amount of food eaten). The included participants (*n* = 2335) were those who self-identified as having type 2 diabetes.

Participants had a mean age of 62.9 years and reported a high prevalence of complications and comorbidities, as evidenced by high prescription medication use (e.g., 75% of participants took medication to control their blood cholesterol). The majority of participants met five of the six clinical monitoring indicators. A high proportion of participants received clinical weight, cholesterol, and blood pressure monitoring, indicating that healthcare professionals recognize the increased risk patients have for cardiovascular diseases. However, less than two-thirds reported having HbA1c monitoring and less than half met the foot monitoring indicator. To meet CDA recommendations, HbA1c measurement and foot examinations should be performed more frequently. Approximately two-thirds of the participants indicated receiving weight management and exercise counselling, with less than half receiving nutritional counselling; these are areas needing improvement in order to meet CDA recommendations. Future studies should consider how to strengthen services, health policies, programs, and strategies to implement CDA CPGs to adequately care for Canadians living with type 2 diabetes.

### Discussion Questions

1. What might be the role of the CHN to address the CDA CPGs currently not being met as identified in the study?

2. Locate the most recent evidence on the experience of living with diabetes (using keywords: diabetes, experience, qualitative research) and determine how the CHN can empower persons with type 2 diabetes to meet the CDA's recommendations for self-monitoring.

3. How would a primary health care (PHC) approach be applied to improve care and health outcomes for persons with type 2 diabetes?

# LONG-TERM CARE: OVER THE CONTINUUM

**Long-term care** is an umbrella term that encompasses a variety of services that are necessary for the physical and psychological needs of patients who are no longer able to function independently. "By definition chronic care is long-term care" (Levine, Halper, Peist, & Gould, 2010, p. 117). In the 1960s the term "long-term care" tended to refer to nursing homes that provided care to persons who could no longer live in their own home (Miller, 2012). Although the notion of institutional care is strongly associated with the concept of long-term care, it is important to note that long-term care services are also provided in the community. It is useful to consider long-term care across a continuum that includes living at home with minimal assistance as one end of the spectrum versus requiring 24-hour care provided in a skilled facility as the other end (Kramer-Kile & Osuji, 2014).

Long-term care may be inevitable as the vast majority of chronic conditions have no cure and patients live with and manage them for the rest of their lives. The transition over the spectrum of long-term care develops as a person ages and chronic conditions progress resulting in increased dependence and reliance on others to accomplish activities of daily living. There are a variety of services available over the long-term care continuum.

## Community-Based Long-Term Care

The provision of **community-based long-term care** is intended as a seamless transition among various types of interventions and services (i.e., preventative, acute, rehabilitative, and supportive) based on the needs of patients. Ideally, long-term care services are put in place to enable patients to remain in their own home for as long as possible (Levine et al., 2010). In Canada, the types and amount of long-term care services available in the community vary with each province and territory (Kramer-Kile & Osuji, 2014). The types of services offered in most parts of Canada include: (a) nursing care; (b) personal support such as self-directed care, housekeeping, or meal preparation; (c) respite or day programs; (d) palliative care; (e) rehabilitative care, such as occupational or physical therapy; and (f) providing necessary medical equipment and supplies (MacAdam, 2009).

The largest component of community-based, long-term care services in Canada is home care. The demand for home care services is increasing. To meet this demand, home care services have shifted to patients with more pressing needs of post-acute or short-term care, leaving fewer resources for long-term patients (Forbes et al., 2003; Levine et al., 2010). The result of this shift has meant that family caregivers and other unpaid caregivers are increasingly responsible for providing long-term care in the community. Family caregivers are further discussed later in this chapter. Home and community-based services are intended to be

utilized for persons who do not yet qualify for admission to a long-term care facility, often with the intent to delay this admission for as long as possible (see Chapter 5). The case study provided above illustrates a very common situation for many older adults and their families who face increasing care needs.

## Facility-Based Long-Term Care

Long-term care services provided in a residential setting are the most intense type of service delivery on the long-term care continuum. In Canada, almost 8% of older adults (i.e., 65 years of age and older) live in a collective dwelling because they are unable to live alone (Statistics Canada, 2012). The most common types of collective dwellings include assisted living centres, nursing homes, and chronic and long-term care hospitals. The three main components of

---

**CASE STUDY**

**M**rs. Helen Anderson is an 82-year-old widow who was recently moved to a private care home. She was given a probable diagnosis of Alzheimer's disease more than three years ago; she also has a 20-year history with diabetes (currently receiving insulin injections twice daily) and mild hypertension, well controlled with a low dose of lasix/ furosemide. She uses Gravol nightly to help her sleep. Helen had required more and more assistance with care and her daughter, who lives in the same city, was becoming concerned for her mother's safety, and thus moved her into the private care home. This move was possible because Helen and her husband had saved sufficient funds in planning for their life after retirement. However, Helen's daughter pays out-of-pocket for services not offered by the private care home; for example, foot care, hair dressing, and transportation to medical appointments.

Since the move, the private care home staff have told the home care nurse (who administers the insulin injections) that Helen has been unable to settle into the home's routine. She is reluctant to shower, is beginning to hide food (e.g., crackers and cookies) in the dresser of her bedroom, and often calls out at night for "David." During the day Helen is in constant motion as if she is looking for something and frequently asks for her coat because she states, "it's time I left." She is easily re-directed if given something to do with her hands.

### Discussion Questions

1. As the home care nurse, how would you share information about Helen with her daughter and primary care physician?

2. What kinds of recommendations would you make to the staff to be able to support Helen (and her daughter) in her new home?

3. What other kinds of community-based services may benefit Helen?

facility-based long-term care include providing accommodations, hospitality services, and health services (Canadian Healthcare Association, 2009). The decision to move from one's own home to a collective dwelling can be made for a variety of reasons. Lack of availability of willing family caregivers, declining health, frailty, and concerns for safety are all motivating factors for admitting older adults to facilities that are able to provide 24-hour supportive services (Kramer-Kile & Osuji, 2014).

Residents in long-term care homes require a great deal of assistance with physical care that is usually provided by unregulated healthcare providers (Canadian Healthcare Association, 2009); unfortunately, the cognitive and psychological needs of residents may be considered less important. In Canada, the titles of these healthcare providers vary among provinces and territories and their work is supervised by registered nurses or licensed practical nurses (Canadian Healthcare Association, 2009). Nurses have a significant leadership role in long-term care facilities; this is particularly important with the increasing complex care that is now required in many facilities (Miller, 2012).

It is important to consider that persons living (and dying) in long-term care facilities tend to be those who are more vulnerable compared to community-dwelling patients (Seitz, Purandare, & Conn, 2010). For example, persons with dementia often present with severe functional limitations, marked cognitive impairment, and problematic behaviours that cause a burden for family caregivers and that precipitate the need for long-term care home admission. Research demonstrates that the prevalence of dementia among long-term care residents may be as high as 95% (Seitz et al., 2010).

## Issues with Long-Term Care

According to the literature, there are a number of issues that impact the delivery of long-term care; specific issues vary within individual provinces and territories (Kramer-Kile & Osuji, 2014). It is imperative for CHNs to be aware of these issues and be politically active in advocating for patients who require and receive long-term care. Concerns range from satisfaction with community-based care services (Forbes et al., 2008), to staffing levels in long-term care facilities (McGregor et al., 2010), and to ethical issues around provision of palliative or end-of-life care (Coventry, Grande, Richards, & Todd, 2005; Peacock, 2008).

According to the World Health Organization (WHO), there is a universal problem in how to meet the increasing demands for long-term care (WHO, 2002a). Changing family demographics, aging populations, and women undertaking paid work contribute to the alterations in social structures that lead to an increased need for long-term care solutions. Many people are living longer and with more chronic conditions than ever before, and a major concern is that little has been done to prepare for the future and the consequences of this increased long-term care. The WHO cautions that the need for long-term care could increase as much as 400% in the coming decades.

# PALLIATIVE CARE IN THE COMMUNITY: GOALS, STANDARDS, AND PRINCIPLES

The terms palliative care, hospice care, and end-of-life care are difficult to define and vary by country and context, but all have a common goal of quality end-of-life care in any setting. The movement to relieve the suffering of dying patients, originally called hospice, was officially started in London, England by Dame Cicely Saunders (Saunders, 1993). Dame Saunders was a nurse, social worker, and physician who opened St. Christopher's Hospice in 1967 and hospice home care services in 1969; the movement found its way to North America shortly after. At a grassroots level, it took hold and flourished where there were strong advocates who believed in the importance of meeting the needs of the dying and their families (Ferris et al., 2002). The term "hospice" is often used interchangeably with "palliative care," a term first proposed in 1974 by a Canadian surgeon, Dr. Balfour Mount (Mount, 1997). The CHPCA has adopted the term hospice palliative care to recognize the convergence of hospice and palliative care into one movement that has the same principles and norms of practice (CHPCA, 2013a). Recently, the CHPCA has led the way by introducing a palliative approach to care (CHPCA, 2013b). This concept can be applied throughout the course of any life-threatening illness trajectory in any setting of care, with the goal of relieving suffering and improving quality of life.

The goals, standards, and principles for palliative care programs and services developed by the WHO in 2002 are an international standard for developing and evaluating palliative care programs and systems of care (WHO, 2002b). Although it was initially established as an essential aspect of the continuum of cancer care, current directions by the WHO (www.who.int/ageing/about/who_activities/en/index1.html) are to include all patients with life-threatening illnesses as both needing and benefitting from palliative care. Specifically, a focus on pain and distress management, support, and integration of palliative care across disease groups and levels of care are needed. The WHO has prioritized palliative care as a global public health problem (Sepúlveda, Marlin, Yoshida, and Ullrich, 2002) requiring a community-based approach (see the box titled "Palliative Care").

## PALLIATIVE CARE

The WHO defines palliative care as an approach focused on improving quality of life for both the patient faced with a life-threatening illness and their family (WHO, 2002b).

Palliative care:
- provides relief from pain and other distressing symptoms;
- affirms life and regards dying as a normal process;
- intends neither to hasten nor postpone death;
- integrates the psychological and spiritual aspects of patient care;

– offers a support system to help patients live as actively as possible until death;

– offers a support system to help the family cope during the patient's illness and in their own bereavement;

– uses a team approach to address the needs of patients and their families, including bereavement counselling, if indicated;

– will enhance quality of life, and may also positively influence the course of illness; and

– is applicable early in the course of illness, in conjunction with other therapies that are intended to prolong life, such as chemotherapy or radiation therapy, and includes those investigations needed to better understand and manage distressing clinical complications.

The WHO guidelines have been widely adopted across the world, including by the CHPCA, which describes the values driving hospice palliative care as including integrity, dignity, and autonomy. Creating a plan of care is guided by quality of life as defined by the individual, and hospice palliative care is only provided when the person and family are prepared to accept it. The CHPCA has developed a definition to guide hospice palliative care norms and practice in Canada (see box titled "Hospice Palliative Care") (CHPCA, 2013a, p. 6).

## HOSPICE PALLIATIVE CARE

Hospice palliative care aims to relieve suffering and improve the quality of living and dying. Hospice palliative care strives to help individuals and families

– address physical, psychological, social, spiritual, and practical issues, and their associated expectations, needs, hopes, and fears;

– prepare for and manage self-determined life closure and the dying process; and

– cope with loss and grief during the illness and bereavement experience.

Hospice palliative care aims to

– treat all active issues;

– prevent new issues from occurring; and

– promote opportunities for meaningful and valuable experiences, personal and spiritual growth, and self-actualization.

Hospice palliative care is appropriate for any person and/or family living with or at risk of developing a life-threatening illness due to any diagnosis, with any prognosis, regardless of age, and at any time they have unmet expectations and/or needs and are prepared to accept care.

Hospice palliative care may complement and enhance disease-modifying therapy or it may become the total focus of care.

The CHPCA advocates for a community response to unique needs. Community action will support and strengthen the community by responding to suffering in appropriate, collaborative, and community-driven approaches. Recognizing unique sociocultural contexts—such as rural settings, urban settings, negative socioeconomic conditions, uncertain access to services and supports, and areas of unique populations—is essential in considering the role of the CHN to provide a socio-environmental approach to health promotion.

## CCHN Standards: Promoting Health and Providing Accessible Palliative Care

The role of the CHN (as described in Chapter 3) is to promote health at all levels, including palliation, building individual and community capacity through strong relationships, and facilitating access and equity. It is important that the CHN evaluate the integration of services and supports for patients and families facing end-of-life care, including accessibility and referrals, identifying gaps, and providing care and support in the home setting. In a recent survey of 283 older adults in Saskatchewan, only 25% had a written advance care plan, suggesting the need for nurses to provide education to promote the autonomy of older adults in the community, based on their readiness to participate (Goodridge, 2013). Following the model in Figure 25.2, the CHN would focus on the illness trajectory. Active treatment often continues while therapy to relieve suffering begins with a focus on improving quality of life. This mix of therapies will depend on the patient's and family's issues, goals, and treatment priorities. Care continues for the family after the person's death, to support positive bereavement outcomes.

## Evidence-Based Practice for Supporting Patients and Families Requiring Palliative Care

Nurses are in an optimal position to identify individuals and families that are facing end-of-life care needs and concerns, based on an in-depth understanding of end-of-life trajectories for various chronic conditions (Lunney, Lynn, Foley, Lipson, & Guralnik, 2003) and astute, holistic assessment skills. Nurses begin by completing a comprehensive, holistic assessment of individuals and families based on the CHPCA's domains of care, which include the following: disease management; physical, psychological, spiritual, social, and practical support; end-of-life care/death management; loss; and grief. Best practice guidelines have been developed to provide evidence-based recommendations for nurses caring for individuals and families facing the end of life (Registered Nurses Association of Ontario, 2011). It is important for CHNs to be aware of their own feelings and

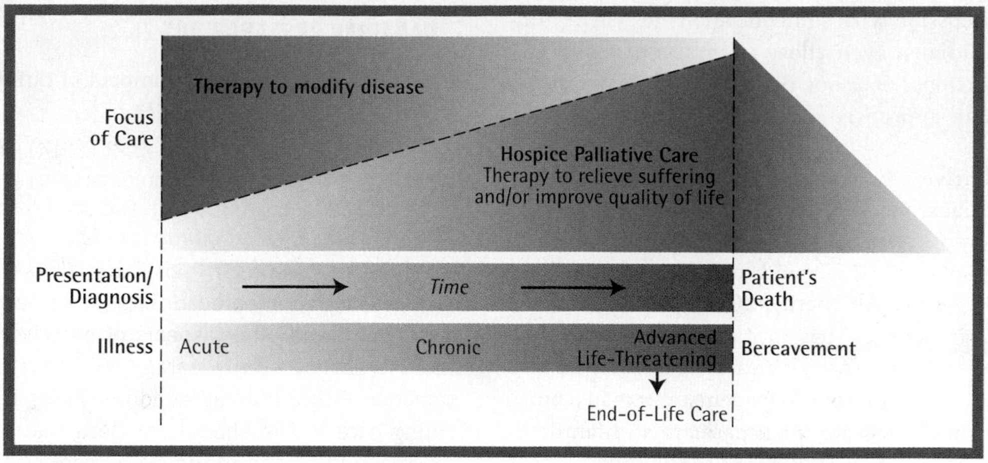

**FIGURE   25.2**   The Role of Hospice Palliative Care throughout the Illness Trajectory

*Source:* Canadian Hospice Palliative Care Association. (2013). *A model to guide hospice palliative care: Based on national principles and norms of practice* (revised and condensed edition, p. 7). Used by permission of Canadian Hospice Palliative Care Association. Retrieved from http://www.chpca.net/media/319547/norms-of-practice-eng-web.pdf

attitudes about death as they provide critical information, support, and practical assistance to individuals and families going through this experience.

## Health Promotion through Primary, Secondary, and Tertiary Prevention

Providing palliative care services requires a continuum of care, across any setting of care, and includes support into bereavement. Primary prevention of negative caregiver outcomes such as strain, burden, or role breakdown includes preparing and supporting family caregivers in their role. Careful assessment and intervention through providing information and support, conducting family meetings to discuss goals of care, and identifying concerns and questions will promote a positive caregiver experience (Hudson & Aranda, 2013).

Secondary prevention involves screening those patients and families most at risk of deleterious outcomes. Most palliative care patients are heavily reliant on the support of family caregivers in order to remain in their homes and communities. It is essential to provide supports for the caregiver, such as offering respite, teaching self-care, and introducing cognitive-behavioural approaches that increase hope and quality of life, such as the "Living with Hope Program," a self-administered intervention. This intervention was tested with rural women caregivers of persons with advanced cancer and was found to increase hope and self-efficacy while decreasing grief (Duggleby et al., 2013). Tertiary prevention focuses on providing excellent palliative care with the goal of a comfortable dying process and excellent support from both formal and informal care providers. In a recent study of 402 patient deaths from cancer in Toronto, Canada, better quality of dying and

death scores were associated with home death that was usually accompanied by better symptom control and an extensive support network (Hales et al., 2014).

## What Is a Palliative Approach?

A palliative approach to support people and families with life-limiting conditions, who may be facing the end of life, has arisen from a need for improved access to end-of-life care across all settings and circumstances (Stajduhar, 2011). Integrating and applying the principles of continuity of care, community capacity building, and promoting access and equity underpin a palliative approach. It is a seamless integration of palliative care services across all healthcare settings for patients with life-limiting conditions and their families (CHPCA, 2012).

Although integration of palliative care is an expected practice in cancer care, it has been neglected in many other situations, such as the care of patients with severe heart disease (Lauck et al., 2014) and a host of other chronic diseases (CHPCA, 2012). There is growing evidence that integrating a palliative approach earlier in the course of a disease, combined with ongoing disease treatment and management, leads to better outcomes for patients and their families. Improved outcomes include better symptom management and quality of life, more appropriate and timely referrals, and less use of futile interventions (Smith et al., 2012). Patients and families need open information about their disease and prognosis, coordination of care, and symptom management, as well as holistic support. Interestingly, a recent survey of 2 976 Canadians, conducted in 2013 through "The Way Forward" initiative of the CHPCA (2013b), revealed a great support for hospice palliative care, coupled with a general reluctance to talk about death or have a discussion with someone about it. The result is that many Canadians, even those with severe, chronic, life-limiting conditions, may not be benefitting from end-of-life planning and appropriate services, information, and support.

Primary palliative care comprises an important set of skills for all clinicians, while **specialist palliative care** for managing more complex and difficult cases can be an optimal solution to meet the growing demand for widespread palliative care services (Quill & Abernethy, 2013). Expanding the role of palliative care so that it is introduced earlier in the course of an illness requires that all healthcare professionals provide expert pain and symptom management and are comfortable engaging in discussions with patients and families about prognosis and goals of care. Referral to the specialist in palliative care is reserved for times of very difficult distress and symptom management, and for conflict resolution regarding goals of treatment within families and among treatment teams. The application of a palliative approach has numerous implications for current healthcare systems, and attention is needed on providing care for caregivers in order to sustain and support them.

# FAMILY CAREGIVERS: CONSEQUENCES, COPING, AND COST

As of 2012, there were 4.5 million **family caregivers** in Canada, an increase of 20% over the previous five years (Sinha, 2013). Over time the number of family caregivers will continue to increase, with the aging of the population, longer life expectancies, and a shift from institutionalized care to community-based care. Women outnumber men as caregivers and tend to provide more of the hands-on personal care, medical treatments, and housework, and they also spend more time caregiving when compared to male caregivers, who typically engage in home maintenance activities and transportation duties (Sinha, 2013). Many key health determinants combine to impact the health of caregivers, such as gender, age, location, education, environment, social support, access to health services, socioeconomic status, and culture. As described in Canadian Research Box 25.2, the type of caregiving greatly impacts caregiver burden and negative impact experienced (Williams, Wang, & Kitchen, 2014).

A family caregiver has been defined as a "relative, friend, or partner who has a significant personal relationship and provides assistance to a person. . . . these individuals may be primary or secondary family caregivers and may or may not reside with the person receiving care" (Hudson et al., 2010, p. 40). Being a caregiver is associated with stress on many levels, including physical, mental, emotional, social, and financial stress. Often caregivers have higher rates of depression and illness and tend to be socially isolated. The suffering and quality of life for family caregivers is an immense public health issue.

---

## CANADIAN RESEARCH BOX 25.2

**What do we know about the impact of different types of family caregiving?**

Williams, A., Wang, L., & Kitchen, P. (2014). Differential impacts of caregiving across three caregiver groups in Canada: End-of-life care, long-term care, and short-term care. *Health and Social Care in the Community, 22*(2), 187–196. Used by permission of John Wiley & Sons, Ltd. doi:10.1111/hsc.12075

This research compared differences in socio-demographics, health, and other aspects of caregiver burden among three types of family caregivers—those caregiving for someone with a chronic condition (long term), those providing care in the short term (less than two years), and those providing end-of-life (EOL) care—from a large sample of Canadian informal caregivers (*n* = 5 574). Data were obtained from Statistics Canada from the 2007 cycle and were analyzed by Canadian researchers in health economics, geography, and environment at McMaster University.

The data revealed that family caregivers across Canada are more likely to be female, married, employed, and living in a Census Metropolitan Area (CMA). More than 50% of all caregivers reported living with at least one chronic condition themselves and stated that their health and social support networks were compromised by caregiving commitments. EOL caregivers were most affected in terms of personal health and in terms of financial and employment costs, as they were incurring extra expenses and giving up job opportunities and hours to be caregivers. EOL caregivers also experienced a more negative impact on their social and activity patterns than other caregivers. EOL caregivers are particularly at risk of negative health outcomes due to the intensity of this type of caregiving. All of this results in a greater amount of caregiver burden on EOL caregivers than on the other two groups.

As women enter the workforce in ever higher numbers, they are increasingly juggling multiple caregiver roles and both paid and unpaid commitments. Female caregivers are more likely to quit their jobs than male caregivers and are more likely to take on the responsibility of caregiving, resulting in negative impacts on their finances, health, and social support networks. More research is needed to explore the extensive diversity found in Canadian family caregivers. Varying personal experiences such as location, culture, socioeconomic status, gender, age, education, and health will greatly impact their unique support needs. However, from this research it can be seen that EOL caregivers are at particular risk of negative outcomes resulting from the burden they are experiencing.

### Discussion Questions

1. Which of the health determinants identified in this report might be most important for the CHN to address to improve health outcomes for caregivers?
2. Choose two strategies for policy makers in order to address to better support family caregivers? (e.g., employment accommodations, financial supports)
3. How would you design a feasible and acceptable social support group for EOL family caregivers? What content would be important to address?

Caregivers face economic costs such as employment consequences, time spent caregiving, and reduced disposable income that may jeopardize some family caregivers' current or future economic security (Fast, Keating, Lero, Eales, & Duncan, 2013). A conservative estimate of the value of unpaid care provided by family caregivers to older adults in Canada is $25 billion annually (Chappell & Hollander, 2011). Without support and preventative care for this population, family caregiver health is at risk and can result in even greater demands on the healthcare system. Family caregivers play a crucial role in community-based care, affecting workplaces and government policy in ways that must be acknowledged, incorporated, assessed, supported, and documented.

Of course, there are many positive aspects of being a caregiver; for instance, the reward of a reciprocal relationship, feeling closer to the care receiver, and finding meaning or a sense of personal growth in the work. It is these positive aspects that may sustain a family caregiver in his or her role for longer than would be expected. It is important to note that the rewards of caregiving should not be exploited as a way of coercing family caregivers to pick up the slack when healthcare services (e.g., community or facility-based care) are reduced or withdrawn (Levine et al., 2010). In a recent Canadian study, caregivers providing end-of-life care described a struggle for survival while hiding their true feelings of isolation, guilt, self-deprecation, sadness, and anger (Ward-Griffin, McWilliam, & Oudshoorn, 2012). Nurses need to build relationships with family caregivers, acknowledging their need for respite and emotional support.

Family caregivers also experience the illness and death of the person they are caring for and must embark on a healing transition through their **bereavement** experience (CHPCA, 2013a). For example, very little research has addressed the needs of family caregivers of persons with dementia at the end of life (Peacock, 2013), and the evidence needed for providing the most effective bereavement support remains lacking (Holtslander, 2008). Bereavement itself has a significant negative effect on the morbidity and mortality of caregivers (Stroebe, Schut, & Stroebe, 2007), and could include risk of suicide (Erlangsen, Jeune, Bille-Brahe, & Vauper, 2004), depression (Holtslander & McMillan, 2011), loneliness, substance abuse, physical and emotional illnesses (Schulz, Hebert, & Boerner, 2008), pain (Kowalski & Bondmass, 2008), sleep disturbance (Carter, 2005), and death (Christakis & Iwashyna, 2003). There is a need to develop interventions that reduce costs and improve the effectiveness of the healthcare system to support family caregiver during caregiving and continuing on into their bereavement.

## CONCLUSION

Nurses are very well positioned to lead the way by improving current healthcare systems; engaging in necessary conversations with patients, families, and communities; and striving to relieve suffering and improve quality of life, based on a holistic person- and family-centred approach that includes a community health focus. Goals for care are shared across a spectrum of care—chronic, long term, and palliative—that aims to support patients and families with open information about their condition(s) and prognosis, the coordination of comprehensive services, symptom management, and holistic support.

## KEY TERMS

## STUDY QUESTIONS

1. What are the major differences between the (Canadian) Expanded Chronic Care Model by Barr and colleagues (2003) and Wagner's Chronic Care Model (1998)?

2. Which specific services are included within long-term care?

3. How can transitions between the community and acute care settings become more seamless and better integrated?

4. Which populations would benefit most from referrals to palliative care services?

5. What is the difference between generalist and specialist palliative care?

> After working through these questions, go to the MyNursingLab at www.pearsoned.ca/mynursinglab to check your answers.

## INDIVIDUAL CRITICAL-THINKING EXERCISES

1. Given the notion of an informed or activated patient being essential to chronic care, how can the CHN support and engage patients in managing their chronic conditions?

2. How do your own cultural beliefs affect your work with others?

3. What experiences of caregiving have you had? How do these experiences shape your work as a nurse?

4. Have you had family who received palliative care services? What was your experience?

# GROUP CRITICAL-THINKING EXERCISES

1. In what ways do social, cultural, and environmental factors affect health and how can they be addressed and acknowledged in the context of chronic care?

2. Considering the scarcity of healthcare resources, how should funding be allocated among acute, long-term, and palliative care?

3. Who should manage palliative care needs in the community setting?

4. What are the challenges and opportunities in implementing a consistent palliative approach to care across Canada?

5. What are your own feelings about death? Your experiences within your own family? How will these experiences impact your work in the community?

# REFERENCES

Alzheimer Society of Canada. (2011). *A new way of looking at dementia*. Retrieved from http://www.alzheimer.ca/~/media/Files/national/Media-releases/asc_factsheet_new_data_09272012_en.ashx

Barr, V., Robinson, S., Marin-Link, B., Underhill, L., Dotts, A., Ravensdale, D., & Salivaras, S. (2003). The expanded chronic care model: An integration of concepts and strategies from population health promotion and the chronic care model. *Hospital Quarterly, 7*(1), 73–82.

Bowen, J., Stevens, D., Sixta, C., Provost, L., Johnson, J., Woods, D., & Wagner, E. (2010). Developing measures of educational change for academic health care teams implementing the chronic care model in teaching practices. *Journal of General Internal Medicine, 25*(Suppl 4), 586–592.

Canadian Academy of Health Sciences. (2010). *Transforming care for Canadians with chronic health conditions: Put people first, expect the best, manage for results*. Retrieved from http://www.cahs-acss.ca/wp-content/uploads/2011/09/cdm-final-English.pdf

Canadian Healthcare Association. (2009). *New directions for facility-based long-term care*. Ottawa, ON: Author.

Canadian Hospice Palliative Care Association. (2012). *Integrating a palliative approach into the management of chronic, life-threatening diseases: Who, how and when. The Way Forward integration initiative*. Retrieved from http://hpcintegration.ca/media/36315/TWF-integrating-palliative-approach-report-Eng_final3.pdf

Canadian Hospice Palliative Care Association. (2013a). *A model to guide hospice palliative care*. Based on national principles and norms of practice - Revised and condensed edition: 2013. Used by permission of Canadian Hospice Palliative Care Association. Retrieved from http://www.chpca.net/media/319547/norms-of-practice-eng-web.pdf

Canadian Hospice Palliative Care Association. (2013b). *What Canadians say: The Way Forward survey draft report*. Retrieved from http://www.hpcintegration.ca/media/51032/The%20Way%20Forward%20-%20What%20Canadians%20Say%20-%20Survey%20Report%20Final%20Dec%202013.pdf

Carter, P. A. (2005). Bereaved caregivers' descriptions of sleep: Impact on daily life and the bereavement process. *Oncology Nursing Forum, 32*(4), E70-E75. doi:10.1188/05.ONF.E70-E75

Chappell, N., & Hollander, M. (2011). An evidence-based policy prescription for an aging population. *Healthcare Papers, 11*(1).

Christakis, N. A., & Iwashyna, T. J. (2003). The health impact of health care on families: A matched cohort study of hospice use by decedents and mortality outcomes in surviving, widowed spouses. *Social Science and Medicine, 57*, 465–475.

Coleman, K., Austin, B., Brach, C., & Wagner, E. (2009). Evidence on the chronic care model in the new millennium. *Health Affairs, 28*(1), 75–85.

Coventry, P., Grande, G., Richards, D., & Todd, C. (2005). Prediction of appropriate timing of palliative care for older adults with non-malignant life-threatening disease: A systematic review. *Age and Ageing, 34*, 218–227.

Delon, S., & MacKinnon, B. (2009). Alberta's systems approach to chronic disease management and prevention utilizing the expanded chronic care model. *Healthcare Quarterly, 13*(Special Issue), 98–104.

Duggleby, W., Swindle, J., & Peacock, S. (2014). Self-administered intervention for caregivers of persons with Alzheimer's disease. *Clinical Nursing Research, 23*(1), 20–35. doi:10.1177/1054773812474299

Duggleby, W., Williams, A., Holtslander, L., Cooper, D., Ghosh, S., Hallstrom, L., . . . Hampton, M. (2013). Evaluation of the living with hope program for rural women caregivers of persons with advanced cancer. *BMC Palliative Care, 12*(1), 1–11. doi:10.1186/1472-684x-12-36

Erlangsen, A., Jeune, B., Bille-Brahe, U., & Vauper, J. W. (2004). Loss of partner and suicide risk among oldest old: A population-based register study. *Age and Ageing, 33*, 378–383. doi:10.1093/ageing/afh128

Fast, J., Keating, N., Lero, D. S., Eales, J., & Duncan, K. (2013). The economic costs of care to family/friend caregivers: A synthesis of findings. Retrieved from http://www.rapp.ualberta.ca/en/~/media/rapp/Publications/Documents/SynthesisCaregiversEconomicCosts_2013Dec.pdf

Ferris, F., Balfour, H., Bowan, K., Farley, J., Hardwick, M., Lamontagne, C., . . . West, P. (2002). *A model to guide hospice palliative care*. Ottawa, ON: Canadian Hospice Palliative Care Association. Retrieved from http://www.chpca.net/marketplace/national_norms/A+Model+to+Guide+Hospice+Palliative+Care+2002-URLUpdate-August2005.pdf

Forbes, D., Markle-Reid, M., Hawranik, P., Peacock, S., Kingston, D., Morgan, D., . . . Jansen, S. L. (2008). Availability and acceptability of Canadian home and community-based services: Perspectives of family caregivers of persons with dementia. *Home Health Care Services Quarterly, 27*(2), 75–98.

Forbes, D., Stewart, N., Morgan, D., Anderson, M., Parent, K., & Janzen, B. (2003). Determinants of home care nursing and home support services. *Canadian Journal of Nursing Research, 35*(4), 14–36.

Goodman, R., Posner, S., Huang, E., Parekh, A., & Koh, H. (2013). Defining and measuring chronic conditions: Imperatives for research, policy, program, and practice. *Preventing Chronic Disease, 10*:120239.

Goodridge, D. (2013). Planning for serious illness amongst community-dwelling older adults. *Nursing Research and*

*Practice,* 2013, 1-7. Retrieved from http://dx.doi.org/10.1155/2013/427917

Hales, S., Chiu, A., Husain, A., Braun, M., Rydall, A., Gagliese, L., . . . Rodin, G. (2014). The quality of dying and death in cancer and its relationship to palliative care and place of death. *Journal of Pain and Symptom Management.* doi:10.1016/j.jpainsymman.2013.12.240

Hollander, M., Liu, G., & Chappell, N. (2009). Who cares and how much? The imputed economic contribution to the Canadian healthcare system of middleaged and older unpaid caregivers providing care to the elderly. *Healthcare Quarterly, 12*(2), 42–49.

Holtslander, L. (2008). Caring for bereaved family caregivers: Analyzing the context of care. *Clinical Journal of Oncology Nursing, 12*(3), 501–506.

Holtslander, L. F., & McMillan, S. (2011). Depressive symptoms, grief and complicated grief among bereaved family caregivers of advanced cancer patients. *Oncology Nursing Forum, 38*(1), 60–65. doi:10.1188/11.ONF.60-65

Hudson, P., & Aranda, S. (2013). The Melbourne Family Support Program: Evidence-based strategies that prepare family caregivers for supporting palliative care patients. *BMJ: Supportive and Palliative Care, 0,* 1–7. doi:10.1136/bmjspcare-2013-000500

Hudson, P., Remedios, C., Zordan, R., Thomas, K., Clifton, D., Crewdson, M., . . . Clarke, D. (2010). *Clinical practice guidelines for the psychosocial and bereavement support of family caregivers of palliative care patients.* Melbourne, Aus: Centre for Palliative Care.

Kowalski, S. D., & Bondmass, M. D. (2008). Physiological and psychological symptoms of grief in widows. *Research in Nursing and Health, 31,* 23–30.

Kramer-Kile, M., & Osuji, J. (Eds.). (2014). *Chronic illness in Canada: Impact and intervention.* Burlington, MA: Jones and Bartlett Learning.

Lauck, S., Garland, E., Achtem, L., Forman, J., Baumbusch, J., Boone, R., . . . Webb, J. (2014). Integrating a palliative approach in a transcatheter heart valve program: Bridging innovations in the management of severe aortic stenosis and best end-of-life practice. *European Journal of Cardiovascular Nursing,* 1–8. doi:10.1177/1474515114520770

Levine, C., Halper, D., Peist, A., & Gould, D. (2010). Bridging troubled waters: Family caregivers, transitions, and long-term care. *Health Affairs, 29*(1), 116–124.

Lunney, J. R., Lynn, J., Foley, D. J., Lipson, S., & Guralnik, J. M. (2003). Patterns of functional decline at the end of life. *Journal of American Medical Association, 289*(18), 2387–2392.

MacAdam, M. (2009). *Moving toward health service integration: Provincial progress in system change for seniors.* Ottawa, ON: Canadian Policy Research Networks. Retrieved from http://www.cprn.org/documents/51302_EN.pdf

McGregor, M., Tate, R., Ronald, L., McGrail, K., Cox, M., Berta, W., & Broemeling, A. (2010). Trends in long-term care staffing by facility ownership in British Columbia, 1996 to 2006. *Health Reports, 21*(4), 1–7.

Miller, C. A. (2012). *Nursing for wellness in older adults* (6th ed.). New York, NY: Lippincott Williams and Wilkins.

Mount, B. (1997). The Royal Victoria Hospital palliative care service: A Canadian experience. In C. Saunders & R. Kastenbaum (Eds.), *Hospice care on the international scene* (pp. 73–85). New York, NY: Springer Publishing.

Peacock, S. (2008). The moral issues involved in palliative end-of-life dementia care. *Canadian Nursing Home, 19*(2), 1–5.

Peacock, S. (2013). The experience of providing end-of-life care to a relative with advanced dementia: An integrative review. *Palliative & Supportive Care, 11*(2), 155–168.

Public Health Agency of Canada. (2011). *Diabetes in Canada: Facts and figures from a public health perspective.* Retrieved from http://www.phac-aspc.gc.ca/cd-mc/publications/diabetes-diabete/facts-figures-faits-chiffres-2011/pdf/facts-figures-faits-chiffres-eng.pdf

Quill, T. E., & Abernethy, A. P. (2013). Generalist plus specialist palliative care—Creating a more sustainable model. *New England Journal of Medicine, 368*(13), 1173–1175. doi:10.1056/NEJMp1215620

Registered Nurses Assocation of Ontario. (2011). End-of-life care during the last days and hours. Retrieved from http://rnao.ca/sites/rnao-ca/files/End-of-Life_Care_During_the_Last_Days_and_Hours.pdf

Saunders, C., & Sykes, N. (Eds.). (1993). *The management of terminal malignant disease.* London, UK: Edward Arnold.

Schulz, R., Hebert, R., & Boerner, K. (2008). Bereavement after caregiving. *Geriatrics, 63*(1), 20–22.

Seitz, D., Purandare, N., & Conn, D. (2010). Prevalence of psychiatric disorder among older adults in long-term care homes: A systematic review. *International Psychogeriatrics, 22*(7), 1025–1039.

Sepúlveda, C., Marlin, A., Yoshida, T., & Ullrich, A. (2002). Palliative care: The World Health Organization's global perspective. *Journal of Pain and Symptom Management, 24*(2), 91–96.

Sinha, M. (2013). *Portrait of caregivers, 2012.* Ottawa, ON: Statistics Canada Catalogue no. 89-652-X — No. 001. Retrieved from http://www.statcan.gc.ca/pub/89-652-x/89-652-x2013001-eng.pdf

Smith, T. J., Temin, S., Alesi, E. R., Abernethy, T. A., Balboni, T. A., Basch, E. M., . . . Von Roenn, J. H. (2012). American Society of Clinical Oncology provisional clinical opinion: The integration of palliative care into standard oncology care. *Journal of Clinical Oncology, 30*(8), 880–887.

Stajduhar, K. I. (2011). Chronic illness, palliative care, and the problematic nature of dying. *Canadian Journal of Nursing Research, 43*(3), 7–15.

Statistics Canada. (2011). *Canada year book 2011.* Retrieved from http://www.statcan.gc.ca/pub/11-402-x/2011000/pdf/seniors-aines-eng.pdf

Statistics Canada. (2012). *Living arrangements of seniors: Families, households and marital status, structural type of dwelling and collectives, 2011 census of population.* Retrieved from http://www12.statcan.gc.ca/census-recensement/2011/as-sa/98-312-x/98-312-x2011003_4-eng.pdf

Statistics Canada. (2013). *Ranking, number and percentage of deaths for the 10 leading causes, Canada, 2000 and 2009.* Retrieved from http://www.statcan.gc.ca/daily-quotidien/120725/t120725b001-eng.htm

Stroebe, M., Schut, H., & Stroebe, W. (2007). Health outcomes of bereavement. *The Lancet, 370,* 1960–1973.

Tsai, A., Morton, S., Mangione, C., & Keeler, E. (2005). A meta-analysis of interventions to improve care for chronic illnesses. *American Journal of Managed Care, 11*(8), 478–488.

Wagner, E. H. (1998). Chronic disease management: What will it take to improve care for chronic illness? *Effective Clinical Practice, 1*, 2–4.

Ward-Griffin, C., McWilliam, C., & Oudshoorn, A. (2012). Relational experiences of family caregivers providing home-based end-of-life care. *Journal of Family Nursing, 18*(4), 491–516.

Williams, A., Wang, L., & Kitchen P. (2014). Differential impacts of caregiving across three caregiver groups in Canada: End-of-life care, long-term care, and short-term care. *Health and Social Care in the Community, 22*(2), 187–196. doi: 10.1111.hsc.12075

World Health Organization. (2002a). *Ethical choices in long-term care: What does justice require?* Retrieved from www.who.int/chp/knowledge/publications/ethical_choices.pdf?ua=1

World Health Organization. (2002b). *WHO definition of palliative care.* Reprinted with permission from World Health Organization. Retrieved from http://www.who.int/cancer/palliative/definition/en

## ABOUT THE AUTHORS

**Lorraine Holtslander**, RN, PhD, CHPCN(C) (University of Saskatchewan), is an Associate Professor in the College of Nursing in Saskatoon, Canada. She teaches family nursing to undergraduate students and an interdisciplinary course in qualitative research methods at the graduate level. Her clinical area of community nursing practice was as a palliative home care nurse for more than 20 years. The focus of her research is in palliative care, grief and loss, and supporting family caregivers during bereavement.

**Shelley Peacock**, RN, BSc, PhD (University of Alberta), is an Assistant Professor with the College of Nursing, University of Saskatchewan, Saskatoon, Canada. Currently, she teaches assessment and components of nursing care to undergraduate students. Her area of interest is with older adults, particularly those with dementia and their family caregivers. Recent research using qualitative methods has involved exploring the experience of bereaved dementia family caregivers.

# Correctional Health

*Cindy Peternelj-Taylor and Phil Woods*

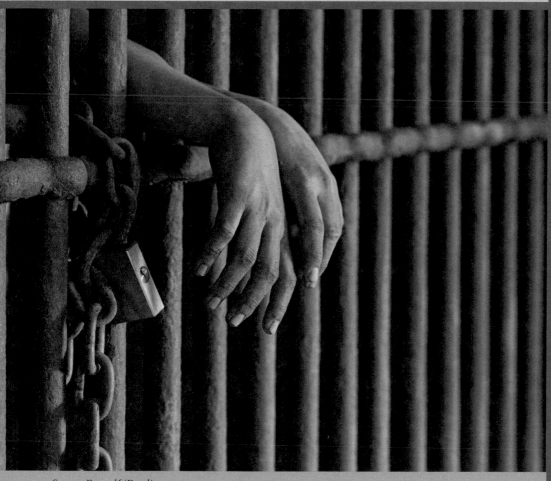

Source: Fresnel6/Fotolia

## LEARNING OUTCOMES

**After studying this chapter, you should be able to:**

1. Discuss the role of the nurse in correctional health.

2. Describe the Canadian offender population.

3. Examine common health challenges seen in correctional settings.

4. Identify the nurse's responsibilities in primary, secondary, and tertiary prevention in correctional health.

5. Analyze professional challenges and ethical responsibilities experienced by nurses in correctional environments.

6. Reflect on ongoing education, research, and practice developments relative to nursing in correctional settings.

## INTRODUCTION

**Correctional nursing** is defined as "the protection, promotion, and optimization of health and abilities; prevention of illness and injury; alleviation of suffering through the diagnosis and treatment of human response; advocacy for and delivery of healthcare to individuals, families, communities, and populations under the jurisdiction of the criminal justice system" (American Nurses Association, 2013, p. 1). Nurses practising in the criminal justice system primarily work in correctional settings, including jails, detention centres, prisons, healing lodges, correctional centres, youth custody facilities, community correctional centres, and halfway houses. They are primarily responsible for providing healthcare services to large and diverse incarcerated populations. The daily practice of correctional nurses "taps the knowledge and skills base of occupational health, emergency room, acute care, community health, maternity care, psychiatric care, geriatrics, and end-of-life nursing domains" (Shelton, Weiskopf, & Nicholson, 2010, p. 299). Through their use of clinical assessment and triage skills, they engage in primary, secondary, and tertiary intervention strategies including early case finding, infection control, treatment and medication administration, health promotion, illness prevention, as well as rehabilitative services (see the box titled "Levels of Prevention in Correctional Health"). As per the Corrections and Conditional Release Act (CCRA), and various provincial and territorial corrections acts, clients incarcerated in correctional facilities are entitled to physical and mental healthcare in accordance with professional and community standards (Canadian Public Health Association, 2004). Nurses represent the largest group of healthcare professionals working with incarcerated individuals, and as such they have a significant role to play. Timely identification, treatment, and management of healthcare

---

## LEVELS OF PREVENTION IN CORRECTIONAL HEALTH

### Primary Prevention

Illness prevention (control of communicable diseases, immunization, suicide prevention, violence prevention)
Health promotion
Provision of education and information
Classification of stressors
Political involvement
Appropriate referrals
Advocacy

### Secondary Prevention

Assessment, evaluation, diagnosis
Health screening
First aid
Community consultation
Crisis intervention
Program planning and implementation
Substance abuse treatment
Sex offender treatment
Aggressive behaviour control
Life and social skills training
Acute inpatient psychiatric nursing
Suicide risk assessment and management
Creation and maintenance of a therapeutic milieu
Short-term therapy
Counselling, psychotherapy
Medication administration and management
Emergency and trauma care

### Tertiary Intervention

Case management
After-care services/community reintegration
Rehabilitation
Vocational training
Relapse prevention
End-of-life/palliative care
Compassionate release
Spiritual care

---

concerns not only contribute to the health of the individual client, but also further contributes to the health and safety of other offenders, facility staff, and the community at large.

Correctional facilities are not generally considered part of the traditional healthcare system; by default they are responsible for the provision of healthcare services to a diverse group of individuals who have come into conflict with the law, including those who are remanded in custody while awaiting trial or sentencing (charged but not yet sentenced), and those found guilty and sentenced by the courts to various periods of time in custody. Federal, provincial, and territorial governments share the administration of correctional services in Canada. Generally, individuals receiving a sentence of two years less a day are the responsibility of either provincial or territorial correctional systems, while those sentenced to two years or longer serve their sentences within the federal system operated by Correctional Service Canada (CSC). Those on remand tend to have greater and more complex healthcare needs than sentenced inmates, who may have had these issues addressed during the remand period.

In the "Correctional Services Key Indicators, 2012/2013" report, Perreault (2014c) has noted that on an average day in 2012/2013 there were on average 40 000 adults in custody. Of this group, approximately 25 600 were in sentenced custody, roughly 14 500 were under federal jurisdiction, and 11 200 were in provincial or territorial custody. During the same time period, another 120 000 offenders were under some form of community supervision (probation, conditional sentences, or parole). Additionally, within provincial and territorial correctional facilities, the number of offenders on remand continues to exceed those in sentenced custody (i.e., about 13 700 offenders on remand versus about 11 200 in sentenced custody). As noted in the "Admissions to Adult Correctional Services in Canada, 2011/2012" report, the majority of those in custody are male; females accounted for 15% of the people admitted to correctional services; and young adults, those under the age of 35 years, represent more than half (55%) of those admitted, even though they only represent 29% of the Canadian population aged 18 and over. On any given day in 2012/2013, there were 73 youth in custody for every 10 000 youth in the general population. This number represents a decline of 5% from the previous year and 31% less than it was in 2002–2003 (Perreault, 2014c). The health and psychosocial issues experienced by this large captive group are extremely complex and contribute to treatment challenges during incarceration and upon release from custody.

## HEALTHCARE OF THE CORRECTIONAL POPULATION

Historically, those who are incarcerated have experienced limited and inconsistent exposure to our healthcare system. They may experience many of the same age- and gender-specific healthcare concerns common to the general population, but morbidity and mortality data suggest higher rates of disease and disability when compared to non-incarcerated populations (American Nurses Association, 2013; Canadian Public Health

Association, 2004). For many individuals, healthcare received while incarcerated may be the first real opportunity that they have had to address their healthcare needs. Numerous opportunities exist for correctional nurses to provide leadership in the provision of health promotion and illness prevention, especially if individuals are motivated to make lifestyle changes that would improve their overall health status.

The correctional system provides care for offenders with all types of acute and chronic illnesses. The lifestyle of many offenders includes substance abuse, which gives rise to various drug and alcohol withdrawal syndromes, diverse infectious diseases, and the need for long-term treatment interventions. Crowded living conditions can result in higher exposure to infectious diseases, a concern of public health officials worldwide, as most clients eventually return to the community (Thomas, 2005). Furthermore, the "deinstitutionalization movement" that began in Canada in the 1960s and continues today has frequently been blamed for the **criminalization of the mentally ill** (Chaimowitz, 2012). Peternelj-Taylor (2008) affirms that prisons were never designed to meet the needs of individuals requiring treatment for mental illness, and much controversy exists around how they can meet these needs. The Mental Health Commission of Canada (MHCC) (2012) concluded that prisons have become the "'asylums' of the 21st century" (p. 60). Finally, it is not uncommon for nurses to care for clients who have intellectual disabilities, including fetal alcohol spectrum disorder, as well as those who have experienced multiple traumas such as sexual assaults, stabbings, beatings, and traumatic brain injuries.

Provincial correctional facilities (and, to a lesser extent, territorial facilities) admit extremely large numbers of offenders on a daily basis. Clearly, the volume, turnover, and lengths of stay, which can range from a few hours to years, definitively impact the professional nursing role. Daily admissions to federal correctional facilities are minimal compared to provincial correctional facilities, and the care they are able to provide is different. Clients presenting with acute healthcare problems are assessed and triaged by nurses, and those requiring acute emergency care are normally transferred to a local community general hospital for further assessment and treatment. Nursing staff, in collaboration with the facilities' physicians, manage other less urgent issues. Nurses frequently assist the clients to bring chronic conditions under better control by attending to treatment protocols, assessing for complications, preventing recurrence of health problems, attending to health-promotion needs, and facilitating transition to the community upon eventual discharge.

## Special Populations in Correctional Settings

The unique needs of offenders who experience mental illness, those who are elderly, women, youth, and those from culturally diverse backgrounds are highlighted here to draw attention to the healthcare concerns and the overall disparities experienced by offender populations.

**Offenders with Mental Illness** Deinstitutionalization has resulted in an influx to correctional facilities of individuals with serious mental illness. Prior to this, police would transport individuals exhibiting bizarre behaviours in public to a mental health facility; now they have little choice but to remand the individual in custody in a local jail or remand centre.

In 2004, the Canadian Public Health Association (CPHA) reported that epidemiological studies in the CSC found high prevalence of mental disorder in inmates, often with two or more coexisting disorders, and higher rates of psychosis, depression, anxiety, and personality disorder when compared to the Canadian population. Since then, the number of those with mental health problems in federal correctional institutions has been on the rise. In fact, since 1997 it is estimated that the number of offenders with mental illness within federal corrections has increased by 60–70% (MHCC, 2012). According to the Office of the Correctional Investigator [OCI] (2013), 13% of male offenders and 29% of female offenders are identified on admission as presenting with mental health problems. In addition, 15% of male offenders and 30% of female offenders had previously been hospitalized because of a psychiatric disorder. In a prevalence study of mental illness in inmates in Ontario correctional facilities, the prevalence of schizophrenia was 4.5%, depression 5.6%, bipolar 5.2%, anti-social personality disorder 4.1%, adjustment disorder 3.4%, anxiety 1.9%, and attention deficit/hyperactivity disorder 1.5% (total 26.2%) (Brown, Girard, & Mathias, 2006). Although these figures are somewhat lower than those identified by the CSC, the discrepancy is most likely due to how mentally ill inmates are assessed and labelled in Ontario facilities. Similar high prevalence rates are reported in other countries. In a survey of psychiatric morbidity among prisoners in England and Wales, Singleton, Meltzer, Gatward, Coid, and Deasy (1998) reported a high prevalence of mental illness and personality disorder in both remanded and sentenced males and females. A study by the U.S. Department of Justice reported that 64% of local jail inmates, 56% of state prisoners, and 45% of federal prisoners have symptoms of serious mental illness (James & Glaze, 2006). In a recent report published by the Vera Institute of Justice, Sabramanian, Delaney, Roberts, Fishman, and McGarry (2015) noted that the rate of serious mental illness in men and women in jail is four to six times higher than the general American population. Finally, in a recent systematic review and meta-analysis of severe mental illness in prisoners worldwide, pooled prevalence of psychosis was 3.6% for males and 3.9% for females, and for major depression, 10.2% for males and 14.1% for females (Fazel & Seewald, 2012).

Generally, correctional facilities are not in a position to provide mental healthcare at the same standard as that found within community mental health systems. Indeed, the OCI (2012, 2013, 2014) has repeatedly emphasized that mental health treatment within federal facilities warrants further development when compared to the community standard. Promoting a mental health agenda in a correctional setting is challenging at best, as the environment is coercive by definition. The MHCC (2012) has observed that without access to appropriate treatment, offenders with serious and complex mental health needs "can get caught up in a vicious cycle of

## KEY ELEMENTS OF THE MENTAL HEALTH STRATEGY FOR CORRECTIONS IN CANADA

Part I

1. Mental health promotion
2. Screening and assessment
3. Treatment, services, and supports
4. Suicide and self-injury prevention and management
5. Transitional services and supports
6. Staff education, training, and support
7. Community supports and partnerships

*Source:* Correctional Services Canada. Federal Provincial/ Territorial Partnership. (2012). *Mental health strategy for corrections in Canada*. Reproduced with the permission of the Minister of Public Works and Government Services Canada, 2015. Retrieved from http://www.csc-scc.gc.ca/health/092/ MH-strategy-eng.pdf

isolation, restraint, and segregation" (p. 47). Since the CPHA (2004) highlighted the need for more proactive standardized mental health intake assessments (rather than reactive, crisis-oriented services), a collaborative venture of the MHCC and federal, provincial, and territorial correctional jurisdictions has resulted in a mental health strategy for corrections in Canada. National consultations with correctional jurisdictions, staff, stakeholders, and offenders resulted in a two-phase strategy. Part I provides a foundation for the strategy and outlines the key elements of the framework (refer to the box titled "Key Elements of the Mental Health Strategy for Corrections in Canada"). Part II builds upon the framework to achieve the best possible mental health and well-being for all prisoners in Canada. Priority areas include knowledge generation and sharing, enhanced service delivery, improved human resource management, and building community supports and partnerships.

All offenders are assessed for suicidal thoughts and plans on admission and reassessed throughout their incarceration as necessary. Suicide may be viewed by inmates as the only way to cope with their charges (and/or their sentence), family responsibilities that cannot be met, fear of the actions of fellow inmates, and the living conditions within the correctional facility. Power and Riley (2010) have identified key suicide risk factors for those in federal custody. Nurses should be particularly concerned with appropriate discharge planning as the days following release from prison are particularly challenging for offenders. While incarcerated, conditions of overcrowding, isolation, and long sentences for violent crimes, coupled with a history of psychiatric disorders and substance abuse, are also identified risk factors. Offenders may be placed on a suicide watch if assessment indicates, and referred to a psychiatrist for further assessment, medication, other treatments, and admission to hospital as necessary. The key components of a suicide prevention program as outlined by the World Health Organization [WHO] (2007) include staff training in suicide prevention programs, intake screening of inmates, post-intake observation and monitoring, and sufficient mental health treatment.

Correctional nurses must conduct mental health assessments on all new admissions and, moreover, be astute to assessing those who may become mentally ill while incarcerated.

While some offenders arrive with overt signs of mental health problems, others will develop mental health problems while incarcerated. Separation from family, friends, and community; and the ever-present potential for violence result in an extremely high-stress environment (MHCC, 2012). Often, those with a mental illness are withdrawn, non-communicative, and suicidal. The nurse requires highly developed assessment and communication skills to elicit data necessary to identify those with mental illness (or mental health problems) and to ensure their safety. It is very important that those with psychosis, or those who have decompensated, are housed in an area where they can be protected from predatory inmates, as those with mental illness can be victimized and "muscled" (i.e., physically bullied) for their medications, canteen items, or other personal belongings. Individuals with mental illness are especially vulnerable within correctional systems due to the pecking order that exists within the prison subculture.

Although policies vary across the country and across jurisdictions, individuals presenting as mentally ill at the time of remand require an advocate to ensure that they move through the justice system as quickly as possible and that appropriate transitional discharge plans are in place; the role of the advocate often falls to the correctional nurse. There is a great opportunity for nurses to work with external community-based organizations in order to meet the treatment and release needs of this vulnerable group. By collaborating with various community agencies, correctional nurses can gain their assistance with the provision of mental health services while the client is in custody, and these same agencies can provide the link to their home community upon release. Increasingly, through the administration of community-based treatment and support services, **diversion programs** and policies have been implemented as a way of redirecting individuals with mental illness who come into conflict with the law from the criminal justice system to appropriate mental health services. In general, there are several types of diversion in Canada: pre-arrest and pre-booking diversion, court diversion, mental health courts, and restorative justice initiatives. Such schemes hold promise for humane treatment and reduced recidivism among this population, but they can only work if there are community-based services, treatments, and resources to support those who have been diverted (Canadian Institute for Health Information, 2008; MHCC, 2012).

In most settings, mentally ill inmates are generally supervised 24 hours per day by correctional staff. Training and experience varies among this group, and minimal training in mental health theory and practice is often the norm. Even though it is recognized that they are primarily responsible for containment and security, the OCI (2014) has recommended that suitable educational programs in particular should be an integral part of the training of all front-line correctional staff. Unfortunately, correctional staff may see suicidal behaviour through a security or disciplinary lens and place offenders in seclusion or segregation, which can be particularly detrimental to their overall well-being and put them at greater risk for suicide. It is important that correctional staff have the necessary skills to identify those with mental health problems, to provide appropriate supervision, and to make referrals to healthcare accordingly (Appelbaum, 2010). However, it is important to remember that correctional officers cannot, and should not, be replacing nurses. In turn, correctional nurses should be advocating for mental healthcare that is consistent with the Mental Health Commission of Canada's Mental Health Strategy.

**The Aging Offender** Unfortunately, for an increasing number of Canadians, growing old in prison is a harsh reality, a trend also experienced in other Western countries (Hayes, Burns, Turnbull, & Shaw, 2012; Human Rights Watch, 2012). Of note, in 2007/2008 offenders aged 50 and over accounted for 9% of admissions to sentenced custody, while in 2011/2012 they accounted for 11% of admissions to sentenced custody (Perreault, 2014a). Offenders over the age of 50 years are among the fastest-growing subgroup found within correctional environments. On average, correctional clients are thought to be 10 to 12 years older physiologically when compared to their chronological age (Beckett, Peternelj-Taylor, & Johnson, 2003). In the most recent report of the OCI (2014), 20%, or one in five offenders, is now age 50 or older.

Common physical healthcare needs experienced by this population include cardiovascular disease, pulmonary disorders, diabetes, arthritis, cancer, and Alzheimer's disease and other dementias (OCI, 2011, 2014). The mental health issues most evident in this group include stress, social isolation, depression, and suicide (CPHA, 2004). Encinares (2007) has reported that offenders with dementia are particularly difficult to place in the community. As a result, correctional nurses are responsible for developing and providing services geared specifically to the elderly, including palliative care services (Beckett et al., 2003; Duggleby, 2005).

"Life in prison can challenge anyone but it can be particularly hard for people whose bodies and minds are being whittled away by age" (Human Rights Watch, 2012, p. 4). Prisons and correctional facilities were never designed for an aging population; subsequently, as a result of this "silver tsunami" (Human Rights Watch, 2012), significant improvements in relation to accommodation planning, program development, palliative care, and reintegration options are required (OCI, 2013, 2014). For many elderly and infirm correctional clients, the fear of dying while imprisoned is a terse reality. Prison models of palliative care, although still very much in their infancy, are based on community-based professional practice standards. For example, CSC's (2009) Hospice Palliative Care Guidelines are based on the national principles and norms of practice of the Canadian Hospice Palliative Care Association (CHPCA) (Ferris et al., 2002). These standards have recently been revised (Canadian Hospice Palliative Care Association, 2013), and will continue to offer guidance to correctional authorities tasked with providing palliative care.

Managing terminally ill offenders within the prison milieu is a time-consuming, resource-intense, exhausting endeavour, one that is fraught with perplexing practical and moral dilemmas not commonly encountered in traditional healthcare settings. And although the CCRA and various pieces of provincial and territorial legislation provide for *parole or release by exception,* also known as *Royal Prerogative of Mercy* (OCI, 2014), it is rarely utilized, or granted, due to ongoing fears about community safety, acute bed shortages in long-term care, and the stigma associated with incarceration. The public in general is not interested in having convicted criminals residing in long-term care facilities (regardless of their health status). Interestingly, between 2008/09 and 2012/13, a total of 11 requests were made to the National Parole Board; seven were granted and four were denied. Sadly, another six inmates died before the application and release planning was completed (OCI, 2014). Transfer of offenders from prison to long-term care requires thorough release planning; nurses are key players in promoting the successful transition of older offenders to community-based long-term care facilities (Loeb, 2013).

**Women's Issues** Women most likely to be incarcerated have grown up in poor communities, have limited education and job skills, are victims as well as perpetrators of crime, and are the primary caregivers for dependent children (Blanchette & Brown, 2006; Fisher & Hatton, 2009; Lewis, 2006). And, like "free" women, they are likely to experience multiple roles, such as mother, daughter, wife, sister, and friend, and to be responsible for the emotional maintenance of the family unit, even when they are not with their families (Breannan, 2014; Harner, 2004). The fear of losing custody of their children is an ever-present reality (Canadian Centre on Substance Abuse, 2006).

Studies indicate that 50–70% of female inmates report physical and/or sexual abuse (Heney & Kristiansen, 2002). Common health concerns experienced by incarcerated women include substance abuse and related sequelae; infectious diseases including HIV, AIDS, and hepatitis B (HBV) and C (HCV); pregnancy-related concerns; gynecological problems; urinary incontinence (especially within the aging population); obesity; and chronic health disorders such as asthma, hypertension, heart disease, and diabetes (Fisher & Hatton, 2009; Maeve, 2003). Blanchette and Brown (2006) report that the mental health needs of women are quantitatively and qualitatively different from their male counterparts. In particular, female offenders experience higher levels of anxiety disorders (including posttraumatic stress disorder), depression, psychopathy, and borderline personality disorder (including self-injurious behaviour), serious mental illness (e.g., schizophrenia and depression), and chronic health disorders. Cloyes, Wong, Latimer, and Abarca (2010), in a study addressing recidivism, community tenure, and illness severity for people with serious mental illness (SMI) released from a state prison, found that women with SMI were at greater risk for repeated incarceration due to factors related to the intersection of gender and mental disorder.

The problem of non-suicidal self-injurious behaviour in women offenders has become a critical issue in correctional facilities. Caring for offenders who engage in self-harming behaviours is a resource-intense, complex, exhausting endeavour; one that can readily split correctional and healthcare staff. Power, Brown, and Usher (2013) found that women engage in self-injurious behaviour for a variety of reasons, including coping with negative emotions (e.g., anger, depression, and anxiety) or interpersonal conflict. Such behaviours are often followed by feelings of relief and regret. Effective treatment of women who engage in self-injurious behaviours needs to focus on the individual's unique experience and treatment needs.

Reproductive issues require considerable attention for women who are pregnant and incarcerated, and nurses are often thrust into a counselling role regarding the woman's choices and decision making surrounding pregnancy. Nurse-to-nurse collaboration with local hospitals is critical, as hospital nurses are often unaware of the extra security precautions that are required during medical transfers. For example, labour and delivery nurses are not generally accustomed to working with women who are in shackles and accompanied by correctional officers (Ferszt, Hickey, & Seleyman, 2013). Following delivery, special provisions must be made so the woman has contact with her child in order to facilitate normal mother–child bonding (Brennan, 2014; Ferszt & Erickson-Owens, 2008; Hufft & Peternelj-Taylor, 2008). The OCI (2014) reports on an innovative pilot project entitled CHILD LINK that allows incarcerated women to visit with their children (who live at a distance) via video conferencing. Preliminary results suggest that the pilot was successful in developing and/or maintaining the bond between mother and child. Nurses are often the ones involved in establishing and evaluating such innovative programming within correctional environments. Incarcerated mothers may require help with parenting skills, and nurses in consultation with community agencies can assist with these skills while the mother is in custody, and again upon her release. If there is a prior history of child abuse or neglect, the newborn may be taken into care as per the authority of provincial or territorial child protection services. In such cases, women may need additional support in relation to the grieving process over the loss of their children. Pregnant women who are addicted to opiates or are involved in a methadone maintenance program will need to have this program either initiated or continued to prevent damage to the fetus from opiate withdrawal.

Women who are incarcerated are often interested in learning more about their health, including family planning services. It is not uncommon for nurses in correctional centres to work with community partners in developing programs that focus on the needs of women related to prenatal, birth, and postpartum issues. Furthermore, nurses have been actively involved in the development and implementation of a number of programs, including those related to self-harming behaviours (Roth & Pressé, 2003), gender-specific substance abuse treatment (Fortin, 2010), the use of storytelling to enhance health promotion among Aboriginal women (Rowan, Auger, Toto, Simpson, & McNab, 2004), and a weight and body image program ("Caring in Corrections," 2010).

Overall, providing safe nursing care to women who are incarcerated requires gender-sensitive strategies and consideration of their vulnerability. Clearly, good correctional healthcare is good public health. As such, strengthening partnerships with community such as re-entry programs, which include healthcare, housing, parenting, education, and employment, are critical (Fisher & Hatton, 2009).

**Youth** Youth ages 12 to 17 residing in youth centres and youth and adult shared facilities are sentenced under the authority of the Youth Criminal Justice Act (YCJA). More often than not, youth in custody present with significant psychiatric morbidity, and partake in risky health behaviours and substance abuse that increase their chances of contracting HIV, hepatitis, and other sexually transmitted infections (STIs). These higher rates are often attributed to inadequate coping skills that are common among incarcerated youth (Griel & Loeb, 2009; Perry & Morris, 2014).

Youth in custody represent a significant portion of the population that is medically underserved yet experiences substantial physical and mental healthcare challenges (Perry & Morris, 2014). In 2004, Shelton observed that youth frequently presented with a variety of symptoms consistent with schizophrenia, anxiety disorders, depression, and behavioural disorders, although they may never have had a formal diagnosis as such. A decade later, Perry and Morris (2014) outline the common health disparities affecting youth who are incarcerated: STIs, teenage pregnancy and parenthood, chronic conditions (asthma, type 2 diabetes), attention deficit/hyperactivity disorder and learning disorders, behavioural problems, post-traumatic stress disorder, mood disorders, substance abuse, and suicidality (p. 693). The first episode of schizophrenia may be seen in this age group and needs to be considered by nurses when conducting mental health assessments. Symptom presentation is often more subtle in this age group. For example, the youth may be withdrawn, display an abnormal affect, and demonstrate a minor thought disorder. A suicide assessment of every youth is also necessary, since studies have found that 11% of non-incarcerated people with a first episode of psychosis have attempted suicide (Tandon & Jibson, 2003). In addition, youth in custody often experience higher rates of fetal alcohol spectrum disorder, significant substance abuse issues, self-harm, suicidal ideation, and high rates of physical, sexual, and emotional abuse, and many are involved with a child protection agency at the time of their arrest (Latimer & Fosse, 2004). Colonialism, residential school systems, and cultural assimilation further contribute to conflict with the criminal justice system among Aboriginal youth (Corrado, Kuehn, & Margaritescu, 2014).

In the most recent report, "Admissions to Youth Correctional Services in Canada, 2011/2012," Perreault (2014b) noted a 7% reduction in admissions to correctional services from the previous year. Aboriginal youth, however, continue to be highly represented in correctional services when compared to their non-Aboriginal counterparts. During 2011/2012, from data supplied by nine jurisdictions, Aboriginal youth accounted for 39% of all youth correctional admissions, whereas 7% of youth were Aboriginal in these same jurisdictions (Perreault, 2014b).

Youth require life skills and substance abuse programs, plus education in prevention of sexually transmitted diseases, family planning, and parenting skills. A recent study on the prevalence of HIV and HCV in youth in secure custody in Ontario found 0% prevalence of HIV and 0.4% of HCV (one case). However, many youth reported engaging in risky behaviours: 33.3% injected drugs with a used needle and 78% engaged in vaginal or anal intercourse without a condom (Calzavara et al., 2007).

Interpersonally, correctional nurses have to be aware of treatment boundaries and the power inherent within their professional roles (Bunner & Yonge, 2006). A participant in Shelton's (2003) study lamented that "the big problem is when patients get attached to staff. For some kids, this is as good as it gets. In many ways you're the parent this kid wished he had" (p. 49).

Clearly, a focus on health promotion and prevention of illness is critical in this age group. Coupled with timely access to services, treatment is necessary, and social supports in the community are critical. Keeping youth out of the criminal justice system through alternative measures and restorative justice initiatives are critical to long-term investment with this group (MHCC, 2012). Correctional nurses, in collaboration with other healthcare professionals across a number of community-based sectors, can make a significant difference in the lives of those at risk of involvement with the criminal justice system through prevention efforts and early intervention strategies.

**Culturally Diverse Offenders** The cultural diversity of Canada as a whole is reflected in the demographic profile of Canadian correctional facilities. Between 2007 and 2012, the foreign-born federal incarcerated population represented 13% of the total incarcerated population. Visible minorities now make up 18% of the federally sentenced offender population. To illustrate further, in 2011/2012, the federal offender population was made up of the following: Caucasian offenders, 62.3%; Aboriginal offenders, 19.3%; Black offenders, 8.6%; Asian offenders, 5.4%; Hispanic offenders, 0.9%; and other visible minority offenders, 3.4% (OCI, 2013). Not surprisingly, the Pacific Region of Correctional Service Canada reflects the greatest diversity of incarcerated offenders when compared to other regions in Canada. As in other Western societies, people of colour are overrepresented within Canadian correctional systems.

Historically, Aboriginal people have been disproportionately represented in provincial, territorial, and federal correctional systems when compared to their representation in the overall population. In 2011/2012, Aboriginal adults accounted for 28% of adult admissions to sentenced custody, even though they represented only 4% of Canada's adult population (Perreault, 2014a). Throughout Canada, the number of Aboriginal adults incarcerated exceeds their representation in the general population. For example, in the Atlantic provinces and Quebec, Aboriginal offenders sentenced to custody were one to three times more likely than the general population to be incarcerated, while in Ontario and the western provinces, their representation is six to nine times higher than their proportion in the overall population (Perreault, 2014a).

The overrepresentation of Aboriginal people within the criminal justice system has been attributed to the commingling of a number of complex factors, including rapid culture change, cultural oppression, marginalization, and the long-term effects of the residential schools (Corrado et al., 2014; Kirmayer, Brass, & Tait, 2000), which together have contributed to high rates of poverty, substance abuse, and victimization within families and communities of origin (CSC, 2010). Perreault (2009) further suggests that a lack of a high school diploma and employment contributes to overall incarceration rates, particularly in the 20 to 34 age group. The OCI (2014) continues to be critical of the federal government's response to Aboriginal offenders, stating, "there is definite room for enhancing Aboriginal cultural competence in the areas of health promotion, peer education, and inmate employment" (p. 44).

There has been a growing awareness in recent years of the need to provide culturally competent care in all areas of healthcare (Srivastava, 2007), and the same can be said for correctional systems. Increasingly, specific cultural practices are incorporated into programming offered within correctional facilities. For example, in collaboration with First Nations, Inuit, and Métis communities, as part of the rehabilitation process, elders, healers, and community leaders often lead traditional activities, including sweet grass ceremonies, smudging, and sweat lodges. Mason (2010) notes that it is important to continue to engage Aboriginal peoples in collaborative dialogue around Aboriginal correctional programming. Clearly, "increased understanding of the culture of incarceration as well as the pre-prison cultural lives of imprisoned [men and women] can serve as a means of establishing relationships and providing culturally congruent care" (Christensen, 2014, p. 230).

## COMMON HEALTH CHALLENGES

For many individuals, healthcare received while incarcerated may be the first real opportunity that they have had to address their healthcare needs. Numerous opportunities exist for correctional nurses to provide leadership in the provision of health promotion and illness prevention, especially if individuals are motivated to make lifestyle changes that would improve their overall health status.

## Substance Abuse

Substance abuse, including alcohol, nicotine, cocaine, opiates, benzodiazepines, cannabis products, and hallucinogens, is a major problem within correctional systems worldwide, and this problem is no different in Canada, although different levels of the problem are reported. The CPHA (2004) has reported that the majority of federally incarcerated inmates meet criteria for substance or alcohol abuse disorders. Likewise, the CSC (2010b) reports that there continues to be a high prevalence of substance abuse within its correctional facilities (80% overall, 95% Aboriginal men, 77% women). The Ontario correctional system has reported that 7.1% of inmates have a definite substance abuse diagnosis (Brown et al., 2006). However, 85% have a substance-abuse note on their correctional files, and the severity of withdrawal syndromes varies, requiring nurses to be astute in their assessments and observations regarding how withdrawal is manifested. Furthermore, nurses have to be alert for drug-seeking attempts and differentiate those who are simply trying to manipulate the system from those who legitimately require medications for health-related problems.

Harm reduction, including methadone maintenance treatment (MMT) and prison needle and syringe programs (PNSP), is the most widely accepted approach for dealing with substance abuse in many correctional institutions worldwide (Canadian HIV/AIDS Legal Network, 2008, 2010; Thomas, 2005). These strategies are not only controversial; they are also generally misunderstood by correctional administrators and healthcare professionals alike. From a public health perspective, such programs are both morally and fiscally responsible, and contribute to the protection of the community at large (Canadian HIV/AIDS Legal Network, 2008). Less than 1% of prisons and correctional facilities worldwide (i.e., only 60 prisons in 10 countries) have adopted a PNSP (Barro et al., 2014). To alleviate some of the fears related to needle stick injuries in Switzerland, retractable needle and syringes were trialled at one prison. To date, no correctional facility in Canada has adopted a PNSP, despite pleas from advocacy groups such as the Canadian HIV/AIDS Legal Network and the Prisoners HIV/AIDS Support Action Network. Of note, a meeting funded by the Canadian Institutes of Health Research was held in 2014 for the purpose of developing PNSP implementation guidelines. A 12-month research consultation project, funded by the Ontario HIV network, is under way to garner the input of former prisoners and healthcare staff. It will be interesting to see if a roll-out of a PNSP will follow (van der Meulen & Ka Hon Chu, 2015). In the interim, bleach kits for the purposes of decontaminating injection equipment are available in some jurisdictions. However, bleach is at best considered a second-line strategy in the absence of clean needles and syringes, as disinfection alone does not kill all viruses such as HBV and HCV (Canadian HIV/AIDS Legal Network, 2010; National Collaborating Centre for Infectious Diseases, 2008; Thomas, 2005).

As of 2002, most Canadian correctional facilities had adopted policies that allowed for the continuation of MMT for those placed in custody while in treatment. And although full access to MMT programs (including initiation and maintenance) has been recommended by both professional and advocacy groups (Canadian HIV/AIDS Legal Network, 2008; Registered Nurses' Association of Ontario, 2009), to date, many jurisdictions do not allow for the initiation of MMT for those already in custody (Canadian HIV/AIDS Legal Network, 2008; Thomas, 2005). MMT, like other harm-reduction strategies, is controversial. As of May 2012, 789 offenders (5.3% of the incarcerated population) were enrolled in an MMT (OCI, 2014). Unfortunately, the lack of understanding among many correctional staff members (including nurses) contributes to the belief that methadone administration simply gives offenders a drug that replaces the illicit drug they were taking prior to arrest. Correctional officers' concerns often stem from the fact that methadone is a highly valued commodity within correctional systems, which can lead to inmate attempts to divert the drug and to bully or muscle other inmates for it. Consequently, the procedure for administration of methadone is tightly supervised, time consuming, and resource intense (OCI, 2014).

The Registered Nurses' Association of Ontario [RNAO] (2009) outlines common MMT-related issues that are specific to correctional environments in its clinical best-practice guideline "Supporting Clients on Methadone Maintenance Treatment." Correctional nurses are often challenged with balancing the goals of harm reduction and MMT with the goals of custody, and, as such, this best-practice guideline is particularly noteworthy as it offers information related to the perceptions of methadone, administration of methadone, discharge or release planning, and related issues specific to correctional environments. In a recent Canadian retrospective study designed to assess the impact of MMT on post-release recidivism among male federal correctional inmates, MacSwain, Farrell-MacDonald, Cheverie, and Fischer (2014) found that offenders who initiated MMT while incarcerated, and who continued with MMT as part of their transition to the community, had a 36% lower risk of returning to custody when compared to the other groups in the study (i.e., those who discontinued MMT upon release, and a non-treated MMT control group). Such findings underscore the importance of correctional nurses collaborating with community-based partners to promote the successful reintegration of opioid-dependent offenders. A variety of community reintegration strategies, including intensive case management, may be required to facilitate positive treatment outcomes and successful reintegration.

## Infectious Diseases

The prevalence of blood-borne infections, STIs, and tuberculosis among offender populations is a real concern for correctional authorities. The prevalence of blood-borne infections such as HIV, HBV, and HCV are higher in the incarcerated population, primarily as a result of the high-risk behaviours demonstrated by offenders before and during incarceration, such as tattooing, ear and body piercing, intravenous drug use, and risky sexual activity. In comparison to non-incarcerated populations, HIV is estimated to be at least 10 times higher in incarcerated populations, while rates of HCV are at least 30 times higher. The picture is even more disconcerting for Aboriginal women, where more than one in 10 federally incarcerated Aboriginal women are living with HIV, and almost one in two live with HCV (van der Meulen & Ka Hon Chu, 2015). Treatment costs associated with HCV are staggering, yet the public health consequences of not treating offenders (not to mention the ethical issues) is even more disconcerting, as untreated HCV clearly will lead to higher rates within the general population. It is unfortunate, indeed, that the federal government continues to reject harm-reduction strategies such as PNSP and safer tattooing projects (Webster, 2012). Such harm-reduction programs, although endorsed by the healthcare community and advocacy groups alike, continue to be deemed controversial and subject to the political whim of governments, as was illustrated in the cancellation of the safe tattooing project that had been piloted in six federal correctional facilities (Canadian Broadcast Corporation, 2006). This is another example where correctional policies (e.g., custody) and healthcare interventions (e.g., caring) often collide.

CSC (2012a) found that in 2007 and 2008 the number of reported infections of hepatitis B in the federal facilities was 18 and 9, respectively. This corresponded to a 0.13% prevalence rate in 2007 and a 0.07% prevalence rate in 2008. The rate in the general population was estimated to be between 0.5% and 1.0% in 2000 (De, 2002). The prevalence of HCV in Canadian federal penitentiaries was 29.6% in 2007 and 30% in 2008. HCV prevalence was higher in adult females for both years, a trend that occurred for previous years as well (CSC, 2012a). HIV prevalence data reported in the same study was 1.84% in 2007 and 1.72% in 2008. Similarly, over the years females have shown higher prevalence rates (CSC, 2012a).

The HIV infection rate in federal facilities is 1.7% for males and 4.7% for females (CSC, 2003). However, as in the Canadian population, true prevalence rates are unknown because screening for HIV and other blood-borne infections is voluntary. It is estimated that up to 70% of federal inmates remain unscreened. Across the country, incarcerated women have a rate of infection 2.5 times that of men, which raises the question whether this difference is due to an actual higher infection rate, or women requesting testing more often than men (National Collaborating Centre for Infectious Diseases, 2008).

In 2008, 130 (1.01%) federal offenders had genital chlamydia, 9 (0.07%) had gonorrhoea, and 21 (0.16%) had syphilis (CSC, 2012a). Previously the highest rates for reported chlamydia and gonorrhoea infection for both men and women were found in the prairie region; the majority of cases of reported syphilis, however, were found among offenders in Quebec (CSC, 2012a), however, the 2008 data report does not report these.

Harm-reduction strategies such as condoms, dental dams, and water-based lubricants are available to offenders who request such products. However, sexual activity between offenders can result in a citation for misconduct. Consequently, they are ambivalent about requesting these products. On the one hand, they are being responsible by using a coping mechanism to prevent spread of disease; on the other hand, by merely requesting these products they are risking misconduct. The Prisoners HIV/AIDS Support Action Network (PASAN) and other advocacy groups such as the Canadian HIV/AIDS Legal Network further recommend that bleach be freely available and that correctional centres introduce PNSPs (Canadian HIV/AIDS Legal Network, 2010). However, many offenders have charges of drug possession and/or trafficking, and governments are loath to be seen as condoning criminal behaviour.

Correctional Service Canada (2012a) released statistics on tuberculosis (TB) infection in their penitentiaries. In summary, participation in TB assessment is high (for a nine-year period between 77.8% and 82% among inmates). The conversion rate for the TB skin test from a previous negative result has consistently remained low over this same period—conversion rates were 1.49% in 2007 and 1.15% in 2008. The latent TB infection rate (LTBI) has been reducing to a rate of 16.6% in 2007 and 15.9% in 2008. Rates in men have been consistently higher over the years. While the number of inmates with LTBI has reduced over the years, those on active treatment have increased. Only a small number of inmates are reported with active TB disease each year (two cases in 2007 and four cases in 2008). TB in crowded correctional settings represents a public health challenge worldwide (CPHA, 2004; Centers for Disease Control and Prevention, 2006), and concerns regarding tuberculin skin test conversion among offenders and staff alike are a real concern for provincial, territorial, and federal correctional authorities (CSC, 2012a).

Nurses are often the first healthcare providers to assess inmates for infectious disease. This assessment is important in case finding and subsequent medical treatment. Nurses also implement infection control precautions to prevent subsequent infection of staff and other inmates. Health education for inmates and staff on the prevention of infection transmission is a good example of a primary prevention strategy.

In 2003, the Ontario government declared a provincial emergency because of severe acute respiratory syndrome (SARS). At that time, not much was known about the disease and its control or treatment. The strategy from the beginning was to prevent offenders or staff with symptoms of SARS from entering the facilities. As a precaution, restrictions were placed on visits to facilities in the greater Toronto area, where SARS cases had been reported. A screening tool was also developed by a group of senior nurse leaders, and correctional nurses in Ontario identified several inmates who required voluntary quarantine as directed by the local public health unit. These inmates were isolated in the province's correctional facilities. Several other inmates, identified with SARS-like symptoms, were sent to hospital and returned to the facility once SARS had been ruled out. As well, several staff members were advised to leave work and consult with public health, Telehealth Ontario, or their family physicians. Approximately 6 000 inmates were screened using this tool.

Similarly, in 2009, the pandemic H1N1 flu virus saw correctional nurses directly involved in the development of policies related to infection prevention and control measures, clinical assessment and management, laboratory testing, antiviral treatment, and outbreak control measures in closed facilities (Public Health Branch, Health Services Sector, 2009). Correctional systems followed Health Canada's guidelines regarding immunization; however, controversies did arise in some jurisdictions when it was discovered that inmates with pre-existing health conditions were immunized before healthy "law-abiding" citizens and correctional staff (Canadian Broadcast Corporation, 2009; Matas, 2009). In total, 56% (8 120) of offenders under the jurisdiction of the CSC received the H1N1 vaccine; a total of 49 laboratory-confirmed cases were reported across the CSC during the 2009–2010 H1N1 influenza pandemic (CSC, 2012b).

In recent years, it has not been uncommon to hear of enteric outbreaks in hospitals, long-term care facilities, cruise ships, schools, and summer camps. And while outbreaks of novovirus-like viruses are likely not considered on the same magnitude as SARS or the H1N1 flu virus, they can cripple an organization's day-to-day operations. Sunil, Holt, Dixon, Dignman, and Noseworthy (2013) report on a norovirus-like outbreak that occurred in a correctional facility located in central east Ontario and illustrate the collaborative coordinated responses of the health and correctional staff of the correctional facility and the local and provincial public health authorities. Recommendations included (1) the implementation of appropriate hand-hygiene supplies that are readily accessible for offenders, visitors, and staff; (2) regular housekeeping and environmental cleaning of high-touch surfaces; (3) routine surveillance of clinical symptoms in the offenders to determine the identification of early outbreaks; (4) regular training of staff to deal with outbreaks; (5) review of policies and procedures to include disease surveillance and outbreak control measures; (6) prompt reporting of outbreaks; and, finally, (7) a coordinated response of correctional and provincial health authorities to manage outbreak investigation and control.

Correctional staff and infectious diseases nurses function within a very narrow margin when addressing staff members' "need to know" and inmates' confidentiality. Nurses cannot provide confidential information regarding diagnoses; however, they must educate and inform correctional staff of infection control and other healthcare procedures. The pressure from staff for confidential healthcare information will continue, as will the need for nurses to protect that confidentiality. Most nurses do find a way to provide health education to correctional staff and alleviate some of their work-related stress. For example, nurses can instruct correctional officers regarding the principles of harm reduction; the use of universal precautions; standard practices; airborne, droplet, and direct-contact isolation procedures; and the need for confidentiality in health-related matters.

## PRACTICE SETTING

The impact of the correctional environment on both offenders and staff members alike can be particularly severe given the interpersonal climate, organizational culture, and social context. The incarceration experience represents a significant stressful life event, as separation from family and friends, limitations on privacy, overcrowding, and the fear of assault can severely impact the offender's health status and quality of life. Furthermore, power, control, and implicit authority are manifested in the physical and interpersonal environments of correctional systems and can be incompatible with the achievement of health-related treatment goals (Lazzaretto-Green, Austin, Goble, Buys, Gorman, & Rankel, 2011; Peternelj-Taylor, 2015).

Nurses working with clients who are incarcerated "face significant challenges in regard to their ability to care in this culture of incarceration" (Christensen, 2014, p. 230). Access to clients can be difficult, depending on the mandate of the institution and the clients' specific healthcare needs. For instance, in many correctional facilities, offenders are housed in units with two-person cells and a common day area. Depending on the institution, they may be allowed out of their cells for up to 12 hours per day, and healthcare must be provided within this time frame. In some settings, assessment of health concerns and provision of minor interventions is provided in the living unit, and more complex care is provided in a centralized ambulatory healthcare clinic. In many facilities a correctional officer accompanies the nurse or supervises the nurse for every offender contact, and this officer must maintain visual contact with the offender at all times. And although the nurse respects the officer's security responsibilities, the nurse must maintain client confidentiality while providing healthcare and eliciting health-related information.

The priorities of the correctional system focus on confinement and security, and matters of security will often take precedence over nursing care. It is not uncommon for nurses to have to wait while the officer completes security-related tasks. And although nurses, as employees of correctional facilities, must abide by the correctional policies that govern all correctional employees, correctional nurses often find themselves in a "Catch-22" position as they face the competing tensions enmeshed in their collective responsibilities. Not only are they responsible to the offender, who is their client; they are also responsible to their profession, to the correctional system which is their employer, and to the community at large (Storch & Peternelj-Taylor, 2009). In order to develop therapeutic relationships and provide professional and ethical care, correctional nurses often are faced with confronting their own reactions to offenders' alleged offences or the crimes for which they have been sentenced. It is also important that they not get caught up in the sensationalism that surrounds a particular offender, or the setting in which nursing practice takes place.

While professional autonomy in practice has often been described as a factor related to job satisfaction in correctional nursing in general ("Caring in Corrections," 2010; Smith, 2005), in practice this often means working alone, and professional isolation is a concern for correctional nursing (LaMarre, 2006; Shelton, 2009). In some instances, there may only be one registered nurse on the day and evening shifts for as many as 200 offenders. This large caseload results in nurses having to set priorities based on assessment of individual client needs. In other settings, nursing practice may reflect a more traditional approach to healthcare, for instance in secure treatment facilities operated by provincial, territorial, and federal correctional agencies.

Regardless of the setting, the therapeutic treatment needs of clients must always be considered within the context of maintaining security. For instance, nurses need to be ever vigilant regarding security awareness. This includes **static security**, the structural environmental features common to correctional facilities (e.g., video monitoring, internal barriers, perimeter fences or walls, personal protection alarms, staffing patterns, policies related to counting offenders, and counting equipment) and **dynamic security**, which addresses such things as institutional policies and procedures related to interpersonal security (e.g., developing professional relationships, "knowing" the client in one's care, managing professional boundaries, and methods of operation). Nurses must be attentive to the materials left with clients, as many could be fashioned into weapons; likewise, in some settings, dental floss may be used (and disposed after use) only in the healthcare clinic, rather than being allowed in the client's living area. Nurses working in other community settings certainly understand the need for innovation; nurses working in a correctional setting require similar "thinking outside the box."

## COMMUNITY CONNECTION

Increasingly, correctional facilities are being identified as a "public health opportunity" (CSC, 2003; Williams, 2007). From a public health perspective, the health of incarcerated population is a reflection of the state of health of the community at large. Offenders come to prison from the community, and they will return to the community upon their release; in short, correctional health affects public health (National Collaborating Centre for Infectious Diseases, 2008). Harm-reduction strategies, as discussed, are recommended for disease prevention and control within correctional facilities, and they have direct implications for the community at large, as the majority of those in custody will eventually reintegrate into the community. Attending to the comprehensive needs of this population requires interdisciplinary and intersectoral collaboration between healthcare, criminal justice, education, social services, non-governmental organizations, and the voluntary sector. Such partnerships need to be established, nurtured, and evaluated (Peternelj-Taylor, 2010).

In 2001, Freudenberg challenged practitioners, researchers, and policy makers to ask new research questions, develop new policies, and implement new programs that improve health and social services, emphasize community reintegration efforts, and support alternatives to incarceration. This agenda is still relevant today and continues to address contemporary concerns. Correctional nurses are in key positions to collaborate with the staff in community-based residential facilities and to ensure a safe release for offenders transitioning to the community. Organizations such as the St. Leonard's Society of Canada (and its affiliate members) and other not-for-profit charitable organizations are excellent resources for correctional nurses as they work with offenders, preparing them for release into the community.

## POLICY DEVELOPMENT

Nurses are especially well situated to influence, develop, and change correctional healthcare policies. For example, nurses have played a huge role in initiating and implementing non-smoking policies in many correctional facilities across the country. Through the implementation of this public health initiative, healthier living and work environments have been created for all concerned. Nurses have also been staunch advocates for the development of policies related to

infection-control courses for delivery in local and regional facilities, prenatal and postnatal program development in women's institutions, resource management (including staffing and scheduling patterns), the introduction of telemedicine and automated external defibrillators, mental healthcare delivery in secure mental health treatment units, and policies regarding palliative care and end-of-life care.

Since the SARS outbreak of 2003 and the emergence of pandemic H1N1 flu virus in North America in 2009, correctional nurses are now at the forefront of policy development in relation to pandemic planning.

## PROFESSIONAL DEVELOPMENT AND RESEARCH IN CORRECTIONAL NURSING

Recognition of correctional nursing as a specialized area of nursing practice is critical to the ongoing growth and development of this specialty area. Prior to the 1960s very few nurses considered a career in correctional nursing. Since then, nurses have slowly and methodically pursued professional nursing practice in the correctional milieu, resulting in significant transformations in professional development. In a recent editorial, Peternelj-Taylor and Panosky (2013) concluded that "nurses represent the largest group of healthcare professionals practising in correctional systems, yet little is known about their work environments, what challenges they experience, or how those challenges impact on the care of those in custody" (p. 1). The essential role of nurses in the provision of offender healthcare in Canadian correctional systems underscores the importance of understanding their professional roles, responsibilities, and learning needs. Refer to Canadian Research Box 26.2.

In 2005, the RNAO Correctional Nurses Interest Group was established by correctional nurses, the first such group in Canada. In 2007, the Forensic Nurses Society of Canada was approved as an emerging special interest group of the Canadian Nurses Association, and represents all forensic nursing specialties, including correctional nursing. However, unlike the American Nurses Association (2013), which published "Corrections Nursing: Scope and Standards of Practice," and the Royal College of Nursing (2009), which published "Health and Nursing Care in the Criminal Justice Service," comparable formal professional nursing documents that provide guidance and direction to nurses working in Canadian correctional facilities are non-existent.

The ongoing evolution of correctional nursing as a specialty is further dependent on the establishment of a nursing culture that supports and nurtures the development of nursing research. And although correctional nursing has undergone significant transformations in professional role development in recent years, the professional literature remains largely anecdotal, as Canadian correctional environments have attracted very few nurse researchers (Ferszt & Hickey, 2013; Peternelj-Taylor, 2005). This has resulted in a severe scarcity of research in correctional nursing in Canada and elsewhere, even though a goldmine of research opportunities exists within correctional environments. Freudenberg (2007), in discussing a research agenda for correctional health, has declared that "correctional research has to be considered a branch of population health research and therefore address the broadest questions that affect the health of the public" (p. 429).

Nursing has a pivotal research role to play in the correctional milieu, both in the translation and interpretation of research relevant to incarcerated populations and in the identification of important nursing research questions that emerge from practice. There are unique issues with this population; for example, ensuring that consent is free, informed, and given without expectation of special favours. Therefore, guidelines are in place that clearly prevent the offer of privileges, early release, or favourable parole assessments in return for participation in a research study during incarceration (Peternelj-Taylor, 2005). Conducting research in correctional facilities however, can be particularly challenging. Ferszt and Hickey (2013) conducted a qualitative study of nurse researchers in correctional environments. Participants described the importance of establishing credibility, the challenges they faced, and the unexpected personal and professional rewards they received. They also provided suggestions to assist others who may be interested in conducting correctional-based research.

Since 1989, the College of Nursing, University of Saskatchewan, in collaboration with the Regional Psychiatric Centre (Prairies), Correctional Service of Canada, has sponsored a biennial nursing conference that showcases the unique contributions nurses make to healthcare within the criminal justice system. This international forum provides opportunities for clinical practitioners, educators, administrators, researchers, and policy makers to learn about matters of interest to correctional nurses. Additionally, correctional environments are being selected more frequently as community and mental health placements for senior nursing students.

Embracing a research agenda with incarcerated populations will provide new insights into nursing practice in this domain. Canadian Research Boxes 26.1 and 26.2 highlight two recent Canadian projects.

## CANADIAN RESEARCH BOX 26.1

**Does cognitive behavioural therapy affect recidivism in adult offenders with diverse backgrounds?**

Usher, A. M., & Stewart, L. A. (2014). Effectiveness of correctional programs with ethnically diverse offenders: A meta-analytic study. *International Journal of Offender Therapy and Comparative Criminology, 58*(2), 209–230. Reprinted by permission of SAGE Publications, Inc. doi:10.1177/0306624X12469507

The authors reported the results from a meta-analysis examining the effectiveness of cognitive behavioural therapy (CBT) on recidivism in Canadian adult offenders from diverse backgrounds. Participants self-identified as Caucasian, Aboriginal, Black and other. The authors searched for all reports published from Correctional Services Canada (CSC) on the effectiveness of their

correctional programming for federal offenders. There were five inclusion criteria:

1. intervention modality–correctional programs were delivered by a CSC institution or parole office and followed the principles and interventions of CBT;
2. participants–treatment and comparison groups comprised male or female offenders serving a federal sentence through CSC and included a range of ethnic groups;
3. outcome measures–readmission to custody followed participation in a correctional program, due either to new offences or failure to comply with conditional release terms;
4. methodology–randomized or matched-control design; and
5. source–CSC published reports.

A total of 21 CSC research reports were identified; eight of these met the inclusion criteria, and their results were entered into the meta-analysis. The authors reported the following overall results:

- regardless of ethnicity, after receiving CBT-based correctional programming, the odds were 1.65 times greater that a Canadian federal offender would not recidivate;
- for Caucasian offenders who had received CBT-based correctional programming, the odds were 1.76 times greater that they would not reoffend;
- for Aboriginal offenders who received the CBT-based correctional programming, odds were 1.45 times greater that they would not reoffend;
- for Black offenders who had received CBT-based correctional programming, odds were 1.36 times greater that they would not reoffend; and
- for other offenders who had received CBT-based correctional programming, odds were 1.53 times greater that they would not reoffend.

Overall, the authors reported that all ethnic groups showed significant gains from participating in the CSC CBT-based correctional programming and were less likely to recidivate following this.

The authors report the following limitations when considering the significance of their results for correctional practice. First, it is not possible to determine the effects of a specific program, as offenders involved in their program may participate in a number of these. Second, there was not any consistent sampling across the included studies. Third, there was variability in follow-up time from one to four years. Fourth, as many studies did not meet the inclusion criteria, including many studies of women offenders, it is not possible to generalize specifically to this group.

### Discussion Questions

1. Based on the results of this study, should it be compulsory for all federal offenders in Canada to complete CBT-based correctional programming?
2. How might nurses incorporate CBT principles into their everyday practice to support such programming?

## CANADIAN RESEARCH BOX 26.2

**What are the work-life issues experienced by nurses working in provincial correctional facilities in Ontario?**

Almost, J., Doran, D., Ogilvie, L., Miller, C., Kennedy, S., Timmings, C., . . . Bookey-Basset, S. (2013). Exploring work-life issues in provincial corrections settings. *Journal of Forensic Nursing, 9,* 3–13. doi:10.1097/JFN.0b013e31827a5613

The authors report the results of a mixed-method study designed to examine the work environment of nurses working in provincial correctional facilities in Ontario. In the first phase of the study, semi-structured interviews were conducted with 13 correctional nurses and healthcare managers from five representative provincial correctional institutions. The purpose of the interviews was twofold: participants were asked to describe issues and challenges within their work environment, which subsequently informed the selection of variables in the study. In the second phase of the study, a convenience sample of all nurses ($n = 511$) working in the 30 correctional facilities in Ontario were invited to participate in the study. Of the 511 nurses eligible to participate in the study, 270 nurses and 27 healthcare managers returned completed surveys, yielding a 56.1% response rate. A variety of well-established self-report instruments were utilized to assess the work environment (i.e., supportive organizational attributes, adequacy in staffing), workplace relationships (i.e., intra-group conflict, bullying, respect), and nurse outcomes (i.e., burnout, job satisfaction, role overload, and intent to leave).

Participants noted several key issues in their work environments:

- inadequate staffing and heavy workloads;
- limited control over practice and scope of practice;
- limited resources; and
- challenging workplace relationships.

The implications of this study are many and include workforce planning, educational and policy initiatives, and attention to interpersonal work relationships. The essential role of nurses in the provision of offender healthcare underscores the importance of understanding their work-life issues. The exploratory nature of this study and its broad findings warrant further investigation in order to improve the lives of correctional nurses. Like nurses in other sectors, nurses in this study valued work environments that provided support for continuing education, positive work relationships, autonomy, control over nursing practice, and adequate staffing.

### Discussion Questions

1. How might a correctional nurse or community health nurse use the information gleaned in this study when planning and implementing a health-promotion program for correctional nurses?

2. How might this research inform a recruitment and retention strategy for correctional nursing?

## CASE STUDY

A 45-year-old male was transferred to a regional treatment centre of a federal penitentiary with end-stage liver failure. The family lives in another province and visit when they can. His pain needs are marginally addressed by the use of a fentanyl patch, which often "disappears" before the next patch change. His family indicated that they saw a news report on "compassionate release" of offenders in the United States and wondered if such options were available in Canada. Visiting has become a real hardship for the family.

### Discussion Questions

1. What are your thoughts and feelings about providing palliative care within a federal penitentiary?

2. What barriers might be encountered when an application for exceptional release is made?

3. What community-based resources are available to assist with caring for this offender?

4. What are the challenges of providing palliative care within a correctional setting?

## CONCLUSION

Correctional nursing, as a specialty area of practice, has undergone significant transformation in role development in recent years. Accepting the challenge to provide nursing care in environments where healthcare delivery is not the primary goal can lead to myriad personal and professional issues for nurses. Correctional nursing is collaborative and interdisciplinary by its very nature; the most successful healthcare outcomes are achieved when nurses and correctional officers share a common vision, one of professionalism in the provision of security and quality nursing care to those in custody (Hufft & Kite, 2003).

## KEY TERMS

correctional nursing  p. 455
criminalization of the mentally ill  p. 457
diversion programs  p. 458
dynamic security  p. 464
static security  p. 464

## STUDY QUESTIONS

1. What are the nursing implications associated with the implementation of a methadone maintenance (MMT) program within a correctional facility?

2. Discuss the reasons why correctional nurses often find themselves in a Catch-22 position when working with offenders in correctional settings.

3. Identify and briefly discuss the common healthcare challenges encountered by incarcerated women.

4. What knowledge, skills, and abilities do nurses need to possess to be successful in their work in secure environments?

5. Increasingly, correctional facilities are being identified as a "public health opportunity." Discuss.

6. What issues need to be considered when implementing harm-reduction strategies in correctional facilities, such as the distribution of condoms, dental dams, and water-based lubricants, and having bleach accessible?

After working through these questions, go to the MyNursingLab at www.pearsoned.ca/mynursinglab to check your answers.

## INDIVIDUAL CRITICAL-THINKING EXERCISES

1. What types of assessment tools would you need in order to assess inmates for their most prevalent health problems?

2. What information would you give to a correctional officer when asked what an inmate's positive TB skin test means?

3. Define "vulnerability" within the context of nursing research. How is this definition relevant to individuals who are incarcerated? What guidelines exist to protect correctional clients as research participants?

4. What would be the advantage of having standards for practice for Canadian nurses who work in correctional facilities?

5. If you were a correctional nurse in your community, what community-based organizations and resources would you collaborate with in meeting the needs of offenders in your care?

## GROUP CRITICAL-THINKING EXERCISES

1. What is the role of the nurse in advocating for individuals with mental illness who find themselves in conflict with the justice system?

2. In comparison to other Western countries, Canadian statistics regarding youth incarceration, especially youth of Aboriginal ancestry, are particularly alarming. What factors contribute to this phenomenon in Canada?

3. Nurses who chose to work in correctional environments are often asked the following questions: "Why would you want to work there?" "How can you stand working with those criminals?" "Aren't you afraid of getting hurt?" What are your initial thoughts about these questions? What do you think is behind such questions?

## REFERENCES

American Nurses Association. (2013). *Correctional nursing: Scope and standards of practice* (2nd ed.). Silver Spring, MD: Author.

Appelbaum, K. L. (2010). The mental health professional in a correctional culture. In C. L. Scott (Ed.), *Handbook of correctional mental health* (2nd ed.). Washington, DC: American Psychiatric Publishing.

Barro, J., Casillas, A., Gétaz, L., Rieder, J-P., Baroudi, M., François, A., . . . Wolf, H. (2014). Retractable syringes in a Swiss prison needle and syringe exchange program: Experiences of drug using inmates and prison staff perceptions. *International Journal of Mental Health Addiction, 12*, 648–659. doi: 10.1007/s11469-014-9498-x

Beckett, J., Peternelj-Taylor, C., & Johnson, R. (2003). Growing old in the correctional system. *Journal of Psychosocial Nursing and Mental Health Services, 41*(9), 12–18.

Blanchette, K., & Brown, S. L. (2006). *The assessment and treatment of women offenders: An integrative perspective.* Chichester, UK: John Wiley & Sons.

Brennan, S. (2014). Canada's mother-child program: Examining its emergence, usage, and current state. *Canadian Graduate Journal of Sociology & Criminology, 3*(1), 1–33. doi: http://dx.doi.org/10.15353/cgjsc-rcessc.v3i1.84

Brown, G., Girard, L., & Mathias, K. (2006, June). *Identifying the psychiatric care needs of adult offenders in the Ontario correctional system.* Paper presented at the 20th Annual Mental Health Centre, Penetanguishene Forensic Conference: Mentally disordered offenders: What have we learned in 20 years? Penetanguishene, ON.

Bunner, K., & Yonge, O. (2006). Boundaries and adolescents in residential treatment settings: What clinicians need to know. *Journal of Psychosocial Nursing and Mental Health Services, 44*(9), 38–44.

Calzavara, L., Ramuscak, N., Burchell, A. N., Swantee, C., Myers, T., Ford, P., . . . Raymond, S. (2007). Prevalence of HIV and hepatitis C virus infections among inmates of Ontario remand facilities. *Canadian Medical Association Journal, 177*, 257–261.

Canadian Broadcast Corporation. (2006, December 4). *Prison tattoo parlours get the axe.* Retrieved from http://www.cbc.ca/news/canada/prison-tattoo-parlours-get-the-axe-1.619060

Canadian Broadcast Corporation. (2009, November 5). Inmates should get priority H1N1 shots: Advocates. *The Canadian Press.* Retrieved from http://www.cbc.ca/news/canada/montreal/inmates-should-get-priority-h1n1-shots-advocates-1.850422

Canadian Centre on Substance Abuse. (2006). *Fact sheet: Self harm among criminalized women.* Retrieved from http://www.ccsa.ca/Resource%20Library/ccsa-011338-2006-e.pdf

Canadian HIV/AIDS Legal Network. (2008). *Opioid substitution therapy in prisons: Reviewing the evidence.* Retrieved from http://www.aidslaw.ca/site/wp-content/uploads/2013/04/OST_brief_08-EN.pdf

Canadian HIV/AIDS Legal Network. (2010). *Under the skin: A people's case for prison needle and syringe programs.* Retrieved from http://www.pasan.org/Toolkits/Under_the_Skin.pdf

Canadian Hospice Palliative Care Association. (2013). *A model to guide hospice palliative care.* Ottawa, ON: Author. Retrieved from http://www.chpca.net/media/319547/norms-of-practice-eng-web.pdf

Canadian Institute for Health Information. (2008). *Improving the health of Canadians: Mental health, delinquency and criminal activity.* Ottawa, ON: Author. Retrieved from https://secure.cihi.ca/estore/productFamily.htm?pf=PFC1007&lang=en&media=1

Caring in Corrections. (2010). *Canadian Nurse, 106*(4), 22–27.

Canadian Public Health Association. (2004). A health care needs assessment of federal inmates. *Canadian Journal of Public Health, 95*(supplement 1), S1–S63.

Chaimowitz, G. (2012). Position Paper: The criminalization of people with mental illness. *The Canadian Journal of Psychiatry, 57*(2), Insert 1–6.

Christensen, S. (2014). Enhancing nurses' ability to care within the culture of incarceration. *Journal of Transcultural Nursing, 25*(3), 223–231. doi:10.1177/1043659613515276

Cloyes, K., Wong, B., Latimer, S., & Abarca, J. (2010). Women, serious mental illness and recidivism: A gender-based analysis of recidivism risk for women with SME released from prison. *Journal of Forensic Nursing, 6*, 3–14. doi:10.1111/j.1939-3938.2009.01060.x

Corrado, R. R., Kuehn, S., & Margaritescu, I. (2014). Policy issues regarding the over-representation of incarcerated Aboriginal young offenders in a Canadian context. *Youth Justice, 14*(1), 40–62. doi:10.1177/1473225413520361

Correctional Service Canada. (2003). *Infectious diseases prevention and control in Canadian federal penitentiaries 2000–01* (Cat. No. 0-662-67144-9). Ottawa, ON: Author.

Correctional Service Canada. (2009). *Hospice palliative care guidelines for Correctional Service Canada.* Ottawa ON: Author.

Correctional Service Canada. (2010, March). *Issues and challenges facing CSC.* Retrieved from http://www.csc-scc.gc.ca/text/pblct/sb-go/pdf/7-eng.pdf

Correctional Service Canada. (2012a). *Infectious diseases surveillance in Canadian federal penitentiaries 2007–2008.* Retrieved from http://www.csc-scc.gc.ca/publications/005007-7602-eng.shtml

Correctional Service Canada. (2012b). *Pandemic H1N1 influenza among CSC inmates 2009–2010: Summary of vaccination campaign, cases, and outbreaks.* Retrieved from http://www.csc-scc.gc.ca/text/pblct/H1N1/p3_scc-eng.shtml

Derkzen D., Booth, L., McConnell, A., & Taylor, K. (2012). Mental health needs of federal women offenders. Research Report R-267. Ottawa, ON: Correctional Service Canada.

Duggleby, W. (2005). Fostering hope in incarcerated older adults. *Journal of Psychosocial Nursing and Mental Health Services, 43*(9), 15–20.

Encinares, M. (2007). Community care of elderly offenders with dementia. *Journal of Chinese Clinical Medicine, 21*(1), 34–41.

Fazel, S., & Seewald, K. (2012). Severe mental illness in 33,588 prisoners worldwide: Systematic review and meta-regression analysis. *British Journal of Psychiatry, 200*(5), 364–373. doi:10.1192/bjp.bp.111.096370

Federal-Provincial-Territorial Partnership. (2012). *Mental health strategy for corrections in Canada.* Retrieved from http://www.csc-scc.gc.ca/health/092/MH-strategy-eng.pdf

Ferris, F. D., Balfour, H. M., Bowen, K., Farley, J., Hardwick, M., Lamontagne, C., . . . . West, P. (2002). *A model to guide hospice palliative care.* Ottawa, ON: Canadian Hospice Palliative Care Association.

Ferszt, G. G., & Erickson-Owens, D. A. (2008). Development of an educational support group for pregnant women in prison. *Journal of Forensic Nursing, 4*, 55–60. doi: 10.1111/j.1939-3938.2008.00010.x

Ferszt, G. G., & Hickey, J. E. (2013). Nurse researchers in corrections: A qualitative study. *Journal of Forensic Nursing, 9*(4), 200–206. doi:10.1097/JFN.0b013e3182970778

Ferszt, G. G., Hickey, J. E., & Seleyman, K. (2013). Advocating for pregnant women in prison: The role of the correc-

tional nurse. *Journal of Forensic Nursing, 9*(2), 108–110. doi:10.1097/JFN.0b013e318281056b

Fisher, A. A., & Hatton, D. C. (2009). Women prisoners: Health issues and nursing implications. *Nursing Clinics of North America, 44*(3), 365–373. doi:10.1016/j.cnur.2009.06.010

Fortin, D. (2010, March). Correctional programs for women offenders. *Let's Talk, 34*(2), 11.

Freudenberg, N. (2001). Jails, prisons, and the health of urban populations: A review of the impact of the correctional system on community health. *Journal of Urban Health: Bulletin of the New York Academy of Medicine, 78*(2), 214–235.

Freudenberg, N. (2007). Health research behind bars: A brief guide to research in jails and prisons. In R. Greifinger (Ed.), *Public health behind bars: From prisons to communities.* New York, NY: Springer.

Griel, L. C., & Loeb, S. J. (2009). Health issues faced by adolescents incarcerated in the juvenile justice system. *Journal of Forensic Nursing, 5*, 162–179. doi: 10.1111/j.1939-3938.2009.01049.x

Harner, H. M. (2004). Relationships between incarcerated women: Moving beyond stereotypes. *Journal of Psychosocial Nursing, 42*(1), 38–46.

Hayes, A. J., Burns, A., Turnbull, P., & Shaw, J. J. (2012). The health and social needs of older male prisoners. *International Journal of Geriatric Psychiatry, 217*, 1155–1162. doi: 10.1002/gps.3761

Heney, J., & Kristiansen, C. (2002). *Working with women in conflict with the law: A trainers' guide.* Toronto, ON: Ministry of Public Safety and Security.

Hufft, A., & Kite, M. M. (2003). Vulnerable and cultural perspectives for nursing care in correctional systems. *The Journal of Multicultural Nursing and Health, 9*(1), 18–26.

Hufft, A., & Peternelj-Taylor, C. (2008). Ethical care of pregnant adolescents in correctional settings. *Journal of Forensic Nursing, 4*, 94–96. doi: 10.1111/j.1939-3938.2008.00015.x

Human Rights Watch. (2012). *Old behind bars: The aging prison population in the United States.* Retrieved from http://www.hrw.org/sites/default/files/reports/usprisons0112webwcover_0.pdf

James, D. J., & Glaze, L. E. (2006, September). Mental health problems of prison and jail inmates. *Bureau of Justice Statistics special report.* U.S. Department of Justice, Office of Justice Programs. Retrieved from http://www.bjs.gov/content/pub/pdf/mhppji.pdf

Kirmayer, L. J., Brass, G. M., & Tait, C. L. (2000). The mental health of Aboriginal peoples: Transformations of identity and community. *Canadian Journal of Psychiatry, 45*(7), 607–616.

LaMarre, M. (2006). Nursing role and practice in correctional facilities. In M. Puisis (Ed.), *Clinical practice in correctional medicine* (2nd ed., pp. 417–418). Philadelphia, PA: Mosby Elsevier.

Latimer, J., & Fosse, L. C. (2004, February). *A one-day snapshot of aboriginal youth in custody across Canada: Phase II.* Department of Justice Canada. Retrieved from http://www.justice.gc.ca/eng/rp-pr/cj-jp/yj-jj/yj2-jj2/yj2.pdf

Lazzaretto-Green, D., Austin, W., Goble, E., Buys, L., Gorman, T., & Rankel, M. (2011). Walking a fine line: Forensic mental health practitioners' experience of working with correctional officers. *Journal of Forensic Nursing, 7*, 109–119. doi: 10.111/j.1939-3938.2011.01107.x

Lewis, C. (2006). Treating incarcerated women: Gender matters. *Psychiatric Clinics of North America, 29,* 773–789.

Loeb, S. J. (2013). Shifting institutions. Preparing for transfers from prison to long-term care facilities. *Journal of Gerontological Nursing, 39*(6), 2–3. doi:3928/00989134-20130318-01

MacSwain, M.-A., Farrell-MacDonald, S., Cheverie, M., & Fischer, B. (2014). Assessing the impact of methadone maintenance on post-release recidivism among male federal correctional inmates in Canada. *Criminal Justice and Behaviour, 41*(3), 380–394. doi:10.1177/0093854813501495

Maeve, K. M. (2003). Nursing care partnerships with women leaving jail: Effects on health and crime. *Journal of Psychosocial Nursing and Mental Health Services, 41*(9), 30–40.

Mason, R. (2010, March). Aboriginal correctional programs. *Let's Talk, 34*(2), 10.

Matas, R. (2009, October 26). B.C. inmates to receive flu vaccine before prison staff. *The Globe and Mail.* Retrieved from http://www.theglobeandmail.com/news/british-columbia/bc-inmates-to-receive-flu-vaccine-before-prison-staff/article4356749

National Collaborating Centre for Infectious Diseases. (2008, April). *Primary HIV prevention interventions in prisons and upon release.* Retrieved from http://librarypdf.catie.ca/PDF/PCatie/24898.pdf

Office of the Correctional Investigator. (2011). *Annual report of the Office of the Correctional Investigator 2010–2011* (No. PS100-2011E-PDF). Ottawa, ON: Her Majesty the Queen in Right of Canada. Retrieved from http://www.oci-bec.gc.ca/cnt/rpt/pdf/annrpt/annrpt20102011-eng.pdf

Office of the Correctional Investigator. (2012). *Annual report of the Office of the Correctional Investigator 2011–2012.* (No. PS100-2012E-PDF). Ottawa, ON: Her Majesty the Queen in Right of Canada. Retrieved from http://www.oci-bec.gc.ca/cnt/rpt/pdf/annrpt/annrpt20112012-eng.pdf

Office of the Correctional Investigator. (2013). *Annual report of the Office of the Correctional Investigator 2012–2013.* (No. PS100-2013E-PDF). Ottawa, ON: Her Majesty the Queen in Right of Canada. Retrieved from http://www.oci-bec.gc.ca/cnt/rpt/pdf/annrpt/annrpt20122013-eng.pdf

Office of the Correctional Investigator. (2014). *Annual Report of the Office of the Correctional Investigator 2013–2014.* No. PS100-2014E-PDF). Ottawa, ON: Her Majesty the Queen in Right of Canada. Retrieved from http://www.oci-bec.gc.ca/cnt/rpt/pdf/annrpt/annrpt20132014-eng.pdf

Perreault, S. (2009, July). The incarceration of Aboriginal people in adult correctional services. *Juristat, 29*(3) (Catalogue no. 85-002-x). Ottawa, ON: Canadian Centre for Justice Studies.

Perrault, S. (2014a). Admissions to adult correctional services in Canada, 2011/2012. *Juristat* (No. 85-002-x). Ottawa, ON: Statistics Canada. Retrieved from http://www.statcan.gc.ca/pub/85-002-x/2014001/article/11918-eng.htm

Perreault, S. (2014b). Admissions to youth correctional services in Canada, 2011/2012. *Juristat* (No. 85-002-X). Ottawa, ON: Canadian Centre for Justice Statistics. Retrieved from http://www.statcan.gc.ca/pub/85-002-x/2014001/article/11917-eng.htm

Perrault, S. (2014c). Correctional services key indicators, 2012/2013. *Juristat* (No.85-002-x). Ottawa, ON: Statistics Canada. Retrieved from http://www.statcan.gc.ca/pub/85-002-x/2014001/article/14007-eng.htm

Perry, C. W., & Morris, R. E. (2014). Health care for youth involved with the correctional system. *Primary Care, 41*(3), 691–705. doi:10.1016/j.pop.2014.05.007

Peternelj-Taylor, C. (2005). Conceptualizing nursing research with offenders: Another look at vulnerability. *International Journal of Law and Psychiatry, 28,* 348–359.

Peternelj-Taylor, C. (2008). Criminalization of the mentally ill. *Journal of Forensic Nursing, 4*(4), 185–187. doi: 10.1111/j.1939-3938.2008.00031.x

Peternelj-Taylor, C. (2010). A new year, a new era, a new page. *Journal of Forensic Nursing, 6*(1), 1–2. doi: 1111/j.1939-3938.2009.01059.x

Peternelj-Taylor, C. (2015). Care of persons under forensic purview. In W. Austin & M. A. Boyd (Eds.), *Psychiatric nursing for Canadian practice* (3rd. ed., pp. 891–905). Philadelphia, PA: Wolters Kluwer.

Peternelj-Taylor, C., & Panosky, D. (2013). Advancing forensic correctional nursing. *Journal of Forensic Nursing, 9*(1), 1–2. doi:10.1097/JFN.0b013e3182867083

Power, J., & Riley, D. (2010). A comparative review of suicide and self-injury investigative reports in a Canadian federal correctional population. *Research at a Glance.* Retrieved from http://www.csc-scc.gc.ca/005/008/092/005008-0221-eng.pdf

Power, J., Brown, S. L., & Usher, A. M. (2013). Non-suicidal self-injury in women offenders: Motivations, emotions, and precipitating events. *International Journal of Forensic Mental Health, 12*(3), 192–204. doi:10.1080/14999013.2013.832442

Registered Nurses' Association of Ontario. (2009). *Supporting clients on methadone maintenance treatment.* Toronto, ON: Author. Retrieved from http://rnao.ca/bpg/guidelines/supporting-clients-methadone-maintenance-treatment

Roth, B., & Pressé, L. (2003). Nursing interventions for parasuicidal behaviors in female offenders. *Journal of Psychosocial Nursing and Mental Health Services, 41*(9), 20–29.

Rowan, J., Auger, S., Toto, H., Simpson, S., & McNab, C. (2004). The use of stories for healing interventions with women. *Forum on Corrections Research, 16*(1), 42–44.

Royal College of Nursing. (2009). *Health and nursing care in the criminal justice service.* London, UK: Author. Retrieved from http://www.rcn.org.uk/__data/assets/pdf_file/0010/248725/003307.pdf

Sabramanian, R., Delaney, R., Roberts, S., Fishman, N., & McGarry, P. (2015). *Incarceration's front door: The misuse of jails in America.* New York, NY: Vera Institute of Justice. Retrieved from http://www.vera.org/sites/default/files/resources/downloads/incarcerations-front-door-report.pdf

Shelton, D. (2003). The clinical practice of juvenile forensic psychiatric nurses. *Journal of Psychosocial Nursing and Mental Health Services, 41*(9), 43–53.

Shelton, D. (2004). Experiences of detained young offenders in need of mental health care. *Journal of Nursing Scholarship, 36*(2), 129–133.

Shelton, D. (2009). Forensic nursing in secure environments. *Journal of Forensic Nursing, 5,* 131–142. doi:10.1111/j.1939-3938.2009.01046.x

Shelton, D., Weiskopf, C., & Nicholson, M. (2010). Correctional nursing competency development in the Connecticut Correctional Managed Health Care Program. *Journal of Correctional Health Care, 16*(4), 299–309. Reprinted by permission of SAGE Publications, Inc. doi:10.1177/1078345810378498

Singleton, N., Meltzer, H., Gatward, R., Coid, J., & Deasy, D. (1998). *Psychiatric morbidity among prisoners in England and Wales.* London, UK: The Stationery Office.

Smith, S. (2005, February). Stepping through the looking glass: Professional autonomy in correctional nursing. *Corrections Today,* 54–56, 70.

Srivastava, R. H. (2007). Understanding cultural competence in health care. In R. H. Srivastava (Ed.), *The healthcare professional's guide to clinical cultural competence* (pp. 3–27). Toronto, ON: Mosby Elsevier.

Storch, J., & Peternelj-Taylor, C. (2009). Ethics for health care providers: Codes as guidance for practice in prisons. In D. Hatton & A. Fisher (Eds.), *Women prisoners and health justice* (pp. 109–116). Oxford, UK: Radcliffe.

Sunil, V., Holt, A. M., Dixon, R., Dingman, D., & Noseworthy, A. L. (2013). Novovirus-like virus outbreak in a correctional facility in Haliburton Kawartha Pine Ridge District Health Unit, March to April 2008. *Journal of Correctional Healthcare, 19,* 269–277. doi:10.1177/1078345813499311

Tandon, R., & Jibson, M. D. (2003). Suicidal behavior in schizophrenia: Diagnosis, neurobiology and treatment implications. *Current Opinion in Psychiatry, 16*(2), 193–197.

Thomas, G. (2005). Harm reduction policies and programs for persons involved in the criminal justice system. *Harm reduction for special populations in Canada.* Canadian Centre on Substance Abuse. Retrieved from http://www.ccsa.ca/Resource%20Library/ccsa-003900-2005.pdf

van der Meulen, E., & Ka Hon Chu, S. (2015, Spring). Harm reduction behind bars: Prison based needle and syringe programs. *CATIE: Canada's Source for HIV and Hepatitis C Information.* Retrieved from http://www.catie.ca/en/pif/spring-2015/harm-reduction-behind-bars-prison-based-needle-and-syringe-programs

Webster, P. C. (2012). Prison puzzle: Treating hepatitis C. *Canadian Medical Association Journal, 184*(9), 1017–1018. doi:10.1503/cmaj.109-4191

Williams, N. H. (2007). Prison health and the health of the public: Ties that bind. *Journal of Correctional Health Care, 13*(2), 80–92. doi:10.1177/1078345807301143

World Health Organization. (2007). *Preventing suicide in jails and prisons.* Retrieved from http://www.who.int/mental_health/prevention/suicide/resource_jails_prisons.pdf

## ABOUT THE AUTHORS

**Cindy Peternelj-Taylor**, RN, BScN, MScN, DE-IAFN (University of Saskatchewan), is a Professor with the College of Nursing, University of Saskatchewan, and a Distinguished Fellow—International Association of Forensic Nurses. She is a graduate of Lakehead University and the University of Saskatchewan and is currently completing doctoral studies with the University of Alberta. Much of Cindy's career has focused on professional role development for nurses who work with vulnerable populations in forensic psychiatric and correctional settings. She is the editor-in-chief of *Journal of Forensic Nursing.* She is currently completing two collaborative research studies: (1) a scoping review exploring palliative care in corrections with Lorraine Holtslander, and (2) together with Phil Woods, a study of the roles, responsibilities, and learning needs of Saskatchewan provincial correctional nurses.

**Phil Woods**, RPN, PhD (Anglia Polytechnic University), is a Professor and Associate Dean of Research, Innovation and Global Initiatives, with the College of Nursing, University of Saskatchewan. He trained as a mental health nurse in the United Kingdom and is a registered psychiatric nurse in Saskatchewan. Phil has a PhD in Nursing Studies. He has an extensive personal portfolio of forensic-related research and is a well-known author of mental health and forensic nursing articles and books. His specific research interests are risk assessment and management, violence prediction, and developing mental health and forensic mental health practice.

# CHAPTER 27

# Environmental and Occupational Health

*Janet Morrison*

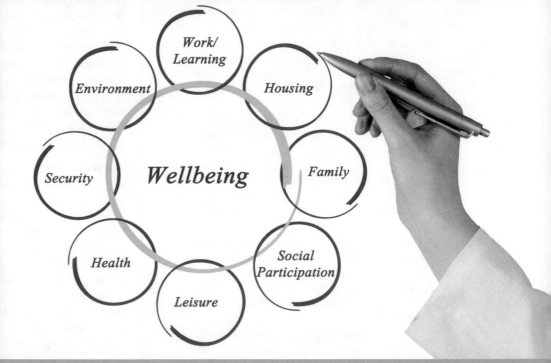

*Source: Arka38/Shutterstock*

## INTRODUCTION

> *"The environment is everything that isn't me."*
> *(Albert Einstein)*

Einstein defined the environment in the broadest of terms. In the context of this chapter, this definition implies that environmental health encompasses all parameters that impact health and that are not the person. The influence of environmental factors on health is receiving increased public, political, scientific, and media attention. Globally, the diseases with the largest absolute burden attributable to modifiable environmental factors include diarrhea, lower respiratory tract infections, malaria, and unintentional injuries (e.g., workplace injuries, industrial accidents, pedestrian and cycling accidents, and radiation exposure), (Prüss-Üstün, 2006). Over the last decade there has been increasing concern over the possible impacts of climate change on health. For example, changing climates increase the risk of temperature-related mortality and morbidity; change the patterns of diseases carried by mosquitoes, ticks, and animals; and result in weather-related natural hazards such as severe storms, floods, and droughts (CDC, 2015).

Compared to other countries, Canada is considered healthy in terms of the environmental burden of disease, although vulnerable and disparate groups may differ from the national average. The World Health Organization (WHO) has estimated that worldwide, 23% of all deaths can be attributed to environmental factors (Prüss-Üstün, 2006). This significant statistic highlights the importance of understanding how the environment influences health.

This chapter will provide an overview of environmental health, including the environmental health assessment process, and environmental health legislation with an emphasis on the role of the occupational health nurse (OHN) and other community health nursing specialties.

## DEFINING ENVIRONMENTAL HEALTH

The WHO defines **environmental health** as all aspects of human health, disease, and injury that are determined by factors in the environment (Prüss-Üstün, 2006). These **environmental factors** include the effects of *chemical, physical, and biological agents* as well as impacts related to the broad physical and social environment (e.g., housing, urban development, land use and transportation, industry, and agriculture) (Prüss-Üstün, 2006). In Canada, a report titled "A New Perspective on the Health of Canadians" was the first documented acknowledgement by a Canadian federal agency that health included environment, genetics, and lifestyle (Lalonde, 1981).

The link between health and environmental factors has underpinned nursing practice for decades. In the mid-1800s Florence Nightingale (1859) stressed the necessity of environmental factors such as good ventilation, pure water, efficient drainage, cleanliness, and light as factors that promoted health. In addition, she urged nurses to modify the environment to promote the "reparative process" of healing the sick and injured. Environmental factors have the potential to impact health at the *individual, family, community, and population levels*, and the ability to initiate, promote, sustain, or stimulate disease and disease conditions. At the individual level, environmental exposures can occur at home, at work, and during social and recreational activities. One or more of the environmental factors an individual is exposed to can produce a range of health effects.

## DEFINING OCCUPATIONAL HEALTH

Working Canadians spend an average of 36.6 hours per week on the job. (Human Resources and Skills Development Canada, n.d.). During that time their working conditions may expose them to heightened levels of chemical, physical, biological, and psychological hazards present in the work environment but that can also occur in other aspects of their life. For example, **workplace exposures** can exacerbate

| Table 27.1 | Sample Occupational Disease Claim Categories and Claims Accepted by WorkSafeBC, 2012 |
|---|---|
| **Category** | **Claims** |
| Repetitive motion | 980 |
| Hearing loss | 459 |
| Infectious diseases | 390 |
| Chemical burns | 246 |
| Respiratory disease | 184 |
| Poisoning | 133 |
| Cancer | 68 |

Source: WorkSafeBC (n.d.). Occupational disease data by type of disease and five-year period; 1988–2012. Retrieved from http://www.worksafebc.com/publications/reports/statistics_reports/occupational_disease/1988-2012/assets/Table1.pdf

existing back pain or cardiovascular conditions, or diminish hearing acuity. **Occupational diseases** can occur from exposures that are unique to the workplace and unlikely to occur in concentrated form in daily life—for example, ionizing radiation, benzene, or asbestos. To give you a sense of the type of occupational diseases suffered by workers, Table 27.1 lists a sample of occupational disease claim categories and the number of accepted claims by WorkSafeBC (WSBC) in 2012. During 2012, WorkSafeBC recorded 86 fatalities due to occupational disease and 63 fatalities due to on-the-job injuries—a total of 149 work-related fatalities (WSBC, 2013). (To see the complete list, go to www.worksafebc.com/publications/reports/statistics_reports/occupational_disease/1988-2012/assets/Table1.pdf.)

In recognition of the importance of workplace health issues, the Joint International Labour Organization (ILO) and the WHO Committee on Occupational Health have defined occupational health as the "promotion and maintenance of the highest degree of physical mental and social well-being of workers in all occupations" by the prevention of injury and disease caused by working conditions, the protection of workers from risks resulting from factors adverse to health, and "the placing and maintenance of the worker in an occupational environment adapted to their physiological and psychological capabilities" (ILO/WHO Committee on Occupational Health, 1995). Figure 27.1 illustrates how exposures from the home, the workplace, and the neighbourhood interact to create an individual's potential exposure profile that makes up the environmental influences on their health.

## A TEAM APPROACH TO ENVIRONMENTAL HEALTH

The complexity of environmental health factors requires a multidisciplinary approach. The role of the multidisciplinary team is to anticipate, recognize, evaluate, and control for environmental factors that arise and have the potential to

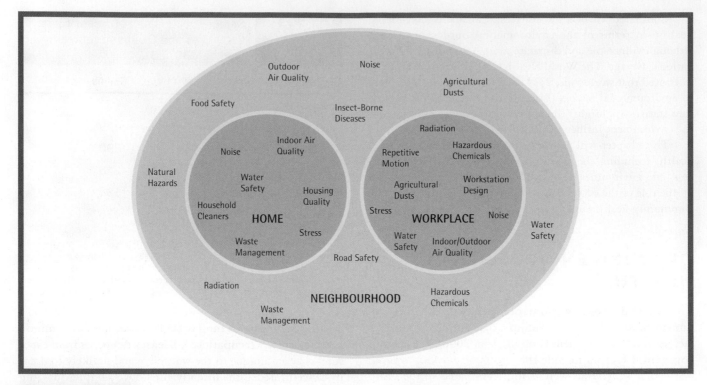

**FIGURE** **27.1** Occupational and Environmental Influences on Health

*Source:* Modified from WHO: Environmental Burden of Disease Series, No. 1 Introduction and methods: Assessing the environmental burden of disease at national and local levels. Figure 2.1 Environmental hazards and risk factors; Myres, A. W., & Betke, K. (2002). Healthy environments = healthy people. *Health Policy Research Bulletin,* Issue 4. Ottawa, ON: Minister of Health: Her Majesty the Queen in Right of Canada, p. 6.

cause impaired well-being at the individual, community, or population level. The team identifies *modifiable environmental factors* that are realistically amenable to change using available technology, policy, prevention, and public health measures. Occupational Health Nurses (OHNs) are one type of community health nurse (CHN), and are part of the multidisciplinary team that may also include physicians, industrial hygienists, toxicologists, engineers, safety professionals, scientists, provincial health and safety officials, workplace safety officials, urban planners, lobbyists, and others. As members of this multidisciplinary team, OHNs must be knowledgeable about how specific factors in the environment (including chemical, physical, and biological hazards) can impact human health. CHNs have the training and background to identify potential health impacts from environmental factors, including the disparate influences on vulnerable and disadvantaged populations.

## OCCUPATIONAL HEALTH NURSING

**Occupational health nursing** is a branch of nursing dealing with health, safety, treatment, care, and prevention of illness or injury in a workplace setting. Whereas CHNs apply the practice of nursing in a wide variety of community settings, OHNs apply the practice of nursing in the workplace to specific populations of workers. OHNs are registered nurses with additional training, skills, and education in occupational health and safety and are often hired by industry to provide services on site or in consulting roles. The Canadian Nurses Association (CNA) offers certification in occupational health nursing. In fact, occupational health nursing was the first nursing specialty in Canada to develop a national certification process. The Canadian Occupational Health Nurses Association (COHNA/ACIIST) is the national association for OHNs in Canada, and provides a national voice to influence health and safety regulations across the country (www.cohna-aciist.ca).

OHNs often work as part of a larger team of occupational health professionals at a workplace. That team might also include industrial hygienists, safety professionals, engineers, management, and physicians. However, on-site physicians are much less common in the workplace than they used to be. It is not unusual for the OHN to be the front-line healthcare provider and emergency response coordinator for a workplace. The experience and scope of practice for an OHN at a workplace can be very broad, encompassing everything from emergency response and first aid to policy planning and prevention initiatives. The Canadian Nurses Association [CNA] (2013) key competencies for the occupational health nursing certification exam can be found here: www.nurseone.ca/en/certification/

what-is-certification/competencies-per-specialty-area. Broadly, they are defined as follows:

- provision of occupational health safety and environmental nursing;
- recognition, evaluation, and control of workplace/environmental health and safety hazards;
- health assessment, planning implementation, monitoring, and evaluation;
- assessment, care, and case management of injuries and illnesses;
- health, safety, and wellness promotion and education; and
- health, safety, and wellness management.

**The many roles of community health nurses** The mission of health professionals in occupational and environmental health is to prevent, anticipate, recognize, evaluate, and control for those environmental exposures that could bring harm to a population. In terms of environmental factors, the most attention has focused on occupational settings and, in particular, manufacturing settings. However, over the past two decades this focus has expanded to include communities, homes, schools, hospitals, offices, and daycares. CHNs practise in all these settings, often as specialists, public health nurses, school nurses, or occupational health nurses (OHNs), and, as such, many are actively involved in addressing exposures to environmental factors.

The environments we live, work, and play in have the potential to impact health. CHNs have a role in preventing exposures to and reducing health risks from environmental factors. The Canadian Nurses Association has developed tools to support nurses in addressing environmental health issues in areas ranging from clinical practice, administration, research, and education through to policy (CNA, 2009). The influence of environment on community health and well-being is an important component of community health nursing practice.

# ENVIRONMENTAL AND OCCUPATIONAL HEALTH FRAMEWORKS

Defining environmental health requires understanding what constitutes an environmental factor. For this purpose, the WHO uses a very broad framework called the **DPSEEA framework** (Driving forces, Pressures, State, Exposures, Effects, and Actions). This framework categorizes environmental health factors into driving forces (D), pressures (P), the state of the environment (S), exposure (E1), defined as the interaction between people and the environment, and resulting health effects (E2) related to the amount of exposure (Briggs, 1999).

- **Driving forces** (D): Driving forces are factors that create pressures, which can influence the state of the environment. Examples include poverty, population density, population growth, age structure, urbanization, and technology.
- **Pressures** (P): The environment can be altered by pressures. Such pressures could include production and consumption of resources as well as waste management. Pressures may be

modifiable environmental factors. For example, public health policy could minimize the extent to which driving forces generate pressures.

- **State of the environment** (S): The state of the environment can be altered in response to pressures (e.g., resource availability, air pollution). However, the environmental state can impact health only following human exposure. Risk assessment determines the environmental hazards important in human health.
- **Exposure and effects** (EE): Exposures occur through inhalation, ingestion, and absorption of hazards (e.g., indoor air pollution, animal and or human waste and by-products, water quality and supply, lead, radiation, communicable diseases, and occupational exposures). The health effects relate to the exposures that occur. Vulnerable, hypersensitive, and disadvantaged populations may have differential health outcomes to similar exposure levels.
- **Actions** (A): The various actions that are undertaken to affect the environmental factor include policy changes, pollution monitoring, environmental improvements, and education or awareness programs (adapted from Briggs, 1999).

**Applying the DPSEEA Framework** Knowledge of all factors in the framework is important to appreciate the complexities related to environmental exposures and health outcomes. The DPSEEA framework can explain how environmental factors of concern will differ locally, regionally, and nationally. For example, driving forces, such as poverty, create pressures, such as poor sanitation and hygiene, which in turn create an environmental state with high risk of diarrhea (Prüss-Üstün, 2006).

## An Occupational Health Framework

Figure 27.2 illustrates Rogers (1994) framework for assessing the occupational health environment. Similar to the DPSEEA framework, Rogers illustrates how driving factors external to the workplace (i.e., economics, politics and legislation, population and health trends, and technology) as well as internal factors (including corporate culture and mission, resources, the work of the organization and its inherent work hazards, and the characteristics of the workforce itself) constitute the occupational environment. As illustrated in the model, these factors are used to focus and direct OHN practice.

# ENVIRONMENTAL FACTORS

## Modelling Environmental Influences on Health

As discussed previously, exposure to individual environmental factors will primarily occur at home, at work, or during recreational activities. These factors have the potential to impact health either individually or in combination. For example, indoor and outdoor air quality are two main environmental factors related to acute lower respiratory infections

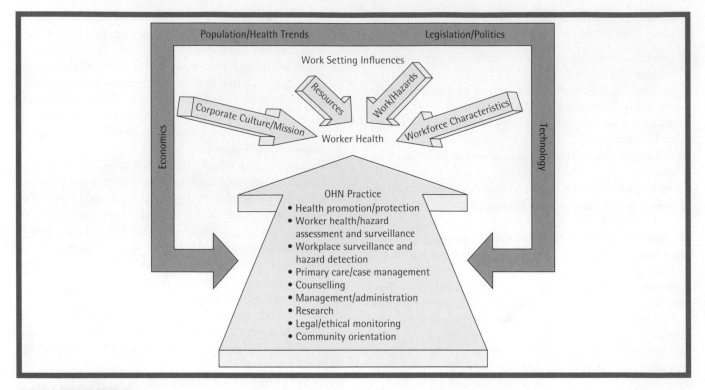

FIGURE 27.2 Rogers' (1994) Conceptual Model of Occupational Health Nursing Practice

*Source:* Rogers, B. (1994). *Occupational health nursing: Concepts and practice.* Philadelphia, PA: WB Saunders. p. 39. Used by permission of American Association of Occupational Health Nurses.

in various parts of the world. Within this context, contributing environmental factors including tobacco smoke, solid fuel use, housing conditions, and possibly hygiene. In recognition of the far-reaching effects of air quality, the International Agency for Research on Cancer (IARC) recently classified air pollution as a Group 1 (known human carcinogen) substance, where it joins other known carcinogens such as asbestos, benzene, formaldehyde, and ionizing radiation (2013). (Please see Photo 27.1. and Canadian Research Box 27.1.)

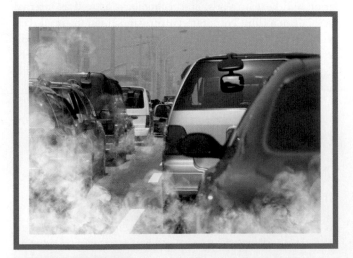

PHOTO 27.1 **Idling vehicles: In an attempt to reduce air pollution, many communities have passed by-laws prohibiting extended vehicle idling.**

*Source: Ssuaphotos/Shutterstock*

### CANADIAN RESEARCH BOX 27.1

**Is there an association between air quality and emergency department visits for asthma?**

Lavigne, E., Villeneuve, P., & Cakmak, S. (2012). Air pollution and emergency department visits for asthma in Windsor, Canada. *Canadian Journal of Public Health, 103*(1), 4–8.

Using a time-stratified case-crossover design, this study correlated data from Environment Canada's network of fixed-site air monitors and emergency department (ED) visits in Windsor, Ontario. Windsor is a city known to have poor air quality in comparison with other Canadian cities. When confounding variables such as ED visits for influenza and weather variables were controlled for, a statistically significant association was observed between ambient air pollution levels (increased levels of sulphur dioxide, nitrogren dioxide, and carbon monoxide) and ED visits for asthma. The effect was particularly noticeable among children from 2 to 14 years of age, between the months of April and September.

The researchers concluded that ambient air pollution appeared to increase the risk of ED visits for asthma, particularly among children, in Windsor.

### Discussion Questions

1. How might a nurse communicate this information to parents of children with asthma?
2. How could parents of children with asthma use this information?
3. How could nurses disseminate this information to the community at large?

## Categorization of Environmental Factors

Individual environmental factors are typically categorized as chemical, physical, biological, psychological, and ergonomic.

- **Chemical factors** are in the form of vapours, gases, dusts, fumes, and mists. Chemicals may be raw materials in original form or by-products of the chemical breakdown or production process.
- **Physical factors** include ionizing and non-ionizing radiation, noise, vibration, and extremes in temperature and pressure.
- **Biological factors** are any living organisms (or their components or properties) that can cause an adverse health effect. Micro-organisms (bacteria, viruses, or fungi), pests and insects, and animals are included in this category.
- **Psychological factors** are individual stress or stressful events that have the ability to impact health. Examples of events that have the potential to be stressful include illness, death, birth, job promotion, or fluctuations in financial status. Recently, the negative effects of bullying and harassment and exposure to violence and traumatic events have gained attention and recognition as interpersonal factors that can have serious effects on health.
- **Ergonomic factors** include factors that influence the compatibility or "fit" between the person and his or her immediate environment, task, job, or activity. Examples of problematic ergonomic factors that could lead to illness or injury include improperly designed or utilized tools or work areas as well as poor work practices, such as improper lifting or reaching, poor visual conditions, or repetitive motion activities.

## Environmental Factors—Routes of Entry

The four common routes of entry for individual environmental factors (chemical, physical, or biological) are inhalation, absorption, injection, and ingestion.

- **Inhalation** involves inhaling agents directly into the respiratory tract and lungs.
- **Absorption** refers to entrance through the skin, regardless of whether the skin is intact or damaged. Some substances may be absorbed by way of openings or through hair follicles, while others may dissolve in fats and oils of the skin (e.g., organic lead compounds, organic phosphate pesticides, and solvents such as toluene and xylene). Some compounds can produce systemic poisoning through direct contact with the skin (cyanides, aromatic amines, amides, and phenols).
- **Injection** can involve accidental or intentional injection of agents from either a high-velocity source (i.e., an agent released under high pressure) or a point source (i.e., needle puncture).
- **Ingestion** includes knowingly or unknowingly eating or drinking a harmful agent and subsequently having a toxic compound absorbed from the gastrointestinal tract into the bloodstream.

## Degree of Hazard

The relationship between the dose of an agent and the response it elicits is a fundamental concept in toxicology (Figure 27.3). The level of harm depends on the level of exposure. The **degree of hazard** from exposure to environmental factors depends on (a) the nature of the agent involved, (b) the intensity of the exposure, and (c) the duration of the exposure. Key elements to consider include (a) how much of the agent is required to produce an effect, (b) the probability of the agent entering the body at levels required to produce an effect, (c) the rate at which the agent is generated or emitted, (d) the total contact time, and (e) the use of any measures that might reduce the level of exposure (e.g., ventilation or personal protective equipment).

When an environmental factor is recognized, three strategies are typically employed to control for exposure; these are known as the "hierarchy of controls." The appropriate type of control will depend on the exposure in question. This is referred to as **hazard control**.

**Engineering controls** are the first line of defence by providing or creating a design, structure, enclosure, or system to engineer the exposure away. Examples of engineering controls include substitution (i.e., replacing a substance of concern with something associated with less or no effects), changing the design of a process so that exposures do not or are less likely to occur (e.g., building enclosures, isolating the hazard from those who may be exposed), and adding ventilation to dilute or remove the agent.

**Administrative controls** are utilized when engineering controls are not feasible, are insufficient, or in the case of sensitive individuals. An example of an administrative control is removing the individual from the source of exposure or limiting contact time with the exposure. In the case of an occupational exposure, this could include changing the job functions of the individual to prevent the exposure from occurring. A classic example of administrative control is limiting time spent performing a repetitive task in order to prevent musculoskeletal injury.

**Personal protective equipment (PPE)** is worn to protect an individual from a known exposure (e.g., respirators to prevent inhalation exposures, gloves to prevent absorption). Although PPE is effective in reducing exposures, individual actions can dictate the effectiveness of the PPE. For example, PPE must be worn properly and fit appropriately to be effective. Due to these limitations, PPE should always be considered a last line of defence; engineering and administrative controls are preferable when feasible.

## Dose–Response

> All things are poisons; there is none which is not a poison. The right dose differentiates a poison and a remedy. (Paracelsus, 1493–1541)

Exposures to an agent may result in a **dose–response** that has no effect, a minimal effect, or an acute or chronic health outcome. Dose–response histograms, such as Figure 27.3, are

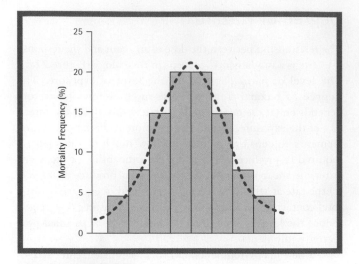

**FIGURE 27.3** The Dose–Response Relationship

*Source:* Casarett, L. J., Doull, J., Klaassen, C. D., & Watkins, J. B. (2007). *Casarett and Doull's toxicology: The basic science of poisons.* New York, NY: McGraw-Hill Companies, p. 21. Used by permission of McGraw-Hill Companies.

often utilized as a means to portray the relationship between the dose of an agent and the elicited responses in a population. The dose–response histogram indicates the frequency of health events associated with varying doses of an agent and forms a bell-shaped curve known as a *normal frequency distribution*. The curve indicates the differences in susceptibility among individuals. In a normally distributed population, the mean ±1 standard deviation (SD) represents 68.3% of the population. The left end of the curve represents hyper-susceptible members of the population, and the right end of the curve represents the resistant population. In other words, those at the left end of the curve experience an effect at lower doses, while those at the right end experience an effect only at high doses. A population will always contain individuals that fall at either end of the curve and at points in between. Individuals at the hyper-susceptible end of the curve may require additional resources to control for exposures, while individuals at the resistant end of the curve might not appear to suffer from above average levels of exposure, though falling in the latter group should not preclude use of appropriate exposure control measures.

# ENVIRONMENTAL HEALTH ASSESSMENT

An **environmental health assessment** is performed to examine possible links between environmental exposures and health outcomes. Some individuals may have a specific environmental exposure concern, such as arsenic in well water or a workplace chemical exposure. Others may have more generalized concerns about environmental exposures or are looking to environmental exposures as the cause of unexplained symptoms. In these cases, a more detailed inventory of possible environmental exposures must be taken. It is not uncommon

for the individual to present with concerns about a potential exposure in the absence of any notable symptoms or health effects. Certain populations might also be considered vulnerable to environmental factors, including children, elderly, pregnant, and immune-compromised individuals.

## Personal Exposure History

An important part of assessing the influence of environmental exposures is the individual interview. The **individual interview** involves asking the individual about the nature of his or her environmental exposures, when and where they occur, the circumstances of how they occur, and whether or not he or she feels any ill effects from those exposures. The impacts of biology (genetics), sociology (habits), occupation, the home environment, and past exposure history must all be considered in the assessment. Specifically, the individual interview includes occupational, residential, and recreational information.

**Occupational information** would include present and past jobs and work exposures, as well as any protective measures related to work exposures. The workplace may be a significant source of chemical, physical, biological, psychological, or ergonomic factors. Duration of exposure, including number of hours a day, days a week, and number of years of exposure are important aspects in the assessment. Source agents of exposure as well as by-products should be included in the assessment. Sources of information include key informants, a review of the Material Safety Data Sheets for the relevant workplace hazardous materials, and the results of any industrial hygiene monitoring conducted in the workplace.

The assessment of the work environment is an essential component in health and safety programming in order to recognize and control for hazards (chemical, physical, biologic, ergonomic, or psychological). An OHN may be involved in the following:

- assessing the work site to identify actual or potential hazards to workers resulting from working conditions, work processes, and materials (raw materials, by-products, and end products);
- conducting health screening and medical assessments for the early detection of occupational diseases (e.g., audiometry, spirometry); and
- advising and making recommendations to those in management positions on occupational injury and disease prevention, and health promotion.

**Residential information** can provide added insights into potential exposures. It includes information about water sources, mould and dampness, and indoor air quality. Those living in rural and remote areas may have adverse exposures because they rely on unprocessed well water, live in non–building code compliant housing, and use alternative fuels resulting in exposure to carbon monoxide. They also have less access to health care services and advice. Refer to Chapter 24 for a further discussion of rural health.

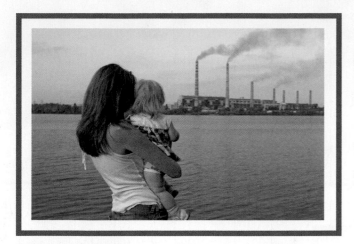

**PHOTO 27.2** Industries impact both workers and their families.

*Source: Sergii Mostovyi/Fotolia*

(c) report on a disease pattern for which there is no causal explanation and where attempts were made to identify potential agents. Cross-sectional, cohort, ecological, case-control, and community intervention study designs, including adaptations to these designs, are utilized in environmental epidemiology studies. Although environmental health is a relatively new field, researchers have been performing environmental epidemiology studies for centuries. In the 1800s, John Snow published his epidemiological work on the transmission of cholera in an essay, "On the Mode of Communication of Cholera." Contrary to common belief at that time, Snow suggested that cholera entered the body via ingestion rather than inhalation. By plotting the position of cholera patients on a map in relation to public water taps, he was able to demonstrate a correlation between contaminated water and cholera outbreaks (Snow, 1860). An in-depth discussion of epidemiology is presented in Chapter 11. The importance of utilizing research evidence is presented in Chapter 10.

Recreational information includes social activities and community-related exposures. Environmental factors associated with industries and processes within the community would be documented during a community assessment, as described in Chapter 13, Community Nursing Process.

Determining whether an individual or a group has experienced an effect from an environmental exposure can be difficult for a variety of reasons. First, environmental exposures may be associated with latent health conditions, highlighting the importance of collecting information from as far back as the individual can provide. Second, the combined effect of one or more exposures from home, work, and social activities can make it difficult to attribute one particular exposure to a particular effect (see Photo 27.2). Third, many environmentally related conditions and illnesses are characterized by signs and symptoms that are very similar to those of more typical "non-environmental" illnesses (e.g., mild respiratory infections can present with symptoms that are sometimes confused with allergy to an environmental agent). Fourth, in cases of low-level environmental exposures and mild or uncertain health effects, attempts to attribute cause to a particular exposure may be extremely difficult. Finally, considerable "background noise" in the form of co-existing health conditions, other exposures (e.g., workplaces, smoking), and inherited factors may be present. The challenge lies in recognizing all potential sources of exposures and factors of influence, then attempting to attribute the cause of illness or symptoms to an exposure.

## OCCUPATIONAL AND ENVIRONMENTAL EPIDEMIOLOGY

**Epidemiology** is utilized to clarify relationships between environmental factors and human health effects. Epidemiological studies might (a) characterize health effects from known exposures, (b) characterize exposures and effects in populations and attempt to determine dose–response relationships, or

## Environmental Indicators

For some environmental factors, **environmental indicators** are monitored to assist in recognizing community and population exposures that have the potential to impact health. Indicators provide a simple way to convey complex environmental information. Through the Canadian Environmental Sustainability Indicators (CESI) initiative, the Canadian federal government reports on three environmental indicators: (a) air quality, (b) water quality, and (c) greenhouse gas emissions.

**Air quality indicators** track ground-level ozone and fine particulate matter ($PM_{2.5}$) (see Figure 27.4). Ground-level ozone has the ability to impact plant, animal, and human health. Fine particulate matter ($PM_{2.5}$) can be inhaled deep into the lungs and can be the cause of **chronic health effects** and **acute health effects**. Long-term high-level exposures may be associated with chronic cardiovascular and respiratory health outcomes, whereas short-term high-level exposures can impact vulnerable populations (e.g., individuals with pre-existing heart or lung disease, infants, or the elderly).

**Water quality indicators** measure the extent and severity of water pollution by tracking a wide range of substances in water across Canada. Water quality is considered a broad reflection of ecosystem health. Health outcomes related to water quality include water-borne illnesses (*E. coli*, *Giardia*, and *Cryptosporidium*) from untreated or undertreated water supplies, infant methemoglobinemia from nitrate exposure in drinking water systems, and mercury poisoning from consuming high amounts of contaminated fish.

**Greenhouse gas indicators** track Canada's greenhouse gas emissions and identify sources. Typical greenhouse gases are carbon dioxide, methane, nitrous oxide, and ozone. Greenhouse gas emissions can be considered a pressure using the DPSEEA model. Greenhouse gases can potentially impact climate, which could influence ecosystems with resultant health outcomes (e.g., changes in disease patterns caused by insects, bacteria, or pathogens).

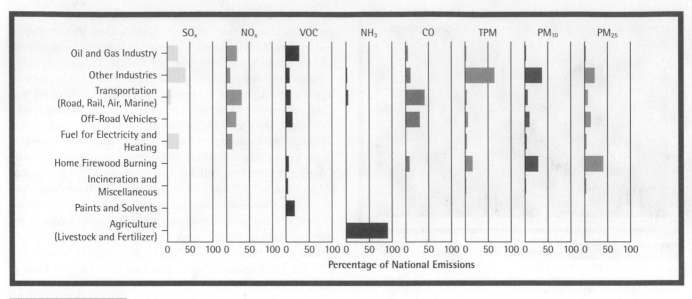

**FIGURE** **27.4** Distribution of Air Pollutant Emissions by Source, Canada, 2011

*Source:* Environment Canada. (n.d.). Distribution of air pollutant emissions by source, Canada, 2011. © Her Majesty The Queen in Right of Canada, Environment Canada, 2013. Reproduced with the permission of the Minister of Public Works and Government Services Canada. Retrieved from http://www.ec.gc.ca/indicateurs-indicators/default.asp?lang=en&n=58DE4720-1#sector

# RISK ASSESSMENT, RISK MANAGEMENT, AND RISK COMMUNICATION

**Risk assessment**, **risk management**, and **risk communication** are tools utilized in environmental health for assessing, managing, and communicating risks associated with environmental factors (see Figure 27.5). Risk assessment is the systematic process for describing and quantifying the level of exposure to particular substances that will result in increased risks to health (Covello & Merkhofer, 1993). Risk assessment typically involves an estimation of risk either through direct association, based on assumptions utilizing the best available information (dose–response curves), or generalizations based on animal models. For example,

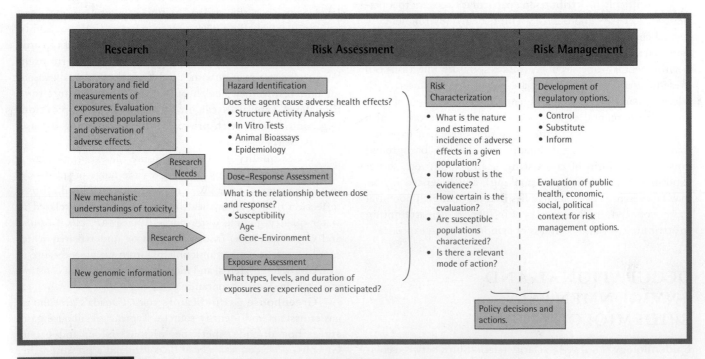

**FIGURE** **27.5** Elements of Risk Assessment and Risk Management

*Source:* Casarett, L. J., Doull, J., Klaassen, C. D., & Watkins, J. B. (2007). *Casarett and Doull's essentials of toxicology*. New York, NY: McGraw-Hill Companies, p. 108, with original text from National Research Council (U.S.). (1983). *Risk assessment in the federal government: Managing the process*. Washington, DC: National Academy Press, pp. 29–33. Used by permission of National Academy of Sciences.

Health Canada is charged with assessing the health risks of many items such as foods, consumer products, medical devices, and drugs. Risk-management options available to Health Canada include minimal intervention (e.g., enhancing public awareness) to maximum intervention (e.g., legislation).

Risk communication is the process of making risk-assessment and risk-management information comprehensible and taking the necessary steps to distribute and present that information (see Canadian Research Box 27.2). CHNs are typically involved in risk communication at the prevention level. Anticipating and recognizing potential environmental factors of concern are important first steps in preventing exposures, while education is a primary preventive strategy in environmental health. Applying the basic principles of disease prevention, including primary, secondary, and tertiary levels of prevention, is important when planning strategies for environmental health.

**Primary prevention** involves promoting activities that prevent the actual occurrence of a specific illness or disease. Such activities might include immunization, counselling about reducing exposures, and supporting development of policy and standards related to occupational and environmental health. In addition, educating about healthy lifestyles related to environmental health (e.g., teaching parents about minimizing exposure to lead during home renovations, in selecting consumer products, or promoting hand washing) are also classified as primary prevention interventions. Furthermore, communicating the health risks of extreme weather conditions as well as supporting and practising positive activities, such as maintaining a healthy work–life balance and maintaining psychological health, are also examples of primary prevention strategies that the CHN may use.

**Secondary prevention** involves promoting early detection or screening of environmentally related disease and limiting disability. Secondary-prevention activities include assessing blood lead levels in at-risk young children and adults, conducting urine testing for arsenic in individuals with arsenic content in their water supply, performing audiometric testing for those exposed to high noise levels, and conducting screening spirometry for those workers exposed to respiratory hazards. **Tertiary prevention** involves recovery or rehabilitation of an environmentally related disease or condition after the disease has developed. Tertiary-prevention activities include assisting in distribution of information as well as taking action (treatment, medical management) in the event of an acute environmental health-related incidence. For example, counselling those with noise-induced hearing loss or exposure to asbestos may be the role of the CHN.

## OCCUPATIONAL AND ENVIRONMENTAL LEGISLATION

Provincial ministries of the environment and health legislate policies for air quality, water quality, and health. For example, provincial legislation often regulates air emissions originating in a given province (e.g., the Clean Air Act [2010] in Saskatchewan) and protects provincial air, land, and water resources by regulating and controlling potentially harmful activities and substances (e.g., the Ontario Environmental Protection Act [1989]). Legislating controls for environmental factors (policy development) is a maximal intervention, as it sets and administrates safe levels of exposure. Due to the complexity of environmental factors, numerous provincial and national government agencies have responsibilities with respect to legislation. The examples that follow are legislation and policies that have been developed in relation to occupational and environmental health.

### Health Canada

The Hazardous Products Act [HPA] (1985) applies limits and conditions on the advertising, sale, and importation of hazardous products. In the workplace, the Hazardous Products Act/Controlled Products Regulations outline the requirements for the Workplace Hazardous Materials Information System (WHMIS)—Canada's national hazard communication system. In 2015 the Hazardous Products Regulations were amended to adopt the Globally Harmonized System of Classification and

---

### CANADIAN RESEARCH BOX 27.2

**How do new mothers perceive the environmental health risks to their children?**

Crighton, E., Brown, C., Baxter, J., Lemyre, L., Masuda, J., & Ursitti, F. (2013). Perceptions and experiences of environmental health risks among new mothers: A qualitative study in Ontario, Canada. *Health Risk & Society. 15*(4), 295–312.

In this study, Canadian researchers set out to explore how new mothers perceive and experience environmental health risks to their children. Qualitative, in-depth interviews with individual new mothers and focus groups of new mothers were conducted. Upon analysis, a wide range of concern was noticed ranging from having no environmental concerns to actively incorporating risk prevention measures into daily life. There appeared to be a common perception that risks in the indoor environment were controllable and of little concern. However, risks that occurred outside of the home were viewed as less controllable and more threatening. Active information-seeking was a common coping strategy. Surprisingly, the researchers also observed an optimistic bias in which new mothers perceived that other children were at greater risk despite similar environmental circumstances. The researchers suggest that when designing strategies around risk-reducing behaviours, attention must be paid to the social and environmental contexts of risk and coping.

#### Discussion Questions

1. What opportunities do nurses have to communicate accurate information about environmental health risks to parents? What sort of information would be most useful to parents?

2. How can nurses assist parents in understanding their environmental health risks?

3. How can nurses address this issue in the community at large?

Labelling of Chemicals (GHS). The Food and Drugs Act [FDA] (1985) ensures the safety of food, drugs, cosmetics, and therapeutic devices. The Pest Control Products Act [PCPA] (2002) governs the importation, manufacture, sale, and use of pesticides.

## Environment Canada

The Canadian Environmental Assessment Act [CEAA] (2012) ensures all new projects with federal involvement include an environmental impact assessment, including an assessment of human health impact. The Canadian Environmental Protection Act (CEPA) (1999) governs pollution prevention and protection of the environment and human health. The Fisheries Act (1985) is administered by the Department of Fisheries and Oceans to control pollutants released into fish-bearing bodies of water.

## Provincial Responsibility

**Workplace Exposure Limits** Provincial labour departments and ministries of labour in Canada (with the exception of British Columbia) are responsible for occupational health and safety legislation and for setting occupational standards for exposure. These are often referred to as **occupational exposure limits** (OELs). In British Columbia, both occupational health and safety legislation and workers' compensation falls under the jurisdiction of WorkSafeBC. Certain industries in Canada—such as air transportation, including airports, aerodromes, and airlines; railroads and grain elevators; feed and

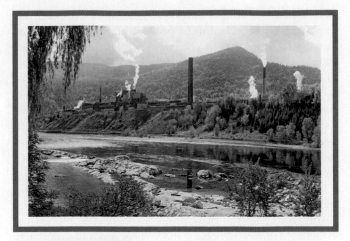

PHOTO   **27.3**   **The smelter overlooks the town of Trail, B.C.**

*Source: Dave Blackey/All Canada Photos/Alamy*

seed mills; banks; and most federal Crown corporations—fall under federal jurisdiction with respect to health and safety legislation. The provinces are responsible for enforcing workplace health and safety legislation and exposure limits for employers within their boundaries who do not fall under federal jurisdiction. Many provincial jurisdictions in Canada rely on the suggested exposure limits published by the American Conference of Governmental Industrial Hygienists (ACGIH) and adopt them as legal OELs (2013).

---

## CASE STUDY

### Community Action on Lead Exposure

The following case study has been adapted from the Canadian Environmental Health Atlas Case Study: Trail, B.C. (http://www.ehatlas.ca/lead/teaching-tools/case-study-trail-bc).

Trail, B.C., is the location of the largest lead-zinc smelter operation in the world. Smelting operations have been conducted there since 1896, so the City of Trail and the surrounding community has a long history of living in the shadow of the smelter (see Photo 27.3). Beginning in 1975, childhood lead poisoning, lead contamination, and other undesirable effects of smelting activities, including the appearance of the smelter operations and the noise and odour they generate, became a cause of concern for the community.

A preliminary study conducted by Neri et al. (1978) reported children in the community aged 12 to 36 months had average blood lead levels of 22mcg/dL. (Canada's current action level is 10mcg/dL.) A study by Hertzman et al. (1991) reported that 40% of children in Trail had blood lead levels above 15 mcg/dL. In 1990 the Trail Community Lead Task Force was established to create a comprehensive childhood lead exposure prevention program. Members of the task force, which included representatives of industry, government, and

the community took several actions to address contamination: they studied exposure pathways, conducted comprehensive education and case-management programs, and monitored blood lead levels in children each year. The task force has five main areas of activity: family health (blood lead testing, education, and support), home and garden (home renovations, garden and yard soil), air quality (emission monitoring, dust control, and air monitoring), parks and wildlands (community greening and ecosystem enhancement), and property development (risk management guidelines and support).

In 1997, the opening of a new state-of-the-art smelter led to a reduction in airborne lead concentrations. Between 1994 and 1999, environmental monitoring data showed that levels of lead in indoor settled dust declined by 50%. At the same time, children's blood lead levels in Trail declined.

The most recent results from the community blood lead monitoring (2012) found that the average blood lead level among children aged 6 to 36 months was 5.4 mcg/dL, a significant reduction from the 1989 levels (Figure 27.6). Still, approximately 3% of children under the age of three in Trail were found to have a blood lead level of 15 mcg/dL or greater, well above Canada's current action guideline of 10 mcg/dL, and considerably higher than the levels of other children in

Canada. Thus, despite success in reducing exposure, some children in Trail are still at risk of lead poisoning.

### Discussion Questions

1. Why might children under age three be more likely to have elevated blood lead levels?

2. Why is childhood exposure to lead a concern?

3. Since the smelter is a major employer in this region, what information do employees need to know about their lead exposures? How can nurses be involved in communicating health information about lead exposures in both children and adults?

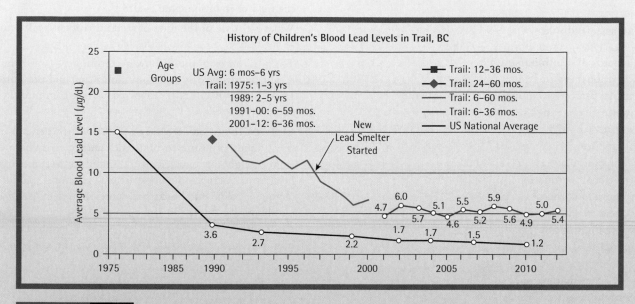

**FIGURE** **27.6** Canadian Environmental Health Atlas

*Source:* Adapted from Trail, BC, in *Canadian environmental health atlas.* Copyright © 2010 by Canadian Environmental Health Atlas. Used by permission of Canadian Environmental Health Atlas. Retrieved from http://www.ehatlas.ca/lead/teaching-tools/case-study-trail-bc

## CONCLUSION

The health of individuals and communities is often closely linked to their environment and to exposures in that environment. Assessing the impact of environmental exposures requires a multidisciplinary approach and a thorough understanding of the factors that influence those exposures and potential health outcomes. Frameworks for categorizing environmental health factors, such as the WHO's DPSEEA framework, are useful for creating a system of factors in a decision-making context. Environmental factors can include chemical, physical, biological, psychological, and ergonomic factors. Typically, personal exposure to such factors occurs through inhalation, absorption, ingestion, or injection. Determining the potential extent of exposure to such factors and possible effects requires careful individual assessment and, where applicable, understanding of dose–response effects and toxicology of the factors in question. Risk assessment, risk management, and risk communication are important tools utilized in environmental health to (a) describe, characterize, and quantify the exposure; (b) intervene as needed for control and prevention; and (c) make the information available to and comprehensible by the general public. Controlling for hazards can occur through engineering, administration (including legislation), and personal protective equipment. Occupational and Environmental Health Nurses play a very important role in preventing

exposures to, and reducing effects from, environmental exposures. As front-line healthcare professionals, nurses may often be the first to encounter those with ill effects from environmental exposures, whether from home, work, or community.

## KEY TERMS

absorption   p. 477
actions   p. 475
acute health effects   p. 479
administrative controls   p. 477
air quality indicators   p. 479
biological factors   p. 477
chemical factors   p. 477
chronic health effects   p. 479
degree of hazard   p. 477
dose–response   p. 478
DPSEEA framework   p. 475
driving forces   p. 475
engineering controls   p. 477
environmental factors   p. 473
environmental health   p. 473
environmental health assessment   p. 478
environmental indicators   p. 479
epidemiology   p. 479
ergonomic factors   p. 477

## STUDY QUESTIONS

1. Using the DPSEEA framework, choose a particular driving force and describe the pressures generated, how these pressures alter the state of environment, what types of hazards may be present, possible routes of exposure, and actions that could improve environmental health issues.

2. What are the five categories of environmental factors? Categorize the environmental influences listed in Figure 27.1 into types of environmental factors.

3. What are the four routes of entry for environmental factors?

4. List the three hazard control strategies for environmental factors in order of preferred use.

5. Describe the three types of information gathered during an individual interview.

6. What are five challenges to environmental health assessments?

7. Describe the three environmental indicators measured by the federal government.

8. Provide examples of primary, secondary, and tertiary prevention in terms of environmental health.

> After working through these questions, go to the MyNursingLab at www.pearsoned.ca/mynursinglab to check your answers.

## INDIVIDUAL CRITICAL-THINKING EXERCISES

1. Name three issues in your local news that relate environment to health. Is there a role for nursing in these issues?

2. What are some of the roles of a community health nurse in the field of environmental health?

3. What are some of the roles of an occupational health nurse in the field of occupational health?

4. Think of an example of how a community health nurse might be involved in risk communication and prevention. How might an OHN be involved in risk communication and prevention?

5. A person living on an acreage presents with general concerns about exposure to pesticides and related chemicals from a neighbouring agricultural (grain) operation. He has been experiencing some unexplained symptoms, including "frequent colds" and headaches, more often than usual. The neighbouring operation has been applying fertilizers and pest-control products by both tractor and aircraft. Describe how you might go about investigating the concern and gathering more information.

## GROUP CRITICAL-THINKING EXERCISES

1. Propose ways of incorporating occupational and environmental health principles into nursing practice, education, research, and policy.

2. Identify policies (including legislation) at the community level (municipal and/or urban level), provincial/territorial level, and national level that have an influence on the health outcomes of clients in your community.

3. Think of an industry in your community. Identify five potential hazards in this industry. For each of the potential hazards, identify at least one control method to reduce or eliminate the hazard.

## REFERENCES

American Conference of Governmental Industrial Hygienists. (2013). *Threshold limit values for chemical substances and physical agents and biological exposure indices.* Cincinnati, OH: ACGIH.

Briggs, D. (1999). *Environmental health indicators: Framework and methodologies for the protection of the human environment occupational and environmental health* (series No. 99.10). Geneva, CH: World Health Organization.

*Canadian Environmental Assessment Act.* (2012). S.C., 2012, c.19, S.52. Retrieved from http://laws-lois.justice.gc.ca/eng/acts/C-15.21/index.html

*Canadian Environmental Protection Act.* (1999). S.C., 1999, c.33. Retrieved from http://laws-lois.justice.gc.ca/eng/acts/c-15.31

Canadian Nurses Association. (2009). *Nursing and environmental health.* Ottawa, ON: Author. Retrieved from http://www.cna-nurses.ca/CNA/issues/environment/default_e.aspx

Canadian Nurses Association. (2013). *Blueprint for the occupational health nursing certification exam.* Ottawa, ON: Author. Retrieved from: http://www.nurseone.ca/docs/NurseOne/Certification/Occupational_Health_Exam_Blueprint_Specialty_Competencies_2013_e.pdf

Centers for Disease Control. (2015). *Climate effects on health.* Retrieved from http://www.cdc.gov/climateandhealth/effects

*Clean Air Act.* (2010). Chapter C-21.1 of the Statutes of Saskatchewan. Retrieved from http://www.qp.gov.sk.ca/documents/English/Statutes/Statutes/C12-1.pdf

Covello, V. T., & Merkhofer, M. W. (1993). *Risk assessment methods: Approaches for assessing health and environmental risks.* New York, NY: Plenum Press.

*Fisheries Act.* (1985). R.S.C., 1985, c. F-14. Retrieved from http://laws-lois.justice.gc.ca/eng/acts/F-14/FullText.html

*Food and Drugs Act.* (1985). R.S.C., 1985, c. F-27. Retrieved from http://laws-lois.justice.gc.ca/eng/acts/f-27

*Hazardous Products Act.* (1985). R.S.C., 1985, c. H-3. Retrieved from http://laws-lois.justice.gc.ca/eng/acts/H-3

Hertzman, C., Ward, H., & Ames, N. (1991). Childhood lead exposure in Trail revisited. *Canadian Journal of Public Health, 82,* 385–391.

Human Resources and Skill Development Canada. (n.d.). *Indicators of well-being–Weekly hours worked.* Retrieved from http://www4.hrsdc.gc.ca/.3ndic.1t.4r@-eng.jsp?iid=19

ILO/WHO Committee on Occupational Health. (1995). *Occupational Health Services and Practice.* Geneva, Switzerland: Author.

International Agency for Research on Cancer. (2013). *Air pollution and cancer.* IARC Scientific Publication no. 161. Geneva, Switzerland: Author.

Lalonde, M. (1981). *A new perspective on the health of Canadians.* Ottawa, ON: Ministry of Supply and Services. Retrieved from http://www.phac-aspc.gc.ca/ph-sp/pdf/perspect-eng.pdf

Neri, L., Johansen, H., & Schmitt, N. (1978). Blood lead levels in children in two British Columbia communities. In D. Hemphill (Ed.), *Trace substances in environmental health – XII.* Proceedings of the University of Missouri's 12th Annual Conference on Trace Substances in Environmental Health, 6–8 June 1978, Columbia, MO: University of Missouri, pp. 403–409.

Nightingale, F. (1859). *Notes on nursing: What it is and what it is not.* London, UK: Harrison.

*Ontario Environmental Protection Act.* (1990). R.S.O., 1990, Chapter E.19, Schedule 7, s.2. Retrieved from: http://www.e-laws.gov.on.ca/html/statutes/english/elaws_statutes_90e19_e.htm

*Pest Control Products Act.* (2002). R.S.C. 1985, c. F-27. Retrieved from http://laws-lois.justice.gc.ca/eng/acts/P-9.01

Prüss-Üstün, A. (2006). In C. Corvalán & World Health Organization (Eds.), *Preventing disease through healthy environments: Towards an estimate of the environmental burden of disease.* Geneva, Switzerland: World Health Organization.

Rogers, B. (1994). *Occupational health nursing: Concepts and practice.* Philadelphia, PA: WB Saunders.

Snow, J. (1860). *On the mode of communication of cholera* (2nd ed.). London, UK: John Churchill.

WorkSafeBC. (2013). *Occupational disease data by type of disease and five-year period; 1988–2012.* Retrieved from http://www.worksafebc.com/publications/reports/statistics_reports/occupational_disease/1988-2012/assets/Table1.pdf

## ABOUT THE AUTHOR

**Janet Morrison**, RN, PhD, M.Ad.Ed., COHN(C), is the Program Head of the Occupational Health Nursing Specialty Program at the B.C. Institute of Technology. Her previous research focused on occupational health and safety issues such as workplace violence and work-related stress. Her recent PhD dissertation research examines the factors that contribute to the successful implementation of complex changes in healthcare using a case study of a successful implementation of a telehealth system in occupational health nursing.

# CHAPTER 28

# Violence in Societies

*Catherine Carter-Snell*

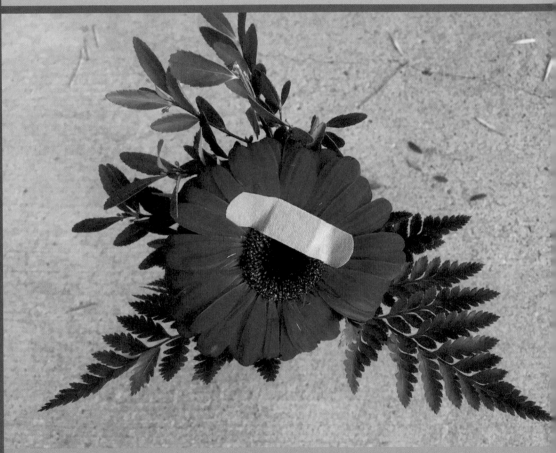

*Source: Courtesy of Catherine Carter-Snell/Mount Royal University*

## INTRODUCTION

Violence has a staggering impact on individuals, families, communities, and society. It is one of the leading causes of death either by suicide or **homicide**, especially for children and young adults. Those who survive violence face significant risk of developing physical or psychological **consequences**, many of which result in increased healthcare visits and chronic illness. These consequences can profoundly impact the individual's family and future generations. The community is therefore impacted, both socially and economically. Violence has been recognized as a public health problem by the World Health Organization (WHO). Community health nurses (CHNs) are in an ideal position to prevent violence as well as to recognize and intervene to limit consequences of existing violence. The focus of this chapter is to develop an understanding of violence in society and the ways in which CHNs can prevent violence or reduce its impact. There are many different types of violence encountered across the lifespan and these are often interrelated. As a result we will explore factors common to most forms of violence, including types of violence, consequences of violence, and theories of violence and violence prevention, with a special focus on interpersonal forms of violence. We will then move into unique considerations with specific forms of violence.

## TYPES OF VIOLENCE

Violence in society appears in many forms. It may be physical or psychological, directed at self or others, and may be initiated by individuals, groups, or whole communities. The consequences of violence are significant for the individual, family, and the community. There are three major groups of violence: self-directed, interpersonal, and collective (Butchart, Phinney, Check, & Villaveces, 2004). **Self-directed violence** includes suicides (attempted or completed) and other forms of self-injury such as cutting behaviour. **Interpersonal violence** is often found in family or relationships and can take the form of child abuse, elder abuse, acquaintance sexual assault, and **intimate partner violence**. Interpersonal violence may also originate from the community by people unrelated to the victim. Examples include physical assaults, bullying and sexting, and stranger sexual assaults. **Collective violence** may be social, political, or economic. Social violence includes acts committed by groups attempting to advance social agendas, such as terrorist organizations or organized groups and mobs. Political violence is seen in the context of military coups, wars, and acts against political groups in power. Economic violence is aimed at disrupting economies or business activities, including blocking access to services.

An individual may experience more than one type of violence at a time, such as physical, emotional, and sexual violence in a relationship. There is also increasing recognition that there are some common risk factors and interrelationships between different types of violence across the lifespan. It is not uncommon to see a victim of child abuse continue on to be a victim of intimate partner violence, and even elder abuse.

## CONSEQUENCES OF VIOLENCE

Violence is a leading cause of death for children and young adults due to either suicide or homicide. **Suicide** is one of the top 10 causes of death for all age groups in Canada, and the second leading cause of death for people between 15 and 34 years of age (Public Health Agency of Canada, 2008; Statistics Canada, 2009). Homicide has been among the top five causes of death for children and young adults for many years, particularly those between 15 and 24 years of age (Public Health Agency of Canada, 2008; Statistics Canada, 2013). Typically, there are 500 to 600 homicides a year in Canada, most often due to shooting, stabbing, or beating. It is important to note that the **perpetrator** in 84% of the solved homicides was someone known to the victim, typically either an acquaintance or a partner (Statistics Canada, 2013).

## Physical Effects on the Individual

The long-term **health effects** of violence are significant for the individual. Healthcare visits are significantly higher for at least three years following intimate partner violence (Bonomi, Anderson, Rivara, & Thompson, 2009), and are also higher after sexual assault (Kapur & Windish, 2011). Abused women have much greater risks than non-abused women of developing both acute and chronic health disorders that may not appear linked to violence (Coker, Hopenhayn, DeSimone, Bush, & Crofford, 2009; Rivara et al., 2007; Sadler, Booth, Mengeling, & Doebbeling, 2004). Acute conditions include not only **injuries** from the assault but other complaints such as somatic pain (pain with no detectable source), contusions or abrasions, or urinary tract infections. Chronic conditions include autoimmune disorders, gastroesophageal reflux, heart disease, headaches, and cancers. Similarly, children who have had adverse experiences such as abuse or neglect are more likely to develop chronic health issues as adults (Chartier, Walker, & Naimark, 2010). Children may also develop somatic pain. The wide range of possible long-term effects often means that health professionals and victims do not link their current health issue to prior violence. Clients may be inappropriately labelled as "frequent flyers," "drug seekers," or "hypochondriacs" without recognition that there are deeper issues. They may be treated or referred for services to remove the consequence (e.g., alcoholism) rather than referrals to treat the root cause, such as how to cope with their abuse history and stress. Their physical disorders are often stress related and are real, even in the case of somatic pain. Females with multiple visits are more likely to have assault and abuse histories, while males with repeat visits most often have histories of physical assault (Kwan, Cureton, Dozier, & Victorino, 2010). Even those who commit violent acts have been found to have increased health risks over time (Stogner, Gibson, & Miller, 2014).

## Psychological Effects on the Individual

Mental health disorders are common after any form of interpersonal violence, particularly with intimate partner violence or sexual assault (Carter-Snell & Jakubec, 2013). Both men and women are at risk of developing **psychological consequences** from interpersonal violence (Iverson et al., 2013). Common psychological reactions to trauma include **post-traumatic stress disorder (PTSD)**, depression, anxiety, substance abuse, eating disorders, risks for re-victimization, and suicide. PTSD is a reaction to a significant event that results in fear or horror and the development of symptoms affecting their daily lives, which persist or begin at least a month after the trauma. Unfortunately, PTSD is one of the most common mental health consequences of violence and brings with it many other consequences. Approximately 40 to 60% of women develop PTSD after sexual assault, compared to rates of 10 to 15% among armed forces personnel or disaster workers (Carter-Snell & Hegadoren, 2003). PTSD symptoms are debilitating and life changing. Adults or children over six years of age with PTSD typically have one or

| Table 28.1 | Symptom Clusters of PTSD |
|---|---|
| **Symptom Cluster** | **Examples** |
| Arousal and reactivity | Exaggerated startle reflex, increased heart rate or blood pressure, anxiety, hypervigilance, difficulty sleeping or concentrating, high risk of aggressive behaviours |
| Negative alterations in affect or mood | Dissociative amnesia, persistent negative beliefs about self-blame or blaming others, seeing world as unsafe, negative emotions (e.g., anger, guilt, shame, fear), feeling alienated from others, difficulty experiencing positive emotions |
| Intrusion | Unwanted and intrusive memories, nightmares, dissociation reactions (e.g., depersonalization, derealization), or flashbacks |
| Avoidance | Avoid reminders of the trauma (e.g., previously enjoyed places, people, activities) or thinking about the trauma |

more symptoms from each of four symptom clusters shown in Table 28.1 (American Psychiatric Association, 2013).

Those who develop PTSD also commonly develop other disorders such as depression and substance abuse at the same time. For instance, at least one-half of sexually assaulted women with PTSD also develop comorbid depression (Pinna, Johnson, & Delahanty, 2013; Taft, Resick, Watkins, & Panuzio, 2009). Women experiencing intimate partner violence have significantly increased risks of developing substance abuse, depression or anxiety, family or social problems, and sexually transmitted infections (Bonomi et al., 2009). Experiencing childhood abuse has been found to be an independent predictor of homelessness and poor physical health (Montgomery, Cutuli, Evans-Chase, Treglia, & Culhane, 2013), with PTSD symptoms and associated disorders often contributing to these consequences.

**Adverse childhood experiences** have also been linked to an increased risk of developing mental illness in adulthood (Greeson et al., 2014; Larkin, Shields, & Anda, 2012) as well as physical health problems (Brown et al., 2009). Children who witness family violence have higher rates of mental health issues including PTSD, traumatic symptoms, and both internalizing and externalizing behaviours (Roustit et al., 2009). Internalizing behaviours may include shyness, depression, anxiety, eating disorders, somatic complaints, or becoming withdrawn. Externalizing behaviours are those in which the child acts out, such as being aggressive, bullying, delinquency from school, or other forms of misconduct. Children who witness intimate partner violence are considered to be victims of emotional child abuse in the Canadian Criminal Code (Sinha, 2012). This means that if a CHN suspects that a child was present when a parent was assaulted then it must be reported to the appropriate child authorities. This may lead to difficult

situations, as intimate partner violence against the parent cannot be reported to police without the assaulted parent's **consent**, but the emotional child abuse must be reported. Children's service agencies and reporting service staff are very helpful in working through dilemmas such as this.

## Effects of Violence on the Family

The effects of violence are also significant for the **family** of the victim. Spouses of sexually assaulted women report a number of negative consequences that affect their relationship to the victims (Connop & Petrak, 2004). Spouses reported difficulty communicating with the victims and experiencing feelings of sadness, anger, and shock. The men also described difficulties with their sexual relationships. Symptoms of PTSD were experienced by at least one-quarter of male partners of assault victims (Christiansen, Bak, & Elklit, 2012). Family or significant others also experienced difficulties providing support to victims. This is a problem, since provision of support from family and friends has been shown to be a valuable part of resilience to the effects of trauma (Ahrens, Cabral, & Abeling, 2009; Carter-Snell & Jakubec, 2013; Ullman & Filipas, 2001a; Ullman & Filipas, 2001b). It may be necessary for the CHN to provide support or to facilitate referrals for support for the family as well as for the client.

Families of victims of abuse may experience **intergenerational transmission** of violence; children who have experienced abuse may become either victims of adult abuse or perpetrators of abuse, compared to non-abused children (Cannon, Bonomi, Anderson, & Rivara, 2009; Manchikanti Gómez, 2011; Smith, Varcoe, & Edwards, 2005). Aboriginal people have often sustained multiple forms of abuse (Andersson & Nahwegahbow, 2010), and the consequences may place their children at risk of abuse as well. Aboriginal families are investigated far more than non-Aboriginal families for child abuse, with multiple points of concern identified for risks to children, including poverty, substance abuse, intimate partner violence, and limited social support (Sinha, Trocme, Fallon, & Maclaurin, 2013). The risk of continued victimization or abuse in future generations is sometimes termed a "legacy of abuse" (Martsolf & Draucker, 2008). It should be emphasized, however, that it is not inevitable for children to abuse or be abused, provided that children and families are provided appropriate support and deficits in the social determinants of health are addressed (Brown et al., 2012), combined with an understanding of the effects of trauma on the family. These will be addressed further in the child abuse section of this chapter.

## Effects of Violence on Society

The economic and societal consequences of the effects of violence are also profound. It is estimated that in 2009 the Canadian government spent $7.4 billion to address the effects of intimate partner violence, $6 billion of which was directly related to healthcare costs and shelters (Zhang, Hoddenbaugh, McDonald, & Scrim, 2012). Another Canadian study extrapolated the costs for caring for women between 19 and 65 years of age who left abusive partners to be $6.9 billion annually, and $3.1 billion for those who left in the last three years (Varcoe et al., 2011). Costs for sexual assault were estimated at $1.9 billion per year (McInturff, 2013). These estimates are mainly related to direct costs of healthcare and services, although some costs are factored in for loss of work to employers and justice costs. What are not typically considered are the costs of the related consequences, such as treatment of addiction or other mental health issues, and the frequent healthcare visits for seemingly unrelated issues. Clearly, there is a significant need for prevention of violence for the health of individuals, their families, their social relationships, and for the health of the community. The impact of prevention for society and costs to the health system are also significant. Prevention of violence was declared a worldwide public health priority in 2002 with the release of the landmark "World Report on Violence and Health" (Krug, Dahlberg, Mercy, Zwi, & Lozano, 2002). The CHN is in a key position to influence violence-prevention and health-promotion initiatives, including developing healthy relationships, addressing determinants of health that impact risk, recognizing violence or risks, collaborating in prevention programs, and facilitating effective intervention for violence. An understanding of theories of violence and risks for violence assists these efforts.

## THEORIES OF VIOLENCE

Theories to explain risks for violence in the past used to follow disciplinary lines. For instance, sociological models focused on how individuals and family or society interacted, with violence resulting from conflicts or discrepancies in social interaction, and factors such as socialization to violence, learned behaviours, and poor social controls or social disorganization (Blume, 1996). Psychological theories focused on altered mental processes or functions such as neurobiology and temperament or the result of a damaged psyche (King, 2012). Political theories of violence relate to the distribution of resources due to political structures, control of people, or resources (Frazer & Hutchings, 2008). It is now recognized that none of these theories on their own is sufficient to explain violence (Hamby, 2011; Hass & Cusson, 2015). For instance, social learning theory would suggest that after witnessing or experiencing child abuse, all abused children would become violent. Although risks are higher to become abusers, the majority of children who have been abused do not abuse (Benz, 2010; Iverson, Jiminez, Harrington, & Resick, 2011) and some perpetrators have never been abused (Iverson et al., 2011). Similarly, psychological theories such as poor anger management do not explain why an abuser can selectively direct anger at his or her intimate partner but not at their employers or coworkers (Klein, Campbell, Soler, & Ghez, 1997).

It is now recognized that we need more complex, multi-dimensional theories to help explain various forms of violence. An example of a complex theory that emerged from a sociological perspective is **intersectionality**. Intersectionality looks particularly at oppression and social structures supporting oppression or discrimination as ways to understand violence by gender, sexuality, class, and race (MacDowell, 2013; Meyer, 2012). This theory deals with how various biological, social, and cultural categories interact to contribute to patterns of oppression that result in systematic injustice and social inequality. Many forms of violence have been linked to power differentials, particularly in gender-based violence such as intimate partner violence, sexual assault, honour killings, sexual trafficking, and femicide (Walby, 2013). It is argued that even this more complex theory is insufficient to explain violence as it is too dichotomous—assuming all victims are disempowered and perpetrators are empowered (Brenner, 2013). Brenner asserts that this position does not allow for other risk factors, contexts, or responses by either party to be considered and that this perspective may further disempower the victim (2013). It would also not describe intimate partner violence situations in which both parties are violent toward each other.

The WHO has developed another complex theory called the "social ecological" or **socioecological** model of violence prevention. This model was first introduced in the WHO's "World Report on Violence and Health" (Krug et al., 2002) and has subsequently been adopted by a number of key organizations working to prevent violence, including the Centers for Disease Control (2009). The model integrates **social determinants of health**, key feminist concepts and theories such as intersectionality, along with concepts from other theories of violence. It has been developed using the public health model of prevention. The socioecological model consists of four major groups or levels of influences that can affect risks for violence (Figure 28.1):

- *individual* factors are the biological, genetic, or personal factors that place one at risk;
- *relationship* factors are those from family, significant others, or peers that influence attitudes or behaviours;
- *community* factors include attitudes, beliefs in organizations, or communities that support or tolerate violence or inequality; and
- *societal* influences include cultural norms, societal values, or policies allowing violence or condoning inequality, such as income distribution or social exclusion of individuals or groups.

The four influences on violence overlap and interact with each other in varying degrees; although some argue that the individual and relationship influences are the most important predictors for violence (Meadows, 2010). An understanding of these four levels of influence on violence assists the CHN in both prevention and early detection of violence as will be discussed later. The WHO emphasizes the need for prevention activities at all four levels of influence and in multiple venues

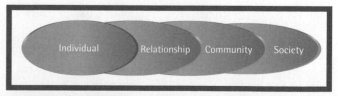

**FIGURE 28.1** Ecological Model of Influences on Violence

*Source:* World Health Report On Violence And Health: Summary. Copyright © 2002 by World Health Organization. Used by Reprinted with permission from World Health Organization.

in order for prevention to be effective. There is a wide range of possible influences for each individual at every level, both within and between categories of influences. This variation and interaction illustrates why it would be possible for one person to resort to violence but another might not, despite similar individual influences. Some influences are protective factors against violence while others are risk factors, further affecting violence risk for violence perpetration or victimization.

## VIOLENCE PERPETRATION

Violence is considered highly predictable based on the presence of a number of key risk or contributing factors, most of which are social determinants of health (WHO, 2004). Some

| Table 28.2 | Risks for Violence Perpetration | |
|---|---|---|
| **Aspect** | **Social Determinants** | **Risk** |
| Individual | Gender | Male |
| | Race/Culture | Minorities, Aboriginal Canadians |
| | Education | |
| | Disability | Limited education, learning disorders |
| | | Poor mental health, substance abuse |
| Relationship/ Family | Early childhood development | Witnessing parental violence |
| | Housing | Experiencing abuse/ aggressive parents |
| | Food insecurity | |
| | | Family attitudes supporting violence |
| | | Low socioeconomic status |
| | | Multiple partners, infidelity |
| Community | Social safety network | Violent peers, peers with weapons |
| | Health services | Community poverty |
| | Unemployment/ job security | High-crime neighbourhoods |
| | | Difficulty accessing social services |
| Society | Income distribution | Income gap/disparity |
| | Social exclusion | Gender norms supporting inequality |
| | | Poor sanctions against violence |
| | | Limited control of weapons, alcohol |
| | | Rapid social change, conflict, disaster |

of the key social determinants that impact a risk for violence are summarized in Table 28.2 (Mikkonen & Raphael, 2010; WHO, 2014a). Other risk factors linked to increases in violence cited by the WHO (2014a) include access to firearms and excessive alcohol use. Various combinations of these factors create an environment that contributes to risks for violence or sustains violence.

Note that deficits in almost all of the social determinants of health are reflected in these risks for violence (Mikkonen & Raphael, 2010). In particular, the determinants of age, gender, Aboriginal status, race, early childhood, education, social isolation, income disparity, and social support networks are most commonly cited risk factors. A few of these factors warrant further exploration in light of the four levels of influence in the socioecological model.

## Individual Influences

Three of the key individual influences for perpetration are age, sex, and substance use (Carnochan, Butchart, Feucht, Mikton, & Shepherd, 2010; WHO, 2010). Adolescents and young adults are at the greatest risk for involvement in violent behaviour. Violent behaviour increases through adolescence, then decreases after reaching adulthood (Stoddard, Zimmerman, & Bauermeister, 2012). Age by itself does not explain risks, however, as there is usually an interaction with other factors, such as age and gender, or age with relationships.

Males are more likely to be involved in violent behaviour than women, although females can be violent offenders (Rossegger et al., 2009). Currently, 95% of the prison population is male (Mikkonen & Raphael, 2010). Gender differences are also seen in specific types of interpersonal violence. In dating relationships, women have higher rates of inflicting emotional abuse or physical abuse such as pushing, hitting, or kicking than men. Males are more likely to perpetrate more serious physical partner abuse (Hickman, Jaycox, & Aronoff, 2004), more often resulting in greater levels of severity and injury on women (Brennan, 2011), while women's partner violence is more often in response to men's violence (Allen, Swan, & Raghaven, 2009). Approximately 80% of sexual assault perpetrators are male (Brennan & Taylor-Butts, 2008).

Aboriginal Canadians (male and female) are overrepresented in the Canadian prison system (Office of the Correctional Investigator, 2013). There are links between minorities, racism, and violence risks (Walcott, Foster, Campbell, & Sealy, 2010). Aboriginal people have been subjected to colonization, to residential schools separating them from family and subjecting them to abuse, and to experiencing systematic racial, cultural, or social disadvantages (Andersson & Nahwegahbow, 2010; Office of the Correctional Investigator, 2013; Smith et al., 2005). The resulting mental health problems, including substance abuse, subsequently become risks for perpetration of violence as well as risks for victimization (Brown et al., 2012).

**Alcohol** use by perpetrators has been linked to increased incidents of sexual assault, intimate partner violence, and other forms of violence (Abbey, Clinton-Sherrod, McAuslan,

Zawacki, & Buck, 2003; Connor, You, & Casswell, 2009; Graham, Bernards, Wilsnack, & Gmel, 2011; McCarroll, Fan, & Bell, 2009; Navarro, Shakeshaft, Doran, & Petrie, 2013; WHO, 2014a), as well as to increased severity of the incidents (Abbey et al., 2003; Graham-Kevan, 2009). Restriction of alcohol and drug use access has been linked to reduced incidents of violence (Cunradi, Mair, Ponicki, & Remer, 2012; Livingston, 2011; Navarro et al., 2013; Schofield & Denson, 2013). Methods included closing bars earlier in the evening or reducing the density of liquor outlets in a community. These findings have implications both for community development as well as for social policy and violence prevention. There is a role for CHNs through involvement in policy and community development initiatives. There is also a reciprocal relationship noted between alcohol and violence—although alcohol use may increase violent behaviour and victimization, experiencing violence may also lead to alcohol use (Browning & Erikson, 2009).

**Mental illness** is often assumed to be a major risk factor for perpetrating violence. In fact, the strongest predictor of violence risk is not having a mental illness but having a history of prior violence (Walters & Crawford, 2013). A U.S. study indicated that less than 5% of crimes are committed by people with mental illness (Applebaum, 2006). Similarly, in Canada, less than 5% of those in correctional services for offences have been found to have mental illness other than substance abuse, or require mental health services (Arboleda-Florez, 2009). A review of the studies on gun violence further demonstrated that only a minority of those with mental illness commit violent acts, and if so, it is typically in combination with alcohol or drug use (Metzl & MacLeish, 2015) or other factors contributing to violence (Canadian Mental Health Association, 2011). The majority of those who are violent are not mentally ill, and the majority of those with mental illness are not violent (Friedman, 2006). Those with mental illness are more likely to be victims than perpetrators of violence. The community often has misconceptions about the risk of violence among those with mental illness. The CHN can help disseminate information about the vulnerability of those with mental illness, and work with communities to reduce stereotypes and decrease the vulnerability of those with mental illness.

## Relationship Influences

Relationships with family and friends also affect risks of violence. Clear links have been established between those who experienced adverse childhood events (ACEs) and health issues as adults (Anda, Tietjen, Schulman, Felitti, & Croft, 2010). The number of ACEs is also linked to risks for committing violent acts (Duke, Pettingell, McMorris, & Borowsky, 2010). Males convicted for assaults and abuse had four times as many ACEs compared to controls (Larkin et al., 2012). Peer relationships can also increase risks of violence, particularly if associating with delinquent peers (Bernat, Oakes, Pettingell, & Resnick, 2012; Henry, Tolan, Gorman-Smith, & Schoeny, 2012) or if peers use weapons (Stoddard et al., 2013). Canadian Research Box 28.1 discusses how ACE might be linked to adult homelessness.

---

### CANADIAN RESEARCH BOX 28.1

**Is there a link between childhood adversity and homelessness?**

Patterson, M. L., Moniruzzaman, A., & Somers, J. M. (2014). Setting the stage for chronic health problems: Cumulative childhood adversity among homeless adults with mental illness in Vancouver, British Columbia. *BMC Public Health, 14,* 350. Epublication April 12, 2014. Retrieved from http://biomedcentral.com/1471-2458/14/350

A study was conducted in Vancouver, British Columbia, with homeless or precariously housed adults with mental illness. The 497 participants were recruited from shelters across the city, as well as from hospitals and other health centres. Participants were given a series of questionnaires to assess their socioeconomic and demographic characteristics, mental health, substance abuse, physical health, quality of life, and the types of services they used. A follow-up interview was conducted 18 months later with 413 participants who returned and received an Adverse Childhood Experiences (ACE) questionnaire with questions about 17 adverse events. Of the participants, 12% did not disclose any ACE events but the remainder had one or more events. Almost half (42%) had five or more ACEs. Household dysfunction was reported by 79%, 65% reported experiencing abuse, and 53% experienced neglect. Analyses showed that those with higher ACE scores were significantly more likely to have incomplete schooling, had children before age 18, and be of Aboriginal ethnicity. The higher scores were also associated with more negative health consequences such as poor health, more infections, more mental health disorders such as post-traumatic stress disorder, depression, and substance use. Both direct and indirect effects were suggested, linking ACEs to homelessness.

#### Discussion Questions

1. How can a community health nurse promote resilience to the effects of ACEs?
2. What strategies could the community health nurse use to reduce the level of household dysfunction?
3. What social changes might help reduce ACEs?

---

## Community Influences

Inequities in access to social safety nets such as income assistance, disability pension, housing, health services, employment, or other social determinants of health can influence risks for violence at multiple levels. Disadvantaged neighbourhoods are those characterized by high levels of economic disadvantage or disparity, low levels of social networks able to establish norms and values (collective efficacy), and transient residents. The rates of violence in disadvantaged Toronto neighbourhoods were higher than non-disadvantaged neighbourhoods, especially if co-occurring with alcohol use (Browning & Erickson, 2009). The influence of the support or collective efficacy of family, schools, and neighbourhood was variable. The effect of neighbourhood disadvantages may also vary by gender—girls living in disadvantaged neighbourhoods were more likely to perpetrate dating violence, while neighbourhood had little influence on male perpetrators (Chang, Foshee, Reyes, Ennett, & Halpern, 2015). In disadvantaged neighbourhoods, violence is used as a means with which to gain respect (Stewart & Simons, 2010).

## Societal Influences

Inequalities in income, power, and resources are key sources of risks for violence perpetration (Owen, Thompson, Shaffer, Jackson, & Kaslow, 2009). These concepts cross all types of violence. We saw that intersectionality focused on imbalances in power between the victim and perpetrator. Inequities in finances, resources, or social determinants of health each create imbalances in power, which in turn is linked to risks for violence or victimization (see Canadian Research box 28.2). Countries and communities with large inequities in income have higher violence rates, including higher homicide rates (Briceno-Leon, Villaveces, & Concha-Eastman, 2008). Social norms contribute to a culture in which violence is acceptable or normalized. An example is the hypersexualized chants and freshmen activities at some Canadian universities (President's Council, 2013). The likelihood that a victim will seek assistance after violence is also affected by social norms and normalization of violence (Amar, Sutherland, Laughon, Bess, & Stockbridge, 2012). A study of 100 junior high aged girls in eastern Canada revealed that they would be unlikely to report sexual violence due to fear of being blamed by others (Hlvala, 2014).

War and political conflict are also socially constructed forms of violence. Differences in political power, policies, access to resources, or disenfranchising of specific groups often result in violent conflict. These also shape social and cultural norms in how others are viewed, which can persist for generations. Violence against entire cultures or religions has been seen as acceptable in many wars across history. Thousands have been raped, mutilated, or killed in mass acts of violence and genocide, such as the Holocaust and the massacres in Rwanda and the Congo (Staub, 2012).

# VICTIMIZATION AND VULNERABLE POPULATIONS

Everyone is at risk of experiencing violence in some form in their lives. There are, however, some who are more vulnerable than others. This vulnerability relates to the social determinants of health, as does violence. Those who have fewer individual resources, more limited relationship support, greater inequities in resources, and fewer societal protections are most vulnerable. Unfortunately, once someone is victimized they are often re-victimized. Another "at-risk" group is those who have previously been victimized. It has been estimated that between 15 and 72% of victims of child sexual abuse and adolescent or adult sexual assault will be assaulted again (Gagne, Lavoie, & Hebert, 2005; Maier, 2008; Mason, Riger, & Foley,

---

### CANADIAN RESEARCH BOX 28.2

**What are the key dimensions of equity-oriented services to guide PHC organizations, and what strategies for operationalizing equity-oriented PHC services could work, particularly for marginalized populations?**

Brown, A. J., Varcoe, C. M., Wong, S. T., Smye, V. L., Lavoie, J., Littlejohn, D., . . . Lennox, S. (2012). Closing the health equity gap: Evidence-based strategies for primary health care organizations. *International Journal for Equity in Health, 11*(1), 59–73.

Throughout this chapter, the role of inequities in resources and supports in increasing risks of violence has been demonstrated. This study was conducted, titled "Closing the health equity gap: Evidence-based strategies for primary healthcare organizations," in which the researchers examined two public healthcare centres in Canada that serve marginalized people, seeking to determine the key dimensions of services that guide "equity-oriented" services and how to put these into operation. An ethnographic approach was used, which included in-depth interviews with patients (73) and staff (41), participant observation (900 hours), and analysis of documents from the organization related to policy and funding. They discovered four key dimensions of equity-oriented services:

- inequity responsive care—incorporation of social determinants of health in routine care;
- trauma and violence-informed care—recognizing that people have experienced systemic and structural inequities and working to empower them through understanding the trauma rather than focusing on trauma treatment;
- contextually tailored care—arranging for services that are unique and appropriate to the population's issues; and
- culturally competent care—considering the cultural meaning of health, and people's experiences of discrimination and how these have shaped their lives.

### Discussion Questions

1. Provide an example of one service that you think could be incorporated into local schools that would help to address context for sexual minority youth at risk for partner violence.

2. Describe the difference and potential impact between trauma-informed approach to services and trauma treatment.

---

2004; Schewe, Riger, Howard, Staggs, & Mason, 2006). There are a number of reasons for this, some of which relate to negative reactions to disclosure with the initial assault, development of mental illness as a result, and substance abuse. A systematic review of risk factors for re-victimization included the following factors: (a) experiencing sexual assault as a child, especially if there were multiple episodes of abuse; (b) severe assaults; (c) greater levels of shame and blame; (d) difficulty in interpersonal relationships; and (e) more recent assaults (Classen, Palesh, & Aggarwal, 2005). Perpetrators seek vulnerable individuals (rather than vice versa). Understanding of vulnerable populations and early intervention are important to break this cycle.

Key **vulnerable** populations discussed here include youth, women, sexual minorities, and those with disabilities. It should be noted that use of the words "victim" and "survivor," while included in this discussion, should be used carefully in practice. Clients may feel stigmatized or labelled and have anecdotally commented that even the use of the term "survivor" makes them feel that violence is defining them.

## Youth

Youth and young adults between 15 and 24 years of age are most often victims of violence in Canada, with 15 times the risk compared to adults over 65 years (Perreault & Brennan, 2010). One of the few General Social Surveys in Canada that focused on sexual assault identified that over 58% of sexual assault victims are under 18 years of age, despite the fact that this age group only accounts for 22% of the Canadian population (Kong, Johnson, Beattie, & Cardillo, 2003). The male victims were more often very young (approximately 29% less than 12 years of age). Self-inflicted deaths are one of the few forms of violence that affect middle adults more often than youth. Males between 40 to 49 years of age accounted for 45% of suicide deaths in 2009, followed by 35% among those between 15 and 39 years (Navaneelan, 2012).

## Women and Gender-Based Violence

Females of any age are at particular risk for violence and the majority of this gender-based violence occurs in the home (Standish, 2013). Standish describes gender-based violence as rooted in culture, kinship, religion, and nationalism, and notes that major community and societal changes would be required to stop it. One of the key forms of violence against women is sexual assault. The vast majority of sexual assaults (70%) reported in the Canadian General Social Survey in 2009 were female (Perreault & Brennan, 2010). Violent victimization was higher in almost all provinces and territories (Vaillancourt, 2010). Only 10% of sexual assaults are reported to police, although approximately 30% of those assaulted will seek healthcare (Johnson, 2006). Women are also at risk during intimate partner violence, in which they are three times more likely to be injured, five times more likely to be hospitalized, and three times more likely to need time off afterward than men (Federal Provincial Territorial Ministers, 2002). Females are also more likely to die from intimate partner violence than men (Vaillancourt, 2010), most often from stabbing (Brennan, 2011).

Aboriginal Canadian women face rates of violence significantly higher than those of non-Aboriginal Canadian women (Dylan, Regehr, & Alaggia, 2008; Lamontagne, 2011; Native Women's Association of Canada, 2007a). Violence within intimate partner relationships was more than twice as high for Aboriginal versus non-Aboriginal women, and almost three times greater outside relationships (Brennan, 2011). At least 17% of victims of homicide are Aboriginal Canadians despite only accounting for 3% of the Canadian population

(Brzozowski, Taylor-Butts, & Johnson, 2006). When compared to non-Aboriginal women's homicides, Aboriginal women were more often killed by casual acquaintances (30% versus 19%) and less often by partners (29% versus 41%) (Royal Canadian Mounted Police [RCMP], 2014). There have been almost 1200 missing and murdered Aboriginal women in Canada since 1980 (RCMP, 2014), and approximately 44% of these occurred in British Columbia and Alberta (Native Women's Association of Canada, n.d.). It is argued that social indifference to the plight of women places them at greater risk of violence (Native Women's Association of Canada, 2007b). The social determinants of health are also key issues in the vulnerability of Aboriginal women to violence. It is well recognized that Aboriginal women have extremely low socioeconomic status, fewer employment options, weaker community structures, more substance abuse, fewer housing options, and more barriers to education than other Canadians (Native Women's Association of Canada, 2007b). Added to these risks are the effects of adverse childhood experiences and intergenerational impact of traumas such as residential schools on the individuals and family (Bombay, Matheson, & Anisman, 2009; Smith et al., 2005).

Conflict and disasters increase the risk for women and children further. Rates of physical and sexual violence have been shown to increase against women after natural disasters such as hurricanes (Anastario, Shehab, & Lawry, 2009), earthquakes (Kolbe et al., 2010) and tsunamis (Pittaway, Bartolomei, & Rees, 2007). In conflict zones, women and female children are often victims of sexual assault, abuse, forced prostitution, forced marriage, and genital mutilation (WHO, 2005).

Women from other cultures may have faced violence in conflict or disaster coming to Canada and may face risks of violence when they arrive. Data on immigrant women, however, have shown that Canadian-born women face higher rates of intimate partner violence than those not born in Canada, unless the immigrant women become sexually active (Silverman, Decker, & Raj, 2007). Their risk may be underestimated, however, as immigrant women often face barriers to accessing or using support services (Guruge & Humphreys, 2009), and thus may not be detected. The danger is increased, however, if their cultural community has beliefs and attitudes that bestow more power and decision making on men and if women do not comply with these beliefs. The term "honour killing" has become sadly more familiar. These are killings of women due to behaviour that is deemed unacceptable (Standish, 2013). Women in the cultures involved in honour killings are seen as property and the killings are, therefore, seen as acceptable and a "private matter." Another culturally sanctioned form of homicide against women is dowry murders; brides are burned to death if the dowry demands of the groom's family are not met (Kumar & Kanth, 2007; Hague & Sardinha, 2010). These killings may be seen in Indian Hindu populations, but have expanded to Christian and Muslim communities as well (Jutla & Heimback, 2004). The basis of these homicides is a deeply rooted belief in the inequality of women, supported by cultural, community, and religious groups.

Canada has vast areas of rural and remote populations. Women in rural and remote areas face greater risks associated with sexual assault and intimate partner violence due to this isolation (Averill, Padilla, & Clements, 2007; Lamont, 2006). Challenges include lack of transportation, difficulties with telecommunication (e.g., poor cellphone service), lack of anonymity in the community, and ready access by abusers to firearms. A review of national U.S. data suggests that separated women face more risks of violence from their ex-partner in rural versus urban communities. Studies have shown that rural women receive reduced levels of services, including healthcare, policing, and counselling, after sexual assault (Lamont, 2006) often due to access, limited resources, and lack of familiarity with protocols. These professionals, however, have expressed a commitment to victims and a desire for further education and strategies to improve services (Jakubec, Carter-Snell, Ofrim, & Skanderup, 2013).

## Sexual Minorities

Rates of violent victimization were higher among Canadians who reported being homosexual (Perreault & Brennan, 2010). Those identifying with sexual minorities of any type are at higher risk for violence in many forms. Over 60% of school students in British Columbia who identified as sexual minorities experienced verbal abuse compared to 29% of heterosexual students (Saewyc et al., 2007). A large Canadian study found that abuse of sexual minority youth was prevalent in all Canadian provinces and that verbal homophobic abuse often preceded physical abuse (Peter, Taylor, & Chamberland, 2015). A comparison of college students who identified as a sexual minority and heterosexual college students in an American university over six months showed that sexual minority students had higher rates of physical intimate partner violence (30% versus 18%) especially if they were female, or experienced more sexual assaults (24% versus 11%), and unwanted pursuits (53% versus 36%) (Edwards et al., 2015).

## People with Disabilities

Those with mental illness or other disabilities are also more vulnerable to victimization. The rates of pre-existing mental health issues among women who were sexually assaulted was significantly high among a large sample of women seeking services after recent sexual assault in Ontario. At least 33% of the women had mental health problems, most often depression or anxiety disorders, followed by bipolar spectrum disorder, suicidal ideation, or substance-abuse problems. These disorders are thought to pose risk factors for the assault. It is also possible that these disorders stemmed from prior assaults and the current visit was from re-victimization. Presence of a physical or mental disability places children at higher risks of physical abuse (Svensson, Bornehag, & Janson, 2011) and sexual abuse (Balogh et al., 2001). Issues of power and vulnerability, as well as increased stress on the family, are potential factors in physical and sexual abuse.

# Perpetration, Victimization, and Intergenerational Violence

There is considerable overlap between risks for becoming a perpetrator and for becoming a victim of violence. Previously, various forms of violence (e.g., child abuse, sexual assault, intimate partner violence) were considered separately. It is argued that we need to stop looking at each form of interpersonal violence separately and begin to understand that all violence is linked, involving the "exercise of power, intimidation, or force that result in hurt, fear or injury" (Tutty et al., 2005, p. 13). The victim of one form of violence may become a victim of another form of violence and/or a perpetrator (Wilkins, Tsao, Hertz, Davis, & Klevens, 2014). For instance, a child who witnesses intimate partner violence at home is more likely to become a victim of bullying or intimate partner violence himself or herself later in life (Duke et al., 2010; Graham-Bermann, Castor, Miller, & Howell, 2012). On the other hand, childhood victims are also more likely than non-victimized children to become bulliers (Espelage et al., 2014), bullies are more likely to abuse their partners (Falb et al., 2011), and partner abusers are more likely to abuse their own children (Duffy, Hughes, Asnes, & Leventhal, 2014). This interrelationship highlights the need for CHNs to use a **trauma-informed perspective** in providing care (Substance Abuse and Mental Health Services Administration [SAMSHA], 2011). While trauma-informed treatment is provision of care based on anticipated consequences, a trauma-informed approach to services, however, requires not only that providers understand the impact of the trauma for the individuals, family, and community, but that there is support from the organization and related services. Examples include a setting conducive to services for traumatized individuals, timing and types of services, and collaborative practice. The behaviours that bring people to seek healthcare or bring the matter to the attention of the justice system are often only symptoms or consequences of underlying histories of violence and trauma. A trauma-informed approach helps to identify those at risk or who are experiencing violence.

# Assessing Victims

There are a number of behavioural and physical responses to trauma that may be seen. Each individual is unique as are the circumstances. An understanding of the range of responses will help the CHN to recognize potential victims of violence and to respond in a positive manner.

**Victim Reactions to Trauma** Indicators of trauma may differ across the developmental stages. Acute stress reactions are normal after experiencing violence or trauma. The neurobiologic response to **stress** involves the locus ceruleus, limbic system (amygdala and hippocampus), the hypothalamic–pituitary–adrenal axis (HPA axis) and the sympathetic nervous system (Charmandari, Tsigos, & Chrousos, 2005; Olson et al., 2011). Stress creates a cascade of reactions that result in the release of norepinephrine, epinephrine, cortisol, and aldosterone to help the body respond. The reactions seen include "fight or flight," which are typically described in the General Adaptation Syndrome (Selye, 1976). There is also a third response known as "freeze," or **tonic immobility**" in which the person cannot move (Bracha, 2004). Tonic immobility is a state of inhibited motor responses resulting in paralysis or "freezing" and an inability to resist (Abrams, Carleton, Taylor, & Asmundson, 2009). This freeze response is more common than previously realized in many forms of assault. Estimates of freeze responses after sexual assault range from 10 to 50% among women (Campbell, 2012) to as high as 89% after sexual assault, particularly if the victims experienced humiliation (Moor, Ben-Meir, Golan-Shapira, & Farchi, 2013). Men have also experienced tonic immobility after sexual assault (Coxell & King, 2010). Immobility may be a form of peritraumatic dissociation. It can be predicted if women have had prior experiences of sexual victimization as a child or adult (Gidycz, Van Wynsberghe, & Edwards, 2008).

The neurobiological response is intended to be self-limiting, with glucocorticoid receptors decreasing production of cortisol when levels become elevated, parasympathetic regulation and oxytocin release to promote calming and connections with others. Severe trauma or sustained and repetitive trauma can damage the neurobiological response. This damage is associated with the development of PTSD and depression after violence. The goal of the CHN with a victim of acute violence is to prevent further trauma or stress.

The victim of violence may have impaired **memory** of the events. The hormonal responses to the trauma, while enhancing focus and attention, can also impair memory encoding and consolidation (Schwabe & Wolf, 2014; Tiller & Baker, 2014). This impairment results in difficulty describing what happened, or in what order, particularly in the first hours or days after an event. Some of this memory may improve, particularly if there was no alcohol or drug use at the time of the event. The normal process of recovery relies upon allowing individuals to alternate between processing the event and avoiding it until they eventually can cope with or face the trauma. Initial avoidance may in fact be a helpful short-term strategy to deal with traumatic events (Bowman, 2007). Where possible, they should be allowed to pace when to disclose and not be pushed to talk about it.

Acute stress responses after trauma may include distress, anxiety, avoidance, re-experiencing, substance abuse, guilt, anger, and shame (Bryant, 2013). If these symptoms persist for more than two to four days after a trauma, then the person may be developing acute stress disorder (American Psychiatric Association, 2013). If they already had PTSD, they may have a worsening of symptoms and re-experience prior traumas or dissociate during the interactions or interview with the CHN. It is not required that the CHN diagnose these stress disorders but referral to counselling may be required. Awareness of prior traumas and risks of dissociation or re-experiencing is also important to help prevent these during the client visit. This can be accomplished by allowing the client to pace disclosure; recognizing signs of distress and making clients comfortable help to prevent dissociation or re-experiencing. Children's responses to stress differ somewhat from adults. Examples of typical stress-related behaviours are shown in Table 28.3 by developmental stage.

**CHN Responses to Disclosure** Victims of violence may never disclose to police or health professionals but often disclose to a peer (Orchowski & Gidycz, 2012; Russell, 2013; Sabina & Ho, 2014).

| Table 28.3 | Trauma Responses by Developmental Stage |
|---|---|
| **Stage** | **Potential Indicators** |
| Birth to 5 years | Clinging to parent, trembling, unexplained crying, inappropriate or regressive behaviours (bedwetting, nail biting, thumb sucking), fear of sleeping, limited social interaction, forgetting how to talk or inability to talk |
| 6 to 11 years | Anxiety, depression, anger, inability to concentrate, disorganization, difficulty socializing, refusal to attend school, sleeping difficulties, headaches, stomach aches (3 times more likely to develop PTSD than adolescents) |
| Adolescents | School difficulties, eating disorders, alcohol abuse, teen pregnancy or high-risk sexual behaviours, suicidality, behavioural problems, loss of family or community connections, may have sense of shortened future, revenge, guilt for not preventing event |
| Adults | Symptoms of post-traumatic stress, depression, hostility, suicidality, substance abuse, high-risk behaviours |

Positive support from family and friends has been found to improve outcomes after trauma, improving **resilience** to the effects of trauma (Glass, Perrin, Campbell, & Soeken, 2007; Littleton, 2010; Ullman, Townsend, Filipas, & Starzynski, 2007). Parenting support is also important to children's resilience. Children have been found to be more resilient if their mother has better mental health and parenting skills (Graham-Bermann, Gruber, Howell, & Girz, 2009) and a stable nurturing environment (Bellis et al., 2014). Victims of sexual assault and intimate partner violence have often had control taken away from them, so efforts to help them regain control over their choices and access to resources, as well as participating in their own recovery, are helpful to reducing risks for PTSD or other mental health issues.

Negative responses to **disclosure** can worsen the risks of victims developing stress disorders such as post-traumatic stress disorder (Flicker, Cerulli, Swogger, & Talbot, 2012; Littleton, 2011; Ullman, 2011). These negative responses are a form of **secondary victimization**. Negative responses include responding with disbelief (e.g., using the term "alleged") or blaming the victim (Sylaska & Edwards, 2014), taking control of the victim's choices, telling them to leave, or treating them differently (Mason, Ullman, Long, Long, & Starzynski, 2009; Ullman, Foynes, & Tang, 2010). Other forms of secondary victimization include making the victim repeat details about the assault too often or when they are not ready to talk about it, focusing on the timing or needs of the professional versus client, or exposing clients to delays in services or incomplete care (Campbell, Wasco, Ahrens, Sefl, & Barnes, 2001; Greeson & Campbell, 2013). These experiences were found to leave victims of violence feeling violated (89%), bad about themselves (87%), and unlikely to seek help again (80%) (Campbell, 2005).

In addition to provision of positive support, the WHO (2011) describes **psychological first aid** (PFA) measures. The steps of PFA include "look," "listen," and "link." Looking refers to ensuring they and the health provider are safe, the environment is safe, and to be aware of other community resources that are available. Listening means to provide comfort, emotional support, believe them, and to actively listen to what the victim needs or expects from the encounter. Asking for details, versus listening, may be retraumatizing; listen if they disclose but do not ask for unnecessary information (Bisson & Andrew, 2009; Kearns, Ressler, Zatzick, & Rothbaum, 2012). Linking the victim to community resources and other professionals is essential to recovery. This includes linkages to both formal agencies and informal support people.

**Physical Indicators of Violence** Physical findings associated with various forms of abuse relate primarily to the mechanisms of injury and anticipated responses. Injuries that do not fit with the events described or activities of the person's developmental age should be suspected. For instance, one would not suspect injuries on the trunk of an infant that is not ambulatory, but bruises to the head or shins of a child beginning to walk would be expected. Patterned injuries, such as circular bruises like finger tips or in the shape of an item, are also suspected. Burns or any other injury that is symmetrical are unusual.

If injuries are present the CHN should document these carefully, including colour, size, shape, and location. Consistent terminology should be used when describing injuries noted in a visit. For instance, the terms "ecchymosis" and "bruise" are not interchangeable—a bruise occurs from trauma while ecchymosis is more often due to aging vessels or to gravitational spread of a bruise (Sheridan & Nash, 2007). Although bruises cannot be accurately dated, there is a pattern of colour progression, so it is important to describe the colour of the bruise. A laceration is from a blunt object, leaving split skin with rough, perhaps bruised or abraded edges and typically cross-bridging of tissues or hair across the wound (Figure 28.2).

| Table 28.4 | BALD STEP Guide to Physical Findings | | |
|---|---|---|---|
| B | BL bleeding | S | SW swelling |
| | BR bruise | | ST stain |
| | BU burn | T | TE tenderness to palpation |
| | BI bite | | |
| A | AB abrasion | | TR trace evidence (specify type) |
| | AV avulsion | | |
| L | LA laceration | E | ER erythema |
| D | DE deformity (acute; e.g., sprain) | P | PA patterned injury (draw shape) |
| | | | PT petechiae |
| | | | PE penetrating injury (add "I" incised, "S" stab, "P" puncture, or "G" Gunshot) |

In contrast, penetrating injuries have cleaner edges and no cross-bridges through the middle. A penetrating stab wound will be deeper than wide, while a penetrating incised cut slashes across skin and so will be wider than it is deep.

The misuse of injury terminology creates difficulty for interpretation of findings and comparison of data. As a result, a standardized terminology has been developed for injuries and other physical findings to be used by any health professional working with victims of trauma such as sexual assault or intimate partner violence (Carter-Snell, 2011). These terms are summarized by the mnemonic **BALD STEP** (Table 28.4). This guide to physical findings is now incorporated in injury documentation nationally with the Royal Canadian Mounted Police sexual assault evidence kits but can be used to guide assessment for any trauma client. Healthcare professionals should use these standardized terms to describe injuries with any victim of trauma. If using body diagrams, the two-letter abbreviations can be used to indicate locations of specific injuries (adding measurements, shape, and colour), as long as the guide is included in the documentation or part of protocols used for charting.

Examples of patterned injuries (that resemble objects) as well as patterns of injury are discussed within each of the various types of abuse and assault in the following section. It is these patterns that will help determine if injuries are abusive. Careful documentation on each visit will help to support victim's histories of assault if they decide to report to police (or if the professional is mandated to report).

## INDICATORS OF SPECIFIC TYPES OF VIOLENCE

The preceding discussion has been focused on risks and resiliency to violence, and the interaction of the various influences as applicable to all forms of violence. There are some considerations that are specific to different types of abuse, such as child abuse, sexual violence, intimate partner violence, and elder abuse. These will be the focus of the remaining discussion.

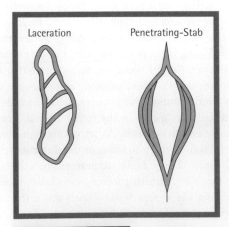

Laceration      Penetrating-Stab

**FIGURE 28.2** Lacerations versus Penetrating Injuries

*Source: Courtesy of Catherine Carter-Snell/ Mount Royal University*

# Violence against Children

**Child Abuse** Children and youth in Canada are entitled to all human rights, including freedom from violence by caregivers and the right to proper care. **Child abuse** includes physical, emotional, or sexual abuse. Precise rates of child abuse are difficult to determine for a number of reasons. A common problem with all abuse data is that many victims of violence do not or cannot report. A General Social Survey in Canada demonstrated that 80% of teens 15 to 17 years old who experience violence do not report their abuse (Sinha, 2013). While children are less likely to be victims of violent offences than adults, police-reported data indicate that children are five times more likely to be victims of sexual offences.

Witnessing intimate partner violence is considered emotional child abuse in Canada and is the most common form of emotional abuse among children (Trocme et al., 2009). The rationale for including witnessing parental violence is found in the ACE study results. Children who experience or witness violence develop increased rates of chronic diseases (e.g., heart disease, fractures, liver disease, cancer, lung disease, AIDS), poor health or risk behaviours (e.g., smoking, alcohol or drug abuse, obesity, somatic symptoms, high prescription drug use), mental illness (depression, panic or sleep disorders, memory issues, poor anger control), high-risk sexual behaviours (e.g., early first intercourse, teen pregnancy, fetal death), social problems (e.g., impaired work performance, relationship problems, and greater likelihood of causing intimate partner violence or being a victim) as well as early mortality (Anda et al., 2010; Lalor & McElvaney, 2010). Neurobiologic studies have shown that pathways are created in the brain as a result of adverse childhood experiences, resulting in greater activation of the hypothalamic–pituitary–adrenal system and inflammatory changes that have been linked to long-term changes to the nervous, endocrine, and immune systems (Danese & McEwen, 2012). Multiple forms of victimization rather than one specific type accounted for the most variability in children developing mental health problems such as depression, anxiety, and anger, or aggression in a study of Quebec children (Cyr, Clément, & Chamberland, 2013).

In the vast majority of cases the abuser is known to the child (Sinha, 2011; Sullivan, Beech, Craig, & Gannon, 2011). Police-reported data show that in 24% of the cases of child abuse, the abuser is a family member or extended family and another 54% of cases are committed by people known by the victim such as friends or acquaintances (Sinha, 2011). Only 21% of violent incidents are by strangers, yet this is where we have devoted much of our prior prevention efforts (e.g., "stranger danger"). Younger children are most likely to be assaulted by family (70% of infants and toddlers, 47% of 3- to 11-year-old victims) compared to 18% of youth victims aged 12 to 17 years (Sinha, 2013). This is due to the fact that older children are more often out in the community and accessible to acquaintances. As the children get older and meet more people outside the family they are more likely to be assaulted by acquaintances. Although

males are responsible for 70% of child abuse in Canada (Sinha, 2011), females are also sometimes abusers, particularly if they were exposed to abuse as a child and an adult (Craig & Sprang, 2007). Contributing factors affecting perpetrators' risk for child abuse include the following (Craig & Sprang, 2007; Peter, 2009):

- individual—substance abuse, lack of understanding of child's needs, prior experience of child abuse, access to younger children, poor parental impulse control;
- relationship—social isolation, family disorganization, parenting stress (younger parents, unemployed, single, many children), intimate partner violence;
- community—community violence, poor neighbourhood, other deficits in social determinants of health; and
- societal—lack of social structures to support the family, inadequate social support or policies to support parenting skills and childcare.

The type of assault also differs by gender and age. Children younger than four years of age and those with special needs, such as illness or disability, are at particular risk of experiencing abuse (Centers for Disease Control, 2014). Boys in Canada under 18 years old are 1.5 times more likely to be victims of physical abuse than females (Ogrodnik, 2010). Studies in both England (Bebbington et al., 2011) and Canada (Ogrodnik, 2010) have indicated that childhood sexual abuse is more common among female children and increases as they reach adolescence. The number of male child sexual assaults is still significant, however, with over one-third of child sexual assaults investigated having male victims (Trocme et al., 2005). Approximately 81% of all child abuse and 75% of sexual assaults are committed by someone well known to the child (Ogrodnik, 2010). Typically, sexual abuse and stalking of females or males is by male perpetrators (Ogrodnik, 2010). Females may also be responsible for sexual abuse; however, it is more often of male children (Tsopelas, Tsetsou, Ntounas, & Douzenis, 2012). Children over 11 years old are more likely to be assaulted by an acquaintance as they are travelling outside on their own more often (Ogrodnik, 2010).

Reporting child abuse of any form, including likelihood of witnessing intimate partner violence, is required of all caregivers by law in Canada (Canadian Child Welfare Research Portal, 2011). It is not necessary to be certain, but only to have a suspicion, of child abuse. Once it is reported to the appropriate agency (social services or police), they have specialized training to follow up and determine the risks and requirement for further action. As previously noted, injuries in unexpected places (e.g., arm for a non-ambulatory child) are suspicious as is inconsistency of history with the injuries. Recurrent injuries may all be suspicious for child abuse (Deans, Thackeray, Groner, Cooper, & Minneci, 2014). Other indicators may be patterned injuries or symmetrical injuries. Burns with a distinct water line are suspicious—if a child is placed feet first into hot water, one would expect kicking and splash burns but if held in the water, a water line can form which gives the burns a stocking or glove-like appearance. Splash burns are usually in a "V" shape, with the narrowest part of the V pointing in the direction of the fluid flow

(Christian, 2011; Giardino & Finkel, 2005). Fractures highly specific for child abuse include those affecting the ribs, scapula, sternum, or metaphyseal regions (Flaherty et al., 2014).

Resiliency to child abuse can be facilitated in a number of ways. Individual resiliency can be supported by aiding children with their social skills and ability to relate to their caregiver. Support of family function and improvement in social determinants of health, such as health services and social services, can improve resilience, as can connecting children with caring adults inside or outside the family as mentors, and facilitating self-esteem and social skills in the child (Afifi & MacMillan, 2011; Wilcox, Richards, & O'Keeffe, 2004).

The community health nurse has many opportunities to prevent child abuse. Key **prevention** interventions for the CHN, regardless of the setting, include the following actions specific to child abuse (Mikton & Butchart, 2009; Mock, Peden, Hyder, Butchart, & Krug, 2008):

- Primary prevention
  - Educate children to facilitate friendships, develop social and emotional skills, and learn healthy relationships
  - Educate parents on skills and links to services
  - Conduct community home visits, looking for risk factors and building on strengths
- Secondary prevention
  - Participate in any surveillance initiatives for adverse childhood experiences
  - Report suspected child abuse to authorities, carefully document physical and behavioural findings, link with key resources, and maintain an attitude of objectivity
- Tertiary prevention
  - Link parents and children with support resources in the community
  - Determine and ensure the immediate safety of the child and the nurse

**Bullying, Cyberbullying, and Sexting** Bullying is the exertion of power and control over another, typically by using vulnerabilities of others to control them. This behaviour continues into adulthood, in gang violence, dating violence, intimate partner violence, child abuse, workplace harassment, and elder abuse (Tutty & Abbott, 2007). Bullying can be in many forms: direct (physical or verbal aggression, intimidation), indirect (social isolation or exclusion, spreading lies), sexual harassment, racial, religious, or electronic (cyberbullying—harassment over social media or Internet, sexting explicit pictures or content). Approximately 40% of adolescents in a Canadian study reported having been both the bully and the victim (Craig & McCuaig, 2012). The most frequent victimization was in the younger grades; it began decreasing by Grade 6 until approximately Grade 9 or 10 when bullying becomes relatively less frequent. Over half of the bullying was indirect or teasing. Boys were more often victims of physical bullying than girls, while sexual harassment and cyberbullying were greater for girls in all grades. Both bullies and victims report physical symptoms such as headaches, difficulty sleeping or stomach aches, and depression or anxiety, especially if they are both bullies and victims (Lamb, Pepler, & Craig, 2009). Bullies also may display alcohol and substance use, suicidal thoughts, or suicide. Victims may begin trying to avoid school, which is where bullying is most likely to occur.

Relationships with parents have been found in a systematic review to be a key risk factor for victims of bullying and those who both bully and are victims (Lereya, Muthanna, & Wolke, 2013). These authors found that bullies are more likely to have experienced abuse or maladaptive parenting before entering school. Warm, affectionate relationships with parents, parental involvement, and supervision were protective for victimization. These findings highlight the need to include families and promote parenting skills in prevention programs. A social risk factor for bullying and victimization is differences in income equality (Elgar et al., 2013). This finding held true in multiple countries. It was also found in wealthier schools where all students came from higher incomes but where some were perceived as having relatively less income than the others. Cyberbullying has been linked to many serious consequences, including academic dropout and mental health problems, gang involvement, and suicide (Notar, Padgett, & Roden, 2013). One of the key differences with cyberbullying as compared to face-to-face bullying is that the teen cannot get away from cyberbullying. The trauma is always there online.

"Sexting" is the sharing of sexually explicit materials (pictures or information) between two people. Data on the prevalence of sexting are in early stages, with most coming from online surveys, which may provide skewed results given that only those online are responding. Data from U.S. surveys suggest that approximately 30% of high school adolescents have received a sexually explicit sext and approximately 10 to 30% have sent them (Lenhart, 2009; McCartan & McAlister, 2012). Rates for adult sexting are even higher (Hewitt, 2009). Almost half of sexts were sent to partners, and in one study 15% said they purposely sent the images to someone online they did not know (Henderson & Morgan, 2009). Teens involved in sexting were typically involved in more high-risk behaviours, were sexually active, and were engaged in high volumes of texting activity (Delevi & Weisskirch, 2013; Lenhart, 2009). The National Center for Exploitation of Missing Children estimates that a quarter of all child pornography victims posted the initial photographs themselves to someone online, 10% of them being self-produced and 14% due to enticement of a third party online (Lenhart, 2009). While these estimates are concerning, almost everyone who received a sext indicated that they forwarded them to other people (Cox Communications, 2009). This forwarding is typically non-consensual and used for cyberbullying.

It is legal for consenting adults in a relationship to transmit texts or photos of a sexual nature between themselves in North America. The law is less clear when teens are involved but tends toward allowing it. The problem arises when the texts or photos ("sexts") are received and distributed by someone not in the relationship or an ex-partner. If these sexts involve children under 18 years old this is considered distribution of child pornography, a Criminal Code offence associated with prison time and a permanent record even if committed by a minor. It is argued that removing sexting from the Criminal Code (decriminalizing it) assumes that the children are not harmed (Slane, 2013) and therefore may decrease the likelihood that it will be further investigated. The distribution of these sexts, however, has even more life-changing consequences for the victims. The first Canadian minor to be charged with child pornography related to sexting was in 2014 (Meissner, 2014).

Until recently we have had little legal recourse for bullying of any form. The only charges available have been charges under the Canadian Criminal Code for assault, stalking or harassment, or distribution of child pornography for emailing or texting inappropriate photographs. In 2013 a working group for the Federal and Territorial Ministers recommended that a new charge be developed (CCSO Cybercrime Working Group, 2013). Approximately 30% of Canadian students are thought to be involved in cyberbullying (Craig & McCuaig, 2012). In 2015 Canada introduced new cyberbullying legislation (Government of Canada, 2015).

Interventions to stop bullying include strategies to promote empathy and prosocial behaviour, and ways to reduce peer reinforcement of bullying behaviour (Lamb et al., 2009). If parents of bullied children are experiencing intimate partner violence they may also need assistance for themselves as well to learn to model healthy relationships. Victims of bullying need assistance in developing assertiveness, as well as in learning friendship skills and having opportunities to interact. Victims of bullying actually develop stronger prosocial skills than children who have never been bullied (Craig & Pepler, 2003).

**Child Exploitation and Human Trafficking** Child exploitation involves sexual abuse, making of pornography, and use of children in prostitution and **trafficking** for purposes of sexual exploitation and sexual tourism. In 2008 there were 1368 incidents of distribution of child pornography reported to police in Canada (Ogrodnik, 2010). This is nine times more than the 1999 data. Some of this may be a function of reporting. It is also in part due to the ease of proliferation of pornography over the Internet and with technology such as smartphones. Sexting has also been linked to risks of child exploitation, facilitating distribution of child pornography, and possession (McCartan & McAlister, 2012; Mitchell, Jones, Finkelhor, & Wolak, 2011). The Internet is often used for child exploitation to meet and engage youth in sexual encounters. Methods include chatrooms, email, and instant messaging programs. The typical perpetrators, according to an American study, were adult males and, contrary to media stereotypes, only 5% pretended to be teens when they met victims (Wolak, Finkelhor, Mitchell, & Ybarra, 2008). Most youth, therefore, knew they were dealing with an adult. The victims were predominantly female and almost three-quarters of victims had face-to-face encounters with the perpetrator more than once. Almost all of the victims of Internet-initiated sex crimes were 13 to 17 years old, which, it is argued, is old enough to have an understanding of the social implications and risks of the Internet and the ability to engage in more complex uses of the Internet (Wolak et al., 2008). The youth involved were often more likely to be risk takers and willing to interact with unknown people. Unfortunately, one of the consequences of child abuse is subsequent high-risk sexual behaviour and risk taking, as well as vulnerability to re-victimization (Lalor & McElvaney, 2010). Child exploitation is a risk for those previously abused. The risk for potential victims is high. Those involved in child exploitation are likely to have prior offences for sexual assault or child pornography, have a history of violence, and have formed partnerships with other offenders (Mitchell et al., 2011). They are typically skilled at "grooming" their prey and at developing trust with the victim (McCartan & McAlister, 2012). Little is known about how to support youth who have been exploited and further research is required.

Human trafficking is an extremely lucrative business, with only drugs and firearm trafficking generating the same amount of money or operating more globally (Government of Canada, 2012). Human trafficking, as opposed to human smuggling, relies upon controlling and exploiting people to generate ongoing income. We may think of trafficking as originating outside of Canada but it happens in Canada with Canadian victims on a daily basis. Victims are often pushed or lured into trafficking through conditions of extreme poverty, lack of education, war, or other determinants of health. The majority of victims are female and most often disadvantaged or at risk, and they are recruited through threats, coercion, abduction, fraud, or use of power to gain control of the person (WHO, 2012). Drug and alcohol use (forced or coerced) is used as a means to control individuals (or as a coping mechanism by victims), as is financial exploitation or control of their funds (WHO, 2012).

Although human trafficking is perhaps seen as something happening elsewhere, the majority of victims in Canada are Canadian citizens or permanent residents of Canada (RCMP, 2010). The average age for exploitation is 13 to 15 years old (Ministry of Public Safety and Solicitor General, 2011). Those most at risk include Aboriginal youth (30 to 50% of exploited youth); lesbian, gay, and bisexual youth; previously abused youth (25% of exploited youth have been abused before); runaways; migrants; and children in protective care (Ministry of Public Safety and Solicitor General, 2011; RCMP, 2010). Non-Canadian victims were found to be most often from Asia (Thailand, Cambodia, Malaysia, and Vietnam) and eastern European countries. The Royal Canadian Mounted Police (RCMP) found a number of women were brought over to work as live-in domestics and were subsequently exploited.

Removing women and girls from human trafficking rings is extremely difficult and dangerous. Many have been threatened as to what will happen to them or their families if police find them or they report. They are understandably fearful of professionals attempting to assist. There is now a network of resources to assist women to get away, one of the most public being that founded by a survivor in the Toronto area, Timea Nagy (Nagy & Rutherford, 2010). CHNs play a key role in early identification of victims. Some key indicators may include repeat visits for sexually transmitted infections, unexplained injuries, fearful behaviour, and perhaps language barriers (Baldwin, Eisenman, Sayles, Ryan, & Chuang, 2011; Crane & Moreno, 2011). Research has shown that almost half of trafficking victims sought healthcare for various reasons (Konstantanopoulos et al., 2013) and yet they were not asked about safety, why they had so many infections, or if they were ever expected to have sexual intercourse when they did not want it (Baldwin et al., 2011; Konstantanopoulos et al., 2013). They may not initially disclose but informants believed they would have done so eventually if asked. Once identified, the next step will be for the CHN to assist them in accessing relevant resources. Toronto and Vancouver have been active centres in developing guidelines for trafficking recognition and interventions, as have the RCMP and Status of Women Canada. Some of the initiatives include training for at-risk groups such as First Nations and refugee communities, training of law enforcement and community service agencies, development of trafficking laws in the Canadian Criminal Code, provision of temporary immigration status and work permits for rescued foreign victims, and international partnerships with police and border service agencies (Government of Canada, 2012).

**Gangs** Gang involvement in Canada has been increasing (Criminal Intelligence Service Canada, 2010). Gangs may be composed of single ethnicities or be heterogeneous, depending on the location. In 2002 it was estimated that there were 434 youth gangs in Canada with over 7000 members (Public Safety Canada, 2013) and they have grown significantly in the subsequent 10 years. Gangs are located in both rural and urban areas across the country, as well as on Aboriginal reservations and in correctional facilities. The highest gang involvement has been in Ontario, Saskatchewan, and British Columbia. Most of the gangs are male, although female gangs have been increasing, especially in British Columbia, Manitoba, and Saskatchewan. At least half the members are under 18 years of age. Public Safety Canada (2013) estimates that 20% of gangs account for 80% of the serious crimes and homicides. Gangs have accounted for at least 95 to 138 homicides a year between 2008 and 2011 (Perreault, 2012). Aboriginal youth gang involvement has been termed an "epidemic" (Public Safety Canada, 2013).

Risks for gang involvement and strategies for prevention are shown in Table 28.5 (Bradshaw, Waasdorp, Goldweber, & Johnson, 2013; Central Intelligence Service Canada, 2010; Public Safety Canada, 2013). Note the similarity of risks and prevention focus to other prevention activities suggested across all violence types.

The implications for the CHN are diverse. Collaboration with community agencies is important. A collective approach is required to determine at-risk populations and local community solutions to reducing the challenges for youth, and programs in which they may become involved.

## Adults and Adolescents

Adolescents and adults may be victims of human trafficking as previously described. Other types of victimization include sexual assault, intimate partner violence and elder abuse or neglect.

| Table 28.5 | Gang Involvement Risks and Prevention | |
|---|---|---|
| **Influence** | **Risks** | **Prevention** |
| Individual | Adverse childhood experiences<br><br>Child welfare involvement | Programs aimed at improving anti-social behaviour, personal challenges, and negative thinking |
| Relationship/ Family | Disconnection from family<br><br>Negative peer influences | Family-oriented approaches to affirm positive values |
| Community | Racism<br><br>Cultural disruption | Opportunities to interact with positive role models, availability to participate in community programs (e.g., Community Cadet Corps) |
| Societal | Factors increasing inequities in determinants of health | Funding for programs and family support |

**Sexual Assault** The term "rape" was replaced with "**sexual assault**" in the Canadian Criminal Code in the 1990s. It was recognized that rape was limited to vaginal-penile penetration. Offences such as penetration with foreign objects, fondling, or oral-penile penetration were not included nor were same-sex assaults. The term "sexual assault" is now used for any form of unwanted sexual contact. The Canadian Criminal Code now includes three levels of sexual assault: section 271, sexual assault; section 272, bodily harm (physical or psychological); and section 273, with use of a weapon, threat, or endangerment (Brennan & Taylor-Butts, 2008). Comments from a victim related to fear for their life, perceived threat, use of a weapon, or findings of significant injury can all increase the level (severity) of the charges police lay against the offender. The CHN's documentation may be valuable to prosecution if these findings are noted.

Young females between 14 and 24 years of age are at highest risk for sexual assault (Johnson, 2006). Teens and college-aged young adults are exposed to social settings, situations, and people associated with increased risks for assault. The rate of male sexual assaults is less clear due to underreporting (Masho & Anderson, 2009; McLean, Balding, & White, 2005). It is estimated that by the age of 16 at least 50% of females will have experienced at least one unwanted sexual experience (Johnson, 2006). Police or hospital statistics may be misleading, as General Social Surveys across Canada have repeatedly demonstrated that only 10% of victims report to police, although 30% will seek healthcare (Johnson, 2006). This provides CHNs with three times as much opportunity to assist victims, and a reminder to look for the 70% in the community who are not reporting.

In 2008, the age of consent for sexual activity in Canada was raised from 14 years of age to 16 years of age, with the addition of "close-in-age" exceptions (Department of Justice, 2013). If someone has intercourse with someone outside of these age exceptions, or with someone who is in a position of responsibility or power (e.g., family, coach, or teacher), then it is considered sexual assault.

- 12- or 13-year-olds can only consent to sexual activity if the person is within two years of their age;
- 14- or 15-year-olds can only consent if the person is within five years of their age (except a person in authority or a family member); and
- 16-year-olds and older can consent to intercourse with anyone (except a person in authority).

Sexual assault in Canada **must** be reported to authorities if a teen has intercourse with anyone in a position of power or authority or who exceeds the close-in-age exceptions, even if they say they consented. If the perpetrator is within the close-in-age exceptions and not in a position of power, then the sexual assault can only be reported to police with the young person's consent, if they have capacity for consent. Some provinces have laws specifying the age at which minors can consent to healthcare. Canada has moved to the concept of a "mature minor" based on a Supreme Court decision. As a result, in Prince Edward Island, the Yukon, Ontario, and the western provinces there is no specific age for children and teens to consent to medical treatment (Jackman & McRae, 2013; Knight, 2014). If the healthcare provider determines that the child or teen understands the options for reporting and the sexual assault examination, as well as the implications of reporting or not reporting, it is the young person's decision. Capacity is generally determined by informing the youth, then asking questions to determine their understanding. Parents cannot overturn the teen's decision. Provincial health information acts also limit who can be informed of the assault, including parents. Child welfare can step in, however, if there is a belief that the minor is at risk with the decision (Harmon, 2010). These considerations are important for the CHN. Consider the situation if a 15-year-old teen seeks support from the CHN without her parents being present. If she does not want her parents informed that she has been assaulted, refuses police reporting, or does not want to go to see the sexual assault team, she may refuse care and notification of her parents as long as she demonstrates capacity for informed consent to healthcare and release of health information. Her parents cannot insist on the exam if they find out. Reporting to police would also not be done against her wishes unless the assailant were not older than the close-in-age exceptions or a person in authority.

Individual risk factors for sexual assault include physical or cognitive disabilities, including temporary effects due to drugs or alcohol use, prior sexual assault or abuse, or the presence of a mental illness such as PTSD (Acierno, Resnick, Kilpatrick, Saunders, & Best, 1999; Felson & Cundiff, 2014; Thrane, Yoder, & Chen, 2011). The most common agent found in approximately 30 to 46% of suspected drug-facilitated assaults is alcohol (Du Mont et al., 2010; McGregor,

Lipowska, Shah, Du Month & De Siato, 2003). The next most commonly found agents are canniboids, cocaine, and prescription anti-anxiety medications. It is relatively rare to find traditionally anticipated agents such as flunitrazepam/rohypnol ("roofies") or gamma hydroxyl butarone (GHB) (Du Mont et al., 2010). A systematic review of drug-facilitated sexual assault research found that less than 2% involved covert administration of agents that could cause sedation or incapacitation (Benyan, McVeigh, McVeigh, Leavey, & Bellis, 2008). College students are at risk, particularly if they are part of sororities (Minow & Einolf, 2009) or consume alcohol and drugs (Hines, Armstrong, Reed, & Cameron, 2012; Krebs, Lindquist, Warner, Fisher, & Martin, 2009). In one U.S. study, 17% of college men gave women alcohol in order to have sex because they knew the women would otherwise say no (Amar, 2013) but only 2% of the men considered this sexual assault. Sexual minorities are also at higher risk for sexual assault, including those in the lesbian, gay, transgendered, or bisexual community (Ard & Makadon, 2011; Hequembourg, Livingston & Parks, 2013; Hines et al., 2012; Raj, 2010).

It is often assumed that perpetrators of sexual assault are usually strangers but this is not the case. The vast majority of sexual assaults are committed by someone known to the victim other than an intimate partner, such as someone recently met at a party, a mutual acquaintance, or a friend (Vaillancourt, 2010). Less than 10% of reported sexual assaults are by strangers, and another 10% are by intimate partners. It is also wrong to assume that most of these assaults are by males who are good people but made a mistake or had too much alcohol (Lisak, 2004). A very small number of males may actually be responsible for a large number of assaults but may go undetected. Some may even commit multiple or serial assaults. In one group of 1882 male college students surveyed (Lisak & Miller, 2002) regarding situations in which they expected sex, 120 were found to have committed acts that could be considered sexual assaults. Of these 120 students, 76 committed an average of 14 assaults each, collectively being responsible for 1225 acts of interpersonal violence. These acts included sexual assault, child abuse, and intimate partner violence. Dr. Lisak refers to these males as "undetected serial rapists" and "predators" (Lisak, 2004). The men are described as having little regard for women and a high sense of control, and are often in traditionally "male" roles. They plan their attacks carefully, such as looking for the most vulnerable or intoxicated female in a bar, and use predatory approaches such as separating the target female from her friends by offering her a ride home and buying her more drinks. These behaviours actually help obscure the offender's role in the assault and shift the perceived blame to the female for becoming intoxicated or going home with him. They also contribute to the victim's self-blame and shame, thus negatively affect their reporting to police or seeking healthcare. A more recent study has indicated that the risk of a male perpetuating sexual assault may be higher and can fluctuate over time (Thompson, Swartout, & Koss, 2013). It is still the minority of men, however, with only 25 to 30% of college men admitting to some form of sexual assault since 14 years of age (Zinzow & Thompson, 2015). Similar to Dr. Lisak's work, the men typically held attitudes that were hostile toward women and some were responsible for multiple sexual assaults. These data have implications for prevention interventions for the CHN.

Victims reporting sexual assault require timely, sensitive treatment and should be treated as victims. One of the most important interventions the CHN can provide to the victim of sexual assault is crisis support and positive responses to disclosure to prevent secondary victimization. The disbelief that victims may encounter from family and friends, healthcare personnel, police, and courts can compound their psychological trauma (secondary victimization). It is estimated that only 2% to 8% of women claiming sexual assault in the United States do so falsely (Lonsway, Archambault, & Lisak, 2009), and in Canada the number is the same as that for false reporting for any crime—less than 4% (Government of Alberta, 2013). Despite this, even healthcare professionals refer to sexual assault as "alleged" and treat the victims with skepticism. Furthermore, the word "alleged" is not used for other types of trauma (e.g., "alleged motor vehicle collision") and can further stigmatize the victim. The term "alleged" should be reserved for the courts and police and remain out of the vocabulary and documentation of health professionals. Many victims, often as a result of the disbelief or self-blame, will not seek help for fear of this treatment or will delay seeking help (Peress et al., 2007; Vertamatti et al., 2012). Victims of sexual assault typically present at least 12 hours or more after the assault—they need time to process what happened or find out from friends if they know, and to consider their actions. If they do seek help and agree to report they may decide later to recant their statements. The recanting may be due to fear of the perpetrator, pressure from family or friends, fear of the legal system, or perceptions of not being believed (Maier, 2014). Approximately 10% of victims recanted in one U.S. study (Spohn, White, & Tellis, 2014). Since many may not be injured and the two parties often know each other, the assault is also difficult to prove, leading to cases being determined "unfounded" (Spohn, White, Tellis, 2014). Unfounded status means only that there was insufficient proof to prosecute, or that the victim withdrew the complaint, not that it was a false allegation or that it did not happen. Skepticism is further compounded if the victim has complained of other sexual assaults. The well-established links between previous sexual assault and risks for re-victimization may not be recognized by professionals or peers.

Sexually assaulted women may not have any injuries, especially if they were unconscious or intoxicated. Those that are present may be very subtle and missed without appropriate examination techniques or examiners with experience detecting these subtle injuries (Carter-Snell, 2011). Injuries are most often what many consider "minor" injuries but which may have significant implications for the victim. Any break in the skin increases a victim's risk of acquiring an infection. The presence of injuries increases the victim's risks of developing PTSD. Presence or absence of injuries can affect legal outcomes as well, as there is an increased likelihood that their case will proceed to court if there is injury present (Kennedy, 2012). There are many reasons why injury may be absent in sexual assault, including intoxication or altered levels of consciousness, relationship to the assailant, inexperience of examiners, and examination techniques (Carter-Snell, 2007). If the victim chooses not to have a sexual assault exam they may have injuries but be unaware of them, particularly in the immediate aftermath of the assault. A median of less than 20% of women with injuries reported pain subjectively, but almost half reported tenderness to palpation during an examination, highlighting the importance of an examination (Carter-Snell, 2007). Those who report to police may also be more likely to have injuries, with injuries present in approximately one in four women who report sexual assault to police (Vaillancourt, 2010). These injuries are most typically lacerations (approximately 0.25 to 5 centimetres) in the posterior fourchette and fossa navicularis region of the genitals, as well as abrasions and bruises.

The number and type of injuries that can be attributed to sexual assault versus consensual intercourse are variable. As more studies are conducted comparing injuries after consensual and non-consensual intercourse, a few patterns are emerging. One of these is that women were more likely to be in the non-consensual group if there were two or more genital injuries (Anderson, McLain, & Riviello, 2006; Lincoln, 2013; McLean, 2011), or if there were particular types of injuries present such as genital abrasions (Anderson, McClain, & Riviello, 2006). Further comparative studies are needed to more fully understand patterns of injuries, both genital and non-genital, after sexual assault. A lack of injury does not mean assault did not occur. Lack of injury is anticipated if the person was intoxicated at the time of the assault or there is no resistance or physical force used (Carter-Snell, 2007). The CHN is encouraged to develop collaborative relationships with these examiners and agencies and to participate in the multidisciplinary collaborative team in the community.

Victims of sexual assault should be evaluated for their risks of sexually transmitted infections and pregnancy as well as drug-facilitated assault. These actions are time sensitive. These factors, combined with the potential for distress in the victim, make the sexually assaulted client fairly high priority in emergency departments. They are considered Level 3 (of 5) on the Canadian triage acuity scale (CTAS) if the assault was more than two hours previous and the client is stable (Bullard, Unger, Spence, & Grafstein, 2008). A Level 3 means they should be seen by a physician within an hour, and sooner if they are distressed, suicidal, in severe pain, or have any significant problems such as bleeding or airway problems (Bullard et al., 2008). Furthermore, the clients need support and counselling. These are key reasons why most sexual assault services are linked to health centres—comprehensive health services are the objective and evidence collection, although important, is secondary to the well-being of the client. The CHN plays a key role in referring clients to the nearest emergency department or sexual assault service, as well as in working with the client when they return to the community. The CHN can play a central role in establishing sexual assault support networks within the community to ensure comprehensive follow-up services. These sexual assault response teams or councils (SART or SARC) typically provide a multidisciplinary network and forum for information sharing among all professionals who provide services. Participants vary in each community but often include representatives from emergency sexual assault health professionals, police, counselling agencies, lawyers, community health services, victim services, and even pastoral services.

Prevention of sexual assault, as with other types of violence, requires a multifaceted approach. Perpetrator-focused prevention is one strategy. It has been recognized that the small minority of men who are most likely to commit sexual assault, known as "predators," are unlikely to change (Lisak, 2004). It is recommended instead that prevention efforts be focused on the majority of men who are less likely to commit sexual assault but may be actively or passively drawn in by these men. They may become involved passively by laughing at their jokes or stories of conquests, being bystanders to the assault, or being pressured into participating. One such prevention program is a media campaign called "Don't Be That Guy," originating in Edmonton in 2010 (Sexual Assault Voices of Edmonton, 2014).

**Victim resistance** or sexual assault avoidance is another strategy used to show women how to avoid risk and how to protect themselves. This includes verbal resistance such as yelling as well as physical resistance if needed. Both verbal and physical resistance are helpful in prevention of the assault itself (Brecklin & Ullman, 2005; Lonsway et al., 2011; Senn et al., 2015) and may result in feelings of greater empowerment (Brecklin & Ullman, 2005). If the assault cannot be prevented, the outcome on injuries is less clear. A theoretical model of factors influencing injury with a large sample of sexually assaulted women showed that perpetrator force and victim resistance during the assault were both linked to greater numbers of body injuries as well as greater severity (Carter-Snell, 2007). Analysis of a large U.S. dataset suggested that there was no significant increase in the number of injuries if the assault could not be prevented with resistance (Tark & Kleck, 2014) although they reported a rate of more serious non-sexual (body) injuries almost twice that of those who did not resist (5% versus 2.8%). Another concern with victim-resistance strategies is that these may lead to greater victim self-blame if they are unable to prevent the assault, and result in no greater attribution of blame to the perpetrator (Brecklin & Ullman, 2005). It also may not be possible to resist, given the number of women likely to experience tonic immobility.

A third type of sexual assault prevention is **bystander prevention**, which has increased in popularity on campuses (Bennett, Banyard, & Garnhart, 2014; McMahon, 2014; Potter, Moynihan, Stapleton, & Banyard, 2009; Warthe, Kostouros, Carter-Snell, & Tutty, 2013). One model used is situational bystander prevention, which relies upon bystanders recognizing there is a risk to the individual, making choices about intervention in that situation, and then acting (Burn, 2009). Another is a peer-facilitated program to raise awareness and initiate discussion of healthy and unhealthy behaviours, and to determine resources and how bystanders might intervene (Warthe & Tutty, 2009).

There is limited evidence as to which method of prevention is most effective: perpetrator change, victim resistance, or bystander prevention. It has been suggested that readiness to change needs to be considered in implementing programs

(Banyard, Eckstein, & Moynihan, 2010). It is not necessary, however, to choose one or the other. Each may be complementary and the use of multiple methods and strategies is consistent with the socioecological model of violence prevention. CHNs can become involved in community prevention initiatives and programs, collaborating with key professionals, and assisting in program evaluation as well as implementation. These teams are often called SART (sexual assault response teams) and represent various agencies that may be required to support victims of assault.

CHNs are also important in secondary prevention of consequences of sexual assault, particularly since at least 70% of victims will not seek healthcare. It is likely that these victims will at some point interact with CHNs for other healthcare reasons directly or indirectly related to their assault. They may seek "morning after" emergency contraception at sexual and reproductive health clinics, request testing for sexually transmitted infections or pregnancy, desire immunization for hepatitis B, seek follow-up from sexual assault centres, or demonstrate behaviours and illness symptoms related to stress. The CHN has a key role in screening clients to detect potential sexual assault or high-risk sexual assault behaviour. The CHN can then provide positive support and collaborate with local professionals knowledgeable about sexual assault services. The collaborative actions with SART or SARC will help the CHN maintain awareness of recommended resources for health examination of acutely assaulted clients, recommended treatment regimens and health follow-up, and guidelines for when to report to police, as well as availability of counselling centres in the area. Some key points include the following recommendations:

- Medical intervention—prophylaxis is typically provided in the first five days post-assault for chlamydia and gonorrhea. This includes a one-time dose of antibiotics according to current national and provincial protocols for sexually transmitted infections (Public Health Agency of Canada, 2014). Alternates for penicillin allergies and pregnancy are recommended in the national and provincial guidelines for sexually transmitted infections. HIV prophylaxis is also considered, particularly if there are injuries, multiple perpetrators, or a perpetrator who is high risk for HIV (e.g., recently incarcerated, intravenous drug user, males who have sex with males, or from an area endemic with HIV). If they have not been immunized for hepatitis B or have had an incomplete series, they may be given hepatitis B vaccine at the assault centre or emergency department and require further immunizations with community health. Check local guidelines.
- Testing—clients may have been tested for baseline sexually transmitted infections even if given prophylaxis. It is usually recommended that they seek further testing if they have signs of sexually transmitted infections a week or more post-treatment, including vaginal discharge and itching.
- Counselling—be familiar with centres or counsellors who are specialized in working with sexually assaulted victims. Trauma-focused interventions are recommended.

Clients may not recognize their symptoms or behaviours as signs of stress or link them to the violence and may need encouragement to seek help. Partners or other family members may also need counselling and support to cope with the assault of their loved one.

**Intimate Partner Violence** There are a number of terms used to refer to intimate partner violence, including intimate partner violence, relationship violence, or dating violence. The term "domestic violence" is problematic as it does not always include dating violence and implies co-habitation. "Relationship violence" implies an established relationship. "Dating violence" infers a newer relationship and until recently was not captured in the intimate partner violence literature (Carter-Snell, 2015). The Canadian government now includes dating violence in their definition of intimate partner violence (Sinha, 2013).

In this chapter the term "intimate partner" is used for any relationship which it is hoped will become intimate (e.g., recent date or meeting someone of interest), a relationship that is intimate, or one which used to be intimate (e.g., ex-husband or partner). Canadian data for intimate partner violence come from two main sources: the General Social Survey (GSS) of the population every five years and police reporting statistics. Both sources are important but offer different information, since only about 22% of women in violent relationships report to police (Brennan, 2011). The GSS data from 2009 indicate that 6% of Canadians reported being abused by a partner—either present or previous (Brennan, 2011). Violence was three times more common among those living common-law and those in blended families. Women between 25 and 34 years of age were in the highest-risk group for violence. Although males were also victims of intimate partner violence, women were three times more likely to be beaten, sexually assaulted, choked, or assaulted with a weapon by their spouse than men (Brennan, 2011), and they were three to four times more likely to be killed by a spouse than men (Taylor-Butts & Porter, 2011). Twice as many in gay or lesbian relationships described partner violence compared to those in heterosexual relationships, and four times as many who were bisexual. Aboriginal people were also twice as likely to describe partner violence. The rates of partner violence were similar among visible minority and immigrants compared to Canadian-born residents or non-minorities.

More than three-quarters of those experiencing partner violence did not report to police (Brennan, 2011). Most of these (82%) believed that it was a private matter, that they were dealing with the matter in another way (81%), or that it was not important enough (70%). They did not report to police until they had been victimized more than once (63%) and 28% had been victimized more than 10 times before reporting to police or were fearful for their lives. Approximately 10% obtained restraining orders but at least 30% of these indicated the partner violated the terms of the restraining order. Women were twice as likely to be injured as compared to males (42%), seven times more likely to be fearful of their partner (23%), and three times more likely to need time away

from work or other activities. Not surprisingly, the police-reported data indicate that the victim was four times more likely to be female than male (Sinha, 2013). The police data indicate reporting was more likely among females who had been sexually assaulted by a partner (53%), or who had experienced other severe forms of violence such as choking, beating, or use of a weapon (60%).

Risks for intimate partner violence include prior experiences of intimate partner violence, age differences between partners with an older abuser, a child in the home who is not the abuser's, living together versus married, and separated (Campbell, Webster, & Glass, 2009). Other risk factors for violent forms of partner violence include being younger (e.g., 15–34 years old), having limited activity, and experiencing emotional or financial abuse (Sinha, 2013). Social determinants of health such as lower education and lower income are also linked to higher rates of violence (Daoud et al., 2012). Pregnancy can increase risks for abuse. A Canadian study of abuse during pregnancy showed that the abuse started during pregnancy for 50% of those women who disclosed abuse (Daoud et al., 2012).

If injuries are present with partner violence they tend to be on the head, face, or neck, and particularly the middle third of the face (Sheridan & Nash, 2007). A systematic review of injuries in women who went to an emergency department following partner violence demonstrated that the majority of injuries affected the head, neck, or face (Wu, Huff, & Bandari, 2010). Attempts at strangulation may be as high as 68% among victims seeking healthcare (Sheridan & Nash, 2007). Asking about loss of consciousness, voice changes, or difficulty breathing is important to detecting damage from strangulation. There may also be small red petechiae (dots) visible above the level of compression, particularly in mucous membranes such as in the sclerae, subconjunctival area, or inside the mouth. There may also be injuries on the arms or legs due to restraint, or genital injuries with sexual assault. Defence injuries, such as on the back of hands while covering the face, may also be seen. As with all forms of potential abuse, look for patterns of injury or inconsistent history and injuries. A woman who falls down the stairs would be expected to have multiple sites of bruising and abrasions, not just bilateral wrist fractures (Sommers et al., 2012). Psychosocial indicators may include isolation from family and friends, financial dependence on the partner, controlling behaviours, and partners providing the answers to screening questions. Canadian data from 2011 illustrate that approximately every six days a woman was killed by a partner or ex-partner (Perreault, 2012). A danger assessment score (DAS) has been developed for women and professionals to determine the risk for femicide (Campbell, 2010; Campbell et al., 2003; Campbell et al., 2009). This tool has been validated and is available online for use. Key risk factors in the DAS are shown in Table 28.6. Scores of 9 to 13 indicate an increased risk of femicide and 14 to 17 suggest severe danger. Women should be aware of these risk factors in order to make informed decisions about whether to stay or to leave.

| Table 28.6 | Danger Assessment Indicators |
|---|---|

- Controls daily activities and contacts
- Violent and constant jealousy
- Following or spying on victim
- Victim has a child that is not perpetrator's
- Threats to harm or kill victim, their children, or animals
- Use of illegal drugs
- Use of or access to a weapon
- Increased severity or frequency of physical violence in last year
- Beating a victim when pregnant
- Leaving threatening notes or destroying victim's property
- Attempted strangulation
- Forced unwanted sex
- Victim threatened or tried to commit suicide
- Leaving perpetrator after living together for a year or more

Females were most often the victims of spousal homicide across all age groups in Canada in 2010 (Sinha, 2013). Homicides in dating relationships were slightly different, with females the more likely victims until middle age, then males over 55 years were up to four times more likely to die than females. Leaving is not always the safest option either. The risk of femicide is even higher at the hands of ex-spouses (Brennan, 2011). The risk for femicide was found to be nine times greater if the victim had left the relationship and if the partner was highly controlling (Campbell et al., 2003). Stalking behaviour is also a risk indicator after leaving a relationship. More than half of femicide victims had previously reported to police that they were being stalked by their partner or ex-partner (Klein, 2008).

A typology of perpetrators has been developed by Johnson and tested in a variety of studies of who are typically involved in one of four types of violence (Table 28.7) (Frye, Manganello,

| Table 28.7 | Intimate Partner Violence Perpetrator Typology |
|---|---|

| Violence Type | Description |
|---|---|
| Intimate terrorism | Pattern of coercive and violent control tactics |
| Situational violence | Crisis results in transient violence, not typically controlling |
| Violent resistance | Violence is in response to or in retaliation for partner's violence |
| Mutual violence | Both partners are violent and attempt to control each other |

Campbell, Walton-Moss, & Wilt, 2006; Johnson & Leone, 2005). The types of violence include intimate terrorism, situational conflict, violent resistance, and mutual violence. Situational violence was found to be most common, while intimate terrorism was found in approximately one-third of abusive relationships (Frye et al., 2006; Johnson & Leone, 2005; Straus & Gozjolko, 2014). Violent resistance to an abuser (23%) and mutual violence and control (3%) were less frequent in Johnson and Leone's work, but have also been described as subtypes of situational violence and intimate terrorism (Straus & Gozjolko, 2014). The perpetrator who relies on intimate terrorism has a high need to control victims (physically, psychologically, and/or financially), abuses more frequently, and is less likely to stop (Johnson & Leone, 2005). Victims of intimate terrorism were found to leave more frequently than with other types, experience more injury and PTSD, and miss more work. Controlling behaviour was identified in the danger assessment as a risk factor for femicide and is seen with the intimate terrorist in Johnson's typologies.

The risks for intimate partner violence are particularly complicated for younger adults due to developmental tasks and pressures from peers, family, and society. One of the social influences on risks for intimate partner violence is the value placed on relationships and having a partner. This expectation is both implicit and explicit in many ways from family, friends, and community members. The media also sends messages of the importance of a partner, and romance messaging. Some of this messaging can be misleading and even place people at risk. Violence in the media is one of the risks for violence identified by the WHO (Krug et al., 2002). Music videos, romance movies, and novels depict one individual as saying "no" and the other as initiating sex, regardless. This may involve restraint, roughness, or further disregard for the feelings or responses of the recipient, and may be associated with fear on behalf of the recipient. These behaviours are viewed as part of a romance narrative rather than being recognized as sexual assault and partner violence (Bonomi, Altenburger, & Walton, 2013). A major developmental task of young adulthood is the struggle to achieve "intimacy versus isolation" (McLeod, 2008). Success in this stage results in experiencing a relationship, love, and intimacy. Failure is predicted to result in isolation and loneliness. The fear of isolation has been found to result in "settling" for a less than ideal mate among Canadian university students (Spielmann et al., 2013). This settling introduces the risk of ignoring behaviours that may signal risks for intimate partner violence. Work with dating violence prevention programs among university students has shown that many students do not recognize risky behaviours (Warthe et al., 2013; Warthe & Tutty, 2009). Stalking or controlling behaviours such as constant texting, needing to know a partner's location, and keeping them away from friends or family are sometimes seen as love rather than risks. Healthy communication and the ability to differentiate healthy from unhealthy behaviours is an essential component of violence prevention.

Primary prevention is aimed at providing conditions for healthy relationships and strategies to foster healthy communication and awareness of resources (Cohen, Davis, & Graffunder, 2005):

■ individual—raise awareness about healthy/unhealthy relationships and gender socialization; screen for risk factors such as witnessing intimate partner violence, alcohol use, weapons in home; and

■ community—raise awareness in the community related to intimate partner violence and bystander roles, dispel myths (e.g., that it is "private" business versus a significant health issue), provide training to other health professionals and collaborative agencies, develop partnerships with community organizations.

Secondary prevention includes screening for intimate partner violence. If someone is identified as experiencing partner violence, the victim should be offered support and resources. In many cases the risk of staying outweighs the risks of leaving or the victim has reached a point of readiness. A key framework for interventions with intimate partner violence was developed and expanded using the stages of change (Weiss, 2003). This framework and subsequent strategies suggested are summarized in Table 28.8 (Kramer, 2002;

Logan & Walker, 2004; Weiss, 2003). It is important to recognize that even if women are prepared to leave, change is a process and it may require repeated efforts before they can permanently separate from the relationship (Weiss, 2003). In addition to increased risks of lethality, separation can worsen the victim's mental health and economic circumstances, add pressure with childcare and changes in children's schools, and remove them from their support systems, all of which may culminate in them returning one or more times to their partner (Logan & Walker, 2004). The principles of this assessment were seen in an example of a home visitation program for low-income, first-time mothers to identify and intervene with partner violence (Jack et al., 2012). If women disclosed violence, they were assessed for severity of abuse and safety. Interventions were then provided relevant to the readiness to address the abuse.

There are challenges with screening during home or clinic visits. Abusers often answer for their partners and hover during assessments. Screening for intimate partner violence should take place with the suspected victim alone, away from

| Table 28.8 | Readiness for Change with Intimate Partner Violence | |
|---|---|---|
| **Stage** | **Signs** | **Interventions** |
| Precontemplation | • Unaware or under-aware of problem<br>• Blame self<br>• Shame, feel others will blame victim for the abuse | • Help explore unhealthy aspects of relationship (e.g., may be revealed after screening tool administered)<br>• Validate/acknowledge disclosure<br>• Inform that abuse is wrong and not victim's fault<br>• May not be willing to accept printed material at this time |
| Contemplation | • Aware of problem<br>• Exploring and weighing options<br>• Not yet committed to action<br>• Emotionally aroused and preoccupied with abuser | • Validate feelings, accept disclosure<br>• Offer information about resources<br>• Affirm they do not have to accept/live with abuse |
| Preparation | • May have taken a few small steps toward leaving<br>• Likely to leave in about six months from beginning this stage | • Link with resources in community<br>• Make aware of dangers of leaving and of escalation<br>• Assist with preparation of safety plan or link to people who can assist |
| Action | • Leave but may relapse numerous times and return<br>• May be fearful of remaining away, be pressured by family/children, need finances<br>• Considered completed once six months pass without relapse | • Discuss safety—may need emergency protection order or restraining order, safe housing<br>• Use stage-based approach to integrating behaviour changes<br>• Focus on listening for readiness to change<br>• Don't expect rapid change or make decision for them<br>• Continue to support if return to spouse |
| Maintenance | • Healing stage | • Listen and validate experience<br>• Continue stage-based approach to change<br>• Assist to become less isolated and more safe |

their partner. Some professionals use policies such as health information regulations to explain why they need to assess the victim without the spouse or parent, even briefly as an opportunity to separate the victim and perform the screening. The person's response to the screening should provide an understanding of their readiness to leave. The table can be used as a guideline for the CHN to intervene appropriately to the victim's level of readiness. Typical guidelines for patient information resources apply, such as reading level and language appropriate to the reader. Some additional considerations are the safety and format of any information provided. The abuser may discover the information and become agitated. Some suggestions include business-sized cards that can be placed in the victim's shoe, information hidden in lipstick tubes or in pens. If a person chooses to remain in the relationship with the abuser they should be aware of the behaviours that are associated with increased risks of death, as described in the danger assessment tool.

If the person is ready to leave, they need a safety plan and resources. Safety plans include seeking formal sources of help, such as shelters, and use of escape plans (Parker & Gielan, 2014). Escape plans include keeping a bag ready with copies of key documents such as birth certificates and passports, some cash, clothing, and extra medications as well as contact numbers for shelters or other resources and any protection or restraining orders. It is recommended that this be kept somewhere safe, such as with a friend, in case they have to leave suddenly or it gets discovered. Their plan to leave should be to go to a place where their partner is unlikely to find them. When they leave, they may seek a restraining order or emergency protection order (the terms vary by province and differ in duration and how it is obtained). Approximately one-third of partners violated their restraining or protection orders in Canada (Brennan, 2011). The benefit of having a restraining order, however, is that if the partner does appear the police can act more quickly to enforce the separation. The CHN can help the victim explore options and safety, and connect them to local community agencies specialized in facilitating emergency plans and protection orders. The collaboration between the CHN and agencies such as women's shelters and counselling centres is vital.

**Elder Abuse and Neglect** Abuse against **elderly** people can be physical, sexual, economic, psychological or emotional, institutional, or spiritual and it includes rights violations. The elderly may also experience neglect. Unfortunately, the majority of elderly live alone or with a family member, which means that abuse or neglect may occur for long periods of time before it is detected. Canadian police-reported data suggest that elders are statistically the lowest-risk group for victimization in 2010 (Sinha, 2012). These data are not likely to reflect the extent of the abuse, however, as many elderly are too vulnerable or unable to report their abuse. Reasons for not reporting or disclosing elder abuse may include reduced physical or cognitive inability, isolation or inability to seek help, and fear of either being forced from their home or having to return to worsened abuse if the perpetrator continues to have access to them. Furthermore, the abuse outside of institutions is more often by a family member, and they may be embarrassed or afraid to report the abuser (Brown, Streubert, & Burgess, 2004; Rinker, 2009).

The elderly have very little societal protection from abuse compared to other vulnerable populations. One of the key interventions that must be considered is reporting to local authorities. Reporting requirements for elder abuse vary across Canada (Canadian Centre for Elder Law, 2011). In virtually all provinces the abuse must be reported if it occurs in a publicly funded institution. This includes hospitals, care homes, or prisons (Canadian Network for the Prevention of Elder Abuse, 2011). If the abuse occurs in a privately owned home, the community health nurse may not be able to report—reporting would be a violation of health information legislation and confidentiality. Most of the Maritime provinces have measures to allow reporting if professionals believe the elderly individual is in need of protection (Canadian Network for the Prevention of Elder Abuse, 2011). There is a gradual movement across Canada to implement reporting measures. It is important that CHNs understand the provincial legislation for persons in care as well as in the home, and the legislation related to elder abuse or dependent adults and health information acts as these vary across provinces. Some provinces have begun to change legislation to mandate reporting as being under the context of "vulnerable" persons, such as the Dependent Adult Act in Alberta. This is an area in which CHNs may choose to advocate for social policy or legislation to protect elders. It should be noted, however, that reporting may place the elderly person at greater risk if the elderly person lives with the abuser and must return to the home. Safety must be considered once reporting is implemented.

The perpetrator characteristics typically vary by the type of abuse, as shown in Table 28.9 (Acierno et al., 2010; Bloom et al., 2009; Brown et al., 2004; Burgess, Watt, Brown, & Petrozzi, 2006; WHO, 2014b).

Victimization of the elderly is more likely with any of the following risk factors (Acierno et al., 2010; Brown et al., 2004):

- individual—dementia or mental disorders of victim or alcohol/substance abuse by offender;
- relationship—shared living arrangements, dependency on the perpetrator, history of poor relationships, particularly with the caregiver (often a male adult child who had been abused by the parent), limited extended family;
- community—social isolation (physical or mental), lack of social support (loss of friends); and
- societal—ageism (seeing elderly as weak, a burden, or dependent), high costs of care, lack of legislation to support elderly.

Elder abuse can also occur in institutions and be perpetrated by caregivers. Data from the U.S. on institutional abuse showed that 36% of staff witnessed at least one episode of physical abuse, 10% committed at least one act of physical abuse, and 40% committed at least one act of psychological abuse (WHO, 2010). Physical acts of violence included use of physical or chemical restraints, deprivation of dignity, aggressive or inappropriate staff–client relationships, over- or under-medicating, crowded or unsanitary conditions, or failure to provide sufficient care or nutrition.

| Table 28.9 | Victim and Perpetrator Characteristics by Type of Abuse | |
|---|---|---|
| **Type of Abuse** | **Victim** | **Perpetrator** |
| Physical and Psychological | "Young" elderly (65–74)<br>Married<br>Poor emotional health<br>Socially isolated<br>Living with others (including abuser)<br>Very few confidantes | Spouses or relatives<br>History of severe mental illness<br>Recent decline in physical health<br>Alcohol or substance abuse, especially during incident<br>Dependent on/living with victim<br>Experienced recent stress<br>Increased legal problems |
| Sexual | Dependence on caregivers, especially for intimate care<br>Living alone<br>Decreased mobility/ability to defend | Almost all male:<br>   11% care providers<br>   26% stranger<br>   23% family<br>   15% partner |
| Material Abuse/ Exploitation | Unmarried or widowed/divorced<br>Older male or female<br>Living alone<br>Problems with money<br>Inadequate social supports<br>Activities limited by health or depression | Younger, distant relatives, or non-relatives<br>Physical or emotional problems<br>Alcohol abuse<br>Do not live with victim but financially dependent on victim |
| Neglect | Older elderly (80 years or older)<br>Widowed<br>Disabled mentally or physically<br>Dependent on caregivers<br>Often live with person neglecting them | Male or female caregivers (family or unrelated)<br>Have experienced losses in own support system<br>See victim as stressor |

The CHN role again centres on prevention. Primary prevention activities may include ensuring that the caregivers have adequate resources to support them, providing the elderly with information about abuse and resources, and reducing the isolation of the elderly (e.g., participation in day programs). Secondary prevention involves screening and supporting their decision making regarding reporting. Recall that reporting may place the elderly person at risk on return home or to the institution, so someone will be required to assist with safety planning. The CHN can play a key role in connecting the elderly with external agencies and supports or by helping them to be placed in a setting which has a strong sense of community and cohesion.

## Disaster, Conflict, Terrorism, and War

Our communities or members of our community may be exposed to **terrorism**, conflict, or other extremely traumatic events. Tragic, high-profile Canadian examples include the shootings on Parliament Hill, the Swiss air crash in Nova Scotia, police shootings such as Mayerthorpe

and Moncton, the Montreal and Taber school shootings, the Slave Lake and Lac-Megantic fires, the Ontario ice storm, and the Calgary flood. Regardless of the disaster, the CHN will be dealing with individuals, groups, and communities in crisis. As noted earlier, violence against women can increase with natural disasters as well as conflict. A key prevention strategy for the CHN is to promote resilience and provide positive support as well as activate available support resources as required. A model of support that can be used by both professionals and lay people has been described and tested in post-disaster situations (Brymer et al., 2006) and is used by the National Center for PTSD and the WHO (2011). Psychological first aid has been found to promote resilience, as it interrupts the stress reaction and helps people reframe their perceptions of dangerousness or continued threat. Key principles to assist any victim of trauma include the following three steps known as "look, listen, and link" (WHO, 2011):

- Look—Initiate contact in a non-intrusive, compassionate, helpful manner; determine immediate safety (yours and theirs); and provide physical and emotional comfort.

- Listen—Calm and orient emotionally distraught survivors; identify immediate needs and concerns; actively listen but refrain from asking about events or making them repeat information, unless the information is necessary to assist; offer practical help to address immediate needs and concerns.
- Link—Reduce distress by connecting to their preferred support persons; provide individuals with information about stress reactions and coping; link individuals to services (e.g., social work, shelter) and inform them of community services they may need to access in future.

The CHN's involvement with victims of terrorism or war is most likely to be with survivors after the violence. Examples would be immigrants or refugees from war zones who have been exposed to killing, torture, and sexual assault. Alternatively, they may have been present during a terrorist action such as a bombing or mass shooting. Terrorism can be either domestic or international (Meadows, 2010). Domestic terrorism is acts initiated within Canada by Canadians. This may come from organized crime, gangs, or other ideological groups acting against governments, policies, businesses, or organizations. In contrast, international terrorism comes from individuals or organizations outside of Canada (or the country in which the violence occurs). Regardless of the source, the result of the terrorist act is fear among the people involved. People can be indirectly affected, as we see in the media with bombings and school shootings.

Refugees from war trauma also come to Canada and may be seen by the community health nurse. They may suffer from significant physical and psychological trauma (Vargas, 2007). Sexual assault is often used as a weapon of war. It is estimated that between 20 000 and 50 000 women were raped and mutilated in Bosnia, as many as 500 000 women in Rwanda, and hundreds of thousands of women continue to be raped in the Democratic Republic of Congo (Hague & Sardinha, 2010). Many women have extensive injuries and mutilations resulting in either major surgery or death. The physical and psychological impact on women is significant, as is the impact on the community. The complexity of symptoms and effects (psychological and physical) will require multidisciplinary services for refugees of war or torture. It is most likely that they will have some symptoms of PTSD and a variety of health disturbances. The CHN plays a key role in linking the victim of war or terror to psychological and other health services in the community. Principles of care for victims of terrorism and war include the following (Coldiron, Liosa, Roederer, Casas, & Moro, 2013; Skjelsbaek, 2006; Vargas, 2007):

- services for nutrition, housing, schooling, physical care, mental healthcare, and employment to support daily functioning;
- access to complementary therapies for those with chronic pain (common after torture or explosions from damaged nerves, muscle, or bones); and
- family-focused, culturally competent support for coping; exploration and support of family strengths in coping.

## VIOLENCE AND THE COMMUNITY HEALTH NURSE

Hearing people's stories of abuse, neglect, and trauma can have serious consequences for those providing assistance. There is the risk of both direct and indirect violence to the CHN. Direct violence may occur as a result of victims re-experiencing the trauma and becoming agitated, or if they are under the influence of drugs or alcohol, or it may come from abusers if they are present. The safety of the CHN has to be a primary consideration. While it is ideal to separate the victim from the abuser for interviews or assessment, this may pose risks. Signs of escalating behaviour include anxiety (increased pacing, fingers drumming, escalated speech rate or volume), defensive manners (challenging postures or attempts to intimidate), and acting out either physically or aggressively.

The CHN may also experience indirect violence, also called "vicarious violence." This results from either witnessing the violence or trauma, or from hearing of the trauma. This form of violence can also result in the mental and physical consequences seen with direct violence, particularly PTSD. It is difficult to deal with violence and its consequences in our clients without some impact. It is important to find ways when dealing with the violence to remain supportive; recall that even the perpetrators have often been victims of violence themselves and the best remediation is to connect them with positive supports in the community. Becoming angry at the child's parent suspected of abuse is not going to be helpful to the parent or you. Signs of secondary stress from vicarious trauma include increased negative emotions, low tolerance for frustration, depression, self-destructive or negative coping mechanisms such as heavy alcohol use, or dread of work (Beck, 2011).

Resilience to vicarious violence is both internal and external to the CHN. Internal mechanisms are related to self-care. Once away from the situation, it is important that the CHN finds ways to place boundaries on the violence and to focus on activities such as sports, hobbies, and laughter (Chouliara, Hutchison, & Karatzias, 2009; VanDeusen & Way, 2006). External factors that promote resilience include accepting the support of peers and allowing time to grieve if required. It may also be necessary to seek professional assistance if the feelings interfere with enjoyment of normal activities or become overwhelming. These strategies can be summarized as the ABCs (American Institute of Stress, n.d.): Awareness of your internal resources and vulnerabilities and seeking help when needed; creating Balance in activities such as work, play, rest, and nutrition; and Connecting with others.

## VIOLENCE PREVENTION AND HEALTH PROMOTION

There was a shift in the 1990s from describing violence to increasing understanding about how to prevent violence (Sleet et al., 2011). In 1996 the WHO called violence a "leading worldwide public health problem" with Resolution WHA 49.25 (Krug, Dahlberg, et al., 2002). By 2000, the Department of Injuries and Violence Prevention was formed. Prevention methods were drawn from social and behavioural sciences, again emphasizing the importance of a combined theory of violence. As noted, the WHO identified that if violent behaviour could be predicted based on certain risk factors, then prevention efforts were possible (Carnochan et al., 2010). Prevention efforts may lead to direct effects, as with removal of risk factors or causes, or have indirect effects, as with policies or programs to reduce exposure to causes. The complex, multifaceted nature of violence requires a multi-dimensional approach to prevention rather than one specific set of activities. The WHO recommended a unified, intersectoral approach, which includes engaging professionals from healthcare, education, social services, police, justice, public safety, liquor licensing, and any other sector who can help remove or reduce underlying causes and risk factors (Carnochan et al., 2010). Together the partners can explore data in their region related to violence, look for factors contributing to risk or resilience, evaluate and implement evidence-based effective prevention strategies, and disseminate these strategies through joint training of the professionals as well as the community.

The World Health Organization (2004) has summarized a series of evidence-based strategies for violence prevention:

1. increase the numbers of safe, stable, and nurturing relationships;
2. reduce availability and misuse of alcohol;
3. reduce access to lethal means;
4. improve skills and opportunities for youth;
5. promote gender equality;
6. change cultural norms that promote violence;
7. improve criminal justice systems;
8. improve social welfare systems;
9. reduce social distance between conflicting groups; and
10. reduce economic inequality and concentrated poverty.

Adoption and dissemination of evidence-based strategies for violence prevention are essential (Sleet et al., 2011). The CHN plays a key role in violence prevention as outlined in the standards of practice (Community Health Nurses of Canada [CHNC], 2011, revised). These include screening and early detection of violence, prevention at all levels, and expanded collaboration across sectors to provide early intervention. The type of collaborative and prevention-focused approach described by the WHO is consistent with the collaborative public health approach well known to CHNs. They can work with community partners to intervene at all levels of prevention and health promotion. We have discussed some specific types of prevention within various types of violence. Examples of general strategies at various levels of intervention in the social ecological model are shown in Table 28.10 (Carnochan et al., 2010; Fagan & Catalano, 2013; Littleton, 2014; WHO, 2010).

| Table 28.10 | Examples of Prevention Activities | |
| --- | --- | --- |
| **Influence** | **Risk Factors** | **Prevention Strategies** |
| Individual | • Attitudes supporting violence<br>• History of abuse or witnessing abuse<br>• Alcohol or drug use<br>• Impulsive behaviour | • Social development programs*<br>• Involvement in recreation programs or community programs (e.g., Community Corps)<br>• Offender prevention programs (e.g., Don't Be That Guy, drug courts)<br>• Victim resistance or resiliency programs |
| Relationship | • Violent or aggressive peers<br>• Violent or patriarchal family<br>• Poor parenting skills<br>• Low socioeconomic status | • Parenting training (non-violent discipline, problem solving)*<br>• Mentoring programs<br>• Healthy relationships (building respect, trust)<br>• Communications training (e.g., Making Waves, Stepping Up) |
| Community | • Tolerance of violence<br>• Lack of police support<br>• Weak sanctions for offenders<br>• High crime rates<br>• High unemployment<br>• Inadequate victim services, supports | • Increased childcare and access to support services<br>• Community engagement activities (e.g., Cadet Corps)<br>• Preschool social enrichment programs (e.g., Roots of Empathy, Seeds of Empathy, Fourth R)<br>• Bystander intervention programs |
| Societal | • Inequality of race, gender, income<br>• Policies supporting access to alcohol or weapons<br>• Limited social policy<br>• Rapid social change<br>• Conflict<br>• Inadequate laws | • Reduced access to alcohol or density of alcohol outlets*<br>• Reduced access to lethal means*<br>• Reduced economic inequality |

*Identified as having strong evidence to support these activities; remainder have emerging evidence.

**Primary prevention programs** focus on health promotion and development of social skills in individuals, such as communication and empathy. There is strong evidence that social development programs reduce youth violence (WHO, 2010). It has been found that social programs with younger children, such as preschool or elementary school age, are more effective than older middle-school aged children (Weir, 2005). Examples of programs include "Roots of Empathy," which is aimed at enhancing empathy in young children (Weir, 2005), and the "Fourth R," which attempts to develop relationship skills in youth (Tutty et al., 2005). There are a large number of programs available, all aimed at various aspects of the influences for violence and with varying effectiveness. School-based programs have also been shown to reduce intimate partner violence and sexual violence if they are aimed at addressing gender norms and attitudes (WHO, 2010). Regardless of the program, key characteristics of effective programs are multifaceted, aimed at primary grades, include interaction and positive messaging, and aimed at promoting norms against violence (Weir, 2005).

Population primary prevention efforts relate to strategies to promote equality and respect in communities and society. Social marketing strategies have also shown promise in modifying social norms related to intimate partner violence and sexual violence. (WHO, 2010).

Selective prevention efforts are primary prevention activities that are focused on high-risk groups and individuals. Examples include parenting programs (e.g., non-violent discipline, problem solving), social or life skills training, and implementation of policies to reduce inequalities. High school and college-aged individuals are high risk for intimate partner violence and sexual assault. Programs are often aimed at sexual health, healthy relationships, and recognition of behaviours or situations that may be high risk for sexual assault or intimate partner violence. Policies and regulations aimed at regulating alcohol access and increasing the cost of alcohol are examples of population-based strategies that have been shown to lead to reductions in all forms of violence (WHO, 2010).

**Secondary prevention** efforts are focused on recognizing potential victims of violence or behaviours that are high risk for violence, and limiting further violence. As many as one-third of women reporting to emergency departments are thought to be victims of intimate partner violence (Feldhaus et al., 1997), but they are not recognized as victims (Rhodes et al., 2011). They typically come with complaints not readily linked to the abuse, such as stomach pain, headaches, depression, substance abuse issues, or gynecologic problems. The variation in illnesses makes it difficult to recognize the patients as victims of violence and to intervene appropriately to address the root cause of their problems. Screening for violence has been advocated for most populations, in particular to detect intimate partner violence, yet it is not uniformly adopted or applied (Allen, Larsen, Javdani, & Lehrner, 2012). Only 13.6% of Canadian emergency departments routinely screen their patients for intimate partner violence (McClennan, Worster, & MacMillan, 2008). Even in departments that do promote screening, there are significant problems with staff being reluctant to ask or assuming they will know who is likely a "victim" (Colarossi, Breitbart, & Betancourt, 2010). In one study of 964 victims of intimate partner violence who had reported to

police, 63.9% had at least one emergency department visit the year they reported, and in the three years following they had an average of 5.65 visits each (Kothari & Rhodes, 2006). Only one-third of these women were screened for intimate partner violence and only 5.8% of the screens were positive. Identification was made instead based on the number of visits to the emergency department for 23% of the victims.

The literature is quite clear now that intimate partner violence screening should be implemented for all women of childbearing age. The level of evidence is described as still insufficient to warrant mandatory screening for other forms of violence, yet the links between child abuse and later risks for victimization are clear (Carnochan et al., 2010; Krug & Sminkey, 2007). Some Canadian agencies have implemented screening across the lifespan. Alberta Health Services in Calgary, for instance, screens all youth, adolescents, and adults, asking if violence is a part of their lives and whether they are safe (Thurston et al., 2009). The need for screening in multiple settings by multiple professionals is consistent both with the population health approach as well as the socioecological model of violence prevention. CHNs can play a key role in screening clients of all ages for violence. One example is a healthcare team of CHNs who state, "We ask all of our clients about violence in their lives as it has such a big effect on their life, health, and safety. Is violence an issue in your life?" If clients say "Yes," then the CHNs ask if they are safe and link them to community resources that can assist. Provision of positive support to disclosure and avoiding secondary victimization are also forms of secondary prevention.

The CHN also has a key role in **tertiary prevention**, working with healthcare institutions and community agencies to identify resources to help clients reduce their violent behaviour or for victims to escape the violence and recover. Some key aspects of the WHO violence prevention model include multidisciplinary collaboration, implementing action on more than one level of intervention (individual, family, community, and population/society), and exposing clients to consistent messages from multiple sources (Carnochan et al., 2010). Multidisciplinary collaboration requires that partnerships be established between professionals in related areas. They can share data and resources, establish collaborative and complementary programs, and engage with key decision makers. There is a risk with multiple agencies working independently within the same market. They are often competing for the same resources and the net result may be reduced resources. This is known as "over-coalitioning" (Campbell, Greeson, Bybee, & Fehler-Cabral, 2012). Collaboration improves the effectiveness of knowledge dissemination (translation) to clients and the community, allocates resources more effectively, and improves uptake of evidence-informed practices among agencies working with the same populations. This also improves consistency of messaging to victims and perpetrators as well as to the community and society.

The multidisciplinary and multifaceted aspects of the WHO's socioecological model are also important given that there is not one prevention program that targets all types of offenders, nor all types of victims. Programs can be aimed at offenders, victims, bystanders, or the general public. The effectiveness of these programs may vary across populations and types of violence. For instance, offender-based programs for sexual assault prevention are shown to be effective only for those males less likely to offend, while those most likely to offend will be unaffected (Stephens & George, 2009). Programs aimed at getting bystanders to intervene have been effective with a number of types of violence, such as dating violence and sexual assault prevention (Amar et al., 2012; Banyard & Moynihan, 2011; Burn, 2009; Lonsway et al., 2011). The willingness to act and the way in which bystanders intervene varies, however, by the assessed risk in the situation.

**Social marketing** is also evolving as a prevention strategy. This involves the use of media to distribute information to the target audience in the hopes of changing norms and attitudes (Anderson & Whiston, 2005). An example of a successful campaign was the "Green Dot" program, aimed at ending sexual violence by increasing bystander intervention (Cook-Craig et al., 2014). The program was found to reduce sexual violence by 50%. Social marketing related to sexual assault aims to increase sexual assault awareness and knowledge. Each of these prevention programs is aimed at a different aspect of risk for sexual assault, has different target audiences (male, female, or both genders), and has different indicators of effectiveness (e.g., attitudes, behaviours, risk reduction). There were some key features of successful programs that helped increase their effectiveness, including the length of the program and the focus. The use of multiple programs, each with different focus, is consistent with the socioecological model of violence prevention.

Factors affecting the success of the prevention programs include the developmental stages of the people involved, the nature or culture within the community, and an understanding of change theory. Development is noted to be dynamic and the effectiveness of interventions may change with different age groups. The research on adolescent violence showed higher risks for violence in mid- to late adolescence; therefore, greater protective factors may be required (Stoddard et al., 2013). Change may be more difficult in a community or society where violence is condoned, especially against certain groups. Change theory is also important for the victim to understand. Different strategies are required if victims do not recognize the behaviours as violence, or if they are hopeless that change is possible. For instance, those who are in the pre-contemplation stage of change may be denying that what they are experiencing is abuse or may be blaming themselves. Providing them with resources for shelters will be more appropriate if they are in the contemplative or preparation phase. Persons in the pre-contemplation stage would need to receive the information that they do not deserve the abuse, that they are not alone, and other positive support.

The role of the CHN and the CHNs' standards of practice (CHNC, 2011, revised) align strongly with the social ecological model of violence prevention. Examples include helping individuals recognize risks to health, using harm reduction principles, providing protection and prevention services, collaborative partnerships for interventions and follow-up, and using epidemiology to plan strategies to reduce violence. The CHN can become involved in violence prevention at many levels.

## CASE STUDY

This afternoon you are visiting a family in the community after the birth of their child. The mother has a 13-year-old son from a previous relationship and this is the couple's first baby after two years together. The mother and father are both present. You ask the mother about how she is sleeping and the father tells you she is doing fine. You note that she looks pale and fatigued. As you hand her an information pamphlet you note some bruises on her wrist. You ask the mother about the baby's health and the father tells you that the baby seems to be very "needy" and perhaps is being fed too often, about every three hours. You ask if there are any concerns with the baby and the father tells you that the baby cries a lot and that his wife is "fussing" too much with the baby, perhaps making the baby too spoiled.

While you are there they receive a phone call from the school. The older child, the 13-year-old, is being sent home for an incident in which he started a fight with another child at the school. He is being suspended for three days. The parents have been asked to come to the school to meet with the principal. When the mother relays this information to the father he gets up from couch and begins pacing. He says to his wife, "It's your fault—you always let him get away with everything. He needs discipline! This is the second time this month he's been suspended. On top of that you know he's sneaking around with those kids who do drugs. You do nothing." He remembers you are in the room and becomes quiet again.

### Discussion Questions

1. What are your concerns for this mother and why?
2. What concerns do you have for the children and why?
3. What actions would you recommend and why?

## CONCLUSION

Violence has been identified as a significant public health problem that must be addressed. We have seen through this chapter that many of the risk factors for the various types of abuse are interrelated. Violence is best explained through a socioecological model due to the complex interplay of factors that may result in violence. Similarly, violence prevention must also be multifaceted and involve multiple professionals and the community. The CHN plays a key role in brokering partnerships and providing links between services to better support victims of violence and perpetrators in their recovery. They need to receive positive support, be linked into networks, and have a sense of control over regaining their lives. The nurse also has a key role in working to effect changes in communities and implementing social policies to reduce inequities and power differentials that may be responsible for violence. The CHN's focus on family-centred care and collaboration are key components to success with violence prevention and early intervention. Their ability to directly interact with both individuals and families allows them opportunities to screen for violence, promote healthy behaviours, and link into the network of community agencies for early and effective intervention.

## KEY TERMS

## STUDY QUESTIONS

1. Caitlin is a 15-year-old high school student. She has come to the public health office looking for the "morning-after pill" (emergency contraception). You explore with her what circumstances led to her requiring this and she reveals that her 19-year-old boyfriend got her drunk and had sex with her. She doesn't want her parents or police to know. She doesn't think it is sexual assault, since they have had sex before. Which of the following statements is correct?

   a. This must be reported to police as it is outside the close-in-age exception.

   b. She requires her parents' permission to have the emergency contraception.

   c. It is her choice whether or not to report and her parents cannot be told.

   d. If they have had sex before it is not considered sexual assault.

2. Bobby is a 2-year-old who is in the home when you do a postpartum home visit. He has a cast on his arm. His mother says that he falls down all the time and is quite clumsy. You see from your files that he has previously had a head injury, another visit to the ER for abdominal bruising (again reportedly from a fall), and has not been kept up to date with his vaccinations. Which statement is correct?

   a. These injuries are understandable given he falls frequently.

   b. Your concerns should be shared with Children's Services.

   c. You should confront the mother about whether she is abusing her child.

   d. You need to be more sure before any authorities are notified.

3. Which statement is correct about injuries and physical findings if intimate partner abuse is suspected?

   a. Bruises of different colours in different locations are normal on the body.

   b. The extremities are most often affected by injuries.

   c. A bruise and ecchymosis mean the same thing.

   d. An open wound with rough edges and hair across it is from blunt objects.

4. A tornado has just come through your community and you are called to assist at a nearby community centre. A number of elderly people have been brought from a nearby seniors' centre that was demolished. Many of the elderly are pacing and agitated, and appear confused or distressed. Which of the following statements is correct?

   a. These are abnormal responses to the trauma and they may need sedation.

   b. Spending time listening to them will be helpful.

   c. Confusion in the elderly is a normal finding.

   d. Asking them specific questions about the trauma will be helpful.

5. A woman is in the public health offices for her flu vaccination. While examining her you note she has multiple bruises on her arms, and bruises on her face. When you screen her for intimate partner violence, she says she is not abused, just clumsy, although sometimes her husband has to give her "heck" because she does "silly" things. Think about the readiness to change. Which would be the most appropriate action for her at this time?

   a. Provide information that no one deserves abuse and describe abusive behaviours.

b. Provide her with a list of printed materials and discuss safety plans.

c. Make her aware of the signs of risks for lethality and link her to community services.

d. Call police to report the abuse and discuss the need for restraining orders.

6. Which of the following statements are correct about stress and consequences of violence?

a. Somatic pain is imagined and likely indicates drug-seeking behaviour.

b. Sustained stress can cause autoimmune and cardiac disorders.

c. The freeze response is very rare with sexual assault.

d. Symptoms of acute stress reactions normally last up to seven days.

---

After working through these questions, go to the MyNursingLab at www.pearsoned.ca/mynursinglab to check your answers.

---

## INDIVIDUAL CRITICAL-THINKING EXERCISES

1. You are going to a home visit for an elderly woman being cared for by her adult daughter in the daughter's home. Think about the following questions:

a. What indicators would you look for to determine the elderly woman's well-being?

b. How might you explore potential caregiver stress with the daughter?

c. What would you do if you suspected abuse?

2. You are working with an elementary school. The teachers are complaining about a particular male student, 10 years old, who is consistently bullying other students. The faculty would like to suspend him.

a. What factors should you consider and what information should you gather about the boy?

b. What type of education might you provide to the teaching staff?

3. You are working with an individual who is a victim of abuse by a same-sex partner. She doesn't want to report the abuse as she is afraid of her partner, especially if the abuser doesn't remain in custody of police. The victim has already had a fractured arm.

a. How will you manage this?

b. What factors should be considered in dealing with this situation?

4. A father of a young infant discloses to you that he was a victim of childhood abuse. He has heard that abused men usually become abusers.

a. What will you tell him?

b. How can you support him in his new role as a father?

c. What community resources are available to you?

5. A fellow student came to you and revealed she was sexually assaulted. She didn't want to have an examination as she is worried the police will be called. It was someone from her dormitory and she sees him often. She was worried if she tells that the school will become involved, and that her education will be affected.

a. What could you tell her?

b. What resources are available to you?

c. How would you know if she needed further assistance?

6. You are providing outreach education to a group of immigrant refugee women from a war zone. The CHN office has information that some of these women may have been victims of sexual assault, forced marriages, and female genital mutilation. You are being asked to provide information related to abuse. A translator is needed.

a. What are some of the considerations involved prior to meeting with them?

b. What considerations do you have for the translator?

## GROUP CRITICAL-THINKING EXERCISES

1. You are working with an inner-city population (think of one in your local area). There are high levels of prostitution, homelessness, mental health problems, and drug use in the area. Your group of students has been invited to come and do some health promotion in the area and you want to focus on reducing their risks for violence.

a. What type of activity might you introduce and why?

b. Think about the information on closing the health equity gap from Canadian Research Box 28.2. Identify at least two other strategies you might use.

2. You have been invited to a local high school to help work with them on a dating violence prevention program for Grade 10 girls. So far you are the only professional who has been invited to set this up.

a. What types of messages would you want to convey and why?

b. What types of activities might you have for the program and why?

c. Who else should be involved in the program and why?

3. The provincial government is trying to establish a family violence prevention network. They have asked for representatives from various sectors to become involved and you are representing CHNs on the advisory group. There are lawyers, policy makers, health services administrators, police, and social workers in attendance.

a. If you only were able to start with one type of violence and/or age group to develop interventions, what would be important for your community and why?

b. What types of funding, laws, or policies do you think would be needed at the provincial level to support the violence prevention efforts?

c. How could you disseminate the information so the public and other professionals will be aware of the efforts (consider the age group, community and existing services in your community)?

# REFERENCES

Abbey, A., Clinton-Sherrod, A., McAuslan, P., Zawacki, T., & Buck, P. O. (2003). The relationship between the quantity of alcohol consumed and the severity of sexual assaults committed by college men. *Journal of Interpersonal Violence, 18*(7), 813–833.

Abrams, M. P., Carleton, R. N., Taylor, S., & Asmundson, G. J. (2009). Human tonic immobility: Measurement and correlates. *Depression & Anxiety (1091–4269), 26*(6), 550–556. doi:10.1002/da.20462

Acierno, R., Hernandez, M. A., Arnstader, A. B., Resnick, H. S., Steve, K., Muzzy, W., & Kilpatrick, D. G. (2010). Prevalence and correlates of emotional, physical, sexual and financial abuse and potential neglect in the United States: The national elder mistreatment study. *American Journal of Public Health, 100*(2), 292–297.

Acierno, R., Resnick, H., Kilpatrick, D. G., Saunders, B., & Best, C. L. (1999). Risk factors for rape, physical assault, and posttraumatic stress disorder in women: Examination of differential multivariate relationships. *Journal of Anxiety Disorders, 13*(6), 541–563.

Afifi, T. O., & Macmillan, H. L. (2011). Resilience following child maltreatment: A review of protective factors. *Canadian Journal of Psychiatry, Revue canadienne de psychiatrie, 56*(5), 266–272.

Ahrens, C. E., Cabral, G., & Abeling, S. (2009). Healing or hurtful: Sexual assault survivors' interpretations of social reactions from support providers. *Psychology of Women Quarterly, 33*(1), 81–F94.

Allen, N., Larsen, S., Javdani, S., & Lehrner, A. (2012). Council-based approaches to reforming the health care response to domestic violence: Promising findings and cautionary tales. *American Journal of Community Psychology, 50*(1), 50–63. http://dx.doi.org/10.1007/s10464-011-9471-9

Allen, C. T., Swan, S. C., & Raghavan, C. (2009). Gender symmetry, sexism, and intimate partner violence. *Journal of Interpersonal Violence, 24*(11), 1816–1834.

Amar, A. (2013). Sexual violence and the campus: Chants and silence. *Aljazeera.* Retrieved from http://www.aljazeera.com/indepth/opinion/2013/09/sexual-violence-campus-chants-silence-2013929121721152931.html

Amar, A. F., Sutherland, M., Laughon, K., Bess, R., & Stockbridge, J. (2012). Peer influences within the campus environment on help seeking related to violence. *Journal of National Black Nurses' Association: JNBNA, 23*(1), 1–7.

American Institute of Stress. (n.d.). Compassion fatigue. Retrieved June 3, 2015, from http://www.stress.org/military/for-practitionersleaders/compassion-fatigue

American Psychiatric Association. (2013). *Diagnostic and statistical manual of mental disorders* (5th ed.). Washington, DC: American Psychiatric Association.

Anastario, M., Shehab, N., & Lawry, L. (2009). Increased gender-based violence among women internally displaced in Mississippi 2 years post-Hurricane Katrina. *Disaster Medicine and Public Health Preparedness, 3*(1), 18–26.

Anda, R., Tietjen, G., Schulman, E., Felitti, V., & Croft, J. (2010). Adverse childhood experiences and frequent headaches in adults. *Headache: The Journal of Head & Face Pain, 50*(9), 1473–1481. doi:10.1111/j.1526-4610.2010.01756.x

Anderson, L. A., & Whiston, S. C. (2005). Sexual assault education programs: A meta-analytic examination of their effectiveness. *Psychology of Women Quarterly, 29*(4), 374–388. http://dx.doi.org/10.1111/j.1471-6402.2005.00237.x

Anderson, S., McClain, N., & Riviello, R. J. (2006). Genital findings of women after consensual and nonconsensual intercourse. *Journal of Forensic Nursing, 2*(2), 59–65.

Andersson, N., & Nahwegahbow, A. (2010). Family violence and the need for prevention research in First Nations, Inuit, and Metis communities. *Pimatisiwin, 8*(2), 9.

Applebaum, P. S. (2006). Violence and mental disorders. *Data and public policy, 163*(8), 1319–1321.

Arboleda-Florez, J. (2009). Mental illness and violence. *Current Opinions in Psychiatry, 22*(5), 475–476. doi:10.1097/YCO.0b013e32832c08fc

Ard, K., & Makadon, H. (2011). Addressing intimate partner violence in lesbian, gay, bisexual, and transgender patients. *JGIM: Journal of General Internal Medicine, 26*(8), 930–933. doi:10.1007/s11606-011-1697-6

Averill, J. B. R., Padilla, A. O., & Clements, P. T. (2007). Frightened in isolation: Unique considerations for research of sexual assault and interpersonal violence in rural areas. *Journal of Forensic Nursing, 3*(1), 42–46.

Baldwin, S. B., Eisenman, D. P., Sayles, J. N., Ryan, G., & Chuang, K. S. (2011). Identification of human trafficking victims in health care settings. *Health and Human Rights, 13*(1), 1–14.

Balogh, R., Bretherton, K., Whibley, S., Berney, T., Graham, S., Richold, P., . . . Firth, H. (2001). Sexual abuse in children and adolescents with intellectual disability. *Journal of Intellectual Disability Research, 45*, 194–201.

Banyard, V. L., & Moynihan, M. M. (2011). Variation in bystander behavior related to sexual and intimate partner violence prevention: Correlates in a sample of college students. *Psychology of Violence, 1*(4), 287–301. Retrieved from http://dx.doi.org/10.1037/a0023544

Bebbington, P. E., Jonas, S., Brugha, T., Meltzer, H., Jenkins, R., Cooper, C., . . . McManus, S. (2011). Child sexual abuse reported by an English national sample: Characteristics and demography. *Social Psychiatry and Psychiatric Epidemiology, 46*(3), 255–262.

Beck, C. T. (2011). Secondary traumatic stress in nurses: A systematic review. *Archives of Psychiatric Nursing, 25*(1), 1–10. http://dx.doi.org/10.1016/j.apnu.2010.05.005

Bellis, M. A., Hughes, K., Leckenby, N., Jones, L., Baban, A., Kacheva, M., . . . Terzic, N. (2014). Adverse childhood experiences and associations with health-harming behaviours in young adults in eight eastern European countries. *Bulletin of the World Health Organization, 92*(9), 641–655. Retrieved from http://www.who.int/bulletin/volumes/92/9/13-129247/en

Bennett, S., Banyard, V. L., & Garnhart, L. (2014). To act or not to act, that is the question? Barriers and facilitators of bystander intervention. *Journal of Interpersonal Violence, 29*(3), 476–496. Retrieved from http://dx.doi.org/10.1177/0886260513505210

Benyan, C. M., McVeigh, C., McVeigh, J., Leavey, C., & Bellis, M. A. (2008). The involvement of drugs and alcohol in drug facilitated sexual assault. *Trauma Violence and Abuse, 9*, 178–188.

Benz, J. L. (2010). *Life experiences of adults who witnessed domestic violence as children.* (Doctoral dissertation). Retrieved from Proquest Dissertations and Theses (Publication number 3419716).

Bernat, D. H., Oakes, J. M., Pettingell, S. L., & Resnick, M. (2012). Risk and direct protective factors for youth violence: Results from the National Longitudinal Study of Adolescent Health. *American Journal of Preventive Medicine, 43*(2), S57–S66. doi:10.1016/j.amepre.2012.04.023

Bisson, J., & Andrew, M. (2009). Psychological treatment of post-traumatic stress disorder (PTSD) (review). *Cochrane Database Systematic Review.* Retrieved from http://onlinelibrary.wiley.com/doi/10.1002/14651858.CD003388.pub3/pdf

Bloom, T., Wagman, J., Hernandez, R., Yrgui, N., Hernandez-Valdovinos, N., Dahlstrom, M., & Glass, N. (2009). Partnering with community-based organizations to reduce intimate partner violence. *Hispanic Journal of Behavioral Sciences, 31*(2).

Blume, T. W. (1996). Social perspectives on violence. *Michigan Family Review, 2*(1), 9–23. Retrieved from http://hdl.handle.net/2027/spo.4919087.0002.102

Bombay, A., Matheson, K., & Anisman, H. (2009). Intergenerational trauma: Convergence of multiple processes among First Nations peoples in Canada. *Journal of Aboriginal Health* (November), 6–47.

Bonomi, A. E., Altenburger, L. E., & Walton, N. L. (2013). "Double crap!" Abuse and harmed identity in Fifty Shades of Grey. *Journal of Women's Health, 22*(9), 733–744.

Bonomi, A. E., Anderson, M. L., Rivara, F. P., & Thompson, R. S. (2009). Health care utilization and costs associated with physical and nonphysical-only intimate partner violence. *Health Services Research, 44*(3), 1052–1067.

Bowman, M. L. (2007). Responding to frightening life events. *Visions: Trauma and Victimization, 3*(3), 6.

Bracha, H. S. (2004). Freeze, flight, fight, fright, faint: Adaptationist perspectives on the acute stress response spectrum. *CNS Spectrum, 9*(9), 679–685.

Bradshaw, C. P., Waasdorp, T. E., Goldweber, A., & Johnson, S. L. (2013). Bullies, gangs, drugs, and school: Understanding the overlap and the role of ethnicity and urbanicity. *Journal of Youth and Adolescence, 42*(2), 220–234. doi:10.1007/s10964-012-9863-7

Brecklin, L. R., & Ullman, S. E. (2005). Self-defense or assertiveness training and women's responses to sexual attacks. *Journal of Interpersonal Violence, 20*(6), 738–762. doi:10.1177/0886260504272894

Brennan, S. (2011). Violent victimization of Aboriginal women in Canadian provinces 2009. Report 85-002-X, *Juristat,* May 17. Retrieved from http://www.statcan.gc.ca/pub/85-002-x/2011001/article/11439-eng.pdf

Brennan, S., & Taylor-Butts, A. (2008). *Sexual assault in Canada: 2004 and 2007.* (No. 85F0033M). Retrieved from http://www.statcan.gc.ca/pub/85f0033m/85f0033m2008019-eng.pdf

Brenner, A. (2013). Resisting simple dichotomies: Critiquing narratives of victims, perpetrators, and harm in feminist theories of rape. *Harvard Journal of Law & Gender, 36*(2), 503–568.

Briceno-Leon, R., Villaveces, A., & Concha-Eastman, A. (2008). Understanding the uneven distribution of homicide in Latin America. *International Journal of Epidemiology, 37,* 751–757.

Brown, D. W., Anda, R. F., Tiemeier, H., Felitti, V. J., Edwards, V. J., Croft, J. B., & Giles, W. H. (2009).

Adverse childhood experiences and the risk of premature mortality. *American Journal of Preventive Medicine, 37*(5), 389–396.

Brown, R., Du Mont, J., Macdonald, S., & Bainbridge, D. (2013). A comparative analysis of victims of sexual assault with and without mental health histories: Acute and follow-up care characteristics. *Journal of Forensic Nursing, 9*(2), 76–83.

Brown, K., Streubert, G. E., & Burgess, A. W. (2004). Effectively detect and manage elder abuse. *Nurse Practitioner, 29*(8), 31.

Brown, A. J., Varcoe, C. M., Wong, S. T., Smye, V. L., Lavoie, J., Littlejohn, D., . . . Lennox, S. (2012). Closing the health equity gap: Evidence based strategies for primary health care organizations. *International Journal for Equity in Health, 11*(1), 59–73.

Browning, S., & Erickson, P. (2009). Neighbourhood disadvantage, alcohol use, and violent victimization. *Youth Violence and Juvenile Justice, 7*(4), 331–349.

Bryant, R. A. (2013). An update of acute stress disorder. *PTSD Research Quarterly, 24*(1), 1–6.

Brymer, M., Jacobs, A., Layne, C., Pynoos, R., Steinberg, A., Vernberg, E., & Watson, P. (2006). *Psychological first aid (PFA) field operations guide* (2nd ed.). Washington, DC: National Center for Posttraumatic Stress. Retrieved from http://resourcecentre.savethechildren.se/library/psychological-first-aid-field-operations-guide-2nd-edition

Brzozowski, J. A., Taylor-Butts, A., & Johnson, S. (2006). Victimization and offending among the Aboriginal population in Canada. *Juristat, 26*(3), 1–31.

Bullard, M. J., Unger, B., Spence, J., & Grafstein, E. (2008). Revisions to the Canadian emergency department triage and acuity scale (CTAS) adult guidelines. *CJEM: Canadian Journal of Emergency Medicine, 10*(2), 136–142.

Burgess, A. W., Watt, M. E., Brown, K. M., & Petrozzi, D. (2006). Management of elder sexual abuse cases in critical care settings. *Critical Care Clinics of North America, 18*(3), 313–319.

Burn, S. (2009). A situational model of sexual assault prevention through bystander intervention. *Sex Roles, 60*(11), 779–792. http://dx.doi.org/10.1007/s11199-008-9581-5

Butchart, A., Phinney, A., Check, P., & Villaveces, A. (2004). *Preventing violence: A guide to implementing the recommendations of the world report on violence and health.* Geneva, Switzerland: Department of Injuries and Violence Prevention, World Health Organization.

Campbell, J. (2010). *Dangerousness assessment.* Retrieved from http://www.dangerassessment.org/WebApplication1/pages/da

Campbell, J., Webster, D. W., & Glass, N. (2009). The danger assessment: Validation of a lethality risk assessment instrument for intimate partner femicide. *Journal of Interpersonal Violence, 24*(4), 653–74. Retrieved from http://dx.doi.org/10.1177/0886260508317180

Campbell, J. C., Sharps, P., Laughon, K., Webster, D., Manganello, J., Schollenberger, J., . . . Frye, V. A. (2003). Risk factors for femicide in abusive relationships: Results from a multisite case control study. *American Journal of Public Health, 93*(7), 1089–1098.

Campbell, R. (2012). Webinar: The neurobiology of sexual assault: Implications for first responders in law enforcement, prosecution, and victim advocacy. Retrieved from nij.gov/multimedia/presenter/presenter-campbell/Pages/welcome.aspx

Campbell, R., Greeson, M., Bybee, D., & Fehler-Cabral, G. (2012). Adolescent sexual assault victims and the legal system: Building community relationships to improve prosecution rates. *American Journal of Community Psychology, 50*(1), 141–154. http://dx.doi.org/10.1007/s10464-011-9485-3

Campbell, R. (2005). What really happened? A validation study of rape survivors' help-seeking experiences with the legal and medical systems. *Violence and Victims, 20*(1), 55–68.

Campbell, R., Wasco, S. M., Ahrens, C. E., Sefl, T., & Barnes, H. E. (2001). Preventing the "second rape": Rape survivors' experiences with community service providers. *Journal of Interpersonal Violence, 16*(12), 1239–1259.

Canadian Centre for Elder Law. (2011). A practical guide for elder abuse and neglect law in Canada. Retrieved from http://www.bcli.org/sites/default/files/Practical_Guide_English_Rev_JULY_2011.pdf

Canadian Child Welfare Research Portal. (2011). Child welfare–Frequently asked questions. Retrieved from http://cwrp.ca/faqs

Canadian Mental Health Association. (2011). *Violence and mental health: Unpacking a complex issue.* Toronto, ON: Canadian Mental Health Association, Ontario. Retrieved from http://ontario.cmha.ca/public_policy/violence-and-mental-health-unpacking-a-complex-issue/#.VXX3d89Viko

Canadian Network for the Prevention of Elder Abuse. (2011). Canadian laws on abuse and neglect. Webpage.

Cannon, E. A., Bonomi, A. E., Anderson, M. L., & Rivara, F. P. (2009). The intergenerational transmission of witnessing intimate partner violence. *Archives of Pediatrics & Adolescent Medicine, 163*(8), 706–708.

Carnochan, J., Butchart, A., Feucht, T., Mikton, C., & Shepherd, J. (2010). *Violence prevention: An invitation to intersectoral action.* Geneva: World Health Organization. Retrieved from http://www.who.int/violenceprevention/about/intersectoral_action.pdf

Carter-Snell, C. (2015). Dating violence: The silent epidemic. In M. Taylor, J. A. Pooley, & R. Taylor (Eds.), *Overcoming domestic violence: Creating a dialogue around vulnerable populations* (pp. 49–65). Australia: Nova Science.

Carter-Snell, C., & Jakubec, S. L. (2013). Exploring influences on mental health after interpersonal violence against women. *International Journal of Child, Youth and Family Studies, 4*(1), 72–99.

Carter-Snell, C. (2011). Injury documentation: Using the BALD STEP mnemonic and the RCMP sexual assault kit. *Outlook, 34*(1), 15–20.

Carter-Snell, C. J. (2007). *Understanding women's risks of injury from sexual assault.* (Doctoral dissertation). Edmonton, AB: University of Alberta. Retrieved from http://www.mtroyal.ca/cs/groups/public/documents/pdf/pdf_womensrisksforinjury.pdf

Carter-Snell, C., & Hegadoren, K. (2003). Stress disorders and gender: Implications for theory and research. *Canadian Journal of Nursing Research, 35*(2), 34–55.

CCSO Cybercrime Working Group, Department of Justice. (2013). *Cyber-bullying and the non-consensual distribution of intimate images.* Retrieved from http://www.justice.gc.ca/eng/rp-pr/other-autre/cndii-cdncii/pdf/cndii-cdncii-eng.pdf

Centers for Disease Control. (2009). *The social-ecological model: A framework for prevention.* Retrieved from http://www.cdc.gov/violenceprevention/overview/social-ecologicalmodel.html

Centers for Disease Control. (2014). *Child maltreatment: Facts at a glance.* Atlanta, GA: Center for Disease Control. Retrieved from http://www.cdc.gov/violenceprevention/pdf/childmaltreatment-facts-at-a-glance.pdf

Chang, L. Y., Foshee, V. A., Reyes, H. L. M., Ennett, S. T., & Halpern, C. T. (2015). Direct and indirect effects of neighbourhood characteristics on the perpetration of dating violence across adolescence. *Journal of Youth and Adolescence, 44,* 727–744.

Charmandari, E., Tsigos, C., & Chrousos, G. (2005). Endocrinology of the stress response. *Annual Review of Physiology, 67,* 259–284.

Chartier, M. J., Walker, J. R., & Naimark, B. (2010). Separate and cumulative effects of adverse childhood experience predicting health and health care utilization. *Child Abuse and Neglect, 34*(6), 454–464. doi: 10.1016/j.chiabu.2009.09.020

Chouliara, Z., Hutchison, C., & Karatzias, T. (2009). Vicarious traumatisation in practitioners who work with adult survivors of sexual violence and child sexual abuse: Literature review and directions for future research. *Counselling & Psychotherapy Research, 9*(1), 47–56. doi:10.1080/14733140802656479

Christian, C. W. (2011). Timing of the medical examination. *Journal of Child Sexual Abuse, 20*(5), 505–520. Retrieved from http://dx.doi.org/10.1080/10538712.2011.607424

Christiansen, D., Bak, R., & Elklit, A. (2012). Secondary victims of rape. *Violence and Victims, 27*(2), 246–262.

Classen, C. C., Palesh, O. G., & Aggarwal, R. (2005). Sexual revictimization: A review of the empirical literature. *Trauma, Violence & Abuse, 6*(2), 103–129.

Coker, A. L., Hopenhayn, C., DeSimone, C. P., Bush, H. M., & Crofford, L. (2009). Violence against women raises risk of cervical cancer. *Journal of Women's Health (2002), 18*(8), 1179–1185.

Cohen, L., Davis, R., & Graffunder, C. (2005). Before it occurs: The primary prevention of intimate partner violence. Washington, DC: Prevention Institute-Center for Disease Control. Retrieved from http://www.preventioninstitute.org/component/jlibrary/article/id-40/127.html

Colarossi, L., Breitbart, V., & Betancourt, G. (2010). Barriers to screening for intimate partner violence: A mixed-methods study of providers in family planning clinics. *Perspectives on Sexual & Reproductive Health, 42*(4), 236–243. Retrieved from http://dx.doi.org/10.1363/4223610

Coldiron, M. E., Llosa, A. E., Roederer, T., Casas, G., & Moro, M.-R. (2013). Brief mental health interventions in conflict and emergency settings: An overview of four Medecins Sans Frontieres—France programs. *Conflict & Health, 7*(1), 1–11. doi:10.1186/1752-1505-7-23

Community Health Nurses of Canada. (2011, revised). *Canadian community health nursing: Professional practice model & standards of practice.* St. John's, NL: Author. Retrieved from https://www.chnc.ca/documents/CHNC-ProfessionalPracticeModel-EN/index.html

Connop, V., & Petrak, J. (2004). The impact of sexual assault on heterosexual couples. *Sexual & Relationship Therapy, 19*(1), 29–38.

Connor, J., You, R., & Casswell, S. (2009). Alcohol-related harm to others: A survey of physical and sexual assault in New Zealand. *The New Zealand Medical Journal, 122*(1303), 10–20.

Cook-Craig, P. G., Millspaugh, P. H., Reckenfeld, E. A., Kelly, N. C., Hegge, L. M., Coker, A. L., & Pletcher, T. S. (2014). From empower to Green Dot: Successful strategies and lessons learned in developing comprehensive sexual violence prevention programming. *Violence Against Women, 20*(10), 1162–1178.

Cox Communications. (2009). Teen online & wireless safety survey. Retrieved from http://www.cox.com/wcm/en/aboutus/datasheet/takecharge/2009-teen-survey.pdf?campcode=takecharge-research-link_2009-teen-survey_0511

Coxell, A. W., & King, M. B. (2010). Adult male rape and sexual assault: Prevalence, re-victimisation and the tonic immobility response. *Sexual and Relationship Therapy, 25*(4), 372–379.

Craig, W., & McCuaig, H. (2012). *Bullying and fighting.* Ottawa, ON: Public Health Agency of Canada. Retrieved from http://www.phac-aspc.gc.ca/hp-ps/dca-dea/publications/hbsc-mental-mentale/bullying-intimidation-eng.php

Craig, C. D., & Sprang, G. (2007). Trauma exposure and child abuse potential: Investigating the cycle of violence. *American Journal of Orthopsychiatry, 77*(2), 296–305. http://dx.doi.org/10.1037/0002-9432.77.2.296

Craig, W. M., & Pepler, D. J. (2003). Identifying and targeting risk for involvement in bullying and victimization. *Canadian Journal of Psychiatry, 48*(9), 577–582.

Crane, P. A., & Moreno, M. (2011). Human trafficking: What is the role of the health care provider? *Journal of Applied Research on Children: Informing Policy for Children at Risk, 2*(1), e-journal.

Criminal Intelligence Service Canada. (2010). *Street gangs in Canada.* Retrieved from http://cisc.gc.ca/annual_reports/annual_report_2010/street_gangs_2010_e.html

Cunradi, C. B., Mair, C., Ponicki, W., & Remer, L. (2012). Alcohol outlet density and intimate partner violence-related emergency department visits. *Alcoholism, Clinical and Experimental Research, 36*(5), 847–853. doi:10.1111/j.1530-0277.2011.01683.x

Cyr, K., Clement, M.-A. V., & Chamberland, C. (2013). Lifetime prevalence of multiple victimizations and its impact on children's mental health. *Journal of Interpersonal Violence, 29*(4), 616–634. doi:10.1177/0886260513505220

Danese, A., & McEwen, B. S. (2012). Adverse childhood experiences, allostasis, allostatic load, and age-related disease. *Physiology & Behavior, 106,* 29–39. doi:10.1016/j.physbeh.2011.08.019

Daoud, N., Urquia, M. L., O'Campo, P., Heaman, M., Janssen, P. A., Smylie, J., & Thiessen, K. (2012). Prevalence of abuse and violence before, during and after pregnancy in a national sample of Canadian women. *American Journal of Public Health, 102,* 1893–1901.

Deans, K. J., Thackeray, J., Groner, J. L., Cooper, J. N., & Minneci, P. C. (2014). Risk factors for recurrent injuries in victims of non-accidental trauma: A retrospective cohort study. *BMC Pediatrics, 31*(14), 217.

Delevi, R., & Weisskirch, R. S. (2013). Personality factors as predictors of sexting. *Computers in Human Behavior, 29,* 2589–2594. doi:10.1016/j.chb.2013.06.003

Department of Justice. (2013). *Age of consent to sexual activity.* Ottawa, ON: Author. Retrieved from http://www.justice.gc.ca/eng/rp-pr/other-autre/clp/faq.html

Duke, N. N., Pettingell, S. L., McMorris, B. J., & Borowsky, I. W. (2010). Adolescent violence perpetration: Associations with multiple types of adverse childhood experiences. *Pediatrics. 5*(4), e778–e786.

Duffy, J. Y., Hughes, M., Asnes, A. G., & Leventhal, J. M. (2014). Child maltreatment and risk patterns among participants in a child abuse prevention program. *Child Abuse and Neglect,* advance online publication. Retrieved from http://www.ncbi.nlm.nih.gov/pubmed/25484318

Du Mont, J., Macdonald, S., Rotbard, N., Bainbridge, D., Asilani, E., Smith, N., & Cohen, M. M. (2010). Drug-facilitated sexual assault in Ontaro, Canada: Toxicological and DNA findings. *Journal of Forensic & Legal Medicine, 17*(6), 333–338.

Dylan, A., Regehr, C., & Alaggia, R. (2008). And justice for all? Aboriginal victims of sexual violence. *Violence Against Women, 14*(6), 678–696.

Edwards, K. M., Sylaska, K. M., Barry, J. E., Moynihan, M. M., Banyard, V. L., Cohn, E. S., . . . Ward, S. K. (2015). Physical dating violence, sexual violence and unwanted pursuit victimization: A comparison of incidence rates among sexual-minority and heterosexual college students. *Journal of Interpersonal Violence, 30*(4), 580–600.

Elgar, F. J., Pickett, K. E., Pickett, W., Craig, W., Molcho, M., Hurrelmann, K., & Lenzi, M. (2013). School bullying, homicide and income inequality: A cross-national pooled time series analysis. *International Journal of Public Health, 58*(2), 237–245. doi:10.1007/s00038-012-0380-y

Espelage, D. L., Low, S., Rao, M. A., Hong, J. S., & Little, T. D. (2014). Family violence, bullying, fighting and substance use among adolescents: A longitudinal mediational model. *Journal of Research on Adolescence, 24*(2), 337–349.

Fagan, A. A., & Catalano, R. F. (2013). What works in youth violence prevention: A review of the literature. *Research on Social Work Practice, 23*(2), 141–156. Retrieved from http://dx.doi.org/10.1177/1049731512465899

Falb, K. L., McCauley, H. L., Decker, M. R., Gupta, J., Raj, A., & Silverman, J. G. (2011). School bullying perpetration and other childhood risk factors as predictors of adult intimate partner violence perpetration. *Archives in Pediatric Adolescent Medicine, 165*(10), 890–894.

Federal Provincial Territorial Ministers. (2002). *Assessing violence against women: A statistical profile.* Ottawa, ON: Government of Canada. Retrieved from https://www.gnb.ca/0037/report/Statusofwomen-e.pdf

Feldhaus, K. M., Koziol-McLain, J., Amsbury, H. L., Norton, I. M., Lowenstein, S. R., & Abbott, J. T. (1997). Accuracy of 3 brief screening questions for detecting partner violence in the emergency department. *JAMA, 277,* 1357–1361.

Felson, R. B., & Cundiff, P. R. (2014). Sexual assault as a crime against young people. *Archives of Sexual Behavior, 43*(2), 273–284.

Flaherty, E. G., Perez-Rossello, J. M., Levine, M. A., Hennrikus, W. L., & American Academy of Pediatrics Committee on Child Abuse and Neglect, Section on Radiology, Section on Endocrinology, Section on Orthopedics, the Society for Pediatric Radiology. (2014). Evaluating children with fractures for child physical abuse. *Pediatrics, 133*(2), e477–e489.

Flicker, S. M., Cerulli, C., Swogger, M. T., & Talbot, N. L. (2012). Depressive and posttraumatic symptoms among women seeking protection orders against intimate partners: Relations to coping strategies and perceived responses to abuse disclosure. *Violence Against Women, 18*(4), 420–436. http://dx.doi.org/10.1177/1077801212448897

Frazer, E., & Hutchings, K. (2008). On politics and violence: Arendt contra Fanon. *Contemporary Political Theory, 7,* 90–108.

Friedman, R. A. (2006). Violence and mental illness—how strong is the link? *The New England Journal of Medicine, 355,* 2064–2066. doi:10.1056/NEJMp068229

Frye, V., Manganello, J., Campbell, J. C., Walton-Moss, B., & Wilt, S. (2006). The distribution of and factors associated with intimate terrorism and situational couple violence among a population-based sample of urban women in the United States. *Journal of Interpersonal Violence, 21*(10), 1286–1313.

Gagne, M. H., Lavoie, F., & Hebert, M. (2005). Victimization during childhood and revictimization in dating relationships in adolescent girls. *Child Abuse & Neglect, 29*(10), 1155–1172.

Giardino, A. P., & Finkel, M. A. (2005). Evaluating child sexual abuse. *Pediatric Annals, 34*(5), 382–394.

Gidycz, C. A., Van Wynsberghe, A., & Edwards, K. M. (2008). Prediction of women's utilization of resistance strategies in a sexual assault situation: A prospective study. *Journal of Interpersonal Violence, 23*(5), 571–588.

Glass, N., Perrin, N., Campbell, J. C., & Soeken, K. (2007). The protective role of tangible support on post-traumatic stress disorder symptoms in urban women survivors of violence. *Research in Nursing & Health, 30*(5), 558–568. Retrieved from http://dx.doi.org/10.1002/nur

Government of Alberta. (2013). *Best practices for investigating and prosecuting sexual assault* (pp. 1–165). Edmonton. Retrieved from http://justice.alberta.ca/programs_services/criminal_pros/documents/sexualassaulthandbook-policecrown.pdf

Government of Canada. (2015). *Get cyber safe.* Retrieved from http://www.getcybersafe.gc.ca/cnt/cbrbllng/prnts/lgl-cnsqncs-en.aspx

Government of Canada. (2012). *National action plan to combat human trafficking.* Retrieved from http://www.publicsafety.gc.ca/cnt/rsrcs/pblctns/ntnl-ctn-pln-cmbt/index-eng.aspx

Graham-Kevan, N. (2009). The psychology of women's partner violence: Characteristics and cautions. *Journal of Aggression, Maltreatment & Trauma, 18*(6), 587–603.

Graham, K., Bernards, S., Wilsnack, S. C., & Gmel, G. (2011). Alcohol may not cause partner violence but it seems to make it worse: A cross national comparison of the relationship between alcohol and severity of partner violence. *Journal of Interpersonal Violence, 26*(8), 1503–1523. doi:10.1177/0886260510370596

Graham-Bermann, S., Castor, L. E., Miller, L. E., & Howell, K. H. (2012). The impact of intimate partner violence and additional traumatic events on trauma symptoms and PTSD in preschool-aged children. *Journal of Traumatic Stress, 25,* 393–400.

Graham-Bermann, S., Gruber, G., Howell, K. H., & Girz, L. (2009). Factors discriminating among profiles of resilience and psychopathology in children exposed to intimate partner violence (IPV). *Child Abuse & Neglect, 33*(9), 648–660.

Greeson, J. K. P., Briggs, E. C., Layne, C. M., Belcher, H. M. E., Ostrowski, S. A., Kim, S., . . . Fairbank, J. A. (2014). Traumatic childhood experiences in the 21st century: Broadening and building on the ACE studies with data from the national child traumatic stress network. *Journal of Interpersonal Violence, 29*(3), 536–556. Retrieved from http://dx.doi.org/10.1177/0886260513505217

Greeson, M. R., & Campbell, R. (2013). Sexual assault response teams: An empirical review of their effectiveness. *Trauma, Violence & Abuse, 14*(2), 83–95.

Guruge, S., & Humphreys, J. (2009). Barriers affecting access to and use of formal social supports among abused immigrant women. *The Canadian Journal of Nursing Research, Revue canadienne de recherche en sciences infirmières, 41*(3), 64–84.

Hague, G., & Sardinha, L. (2010). Violence against women: Devastating legacy and transforming services. *Psychiatry, Psychology and Law, 17*(4), 503–522. doi:10.1080/13218711003709410

Hamby, S. (2011). The second wave of violence scholarship: Integrating and broadening theories of violence. *Psychology of Violence, 1*(3), 163–165.

Harmon, S. (2010). Body blow: Mature minors and the Supreme Court of Canada's decision in A.C. v. Manitoba. *McGill Law Journal, 4*(1), 84–95.

Hass, H., & Cusson, M. (2015). Comparing theories' performance in predicting violence. *International Journal of Law and Psychiatry.* Online publication. Retrieved from http://www.sciencedirect.com/science/article/pii/S0160252715000114

Henderson, L., & Morgan, E. (2009). Sexting and sexual relationships among teens and young adults. *McNair Scholars Research Journal, 7*(1), 31–39.

Henry, D. B., Tolan, P. H., Gorman-Smith, D., & Schoeny, M. E. (2012). Risk and direct protective factors for youth violence: Results from the Centers for Disease Control and Prevention's Multisite Violence Prevention Project. *American Journal of Preventive Medicine, 43,* S67–75. doi:10.1016/j.amepre.2012.04.025

Hequembourg, A. L., Livingston, J. A., & Parks, K. A. (2013). Sexual victimization and associated risks among lesbian and bisexual women. *Violence Against Women, 19,* 634–657.

Hewitt, B. (2009). The dangers of "sexting": *People. 71*(12), 111.

Hickman, L. J., Jaycox, L. H., & Aronoff, J. (2004). Dating violence among adolescents. *Trauma, Violence & Abuse, 5*(2), 123–142. doi:10.1177/1524838003262332

Hines, D. A., Armstrong, J. L., Reed, K. P., & Cameron, A. Y. (2012). Gender differences in sexual assault victimization among college students. *Violence & Victims, 27*(6), 922–940.

Hlvaka, H. R. (2014). Normalizing sexual violence: Young women account for harassment and abuse. *Gender & Society, 28*(3), 337–358. doi:10.1177/0891243214526468

Iverson, K. M., Dick, A., McLaughlin, K. A., Smith, B. N., Bell, M. E., Gerber, M. R., . . . Mitchell, K. S. (2013). Exposure to interpersonal violence and its associations with psychiatric morbidity in a U.S. national sample: A gender comparison. *Psychology of Violence, 3*(3), 273–287. Retrieved from http://dx.doi.org/10.1037/a0030956

Iverson, K. M., Jimenez, S., Harrington, K. M., & Resick, P. A. (2011). The contribution of childhood family violence on later intimate partner violence among robbery victims. *Violence and Victims, 26*(1), 73–87. doi:10.1891/0886-6708.26.1.73

Jack, S. M., Ford-Gilboe, M., Wathen, C. N., Davidov, D. M., McNaughton, D. B., Cohen, J. H., Olds, D. L., Macmillan, H. L., & NFP IPV Research Team. (2012). Development of a nurse home visitation intervention for intimate partner violence. *BMC Health Services Research, 19,* 50. Retrieved from http://www.biomedcentral.com/1472-6963/12/50

Jackman, M., & McRae, A. (2013). Medical decision-making and mature minors. *Royal College of Physicians and Surgeons of Canada.* Retrieved from http://www.royalcollege.ca/portal/page/portal/rc/common/documents/bioethics/section1/case_1_5_2_e.html

Jakubec, S., Carter-Snell, C., Ofrim, J., & Skanderup, J. (2013). Identifying rural sexual assault service strengths, concerns and educational needs in rural and Aboriginal communities in Alberta, Canada. *Enfermeria Global, 12*(31), 427–442.

Johnson, H. (2006). *Measuring violence against women: Statistical trends 2006*. Ottawa, ON: Statistics Canada.

Johnson, M. P., & Leone, J. M. (2005). The differential effects of intimate terrorism and situational couple violence: Findings from the national violence against women survey. *Journal of Family Issues, 26*(3), 322–349.

Jutla, R. K., & Heimback, D. (2004). Love burns: An essay about bride burning in India. *Journal of Burn Care & Rehabilitation, 25*(2), 165–170.

Kapur, N., & Windish, D. (2011). Health care utilization and unhealthy behaviors among victims of sexual assault in Connecticut: Results from a population-based sample. *JGIM: Journal of General Internal Medicine, 26*(5), 524–530. http://dx.doi.org/10.1007/s11606-010-1614-4

Kearns, M. C., Ressler, K. J., Zatzick, D., & Rothbaum, B. O. (2012). Early interventions for PTSD: A review. *Depression & Anxiety (1091–4269), 29*(10), 833–842. Retrieved from http://dx.doi.org/10.1002/da.21997

Kennedy, K. M. (2012). The relationship of victim injury to the progression of sexual crimes through the criminal justice system. *Journal of Forensic and Legal Medicine, 19*(6), 309–311.

King, B. (2012). Psychological theories of violence. *Human Behavior in the Social Environment, 22*(5), 553–571.

Klein, A. R. (2008). *Practical implications of current domestic violence research part iii: Judges*. (Award No. 2007 M-07032). Washington: U.S. Department of Justice. Retrieved from https://www.ncjrs.gov/pdffiles1/nij/grants/222321.pdf

Klein, E., Campbell, J., Soler, E., & Ghez, M. (1997). *Ending domestic violence: Changing public perceptions/halting the epidemic*. Thousand Oaks, CA: Sage Publications.

Knight, K. (2014). *Consent of minors to medical treatment*. Retrieved from http://www.siskinds.com/consent-of-minors-to-medical-treatment

Kolbe, A. R., Hutson, R. A., Shannon, H., Trzcincksi, E., Miles, B., Levitz, N., . . . Muggah, R. (2010). Mortality, crime and access to basic needs before and after the Haiti earthquake: A random survey of Port-au-Prince households. *Medicine, 26*(4), 281–297.

Kong, R., Johnson, H., Beattie, S., & Cardillo, A. (2003). Sexual offences in Canada. *Juristat, 23*(6), 1–26.

Konstantanopoulos, W. M., Ahn, R., Alpert, E. J., Cafferty, E., McGahan, A., Williams, T. P., . . . Burke, T. F. (2013). An international comparative public health analysis of sex trafficking of women and girls in eight cities: Achieving a more effective health sector response. *Journal of Urban Health: Bulletin of the New York Academy of Medicine, 90*(6), 1194–1204.

Kothari, C. L., & Rhodes, K. V. (2006). Missed opportunities: Emergency department visits by police-identified victims of intimate partner violence. *Annals of Emergency Medicine, 47*(2), 190–199. doi:10.1016/j.annemergmed.2005.10.1016

Kramer, A. (2002). Domestic violence: How to ask and how to listen. *Nursing Clinics of North America, 37*(1), 189–209.

Krebs, C. P., Lindquist, C. H., Warner, T. D., Fisher, B. S., & Martin, S. L. (2009). The differential risk factors of physically forced and alcohol- or other drug-enabled sexual assault among university women. *Violence & Victims, 24*(3), 302–321.

Krug, E. G., Dahlberg, L. L., Mercy, J. A., Zwi, A. B., & Lozano, R. (2002). *World report on violence and health*. Geneva, Switzerland: World Health Organization. Retrieved from http://www.who.int/violence_injury_prevention/violence/world_report/en/full_en.pdf?ua=1

Krug, E. G., & Sminkey, L. A. (2007). The role of the ministry of health in preventing injuries and violence. *International Journal of Injury Control and Safety Promotion, 14*(3), 199–201.

Kumar, V., & Kanth, S. (2007). Bride burning in India. In P. M. Verity (Ed.), *Violence and aggression around the globe* (pp. 147–148). New York, NY: Nova Science Publishers Inc.

Kwan, R. O., Cureton, E. L., Dozier, K., & Victorino, G. (2010). Gender differences among recidivist trauma patients. *Journal of Surgical Research, 165*, 25–29.

Lalor, K., & McElvaney, R. (2010). Child sexual abuse, links to later sexual exploitation/high-risk sexual behavior, and prevention/treatment programs. *Trauma, Violence & Abuse, 11*(4), 159–177. doi:10.1177/1524838010378299

Lamb, J., Pepler, D. J., & Craig, W. (2009). Approach to bullying and victimization. *Canadian Family Physician Medecin de Famille Canadien, 55*, 356–360.

Lamont, W. (2006). *Sexual assault services in Alberta: A framework of service delivery for sexual assault survivors living rural, remote and northern communities*. Calgary, AB: Alberta Association of Sexual Assault Centres.

Lamontagne, M. (2011). *Violence against Aboriginal women: Scan and report*. Canadian Women's Foundation.

Larkin, H., Shields, J. J., & Anda, R. F. (2012). The health and social consequences of adverse childhood experiences (ACE) across the lifespan: An introduction to prevention and intervention in the community. *Journal of Prevention & Intervention in the Community, 40*(4), 263–270. Retrieved from http://dx.doi.org/10.1080/10852352.2012.707439

Lenhart, A. (2009). *Teens and sexting: How and why minor teens are sending sexually suggestive nude or nearly nude images via text messaging*. Washington, DC: Pew Research Center. Retrieved from http://pewresearch.org/files/old-assets/pdf/teens-and-sexting.pdf

Lereya, S. T., Muthanna, S., & Wolke, D. (2013). Parenting behaviour and the risk of becoming a victim and a bully/victim: A meta-analysis study. *Child Abuse & Neglect, 37*(12), 1091–1108.

Lincoln, C., Perera, R., Jacobs, I., & Ward, A. (2013). Macroscopically detected female genital injury after consensual and non-consensual vaginal penetration: A prospective comparison study. *Journal of Forensic and Legal Medicine, 20*, 884–901.

Lisak, D. (2004). Predators. *Connection: The Journal of the New England Board of Higher Education, 19*(1), 19–20.

Lisak, D., & Miller, P. M. (2002). Repeat rape and multiple offending among undetected rapists. *Violence & Victims, 17*(1), 73–84.

Littleton, H. (2010). The impact of social support and negative disclosure reactions on sexual assault victims: A cross-sectional and longitudinal investigation. *Journal of Trauma & Dissociation, 11*(2), 210–227. Retrieved from http://dx.doi.org/10.1080/15299730903502946

Littleton, H. (2011). Talking about sexual assault: Society's response to survivors. *Psychology of Women Quarterly, 35*(1), 167–167. http://dx.doi.org/10.1177/0361684310388740

Littleton, H. (2014). Interpersonal violence on college campuses: Understanding risk factors and working to find solutions. *Trauma, Violence & Abuse, 15*(4), 297–303.

Livingston, M. (2011). A longitudinal analysis of alcohol outlet density and domestic violence. *Addiction, 106*(5), 919–925. doi:10.1111/j.1360-0443.2010.03333.x

Logan, T. K., & Walker, R. (2004). Separation as a risk factor for victims of intimate partner violence: Beyond lethality and injury: A response to Campbell. *Journal of Interpersonal Violence, 19*, 1478–1486. Retrieved from http://dx.doi.org/10.1177/0886260504269699

Lonsway, K. A., Archambault, J., & Lisak, D. (2009). False reports: Moving beyond the issue to successfully investigate and prosecute non-stranger sexual assault. *The Voice, 3*(1), 1–12.

Lonsway, K. A., Banyard, V. L., Berkowitz, A. D., Gidycz, C. A., Katz, J. T., Koss, M. P., . . . Ullman, S. E. (2011). *Rape prevention and risk reduction: Review of the research literature for practitioners.* Harrisburg, PA: Violence Against Women. Retrieved from http://www.vawnet.org/applied-research-papers/print-document.php?doc_id=1655

MacDowell, E. L. (2013). Theorizing from particularity: Perpetrators and intersectional theory on domestic violence. *Journal of Gender, Race and Violence, 16*(2), 531–576.

Maier, S. L. (2014). *Rape, victims, and investigations: Experience and perceptions of law enforcement officers responding to reported rapes.* New York, NY: Routledge.

Maier, S. L. (2008). "I have heard horrible stories . . .": Rape victim advocates' perceptions of the revictimization of rape victims by the police and medical system. *Violence Against Women, 14*(7), 786–808.

Manchikanti Gómez, A. (2011). Testing the cycle of violence hypothesis: Child abuse and adolescent dating violence as predictors of intimate partner violence in young adulthood. *Youth & Society, 43*(1), 171–192. Retrieved from http://dx.doi.org/10.1177/0044118X09358313

Martsolf, D. S., & Draucker, C. B. (2008). The legacy of childhood sexual abuse and family adversity. *Journal of Nursing Scholarship, 40*(4), 333–340.

Masho, S. W., & Anderson, L. (2009). Sexual assault in men: A population-based study of Virginia. *Violence & Victims, 24*(1), 98–110.

Mason, G. E., Riger, S., & Foley, L. A. (2004). The impact of past sexual experiences on attributions of responsibility for rape. *Journal of Interpersonal Violence, 19*(10), 1157–1171. doi:10.1177/0886260504269094

Mason, G. E., Ullman, S., Long, S. E., Long, L., & Starzynski, L. (2009). Social support and risk of sexual assault revictimization. *Journal of Community Psychology, 37*(1), 58–72. Retrieved from http://dx.doi.org/10.1002/jcop.20270

McCarroll, J. E., Fan, Z., Bell, N. S. (2009). Alcohol use in nonmutual and mutual domestic violence in the U.S. Army: 1998-2004. *Violence and Victims, 24*(3), 364–379.

McCartan, K. F., & McAlister, R. (2012). Mobile phone technology and sexual abuse. *Information & Communications Technology Law, 21*(3), 257–268. doi:10.1080/13600834.2012.744223

McClennan, S., Worster, A., & MacMillan, H. (2008). Caring for victims of intimate partner violence: A survey of Canadian emergency departments. *CJEM: Canadian Journal of Emergency Medicine, 10*(4), 325–328.

McGregor, M. J., Lipowska, M., Shah, S., Du Mont, J., & De Siato, C. (2003). An exploratory analysis of suspected drug-facilitated sexual assault seen in a hospital emergency department. *Women's Health, 37*(3), 71–80.

McInturff, K. (2013). Preventing violence a good investment. *Herizons, 27*(2), 11–12.

McLean, I. A., Balding, V., & White, C. (2005). Further aspects of male-on-male rape and sexual assault in greater Manchester. *Medicine, Science & the Law, 45*(3), 225–232.

McLean, I., Roberts, S. A., White, C., & Paul, S. (2011). Female genital injuries resulting from consensual and non-consensual vaginal intercourse. *Forensic Science International, 204*(1–3), 27–33. doi:10.1016/j.forsciint.2010.04.049

McLeod, S. A. (2008). Simply Psychology: Erik Erikson. Web Page. Retrieved from http://www.simplypsychology.org/Erik-Erikson.html

McMahon, S. (2014). Participation in high school sports and bystander intentions, efficacy to intervene, and rape myth beliefs. *Journal of Interpersonal Violence.* Epublication. doi:10.1177/0886260514555009

Meadows, R. J. (2010). *Understanding violence and victimization* (Vol. 5). New Jersey: Prentice Hall.

Meissner, D. (2014). Sexting B.C. teen found guilty of child pornography. Retrieved from http://bc.ctvnews.ca/sexting-b-c-teen-found-guilty-of-child-pornography-1.1633678

Metzl, J. L., & MacLeish, K. T. (2015). Mental illness, mass shootings, and the politics of American firearms. *American Journal of Public Health, 105*(2), 240–249.

Meyer, D. (2012). An intersectional analysis of lesbian, gay, bisexual, and transgender (LGBT) people's evaluations of anti-queer violence. *Gender & Society, 26*(6), 849–873. doi:10.1177/0891243212461299

Mikkonen, J., & Raphael, D. (2010). *Social determinants of health: The Canadian facts.* Toronto, ON: The Canadian Facts Organization. Retrieved from http://www.thecanadianfacts.org/The_Canadian_Facts.pdf

Mikton, C., & Butchart, A. (2009). Child maltreatment prevention: A systematic review of reviews. *Bulletin of the World Health Organization, 87*(5), 353–361. doi:10.2471/BLT.08.057075

Minow, J. C., & Einolf, C. J. (2009). Sorority participation and sexual assault risk. *Violence Against Women, 15*(7), 835–851.

Ministry of Public Safety and Solicitor General (2011). *Stopping the sexual exploitation of children and youth.* Retrieved from http://www.pssg.gov.bc.ca/crimeprevention/shareddocs/pubs/crime-prev-series2-sexual-exploitation-children-youth.pdf.

Mitchell, K. J., Jones, L. M., Finkelhor, D., & Wolak, J. (2011). Internet-facilitated commercial sexual exploitation of children: Findings from a nationally representative sample of law enforcement agencies in the United States. *Sexual Abuse: A Journal of Research & Treatment, 23*(1), 43–71. doi:10.1177/1079063210374347

Mock, C., Peden, M., Hyder, A. A., Butchart, A., & Krug, E. (2008). Child injuries and violence: The new challenge for child health. *Bulletin of the World Health Organization, 86*(6), 420–420.

Montgomery, A. E., Cutuli, J. J., Evans-Chase, M., Treglia, D., & Culhane, D. P. (2013). Relationship among adverse childhood experiences, history of active military service, and adult outcomes: Homelessness, mental health, and physical health. *American Journal of Public Health, 103,* S262–S268. http://dx.doi.org/10.2105/AJPH.2013.301474

Moor, A., Ben-Meir, A., Golan-Shapira, D., Farchi, M. (2013). Rape: A trauma of paralyzing dehumanization. *Journal of Aggression, Maltreatment & Trauma, 22*(10), 1051–1069.

Nagy, T., & Rutherford, M. (2010). Memoirs of a sex slave survivor. Toronto, ON: Perfect Paperback.

Native Women's Association of Canada. (2007a). Aboriginal women too often the victims of racialized sexualized violence. *Network Magazine of the Canadian Women's Health Network, 9*(3–4), 4–5. Retrieved from http://www.cwhn.ca/en/node/39430

Native Women's Association of Canada. (2007b). Violence against Aboriginal women and girls. Paper presented at the National Aboriginal Women's Summit, June 20–22, Cornerbrook, NL, Canada. Retrieved from www.laa.gov. nl.ca/laa/naws/pdf/nwac-vaaw.pdf

Native Women's Association of Canada (n.d.). Fact sheet: Missing and murdered Aboriginal women and girls. Retrieved from www.nwac.ca/files/download/NWAC_3D_ Toolkit_e_0.pdf

Navaneelan, T. (2012). Suicide rates: An overview. (Vol. 82-624-X). Ottawa, ON: Statistics Canada. Retrieved from http://www.statcan.gc.ca/pub/82-624-x/2012001/ article/11696-eng.htm

Navarro, H., Shakeshaft, A., Doran, C. M., & Petrie, D. J. (2013). Does increasing community and liquor licensees' awareness, police activity, and feedback reduce alcohol-related violent crime? A benefit-cost analysis. *International Journal of Environmental Research and Public Health, 10*(11), 5490–5506. doi:10.3390/ijerph10115490

Notar, C. E., Padgett, S., & Rodern, J. (2013). Cyberbullying: A review of the literature. *Universal Journal of Educational Research, 1*(1), 1–9.

Office of the Correctional Investigator. (2013). *Aboriginal offenders: A critical situation.* Ottawa: Government of Canada. Retrieved from http://www.oci-bec.gc.ca/cnt/rpt/oth-aut/ oth-aut20121022info-eng.aspx

Ogrodnik, L. (2010). *Child and youth victims of police-reported violent crime, 2008.* Ottawa, ON: Statistics Canada. Retrieved from www.statcan.gc.ca/pub/85f0033m/ 85f0033m2010023-eng.pdf

Olson, K. L., Marc, D. T., Grude, L. A., McManus, C. J., & Kellerman, G. H. (2011). Chapter 10: The hypothalamic-pituitary-adrenal axis: The actions of the central nervous system and potential biomarkers. In R. Klatz & R. Goldman (Eds.), Anti-aging therapeutics, XIII (pp. 91–100). Chicago, IL: American Academy of Anti-Aging Medicine.

Orchowski, L. M., & Gidycz, C. A. (2012). To whom do college women confide following sexual assault? A prospective study of predictors of sexual assault disclosure and social reactions. *Violence Against Women, 18*(3), 264–288. http://dx.doi.org/10.1177/1077801212442917

Owen, A., Thompson, M., Shaffer, A., Jackson, E., & Kaslow, N. (2009). Family variables that mediate the relation between intimate partner violence (IPV) and child adjustment. *Journal of Family Violence, 24*(7), 433–445. doi:10.1007/s10896-009-9239-2

Parker, E. M., & Gielen, A. C. (2014). Intimate partner violence and safety strategy use: Frequency of use and perceived effectiveness. *Women's Health Issues, 24*(6), 584–593.

Peress, D. A., Ward, M. F., Rudolph, G., Ayan, J., Wectawski, J., Dubon, M. E., . . . Sama, A. E. (2007). 426: Factors associated with prompt vs. delayed treatment-seeking among sexual assault victims. *Annals of Emergency Medicine, 50*(3), S134.

Perreault, S. (2012). *Homicide in Canada, 2011.* (No. 85-002-X). Ottawa, ON: Canadian Centre for Justice Statistics. Retrieved from http://www.statcan.gc.ca/pub/85-002-x/2012001/article/11738-eng.htm

Perreault, S., & Brennan, S. (2010) *Criminal victimization in Canada 2009* (Vol. 85-002-X). Ottawa, ON: Statistics Canada. Retrieved from http://www.statcan.gc.ca/pub/ 85-002-x/2010002/article/11340-eng.htm

Peter, T., Taylor, C., & Chamberland, L. (2015). A queer day in Canada: Examining Canadian high school students' experiences with school-based homophobia in two large-scale studies. *Journal of Homosexuality, 62,* 186–206.

Peter, T. (2009). Exploring taboos: Comparing male- and female-perpetrated child sexual abuse. *Journal of Interpersonal Violence, 24*(7), 1111–1128. Retrieved from http://dx.doi. org/10.1177/0886260508322194

Pinna, K. L. M., Johnson, D. M., & Delahanty, D. L. (2013). PTSD, comorbid depression, and the cortisol waking response in victims of intimate partner violence: Preliminary evidence. *Anxiety, Stress, and Coping, 27*(3), 253–269.

Pittaway, E., Bartolomei, L., & Rees, S. (2007). Gendered dimensions of the 2005 tsunami and a potential social work response in post-disaster situations. *International Social Work, 50,* 307–319.

Potter, S. J., Moynihan, M. M., Stapleton, J. G., & Banyard, V. L. (2009). Empowering bystanders to prevent campus violence against women: A preliminary evaluation of a poster campaign. *Violence Against Women, 15*(1), 106–121. Retrieved from http://dx.doi.org/10.1177/1077801208327482

President's Council. (2013). *Promoting a culture of safety, respect and consent at Saint Mary's University and beyond.* Halifax, NS: St. Mary's University.

Public Health Agency of Canada. (2008). *Leading causes of death and hospitalization in Canada.* Retrieved from http://www. phac-aspc.gc.ca/publicat/lcd-pcd97/table1-eng.php

Public Health Agency of Canada. (2014). *Canadian guidelines on sexually transmitted infections.* Retrieved from http://www. phac-aspc.gc.ca/std-mts/sti-its/cgsti-ldcits/index-eng.php

Public Safety Canada. (2013). *Youth gangs in Canada: What do we know?* Retrieved from http://www.publicsafety.gc.ca/cnt/ rsrcs/pblctns/gngs-cnd/index-eng.aspx

Raj, S. (2010). Que(e)rying violence: Rethinking pleasure, harm and intimacy in lesbian sadomasochism. *Gay & Lesbian Issues & Psychology Review, 6*(3), 122–131.

Raj, A., & Silverman, J. G. (2003). Immigrant South Asian women at greater risk for injury from intimate partner violence. *American Journal of Public Health, 93*(3).

Royal Canadian Mounted Police (RCMP). (2014). *Missing and murdered Aboriginal women: A national operational overview.* Ottawa. ON: Royal Canadian Mounted Police. Retrieved from www.rcmp-grc.gc.ca/pubs/ mmaw-faapd-eng.pdf

Rhodes, K. V., Kothari, C. L., Dichter, M., Cerulli, C., Wiley, J., & Marcus, S. (2011). Intimate partner violence identification and response: Time for a change in strategy. *JGIM: Journal of General Internal Medicine, 26*(8), 894–899. doi:10.1007/ s11606-011-1662-4

Rinker, A. G. (2009). Recognition of elder abuse by prehospital and hospital-based care providers. *Archives in Gerontology and Geriatrics, 48*(1), 110–115.

Rivara, F. P., Anderson, M. L., Fishman, P., Bonomi, A. E., Reid, R. J., Carrell, D., & Thompson, R. S. (2007). Healthcare utilization and costs for women with a history of intimate partner violence. *American Journal of Preventive Medicine, 32*(2), 89–96.

Rossegger, A., Wetli, N., Urbaniok, F., Elbert, T., Cortoni, F., & Endrass, J. (2009). Women convicted for violent offenses: Adverse childhood experiences, low level of education and poor mental health. *BMC Psychiatry, 9*, 81–81.

Roustit, C., Renahy, E., Guernec, G., Lesieur, S., Parizot, I., & Chauvin, P. (2009). Exposure to interparental violence and psychosocial maladjustment in the adult life course: Advocacy for early prevention. *Journal of Epidemiology and Community Health, 63*(7), 563–568.

Russell, K. (2013). Supporting young people who disclose rape and sexual assault. *British Journal of School Nursing, 8*(8), 376–377.

Sabina, C., & Ho, L. Y. (2014). Campus and college victim responses to sexual assault and dating violence: Disclosure, service utilization, and service provision. *Trauma, Violence & Abuse, 15*(3), 201–226.

Sadler, A. G., Booth, B. M., Mengeling, M. A., & Doebbeling, B. N. (2004). Life span and repeated violence against women during military service: Effects on health status and outpatient utilization. *Journal of Women's Health (2002), 13*(7), 799–811.

Saewyc, E., Poon, C., Wang, N., Homma, Y., Smith, A., & the McCreary Centre Society. (2007). *Not yet equal: The health of lesbian, gay, & bisexual youth in BC*. Vancouver, BC: McCreary Centre Society. Retrieved from http://www.mcs.bc.ca/pdf/not_yet_equal_web.pdf

Substance Abuse and Mental Health Services Administration (SAMHSA). (2011). *Trauma-informed approach and trauma-specific interventions*. Rockland, MD: Substances Abuse and Mental Health Services Administration. Retrieved from http://www.samhsa.gov/nctic/trauma-interventions

Schewe, P., Riger, S., Howard, A., Staggs, S., & Mason, G. (2006). Factors associated with domestic violence and sexual assault victimization. *Journal of Family Violence, 21*(7), 469.

Schofield, T. P., & Denson, T. F. (2013). Alcohol outlet business hours and violent crime in New York State. *Alcohol & Alcoholism, 48*(3), 363–369. doi:10.1093/alcalc/agt003

Schwabe, L., & Wolf, O. T. (2014). Timing matters: Temporal dynamics of stress effects on memory retrieval. *Cognitive, Affective & Behavioral Neuroscience, 14*(3), 1041–1048.

Selye, H. (1976). *Stress in health and disease*. Reading, MA: Butterworth's.

Senn, C. Y., Eliasziw, M., Barata, P. C., Thurston, W. E., Newby-Clark, I. R., Radtke, L., & Hobden, K. L. (2015). Efficacy of a sexual assault resistance program for university women. *New England Journal of Medicine, 372*, 2326–2335.

Sexual Assault Voices of Edmonton. (2014). *"Don't Be That Guy" campaign*. Retrieved from http://www.savedmonton.com

Sheridan, D. J., & Nash, K. R. (2007). Acute injury patterns of intimate partner violence victims. *Trauma, Violence & Abuse, 8*(3), 281–289.

Silverman, J. G., Decker, M. R., & Raj, A. (2007). Immigration-based disparities in adolescent girls' vulnerability to dating violence. *Maternal & Child Health Journal, 11*(1), 37–43.

Sinha, M. (2011). *Family violence against children and youth: Family violence in Canada—A stastistical profile* (No. 85-224-X). Ottawa, ON: Statistics Canada.

Sinha, M. (2012). *Family violence in Canada: A statistical profile, 2010*. (No. 85-002-X). Ottawa, ON: Statistics Canada. Retrieved from www.statcan.gc.ca/pub/85-002-x/2012001/article/11643-eng.pdf

Sinha, M. (2013). *Measuring violence against women: Statistical trends*. Ottawa, ON: Statistics Canada. Retrieved from http://search.proquest.com/docview/1324040258/fulltextPDF/embedded/61W1TCW798BW91QK?source=fedsrch

Sinha, V., Trocmé, N., Fallon, B., & Maclaurin, B. (2013). Understanding the investigation-stage overrepresentation of First Nations children in the child welfare system: An analysis of the First Nations component of the Canadian incidence study of reported child abuse and neglect 2008. *Child Abuse & Neglect, 37*(10), 821–831.

Skjelsbaek, I. (2006). Therapeutic work with victims of sexual violence in war and postwar: A discourse analysis of Bosnian experiences. *Peace & Conflict, 12*(2), 93–118. doi:10.1207/s15327949pac1202_1

Slane, A. (2013). Sexting and the law in Canada. *Canadian Journal of Sexuality, 22*(3), 117–122. doi:10.3138/cjhs.22.3.C01

Sleet, D. A., Dahlberg, L. L., Basavaraju, S. V., Mercy, J. A., McGuire, L. C., & Greenspan, A. (2011). Injury prevention, violence prevention, and trauma care: Building the scientific base. *Morbidity and Mortality Weekly Report. Surveillance Summaries (Washington, D.C.: 2002), 60 Suppl 4*, 78–85.

Smith, D., Varcoe, C., & Edwards, N. (2005). Turning around the intergenerational impact of residential schools on Aboriginal people: Implications for health policy and practice. *Canadian Journal of Nursing Research, 37*(4), 38–60.

Sommers, M. S., Brown, K. M., Buschur, C., Everett, J. S., Fargo, J. D., Fisher, B. S., . . . Zink, T. M. (2012). Injuries from intimate partner and sexual violence: Significance and classification systems. *Journal of Forensic and Legal Medicine, 19*(5), 250–263.

Spielmann, S. S., Macdonald, G., Maxwell, J. A., Joel, S., Peragine, D., Muise, A., & Impett, E. A. (2013). Settling for less out of fear of being single. *Journal of Personality and Social Psychology, 105*(6), 1049–1073. doi:10.1037/a0034628

Spohn, C., White, C., & Tellis, K. (2014). Unfounded sexual assault: Examining the decision to unfound and identifying false reports. *Law & Society Review, 48*(1), 161–191.

Standish, K. (2013). Understanding cultural violence and gender: Honour killings; dowry murder, the zina ordinance, and blood-feuds. *Journal of Gender Studies, 23*(2), 111–124.

Statistics Canada. (2009). *Leading causes of death in Canada, 2009*. Retrieved from http://www.statcan.gc.ca/pub/84-215-x/84-215-x2012001-eng.htm

Statistics Canada. (2013). Homicide in Canada, 2012. *The Daily*, December 1(11), 1–4. Retrieved from http://www.statcan.gc.ca/pub/85-002-x/2013001/article/11882-eng.htm?fpv=2693

Staub, E. (2012). The roots and prevention of genocide and related mass violence. *Zygon: Journal of Religion & Science, 47*(4), 821–842. Retrieved from http://dx.doi.org/10.1111/j.1467-9744.2012.01302.x

Stephens, K. A., & George, W. H. (2009). Rape prevention with college men: Evaluating risk status. *Journal of Interpersonal Violence, 24*(6), 996–1013.

Stewart, E. A., & Simons, R. L. (2010). Race, code of the street, and violent delinquency: A multilevel investigation of neighborhood street culture and individual norms of violence. *Criminology: An Interdisciplinary Journal, 48*(2), 569–605.

Stoddard, S. A., Whiteside, L., Zimmerman, M. A., Cunningham, R. M., Chermack, S. T., & Walton, M. A. (2013). The relationship between cumulative risk and promotive factors and violent behavior among urban adolescents. *American Journal of Community Psychology, 51*(1–2), 57–65. doi:10.1007/s10464-012-9541-7

Stoddard, S. A., Zimmerman, M. A., & Bauermeister, J. A. (2012). A longitudinal analysis of cumulative risks, cumulative promotive factors, and adolescent violent behavior. *Journal of Research on Adolescence, 22*(3), 542–555. doi:10.1111/j.1532-7795.2012.00786.x

Stogner, J., Gibson, C. L., & Miller, J. M. (2014). Examining the reciprocal nature of the health-violence relationship: Results from a nationally representative sample. *JQ: Justice Quarterly, 31*(3), 473–499. Retrieved from http://dx.doi.org/10.1080/07418825.2012.723029

Straus, M., & Gozjolko, K. (2014). Intimate terrorism and gender differences in injury of dating partners by male and female university students. *Journal of Family Violence, 29*(1), 51–65. http://dx.doi.org/10.1007/s10896-013-9560-7

Sullivan, J., Beech, A. R., Craig, L. A., & Gannon, T. A. (2011). Comparing intra-familial and extra-familial child sexual abusers with professionals who have sexually abused children with whom they work. *International Journal of Offender Therapy & Comparative Criminology, 55*(1), 56–74. doi:10.1177/0306624X09359194

Svensson, B., Bornehag, C.-G., & Janson, S. (2011). Chronic conditions in children increase the risk for physical abuse—but vary with socio-economic circumstances. *Acta Paediatrica, 100*(3), 407–412. doi:10.1111/j.1651-2227.2010.02029.x

Sylaska, K. M., & Edwards, K. M. (2014). Disclosure of intimate partner violence to informal social support network members: A review of the literature. *Trauma, Violence & Abuse, 15*(1), 3–21. doi:10.1177/1524838013496335

Taft, C., Resick, P., Watkins, L., & Panuzio, J. (2009). An investigation of posttraumatic stress disorder and depressive symptomatology among female victims of interpersonal trauma. *Journal of Family Violence, 24*(6), 407–415.

Tark, J., & Kleck, G. (2014). Resisting rape: The effects of victim self-protection on rape completion and injury. *Violence Against Women, 20*(3), 270–292.

Taylor-Butts, A., & Porter, J. (2011). *Family violence in Canada: A statistical profile* (Vol. 85-224-X). Ottawa, ON: Statistics Canada.

Thompson, M., Swartout, K., & Koss, M. P. (2013). Trajectories and predictors of sexually aggressive behaviors during emerging adulthood. *Psychology of Violence, 3*(3), 247–259. doi:http://dx.doi.org/10.1037/a0030624

Thrane, L. E., Yoder, K. A., & Chen, X. (2011). The influence of running away on the risk of female sexual assault in the subsequent year. *Violence & Victims, 26*(6), 816–829.

Thurston, W. E., Tutty, L. M., Eisener, A. C., Lalonde, L., Belenky, C., & Osborne, B. (2009). Implementation of universal screening for domestic violence in an urgent care community health center. *Health Promotion Practice, 10*(4), 517–526. doi:10.1177/1524839907307994

Tiller, J., & Baker, L. (2014). *The neurobiology of sexual assault.* Learning Network Brief (14) January. London, ON: Learning Network, Centre for Research and Education on Violence Against Women and Children. Retrieved from http://www.vawlearningnetwork.ca/social-marketing-publiceducation

Trocme, N., Fallon, B., MacLaurin, B., Daciuk, J., Felstiner, C., Black, T., . . . Cloutier, R. (2005). *Canadian incidence study of reported child abuse and neglect 2003: Major findings.* Ottawa, ON: Minister of Public Works and Government Services Canada.

Trocme, N., Fallon, B., MacLaurin, B., Sinha, V., Black, E., Fast, E., . . . Holroyd, J. (2009). *Canadian incidence study of reported child abuse and neglect 2008.* Ottawa, ON: Public Health Agency of Canada. Retrieved from http://www.phac-aspc.gc.ca/cm-vee/csca-ecve/2008/cis-eci-08-eng.php#c4-5

Tsopelas, C., Tsetsou, S., Ntounas, P., & Douzenis, A. (2012). Female perpetrators of sexual abuse of minors: What are the consequences for the victims? *International Journal of Law and Psychiatry, 35*(4), 305–310. doi:10.1016/j.ijlp.2012.04.003

Tutty, L. M., & Abbott, P. (2007). *An evaluation of phases one and two of the Action Committee against Bullying and Harassment.* Calgary. Retrieved from http://www.ucalgary.ca/resolve-static/reports/2006/2006-07.pdf

Tutty, L. M., Bradshaw, C., Thurston, W. E., Barlow, A., Marshall, P., Tunstall, L., . . . Nixon, K. (2005). *School-based violence prevention programs: A resource manual.* Calgary, AB: RESOLVE Alberta.

Ullman, S. E., Foynes, M. M., & Tang, S. S. (2010). Benefits and barriers to disclosing sexual trauma: A contextual approach. *Journal of Trauma & Dissociation, 11*(2), 127–133. http://dx.doi.org/10.1080/15299730903502904

Ullman, S. E. (2011). Is disclosure of sexual traumas helpful? Comparing experimental laboratory vs. field study results. *Journal of Aggression, Maltreatment & Trauma, 20*(2), 148–162.

Ullman, S. E., & Filipas, H. H. (2001a). Correlates of formal and informal support seeking in sexual assault victims. *Journal of Interpersonal Violence, 16*(10), 1028–1047.

Ullman, S. E., & Filipas, H. H. (2001b). Predictors of PTSD symptom severity and social reactions in sexual assault victims. *International Society for Traumatic Stress Studies, 14*(2), 369–389.

Ullman, S. E., Townsend, S. M., Filipas, H. H., & Starzynski, L. L. (2007). Structural models of the relations of assault severity, social support, avoidance coping, self-blame and PTSD among sexual assault survivors. *Psychology of Women Quarterly, 31*(1), 23–37.

Vaillancourt, R. (2010). *Gender differences in police-reported violent crime in Canada, 2008.* (Vol 85F0033M, no.24). Ottawa, ON: Statistics Canada.

VanDeusen, K. M., & Way, I. (2006). Vicarious trauma: An exploratory study of the impact of providing sexual abuse treatment on clinicians' trust and intimacy. *Journal of Child Sexual Abuse, 15*(1), 69–85.

Varcoe, C., Hankivsky, O., Ford-Gilboe, M., Wuest, J., Wilk, P., Hammerton, J., & Campbell, J. (2011). Attributing selected costs to intimate partner violence in a sample of women who have left abusive partners: A social determinants approach. *Canadian Public Policy, 37*(3), 359–380.

Vargas, C. M. (2007). War trauma in refugees: Red flags and clinical principles. *Visions Journal, 3*(3), 12–13.

Vertamatti, M. A. F., de Abreu, L. C., Otsuka, F. C., Costa, P. R. F., Ferreira, J. D., Tavares, C., & Barbosa, C. P. (2012). Factors associated to time of arrival at the health service after sexual violence. *HealthMed, 6*(1), 37–41.

Walby, S. (2013). Violence and society: Introduction to an emerging field of sociology. *Current Sociology, 61*(2), 95–111.

Walcott, R., Foster, C., Campbell, M., & Sealy, D. (2010). *Review of the roots of youth violence: Research papers, volume 4: Racial minority perspectives on violence.* Toronto, ON: Queen's Printer for Ontario. Retrieved from http://www.children. gov.on.ca/htdocs/English/topics/youthandthelaw/roots/ volume4/minority_perspectves.aspx

Walters, G.D., & Crawford, G. (2013). Major mental illness and violence history as predictors of institutional misconduct and recidivism: Main and interaction effects. *Law and Human Behavior, 38*(3), e-publication. doi:10. 1037/lhb0000058

Warthe, D. G., Kostouros, P., Carter-Snell, C., & Tutty, L. M. (2013). Stepping up: A peer-to-peer dating violence prevention project on a postsecondary campus. *International Journal of Child, Youth and Family Studies, 4*(1), 100–118.

Warthe, D. G., & Tutty, L. M. (2009). *College dating violence: Correlations with health and risk behaviours.* Paper presented at the International Conference on Violence, Abuse and Trauma.

Weir, E. (2005). Preventing violence in youth. *CMAJ, 172*(10), 1291–1292.

Weiss, E. (2003). Leaving is a process: Supporting victims of domestic violence. *On the Edge, 9*(2), 1, 19–22.

Wilcox, D. T., Richards, F., & O'Keeffe, Z. C. (2004). Resilience and risk factors associated with experiencing childhood sexual abuse. *Child Abuse Review, 13*(5), 338–352. doi:10.1002/car.862

Wilkins, N., Tsao, B., Hertz, M., Davis, R., & Klevens, J. (2014). Connecting the dots: An overview of the links among multiple forms of violence. Washinton, DC: Centers for Disease Control. Retrieved from http://www.cdc.gov/ violenceprevention/pdf/connecting_the_dots-a.pdf

Wolak, J., Finkelhor, D., Mitchell, K. J., & Ybarra, M. L. (2008). Online "predators" and implications for prevention and treatment. *American Psychologist, 63*(2), 111–128.

World Health Organization. (2014a). *Global status report on violence prevention.* Geneva, Switzerland: Author. Reprinted with permission from World Health Organization. Retrieved from www.who.int/violence_injury_prevention/ violence/status_report/2014

World Health Organization. (2014b). Elder abuse: Fact sheet 357. Retrieved from http://www.who.int/mediacentre/ factsheets/fs357/en

World Health Organization. (2012). Human trafficking. Geneva: Author. Reprinted with permission from World Health Organization. Retrieved from http://apps.who.int/ iris/bitstream/10665/77394/1/WHO_RHR_12.42_eng.pdf

World Health Organization. (2011). *Psychological first aid: Guide for field workers.* Geneva: Author. Retrieved from http://www.who.int/mental_health/publications/ guide_field_workers/en

World Health Organization. (2010). *Violence prevention: The evidence.* Geneva: World Health Organization.

World Health Organization. (2005). *Violence and disasters.* Geneva: Author. Retrieved from www.who.int/violence_ injury. . ./violence/violence_disasters.pdf

World Health Organization (2004). Preventing violence: A guide to implementing the recommendations of the World report on violence and health. Retrieved from http://www.who.int/ violence_injury_prevention/media/news/08_09_2004/en

Wu, V., Huff, H., & Bhandari, M. (2010). Pattern of physical injury associated with intimate partner violence in women presenting to the emergency department: A systematic review and meta-analysis. *Trauma, Violence and Abuse, 11*(2), 71–82.

Zhang, T., Hoddenbaugh, J., McDonald, S., & Scrim, K. (2012). *An estimation of the economic impact of spousal violence in Canada, 2009.* (No. rr12-07-e). Ottawa, ON: Department of Justice Canada.

Zinzow, H. M., & Thompson, M. (2015). A longitudinal study of risk factors for repeated sexual coercion and assault in U.S. college men. *Archives of Sexual Behavior, 44*(1), 213–222.

## ABOUT THE AUTHOR

**Dr. Catherine Carter-Snell**, RN, BScN, MN, PhD, ENC-C, SANE-A, is an Associate Professor and Nurse Education Scholar for the School of Nursing and Midwifery, Faculty of Health, Community and Education at Mount Royal University in Calgary Alberta. Her clinical background is in Emergency and Intensive Care Nursing and as a nurse examiner with victims of sexual assault and intimate partner violence. Dr. Carter-Snell's research focus is on reducing violence or its effects. Project examples include a student dating violence prevention program and multidisciplinary programs to improve sexual assault services in Prince Edward Island and western Canada. She co-founded the Canadian Forensic Nurses' Association, co-developed the core curriculum and standards for forensic nurses with the International Association of Forensic Nurses, and works with a number of community agencies related to violence and recovery. She has been recognized as an expert on sexual assault in court multiple times and has received a number of awards for her research, teaching, and contributions to forensic nursing.

# Poverty, Homelessness, and Food Security

*Lynnette Leeseberg Stamler and Aaron Gabriel*

## LEARNING OUTCOMES

**After studying this chapter, you should be able to:**

1. Outline the consequences of multiple definitions of and poor data related to homelessness on understanding the scope of the issue.

2. Apply at least one definition and source of data to describing the issue of poverty and homelessness in your own geographic area.

3. Use the determinants of health framework to assess the influence of poverty and/or homelessness on an individual's or family's health.

4. Identify at least two health issues that are specifically impacted by poverty and homelessness.

5. Describe the concept of food security and how it may impact family health even in populations of working poor.

6. Describe the community health nurse (CHN) role in advocating for groups and populations affected by food insecurity, poverty, and homelessness.

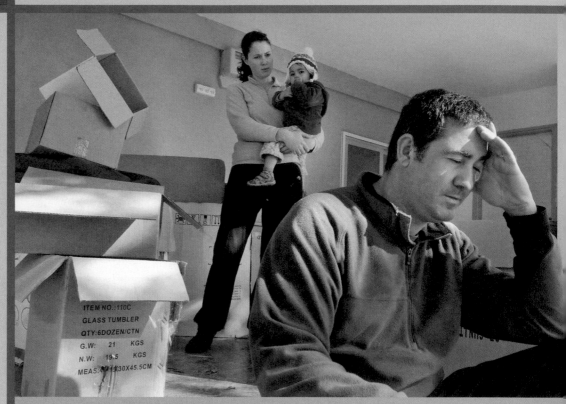

*Source: ChameleonsEye/Shutterstock*

## INTRODUCTION

Many factors contribute to homelessness, poverty being significant among them. A concept related to poverty and homelessness is food insecurity or security. Because there is ongoing interest in poverty and homelessness in the media, it is disheartening and perhaps surprising to realize that few firm statistics that demonstrate the scope of the issues are available. For example, the data collection methods for homelessness are most often done using snowball sampling, point in time "guesstimates," and indirect estimations; and while poverty statistics are a bit more fulsome, the varying definitions of poverty contribute to a lack of clarity. Food security statistics are even more difficult to demonstrate. Despite the absence of definitive statistics, it is clear from the data available that poverty, homelessness, and food security are continuing problems in Canada, albeit with some bright glimpses of progress.

■ It is estimated that at least 30 000 Canadians are homeless on a given night, that 200 000 Canadians experience homelessness in a year, that during the past five years 1.3 million Canadians have experienced homelessness or extremely insecure housing, and that there are up to 50 000 hidden homeless on any given night (Gaetz, Donaldson, Richter, & Gulliver, 2013).

- In the downtown core of Toronto, Canada, it has been estimated that between 900 and 1 100 visible individuals are homeless on the street (Berry, 2007).
- The Salvation Army alone reports over 6 000 "shelter, addictions, detox and mental health beds [are] provided each night for vulnerable men, women and families" (The Salvation Army, 2012/2013, p. 3).
- Homeless Aboriginal people are over-represented in terms of the Canadian population. Aboriginals make up 3% of the Canadian population, but they account for 10% of the country's entire homeless population (Regroupement des centres d'amitiéautochtones du Québec, 2008).
- Belanger, Awosoga, and Head (2013) estimate that "on any one given night, 6.97 percent of the urban Aboriginal population in Canada is homeless, as compared to a national average of .78 percent" (p. 4).
- In 2008, the City of Calgary launched a 10 Year Plan to End Homelessness. In 2014, they reported that a "Point-in-Time Count" indicted 3 533 people were homeless on one night, which was relatively unchanged since 2012. This represents a positive move forward (Calgary Homeless Foundation, 2014, p. 2).
- In Ontario, there are over 168 711 households on waiting lists for social housing (Ontario Non-Profit Housing Association, 2015).
- Habitat for Humanity, Canada, a volunteer non-profit organization that partners with communities to build and promote homeownership as a means of breaking the cycle of poverty, has successfully completed more than 2 200 safe, decent, and affordable homes for low-income Canadian families (Habitat for Humanity, 2013).

In this chapter, we will consider the scope of poverty and homelessness in Canada, and the demographic composition of these populations. Using the Health Canada determinants of health as a framework, we will examine the effects of poverty and homelessness on the health of Canadians and the role of CHNs who work with these populations. Finally, we will discuss food security, recognizing that it is a related but not necessarily a causal companion to poverty and homelessness.

## POVERTY

One difficulty inherent in discussing poverty is the fact that we have no universally accepted definition of poverty. The measurement of a societal condition (such as poverty) is an essential precondition to taking corrective policy action. It seems that in modern societies, unless a societal condition has some statistical visibility, it is deemed not to exist. For example, even the census does not represent the most deprived citizens in Canada. At least three common definitions of poverty are used by policy makers; the two most often used are government developed.

The **basic needs** approach defines **poverty** as lacking food, clothing, and shelter plus other necessities that would be required to maintain physical health in the long term (Parliament of Canada, 2008), and was first defined by the Fraser Institute. The author of a basic-needs measure arbitrarily determines the basic necessities and costs them out. Those who cannot afford these items are, by definition, poor. The **market basket measure (MBM)**, created by Human Resources Development Canada, is similar except that the contents of measure include a non-defined category of essentials in addition to food, clothing, and shelter. Thus, the MBM looks at needs beyond purely physical needs. In both measures, the reference family includes two adults and two children. Inferences for other family configurations must be drawn by the users of the measure.

The **low-income cut-off measure (LICO)** is based on family income rather than family costs. It is based on the premise that the average Canadian family spends half its income on food, clothing, and shelter. Researchers at Statistics Canada therefore concluded that any family that had to spend more than 70% of its income on those three items would have little disposable income to spend on other things, such as transportation. The LICO is divided into family sizes ranging from one to seven and more, and is also referenced against the number of people in that family's place of residence. As such, the LICO is able to capture how the family rates economically in relation to changing geography and a corresponding change in cost of living (Statistics Canada, 2009). One of the advantages of the LICO is that it reflects the community of residence and the composition of the family. This measure assumes that it takes more income to live in a larger centre and to support a larger family. Although Statistics Canada denies that this is a measure of poverty, it is a commonly used measure to describe that segment of our population that is worst off in economic terms, which some policymakers believe to be synonymous with poverty. Thus, families with lower incomes than those in Table 29.1 are considered to be living in poverty.

The LICO provides a unique view of poverty in Canada by looking at the issue from the local level and then comparing the incomes with those in other centres. Economic growth is not equally divided among the constituents of a country. As the economy grows and communities prosper, the numbers living in poverty also grow, although at different rates.

People can have working income and still be considered poor. A working-poor person has been defined as "someone who works the equivalent of full-time for at least half of the year but whose family income is below a low-income threshold" (Human Resources and Skills Development Canada, 2007, p. 13). Rothwell and Haveman (2013) suggest that "a household is 'asset poor' if it does not own sufficient assets to survive at the low-income cutoff for three months" (p. 1). In fact, the Conference Board of Canada notes that Canada is 12th in ranking for income inequality and indicates Canada has the third-highest increase compared to peer countries in rates of working-age poverty (Conference Board of Canada, 2013). Several factors contribute to a perception of working poor moving into middle class:

- recent tax policies have shifted the burden of federal and provincial income taxes onto lower-income workers;
- a second tax is the consumption tax, such as the sales tax. The required outlay for basic necessities takes a larger

| Table 29.1 | Low-Income Cut-Offs (LICOs), After Tax, 2012 | | | | |
|---|---|---|---|---|---|
| | | Urban Areas Size of Communities | | | |
| Size of Family Unit | Rural Areas | Less than 30 000 | 30 000–99 999 | 100 000–499 999 | 500 000 and over |
| 1 person | $12 819 | $14 671 | $16 366 | $16 573 | $19 597 |
| 2 people | 15 602 | 17 857 | 19 920 | 20 170 | 23 850 |
| 3 people | 19 429 | 22 233 | 24 804 | 25 117 | 29 699 |
| 4 people | 24 237 | 27 739 | 30 945 | 31 335 | 37 052 |
| 5 people | 27 600 | 31 587 | 35 238 | 35 681 | 42 191 |
| 6 people | 30 609 | 35 031 | 39 080 | 39 571 | 46 191 |
| 7 or more people | 33 618 | 38 475 | 42 291 | 43 461 | 51 391 |

Source: Statistics Canada. (2013). Low income cut-offs (1992 base) after tax. Retrieved from http://www.statcan.gc.ca/pub/75f0002m/2013002/tbl/tbl01-eng.htm

percentage of the poor family's income; thus, they bear a higher burden from consumption taxes; and

■ wages, including low-income wages, have only been increasing at or below the rate of inflation. Thus, relative income is stagnant or decreased across all but the higher incomes.

Many factors can place people at risk for living in poverty. Human Resources and Skills Development Canada (2008) completed a report on low income in the years 2000 to 2006. This report identifies five "high-risk" groups for low income:

■ lone parents with at least one child under 18 years of age;
■ unattached individuals between the ages of 45 and 64;
■ people with physical or mental disabilities that impede working;
■ recent (within the past 10 years) immigrants to Canada; and
■ Aboriginal Canadians living off-reserve.

It is important to note that the above list does not refer to children or the elderly, who are often represented in the low-income ranges. This was likely because the family or household income status includes these two groups, as children and the elderly often live in shared accommodations, or "households." To this end, it is important to note that if the main income earner of a family falls under any of the above categories, the family would therefore also be considered "high-risk" for low income and would have three times the risk of being low income compared to families whose main earner did not fall into the risk categories, and also experience persistent low income more often (Human Resources and Skills Development Canada, 2008).

## HOMELESSNESS

As with poverty, the definitions of homelessness are many and varied (see Figure 29.1). Over the years, several definitions have been used, but the Canadian Homelessness Research Network recently released a Canadian definition of **homelessness** described as "the situation of an individual or family without stable, permanent, appropriate housing, or the immediate prospect, means and ability of acquiring it" (Canadian Homelessness Research Network, 2015). This definition takes into account that the state of homelessness is not static and that it can change frequently and dramatically. This definition recognizes four types of physical living conditions:

■ unsheltered—individuals living on the streets or in places never intended for habitation;
■ emergency sheltered—individuals staying overnight in shelters designated for the homeless and those seeking refuge from family violence;

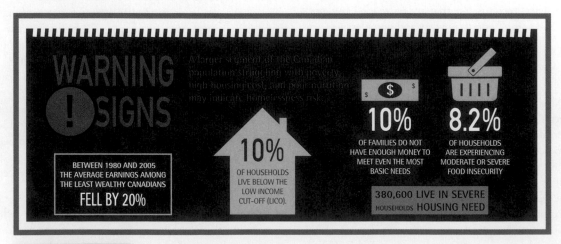

**FIGURE 29.1** Homelessness in Canada

*Source:* Gaetz, S., Donaldson, J., Richter, T., & Gulliver, T. (2013). *The State of Homelessness in Canada.* Toronto, ON: Canadian Homelessness Research Network Press. Used by permission. Retrieved from http://www.homelesshub.com

- provisionally accommodated—individuals with temporary, insecure accommodation, such as hotels, temporary housing for new refugees or immigrants, penal institutions, friend/family "couch surfing," hospitals, and group homes; and
- at risk of homelessness—individuals who are not homeless but in a precarious situation, housing or economic, where they cannot meet public health or safety standards.

Once a working definition of homelessness has been chosen, the next step is to ascertain how many people fall into that category. However, this presents significant difficulties. The data are incomplete because most population descriptions are a snapshot of time, and many survey methodologies are based on the ability to contact the population in order to count them. In other words, telephone surveys and census surveys assume a fixed address or telephone number. While this has changed somewhat with the advent of cellphones and the efforts of organizations to supply these to low-income and homeless persons, difficulties remain. Thus, the provisionally accommodated and at-risk homeless may well be absent in any given counting. The unsheltered and emergency sheltered, unless they happen to be in a shelter during census time, likewise may be completely missed. Given these difficulties, it is not surprising that agencies like Statistics Canada are unable or unwilling to publish complete statistics on Canada's homeless population. At best, they can suggest inferences from other data. Murphy (2000) contends that this inability to be precise is a grave difficulty because "overestimating (the number of homeless) invites public cynicism, [and] underestimating incurs the wrath of service agencies that rely on public funding" (p. 11). She acknowledges that counting people in shelters misses "Canadians whose incomes force them to live in substandard housing with constant fear of eviction if their meager incomes should temporarily disappear. Nor does it address the growing number of poor who must spend up to 70% of their incomes on rent, leaving very little for food, nor those doubling up in accommodations" (pp. 12–13). She notes that some studies have estimated that for every person in a shelter on a given night, there are one to two people living on the street on the same night.

A relatively new technology available to community stakeholders is the Homeless Individuals and Families Information System (HIFIS) initiative, which collects information related to the population using shelter services. This initiative has been implemented in many of the known shelters in Canada, and was created with the purpose of providing a national understanding of homelessness in Canada which can help communities plan for their local challenges. The HIFIS provides software and training to shelter staff that enables the staff to collect a comprehensive set of data on individuals using the services (Human Resources and Skills Development Canada, 2013).

But what does being homeless really mean? Is it more than not having a roof over one's head? Murray (1990) used Tognoli's (1987) framework to examine the concept of "homefullness" in light of the homeless population. Tognoli (pp. 657–665) suggested that many aspects are missing for those persons who are homeless. They include a place for social and family relations, privacy, continuity, order, identity, rootedness, ownership, and security. Lastly, Tognoli suggests that a home is a sociocultural context. It is clear that the homeless are missing much more than a roof. Rather, many of the connections in their life that link them to mainstream society are decreased or absent.

Gaetz et al. (2013, p. 13) summarized the causes of homelessness as follows:

- structural issues (e.g., inadequate income, discrimination, lack of access to affordable housing);
- systems failures (e.g., failed support for refugees and immigrants, discharges from institutions); and
- individual and relational factors (e.g., personal crises, extreme poverty, family violence).

The issue of homelessness is not confined to large urban centres. Remarkably, for the majority of Canadians who become homeless the experience is a short, one-time event of approximately less than a month in length, and they manage to leave homelessness with little support (Gaetz et al., 2013). In 2014, the implementation of the federal Homelessness Partnering Strategy was begun. A cornerstone of this plan is Housing First, "an evidence-based approach that aims to stabilize the lives of homeless individuals for the long-term by first moving them into permanent housing, and then providing additional support for underlying issues, such as

> **"RAISING THE ROOF"**
>
> You may have noticed commercials on TV showcasing "Raising the Roof" toques as a fundraiser to stop youth homelessness. Raising the Roof is a charity created in 1998 by members of the Canadian Non-Profit Housing Foundation as a means of focusing on long-term solutions to homelessness. The charity's mission is to "provide leadership on long-term solutions to homelessness through partnerships and collaboration with diverse stakeholders, investment in local communities, and public education" (www.raisingtheroof.org/Our-Programs/Toque-Campaign.aspx). (See Figure 29.2.)

 **1 Toque** = a bus pass or some clothing for a youth's all-important first job interview

 **10 Toques** = supportive housing for one youth for a week, allowing him or her to learn essential life skills to help break away from street culture

 **200 Toques** = enough to support a youth to go back to school for a year or enroll in an apprenticeship program for two months

**FIGURE  29.2  Raise the Roof**

addiction and mental health" (Government of Canada, 2014). This program represents a significant shift in priorities for assistance of homeless people.

# POVERTY, HOMELESSNESS, AND THE DETERMINANTS OF HEALTH

In 2003, Health Canada, based on evidence, identified 12 key determinants of health, sometimes known as the social determinants of health. The World Health Organization (WHO) (2015) described the social determinants of health as "the conditions in which people are born, grow, live, work and age. These circumstances are shaped by the distribution of money, power, and resources at global, national and local levels. The social determinants of health are mostly responsible for health inequities—the unfair and avoidable differences in health status seen within and between countries" (par. 1). In 2005 to 2008, the WHO established a commission to study health inequities on a global scale and report on the best way to reduce the inequities. The commission reported that "closing the health gap" would require "concerted actions across sectors," and presented three recommendations: (1) improving daily living conditions; (2) tackling inequitable distribution of power, money, and other resources; and (3) measuring and understanding the problem and assessing the impact of action (WHO, 2009). Raphael, Curry-Stevens, and Bryant argue that "Despite Canada's reputation as a leader in health promotion and population health, implementation of public policies in support of the social determinants of health has been woefully inadequate" (2009, p. 222). Recently, videos have been produced that discuss determinants of health; they are referenced in the MyLab online resources. In this chapter, we do not reiterate the data that produced these determinants; rather, we discuss how poverty and homelessness affect each determinant and mention a few of the programs in place to mitigate the effects of poverty and homelessness. (See Photo 29.1.)

**Income and Social Status** Our income often dictates where we can afford to live, what we can afford to eat, and the activities we enjoy. The 2011 census indicates that the percentage of Canadians living in urban areas continues to grow (Statistics Canada, 2012). A research group studied the results of the 2001 census to determine links between health outcomes and living in five urban centres in Canada (Canadian Population Health Initiative, 2006). Findings included the fact that more people living in high-income neighbourhoods tended to rate their health as excellent or very good, report more leisure-time activity, and be non-smokers. The chief public health officer's report on the state of public health in Canada 2008 indicated that if all the population had the same income levels and mortality rates as our highest-income neighbourhoods, the potential for years lost (see Chapter 11) to urban populations would decrease by almost 20% (Minister of Health, 2008). Some provincial governments have put programs in place to assist low-income families with early kindergarten programs, subsidized housing, and child benefits; however, families with no fixed address may still have difficulty accessing these programs. People who perceive their health as poor may be less likely or less able to overcome barriers to seeking healthcare. While LICO recognizes that less income is needed in rural areas, transportation costs are higher and healthcare services may be less available in these areas due to consolidation of services in urban centres.

**Social Support Networks** Historically, Canadians have looked out for each other. This is evident in the way our healthcare and social support systems have evolved. However, the poor and the homeless are less able to meet this determinant of health in several ways.

- Many of these networks are not available to them. A poor family's circle of friends and relatives may have exhausted the assistance they are able to give, putting strain on the relationships. This absence may come just at a time when the family needs the support desperately. See Canadian Research Box 29.1.
- Obtaining money for travel or long-distance communication to continue the relationships may be problematic. Not having a fixed address makes it very difficult to receive mail or other communication from family and friends.
- Establishing new and meaningful relationships while living in shelters or when moving frequently is difficult.
- Poor people may perceive they have nothing to offer in a relationship and begin to withdraw, increasing a sense of low self-esteem. Children who live in poverty may not learn to access and build social support networks.

**Education and Literacy** People who are poorly educated are less likely to qualify for high-paying jobs. As our use of technology increases, literacy requirements for many jobs are increasing. Persons with undiagnosed or untreated learning disabilities are more likely to drop out of school, again decreasing the opportunities available. Even if upgrading classes are subsidized and can be reached with affordable transportation,

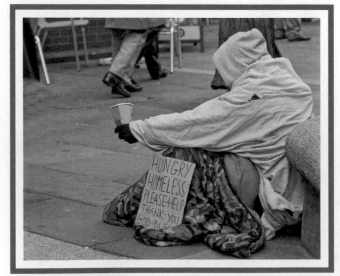

**PHOTO 29.1** It is estimated that 150 000 to 300 000 people are homeless in Canada.

*Source: Urbanbuzz/Shutterstock*

**CANADIAN RESEARCH BOX 29.1**

**What is the effect of hidden homelessness on family relationships?**

Peterson, E., (2012). "I like to let them have their time." Hidden homeless First Nations people in the city and their management of household relationships. *Social & Cultural Geography, 13*(4), 321–338. Copyright © 2012 by Taylor & Francis Group. Reprinted by permission of the author. doi:10.1080/14649365. 2012.683805

Nurses have completed little research on homelessness. This study, completed by a geographer, examined the experiences of the hidden homeless—people who are living with someone else in their social network. Prior research indicates that immigrant and Aboriginal persons are less likely to access mainstream options (e.g., shelters) as a solution to housing issues, but prefer to utilize opportunities through families and friends. Many of these are precarious solutions, as there is no permanency and one is dependent on the willingness of others to share. This researcher interviewed 56 Aboriginal people, including males, females, individuals, couples, and adults with dependent children. All had spent over 50% of the previous 18 months living with family or friends. The qualitative data demonstrated that each individual had to develop strong insights into when they were no longer welcome, and strategies to delay that circumstance as long as possible. Five themes that illustrate the strategies were identified, including minimizing one's presence in the household, providing household and personal services for others, moving frequently, contributing as much as possible to the household budget, and eating as little of the household food as possible. Because of the dearth of research with hidden homeless individuals and families, it is difficult to compare experiences of the hidden homeless.

### Discussion Questions

1. What would be the effect of using these "welcome" strategies on other necessary tasks (e.g., returning to school, getting a job)?
2. How might public policy contribute to the numbers of hidden homeless?

these people may not be able to afford the simplest of supplies to go to school or the childcare required in order to attend.

**Employment or Working Conditions** Persons with no fixed address and little or no income have difficulty getting identification papers, applying for jobs, or maintaining employment. The jobs they do get are often transitory, hourly wage jobs with few benefits; for example, they may be forced to choose between going to a health professional for a personal or family health problem and going to work. Further, people working in low-paying jobs may be more susceptible to workplace injury, thus further limiting opportunities. While Canada enjoyed a relatively low unemployment rate as late as 2008, the global financial events in 2008 and onward have increased the numbers of families affected by unemployment.

**Social Environments** Poverty can be viewed as a social exclusionary factor. Many people who are poor or homeless are victims of violence or have been deinstitutionalized. Thus, social supports previously available may not be in place. Further, the social definition of poverty can be internalized, contributing to a sense of stigma, feelings of shame and inferiority, and low self-esteem (Reutter et al., 2009).

**Physical Environments** Some cities and neighbourhoods are in geographic areas of high pollution, where whole populations are exposed to additional health risks. However, within specific geographic locations there might be housing that is affordable to the poor family. Although it is not subsidized, it is frequently substandard, may be unsafe, and is often crowded. Overcrowding, combined with poor hygiene, can contribute to the spread of contagious diseases, including tuberculosis. Further, low-income housing is more likely to be in an unsafe neighbourhood, exposing the inhabitants to increased violence and fewer supports such as law enforcement. Over the last several years, national and local organizations such as Habitat for Humanity have worked to ensure affordable and safe housing for low-income families. While poverty can be less visible in rural communities, inability to maintain or enhance the physical environment (e.g., house, outbuildings) can lead to increased accidents and disease.

**Personal Health and Coping Skills** The facilities and opportunities available for basic personal hygiene, much less optimal health practices, are more difficult for the poor and the homeless populations. While biology and genetics may account for vision, hearing, and dental problems, poverty may ensure that those problems remain untreated. Poor people may delay seeking help due to their inability to pay for medication or other treatment not covered by the healthcare system. Mortality rates in poorer neighbourhoods are higher than in the general population. Votta and Manion (2003) found that homeless male youth reported more substance abuse, family dysfunction, difficulties in school, legal problems, and suicide attempts than non-homeless youth. Further, these youth reported less parental support, greater depressive episodes, and increased use of disengagement as a coping style.

**Healthy Child Development** One of the greatest concerns with poverty and homelessness is their effect on children. An obvious issue here is food insecurity, or the lack of access to sufficient nutritious food, which is discussed later in the chapter. This can result in children experiencing difficulties with memory, concentration, energy, problem-solving skills, and creativity (Minister of Health, 2008). Food banks, before-school breakfast programs, and other social activities to encourage healthy eating are making some inroads to better food security in Canada where they are available. Other issues to consider are poor hygiene and increased exposure to hazards and violence, resulting in lower life expectancy for persons who grow up in poverty. One of the less-obvious results of poverty is that families with little or no disposable income have difficulty ensuring their children have access to activities that would enhance their development. Even reading to a child at night becomes problematic when one cannot afford books and cannot access a library card due to the lack of a fixed address. Constant moving can also interfere with normal progress through public education. Further, poor children who do not dress like other children or have the same type of school supplies may feel more ostracized and victimized by peer bullying.

**Health Services** While geography is frequently a barrier to health services for all Canadians, the poor family faces additional barriers. Despite a strong universal healthcare system, income is required for services such as dental care and pharmaceuticals. Unemployment makes access that much more difficult. The lack of a fixed address can wreak havoc with making healthcare appointments or registering for services. The family seeking care may be faced with health professionals who do not provide culturally safe care, thus discouraging the family from returning for follow-up care. When a poor or homeless person is hospitalized, assumptions may be made about the care that can be delivered after discharge—a challenge even for families with adequate income. Mobile health units and the use of technology such as telehealth has increased access for many people, but still it does not always meet the needs of the poor and homeless.

**Gender** Women generally live longer than men and experience greater incidences of depression, stress overload, and some chronic conditions. When rates of physical activity (often part of leisure time) are included in the equation, risk for chronic illnesses among women increases. Women are more likely to be the victims of family violence. As well, they are more likely to be in the lower employment categories. Lone-parent families continue to experience the lowest levels of family income in Canada, with the majority of these headed by women (Statistics Canada, 2008). Further, women who become lone-parent heads of households while still under the age of 40 tend to remain in poverty (Gadalla, 2008). All these factors contribute to inclusion in the populations of poverty and homelessness.

**Culture** Each person belongs to several different cultures, including ethnic, neighbourhood, work, club (e.g., the Legion), and religious groups. Part of belonging to any given culture is the desire to meet that culture's expectations. The Canadian Homelessness Research Network (2012) further suggests that in Canada the over-representation of Aboriginal peoples (First Nations, Métis, and Inuit) among the homeless population indicates that there is a need to recognize historical, experiential (i.e., experiences with colonization and racism), and cultural differences when considering Canadian homelessness. Poverty and homelessness for many of the reasons already stated may increase the barriers to meeting one's cultural tasks, thereby contributing to decreases in a sense of self-worth and failure to engage in healthy behaviours when possible.

This limited discussion on the effects of poverty and homelessness on the determinants of health demonstrates that both poverty and homelessness increase the barriers to meeting the determinants, and reinforces their interrelatedness. A barrier is anything that prevents the person or family from accomplishing a health task. Barriers may be actual (lack of address or identification resulting in refusal of services) or perceived (belief that as a poor or homeless person I have nothing to offer a relationship). In the case of poverty and homelessness, we have now identified multiple barriers to each of the determinants of health. When there is a barrier to one determinant of health, that barrier influences several other determinants as well. In the next section, we will consider specific health issues for these populations.

## SPECIFIC HEALTH ISSUES OF THE HOMELESS AND POOR

Health issues of the homeless do not differ from those of the general population. Hwang's (2001) seminal work identified that disease severity is related to a number of factors: poverty, cognitive impairment, delays in seeking treatment, non-adherence to therapy, and the adverse health effects of homelessness itself. Adverse health effects of homelessness include, but are not limited to, skin and foot disorders, poor oral hygiene, respiratory tract infections, and hypertension (Hwang, 2001; Khan et al., 2011, Kulik, Gaetz, Crowe, & Ford-Jones, 2011). Foot disorders, for example, can be related to improperly fitted footwear or wearing the same footwear for prolonged periods of time. Shoes are sometimes used as pillows, which also allows the feet to breathe. Socks also may be worn for extended periods of time. All of these factors can impact the treatment of specific foot disorders such as fungal infections, plantar warts, ulcers, and large calluses.

Diseases and conditions often seen by clinicians whose practice includes homeless individuals reflect environmental factors, lifestyle choices, and the impact of poverty on health. Hypertension, cardiovascular disease, diabetes, asthma, renal disease, mental illness, cancer, HIV infection, AIDS, sexually transmitted infections, infant mortality, trauma caused by violence, and substance abuse are some of the conditions experienced by people who are homeless. An obvious correlation can be found between some of the diagnoses and life on the street. For example, a person sleeping on heating grates may be burned. One area that has received little attention has been end-of-life care for homeless persons (see Canadian Research Box 29.2).

To find the relationships between an adverse health effect and a homeless person, the healthcare provider needs to assess the lifestyle of the client. Assessment should include sleeping patterns and where sleep is obtained as well as information regarding food, smoking, substance use, support networks, and income. A thorough assessment of the daily routine of the client is important because it may reveal the relationships. A good understanding of the determinants of health and their application is important when doing the assessment. Other relationships or the weight these relationships place on the health of the person may not be so obvious to the novice clinician.

**CANADIAN RESEARCH BOX 29.2**

**What can be done to improve end-of-life care for homeless populations?**

McNeil, R., Guirguis-Younger, M., & Dilley, L. (2012). Recommendations for improving the end-of-life care system for homeless populations: A qualitative study of the views of Canadian health and social services professionals. *BMC Palliative Care, 11*(14), 1–8. Retrieved from http://www.biomedcentral.com/content/pdf/1472-684X-11-14.pdf. doi:10.1186/1472-684X-11-14

Homeless populations have diverse and complicated care needs. Compared with housed populations, it has been shown that the homeless suffer disproportionately from poor health in terms of chronic conditions, mental illness, substance abuse, and infectious diseases. The homeless are faced with daily physical challenges (i.e., exposure to the elements and food scarcity), and barriers to accessing healthcare services (i.e., lack of insurance, discrimination), which make it difficult to manage their healthcare needs and may actually lead to further health deterioration. As such, homeless populations have the highest "all-cause" mortality rates of any population in Canada, indicating that this population also has a high level of need for end-of-life care services.

McNeil, Guirguis-Younger, and Dilley noted that the homeless population is aging in time with the general population of Canada, and suggested that in the homeless population the "natural" health challenges faced in conjunction with advancing age will likely lead to an increased demand for end-of-life services. They also noted that the Canadian end-of-life care system is largely based on social assumptions that do not reflect the homeless (or precariously housed) person's experiences and limited access to such services. For example, the Canadian healthcare system generally expects that individuals are housed, have supportive friends and families, and can afford to pay for supplementary services.

These researchers noted that system-level recommendations for improving end-of-life care services for the homeless populations are urgently needed. They conducted qualitative interviews of health and social services professionals in six Canadian cities (Ottawa, Halifax, Hamilton, Toronto, Thunder Bay, and Winnipeg) with the objectives of identifying barriers to services and identifying recommendations to improve the system for the terminal homeless population.

The results indicated that there were three barrier themes to accessing end-of-life care services in these cities:

- lack of caregiver support and/or financial resources (i.e., having no family to help with care, inability to afford assisted living facilities, and inability to afford medications);
- exclusionary operating policies for community service providers (e.g., anti-drug policies, codes of conduct) on the basis of a range of conditions common in homeless populations (e.g., mental illness and substance abuse); and
- lack of continuity of care (e.g., no follow-up, poor discharge planning) that hastens the need for end-of-life care in those with chronic diseases and places undue burden on community agencies ill-equipped to provide palliative services.

The results of this research indicated four main recommendations:

- healthcare systems adopt "low-threshold" approaches for admission and care (i.e., change the rules and regulations regarding alcohol and drug abstinence and integrate harm-reduction strategies);
- formal partnering of health and social services agencies accessed by homeless people with end-of-life care systems, because this fosters trust; trusted staff could monitor changes in health status and through this mediate access to needed end-of-life services;
- patient advocates could play a role in liaising between community agencies and the end-of-life care system to strengthen partnerships; and
- increased training to strengthen the capacity of healthcare professionals to address the complex and diverse needs of homeless populations at the end of life, and decrease discrimination.

### Discussion Questions

1. As a CHN working at an emergency shelter, you are asked to help with research designed to develop an end-of-life program for the homeless population in your community. This would be an excellent opportunity for inter-professional collaboration. What types of informants and professionals would best suit this research endeavour? What types of information might you be interested in gathering?

2. Would harm-reduction strategies for the homeless be a feasible option in your community's healthcare facilities? Why or why not?

3. What kinds of training would strengthen your ability as a CHN to provide culturally competent end-of-life care to the homeless population in your community?

# FOOD INSECURITY

Food insecurity is a relatively invisible issue except among the most poverty-stricken individuals. In other words, food crisis is a poverty issue. Household **food insecurity** is defined as "the inability to acquire or consume an adequate diet quality or sufficient quantity of food in socially acceptable ways, or the uncertainty that one will be able to do so" (Health Canada, 2012). It is a problem that continues to affect an estimated one in 12 Canadian households (Tarasuk, McIntyre, & Power, 2012). (See Figure 29.3.) In Canada, factors including remote geographic locations, changing seasons, and insecure financial resources make the acquisition of food through acceptable sources difficult. Food insecurity predicts poorer overall physical and mental health and can lead to nutrient deficiencies and chronic diseases. The number-one response to food insecurity in Canada has been the development of food banks. The first food bank was developed in Edmonton in 1981 as a temporary measure, but the issue of food scarcity has continued to grow (Food Banks

Canada, 2013a). Today there are over 800 food banks and 3 000 food programs in Canada that provide services to approximately 850 000 Canadians (36.4% are children and youth) each month (Food Banks Canada, 2013b).

Significant predictors of food insecurity are as follow:

- low income (Canadians on social assistance are at a higher risk than those who rely on employment income, however they comprise only one-quarter of the food insecure households in Canada);
- Aboriginal status;
- renting instead of owning one's domicile; and
- being a lone-parent, female-led family (Tarasuk, McIntyre, & Power, 2012). See Figure 29.3 for food insecurity across Canada.

## CASE STUDY

Case study inspired by Loopstra, R., & Tarasuk, V. (2013). Perspectives on community gardens, community kitchens and the Good Food Box program in a community-based sample of low-income families. *Canadian Journal of Public Health, 104*(1), e55–e59.

Several noteworthy programs have been developed in response to the awareness that food security has become a major issue for the health of Canadians, especially those struggling with fewer resources. These programs include (but are not limited to) collective kitchens, community gardens, and the Good Food Box. However, there has been speculation as to whether these types of programs are an effective means of bettering the food scarcity in communities. You are a CHN looking into the viability of expanding a food security program (choose one of the three mentioned above) in your community; you decide to do a bit of reading and come across research by Loopstra and Tarasuk. In their study, they randomly selected participants (a total of 371 families) from 23 "high poverty" census tracts in Toronto to be interviewed at baseline and then re-interviewed one year later, inquiring as to why food programs were not used. Their results indicated that over the 12-month period only 12 families (3.2%) indicated participation in a community garden, 16 families (4.3%) indicated participation in a community kitchen, and 4 families (1.1%) participated in the Good Food Box program. Further, the results of these interviews divided the lack of participation into two themes: the "programs were not accessible" and a "lack of program fit."

### Discussion Questions

1. Understanding that these results may shed light on the effectiveness of your program(s), what might you try doing to increase accessibility and fit in your community?

2. How might the culture within your community play a role or affect the changes you propose?

3. What role(s) do the social determinants of health play in terms of increasing community participation? Please give examples.

## MATCHING NEED WITH RESOURCES

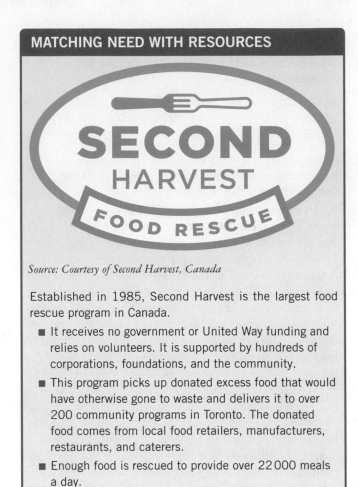

*Source: Courtesy of Second Harvest, Canada*

Established in 1985, Second Harvest is the largest food rescue program in Canada.

- It receives no government or United Way funding and relies on volunteers. It is supported by hundreds of corporations, foundations, and the community.

- This program picks up donated excess food that would have otherwise gone to waste and delivers it to over 200 community programs in Toronto. The donated food comes from local food retailers, manufacturers, restaurants, and caterers.

- Enough food is rescued to provide over 22 000 meals a day.

## CHILDHOOD: PUTTING IT ALL TOGETHER

Childhood represents a unique, time-sensitive, and vulnerable period in which individuals grow and develop. To this end, the government of Canada recognizes that every child has rights and that among those rights it is understood that adults must make decisions with the child's best interests as a priority; and that the government has a responsibility to protect and assist families in the nurturing of children (UNICEF, 2002). UNICEF Canada reports that governments that are most successful in protecting children from poverty are those that work to decrease the number of low-income households (e.g., through benefits and tax credits) and assist in providing services and opportunities for good childhood development. UNICEF Canada also suggests that industrialized countries that accept higher levels of child poverty do so as a function of policy and budgetary priority, which has the negative impact of limiting individual potential and prosperity and increasing social costs. Unfortunately, during UNICEF's most recent report card on childhood poverty, Canada ranked 18th of 35 industrialized nations in terms of the gap between childhood poverty (14%) and population poverty (12%), after taxes, indicating that in Canada children are more likely to live in poverty than the overall population (UNICEF Canada, 2012). (See Figure 29.4 for Canadian childhood poverty rates across time.)

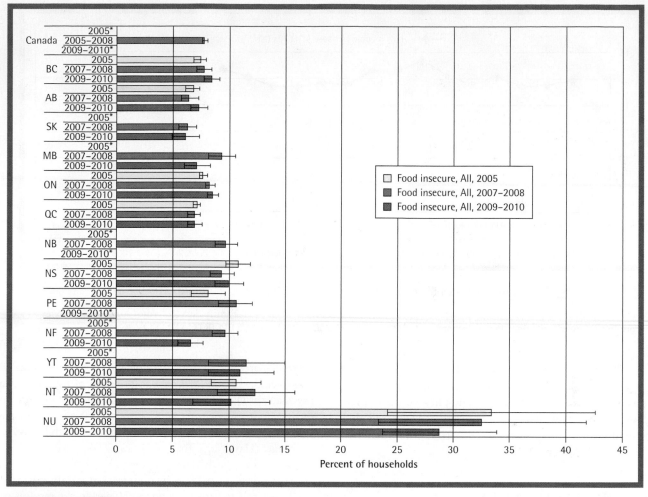

Being "poor" can have many broad socially exclusionary consequences for adults, but also for children who have little understanding or control of choices or life experiences. The choices adults make and the chance events in a child's experience can affect physical and mental development as well as their future roles in society. Research indicates that socioeconomic settings impact the physical and social aspects of neighbourhoods, families, and children, often with health implications (Schreier & Chen, 2013). By looking at childhood through the determinants of health (discussed earlier in this chapter), a CHN can easily recognize how low income can negatively affect family life as well as an individual's development. For example, a single-parent family may only be able to afford rent in a "sketchy" neighbourhood, may only be able to afford sporadic amounts of high-nutrition foods, and may not be able to afford childcare services. These living conditions can be perceived as stressful by the whole family, which may impair physical and mental health,

academic or work performance, ability to parent, and ability to improve income and living situations, essentially creating a cycle of continued poverty for the entire family.

- The sharpest increase in use of Canadian shelters has been for families, more specifically, children. Statistics indicate that although families account for only 4% of shelter stays, they use 14% of total bed nights (Gaetz et al., 2013).
- Roustit, Hamelin, Grillo, Martin, and Chauvin (2010) indicated a relationship between food insecurity in Québécois adolescents and poor academic performance, and suggested that attending schools with food assistance programs could act as a moderating factor.
- Adverse childhood events are early risk factors for adult health and psychiatric problems, which are over-represented in adult homeless populations. Self-reported childhood learning disabilities predicted longer durations of

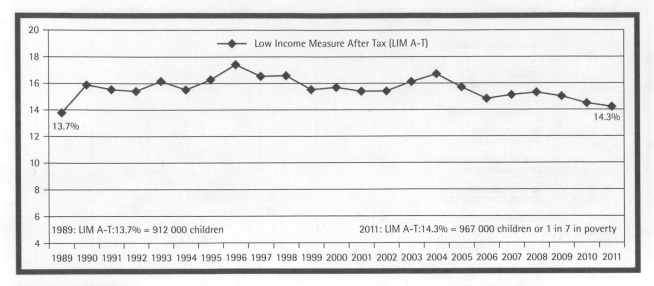

**FIGURE 29.4** Poverty Rates for Children in Low-Income Families in Canada, 1989–2011

*Source:* 2013 Campaign 2000 Report Card on Child and Family Poverty in Canada. Family Services Toronto, page 3. Retrieved from http://www.campaign2000.ca/reportCards/national/2013C2000NATIONALREPORTCARDNOV26.pdf

homelessness, less-severe mental disorders but multiple mental disorders and higher suicidal ideation, early and severe substance abuse problems, and physical health problems for homeless adults in Vancouver who rated their overall health as "fair or poor" (Patterson, Moniruzzaman, Frankish, & Somers, 2012).

## ACCESS TO HEALTHCARE

Challenging economic, social, and environmental conditions often result in poor health. Unfortunately, some populations in urban, rural, remote, and northern environments have difficulty accessing mainstream healthcare services. Canadians living in urban and non-urban areas face different difficulties in accessing the care they require, as such community-based front-line health services need to be able to provide necessary care while addressing the local determinants of health. Individuals living in non-urban areas often experience more challenges when accessing healthcare services compared to those living in cities. Rural, remote, and northern areas often struggle with attracting healthcare professionals, leading to a decreased selection in healthcare services. For example, many rural hospitals are staffed by family doctors and there are few specialists. Further, patients seeking health services outside of their community often must travel great distances and usually incur further costs such as taking time off work, having decreased social support from family and friends, and expenses for travel, lodging, and food (Hay, Varga-Toth, & Hines, 2006).

The most common access points for healthcare in rural areas are family doctors or nurse practitioners, small rural hospitals, community health centres or clinics, nursing stations, and mobile health units. However, the use of telehealth is an option explored in these areas to allow specialists to consult with the local healthcare providers as well as to provide an avenue for training. Essentially, telehealth involves use of a telephone,

written materials, and a video or Web-based program. For example, Dr. Patrick McGrath, a professor of psychology and psychiatry at Dalhousie University, and colleagues are providing mental health services to rural persons being treated for postpartum depression and for parents of children with behavioural challenges (Hay, Varga-Toth, & Hines, 2006, p. 18).

Travelling healthcare providers, particularly those who are specialized, may stop in underserved communities and rural hospitals to provide services. However, the services may be few and far between due to time constraints, waiting list times, lack of medical resources and supplies, and distances of travel for the healthcare provider. For this reason a proactive form of healthcare services was created wherein the service is brought to those who need it. For example, in Saskatoon, Saskatchewan, a mobile health bus has been staffed with a nurse practitioner and a paramedic in order to provide primary healthcare services closer to home for members of the core community. The services provided on the bus are health checks, blood pressure and sugar checks, chronic disease management, disease prevention, health education, wound care, and follow-up care. The staff also link clients to youth, addiction, and mental health services, and to community-based organizations and programs (Saskatoon Health Region, 2015).

This chapter has previously discussed how homelessness is associated with many negative health and social outcomes, but what is perhaps more astonishing is the type and severity of encounters they have with higher-level healthcare services, mostly due to barriers in accessing primary and preventative healthcare. Hwang et al. (2013) studied the type and number of healthcare utilizations of 1 165 homeless participants and matched low-income control participants from Toronto, Ontario, over an observation period of approximately 3.9 years. The results indicated that 95.5% of homeless participants had at least one encounter with health services, 92.5% visited a doctor's office, 76.6% visited an emergency department, 19.5% were hospitalized in a medical-surgical bed, and 11.5% were hospitalized in a psychiatric bed. By comparison, among the control participants, 84.2% had at least one encounter with health services, 83.3% visited a doctor's office, 35.6% visited an emergency department, 7.1% were hospitalized in a medical-surgical bed, and 1.6% were hospitalized in a psychiatric bed. On average, this research indicated that in a year the control participants accessed health services 6 220 times, whereas the homeless participants had approximately made 13 240 encounters with health services! Interestingly, the frequent users of each type of healthcare service represented only 10% of the homeless population studied, but these 10% accounted for 43% of the total ambulatory care encounters, 60.3% of the emergency department encounters, 79.9% of the medical-surgical encounters, and 85.9% of the psychiatric hospitalizations. Overall, this research indicated that in a universally insured healthcare system, people who are homeless are more intensive users of the healthcare system than a matched low-income control group, and that within the homeless population there was a subset of persons who were extremely frequent health service users. These findings could be an indicator that the frequent service users are encountering more barriers to appropriate healthcare and that interventions focusing on more-effective healthcare for this group may have the potential to improve their health as well as free up resources within a busy healthcare system.

## COMMUNITY HEALTH NURSES' ROLE

CHNs act to provide community empowerment through their public health functions, with the goal of providing services to the population, community, families, and individuals in terms of outcomes such as protection, promotion, prevention, and access. By increasing their clinical acumen within their population, CHNs learn or take on new roles. One role is that of an advocate through political action (e.g., Cathy Crowe). Another is enabling clients to empower themselves.

Cathy Crowe is an example of a CHN who is committed to this high-risk population. It is fitting that she works in the Canadian city with one of the highest populations of poor, although there are now CHNs in most major cities working with this population. Ms. Crowe advocates through strong political action for the rights of the homeless. She is noted for legal action she has brought against the Province of Ontario to increase affordable housing, to reduce the number of deaths related to homelessness, and to hold the province accountable for its policies. Ms. Crowe received the first-ever Woodsworth Award for Social Advocacy in recognition of her commitment to social advocacy. Further, in 2004 she received an Atkinson Fellowship award, which was extended in both 2007 and 2009, to help fight homelessness during the economic recession. In 2009, she published a book called *Dying for a Home*, and has continued to travel to other Canadian cities to offer support while advocating for the homeless (see Crowe, 2009).

Toronto Public Health developed a project for supporting at-risk homeless pregnant and parenting women. Two nurses worked on this project. One nurse worked in the downtown area of Toronto and the other in the suburbs where there were hotels serving homeless families. These nurses received referrals from shelters, drop-in health centres, and street hangouts. The nurses coordinated care involving several community services, provided home visits, and made telephone follow-ups. The nurses also accompanied clients to prenatal visits until they were comfortable going alone (Little, Gorman, Dzendoletas, & Moravac, 2007).

## TECHNOLOGY AND HOMELESSNESS

Technology is a part of everyday living in Canada, and it has been suggested that technology has the capacity to improve the quality of life that people enjoy. However, most people do not reflect on how the technology in their environments affects their lives, or how the lack of that technology may put people at a disadvantage. Although the development of technology is not to blame for poverty or homelessness, it does play an integral role in how everyone interacts with society as a whole.

Le Dantec and Edwards (2008) suggested that "the factors that disadvantage developing nations are also present among the homeless population in industrialized nations and affect the relationship of this population with technology; lower levels of education and literacy restrict access to information, a lack of economic independence restricts access to computers and Internet resources, and limited access to training hinders the uptake of digital technology when it is made available" (p. 628). A qualitative study by Le Dantec and Edwards (2008) used one-on-one interviews from which several themes were developed about the relationship homeless people have with technology. They suggested that the homeless use technology regularly, especially if there is a perceived benefit. This research indicated that the homeless place great value in being able to stay connected with family, friends, and important contacts or resources whether by phone, Internet, or in person. This research also indicated that homeless people utilize computers and the Internet to find resources (such as where they can go for a shower, meals, and job postings), to access information or give tips on how to survive on the streets, and to do social networking on sites without feeling the stigma associated with homelessness. Incidentally, research by Guadagno, Muscanell, and Pollio (2013) indicated that there is only a minor "digital divide" between undergraduates and young adult homeless persons in terms of access to the Internet, but that there was a marked difference in the use of the Internet. The proportion of homeless young adults and undergraduate students utilizing social networking sites were found to be similar, but undergraduates were more likely to use the sites for games and locating others whereas homeless young adults were more likely to use social networking sites for private messaging and blogging. This demonstrates that the young homeless population is interacting on similar social levels as housed persons, that they are not "cut off" from Internet resources, and that research into types of Internet usage, quality of access points or equipment, and fee-for-service sites may be of interest to individuals working with the homeless population.

Several difficulties related to technology use and the homeless were reported by Le Dantec and Edwards, including finding an affordable or available telephone or computer, being able to receive or respond to messages on the telephone, the availability of electricity to recharge batteries, literacy and understanding how to use technology, and the time involved in finding sources of technology (e.g., waiting in line for a public phone or computer, taking public transit).

Le Dantec and Edwards's research suggests that thoughtful technologies that are socially relevant could be used as an intervention to reduce homelessness while helping those already at risk. This is a belief shared by several networking sites, such as "Homeless Nation," which describes itself as a website for and by the street community. This website was developed in 2003 by a Montreal-based documentary filmmaker and friends who were interested in the stories of the homeless. This site was created as an access point for online media, a place to share stories and information, a social networking site, a place to locate friends who have gone missing, and most importantly, to create social awareness and positive change. Nearly 4 500 people have joined the site and it has received several awards; most recently, this site was recognized by receiving the UN-based 2009 World Summit Award (Pinchin, 2009).

In Vancouver, B.C., the Lu'ma Native Housing Society began a program to provide free phone numbers and voicemail to the homeless. This voicemail acts as a means to contact the homeless individual, whether that person is a landlord, prospective employer, healthcare provider, or loved one (Paulsen, 2010). This service provides persons in crisis or transition a reliable way to maintain contact. Clients can manage their own appointments by dialling into the system. Community voicemail is also available in Calgary and Prince George (Lu'ma Native Housing Society, 2010).

# RESEARCH

Research in the area of homelessness can be difficult for a number of reasons. Not knowing who the homeless people are or where to find them is the most obvious. Other reasons may include, but are not limited to, competing priorities of the client (finding food may take precedence over participation in research), the perception that the endpoint of the research does not make a difference in the daily life of the homeless, and the inability of the researcher to find a funding agency. To overcome some of these barriers, researchers have begun to use the community participation approach to their research. Community participatory research is characterized by using community leaders in partnership with the researchers through the entire research process. That is, the community is involved from the inception, when the gap is identified, to the endpoint of writing the report and disseminating the information. Through this process the community has the opportunity to see a difference in their daily lives as a result of the research process.

Research contributing to the understanding of these populations is limited. It is interesting to note that in a recent search of professional literature, nursing literature was sparse in the areas of homelessness and poverty, and other Canadian researchers appear more likely to study these topics elsewhere in the world rather than at home.

# CONCLUSION

In this chapter we have explored the definitions and scope of poverty and homelessness in Canada. Recognition of the difficulty in defining and describing these populations separately or together has informed the process. Using the determinants of health as a framework, we have explored the effect of poverty and homelessness on the determinants. Food security as an issue frequently related to poverty and homelessness was also explored. Specific health issues for these populations and the CHN's role were explored.

The CHN is the healthcare provider who may have first access to poor or homeless persons through community outreach activities. By initiating communication and making a determined effort to understand their world, the CHN may be able to establish a trusting relationship that enables the nurse and the client to co-create a higher level of health.

## KEY TERMS

basic needs   p. 527
food insecurity   p. 533
homelessness   p. 528
low-income cut-off measure (LICO)   p. 527
market basket measure (MBM)   p. 527
poverty   p. 527

## STUDY QUESTIONS

1. Discuss the five descriptions of homelessness; how are they similar and different?

2. What is the difference between families in poverty and the working poor?

3. Identify three ways that a CHN can contribute to ensuring food security in a given community.

4. Discuss the assumption that it is less expensive to live in rural areas.

5. What factors contribute to the statistic that female-headed, lone parent families are more likely to live in poverty than those headed by males? Consider all the determinants of health.

6. There are increasing advertisements or other media that look at free cellphones and/or texting opportunities for low-income or homeless people. How would this intervention affect the factors of homefullness that Tognoli (1987) identified (see page 529)?

After working through these questions, go to the MyNursingLab at www.pearsoned.ca/mynursinglab to check your answers.

## INDIVIDUAL CRITICAL-THINKING EXERCISES

1. In 1990, the Canadian Public Health Association described the advocacy role of public health nursing as one of helping the socially disadvantaged to become aware of issues relevant to their health and promoting the development of resources that will result in "equal access to health and health-related services." As a nurse working in the community, how would you develop a plan of care for a person living in a shelter? Use the above statement as a guide, paying close attention to accessing healthcare services.

2. Consider how many times a day you are asked for some form of identification. What activities would you be unable to perform if you did not have this identification? How might this affect your health and healthcare?

3. List 10 personal, everyday activities that require money for participation, and add up the total. What activities would you need to delete if your income were below the LICO level? Would the removal of any of these activities affect your health status? How?

4. There is evidence that homeless children have more health problems, more hospitalizations, and more developmental problems than poor children who have never been homeless. Using the determinants of health as your guide in the discussion, comment on this quotation and discuss its validity.

5. Consider how a CHN might need to reframe his or her perceptions of healthcare service delivery when working with the homeless populations.

6. As a CHN, what can you do to address food scarcity in your community?

7. As a CHN, what kind of personal preparation/reflection must you do to best serve the homeless population?

## GROUP CRITICAL-THINKING EXERCISES

1. Recent extreme heat waves in the summer months have led to growing public health concern regarding the elderly, people with chronic and debilitating health conditions, and people living in poverty and inadequate housing such as rooming houses. Existing public health measures seem to rely on public service announcements that encourage the public to drink lots of fluids and go to air-conditioned spaces such as libraries. Provide a critique of these measures and consider possible solutions and advocacy measures.

2. The working poor live on a precipice that can tumble them into homelessness at any time. An illness or an unexpected layoff brings missed paycheques, which leads to skipped utility or rent payments, which snowballs into penalties, which ends in shutoffs or evictions. Discuss how a CHN would interact with a person in this situation. Consider advocacy measures and possible research questions that would assist this high-risk clientele.

3. You are a CHN and you receive a phone call from the TB nurse regarding Henry. Henry is an 85-year-old homeless man who has chosen not to stay in hospital and instead to reside in a men's shelter that you visit weekly. Henry refuses to wear personal protective equipment and is often difficult to locate for TB medication administration. What can you do to best assist Henry? What can you do to best advocate for your community? As a CHN, is your primary responsibility for the individual or for the community?

## REFERENCES

Belanger, Y. D., Awosoga, O., & Head, G. W. (2013). Homelessness, urban Aboriginal people, and the need for a national enumeration. *Aboriginal Policy Studies, 2*(2), 4–33. doi:http://dx.doi.org/10.5663/aps.v2i2.19006

Berry, B. (2007). A repeated observation approach for estimating the street homeless population. *Evaluation Review, 31*(2), 166–199. doi:10.1177/0193841X06296947

Calgary Homeless Foundation. (2014). *Working together to build a better homeless-serving system annual report 2014.* Retrieved from http://calgaryhomeless.com/wp-content/uploads/2014/06/CHF-2014-Annual-Report.pdf

Canadian Homelessness Research Network. (2015). Canadian definition of homelessness. Retrieved from http://homelesshub.ca/about-homelessness/homelessness-101/homelessness-glossary

Canadian Population Health Initiative. (2006). *Improving the health of Canadians: An introduction to health in urban places.* Ottawa, ON: The Canadian Institute of Health Information.

Conference Board of Canada. (2013). *Canada failing to close the income inequality gap.* Retrieved from http://www.conferenceboard.ca/press/newsrelease/13-02-04/canada_failing_to_close_the_income_inequality_gap.aspx

Crowe, C. (2009). *Cathy Crowe newsletter,* #57, summer 2009. Retrieved from http://tdrc.net/uploads/file/Cathy/newsletter/ccnews_summer09.pdf

Food Banks Canada. (2013a). *Food banking in Canada.* Retrieved from http://www.foodbankscanada.ca/Learn-About-Hunger/Food-Banking-in-Canada.aspx

Food Banks Canada. (2013b). *About hunger in Canada.* Retrieved from http://www.foodbankscanada.ca/Learn-About-Hunger/About-Hunger-in-Canada.aspx

Gadalla, T. M. (2008). Gender differences in poverty rates after marital dissolution: A longitudinal study. *Journal of Divorce and Remarriage, 49*(3–4), 225–238. doi:10.1080/10502550802222493

Gaetz, S., Donaldson, J., Richter, T., & Gulliver, T. (2013). *The state of homelessness in Canada 2013.* Retrieved from http://homelesshub.ca/SOHC2013

Government of Canada. (2014). *Minister Bergen highlights Canada's progress and leadership with Housing First at national conference on ending homelessness.* Retrieved from http://news.gc.ca/web/article-en.do?nid=899589

Guadagno, R., Muscanell, N., & Pollio, D. (2013). The homeless use Facebook?! Similarities of social network use between college students and homeless young adults. *Computers in Human Behavior, 29*(1), 86–89. doi:10.1016/j.chb.2012.17.019

Habitat for Humanity. (2013). *Our history.* Retrieved from http://www.habitat.ca/en/about/history

Hay, D., Varga-Toth, J., & Hines, E. (2006). *Frontline health care in Canada: Innovations in delivering services to vulnerable populations.* Canadian Policy Research Networkers INC. Retrieved from http://www.cprn.org/documents/45652_en.pdf

Health Canada. (2012). *Household food insecurity in Canada: Overview.* Adapted and reproduced with permission from the Minister of Health, 2015. Retrieved from http://www.hc-sc.gc.ca/fn-an/surveill/nutrition/commun/insecurit/index-eng.php

Homelessness Action Week. (2013). *Media advisory: 8th annual homelessness action week to draw attention to major issue of in visible homelessness in metro Vancouver.* Retrieved from http://stophomelessness.ca/wp-content/uploads/2008/09/24.9.13-Release_HAW_Final.pdf

Human Resources and Skills Development Canada. (2007). *When working is not enough to escape poverty: An analysis of Canada's working poor.* August 2006. Retrieved from http://publications.gc.ca/site/eng/294745/publication.html

Human Resources and Skills Development Canada. (2008). *Low income in Canada: 2000–2006 using the market basket measure.* Retrieved from http://www.servicecanada.gc.ca/eng/cs/sp/sdc/pkrf/publications/research/SP-630-06-06/page06.shtml

Human Resources and Skills Development Canada. (2013). *National homelessness information system.* Retrieved from http://hifis.hrsdc.gc.ca/index-eng.shtml

Hwang, S. W. (2001). Homelessness and health. *Canadian Medical Association Journal, 164*(2), 229–233.

Hwang, S., Chambers, C., Chiu, S., Katic, M., Kiss, A., Redelmeier, D., & Levison, W. (2013). A comprehensive assessment of health care utilization among homeless adults under a system of universal health insurance. *American Journal of Public Health, 103*(S2), S294–S301. doi:10.2105/AJPH.2013.301369

Khan, K., Rea, E., McDermaid, C., Stuart, R., Chambers, C., Wang, J., . . . Hwang, S. (2011). Active tuberculosis among homeless persons, Toronto, Ontario, Canada, 1998–2007. *Emerging Infectious Diseases, 17*(3), 357–365. doi:10.3201/eid1703.100833

Kulik, D. M., Caetz, S., Crowe, C., & Ford-Jones, E. (2011). Homeless youth's overwhelming health burden: A review of the literature. *Paediatrics Child Health, 16*(6), e43–e47.

Le Dantec, C., & Edwards, K. (2008). Designs on dignity: Perceptions of technology among the homeless. *Conference on Human Factors in Computing Systems—Proceedings*, 627–636. Retrieved from http://www.cc.gatech.edu/~keith/pubs/chi2008-homeless.pdf

Little, M., Gorman, A., Dzendoletas, D., & Moravac, C. (2007). Caring for the most vulnerable: A collaborative approach to supporting pregnant homeless youth. *Nursing for Women's Health, 11*(5), 458–466. doi:10.1111/j.1751-486X.2007.00213.x

Loopstra, R., & Tarasuk, V. (2013). Perspectives on community gardens, community kitchens and the Good Food Box program in a community-based sample of low-income families. *Canadian Journal of Public Health, 104(1)*, e55–e59.

Lu'ma Native Housing Society. (2010). *Community voice mail.* Retrieved from http://lnhs.ca/community-voice-mail

Minister of Health. (2008). *The chief public health officer's report on the state of public health in Canada 2008.* Retrieved from http://www.phac-aspc.gc.ca/cphorsphc-respcacsp/2008/fr-rc/index-eng.php

Murphy, B. (2000). *On the street: How we created homelessness.* Winnipeg, MB: J. G. Shillingford.

Murray, A. (1990). Homelessness: The people. In G. Fallis & A. Murray (Eds.), *Housing the homeless and poor: New partnerships among the private, public and third sectors.* Toronto, ON: University of Toronto Press.

Ontario Non-Profit Housing Association. (2015). *2015 waiting lists survey.* Retrieved from http://onpha.on.ca/onpha/web/Policyandresearch/Waiting_lists_2015/Content/PolicyAndResearch/Waiting_Lists_2015/2015_Waiting_Lists_Survey.aspx?hkey=64634a36-b6de-46b2-b76b-39541b2ea497

Parliament of Canada. (2008). *Measuring poverty: A challenge for Canada.* Retrieved from http://www.parl.gc.ca/Content/LOP/ResearchPublications/prb0865-e.htm

Patterson, M., Moniruzzaman, A., Frankish, C., & Somers, J. (2012). Missed opportunities: Childhood learning disabilities as early indicators of risk among homeless adults with mental illness in Vancouver, British Columbia. *BJMOpen, 2*(e001586). Retrieved from http://bmjopen.bmj.com/content/2/6/e001586.full.pdf+html

Paulsen, M. (2010, April). *Giving voice(mail) to the homeless.* Retrieved from http://thetyee.ca/Blogs/TheHook/Housing/2010/04/30/Giving-voicemail-to-the-homeless

Pinchin, K. (2009, September). Technology for tomorrow: Homeless find hope through technology, Internet. *The Globe and Mail.* Retrieved from http://www.theglobeandmail.com/news/technology/homeless-find-hope-through-technology-internet/article1296491

Raphael, D., Curry-Stevens, A., & Bryant, T. (2009). Barriers to addressing the social determinants of health: Insights from the Canadian experience. *Health Policy, 88*(2–3), 222–235. Used by permission of School of Health Policy & Management. doi:10.1016/j.healthpol.1008.03.015

Regroupement des centres d'amitié autochtones du Québec. (2008). *Brief concerning urban Aboriginal homelessness in Quebec.* Retrieved from http://www.reseaudialog.qc.ca/DocsPDF/URBANABORIGINALHOMELESSNESS.pdf

Reutter, L., Stewart, M. J., Veenstra, G., Love, R., Raphael, D., & Makwarimba, E. (2009). Who do they think they are, anyway? Perceptions of and responses to poverty stigma. *Qualitative Health Research, 19*(3), 297–311. doi:10.1177/1049732308330246

Rothwell, D. W., & Havemen, R. (2013). *Definition and measurement of asset poverty in Canada.* Retrieved from http://papers.ssrn.com/sol3/papers.cfm?abstract_id=2367057

Roustit, C., Hamelin, A., Grillo, F., Martin, J., & Chauvin, P. (2010). Food insecurity: Could school food supplementation help break the cycles of intergenerational transmission of social inequities? *Pediatrics, 126*(6), 1174–1181. doi:10.1542/peds.2009-3574

Saskatoon Health Region. (2015). Primary health bus. Retrieved from https://www.saskatoonhealthregion.ca/locations_services/Services/Primary-Health/Pages/HealthBus.aspx

Schreier, H., & Chen, E. (2013). Socioeconomic status and the health of youth: A multilevel, multidomain approach to conceptualizing pathways. *Psychological Bulletin, 139(3),* 606–654. doi:http://dx.doi.org/10.1037/a0029416

Statistics Canada. (2008). *Earnings and incomes of Canadians over the past quarter century, 2006 census: Findings.* Retrieved from http://www12.statcan.gc.ca/english/census06/analysis/income/index.cfm

Statistics Canada. (2009). *Low income cut-offs for 2008 and low income measures for 2007.* Retrieved from http://www.statcan.gc.ca/pub/75f0002m/75f0002m2009002-eng.pdf

Statistics Canada. (2012). *The Canadian population in 2011: Population counts and growth.* Retrieved from http://www12.statcan.gc.ca/census-recensement/2011/as-sa/98-310-x/98-310-x2011001-eng.pdf

Tarasuk, V., McIntyre, L., & Power, E. (2012). *Report to Olivier De Schutter, the United Nations Special Rapporteur on the right to food mission to Canada: Submission on civil society priority issue #1: Hunger, poverty and the right to food.* Retrieved from http://nutritionalsciences.lamp.utoronto.ca/wp-content/uploads/2012/07/Special-Rapporteur-submission-on-household-food-insecurity-01MAY2012-final-copy.pdf

The Salvation Army. (2013). *Annual review 2012/2013.* Retrieved from http://www.salvationarmy.ca/wp-content/uploads/2013/09/AnnualReview2012-13_web-final.pdf

Tognoli, J. (1987). Residential environments. In D. Stokols & I. Altman (Eds.), *Handbook of environmental psychology.* New York, NY: Wiley Interscience.

UNICEF. (2002). *Fact sheet: A summary of the rights under the convention on the rights of the child.* Retrieved from http://www.unicef.org/crc/files/Rights_overview.pdf

UNICEF Canada. (2012). *Report card 10: Measuring child poverty, Canadian companion.* Retrieved from http://www.unicef.ca/sites/default/files/imce_uploads/TAKE%20ACTION/ADVOCATE/DOCS/canadian_companion_updated.pdf

Votta, E., & Manion, I. G. (2003). Factors in the psychological adjustment of homeless adolescent males: The role of coping style. *Journal of the American Academy of Child and Adolescent Psychiatry, 42*(7), 778–785. doi:10.1097/01.CHI.0000046871.56865.D9

World Health Organization. (2009). *Closing the gap in a generation—how?* Reproduced with the permission of World Health Organization. Retrieved from http://www.who.int/social_determinants/thecommission/finalreport/closethegap_how/en/print.html

World Health Organization. (2015). *The social determinants of health.* Reproduced with the permission of World Health Organization. Retrieved from http://www.who.int/social_determinants/sdh_definition/en

## ABOUT THE AUTHORS

**Lynnette Leeseberg Stamler**, RN, PhD, FAAN, is Professor and Associate Dean for academic programs at the College of Nursing, University of Nebraska Medical Center. From 1984 to 2012 she taught in Canadian schools of nursing, and was a VON nurse prior to her teaching career. She completed her BSN at St. Olaf College, Minnesota; her MEd in health education at the University of Manitoba; and her PhD in nursing at the University of Cincinnati. Her research interests include patient/health education, diabetes education, nursing education, and quality care. She is active in national and international nursing organizations, including Sigma Theta Tau International and the Nursing Honor Society, and was president of the Canadian Association of Schools of Nursing from 2008 to 2010. In 2011 she was inducted into the American Academy of Nursing.

**Aaron Gabriel**, RN, BA, BSN, MSN, is employed as a full-time medical-surgical floor nurse and casually as a clinical educator for the College of Nursing at the University of Saskatchewan. She completed a BA in psychology prior to completing her BSN and MSN in nursing.

# CHAPTER 30

# Substance Use, Abuse, and Addictions

*Hélène Philbin Wilkinson*

## LEARNING OUTCOMES

**After studying this chapter, you will be able to:**

1. Explore the reasons why people use psychoactive substances.

2. Differentiate between substance use, abuse, dependency, and addiction.

3. Describe the incidence and prevalence of substance use, abuse, and addiction in Canada and their implications.

4. Examine the relationship between substance abuse and the social determinants of health.

5. Discuss the public health philosophy and strategy of harm reduction.

6. Formulate comprehensive and integrated community interventions the community health nurse can apply within the context of primary, secondary, and tertiary prevention.

7. Examine components of Canada's Federal Drug Strategy and other substance abuse frameworks.

8. Reflect on your own values and beliefs about the use of psychoactive substances and the role of the community health nurse.

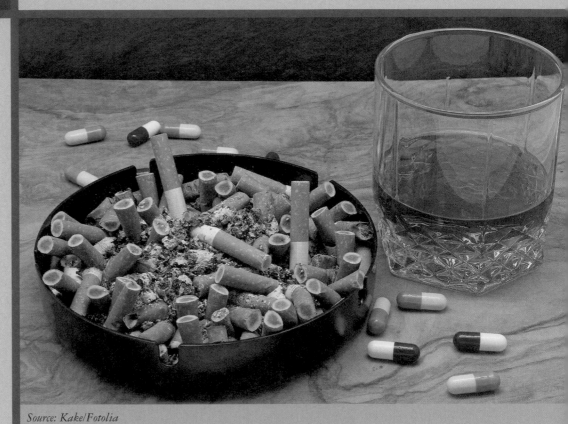

*Source: Kake/Fotolia*

## INTRODUCTION

Substance abuse is a complex public health issue that spans the life cycle and can have severe and permanent consequences for individuals, families, and communities. The overall cost of substance abuse (including alcohol, tobacco, and illicit drugs) to Canadians is estimated at approximately $40 billion, with tobacco and alcohol accounting for almost 80% of the total (Rehm et al., 2006). The recent surge in the abuse of prescription opioid pain relievers can also cost up to $50 billion a year, mostly in lost productivity and crime, according to the CCSA 2013. As such, substance abuse has a significant and direct impact on our healthcare, social service, and judicial systems. It is also a significant risk factor for a number of chronic health conditions such as HIV/AIDs, several types of cancers, as well as acute problems related to injuries, violence, and suicide. Considerable non-monetary costs to Canadian society also exist, such as the pain, suffering, and bereavement experienced by families, friends, and victims, which can have profound and lasting effects that cannot be measured in dollars.

Evidence from various fields of inquiry strongly suggests that substance abuse is multi-factorial—that familial, genetic, psychological, and socioeconomic factors are all determinants of this problem. Other factors that may influence alcohol and drug consumption include gender, culture, education, income, and employment status. The community health nurse (CHN) should therefore understand the social context of substance use and abuse, and the social conditions that can influence the initiation of drug use. It is also essential for CHNs to recognize patterns of ongoing use, cessation, abstinence, and relapse (Galea, Nandi, & Vlahov, 2004). Using a socio-environmental perspective calls for the development of comprehensive community health nursing interventions that acknowledge the interdependence among the person, the substance, and the environment. The impact of substance abuse on the individual or collective is often seen first-hand by the CHN. Traditionally, nurses have often been described as sentinels on the riverbanks, responding to a problem occurring upstream (Butterfield, 1997). This chapter is therefore intended to challenge you to make those critical connections to what is happening upstream in your community and the reasons why people use drugs.

## WHY DO PEOPLE USE DRUGS?

People use different drugs for different reasons, and the reasons vary from drug to drug, from person to person, and from circumstance to circumstance. While certain psychoactive drugs may be prescribed to relieve anxiety, tension, stress, or insomnia, some people may self-medicate to improve performance or to resolve physical or emotional discomfort. For example, people who use a depressant like alcohol may be trying to get relief from feelings that are overwhelming or painful (Health Canada, 2000). The mere availability of a drug may also cause individuals to be curious enough to experiment. Although experimenting does not mean a person will become a regular user, it does remove the barriers against trying again. However, it is important to note that people who start smoking and drinking early in adolescence may be more likely to develop drug problems in later life compared to those who begin later in adolescence (Leyton & Stewart, 2014).

Studies have found that some people may take drugs to boost their self-confidence or as a way to cope with traumatic life events or situations. Immediate gratification from drugs may also make others feel good or quickly reduce or eliminate uncomfortable emotions, albeit temporarily. Social pressures to use drugs can be very strong. Children are especially vulnerable as they may imitate and interpret their parents' or role models' use as a necessary part of having fun or relaxing (Health Canada, 2000). The evidence suggests that young people may also use drugs to rebel against unhappy situations or because they feel alienated, have an identity crisis, or need to be accepted by their peers. Dahl (2004) suggests that drinking by young people may also be a response to developmental issues such as risk taking and sensation seeking, which are biologically linked with puberty. The media, including popular music and videos, are also considered a powerful source of influence. Advertisements often promote drinking or smoking as an essential social activity or as a factor in the achievement of success (Health Canada, 2000). Canadian Research Box 30.1 illustrates the importance of analyzing patterns of use which inevitably helps to develop more effective interventions.

## TERMINOLOGY

Like many other areas of clinical practice, the field of addiction includes a number of terms that may be incorrectly used, as illustrated in Photo 30.1. This section is intended to familiarize the CHN to terms that have distinct clinical significance. The term **drug** refers to a **psychoactive substance** that affects a person's physiological or psychological state or behaviour. In this chapter, *drugs* will indicate substances consumed for medicinal and non-medicinal purposes, legally or illegally, and the term will be used interchangeably with the term *psychoactive substances*.

Most people do not think of **alcohol** as a drug, but it is. Ethyl alcohol (usually made from grain) is present in beer, wine, spirits, and liqueurs. Methyl alcohol (made from wood) is found in solvents, paint removers, antifreeze, and other household and industrial products. The distinction between the two types is important to make when referring to or defining the term and its consumption. At low doses, ethyl alcohol acts as a central nervous system depressant, producing relaxation and a release of inhibitions. At higher doses, it can produce intoxication, impaired judgment and co-ordination, even coma and death (Health Canada, 2000). Methyl alcohol must never be consumed; it is poisonous to the central nervous system. When ingested, it can be lethal. Even when it is not, it can result in blindness and coma (Canada Safety Council, 2013).

**Tobacco** leaves, which are shredded and dried, can be smoked in cigarettes, cigars, or pipes. They may also be chewed, inhaled, or "dipped" (tucked between the gum and lip). More than 4000 chemicals are found in tobacco, including nicotine, the main psychoactive component that stimulates the central nervous system (Health Canada, 2000).

**Licit drugs** (legal drugs) refer to drugs that are used for medicinal purposes. Licit drugs are available by prescription or sold over the counter to relieve common symptoms such as pain, anxiety, or insomnia. Some of these drugs are regulated by the Controlled Drugs and Substances Act 1996 (CA). They have practical, legitimate uses; however, they may also be used unlawfully. Non-medicinal licit drugs include alcohol and tobacco, both of which can be legally purchased and used by those who are of legal age.

**Illicit drugs** (illegal drugs) include cannabis (marijuana and hashish), phencyclidines (PCP, ketamine), hallucinogens (LSD, mescaline, psilocybin, MDA), stimulants other than caffeine and nicotine (amphetamines, cocaine, crack), depressants (barbiturates, methaqualone, benzodiazepine), and opiates (heroin, morphine, methadone, codeine).

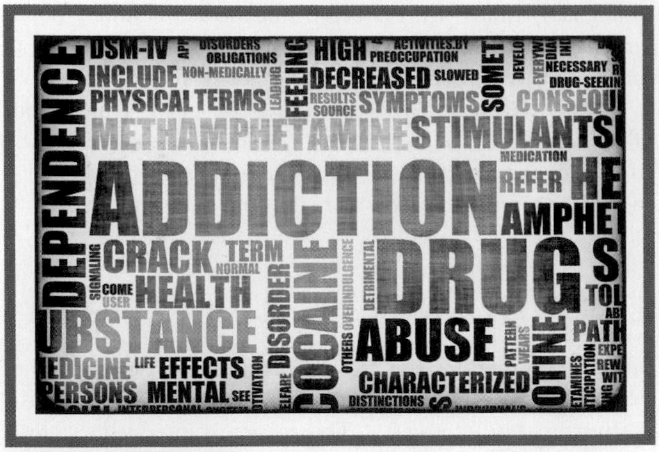

**PHOTO** **30.1** The field of addiction includes several terms that may be used incorrectly.

*Source: Kentoh/Shutterstock*

**Inhalants**, also known as volatile solvents, are depressant drugs that produce feelings of euphoria, exhilaration, and vivid fantasies. These products have no medical use and are intended for commercial and household use. Inhalants such as gasoline can cause immediate and serious problems regardless of how they are taken, or how much is taken. They are known to cause kidney, liver, and brain damage, and it is not known to what extent the damage is reversible (Health Canada, 2000).

**Substance use** refers to any consumption of psychoactive drugs that can either be beneficial or harmful, whereas **substance abuse** is a maladaptive pattern of substance use characterized by resulting in harmful consequences due to repeated use, as defined by the American Psychiatric Association [APA] (2013). It can lead to adverse physical, psychological, legal, social, or interpersonal consequences, which may or may not involve dependence. **Dependence** is progressive in nature and affects the physiological, cognitive, behavioural, and psychological dimensions of a person's health. It is manifested by continuous use despite the presence of problems caused by use. Dependence results in tolerance, withdrawal, and compulsive substance-taking behaviour (APA, 2013). Dependence can be physical or psychological, and sometimes both. **Physical dependence** occurs when an individual's body reacts to the absence of a drug with withdrawal symptoms. **Psychological dependence** occurs when drug use becomes central to a person's thoughts and emotions. Other forms of dependence such as gambling, Internet social networking, sex, and binge eating are becoming increasingly prevalent and have implications for community health nursing. **Addiction** is characterized by patterns of heavy use, primarily taken for the effects on consciousness, mood, and perception. The term "addiction" is often equated with physical dependence but it is also used to define non-substance-related behavioural addictions like a gambling disorder (APA, 2013). The terms "substance abuse" and "addiction" are also used interchangeably with the term **substance use disorder**.

## PATTERNS OF SUBSTANCE USE AND ABUSE IN CANADA

The following section is a brief and general overview of the most common prevalence patterns of substance use and abuse in Canada. CHNs can use this type of epidemiologic data to inform community health nursing interventions. This type of information may also be used to leverage broader stakeholder involvement when working to address individual or community-based issues related to substance use and abuse. The data in this chapter are by no means comprehensive; however, should you wish to further explore epidemiologic data related to substance use, abuse, and addictions, you are encouraged to consult the federal and provincial websites listed as additional resources in MyNursingLab. Some of these additional resources will provide you with more detailed information about consumption patterns in various regions across Canada and among specific vulnerable population groups.

## TOBACCO

Tobacco use is the leading cause of preventable death in Canada. Smoking kills more Canadians than obesity or being overweight, physical inactivity, and high blood pressure. The most recent analysis of tobacco prevalence in Canada indicates 37 000 Canadians die prematurely each year, with 100 dying every day of a smoking-related illness (Reid, Hammond, Burkhalter, Rynard, & Ahmed, 2013). Although the prevalence of smoking in our country has decreased considerably over the past decade, the decrease has somewhat stalled. As demonstrated in Table 30.1, smoking rates are below the national average in Ontario and British Columbia, and highest in Quebec. Rates also vary by age, sex, and educational level. For example, the prevalence of smoking is currently highest among young adults, males continue to smoke more than females, and university graduates have the lowest rates of smoking (Reid et al., 2013).

### Alcohol

The consumption of alcohol in Canada has risen by 14% since 1996 (Statistics Canada, 2001, 2005, 2009), and it is higher than in the United States (see Figure 30.1). The average age of first alcohol use among youth is approximately 15 years and consumption rates among high school students increase substantially with each grade level (Health Canada, 2011, 2012). Alcohol consumption by underage youth appears to have declined in 2010 but remains constant among young adults and adults (Figure 30.1). Although men typically drink more than women, female post-secondary students drink more than their male counterparts (Adlaf, Demers, & Gliksman, 2005). Drinking patterns also vary across our country. Maritimers tend to drink more per occasion and men largely prefer beer. In the Prairies, people are more likely to favour spirits. They also tend to drink smaller amounts, drink less frequently, and drink less often with a meal. In Quebec, Ontario, and British

| Table 30.1 | Adult (Age 15+) Smoking Prevalence* by Province, 1999–2013 |

| Year | 1999 | 2000 | 2001 | 2002 | 2003 | 2004 | 2005 | 2006 | 2007 | 2008 | 2009 | 2010 | 2011 | 2012 | 2013 |
|---|---|---|---|---|---|---|---|---|---|---|---|---|---|---|---|
| Canada | 25.2 | 24.4 | 21.7 | 21.4 | 20.9 | 19.6 | 18.7 | 18.6 | 19.2 | 17.9 | 17.5 | 16.7 | 17.3 | 16.1 | 14.6 |
| British Columbia | 20.0 | 19.6 | 16.7 | 16.5 | 16.4 | 15.2 | 14.7 | 16.4 | 14.4 | 14.7 | 14.9 | 14.3 | 14.2 | 13.2 | 11.4 |
| Alberta | 26.0 | 22.6 | 25.1 | 22.8 | 20.0 | 20.1 | 20.6 | 21.3 | 21.0 | 20.4 | 18.0 | 18.8 | 17.7 | 17.4 | 16.0 |
| Saskatchewan | 25.9 | 28.1 | 25.4 | 21.2 | 24.1 | 21.7 | 22.0 | 23.7 | 24.0 | 20.4 | 22.3 | 21.1 | 19.2 | 18.5 | 17.6 |
| Manitoba | 23.3 | 25.7 | 25.9 | 21.1 | 20.9 | 20.6 | 22.3 | 20.1 | 19.9 | 20.8 | 18.9 | 20.5 | 18.7 | 17.9 | 17.4 |
| Ontario | 23.2 | 23.1 | 19.7 | 19.7 | 19.6 | 18.7 | 16.4 | 16.6 | 18.3 | 16.8 | 15.4 | 15.2 | 16.3 | 15.7 | 12.6 |
| Quebec | 30.3 | 28.2 | 24.1 | 25.8 | 24.6 | 22.2 | 22.2 | 20.1 | 21.7 | 19.1 | 20.7 | 17.8 | 19.8 | 17.1 | 17.1 |
| New Brunswick | 26.5 | 26.6 | 25.0 | 21.1 | 24.3 | 24.2 | 21.8 | 22.6 | 21.2 | 19.9 | 21.3 | 19.3 | 18.8 | 17.3 | 19.6 |
| Nova Scotia | 28.9 | 29.8 | 24.9 | 25.3 | 22.1 | 20.2 | 21.0 | 21.8 | 20.4 | 19.7 | 19.8 | 20.8 | 18.1 | 15.6 | 19.4 |
| Prince Edward Island | 25.6 | 25.7 | 25.6 | 23.1 | 21.4 | 21.2 | 19.9 | 19.2 | 18.4 | 19.2 | 17.7 | 16.2 | 19.1 | 15.2 | 17.3 |
| NewFoundland & Labrador | 28.5 | 27.7 | 25.7 | 24.1 | 23.0 | 21.8 | 20.6 | 21.7 | 21.2 | 20.2 | 20.7 | 20.0 | 19.0 | 19.7 | 19.5 |

*Includes daily and non-daily smokers

Source: Reid, J. L., Hammond, D., Rynard, V. L., & Burkhalter, R. (2015). *Tobacco Use in Canada: Patterns and Trends*, 2015 Edition. Waterloo, ON: Propel Centre for Population Health Impact, University of Waterloo. With data from the Canadian Tobacco use Monitoring Survey (1999–2012) and the Canadian Tobacco, Alcohol and Drugs Survey (2013).

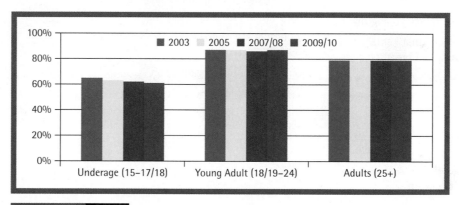

**FIGURE 30.1** Prevalence of Self-Reported Alcohol Use among Canadians by Age in the Past Year

*Source:* Statistics Canada. (n.d.). *Canadian Community Health Survey, 2003–2010.* Reproduced with permission.

Columbia, people drink more often, drink wine more often than spirits, and drink more often with a meal compared to other parts of Canada (Paradis, Demers, & Picard, 2010).

## Energy Drinks and Alcohol

**Caffeinated alcoholic beverages** can either be pre-mixed and purchased in liquor stores or licensed establishments or hand-mixed by consumers. Brache (2014) reports that the motivation for drinking caffeinated alcoholic beverages include feeling more energetic, being able to stay awake, being able to party longer when drinking, and getting a quicker buzz. Brache suggests that these reasons represent higher-risk drinking patterns. Because the effects of these beverages can decrease one's awareness of intoxication (caffeine

masks the effects of alcohol), they can lead to longer and more active drinking sessions, and greater overall alcohol intake (Brache, 2014).

## Licit Drugs

**Prescription drugs**, normally prescribed for therapeutic purposes, have the potential to be abused due to their psychoactive properties. In Canada, opioid pain relievers such as Oxycontin®, stimulants such as Ritalin®, and sedatives and tranquilizers like Valium® are the most commonly used. Health providers in many parts of Canada are reporting recent problems associated with the abuse of fentanyl. According to Health Canada (2011), the abuse of opioid pain relievers is about six times higher among youth compared to adults. In

## CANADIAN RESEARCH BOX 30.1

**What are the reasons for teenage smokers wanting to quit, and are there gender differences for their reasons?**

Struik, L. L., O'Loughlin, E. K., Dugas, E. N., Bottorff, J. L., & O'Loughlin, J. L. (2014). Gender differences in reasons to quit smoking among adolescents. *Journal of School Nursing, 34*(4), 303–308. doi:10.1177/1059840513497800

Over the past 30 years, smoking rates among youth have declined. Despite this decline, current smoking rates among young people remain high. While the literature on adult smoking cessation is relatively well developed, little is known about youth cessation. Smoking cessation success among youth is infrequent and few cessation interventions aimed at youth have been effective, especially in the long term. Without sufficient research on how to motivate, facilitate, and support adolescent smoking cessation, the authors of this research focused their efforts on studying the reasons adolescents want to quit and if their reasons to quit are influenced by gender-related factors. They hypothesized that reasons to quit would differ between genders.

Data on the Adolescent Reasons for Quitting (ARFQ) scale (see below) were collected in a mailed self-reported questionnaire in 2010 and 2011 from 113 females and 83 male smokers between the ages of 14 and 19 years in Montreal, Quebec. The ARFQ is a scale used by respondents to rate the level of importance on 16 reasons to quit smoking.

### Adolescent Reasons for Quitting Scale

| Short-Term Consequences | Social Disapproval | Long-Term Concerns |
| --- | --- | --- |
| I walk up stairs and I'm out of breath. | People I date/go out with don't like me smoking. | I don't want to get sick when I'm older if I still smoke (get cancer). |
| I'm coughing up stuff every day. | I don't want my parents to find out. | I don't want to be smoking when I get older. |
| I can't breathe when exercising (jogging, working out). | My friends who don't smoke give me a hard time. | |
| I feel like cigarettes are controlling my life. | My parents are really upset about me smoking. | |
| Other people are thinking that I smell or look bad (yellow teeth/nails, bad breath, etc.). | I joined a group or organization (church, youth group) that didn't like my smoking. | |
| I get sick more often because of smoking. | | |
| Smoking gets me in trouble at school or with the police (citations, etc.). | | |
| My stuff gets damaged because of my smoking (burns on clothes, in car, etc.). | | |
| I keep smoking cigarettes out of habit even though I don't want to. | | |

Overall, the findings of this study indicated that reasons to quit between boys and girls appear to be similar. Both boys and girls rated long-term concerns as the most important reason to quit smoking, followed by short-term consequences and social disapproval. However, girls rated "I don't want my parents to find out" as more important than boys did, and although only minimally statistically significant, girls rated "I don't want to be smoking when I am older" as more important than boys did. Boys, on the other hand, rated "I walk up stairs and I'm out of breath" as a short-term consequence more often than girls. There were no other statistically significant differences in the other items of the ARFQ scale.

The results of this study revealed that there were not many gender differences, but the differences identified between boys and girls are consistent with other research discussed in this article. For example, reasons for smoking uptake differ between boys and girls. Girls are more influenced by social relationships, body image, weight control, and enhancing their social identity and status. Boys are influenced by the appearance of masculinity and the denial of risk. Reasons to quit may not be similarly rooted in these factors and while the ARFQ scale used in this study may not have been robust enough to detect many gender differences, the authors make very interesting points about their findings.

According to the authors, the higher rating girls gave to the factor "I don't want my parents to find out" is consistent with other research available in the literature. This finding confirms that smoking behaviours in girls may be more influenced by the attitudes and smoking behaviours of family members. If adolescent girls have closer family bonds than boys, they may be more influenced by their parents. This notion is supported by other evidence that confirms that parents can have an influential role in the prevention and disruption of youth smoking behaviour, especially in girls. The authors highlight that the higher rating girls gave to the long-term concern "I don't want to be smoking when I am older" is consistent with feminine ideals that position women as nurturing and caring for others, being more responsible health consumers, and more attuned to and concerned about their future health than are boys. As for the boys, their higher rating of "I walk up the stairs and I'm out of breath" suggests an alignment with masculine ideals that are related to physical endurance. This finding is also consistent with other studies in the literature that report that boys frequently endorse performance-related reasons to quit smoking.

The similarities in the reasons to quit between genders in this study raise important considerations about youth tobacco cessation efforts. Because adolescents tend to focus on the immediate pleasure of smoking, some researchers have suggested that the content of cessation messages should focus on short-term concerns. Others have argued that a focus on long-term consequences may lead to more desirable outcomes. This study supports recommendations that long-term health concerns should be considered in any tobacco control interventions aimed at youth, regardless of gender. The authors suggest that nurses and other practitioners who provide smoking cessation programs to adolescents may need to consider the relevance of incorporating long-term concerns into their smoking cessation strategies. They also encourage the development of resources for parents, including cessation strategies that involve parents to positively influence the smoking behaviours of girls, and cessation programs with a focus on physical endurance to further motivate boys in their cessation efforts.

### Discussion Questions

1. Are smoking cessation initiatives effective for teens?
2. How might you assess a teen's readiness to quit?
3. What are some effective cessation strategies for teens?

fact, Canadians are the second-largest per capita consumer of prescription opioids in the world (International Narcotics Control Board, 2013). The Royal Canadian Mounted Police (2010) also reports a significant increase in criminal activity related to diverting prescription drugs from legal and regulated supply routes. In Ontario, the number of emergency room visits for narcotic withdrawal, overdose, intoxication, psychosis, and harmful use increased by 250% between 2005 and 2011. Visits for opioid-related mental and behavioural disorders also climbed. Other licit drugs known to be abused for their psychoactive effects include "over-the-counter" medications such as cough medicines, sleep aids, antihistamines, and diet pills. The use of over-the-counter and prescription drugs by older people may present unique challenges. The aging process is frequently accompanied by an increase in chronic and acute illnesses and corresponding increases in the total number of prescribed drugs. Older adults are therefore at higher risk for medication interactions. Older adults may also experience the effects of drugs at much lower levels of drug consumption because of the changes in kidney and liver functions related to aging. Some older adults may be socially isolated, which may make them less likely to be identified as misusing drugs. The signs of substance abuse in older adults include confusion, falls, or lack of self-care that could be mistakenly attributed to the natural course of aging (Steinhagen, 2008).

## Illicit Drugs

Cannabis is the most widely used illicit drug in Canada and the second-most used substance among youth (Table 30.2). Studies indicate that the average age of first illicit drug use is approximately 15 years of age. The next most widely used class of illicit drugs is hallucinogens, followed closely by cocaine and crack, and ecstasy. The rate of illicit drug use by young people is much higher than adults. For example, young people are three times more likely to use cannabis, and nine times more likely to have used any one of five other types of illicit drugs, including cocaine or crack, speed, hallucinogens, ecstasy, or heroin in the past year (Health Canada, 2011).

**Bath salts** are a classification of products containing synthetic amphetamine-type stimulants also known as cathinones. According to the CCSA (2012), these substances are prepared in illicit drug labs and sold by dealers via the Internet or in drug paraphernalia shops. They can be swallowed, snorted, smoked, or injected and, although little is known about how many people use bath salts, some evidence suggests that they are becoming more popular as a result of their widespread availability and sensationalist media coverage (Prosser & Nelson, 2011). People under the influence of these substances report hallucinations, paranoia, chest pain, and blurry vision. They may also become agitated and combative and can therefore pose a danger to themselves and others.

| Table 30.2 | Top Five Substances Used in the Past Year by Canadians | | | | |
|---|---|---|---|---|---|
| | **#1** | **#2** | **#3** | **#4** | **#5** |
| General Population | Alcohol (78%) | Cannabis (9.1%) | Hallucinogens (0.6%)* | Cocaine/Crack (0.9%)* | Ecstasy (0.7%)* |
| Youth (15–24) | Alcohol (70.8%) | Cannabis (21.6%) | Hallucinogens (2.0%) | Ecstasy (2.6%)* | N/A (suppressed) |
| Adults (25+) | Alcohol (79.3%) | Cannabis (6.7%) | Cocaine/Crack (0.7%)* | N/A (suppressed) | N/A (suppressed) |

Note: Figures identified with an asterisk should be interpreted with caution because of small sample size.

Source: Health Canada. (2011). Canadian Alcohol and Drug Use Monitoring Survey (CADUMS), as cited in Canadian Centre on Substance Abuse (2013). Cannabis (Canadian Drug Summary).

The abuse of **injectable drugs** is an illegal activity and therefore difficult to measure; however, the CCSA (2005) reports that the most commonly injected drugs in Canada include cocaine, heroin, combinations of heroin and cocaine, amphetamines, Talwin® and Ritalin®, pharmaceutical opioids (i.e., morphine), and anabolic steroids. In the past, injection drug use was thought to be limited to Canada's largest urban centres but the numbers are increasing across the county and the problem also exists in rural areas. Additionally, the CCSA (2005) suggests that women make up approximately one-third of the injectable-drug user population, and about 20% of injectable-drug users are injecting performance-enhancing drugs. Steroid use is more frequent among males, who indicate performance-related reasons for using.

The abuse of inhalants, such as gasoline and glue, is highest among children and youth. Some studies involving inmates in detention centres reveal that inhalants were the first drugs ever used by this population. According to Baydala (2010), there are several studies that report higher rates of inhalant abuse by people living in rural and isolated areas, in Inuit and First Nations communities, and in communities with high rates of unemployment, poverty, and violence. The low cost of and ease of access to these substances are significant factors that contribute to their abuse.

While **gambling** is a form of entertainment for most Canadians, it has become a problem for a high percentage of people. The Canadian Public Health Association (2000) defines problem gambling as a progressive disorder characterized by continuous or periodic loss of control over gambling; preoccupation with gambling and money with which to gamble; irrational thinking; and continuation of the activity despite adverse consequences. Approximately 3.2% of Canadian adults (Wood & Williams, 2009) and 2.2 % of youth between the ages of 15 and 24 (Huang & Boyer, 2007) are affected by varying levels of problem gambling. Provincial surveys conducted between 2001 and 2006 indicate that the highest rates of moderate risk and problem gambling are found in Saskatchewan and Manitoba, and the lowest in Quebec and New Brunswick (Canadian Partnership for Responsible Gambling, 2009).

# HARMFUL EFFECTS OF SUBSTANCE USE, ABUSE, AND ADDICTIONS

## Concurrent Disorders

Although previously covered in Chapter 23, this chapter would be incomplete if we failed to present information about **concurrent disorders**. A concurrent disorder refers to co-occurring mental health and substance use problems within the same person. In diagnostic terms, a concurrent disorder refers to any combination of mental health and substance use disorders, as defined on either Axis I or Axis II of the DSM-5 (APA, 2013). More than 50% of people seeking help for an addiction also have a mental illness, and 15% to 20% seeking help from mental health services are also living with an addiction (CCSA, 2009a). People with concurrent disorders who may come to your attention will often have multiple problems. Rush, Urbanski, Bassani, Castel, and Wild (2010) suggest that those

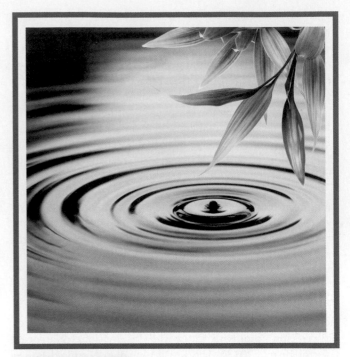

with concurrent disorders are at higher risk for poor physical health, family conflict, arrest, incarceration, victimization, homelessness, and suicide. They experience frequent relapses and recurring crises, and their cases are complex (CCSA, 2009a).

## Harmful Consequences of Substance Abuse

All drugs are known to have adverse and undesirable effects when abused. For example, long-term tobacco use can cause lung damage. Every year in Canada, more than 37 000 people prematurely of tobacco-related disorders (Reid et al., 2013). Smoking is the leading preventable cause of death in our country (Baliunas et al., 2007). Nicotine dependence or tobacco addiction is commonly known as a lethal form of addiction, often characterized by being a chronic and relapsing disorder. Exposure to second-hand smoke among neonates, infants, children, and adults is associated with an increased risk of a number of acute and chronic conditions. Alcohol abuse can cause liver damage and sniffing cocaine can damage nasal passages. People who inject drugs can become infected with blood-borne pathogens such as HIV and hepatitis B and C.

Significant social implications associated with the abuse of alcohol in our country include driving under the influence of alcohol and domestic and interpersonal violence. Although impaired driving rates have dropped over the last couple of decades, the percentage of all motor vehicle deaths caused by drinking drivers in Canada has increased (Traffic Injury Research Foundation, 2013). Young Canadian males are over-represented in alcohol-related driving fatalities. Alcohol is also frequently involved in snowmobiling and boating accidents in this country. Almost 40% of boating deaths have alcohol involvement, and at least one-half of all fatally injured snowmobilers in Canada have been drinking (TIRF, 2009). Although alcohol remains the primary cause of motor vehicle fatalities in Canada, traffic injury experts and police officials report a growing concern about drug use while driving. The CCSA (2009b) confirms that, after alcohol, cannabis is the most common substance found in young fatally injured drivers.

Other associated harms of alcohol abuse can include an increase in crime and violent acts, strained relationships, accidents at home and work, familial neglect and discord, and workplace and school absenteeism. Alcohol abuse can also cause significant health problems, including ulcers, liver and kidney damage, pancreatic diseases, heart disease, cancer, sexual and reproductive issues, and pre- and postnatal complications. Alcohol is the most commonly used psychoactive substance among people over the age of 65 years. Although seniors consume lower levels of alcohol than younger people, they have high rates of prescription drug use, especially older women. The CHN is cautioned not to overlook problems with prescription drugs among seniors.

There has been a long-held belief that drinking a glass of red wine a day can help protect against heart disease. Although experts confirm this association exists, they recommend that caution be exercised; this association cannot be assumed for all drinkers, even at small levels of intake. It is important to note that the relationship between alcohol and heart disease cannot be isolated from other individual risk factors or disease outcomes. For example, even one drink a day increases risk of breast cancer. With as little as one drink a day, the net effect on mortality is beneficial but beyond that, the net risk increases with every drink (Roerecke & Rehm, 2012).

The consumption of alcohol during pregnancy can result in **fetal alcohol spectrum disorder** (FASD), which is manifested by developmental, neurological, and behavioural delays in infants and young children that persist into adulthood (Chudley et al., 2005). Although FASD is related to the frequency and volume of an expectant mother's alcohol intake, other contributing factors to consider include genetic predisposition, poor nutrition, age, the lack of prenatal care, and the use of other drugs. Since a safe level of alcohol consumption during pregnancy or while breastfeeding has not been established, public health professionals advise expectant and breastfeeding mothers not to drink alcohol, even in moderation. Consult your maternity and pediatric nursing texts for more information about the incidence and clinical symptoms of FASD.

People who use drugs that have been obtained illegally can never really know what they are taking. For example, ecstasy and crystal meth, both of which belong to the amphetamine family, can be easily manufactured in clandestine or unregulated illegal labs. Non-prescription opioids are famous for having been "cut," often repeatedly, as the drug makes its way to the eventual consumer. As a result, the chemicals and processes vary affecting the strength, purity, and effect of the final product. The consequences can be devastating and include severe dependency, drug reactions, and fatal overdoses, which is evidenced by the sharp increase of mortality rates due to opioids in Canada (Dhalla et al., 2009).

The harms of illicit drug use are made worse in certain social conditions. The harmful consequences to one's health and well-being are magnified when homeless or living in poverty (Galea, Nandi, & Vlahov, 2004). In a study of illicit drug use in five Canadian cities, Fischer and colleagues (2005) found that many people who injected illicit drugs experienced increased physical and mental health problems. They also lacked permanent housing, did not have access to treatment, and experienced social marginalization (Fischer et al., 2005).

Injecting drugs has a number of inherent risks including overdose and suicide; contracting infections such as HIV, hepatitis C, and other blood-borne infections; developing abscesses, poor nutritional status, and endocarditis; and experiencing adverse drug interactions. Many injection drug users report a history of physical, emotional, or sexual abuse during their time of drug use. Using injection drugs may further marginalize individuals, making it very difficult for them to access supports in the community (CCSA, 2011). As well, injection drug users may share needles and drug injection equipment, and engage in unprotected sex for money or drug exchange. Women who inject drugs also face unique challenges because they may have links to the sex trade industry and become reluctant to access services for fear of having their children taken away (CCSA, 2011).

The use of opioid drugs during pregnancy can result in **neonatal abstinence syndrome** (NAS). In-utero exposure to these substances results in infants born with physical dependence and withdrawal symptoms. They present with neurological, gastrointestinal, and respiratory difficulties, including a high-pitched cry, poor feeding, sleep-wake abnormalities, poor weight gain, tremors, and seizures—all of which require prolonged hospitalizations and treatment in a special-care nursery. NAS also often leads to the development of life-long issues that may include FASD, behaviour problems, and developmental delays. Stigmatization may cause an underestimation of the prevalence of NAS; however, the Canadian Institute for Health Information has reported that its incidence has more than doubled from 2004 to 2010 (Dow et al., 2012).

The National Advisory Committee on Prescription Drug Misuse (2013) reports that certain populations in Canada, such as women, youth, seniors, First Nations, and Inuit people, can have higher rates of prescription drug use or abuse, or experience greater related harms than the general population. While further research is needed to confirm prevalence rates and related harms, a number of other groups may also be at risk for prescription drug abuse, including military personnel and veterans, incarcerated offenders, homeless people, individuals with concurrent disorders, and healthcare professionals.

The Canadian Women's Foundation (2011) reports that women who experience violence have increased rates of drug use. Women who are impacted by violence are more likely to use multiple substances and consume higher levels of substances than people who have not experienced violence. Substance use may be a coping strategy for women who experience violence. Please refer to Chapter 28 for more information about violence.

The CCSA (2008) reports that for many First Nations, Inuit, and Métis Canadians, a loss of culture, the intergenerational impacts of colonization and residential schools, poverty, low education, unstable family structure, and poor social support networks increase their vulnerability to drug abuse. Recent studies confirm the alarmingly high rates of injection drug use among urban Canadian Aboriginal youth, especially women (Miller et al., 2011). The rate of prescription drug abuse is twice to three times higher among urban Aboriginal youth than among non-Aboriginal youth (Webster, 2012). Please refer to Chapter 22 for a more detailed discussion about Aboriginal health.

As you can see, the harmful consequences of substance abuse extend far beyond the individual using psychoactive substances. It is both a response to social breakdown and an important factor in worsening the inequities of one's health (World Health Organization, 2003). Substance abuse can have lasting effects on individuals, families, and communities, impacting their health, safety, and quality of life. This ripple effect is nicely captured in Photo 30.2. The World Health Organization [WHO] (2003) recommends that we must address the complexities of the social circumstances and context(s) that are responsible for drug use. As such, the response to substance abuse problems in a community must be broad and include different interventions at the most appropriate level of action (individual, family, community, system, or population).

# SUBSTANCE ABUSE COMMUNITY HEALTH INTERVENTIONS

Given the wide range of individual, social, and cultural factors that can influence patterns of drug use, we now understand that substance abuse is not merely due to individual psychological or moral factors. Substance abuse is a chronic, multifaceted social problem that requires a broad range of community health nursing interventions that are both timely and relevant.

## Canada's Federal Drug Strategy

Recognizing that a wide range of tools and solutions are needed, experts in Canada have developed a framework that combines the elements of health promotion with prevention, treatment, harm reduction, and enforcement. These elements were coined the "pillars" of **Canada's Federal Drug Strategy**, which recognizes the need for a balanced approach to address these problems. This "four-pillar" approach was considered a best-practice model, ensuring that any substance abuse strategy would be comprehensive and coordinated. In 2007, Canada's Drug Strategy was renamed the National Anti-Drug Strategy with a focus on only three pillars: preventing illicit drug use, treating illicit drug dependency, and combatting the production and distribution of illicit drugs. The fourth pillar of harm reduction was removed and became reassigned to a collaborative effort involving multiple other ministries. In light of an international shift toward public health and harm-reduction approaches, critics have described our new national policy as regressive, with an overemphasis on enforcement strategies to combat the production and distribution of illicit drugs, rather than a focus on effective harm-reduction programs. There is recognition that Canada's strategy could also include more emphasis on widely harmful substances, including tobacco, alcohol, and prescription drugs. Critics claim that our country now has an Americanized strategy, or a Canadianized version of the U.S. "war on drugs."

For the purpose of this chapter, the fourth pillar, harm reduction, will be discussed, as it must continue to be viewed by CHNs as a complementary component of a comprehensive response to substance abuse. Not doing so would disaffirm the social context of substance abuse and would be incongruent with the practice of addressing the determinants of health. The CHN is therefore encouraged to be concerned about the advocating for strategies that reflect a broadly defined concept of health. There are numerous examples in history of CHNs assisting with the advancement of harm-reduction programs. Please refer to Chapters 8 and 31 for a more in-depth discussion of harm reduction. The CHN is poised to influence and further advance comprehensive and complementary prevention strategies.

## Primary Prevention

Health-promotion and primary-prevention activities consist of interventions that seek to prevent or delay the onset of substance use as well as to avoid problems before they occur. **Health promotion** is more than health education. It also includes strengthening the health, social, and economic elements that can reduce the risk of substance use; for example, creating alternative activities for youth groups. The main focus is to help people avoid the use of harmful substances. In the case of those individuals who do use substances, **primary prevention** of substance abuse is focused on enhancing their ability to control their use and prevent the development of substance abuse (harmful use) and addictions. An example of a primary prevention initiative is Canada's **Low-Risk Drinking Guidelines (LRDG)**. These guidelines were developed to promote a culture of moderation for people of legal drinking age. The guidelines help individuals to identify what is considered a standard drink in terms of alcohol content rather than volume (see Figure 30.2). The standard drink definition is also intended to help people monitor their individual alcohol intake against the recommended guidelines. High-risk drinking practices are presented in Figure 30.3. This information helps Canadians make better decisions about their drinking habits to avoid long-term health risks. Being aware of the guidelines may also promote individuals to limit their consumption at special occasions, reinforce when zero consumption should be the limit (i.e., when operating a vehicle and when pregnant or breastfeeding) and promote the value of delaying drinking for adolescents (Butt, Beirness, Gliksman, Paradis, & Stockwell, 2011). For a more detailed overview of LRDG, consult the CCSA website in the online resources listed in MyNursingLab.

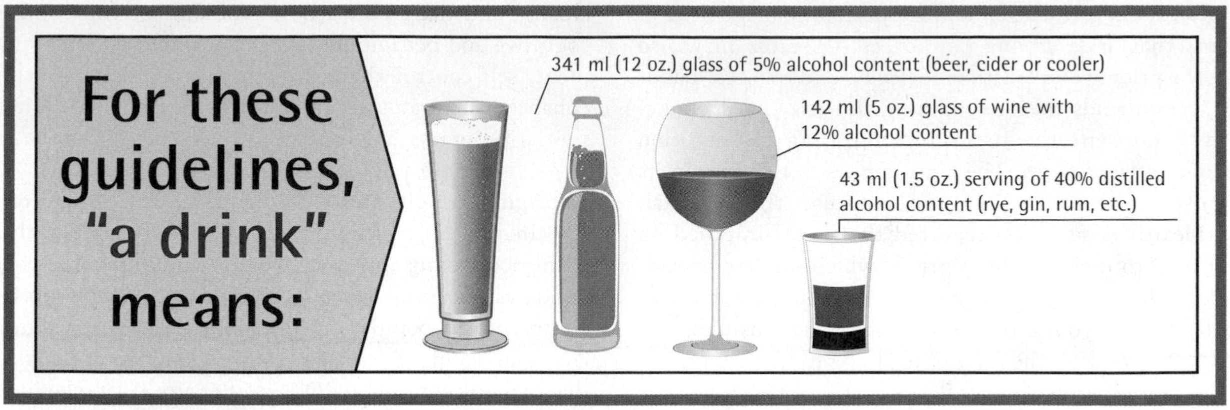

**FIGURE 30.2** What Is a Standard Drink?

*Source:* Canadian Centre on Substance Abuse. (2013). *Canada's low risk alcohol drinking guidelines.* Reproduced with permission of Canadian Centre on Substance Abuse.

*Twelve Risky Drinking Practices:*

1. Drinking more than 10 to 15 standard drinks a week
2. Drinking more than 3 drinks a day for men and 2 drinks a day for women
3. Drinking more than one standard drink an hour
4. Drinking and driving
5. Drinking before or during work
6. Drinking before or during sports or other physical activities
7. Drinking during pregnancy
8. Drinking while on medication or with other drugs
9. Drinking with the intention of becoming intoxicated
10. Drinking to cope with difficulties or negative outlook
11. Drinking out of habit
12. Drinking underage

**FIGURE 30.3** Twelve Risky Drinking Practices Addressed by Canada's Low-Risk Drinking Guidelines

*Source:* Canadian Centre on Substance Abuse, (2007). *Reducing alcohol related harm in Canada: Toward a culture of moderation.* Adapted and Reproduced with permission from the Minister of Health, 2015. Recommendations for a National Alcohol Strategy.

The Simcoe Muskoka Health Unit in Ontario launched a multi-year campaign in 2011 to increase awareness about the risks associated with alcohol and Canada's LRDG. Several approaches were planned to focus on different stakeholders, community groups, and sectors. These approaches included how to work with health professionals, advocacy for workplace alcohol policies, developing strategies with local partners to address alcohol use, and a generic campaign to raise public awareness about the LRDG.

As discussed in Chapter 8, social marketing is a health-promotion activity. In the substance abuse context, social media campaigns are typically designed to impart knowledge about substances and help develop refusal skills. They can be developed to focus on the whole community or specific at-risk or high-risk populations like early intervention programs for elementary schools or students living on university or college campuses. Consult Chapter 17 for more information about school health nursing. As you work through the Individual and Group Critical-Thinking Exercises, keep in mind that health-promotion activities should be tailored to the needs and characteristics of the sector and stakeholder group whose attitudes, behaviours, or health status you are hoping to influence. Although social media campaigns are designed to produce positive changes or prevent negative changes in health-related behaviours across large populations (Wakefield, Loken, & Hornik, 2010), recent observations have been made about the ethics of some strategies that de-normalize substance use. For example, some campaigns stigmatize smoking. And while they may be effective in ultimately reducing its prevalence, some researchers suggest that they will not help to reduce smoking rates among people who are socially and economically disadvantaged and who also represent the majority of tobacco users (Bell, Salmon, Bowers, Bell, & McCullough, 2010). The CHN is encouraged to work on health-promotion activities from a determinants of health perspective.

Health-promotion activities may also include regulations, policies, health warning labels, and even elements of harm reduction. In fact, it is best practice to combine education and harm reduction with policy changes and environmental supports, as they are complementary and strengthen the overall impact of prevention activities. **Policies** such as tobacco by-laws, secondary school and campus alcohol and drug use policies, or alcohol and drug legislation can create healthy social and physical environments. They can create an environment that is conducive to healthy practices by making it easier to adopt healthy behaviours and more difficult to adopt unhealthy ones. **Environmental support and controls** help to ensure healthy conditions, practices, and policies that make it easier for people to achieve and maintain their health. For example, the presence of recreational activities and self-help groups can provide important environmental supports for a community. Environmental supports are also present in the workplace. While some workplaces in Canada have instituted drug testing programs, many have put in place comprehensive alcohol and drug human resource policies that include strategies for the prevention and supportive management of problems that arise among employees. Controls may also include the pricing and taxation of alcohol and tobacco. Babor (2010) recommends that maintaining the price of alcohol is one of the most effective means of controlling consumption and alcohol-related harm. The same applies to tobacco. In its 2011 position paper on ending tobacco use, the Canadian Public Health Association reported that taxes imposed on tobacco help to maintain high prices, which are also considered one of the most effective measures to reduce tobacco use, especially among young people who are price sensitive, and that a 10% increase in the price of tobacco products can result in a consumption drop of about 8%, with the greatest decrease among youth (Canadian Public Health Association, 2011).

## Secondary and Tertiary Prevention

**Screening**, **early identification**, treatment, enforcement, and harm-reduction programs are components of **secondary prevention** and **tertiary prevention** activities for people who have started to experience problems related to their substance use. The emphasis of screening and early identification is on the detection of signs and symptoms in order to intervene, reduce consumption levels, and effectively minimize or interrupt and manage the progression of problems that have started to develop.

**Treatment** is intended to assist people with substance abuse problems as their consumption is considered to be "high risk." These individuals should be provided with a range of options in order to match their recovery needs and personal circumstances with appropriate treatment options. Essentially, the purpose of treatment is to prevent further deterioration and reduce the harms that have resulted from a problematic consumption pattern. To some extent, treatment is focused on slowing down the addiction trajectory or controlling related harms and disabilities. The CHN should also be aware that the **stigma** associated with substance abuse can restrict access to healthcare and have a negative impact on the health and well-being of individuals. For example, research indicates that women experience different barriers to treatment services and lower rates of service access than men (Pirie, Jesseman, & National Treatment Indicators Working Group, 2013). Be aware of your own views and attitudes; nurses and other healthcare providers have been found to hold negative attitudes about people who use substances, especially illicit drugs (McLaughlin, McKenna, Leslie, Moore, & Robinson, 2006), falling into the "well they could just quit" over-simplification. Later in this chapter, you will have the opportunity to reflect on your own attitudes, which may reflect some of society's most common misconceptions about people who have substance use, abuse, and addictions problems.

Community treatment services typically include detoxification services, screening, assessment, inpatient and outpatient treatment, and aftercare and follow-up. Non-residential treatment services, such as day treatment, make up the majority of all substance use treatment episodes (Pirie et al., 2013). The most common treatment services used in Canada include

alcohol and drug education, problem-solving counselling, cognitive and behavioural skills training (i.e., stress management, self-control therapy), motivational interviewing and enhancement strategies, and 12-step approaches. Additionally, special programs have been designed to address the unique needs of certain population groups, such as women, youth, Aboriginal people, inmates of correctional institutions, and impaired driving and drug offenders. For example, the great number of young males in driving-while-impaired programs validates the need for effective education and prevention efforts for this population (Pirie et al., 2013). Although they use some elements of coercion, diversion programs such as **drug treatment courts** (DTCs) offer alternatives to incarceration of repeat drug-involved offenders. These programs facilitate access to treatment and help reduce the harms and risk of ongoing dependence and criminal recidivism. These special courts are working to reduce the number of crimes committed to support drug dependence by providing judicial supervision, comprehensive substance abuse treatment, random and frequent drug testing, incentives and sanctions, clinical case management, and social support services (CCSA, 2007).

The treatment and rehabilitation system in many communities is often structured as a set of individual services rather than as a continuum. Services are often not integrated or coordinated. This can create access barriers for appropriate and timely treatment. A **treatment service continuum** should be coordinated, provide services that are based on best practices, have medically appropriate care, provide continuity of care among programs and organizations, and meet the diverse needs of individuals, including those with concurrent disorders. Key features of an effective treatment service continuum include services that are facilitated by different means (i.e., telehealth); have standardized screening and assessment tools that respect individual considerations, including culture and language; and offer choices (National Treatment Strategy Work Group, 2008). Research has demonstrated that treatment services and programs are far more effective and efficient when integrated within various sectors, including health, mental health social services, education, and the criminal justice system. For instance, screening, when conducted in various points of entry or agencies across multiple sectors, is a good example of integrating access to services throughout the system.

CHNs practising in health centres, homes, schools, and other community-based settings should be aware of the available treatment options in their communities. It is imperative that CHNs become familiar with screening and care planning in order to appropriately refer individuals who need additional support, counselling, or treatment. CHNs must have the skills to recognize the signs and symptoms of substance abuse and dependence, and be comfortable raising the topic with all clients as a matter of course. Screening can be conducted in a variety of settings, by a variety of individuals, and under a variety of conditions. In fact, health professionals such as CHNs are significantly more likely to be involved in screening than substance abuse specialists. Additionally, the CHN, in collaboration with professionals from other disciplines, should strive to advocate for and develop treatment options that acknowledge and integrate concurrent disorders, thus "making every door the right door" along the service continuum in their community. For this reason, it is important that CHNs understand that they can play a key role as primary screening agents in the community. Training to administer screening tools is recommended, and CHNs are encouraged to consult local substance abuse specialists in their community or province. You are encouraged to explore additional training in **motivational interviewing**, which is a powerful technique that can help people make a variety of lifestyle and behaviour changes. It centres on motivational processes within the person, moving the individual away from feelings of ambivalence, which tends to be the key stumbling block toward making constructive change. This approach was first developed in the 1980s in response to concerns about the traditional confrontational approach that was commonly used in addiction treatment at that time (Bailey, Colautti, & Parker, 2012). It has been used extensively in smoking cessation (Heckman & Egleston, 2010) and for the treatment of other substance use problems (Burke, Arkowitz, & Menchola, 2003).

The goal of **enforcement** is to strengthen community health and safety by responding to the crimes and community disorder issues associated with the supply (importation, manufacturing, cultivation), distribution, possession, and use of legal and illegal substances. Effective enforcement also means being visible in communities, understanding local issues, being aware of existing community resources, and participating in improving social conditions and attitudes while upholding public safety. Enforcement interventions must be linked to the three other "pillars" of Canada's original drug strategy to ensure that social, economic, and emotional complexities of substance abuse are recognized and addressed. Although the failure of some law enforcement efforts to counteract illicit drugs has led to recent debates over the decriminalization and/or the legalization of illicit substances, it has also led to the introduction of innovative harm-reduction strategies such as drug treatment courts that focus on treating rather than charging and incarcerating the substance abuser (Collin, 2006).

Harm-reduction strategies should be viewed as part of a continuum of prevention and treatment strategies. It is important to understand that abstinence is the best goal for those who are dependent on drugs. Although ideal in these circumstances, it may not always be achievable. **Harm reduction** is a powerful tool to minimize the harms associated with substance abuse. It offers a wide spectrum of opportunities for the CHN to help strengthen the capacity of individuals and communities experiencing the adverse effects of substance abuse.

As explained previously in this chapter and in Chapter 8, harm reduction is a public health philosophy that gained popularity in the last two decades; however, some claim that it is a new name for an old concept. It is described as a program or policy designed to reduce drug-related harms without requiring the cessation of drug use (Beirness, Jesseman, Notarandrea, & Perron, 2008). Examples of interventions include the availability of "light" alcoholic beverages, moderated use, alcohol server training programs, and impaired driving countermeasures. A harm-reduction message to the public is different from other types of prevention messages. Harm-reduction

messages may include statements such as "avoid problems when you drink" compared to "drinking less is better." As you work through the case study in this chapter, you will learn that many policies, such as the promotion of low-alcohol beverages, are based on harm-reduction principles. In the treatment field, the most pre-eminent harm-reduction strategies are medically supervised injection sites, street outreach, needle exchange, and methadone maintenance treatment programs, all of which allow the individual to live with a certain level of dependency while minimizing risks and other disruptive effects to the person and community.

**Medically supervised injection sites**, such as the InSite facility in Vancouver, offer a safe place where people inject their own drugs, supported by and connected to healthcare services. Health professionals are on site to prevent harmful consequences, such as overdose, and to provide users with information about health, treatment, and rehabilitation programs.

**Street outreach programs** tend to target marginalized populations such as street-involved youth, homeless people, sex-trade workers, and injection drug users. As part of street outreach, counselling and health services as well as information about additional services that are available in the community are provided.

**Needle exchange programs** have been developed to reduce the transmission of blood-borne pathogens. Needle exchange programs also reduce the circulation of contaminated needles between users and their unsafe disposal in public places. Such programs provide injection drug users with clean needles and syringes, health counselling, and social support and services. In Halifax, Nova Scotia, the Mainline Needle Exchange program has reported an unprecedented increase in the demand for sterile needles in recent years, attributing the jump to more awareness about the importance of safer use.

**Methadone maintenance treatment** (MMT) programs were introduced across Canada in response to the increasing use of opioids and the extensive cycle of this devastating drug dependency. Methadone alleviates the symptoms of opioid withdrawal by creating stable and sufficient blood levels of methadone. MMT has been demonstrated to improve physical and mental health status, reduce illicit drug use, decrease infectious disease risks, and reduce crime involvement among those involved in treatment. MMT offers a significant cost benefit to the community, given the costs associated with untreated opioid dependency. Supportive programs for opioid users have also arisen, using buprenorphine and suboxone; in some cases, these substances can have advantages over methadone. Harm reduction stands in contrast to other models and philosophies such as zero tolerance and abstinence-based health-promotion initiatives.

Harm reduction focuses on lowering the risk and severity of adverse consequences without necessarily reducing or eliminating use (International Harm Reduction Association, 2010). Although different, these approaches are complementary and all have an important role in addressing substance abuse problems in our communities. It is often said that harm reduction is not "what's nice, it's what works." The focus is therefore not on the use or the extent of use, but on the harms associated with the use. While becoming drug free may be the ultimate goal, it is not required. The goal is to reduce the more immediate and tangible harms. Providing nursing care in the context of harm reduction can raise ethical questions for the CHN, and community debates. Some may argue that harm reduction cannot be applied to tobacco since even small quantities of tobacco can be harmful. But consider the recent harm-reduction measures that have been put in place and have created protection for non-smokers in public places.

The CHN should be prepared for the controversy and debates harm reduction may elicit. Strong community stakeholder endorsement is essential as there may be public outcries about the appropriateness of harm-reduction programs. Be aware that this can inadvertently polarize the community and shift the focus from the program's intended purpose to a debate about social, moral, or criminal issues. On the other hand, such a dialogue may be essential to produce a shift in knowledge, attitudes, and values. Harm-reduction programs exist in most provinces, but generally speaking, federal political support is weak. Harm-reduction approaches are still considered unconventional. They force people to move away from the comfortable but failed "just say no" approach and are therefore met with ambivalence or resistance despite being epidemiologically relevant and highly effective. For example, Saskatchewan's rates of HIV/AIDS are currently the highest in Canada. Its provincial government wanted to halt unlimited needle distribution despite an earlier government-ordered review that found reductions in disease and healthcare costs. As such, new funding has not been offered despite the fact that the return rate of used needles in Regina is one of the highest in the world (Cavalieri & Riley, 2012). As a consequence, the cost in harms to individuals and the community is severe.

Consider the highly publicized debate about the InSite facility in Vancouver. In 2003, it was originally opened for research purposes with a three-year exemption from the federal Controlled Drugs and Substances Act 1996 (CA), permitting users to bring illicit drugs into the centre and inject themselves while under medical supervision. The exemption was extended to 2008, at which time a new government indicated that it would not support what it considered a "failed experiment," despite the strong body of research demonstrating the success of such programs. The matter was heard by the Supreme Court of B.C., which ordered the federal government to abandon its efforts to close the facility and requested an exemption be granted to protect InSite staff from prosecution for drug possession or trafficking charges. The government refused. The facility currently operates under a constitutional exception to the Controlled Drugs and Substances Act 1996 (CA).

Harm-reduction programs may not necessarily be available to all groups. For example, models of abstinence and prohibition in some Aboriginal communities may not allow moderate or reduced consumption or use, and many Aboriginal treatment programs and communities adhere to models of abstinence. However, harm reduction may not be entirely incompatible in some jurisdictions that have supported harm-reduction programs for Aboriginal drug users, offering abstinence as the potential but not required goal (Dell & Lyons, 2007). As with any community group, regardless of its cultural affiliation or diversity, the CHN should ensure that any harm-reduction service is developed in full partnership with members of the community.

While highly political and debated, the values of harm reduction are consistent with those of nursing (Canadian Nurses Association, 2011). While it is important for you to be aware of the controversial landscape of harm reduction, it is equally important to consider how you will advocate for system improvements in your community or at the broader levels. Nurses have long been successful advocates for their patients. The Discussion Questions presented as part of Canadian Research Box 30.2 will help you identify common misconceptions about harm reduction that often result in ethical debates about its role in healthcare.

# DEVELOPING COMMUNITY NURSING HEALTH INTERVENTIONS

No single type of community intervention can resolve a community's substance abuse problems. Communities should have a combination of **complementary interventions**, blending elements of all three levels of prevention. Although some of the frameworks and models presented in this section come from the substance-abuse field, they are grounded in the same principles of the population health-promotion model that is used throughout this text. Developing interventions should be informed by evidence, best practices, existing community knowledge, and the insight and experiences of those affected by the issue. For example, research shows that preventing adolescents from consuming alcohol and tobacco is difficult and that the impact is usually short term. Delaying the onset of substance use and preventing or minimizing harm is much more feasible. Interventions should also integrate principles of **cultural safety and competency** (please refer to Chapter 9, Cultural Care, for more details). CHNs should be culturally aware and sensitive to the needs of cultural, immigrant, and ethnic groups. Additionally, CHNs should acknowledge, reflect, and act upon the structural differences and power relationships within the addiction services they provide to ensure that access is barrier free and outcomes are achievable. The needs of Canada's Aboriginal population are not homogeneous. As such, the CHN should keep in mind that substance-abuse problems are manifested differently among First Nations, Inuit, and Métis people; people belonging to various ethnocultural groups; LGBTQ (lesbian, gay, bisexual, transgendered, and queer or questioning) people; and people with mental and physical challenges.

Responding to substance abuse–related problems cannot be done in isolation of the social determinants of health. Taking stock of the community, its cultural and ethnic profile, and its unique strengths and challenges, is essential to

## CANADIAN RESEARCH BOX 30.2

### Can accidental fatal overdose rates among injecting drug users be reduced by providing medically supervised safer injecting facilities?

Marshall, B. D. L., Milloy, M. -J., Wood, E., Montaner, J. S. G., & Kerr, T. (2011). Reduction in overdose mortality after the opening of North America's first medically supervised safer injecting facility: A retrospective population-based study. *The Lancet, 377,* 1429–1437.

Accidental drug overdose is a leading cause of death among injecting drug users. It contributes substantially to the mortality rate in communities where injection drug use is prevalent. Although risk factors for fatal overdose have been well documented in the literature, there are few evidence-based strategies to reduce the risk of overdose mortality that have proven to be effective. In Vancouver, high rates of overdose mortality in the 1990s led to the establishment of North America's first medically supervised safer injecting facility (SIF) in the city's Downtown Eastside, a community known for its large open drug market and well-described HIV epidemic. The local drug scene is characterized by high rates of polysubstance use, including heroin, cocaine, and methamphetamine injection in addition to crack cocaine smoking. The local neighbourhood is branded by a concentration of low-cost housing (e.g., single room occupancy hotels), high rates of homelessness, and drug-related disorders, including public drug injecting. The SIF is centrally located in this neighbourhood and aims to reduce public drug injection, decrease drug overdose, reduce the risk of infectious disease transmission, and improve access to healthcare services. Vancouver's SIF operates at capacity with over 500 supervised injections per day on average, with only 12 injection seats in a neighbourhood with about 5000 injection drug users. Waiting times and travel distance to the facility are barriers to SIF use. Similar to several other SIFs that exist around the world, injecting drug users in Vancouver consume pre-obtained illicit drugs under the supervision of healthcare professionals, who provide sterile syringes and referrals to primary health services as well as emergency care in the event of an overdose. Although SIFs have been associated with public health and community benefits in several international settings, they remain controversial. In Canada, although the Vancouver facility garnered broad public and local support, it continues to meet opposition by the federal government. Critics argue that objective outcomes are required to definitively establish the true effectiveness of SIFs. Moreover, the authors agreed there is an absence of rigorous assessments of SIFs and their impact on overdose mortality. To address the evidence gap and the need for more objective outcomes, the authors undertook a population-based study of drug-related overdose mortality rates before and after the establishment of North America's first SIF in Vancouver.

Data were drawn from review of files obtained from a central registry maintained by British Columbia's Coroners Service (BCCS). The registry is highly accurate as the BCCS is responsible for investigating and documenting all unnatural, unexpected, unexplained, or unattended deaths. Coroners are required to determine the identity of the deceased and record the manner, location, and cause of death. All deaths deemed to be caused by an accidental illicit drug overdose were eligible for inclusion in the analysis. The authors reviewed case files for all illicit drug overdose deaths that occurred in the City of Vancouver between January 1, 2001, and December 31, 2005, and found 290 accidental illicit drug overdoses occurred within the city's boundaries—an average of one per week. Men accounted for 229 (79%) deaths and the median age at death was 40 years. Overdoses did not vary significantly across seasons. There were no significant differences regarding the types of drugs implicated in the cause of death but one-third of the fatal overdoses were attributed to multiple combinations of drugs.

Data were analyzed according to proximity to the SIF. The locations of death were heavily concentrated in the city's Downtown Eastside with one-third occurring within 500 metres of the SIF. Decedents in city blocks farther than 500 metres from the facility were more likely to be female and of First Nations ancestry during the post-SIF period. Reductions in overdose rates were most evident within close vicinity of the facility. In city blocks within 500 metres of the facility, the overdose rate decreased by 35% after the opening of the facility. By contrast, the fatal overdose rate in other areas of the city during the same period declined by only 9%. There were no significant reductions in overdose mortality further than 500 metres from the SIF. This was not surprising to the authors, since over 70% of frequent SIF users reported living within four blocks of the facility.

The rise in the proportion of female and First Nations deaths in areas further than 500 metres from the facility is concerning, given previous evidence showing an increased drug-related vulnerability in these subpopulations. Because the SIF is well received by women and First Nations individuals, the authors recommend efforts should be made to expand services to reach vulnerable injecting drug users who reside outside of the Downtown Eastside area. Given that a significant percentage of the fatal overdoses were attributed to multiple combinations of drugs, the authors recommend a range of innovative public health responses be developed to address the risks associated with polydrug use. Consistent with earlier evidence that SIFs are not associated with higher rates of injecting, the findings of this study indicate that such facilities are safe and effective public health harm-reduction interventions. Therefore, SIFs should be considered in settings with a high rate of overdose related to injection drug use. Larger reductions in community overdose mortality would probably require an expansion of this SIF, given its limited number of seats and the high density of this community's rate of overdose and drug-injecting population.

### Discussion Questions

1. Why should harm-reduction supplies be available to people who use illicit drugs?

2. What might be some of the barriers for pregnant women seeking out harm-reduction services?

3. Do harm-reduction programs make it easier for people to use substances?

understand the context of any problematic substance use and abuse pattern. Social and economic conditions such as limited income, living in unsafe neighbourhoods, and lack of leisure, recreation, job, and training opportunities are known to increase the risk of substance use and abuse. Strategies based on sensationalism and shock value should be avoided. Research has shown that while they may produce some deterrence, benefits are short lived and cannot be sustained over time. Taking the time to assess the community's condition is the first step the CHN should take before defining, supporting, or moving ahead with any intervention. The application of the resiliency theory is especially valuable because it identifies a community's predominant risk and protective factors, and facilitates planning efforts that integrate the determinants of health and connect individuals, families, and the community to their sociocultural and economic environment. Strategies developed within this framework will address the root causes of a community's substance abuse problems. **Resiliency** is described as the capability of individuals, families, groups, and communities to cope successfully in the face of significant adversity or risk (Mangham, McGrath, Reid, & Stewart, 1995). The theory of resiliency consists of two fundamental concepts—risk and protective factors—both of which contribute to one's sense of resistance or resiliency. Mangham et al. (1995) describe **risk factors** as stressors that

challenge individuals, including their own personal and environmental characteristics. When a stressor is greater than one's protective factors, even among those who have been resilient in the past, the person may become overwhelmed. **Protective factors** (Mangham et al., 1995) are defined as skills, personality factors, and environmental supports that act as buffers when people are faced with stressful events. These may include literacy and interpersonal skills. Community-based protective factors may consist of a strong economic base and access to affordable and safe housing. Assessing factors such as poverty or social isolation, which may lead to maladaptive patterns of drug use, can help the CHN understand why some individuals and communities respond differently to adversity and have different levels of consumption and substance abuse patterns. In essence, the theory helps pinpoint predominant risk factors that need to be addressed as well as the protective factors that need to be optimized as part of any community assessment and substance abuse intervention strategy (Figure 30.4). CHNs must be innovative in their approaches that promote partnerships among community members. This maximizes knowledge exchange, a community's assets, and its leverage to acquire additional resources. A multi-pronged approach involving multiple sectors ensures that interventions are relevant and result in optimal outcomes.

| **Community Risk Factors** | | |
| --- | --- | --- |
| Social | Environmental | Behavioural |
| Economic disadvantage | Isolation | Communal apathy |
| Unemployment | - geographical | Community anger |
| Educational disadvantage | - social | Low participation in |
| Cultural barriers | Disasters | community development |

+

| **Community Protective Factors** | | | |
| --- | --- | --- | --- |
| Social Support | Empowerment | Community Connectedness | Communal Coping |
| Communal support | Communal responsibility | Shared history and culture | Problem focused |
| Family and friends | and action | Residents "know everyone" | Emotion focused |
| Volunteers | Retraining | Schools and churches | |
| Lay support | Educational services | | |
| Community organizations | | | |

↓

| **Community (Positive) Resilient Outcomes** | | | |
| --- | --- | --- | --- |
| Growth | Residents' Health | Community Tone/Outlook | Community Development |
| New economic and | Physical health | Hope | Community participation |
| cultural initiatives | Mental health | Optimism | and connectedness |
| | Healthy behaviours | Embrace opportunities | Organizations survive |
| | | | Acquire resources |

**FIGURE 30.4** Framework of Community Resilience

*Source:* Reproduced with the permission of the Minister of Public Works and Government Services Canada, 2007.

## CASE STUDY

### Testing Website Accessibility

A local junior hockey team plays in your community's municipally owned arena. Team officials have been selling beer during home games as a means of generating much-needed revenue for the team. There have been recent and well-publicized complaints about people becoming intoxicated and creating disturbances during and after games. Community officials and private entrepreneurs are looking for the support of the local police department and your public health unit in order to effectively address this issue and prevent further disturbances. The well-attended hockey games represent the main source of entertainment for many families during the long winter season. Your public health board has requested a substance abuse program to explore this issue and develop an appropriate strategy to reduce these emerging alcohol-related problems.

### Discussion Questions

1. Discuss the health, social, and legal risks that are commonly associated with the practice of serving alcohol during sports events in municipally owned facilities.

2. Explore various prevention and enforcement strategies that can be adopted to minimize the risks that are associated with the serving of alcohol.

3. Identify the various groups of stakeholders that should be targeted as part of these strategies.

## CONCLUSION

CHNs have the leadership, knowledge, and skills to influence and leverage support and resources that will optimize and support healthy individuals, families, communities, and populations. Doing so requires a good understanding of the interconnectedness between the use and abuse of substances and the determinants of health. Paying attention to issues that impact a community and the factors that may influence individuals who need information and/or professional assistance for a substance abuse–related problem is paramount to finding the right solution, for the right people, and at the right place and time. The application of the conceptual frameworks and models presented in this chapter can serve to guide the CHN in the advocacy and development of relevant interventions that are based on evidence; make important linkages between the individual, the drug, and the environment; and reflect the values and practice standards of community health nursing.

## KEY TERMS

## STUDY QUESTIONS

1. Why do people use drugs?

2. What is drug dependence? Distinguish between physical and psychological dependence.

3. What are the harmful consequences of substance abuse?

4. Describe important aspects of developing interventions to address substance abuse issues in communities.

5. Describe the "four pillars" of Canada's Federal Drug Strategy.

6. What are the six principles that should guide a CHN's work in community-based substance abuse interventions?

7. What are the limitations of exclusively focusing on law-enforcement interventions?

8. Explain two harm-reduction programs available in Canada.

After working through these questions, go to the
MyNursingLab at www.pearsoned.ca/mynursinglab
to check your answers.

# INDIVIDUAL CRITICAL-THINKING EXERCISES

1. RNs and other healthcare providers have been found to hold negative attitudes concerning people who use substances, particularly illegal drugs (Carroll, 1995; McLaughlin & Long, 1996; McLaughlin, McKenna, Leslie, Moore, & Robinson, 2006). Privately explore the first thing that comes to mind when you read each of the following expressions. Then, explore your reactions to each expression. Do they differ from each other? If so, consider the reasons why. Did any of your reactions surprise you? If yes, reflect on how your personal values may influence your professional practice.

   - a homeless alcoholic
   - needle exchange program
   - abstinence-based treatment
   - problem drinker
   - methadone treatment
   - parent with hangover
   - IV drug user
   - crack dealer
   - professor smoking marijuana
   - pregnant methadone client
   - crystal meth addict
   - chain (tobacco) smoker
   - female cocaine user
   - drunk driver
   - 20-year-old buying booze for underage sibling
   - person with HIV
   - gas sniffer
   - underage drunk
   - coffee drinker

2. Read your local newspaper or a magazine, or watch the news, a television program, or a movie. Pay attention to the images and messages about the consumption of alcohol, tobacco, and illicit or licit drugs. Who are these messages aimed at? What are they portraying? Consider the degree of influence that these images and messages have on drug consumption patterns in society.

3. Think of a community you have lived in and consider the factors that were attributed to that community's health status. What was the prevalence of psychoactive substances in that community? You may want to focus on one or more substances. Explore the factors that placed that community at risk and those that protected it or acted as buffers.

4. In the community you are living in now, think about where screening for the use of psychoactive substances might take place. As a CHN, how might you introduce the concept of screening in a primary health clinic?

5. Thinking of your university or college, consider the activities that should be provided to reduce the abuse of alcohol on campus.

# GROUP CRITICAL-THINKING EXERCISES

1. Select a particular issue or harm that is associated with substance abuse in your community (e.g., the misuse and abuse of opioid prescription drugs, impaired driving, FASD). What sources of information (local, regional, provincial, and national) can be used to help your group accurately define the problem?

2. For the issue identified in Question 1, have your group map your community's current capacity in terms of substance abuse prevention and treatment (health promotion and health recovery/rehabilitation) services and programs. You may use the telephone directory or contact local health and social service agencies. For example, you should highlight any screening and prevention programs, how people access general information about the issue, and, if appropriate, where people access treatment services. Make note of any service or program gaps your group observes.

3. Using the results of the mapping exercise in Question 2 and referring to the Framework for Community Resilience, discuss and analyze as a group the risk factors that you believe have contributed to the development of the issue or harm identified in Question 1. Additionally, your group should explore the protective factors that have acted as buffers or that will have the capacity to create positive outcomes for your target population or for the community.

# REFERENCES

Adlaf, E., Demers, A., & Gliksman, L. (Eds.). (2005). *Canadian Campus Survey 2004*. Toronto: Centre for Addiction and Mental Health. Retrieved from http://www.camh.ca/en/research/research_areas/community_and_population_health/Documents/CCS_2004_report.pdf

American Psychiatric Association. (2013). *Diagnostic and statistical manual of mental disorders* (5th ed.). Washington, DC: Author.

Babor, T. (2010). *Alcohol: No ordinary commodity: Research and public policy* (2nd ed.). New York, NY: Oxford University Press.

Bailey, A., Colautti, L., & Parker, A. (2012). *Evidence Summary: The effectiveness of motivational interviewing for young people engaging in problematic substance use*. Headspace, National Youth Mental Health Foundation: Orygen Youth Health Research Centre, Australia.

Baliunas, D., Patra, J., Rehm, J., Popova, S., Kaiserman, M., & Taylor, B. (2007). Smoking-attributable mortality and expected years of life lost in Canada 2002: Conclusions for prevention and policy. *Chronic Diseases in Canada, 27*(4), 154–162.

Baydala, L. (2010). Inhalant abuse. *Paediatrics & Child Health 15*(7), 443–448.

Beirness, D. J., Jesseman, R., Notarandrea, R., & Perron, M. (2008). *Harm reduction: What's in a name?* Ottawa, ON: Canadian Centre on Substance Abuse.

Bell, K., Salmon, A., Bowers, M., Bell, J., & McCullough, L. (2010). Smoking, stigma and tobacco "denormalization": Further reflections on the use of stigma as a public health tool. A commentary on social science & medicine's stigma, prejudice, discrimination and health. *Social Science & Medicine, 70*(6), 795–799.

Brache, K. (2014). Alcohol and energy drinks: Motivations, drinking behaviours and associated risks (Doctoral dissertation). University of Victoria. Retrieved from https://dspace.library.uvic.ca:8443/bitstream/handle/1828/5727/Brache_Kristina_PhD_2014.pdf?sequence=3&isAllowed=y

Burke, B., Arkowitz, H., & Menchola, M. (2003). The efficacy of motivational interviewing: A meta-analysis of controlled clinical trials. *Journal of Consulting and Clinical Psychology, 71*(5). 843–61.

Butt, P., Beirness, D., Gliksman, L., Paradis, C., & Stockwell, T. (2011). *Alcohol and health in Canada: A summary of evidence and guidelines for low risk drinking.* Ottawa, ON: Canadian Centre on Substance Abuse.

Butterfield, P. (1997). Thinking upstream: Conceptualizing health from a health population perspective. In J. Swanson & M. Nies (Eds.), *Community health nursing: Promoting the health of the aggregate* (pp. 69–92). Philadelphia, PA: W. B. Saunders.

Canada Safety Council. (2013). *Safety Info on Methanol.* Retrieved from https://canadasafetycouncil.org/workplace-safety/methanol

Canadian Centre on Substance Abuse. (2005). *Supervised Injection Facilities (SIFs): Frequently asked questions.* Retrieved from http://www.ccsa.ca/Resource%20Library/ccsa-010657-2004.pdf

Canadian Centre on Substance Abuse. (2007). *Drug treatment court: Frequently asked questions.* Retrieved from http://www.ccsa.ca/Resource%20Library/ccsa-011348-2007.pdf

Canadian Centre on Substance Abuse. (2008). *Canada's North.* Retrieved from http://www.archive-ca-2012.com/open-archive/1070800/2012-12-26/cd1989fd8af-7315f7acd1eb68999d0c4

Canadian Centre on Substance Abuse. (2009a). *Substance abuse in Canada: Concurrent disorders.* Retrieved from http://www.ccsa.ca/Resource%20Library/ccsa-011811-2010.pdf

Canadian Centre on Substance Abuse. (2009b). *Clearing the smoke on cannabis: Cannabis use and driving.* Retrieved from http://www.ccsa.ca/Resource%20Library/CCSA-Cannabis-Use-and-Driving-Report-2015-en.pdf

Canadian Centre on Substance Abuse (2011). Injection Drug Users Overview.

Canadian Centre on Substance Abuse. (2012). Prepared by the Canadian Community Epidemiology Network on Drug Use. *CCENDU drug alert – Bath salts.* Retrieved from http://www.ccsa.ca/Resource%20Library/CCSA-CCENDU-Drug-Alert-Bath-Salts-2012-en.pdf#search=bath%20salts

Canadian Centre on Substance Abuse. (2013). *Prescription sedatives and tranquilizers.* Canadian Drug Summary. Retrieved from http://www.ccsa.ca/Resource%20Library/CCSA-Prescription-Sedatives-and-Tranquilizers-2013-en.pdf

Canadian Nurses Association. (2011). *Harm reduction and currently illegal drugs: Implications for nursing policy, practice, education and research – discussion paper.* Ottawa, ON: Author.

Canadian Partnership for Responsible Gambling. (2009, April). *Canadian gambling digest 2007–2008.*

Canadian Public Health Association. (2000). *Gambling expansion in Canada: An emerging public health issue, 2000.* Retrieved from http://www.cpha.ca/uploads/resolutions/2000-1pp_e.pdf

Canadian Public Health Association. (2011). *The winnable battle: Ending tobacco use in Canada, a position paper.* Ottawa, ON: Author.

Canadian Women's Foundation. (2011). *Report on violence against women, mental health and substance use.* Canadian Women's Foundation and BC Society of Transition House. Retrieved from http://www.canadianwomen.org/sites/canadianwomen.org/files/PDF%20-%20VP%20Resources%20-%20BCSTH%20CWF%20Report_Final_2011_%20Mental%20Health_Substance%20use.pdf

Cavalieri, W., & Riley, D. (2012). Harm reduction in Canada: The many faces of regression. In R. Pates & D. Riley (Eds.), *Harm reduction in substance use and high risk behaviour: International policy and practice* (pp. 382–394). London, UK: Blackwell.

Chudley, A. E., Conry, J., Cook, J. L., Loock, C., Rosales, T., & LeBlanc, N. (2005). Fetal alcohol spectrum disorder: Canadian guidelines for diagnosis. *Canadian Medical Association Journal, 172*(5 suppl), S1–S21.

Collin, C. (2006). *Substance abuse issues and public policy in Canada: Canada's federal drug strategy.* Parliamentary Information and Research Service: Political and Social Affairs Division. Retrieved from http://www.parl.gc.ca/information/library/PRBpubs/prb0615-e.pdf

*Controlled Drugs and Substances Act, 1996* (CA). (n.d.). Retrieved from http://laws-lois.justice.gc.ca/PDF/C-38.8.pdf

Dahl, R. E. (2004). Adolescent brain development: A period of vulnerabilities and opportunities. *Annals of the New York Academy of Sciences, 1021,* 1–22.

Dell, C. A., & Lyons, T. (2007). *Harm reduction for special populations in Canada: Harm reduction policies and programs for persons of Aboriginal descent.* Canadian Centre on Substance Abuse. Retrieved from http://www.addictionresearchchair.ca/wp-content/uploads/Harm-Reduction-Policies-and-Programs-for-Persons-of-Aboriginal-Descent.pdf

Dhalla, I. A., Mamdani, M. M., Sivilotti, M. L. A., Kopp, A., Qureshi, O., & Juurlink, D. N. (2009). Prescribing of opioid analgesics and related mortality before and after the introduction of long-acting oxycodone. *Canadian Medical Association Journal, 181,* 891–896.

Dow, K., Ordean, A., Murphy-Oikonen, J., Pereira, J., Koren, G., Roukema, H., . . . Turner, R. (2012). Neonatal abstinence syndrome: Clinical practice guidelines for Ontario. *Journal of Popular Clinical Therapies and Pharmacology, 19*(3), 488–506.

Fischer, B., Rehm, J., Brissette, S., Brochu, S., Bruneau, J., El-Guebaly, N. . . . Baliunas, D. (2005). Illicit opioid use in Canada: Comparing social, health, and drug use characteristics of untreated users in five cities (OPICAN study). *Journal of Urban Health: Bulletin of the New York Academy of Medicine, 82*(2), 250–266.

Galea, S., Nandi, A., & Vlahov, D. (2004). The social epidemiology of substance use. *Epidemiological Reviews, 26,* 36–52.

Health Canada. (2000). *Straight facts about drugs and drug abuse.* Retrieved from http://www.cds-sca.com

Health Canada. (2011). *Canadian alcohol and drug use survey (CADUMS).* Retrieved from http://www.hc-sc.gc.ca/hc-ps/drugs-drogues/stat/_2010/summary-sommaire-eng.php

Health Canada. (2012). *Youth smoking survey 2010–11 data tables.* Retrieved from http://www.yss.uwaterloo.ca/results/YSS2010-2011_supplementary_tables_en.pdf.

Heckman, C. J., & Egleston, B. L. (2010). Efficacy of motivational interviewing for smoking cessation: A systematic review and meta-analysis. *Tobacco Control, 19*(5), 410–16.

Huang, J. H., & Boyer, R. (2007). Epidemiology of youth gambling problems in Canada: A national prevalence study. *The Canadian Journal of Psychiatry, 52*(10), 657–664.

International Harm Reduction Association. (2010). *What is harm reduction? A position statement from the International Harm Reduction Association*. London, UK. Retrieved from http://www.ihra.net/what-is-harm-reduction

International Narcotics Control Board. (2013). *Narcotic drugs: Estimated world requirements for 2013—Statistics for 2011*. New York, NY: United Nations.

Leyton, M., & Stewart, S. (Eds.). (2014). *Substance abuse in Canada: Childhood and adolescent pathways to substance use disorders*. Ottawa, ON: Canadian Centre on Substance Abuse.

Mangham, C., McGrath, P., Reid, G., & Stewart, M. (1995). *Resiliency: Relevance to health promotion: Discussion paper*. Ottawa, ON: Health Canada.

McLaughlin, D., McKenna, H., Leslie, J., Moore, K., & Robinson, J. (2006). Illicit drug users in Northern Ireland: Perceptions and experiences of health and social care professionals. *Journal of Psychiatric and Mental Health Nursing, 2006*(13), 682–686.

Miller, C. L., Pearce, M. E., Moniruzzaman, A., Thomas, V., Schechter, M. T., & Spittal, P. M. (2011). The Cedar Project: Risk factors for transition to injection drug use among young, urban Aboriginal people. *Canadian Medical Association Journal, 183*(10), 1147–1154.

National Advisory Committee on Prescription Drug Misuse. (2013). *First do no harm: Responding to Canada's prescription drug crisis*. Ottawa: Canadian Centre on Substance Misuse. Retrieved from http://www.ccsa.ca/resource%20library/canada-strategy-prescription-drug-misuse-report-en.pdf

National Treatment Strategy Working Group. (2008). *A systems approach to substance use in Canada: Recommendations for a national treatment strategy*. Ottawa: National Framework for Action to Reduce the Harms Associated with Alcohol and Other Drugs and Substances in Canada. Retrieved from http://www.ccsa.ca/Resource%20Library/nts-systems-approach-substance-abuse-canada-2008-en.pdf

Paradis, C., Demers, A., & Picard, E. (2010). Alcohol consumption: A different kind of Canadian mosaic. *Canadian Journal of Public Health, 101*(4), 275–80.

Pirie, T., Jesseman, R., & National Treatment Indicators Working Group. (2013). *National Treatment Indicators Report: 2010–2011 Data*. Ottawa, ON: Canadian Centre on Substance Abuse.

Prosser, J. M., & Nelson, L. S. (2011). The toxicology of bath salts: A review of synthetic cathinones. *Journal of Medical Toxicology, 8*(1), 33–42.

Rehm, J., Ballunas, D., Brochu, S., Fischer, B., Gnam, W., Patra, J., & Taylor, B. (2006). *The costs of substance abuse in Canada, 2002 highlights*. Retrieved from http://www.ccsa.ca/Resource%20Library/ccsa-011332-2006.pdf

Reid, J. L., Hammond, D., Burkhalter, R., Rynard, V. L., & Ahmed, R. (2013). *Tobacco use in Canada: Patterns and trends, 2013 Edition*. Waterloo, ON: Propel Centre for Population Health Impact, University of Waterloo. Retrieved from http://www.tobaccoreport.ca/2013

Roerecke, M., & Rehm, J. (2012). The cardioprotective association of average alcohol consumption and ischaemic heart disease: A systematic review and meta-analysis. *Addiction, 107*(7), 1246–1260.

Royal Canadian Mounted Police. (2010). *Report on the illicit drug situation in Canada, 2009*. Ottawa, ON: Royal Canadian Mounted Police.

Rush, B. R., Urbanski, K. A., Bassani, D. G., Castel, S., & Wild, T. C. (2010). The epidemiology of co-occurring substance use disorders and other mental disorders in Canada: Prevalence, service use and unmet needs. In J. Cairney & D. L. Streiner (Eds.), *Mental disorders in Canada: An epidemiological perspective* (pp. 170–204). Toronto, ON: University of Toronto Press.

Statistics Canada. (2001). The control and sale of alcoholic beverages in Canada, 2001. *The Daily*. Catalogue no. 63-202-XIB. Ottawa, ON: Minister of Industry.

Statistics Canada. (2005). The control and sale of alcoholic beverages, fiscal year ending March 31, 2005. *The Daily*. Catalogue no. 63-202-XIE. Ottawa, ON: Minister of Industry.

Statistics Canada. (2009). The control and sale of alcoholic beverages, fiscal year ending March 31, 2008. *The Daily*. Retrieved from http://www.statcan.gc.ca/daily-quotidien/090420/t090420b2-eng.htm

Steinhagen, K. A. (2008). Substance abuse and misuse in older adults. Aging Well, 3, p. 20. Retrieved from http://www.todaysgeriatricmedicine.com/archive/071708p20.shtml

Traffic Injury Research Foundation. (2009). *The alcohol crash problem in Canada: 2006*. Ottawa, ON: Author.

Traffic Injury Research Foundation. (2013). *The alcohol crash problem in Canada: 2010*. Canadian Council of Motor Transport Administrators and the Minister of Public Works and Government Services, represented by the Minister of Transport. Retrieved from http://www.tirf.ca/publications/publications_show.php?pub_id=292

Wakefield, M. A., Loken, B., & Hornik, R. C. (2010). Use of mass media campaigns to change health behavior. *The Lancet, 376*(9748), 1261–1271.

Webster, P. C. (2012). Prescription drug abuse rising among Aboriginal youths. *Canadian Medical Association Journal, 184*(12), 647–648.

Wood. R. T., & Williams, R. J. (2009, January). Internet gambling: Prevalence, patterns, problems, and policy options. Final report for the Ontario Problem Gambling Research Centre; Guelph, Ontario.

World Health Organization. (2003). *Social determinants of health: The solid facts* (2nd ed.). R. Wilkinson & M. Marmot (Eds.). WHO: Copenhagen, Denmark.

## ABOUT THE AUTHOR

**Hélène Philbin Wilkinson**, RN, BScN, MN. After spending the early part of her nursing career in hospital and public health nursing, Hélène turned to the community, working at the Centre for Addiction and Mental Health as a senior program consultant in policy and service development, and applied research and program evaluations projects in both substance abuse and mental health. In 1999, she joined the Northern Shores District Health Council as a senior health systems planner overseeing the planning portfolios of addiction, mental health, and French-language health services. Following the closure of the Ontario District Health Councils in 2005, Hélène returned to the hospital sector where she is currently working as the Administrate Director of the Mental Health and the Law Service at the North Bay Regional Health Centre. She dedicates her chapter to her godmother Ella, who was a pioneer public health nurse in Northeastern Ontario.

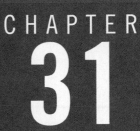

# CHAPTER
# 31

# Sexually Transmitted Infections and Blood-Borne Pathogens

*Wendi Lokanc-Diluzio and Tammy Troute-Wood*

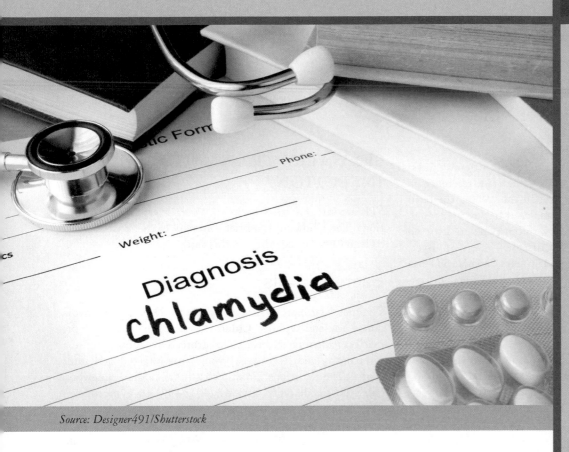

*Source: Designer491/Shutterstock*

## INTRODUCTION

**Sexually transmitted infections (STIs)** and **blood-borne pathogens (BBPs)** are significant public health issues in Canada. STIs are infections that are spread through insertive and receptive sexual practices (vaginal, anal, or oral) with an infected person. In addition, some viral STIs, such as genital herpes and human papillomavirus, can be transmitted by intimate skin-to-skin contact (Government of Alberta, 2012). BBPs are infections that are carried and transmitted by blood (Public Health Agency of Canada, 2003).

In Canada, some STIs and BBPs are notifiable (or reportable) diseases. The Public Health Agency of Canada (PHAC) (PHAC, 2013–2014) stipulates which STIs and BBPs are reportable nationally and each province or territory can add diseases to be reported in that jurisdiction. The need for partner notification, contact tracing, testing, and treatment can differ between jurisdictions and are important considerations of the notifiable disease program.

People affected by STIs and BBPs have encountered stigmatization and discrimination. STIs and BBPs often elicit emotional reactions such as anxiety, fear, and shame.

The stigma of STIs and BBPs may impede people from protecting themselves as well as from seeking testing and treatment. Societal reactions of intolerance toward people at risk for contracting STIs and BBPs, as well as those living with **human immunodeficiency virus (HIV)** and **acquired immune deficiency syndrome (AIDS)** may further marginalize populations who already experience health inequities.

In this chapter, you will learn how community health nurses (CHNs) are challenged to promote health, build capacity, and facilitate access and equity through innovative community strategies to address STIs and BBPs. Historical and current challenges regarding the prevention of STIs and BBPs and the development of healthy public policies are discussed. An overview of common STIs and selected BBPs, their incidence, and/or their prevalence in Canada are presented. Prevention and risk- and harm-reduction strategies are discussed and examples of innovative prevention strategies are offered.

## HISTORY OF STIs AND BBPs AND THEIR EFFECTS ON HEALTHY PUBLIC POLICY

Over the years, STIs have been labelled in different ways, including **venereal disease** (VD), which is a reference to Venus, the Roman goddess of love. In the 1970s, the term VD was viewed as inaccurate and replaced by sexually transmitted disease (STD), because "love often plays little or no role in the transmission of such diseases" (Shriver, Byer, Shainberg, & Galliano, 2002, p. 136). In Canada, STI has become the preferred term, as STI is viewed as an encompassing term that includes infections which may be asymptomatic (PHAC, 2013a). Recently, the acronym STBBI (sexually transmitted and blood-borne infections) is used when referring to both STIs and BBPs.

Healthy public policies and guidelines are revisited and updated based on research to assist in protecting the public from the consequences of infection. There is a complex relationship between STI and HIV. STI and HIV infections often co-exist. A person with HIV who also has an STI is more likely to transmit HIV to an unaffected sexual partner. Conversely, any person who has an STI is more likely to acquire HIV if exposed (PHAC, 2013–2014). Community health nursing interventions that support people to take precautions to prevent STI may also reduce the risk of HIV infection. However, it is important to note that although HIV can be sexually transmitted (semen, vaginal, and rectal fluids), HIV is also transmitted in other ways, such as exposure to infected blood or items contaminated with blood (needles) and vertical transmission from mother to infant (PHAC, 2013b).

Prior to the discovery of bacterial antibiotics, STIs were not treatable and caused serious illness. Historically, public policies were implemented to test men and women for syphilis prior to marriage and to test women during pregnancy to prevent neonatal infection through **vertical transmission**. With the advent of antibiotic treatment, new policies were developed. For example, for more than 100 years, silver nitrate eye drops, or more recently other antibiotics such as erythromycin, have been recommended by the Canadian Paediatric Society (CPS) for all newborns to prevent blindness from gonorrhea (CPS, 2008a). Currently, all Canadian provinces and territories have developed recommendations and/or guidelines for prenatal HIV testing to promote informed decision making related to neonatal HIV prevention (PHAC, 2013–2014). Healthy public policies have also been developed in response to community action. The Canadian Red Cross became entrenched in public health scandal when it was discovered that over 1000 Canadians had become infected with HIV from blood transfusions. Although the medical community had become aware of a new blood-borne infection in the late 1970s and early 1980s, strict HIV blood surveillance guidelines were not implemented until 1985. People infected with HIV from blood transfusions launched class actions and other compensation programs were established. The risk of HIV transmission via blood transfusion decreased during 1985 to 2003, from roughly 1 in 16 000 to 1 in greater than a million (PHAC, 2009).

## SEXUALLY TRANSMITTED INFECTIONS

STIs are categorized as bacterial, viral, or ectoparasitic infections. The following is a brief summary of the most common STIs in Canada, according to this categorization.

### Bacterial STIs

The most common reportable **bacterial STIs** are chlamydia, gonorrhea, and syphilis. **Chlamydia** and **gonorrhea** are primarily transmitted through unprotected vaginal and anal intercourse, and less often through unprotected oral intercourse. The infections can also pass from mother to newborn baby during delivery (PHAC, 2013–2014). Symptoms in females may include abnormal vaginal discharge or bleeding, lower abdominal pain, pain during intercourse, or burning during urination (PHAC, 2013–2014). Symptoms in males may include unusual penile discharge, burning while urinating, or pain or swelling of the testes. Additionally, rectal pain and discharge may indicate infection through anal intercourse. Pharyngeal infection may present as a sore throat. Most often, however, individuals may not experience any symptoms, resulting in the ongoing spread of infection or serious complications (PHAC, 2013–2014). In women, untreated chlamydia and gonorrhea infections may lead to pelvic inflammatory disease (PID), which is an inflammation of the upper female genital tract. Complications of PID may include chronic pelvic pain, infertility, and ectopic pregnancy. In men, untreated infections may lead to infections of the testicle, scrotum, infertility, and chronic pelvic pain (PHAC, 2013–2014).

Many people avoid being tested for STIs because of their fear of pain or embarrassment. Chlamydial and gonorrheal infections are detected via urine testing or cervical, penile, anal, or throat swabbing. Both infections are treatable with antibiotics (PHAC, 2013–2014). An uncomplicated chlamydia infection can be treated with a single dose of azithromycin. In recent years, gonorrhea has become increasingly resistant to antibiotics, and treatment with penicillin, tetracycline, and quinolones are no longer recommended. People with gonorrheal infections should be treated with combination therapy of cephalosporin and azithromycin and be re-screened in six months post treatment (PHAC, 2013–2014).

In Canada, chlamydia is the most prevalent reportable STI. From 2000 to 2012, the chlamydia rate increased from 149.7 to 298.7 per 100 000 persons (PHAC, 2014a). A disproportionate number of youth between the ages of 15 and 24 and females are infected with chlamydia (PHAC, 2014a). Gonorrhea is the second-most prevalent reportable STI in Canada. From 2000 to 2008, the reported rate increased from 20.2 to 38.1 per 100 000 people (PHAC, 2014a). The gonorrhea rate declined to 33.2 in 2009; however, it has steadily increased to 36.2 per 100 000 people in 2012 (PHAC, 2014a). Males tend to have higher rates of gonorrhea than females (PHAC, 2014a). See Table 31.1 for rates of chlamydia and gonorrhea in Canada. **Syphilis** is primarily transmitted via unprotected vaginal, oral, or anal sexual contact (PHAC, 2013–2014). The signs and symptoms of syphilis are often overlooked because in the early stages it manifests as painless sores (chancres) with flu-like symptoms. Diagnosis is often delayed until later stages, when there is already extensive damage to the central nervous or cardiovascular systems, resulting in complications such as paralysis or mental illness (PHAC, 2013–2014). Syphilis is diagnosed through blood tests, swabs with dark-field microscopy, and clinical symptoms (e.g., chancres and rash that can appear anywhere including trunk, palms of the hands, or soles of the feet) (PHAC, 2013–2014). Syphilis infections are treated with antibiotics, and negative

long-term outcomes are reduced with early diagnosis (PHAC, 2013–2014). Syphilis can also be passed from mother to baby during pregnancy or childbirth, resulting in congenital syphilis or even fetal death (PHAC, 2013–2014). The Canadian Guidelines on Sexually Transmitted Infections (PHAC, 2013–2014) recommend that all pregnant women be screened for infectious syphilis during the first trimester of pregnancy. Women who are considered "high risk" should also be re-screened at 28–32 weeks and again at delivery (PHAC, 2013–2014).

In Canada, syphilis is the least common of the reportable STIs. That said, from 2000 to 2006 the syphilis rate increased from 1.8 to 10.8 per 100 000 population (PHAC, 2014a). From 2007 to 2012, the rate has fluctuated between 8.3 and 8.9 (PHAC, 2014a). Over the past decade, there have been several syphilis outbreaks across Canada, including in Montreal, Ottawa, Toronto, Winnipeg, Calgary, Edmonton, Vancouver, Yukon, and Northwest Territories (PHAC, 2011). The majority of the outbreaks have been linked to men who have sex with men (MSM) and sex-trade worker populations (PHAC, 2013–2014). See Table 31.1 for rates of infectious syphilis.

In 2010, the Government of Alberta (2010) stated that Alberta had experienced a "sustained outbreak of syphilis, which shows no sign of abating" (p. 2). From 2000 to 2009, the infectious syphilis rate in Alberta increased from 0.5 to 7.7 per 100 000 persons (Government of Alberta, 2014) (see Photo 31.1). Furthermore, 26 Albertan babies were diagnosed with congenital syphilis during this time. This has changed prenatal screening practices in Alberta. It is recommended that all pregnant Albertan women are screened for syphilis during their first trimester or during their first prenatal visit, and re-screened again at delivery (Alberta Health Services & ProvLab Alberta, 2012). Although the syphilis rate has steadily declined from 7.7 in 2009 to 2.9 in 2013 (Government of Alberta, 2014), the prenatal syphilis screening practices in Alberta continue.

| Table 31.1 | Chlamydia, Gonorrhea, and Syphilis Rates per 100 000 People in Canada: 2000, 2004, 2008, and 2012 Comparisons | | | | |
|---|---|---|---|---|---|
| | | **2000** | **2004** | **2008** | **2012** |
| **Chlamydia** | Total | 149.7 | 200.9 | 244.8 | 298.7 |
| | Male | 87.8 | 131.9 | 166.0 | 212.0 |
| | Female | 210.1 | 268.4 | 321.7 | 383.5 |
| **Gonorrhea** | Total | 20.2 | 27.5 | 38.1 | 36.2 |
| | Male | 25.2 | 34.6 | 41.5 | 41.4 |
| | Female | 15.2 | 20.5 | 32.4 | 31.0 |
| **Syphilis** | Total | 1.8 | 5.6 | 8.9 | 8.9 |
| | Male | 2.2 | 9.0 | 13.1 | 14.9 |
| | Female | 1.5 | 2.2 | 4.8 | 2.8 |

Source: Public Health Agency of Canada (PHAC). (2014a). *Notifiable diseases on-line.* Retrieved from http://dsol-smed.phac-aspc.gc.ca/dsol-smed/ndis/index-eng.php

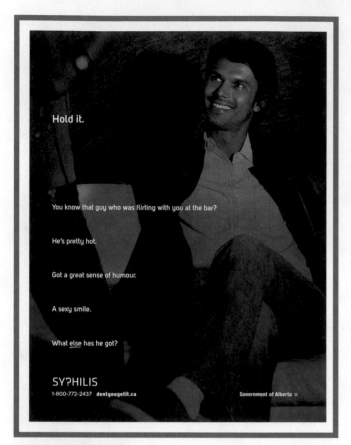

Hold it.

You know that guy who was flirting with you at the bar?

He's pretty hot.

Got a great sense of humour.

A sexy smile.

What _else_ has he got?

SY?HILIS
1-800-772-2437 dontyougetit.ca          Government of Alberta

**PHOTO  31.1**  The "Don't You Get It" Syphilis
Awareness Campaign

*Source: Courtesy of Alberta Health Services*

## Viral STIs

**Genital herpes** and **human papillomavirus (HPV)** are highly prevalent **viral STIs**. These viruses spread easily, are difficult to prevent and detect, and are non-reportable. Genital herpes and HPV are transmitted through vaginal, oral, and anal sexual intercourse, but mostly through intimate skin-to-skin sexual contact. Herpes can also be spread from mother to baby through childbirth and can cause serious complications such as abnormal development or death (PHAC, 2013–2014).

Genital herpes often appears as one or a group of painful, itchy, fluid-filled blisters in or around the genitals, buttocks, and/or thighs. People may experience burning during urination, fever, flu-like symptoms, and swollen glands. Some people experience only one outbreak of herpes; others may experience recurrent outbreaks. Recurrent outbreaks tend to be short lived and less severe than first outbreaks (PHAC, 2013–2014). It is important to note that of new genital herpes infections, 60% are asymptomatic (PHAC, 2013–2014).

Herpes is diagnosed through clinical examination or a culture of the fluid drawn from a sore (PHAC, 2013–2014). There are two types of herpes: type 1 (most commonly found as cold sores around the mouth) and type 2 (most commonly found on the genitals) (PHAC, 2013–2014). Both types 1 and 2 are found on the genitals or mouth due to oral sex. There is no cure for herpes; however, outbreaks can be managed through antiviral medication (PHAC, 2013–2014). The

incidence and prevalence of genital herpes is unknown, however the PHAC (2013–2014) reports that genital herpes is increasing worldwide. Condom use decreases genital herpes transmission by 50% (PHAC, 2013–2014).

Many people infected with HPV also have no symptoms. There are more than 130 strains of HPV with about 40 strains affecting the anogenital tract (PHAC, 2013–2014). Some HPV strains cause genital warts; other carcinogenic strains cause abnormal cell changes on the cervix. This may lead to cervical cancer if left untreated. Abnormal cervical changes as a result of HPV infection are detected through having Pap tests on a regular basis (PHAC, 2013–2014). Abnormal cervical changes may be monitored by repeat Pap tests, or through referral for colposcopy for more intensive diagnostic testing and treatment. Genital warts appear as groups of cauliflower-like growths in the genital area. Clinical examinations and special testing are used to visualize genital warts. Freezing, burning, or laser therapies are used to treat genital warts. HPV is also linked to oral, penile, and anal cancers (PHAC, 2013–2014). Because HPV is non-reportable, its incidence is unknown. However, the PHAC carries out studies to assess the prevalence of the virus and the incidence of HPV types associated with cancer. It is estimated that 70% of adults will experience at least one type of HPV infection in their lifetime. This viral infection usually clears up on its own within two years; however, for some people the virus persists (PHAC, 2013–2014).

## Ectoparasites

**Ectoparasites** include pubic lice (crabs) and scabies. Both can be transmitted through sexual or non-sexual (e.g., contact with infected towels or bed linens) contact. **Pubic lice** are most commonly found in genital and surrounding hair; however, they can also be found in chest, armpit, or facial hair (PHAC, 2013–2014). The adult louse lays eggs in the hair, and within 5 to 10 days they hatch. Symptoms of lice include itching and skin irritation.

**Scabies** are parasites that burrow under the skin, leaving red bumps that cause irritation and itchiness (PHAC, 2013–2014). Scabies can be found on any part of the body; however, they prefer warm, moist places such as the genital area. Both conditions, ectoparasites and scabies, are diagnosed through careful examination of infected areas and are treated with OTC (over-the-counter) products containing insecticides such as permethrin (PHAC, 2013–2014).

## Vaginal Infections

Vaginal infections are often called **vaginitis**. Vaginitis is the most common reason for gynecological visits. Depending on the etiology, they may or may not be classified as an STI. Vaginal infections are characterized by one or more of the following: vaginal discharge, rash, itching, irritation, and vaginal odour. The three most common vaginal infections include **trichomoniasis, bacterial vaginosis (BV)**, and **candidiasis** (yeast) (PHAC, 2013–2014). Treatment for the most common types of vaginitis differ according to the cause, therefore first-time sufferers should avoid self-diagnosis and seek medical assessment as diagnosis is based on laboratory testing.

Trichomoniasis is an STI caused by the protozoa *Trichomonas vaginalis*. Trichomoniasis symptoms include foamy yellow or green vaginal discharge that may be musty or foul smelling, itching or burning around the vagina, and pain with urination or sexual intercourse. The preferred treatment is the antibiotic metronidazole. Men usually do not have symptoms or may have mild discharge or pain with urination (PHAC, 2013–2014).

Bacterial vaginosis (BV) is the most common cause of vaginitis and is not usually sexually transmitted. BV is associated with a depletion of lactobacilli and an overgrowth of genital tract organisms. BV is associated with increased acquisition of HIV. BV symptoms include white or grey, thin vaginal discharge; fishy smelling vaginal discharge; and burning or itching around the vagina. The preferred treatment is the antibiotic metronidazole (PHAC, 2013–2014).

Candidiasis infections are commonly referred to as yeast infections. The majority of infections are caused by candida albicans and is not usually sexually transmitted. Antifungal medications are available over the counter (PHAC, 2013–2014).

## BLOOD-BORNE PATHOGENS

BBPs such as HIV, hepatitis B, and hepatitis C need special consideration as they are not solely transmitted by sexual activity. Transmission can also occur by reusing drug, tattooing, or piercing equipment that has residual traces of infected blood, and from mother to neonate during pregnancy or birth (PHAC, 2013–2014). Additionally, HIV can be transmitted through breast milk, and hepatitis B and hepatitis C can be transmitted by sharing razors or toothbrushes with an infected person (PHAC, 2013–2014).

## HIV/AIDS

Advances in HIV treatment and antiviral therapies have slowed the progression of HIV to a point where the disease is accepted to be a manageable, chronic condition (PHAC, 2013b). However, in 2011, 25% of people in Canada infected with HIV were unaware of their status (PHAC, 2013b). Undiagnosed cases of HIV are a public health concern and represent a missed opportunity to improve the prognosis for people living with HIV and reduce rates of transmission. It is estimated that up to 90% of those infected experience primary or acute HIV symptoms, which occur two to six weeks after infection (PHAC, 2013–2014). Symptoms are generally mild and may include sore throat, fatigue, fever, headache, rash, nausea, diarrhea, and vomiting (PHAC, 2013–2014). The chronic symptomatic phase occurs when the HIV weakens the immune system and the body exhibits long-term symptoms such as swollen lymph nodes, skin lesions, fever, and diarrhea. AIDS is diagnosed when a person with HIV experiences one or more AIDS-defining illnesses including opportunistic infections (e.g., recurrent bacterial pneumonia, fungal infections), or malignancies (e.g., lymphomas, Kaposi's Sarcoma), or neurological diseases (e.g., AIDS dementia) (PHAC, 2013–2014).

HIV is diagnosed through a blood test. In Canada, testing first became available in 1985 (PHAC, 2012a). There is a period of time, or window, after acquisition of HIV infection when the person is highly infectious but antibody tests are negative. This window period has changed as screening tests have improved. Testing is recommended at baseline, three weeks, and three months after exposure (PHAC, 2013b). It is now recommended that HIV testing be made a component of routine medical care, whenever a person requests one, has symptoms of HIV infection or weakened immune system, is pregnant or planning to be pregnant, or is the victim of sexual assault (PHAC, 2013b). Pre- and post-test counselling by CHNs is important because they can engage clients, prepare them for the potential impact of test results, and raise awareness of risk-reduction practices such as condom use. The minimum requirement for HIV testing is informed verbal consent and an understanding of the testing procedures and results (PHAC, 2013b).

In 2012, there were 2062 positive HIV tests reported in Canada, for a national rate of 5.9 per 100 000 persons (PHAC, 2013c). According to PHAC (2013c), this is the lowest rate reported to date. From 1985 to 2012, there were 76 275 positive HIV tests reported in Canada (PHAC, 2013c). In 2012, 50.3% of all positive adult HIV tests were identified as exposure through the men who have sex with men (MSM) population, 32.6% were identified as exposure through heterosexual contact, and 14.0% were identified as exposure through injection drug use (PHAC, 2013c).

## Hepatitis B

Many people who are infected with hepatitis B do not know it because they are asymptomatic. Approximately 50% of adults infected with hepatitis B will show non-specific symptoms, including fatigue, nausea, vomiting, jaundice (yellowing of the skin or whites of the eyes), decreased appetite, and joint swelling or pain (PHAC, 2013d). Most people infected with hepatitis B recover; however, some people become chronic carriers. Most carriers have no symptoms but can infect others. Carriers may eventually develop liver cancer or cirrhosis (PHAC, 2013d). Hepatitis B is diagnosed through blood testing. Combination antiviral drugs are available for those with chronic active hepatitis B (PHAC, 2013–2014).

It is estimated that fewer than 5% of Canadians show signs of past hepatitis B infection, and fewer than 1% are carriers of hepatitis B (PHAC, 2013d). Certain sub-populations tend to be at greater risk for the virus, including those who were born in endemic areas, men who have sex with men, sex-trade workers, and injection drug users (PHAC, 2013d). The widespread availability of hepatitis B vaccine has assisted in prevention of the infection. Publicly funded vaccination programs are offered in all Canadian provinces and territories. Hepatitis B vaccine is routinely offered to all Canadian children and adolescents. If parents are hepatitis B carriers or they were born in endemic areas, the vaccination is offered to children during the first year of life (PHAC, 2013d). From 2002 to 2009, the rate of hepatitis B increased from 1.8 to 10.5 per 100 000 persons. From 2009 to 2012, the rate declined from 10.5 to 9.4 (PHAC, 2014a).

## Hepatitis C

Hepatitis C (HCV) is a chronic liver disease caused by the hepatitis C virus. The majority of HCV cases in Canada are among people who inject drugs, accounting for 61% of new infections. Sexual transmission of HCV is uncommon in the general population; however, HCV is recognized as a growing public health concern among HIV-infected individuals. Co-infection with HIV and other STIs increase the risk of HCV transmission (PHAC, 2012b). From 2000 to 2011, the HCV rate declined from 57.8 to 28.9 per 100 000 persons (PHAC, 2014a). In 2012, there were 10 180 newly reported cases of HCV in Canada for a rate of 29.3 per 100 000 persons in 2012 (PHAC, 2014a).

## COMMUNITY HEALTH NURSING IMPLICATIONS OF STI AND BBP

All STIs and BBPs are under reported as many Canadians do not go for testing or do not know that they are infected (PHAC, 2013–2014). There are large numbers of people living with viral, non-reportable STIs such as herpes and HPV. Rates of reportable STIs and BBPs provide CHNs with some understanding regarding the scope of the problem. If STIs and BBPs remain inadequately addressed and treated, they can lead to ongoing spread of the infection, infertility, neonatal complications, pelvic inflammatory disease, or even death (PHAC, 2013–2014). STIs can negatively impact a person's relationships, self-esteem, mental health, coping abilities, and work productivity. Additionally, there are societal economic implications due to the medical costs associated with diagnosis and treatment (McKay, 2006), especially if there are complications such as infertility and neonatal infection.

CHNs must attempt to address not only medical issues such as testing and treatment, but also the social and economic issues. For example, CHNs can advocate for the development of support groups that can assist people to cope with their diagnosis of herpes or HIV while supporting them to pursue loving, sexual relationships with an understanding partner. Additionally, CHNs can raise awareness in the workplace and community to increase the funding for HIV medication, research, and alternative employment during times of intense treatment.

## STI AND BBP PREVENTION AND RISK AND HARM REDUCTION

Accurate and consistent use of **male condoms** or **female condoms** (see Photos 31.2a and 31.2b) is important to decrease the transmission of STIs (PHAC, 2013–2014). A male condom is a disposable latex or polyurethane sheath worn on the penis (Society of Obstetricians and Gynaecologists of Canada [SOGC], 2012). A female condom is a disposable polyurethane sheath placed inside the vagina (SOGC, 2012). (See Canadian Research Box 31.1.) Both male and female condoms prevent direct contact between the genitals, inhibiting the exchange of bodily fluids such as semen, pre-ejaculate fluid, and vaginal secretions. Condoms help to protect against pregnancy, STIs, and BBPs (SOGC, 2012).

It is important to note that condoms are not 100% effective in protecting against herpes or HPV (e.g., genital warts on the testicles or labia). Abstinence from all types of sexual activity (e.g., genital-to-genital contact) is the only 100% effective method of preventing these STIs. Between 2006 and 2015, Health Canada approved three HPV vaccines that will prevent between two and nine types of HPV infections. More information on HPV vaccine is discussed further in this chapter. Infection by BBPs, such as HIV, hepatitis B, and hepatitis C, are prevented by condom use and by using clean needles and equipment for tattooing, piercing, and injecting drugs. Condoms and dental dams (Photo 31.3) should always be used for oral sex (PHAC, 2013–2014). As mentioned previously, hepatitis B is also prevented through vaccination.

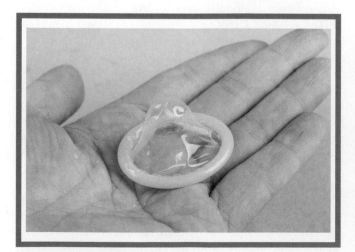

**PHOTO** **31.2a** Male Condom

*Source: Xuejun li/Fotolia*

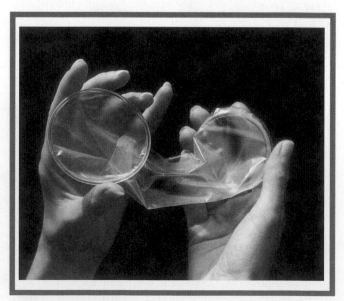

**PHOTO** **31.2b** Female Condom

*Source: Scott Camazine/Science Source*

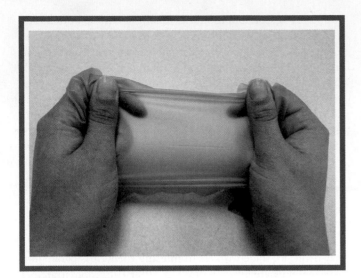

**PHOTO 31.3** Dental Dam

*Source: Courtesy of Tammy L Troute-Wood*

CHNs face challenges when attempting to promote and protect the sexual health of Canadians. **Safe sex fatigue** refers to an individual's apathy regarding hearing about and complying with safer-sex messages, resulting in risky behaviour (PHAC, 2013–2014). **Treatment optimism**, on the other hand, refers to not feeling too worried about contracting HIV because of the medications available to decrease HIV associated morbidity and mortality (Rowniak, 2009).

CHNs can consider interventions that include **sexual health education** and **harm reduction**. Sexual health education is defined as "the process of equipping individuals, couples, families, and communities with the information and motivation needed to enhance sexual health and avoid negative sexual health outcomes" (PHAC, 2008, p. 5). Harm reduction, on the other hand, can be defined as a strategy targeted at groups or individuals that endeavours to reduce the harms related to certain behaviours (CPS, 2008b). Examples of harm-reduction strategies include educating sex-trade workers about male and female condoms. Although these types of interventions are important, they must be timely and relevant to the target population in order to have an impact. It is vital to find innovative ways to promote the use of male and female condoms and dental dams. CHNs must "think upstream" and use health-promotion approaches that address the issues of their target population. CHNs can reach individuals through street outreach, counselling, and peer mentoring programs. Furthermore, CHNs can explore innovative ways to make these risk- and harm-reduction measures appealing to groups or communities through poster and social marketing campaigns. CHNs can work with other sectors and multidisciplinary groups to develop healthy public policy to address STI and BBP issues. Offering chlamydia urine testing in outreach vans and putting condom machines in schools are examples of health promotion activities resulting from healthy public policies.

---

### CANADIAN RESEARCH BOX 31.1

**What are the condom use behaviours among youth aged 15 to 24?**

Rotermann, M. (2012). Sexual behaviour and condom use of 15- to 24-year-olds in 2003 and 2009/2010. *Health Reports, 23*(1). Retrieved from Statistics Canada Catalogue no. 82-003-X.

The objective of the research was to investigate if sexual behaviours and condom utilization among youth aged 15 to 24 years changed from the years 2003 to 2009/2010. The researcher analyzed data from the Canadian Community Health Survey (CCHS), which consists of cross-sectional surveys conducted in 2003 and 2009/2010. The CCHS collects information from individuals aged 12 and over living in private residences. Data were collected either in person or over the phone. In this study, the researcher included respondents between the ages of 15 and 24. A total of 18 084 and 15 966 participants were included in 2003 and 2009/2010, respectively.

In terms of sexual behaviours, the findings revealed the following:

(a) In 2009/2010, 66% of youth aged 15–24 had sexual intercourse at least one time, which was not significantly different in 2003.

(b) In 2009/2010, 30% of teens aged 15–17, 68% of teens aged 18–19, and 86% of youth aged 20–24 had sexual intercourse at least one time, which was not significantly different in 2003.

(c) In 2009/2010, 32.5% of sexually active youth reported having sex with more than one partner, with males (39.0%) more likely to have multiple partners than females (25.4%), which was not significantly different in 2003.

With regards to condom use, the findings revealed the following:

(a) In 2009/2010, 67.9% of youth ages 15–24 used condoms during their last sexual intercourse compared to 62.2% in 2003, which was significantly different.

(b) In 2003 and 2009/2010, condom use decreased with age. For example, in 2009/2010, 79.9% of teens aged 15–17 used condoms during their last intercourse compared to 78.5% in 2003 (not significantly different). In 2009/2010, 73.7% of teens aged 18–19 used condoms during their last intercourse compared to 67.6% in 2003 (significantly different). Finally, 62.8% of youth aged 20–24 used condoms during their last intercourse compared to 56.4% in 2003 (significantly different).

(c) In 2009/2010, 72.5% of males and 62.5% of females aged 15–24 used condoms during their last intercourse compared to 67.3% of males and 56.5% of females in 2003 (significantly different).

**Discussion Questions**

1. What should a CHN consider when counselling youth with regard to condom use?
2. How can a CHN use the Internet to promote the use of condoms with youth?
3. What factors might inhibit the use of condoms?

# SPECIFIC POPULATIONS AT A HIGHER RISK FOR ACQUIRING STIs OR BBPs

Individuals who may be at a higher risk for acquiring an STI or BBP include but are not limited to people who are sexually active under the age of 25, report more than two new sexual partners in the past year, report the use of non-barrier methods of contraception, report unprotected anal or vaginal intercourse, report injection or other drug use, report anonymous sexual partnering, and are those who are victims of sexual abuse or assault (Government of Alberta, 2012). Specific at risk populations are discussed below.

## Men who have Sex with Men

The **men who have sex with men (MSM)** population in Canada has the highest proportion of HIV/AIDS when compared to other sub-populations (PHAC, 2013–2014, 2012a). A survey of Ontario self-identified gay and bisexual MSM determined that 35% to 40% of respondents had participated in unprotected anal intercourse within the last year, approximately 17% had unprotected anal intercourse with a partner whose HIV status was unknown, and 4% had unprotected anal intercourse with a partner who tested positive for HIV (Myers et al., 2004).

Although health education messages addressing condom use are constantly being reinforced, it is clear from this study that certain cohorts of MSM are still not being reached with current prevention strategies. It is important for CHNs to *work with* the MSM population to develop messaging that is accessible, innovative, and relevant. Additionally, it is important for CHNs to deliver messaging at venues frequented by the MSM population. For example, Myers et al. (2004) noted that MSM search for sexual relations in a number of different sites, including gay bars (60.3%), the Internet (35.3%), and bath houses (31.4%). These sites can therefore serve as venues for prevention messaging.

## Sex-Trade Workers

Sex-trade workers are at increased risk for contracting and spreading STIs and BBPs for several reasons. These reasons include having a high number of sexual partners; limited ability to access social, health, and legal services; lifestyle risks such as substance use; and limited economic resources (PHAC, 2013–2014). Condom use varies among sex-trade workers and the choice to use condoms may be controlled by the customer (Comack & Seshia, 2010). Customers often refuse to use condoms or offer additional money for "condomless" sex (HIV Prevention Research Team University of Ottawa, Provincial Women and HIV Group, & Ontario Women's Study Research Design Committee, 2007). Sexual violence is prevalent among sex-trade workers. In a study of Winnipeg sex-trade workers, 58% of "bad date reports" included some form of sexual violence (e.g., refusal to use a condom, unwanted touching, or sexual assault) (Comack & Seshia, 2010).

CHNs working with this group can promote a variety of risk-reduction strategies (e.g., correct use of male or female condoms) to prevent this population from acquiring or spreading STIs and BBPs. Since access to and the cost of condoms may deter sex-trade workers from using them, it is paramount that condoms are available for free. Peer education strategies have proven promising in terms of increasing knowledge related to STIs and HIV and safer sex practices (PHAC, 2013–2014; Rekart, 2005). CHNs can work with sex-trade workers to educate their peers regarding risk-reduction strategies such as condom negotiation. Overall, it is important that the services developed for sex-trade workers (e.g., peer education, hepatitis B vaccinations, STI testing and treatment) are delivered innovatively (e.g., from a mobile van, hotel room, community centre) and with the workers' input (PHAC, 2013–2014; Rekart, 2005).

## Street-Involved Youth

It is estimated that approximately 150000 youth in Canada live on the streets on any given day (PHAC, 2006a). This population is extremely vulnerable because, for many, addressing the basic necessities of life is of greater priority than preventing or addressing potential health risks (PHAC, 2006b). As a result, youth involved in street culture often do not take effective action in preventing STIs and BBPs (PHAC, 2006b).

In an Ottawa study, street youth aged 15 to 24 reported inconsistent use of condoms. For example, approximately 50% of street youth reported use of condoms during their last vaginal or anal sexual encounter, and 15% stated they used condoms for their last oral sexual encounter (Ottawa Public Health, 2011). Other factors that impact STIs and BBPs in street youth is their use of drugs. In 2009, 93% of Ottawa street youth reported use of non-injection drugs and 19% reported use of injection drugs (Ottawa Public Health, 2011).

STIs and BBPs are higher among street youth in comparison to mainstream youth. In the Ottawa study, 8.8% of youth were infected with chlamydia and 0.59% were infected with gonorrhea. Among non-injection drug users, 5% were infected with hepatitis C and 2% were infected with HIV. Among youth who used injection drugs, 24% were infected with hepatitis C and 4% were infected with HIV (Ottawa Public Health, 2011). Resources must be allocated for both sufficient outreach with this population and comprehensive programming that entails prevention, screening, and treatment services (PHAC, 2006b).

## Injection Drug Users

Injection drug users represent a growing concern for CHNs, as the craving for "another hit" overrides the importance of using a clean needle to prevent the transmission of HIV, hepatitis B, or hepatitis C. Offering better access to condoms and clean needles or drug equipment via needle exchange programs and safer injection facilities may help these populations lower their risk of contracting HIV while they search for effective treatment (PHAC, 2013–2014). Needle exchange programs and safer injection facilities are discussed later in this chapter.

## New Immigrants

In 2013, nearly 259 000 immigrants became permanent Canadian residents (Government of Canada, 2014). Citizenship and Immigration Canada (CIC) requires syphilis and HIV testing for immigrants and refugees over the age of 15 seeking Canadian citizenship. HIV testing is also required for children born to a mother infected with HIV, those with blood or blood product exposure, or those who may be an international adoptee (PHAC, 2013–2014). Presently, syphilis and HIV testing are the only compulsory STI tests for immigrants and refugees applying to become citizens (PHAC, 2013–2014). According to the Immigration and Refugee Protection Act (Minister of Justice, 2014), immigrants are inadmissible to Canada if they have conditions or illnesses that pose a danger to Canadians or are very expensive to treat in Canada.

Language, cultural, socioeconomic, and educational barriers may deter certain immigrant sub-populations from seeking health services (PHAC, 2013–2014). New immigrants are overwhelmed with adapting to new cultural and healthcare practices. Many come from countries where HIV, hepatitis, and other STIs are more prevalent and treatment is inaccessible (PHAC, 2013–2014). Cultural beliefs may also influence a person's motivation to access health services. Some may try a variety of herbs or culturally accepted medications before seeking medical treatment for an STI or HIV. Many Canadian provinces lack services and resources that are translated, culturally safe, and accessible to newcomers. It is important that CHNs be attentive to the stressful and complex issues faced by immigrants as they integrate into Canadian culture (PHAC, 2013–2014).

## Unwilling or Unable Population

Researchers have identified that some HIV-positive individuals are recalcitrant or "unwilling or unable" (e.g., refuse to disclose HIV-positive status to sexual partners) to prevent the spread of HIV (Government of Alberta, 2011). The research has determined that these individuals often present with one or more of the following issues: psychiatric issues (e.g., depression, fetal alcohol spectrum disorder), addictions, social deficits (e.g., lack of support and housing, involvement in the sex-trade), and health deficits (e.g., lack of HIV knowledge) (Calgary Coalition on HIV/AIDS, 2004). Researchers believe

these variables contribute to higher-risk activities (e.g., having sex without a condom) and can impede a person's efficacy at implementing risk- or harm-reduction practices. Health regions across Canada are addressing this issue in different ways, ranging from implementing comprehensive referral systems to providing housing and treatment.

## Inmates in Correctional Facilities

Inmates in Canada's correctional facilities have disproportionately high rates of STIs and BBPs including HIV, hepatitis B, and hepatitis C (PHAC, 2013e). People in corrections facilities may be from populations participating in high-risk behaviours such as injection drug use, other substance abuse, and unprotected sex. Also, those inmates who have consensual or non-consensual sexual contact, or participate in practices such as injection drug use or tattooing or piercing while incarcerated, are at risk for becoming infected and contributing to disease transmission (PHAC, 2013–2014). At the end of 2008, in Canadian federal penitentiaries, 1.7% of the population were known to be living with HIV, and 30.2% were known to be infected with hepatitis C (PHAC, 2012c). However, lack of routine screening for STIs and BBPs are likely to result in underestimates of the actual infection rates (PHAC, 2013–2014).

The time of incarceration represents a public health opportunity. Upon admission and during the period of incarceration, Correctional Services Canada (CSC) offers voluntary infectious disease testing, pre- and post-test counselling, treatment, and access to medical specialists. STI prevention programs offering education, voluntary testing and counselling, drug-dependence treatment, and harm-reduction strategies (distribution of condoms and clean needles) have been proven to reduce STI/HIV risk in prisons (PHAC, 2013–2014). Since most inmates return to the community, CHNs are positioned to coordinate STI prevention and discharge strategies to support healthy transition back to public life.

## Aboriginal People

It is estimated that 4.3% of the Canadian population self-identify as an Aboriginal person (Statistics Canada, 2011). Aboriginal is a broad term that comprises First Nations, Inuit, and Métis people. Despite the small population size, Aboriginal people have disproportionately high rates of HIV/AIDS and STIs compared to non-Aboriginal people in Canada (PHAC, 2010).

From 1998 to 2008, reports that included ethnicity data indicate that Aboriginal people represented 24.0% of all new HIV test reports and 8% of all Canadian persons living with HIV. In addition, Aboriginal persons who are diagnosed with HIV infection are younger than infected non-Aboriginal people. As reported from 1998 to 2006, 32.4% of Aboriginal persons diagnosed with HIV were less than 30 years old, compared to 21.0% of non-Aboriginal persons. During this timeframe, injection drug use (IDU) was the main HIV exposure risk for Aboriginal people, with 53% of new infections due to IDU compared to 14% of new infections for non-Aboriginal person where IDU was identified as the main exposure risk. IDU is also the main exposure risk for hepatitis C. Rates of acute HCV infection from 2004 to 2008 were reported as 5.5 times higher in Aboriginal people than in non-Aboriginal people (PHAC, 2010).

Although ethnicity data is not reported for the majority of STI cases, in 2006, in the four jurisdictions that report ethnicity data, Aboriginal people accounted for 15.0% of reported genital chlamydia cases, 27.4% of reported gonorrhea cases, and 19.7% of reported infectious syphilis cases (PHAC, 2010).

With any of the specific populations we have discussed, it is important for CHNs to forge new partnerships with the agencies these populations access. For example, to promote the health of new immigrants, CHNs can partner with cultural organizations, public health centres, community groups, or religious centres. For street-involved youth, CHNs can collaborate with sexual and reproductive health centres, mental health services, social services, detox or drug treatment programs, and community groups. Moreover, it is important to actively involve clients in the development, dissemination, and evaluation of promotion and prevention programs.

## INNOVATIVE STI AND BBP PREVENTION INTERVENTIONS IN CANADA

The population health promotion model (Hamilton & Bhatti, 1996) provides a comprehensive tool for CHNs to utilize when planning STI and BBP prevention interventions with individuals, families, communities, and populations. (Please refer to Chapter 8 for more information on the population health promotion model.) Novel and innovative strategies are being implemented across Canada in an attempt to lower the prevalence of STIs and BBPs.

## Needle Exchange Programs and Safer Injection Facilities

IDU is a mounting public health concern in Canada. Individuals who participate in high-risk drug injection behaviours (e.g., sharing needles) pose a number of potential health risks to themselves and others, such as transmission of HIV/AIDS and hepatitis B and C (PHAC, 2013–2014). Some Canadian communities have addressed the issue of needle sharing with harm-reduction strategies such as needle-exchange programs and safer injection facilities. The harm-reduction model acknowledges that abstinence from all drugs is not realistic for all people and, therefore, although drug use is not condoned, it is seen as essential to implement risk-reduction strategies to reduce harmful outcomes related to drug use (Elliott, Malkin, & Gold, 2002).

**Needle exchange programs (NEPs)**, also called needle and syringe programs (NSPs), provide injection drug users with free, sterile injecting equipment to reduce their risk of

contracting and spreading infection (Elliott et al., 2002). This harm-reduction strategy is endorsed by the World Health Organization as well as health authorities across Canada. However, NEPs are considered controversial among policy makers and the general public. Although research supports that NEPs decrease HIV among injection drug users (IDUs), there are concerns that they may "enable or encourage injection drug use, prolong the injection drug use of their clients, and/or discourage clients from seeking addiction treatment" (Werb et al., 2013, p. 535). Werb and colleagues (2013) investigated NEPs in Vancouver from 1996 until 2010. During that time, the number of NEPs increased from 1 to 29. Their research suggests that as the number of NEPs increased, the proportion of injection drug users reporting cessation increased as well.

**Safer injection facilities (SIFs)** provide a safe location for drug users to inject their own drugs with clean equipment under the supervision of medically trained professionals (Small et al., 2011). SIFs aim to decrease the spread of infectious disease, improve contact between the healthcare system and injection drug users, decrease the use of drugs in public places, decrease fatal and non-fatal drug overdoses, and increase enrolment of injection drug users into addiction treatment and rehabilitation programs (Small et al., 2011; Wood et al., 2004a). Although SIFs are an innovative public health intervention, they are extremely controversial in various countries, including Canada.

In 2003, healthcare providers in Vancouver piloted the first medically supervised SIF in North America (Kerr, Tyndall, Montaner, & Wood, 2005). Evaluation research of this

---

### CASE STUDY

During the last two decades, Canada's population of Aboriginal people living in urban centres has dramatically increased. In the fictitious community called WinnCity, the urban Aboriginal population represents nearly 10% of the city population. Aboriginal families living in this city tend to be young families and may be at risk for unstable housing, with some families moving residences yearly or more often. The CHNs understand through a review of the literature, talking with community advocates, and by examining local communicable disease surveillance data that within WinnCity Aboriginal people have low rates of accessing sexual and reproductive healthcare and even lower rates of screening for HIV and STIs. The CHNs want to improve the accessibility to sexual and reproductive healthcare, including HIV and STI testing and treatment for Aboriginal youth living in WinnCity.

#### Discussion Questions

1. What determinants of health will the CHNs need to be aware of when planning youth services?

2. Discuss the importance of performing a community assessment.

3. What health-promotion strategies can the CHNs implement to improve accessibility?

program indicated several positive outcomes, including decreased syringe sharing (Kerr et al., 2005), decreased injection-related litter, decreased numbers of individuals injecting in public, and decreased numbers of syringes discarded in public (Wood et al., 2004b).

## SOCIAL MARKETING CAMPAIGNS

**Social marketing** can be defined as "a program-planning process that applies commercial marketing concepts and techniques to promote voluntary behavior change" (Grier & Bryant, 2005, p. 319). In Canada, these types of campaigns are becoming more innovative as they provide blatant and, at times, provocative messages to different segments of the population. Unfortunately, many of these campaigns are not properly evaluated for their short- or long-term impact on the target population. Please refer to Chapter 8 for an in-depth discussion of social marketing.

One Alberta STI campaign that had evaluated results was launched by Alberta Heath Services from mid-September through mid-November 2013. The purpose of the "Sex Germs" campaign was to raise awareness and provide information about STIs and BBPs, and encourage safer sexual practices among 16- to 29-year-olds. The campaign was an extension of the previous 2011 Alberta Syphilis awareness campaigns

"Don't You Get It" and "Plenty of Syph," but was expanded to include STIs and BBPs in response to continued high infection rates in Alberta (Howard Research & Management Consulting Inc., 2014).

A variety of English-only campaign materials (e.g., posters; bar coasters; matchbook condom covers; bar stamps; washroom video boards; and television, radio, and cinema pre-roll ads), social media tools (e.g., Twitter and Facebook), and guerrilla tactics (penis mascot in bars and on the street) captured attention and directed viewers to the www.sexgerms .com website. Campaign images featured attractive individuals displaying graphic flu-like symptoms (e.g., runny nose, red eyes) with the slogan "A cold isn't the only thing you could catch." A second group of posters displayed made-up words combining sexual body parts and disease suffixes such as "vagfluenza" and "dickgitis." (See Photos 31.4a and 31.4b.) The images and words were meant to capitalize on public awareness about flu and other germs and the need for good hygiene, creating a parallel to awareness about STI and the need for safer sexual practices. The primary messaging focused on behaviour change to safer sexual practices with the website providing secondary messages and resources for getting tested.

The campaign was evaluated using online surveys. A total of 1152 persons completed the survey. Over three-quarters of the survey participants reportedly had seen or heard at least

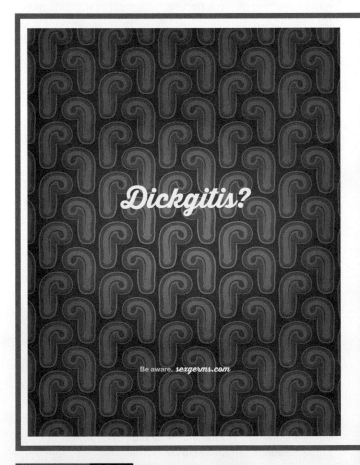

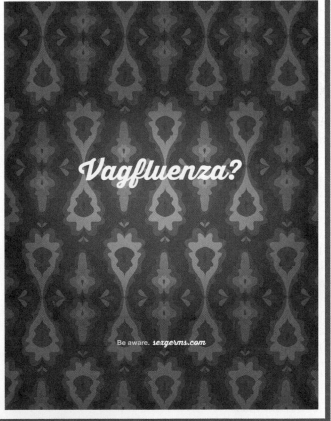

**PHOTO** **31.4a** The "Sex Germs" Campaign

*Source: Courtesy of Alberta Health Services*

**PHOTO** **31.4b** The "Sex Germs" Campaign

*Source: Courtesy of Alberta Health Services*

one component of the campaign (Howard Research & Management Consulting Inc., 2014). Overall, 55% of the respondents reported that seeing or hearing the campaign or visiting the sexgerms.com website made them wonder "a little" or "a lot" if they might be at risk for having an STI. Of the respondents who had seen or heard at least one component of the campaign or visited the website, 73% reported that the information made them think they ought to practise safer sex, 64% indicated that they expected to use safer sexual practices in the future, and 41% reported they had already practised safer sex.

## Capacity Building

As discussed in Chapters 7 and 8, **capacity building** is a process that increases the ability of an individual, a community, or an organization to promote health. CHNs "build individual and community capacity by actively involving and collaborating with individuals, families, groups, organizations, populations, communities, and systems. The focus is to build on strengths and increase skills, knowledge, and willingness to take action in the present and in the future" (Community Health Nurses of Canada, 2011, revised, p. 18).

In one Canadian study, face-to-face and online training programs were used as a means for capacity building of service providers (Lokanc-Diluzio, 2014). As identified in this chapter, street youth are at risk for STIs and BBPs. Service providers (e.g., CHNs, social workers, youth workers, and teachers) working with street youth represent a valuable resource for sexual health protection and promotion. Although service providers are well positioned to make a difference in the sexual health outcomes of street youth, their lack of knowledge and comfort may impede their ability to do so. The study explored the effectiveness of face-to-face and online training programs for building the capacity of service providers to protect and promote the sexual health of street youth. Knowledge related to several topics (including STIs, BBPs, and condoms) was measured three times (prior to the training programs, immediately after the training programs, and six weeks after the training programs). Participants in both training programs experienced significant increases in knowledge immediately after the training programs and six weeks later. Self-reported comfort discussing sexual-health topics such as STIs, HIV, male condoms, and female condoms were also measured three times. The face-to-face participants experienced a significant increase in comfort addressing those topics immediately after the training; however, the comfort was not sustained at six weeks later. The online participants, on the other hand, experienced significant increases in comfort addressing those topics immediately after the training program and six weeks later.

## Telehealth

**Telehealth** has become important in terms of health education and prevention of STIs and BBPs as well as support for those living with HIV or AIDS (Kalichman et al., 2003;

Shoveller et al., 2012; White & Dorman, 2001). Telehealth is "the use of information and communication technology to deliver health services, expertise, and information over distance" (Health Telematics Unit, University of Calgary as cited in Canadian Nurses Association, 2007). Telephone, email, and the Internet are means of providing telehealth services to those seeking information about STIs and BBPs (Canadian Nurses Association, 2007; Shoveller et al., 2012). Individuals may experience increased comfort utilizing these vehicles as ways of communicating, especially if their questions or concerns are personal or sensitive in nature (Care, Gregory, Whittaker, & Chernomas, 2003). (See Canadian Research Box 31.2.)

---

### CANADIAN RESEARCH BOX 31.2

**What are youth's perspectives regarding online sexual health services?**

Shoveller, J., Knight, R., Davis, W., Gilbert, M., & Ogilvie, G. (2012). Online sexual health services: Examining youth's perspectives. *Canadian Journal of Public Health, 103*(1), 14–18.

STIs, particularly in youth ages 15–24, are a growing public health concern in Canada. Contemporary interventions are utilizing technology, such as the Internet, to reach populations most at risk. The purpose of this qualitative study was to examine youth's perspectives regarding online sexual health services.

Fifty-two (38 male, 14 female) Metro Vancouver youth aged 15–24 participated in in-depth semi-structured interviews, approximately 60–90 minutes in length. The researchers employed a purposive sampling plan in order to recruit youth with diverse sexual identities and from diverse cultural and socioeconomic backgrounds.

Participants were asked to provide their opinion regarding (1) online STI/HIV testing (e.g., downloading a lab requisition form specifying a specimen collection protocol) and risk assessment (e.g., a sexual history questionnaire); and (2) online education and counselling services (e.g., email with a nurse, live chat with a nurse, moderated forums).

**1.** Online STI/HIV testing and risk assessment

Most of the participants indicated that online testing and risk assessment provides (a) the convenience of circumventing clinic visits, particularly for routine or asymptomatic testing; (b) the ability to attain testing options privately and instantly, particularly for urgent testing needs (e.g., those presenting with symptoms); and (c) an alternative to an in-person clinical appointment, enhancing privacy and reducing anxiety. However, a small number of participants, who routinely accessed clinic testing, were not certain that online risk assessment could be as effective as risk assessment within an in-person setting. In person, the clinician has the ability to read body language and probe. Additionally, "despite online services' general appeal, in order to realize their full potential (and therefore attain/retain saliency and credibility), online services must fully 'harness' online technological capabilities" (p. 16). For example, it is inconvenient to print downloadable requisition forms.

**2.** Online counselling and education

Most participants viewed the ability to ask questions to clinicians online as positive. They deemed nurses as valuable and trusted resources. Many participants had positive feelings regarding live, one-to-one online discussions with a nurse. Online discussions provided the benefit of obtaining answers fast and in an anonymous manner. The discussion format provided the opportunity for clarification if needed. Participants were less positive toward communicating with a nurse via email because it was perceived that email lacks expediency. Participants had mixed views regarding a clinician-moderated online forum. Although participants might read a forum, they were less likely to post questions.

### Discussion Questions

1. What are the advantages of any online health service?
2. What are the disadvantages of any online health service?
3. What should a CHN consider when designing an online sexual health service?

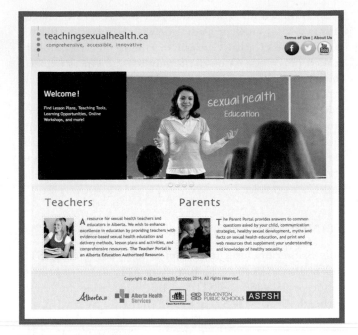

**PHOTO 31.5** Website that promotes sexual health

*Source: Courtesy of Alberta Health Services*

Although telehealth is promising for sexual health promotion, CHNs need to acknowledge its downfalls. First, it is important for CHNs to consider the legal implications associated with potential misdiagnoses when offering services online (Care et al., 2003). Second, this technology may be inaccessible to those who cannot afford computers. Finally, when communication is conducted electronically, the contextualization of the client's situation may be lost.

Internet sites can also be used to disseminate information on STI and BBP signs and symptoms, prevention, treatment, and referral. For example, www.teachingsexualhealth.ca (see Photo 31.5) was developed to provide accurate, relevant, and timely resources for Alberta-based sexual health educators, parents, and students. As a provincial Alberta Education (Ministry of Education) approved learning resource, coordinated by Alberta Health Services, the Internet resource provides educators with teaching strategies while considering diversity issues such as ethnicity, differing abilities, and gender in the learning setting.

## Human Papillomavirus (HPV) Vaccination

In 2006, Health Canada approved a vaccine (**Gardasil**) that protects against four strains of HPV (National Advisory Council on Immunization, 2012). According to the National Advisory Council on Immunization (NACI), two of the strains are responsible for approximately 70% of cervical cancer cases (HPV 16 and 18), whereas the other two strains are responsible for around 90% of genital warts

cases (HPV 6 and 11) (NACI, 2012; Shier & Bryson, 2007). In 2010, a second HPV vaccine, **Cervarix**, was approved by Health Canada (GlaxoSmithKline, 2010; NACI, 2012). Cervarix was designed to protect against two strains of HPV (HPV 16 and 18) causing cervical cancer. It also provides some protection from two additional strains (HPV 45 and 31). Together, the four strains account for 80% of cervical cancer cases (GlaxoSmithKline, 2014). Although Cervarix does not protect against genital warts, it may offer longer-term protection against HPV causing cervical cancer (GlaxoSmithKline, 2010). In 2015, a third vaccine, Gardasil 9 was approved by Health Canada. Gardasil 9 protects against nine HPV strains (HPV 6, 11, 16, 18, 31, 33, 45, 52, and 58). These nine strains cause around 80% of cervical pre-cancers, 90% of cervical cancers, 75% of HPV related anal, vulvar, and vaginal pre-cancers and cancers, and more than 90% of genital warts (SOGC, n.d.). HPV vaccination is considered a medical milestone in terms of cancer prevention. It is anticipated that the long-term implications of the vaccine will result in a reduction of cervical cancer cases, although the need for women to have regular Pap tests will continue (Shier & Bryson, 2007). The NACI (2007, 2012) released statements on HPV immunizations in 2007 and 2012 to inform Canadian healthcare providers regarding appropriate use of HPV vaccine. The Society of Obstetricians and Gynaecologists of Canada (n.d.) has developed a website (www.hpvinfo.ca) to provide up-to-date HPV information to teens, adults, parents, teachers, and health professionals.

Gardasil and Gardasil 9 HPV vaccines are available for females ages 9–45 and males ages 9–26 (NACI, 2012). Cervarix HPV vaccine is available for females ages 9–45 (GlaxoSmithKline, 2014). Currently, all Canadian provinces have publicly funded vaccination strategies in place for school-aged girls in Grades 5 to 9, depending on where they reside (PHAC, 2014b). The original Gardasil vaccine is used for publicly funded programs. As of 2014, only two provinces (Alberta and Prince Edward Island) have also implemented publicly funded vaccination programs for boys (PHAC, 2014b). For females and males who do not qualify for the publicly funded programs but are within the recommended age group, the vaccination is available for a cost for the three doses. Women older than 45 and men older than 26 who are interested in HPV vaccination should be encouraged to speak to their healthcare provider.

## CONCLUSION

This chapter discusses the complex issues surrounding STIs and BBPs in Canada. The history of STIs and how healthy public policy addresses STI and BBP prevention are briefly outlined. A review of STI and BBP statistical trends and epidemiology are presented. The needs of specific populations who may present unique challenges to CHNs related to STIs and BBPs are illustrated. Finally, suggestions on how CHNs can use the PHP model to plan innovative prevention strategies are made.

## KEY TERMS

acquired immune deficiency syndrome (AIDS)   p. 562
bacterial STIs   p. 562
bacterial vaginosis (BV)   p. 564
blood-borne pathogens (BBPs)   p. 561
candidiasis   p. 564
capacity building   p. 572
Cervarix   p. 573
chlamydia   p. 562
ectoparasites   p. 564
female condoms   p. 566
Gardasil   p. 573
genital herpes   p. 564
gonorrhea   p. 562
harm reduction   p. 567
human immunodeficiency virus (HIV)   p. 562
human papillomavirus (HPV)   p. 564
male condoms   p. 566
men who have sex with men (MSM)   p. 568
needle exchange programs (NEPs)   p. 571
pubic lice   p. 564
safe sex fatigue   p. 567
safer injection facilities (SIFs)   p. 571
scabies   p. 564
sexual health education   p. 567
sexually transmitted infections (STIs)   p. 561
social marketing   p. 571
syphilis   p. 563
telehealth   p. 573
treatment optimism   p. 567
trichomoniasis   p. 564
vaginitis   p. 564

venereal disease   p. 562
vertical transmission   p. 562
viral STIs   p. 564

## STUDY QUESTIONS

1. When developing an information sheet on STIs, what are the three most common bacterial STIs and their symptoms that a CHN would need to include?

2. What three key messages about HIV transmission would a CHN want to include in a community presentation on "Protecting Your Children from HIV"?

3. When working in a community sexual health clinic, what are three main points plus supporting evidence that a CHN could integrate into client counselling guidelines to potentially reduce the transmission of STIs and BBPs?

4. What measures can a CHN ensure are in place within primary health services to prevent the consequences of congenital syphilis?

5. How would a CHN describe safer injection facilities when planning a community harm-reduction strategy?

6. When writing an Internet article on HPV vaccine, how would a CHN answer the question "What is Cervarix?"

After working through these questions, go to the MyNursingLab at www.pearsoned.ca/mynursinglab to check your answers.

## INDIVIDUAL CRITICAL-THINKING EXERCISES

1. Go to www.teachingsexualhealth.ca and complete the your values exercise (http://teachers.teachingsexualhealth.ca/teaching-tools/your-values). What did you learn from completing the exercise? How do personal values impact sexual health education provided by CHNs?

2. STI rates are increasing in males 15–24 years old. The Public Health Agency of Canada states that testing and education are important to prevent STIs. Unfortunately, many youth at risk for STIs leave school early and become street involved, thus missing the benefit of sexual health education opportunities. What determinants of health could be addressed by CHNs related to the issues of street youth and STIs?

3. Search the Internet and find one STI prevention resource that can be used with teens. How can CHNs use this resource in a teen clinic?

4. The recommendation to vaccinate elementary school girls against HPV has caused controversy in Canada. What can CHNs say to parents who are uncertain of whether or not to have their daughters vaccinated?

5. Women involved in the sex trade participate in high-risk sexual behaviours (e.g., sex without a condom, sex with

multiple partners), placing them at risk for STIs and HIV. How can CHNs protect and promote the sexual health of this population?

## GROUP CRITICAL-THINKING EXERCISES

1. Gay youth often face rejection from significant support systems such as family and friends when they "come out." Some youth quit school and leave home to live on the street. Some rely on panhandling and prostitution to support themselves or to pay for drugs that help them cope. High-risk activities and a lack of resources increase gay youths' risk for STIs and HIV. How can a CHN use the Canadian Community Health Nursing Standards of Practice (CCHNSP) to plan care for gay youth within a sexual health clinic?

2. To address the complications associated with STIs and HIV, healthy public policy has been initiated and developed by policymakers and health professionals, but often with little input from the public. How can CHNs use primary health care's principle of public participation to inform the development of healthy public policy related to STIs and HIV?

3. Social marketing campaigns can be effective in raising awareness about public health issues, such as STIs and HIV.

   a) Create an idea for a social marketing campaign addressing STIs and/or HIV.

   b) What is the objective(s) of the campaign?

   c) What is the message of the campaign?

   d) How will the message be delivered?

## REFERENCES

Alberta Health Services & ProvLab Alberta. (2012). *Laboratory bulletin: Discontinuation of second trimester syphilis screening on pregnant women.* Retrieved from http://www.provlab.ab.ca/partner_updates.htm

Calgary Coalition on HIV/AIDS. (2004). *Phase two: Guidelines for working with U2 clients.* Calgary, AB: Author.

Canadian Nurses Association. (2007). *Telehealth: The role of the nurse.* Ottawa, ON: Author.

Canadian Paediatric Society. (2008a). *Position statement: Recommendations for the prevention of neonatal ophthalmia.* Retrieved from http://www.cps.ca/english/statements/ID/ID02-03.htm

Canadian Paediatric Society. (2008b). Harm reduction: An approach to reducing risky health behaviours in adolescents. *Paediatric Child Health, 13*(1), 53–56.

Care, W. D., Gregory, D., Whittaker, C., & Chernomas, W. (2003). Nursing, technology, and informatics: An easy or uneasy alliance? In M. McIntyre & E. Thomlinson (Eds.), *Realities of Canadian nursing: Professional, practice and power issues* (pp. 243–261). Philadelphia, PA: Lippincott Williams & Wilkins.

Comack, E., & Seshia, M. (2010). Bad dates and street hassles: Violence in the Winnipeg street sex trade. *Canadian Journal of Criminology and Criminal Justice,* 203–214.

Community Health Nurses of Canada. (2011). *Canadian community health nursing: Professional practice model & standards of practice – Revised March 2011.* St. John's, NL: Author. Reprinted with permission. Further reproduction prohibited. Retrieved from https://www.chnc.ca/documents/CHNC-ProfessionalPracticeModel-EN/index.html

Elliott, R., Malkin, I., & Gold, J. (2002). *Establishing safe injection facilities in Canada: Legal and ethical issues.* Ottawa, ON: Canadian HIV/AIDS Legal Network.

GlaxoSmithKline. (2010). *Health Canada approves Cervarix, new GSK cervical cancer vaccine.* Retrieved from http://www.gsk.ca/english/docs-pdf/FINAL_Press_Release_Cervarix_EN.pdf

GlaxoSmithKine. (2014). *Product monograph: Cervarix.* Retrieved from http://www.gsk.ca/english/docs-pdf/product-monographs/Cervarix.pdf

Grier, S., & Bryant, C. A. (2005). Social marketing in public health. *Annual Review of Public Health, 26,* 319–339. Published by Annual Reviews, Inc.

Government of Alberta. (2010). *The syphilis outbreak in Alberta.* Retrieved from http://www.health.alberta.ca/documents/STI-Syphilis-Report-2010.pdf

Government of Alberta. (2011). *Alberta health and wellness public health notifiable disease management guidelines: Acquired immunodeficiency syndrome (AIDS).* Retrieved from http://www.health.alberta.ca/documents/Guidelines-Acquired-Immunodeficiency-Syndrome-2011.pdf

Government of Alberta. (2012). *Alberta treatment guidelines for sexually transmitted infections (STI) in adolescents and adults.* Retrieved from http://www.health.alberta.ca/documents/STI-Treatment-Guidelines-2012.pdf

Government of Alberta. (2014). *Health and wellness interactive health data application.* Retrieved from http://www.ahw.gov.ab.ca/IHDA_Retrieval

Government of Canada. (2014). *Facts and figures 2013 – Immigration overview: Permanent residents.* Retrieved from http://www.cic.gc.ca/english/resources/statistics/facts2013/index.asp

Hamilton, N., & Bhatti, T. (1996). *Population health promotion: An integrated model of population health and health promotion.* Ottawa, ON: Public Health Agency of Canada, Health Promotion Development Division. Retrieved from http://www.phac-aspc.gc.ca/ph-sp/php-psp/index-eng.php

HIV Prevention Research Team University of Ottawa, Provincial Women and HIV Group, & Ontario Women's Study Research Design Committee. (2007). *Women and HIV prevention: A scoping review.* Retrieved from http://www.med.uottawa.ca/epid/assets/documents/women_hivprevention.pdf

Howard Research & Management Consulting, Inc. (2014). *Evaluation of the sexually transmitted infection (STI) awareness campaign.* Calgary, AB: Author.

Kalichman, S. C., Benotsch, E. G., Weinhardt, L., Austin, J., Luke, W., & Cherry, C. (2003). Health-related Internet use, coping, social support, and health indicators in people living with HIV/AIDS: Preliminary results from a community survey. *Health Psychology, 22*(1), 111–116.

Kerr, T., Tyndall, M., Montaner, J., & Wood, E. (2005). Safer injection facility use and syringe sharing in injection drug users. *The Lancet, 366,* 316–318.

Lokanc-Diluzio, W. (2014). *A mixed methods study of service provider capacity development to protect and promote the sexual and reproductive health of street-involved youth: An evaluation of two training approaches*. (Doctoral dissertation). Retrieved from http://hdl.handle.net/11023/1507

McKay, A. (2006). Chlamydia screening programs: A review of the literature. Part 1: Issues in the promotion of chlamydia testing of youth by primary care physicians. *The Canadian Journal of Human Sexuality, 15*, 111.

Minister of Justice. (2014). *Immigration and refugee protection act.* Retrieved from http://laws-lois.justice.gc.ca/PDF/I-2.5.pdf

Myers, T., Allman, D., Calzavara, L., Maxwell, J., Remia, R., Swantee, C., & Travers, R. (2004). *Ontario's men survey final report.* Retrieved from http://library.catie.ca/PDF/P15/21334.pdf

National Advisory Council on Immunization. (2007). Statement on human papillomavirus vaccine. *Canadian Communicable Disease Report, 33*(ACS-2), 1–32.

National Advisory Council on Immunization. (2012). Update on human papillomavirus (HPV) vaccines. *Canadian Communicable Disease Report, 38*(ACS-1), 1–62. Retrieved from http://www.phac-aspc.gc.ca/publicat/ccdr-rmtc/12vol38/acs-dcc-1/index-eng.php

Ottawa Public Health. (2011). *Enhanced street youth surveillance in Ottawa 2011.* Ottawa, ON: Author. Retrieved from http://ottawa.ca/calendar/ottawa/citycouncil/obh/2011/11-21/F%205788%20OPH%20E%20SYS%20Report%20Eng%20WEB%20Tagged%20Nov14-11.pdf

Public Health Agency of Canada. (2003). *Bloodborne pathogens section.* Ottawa, ON: Author. Retrieved from http://www.phac-aspc.gc.ca/hcai-iamss/bbp-pts/index-eng.php

Public Health Agency of Canada. (2006a). *Street youth in Canada: Findings from enhanced surveillance of Canadian street youth, 1999–2003.* Ottawa, ON: Author. Retrieved from http://www.phac-aspc.gc.ca/std-mts/reports_06/pdf/street_youth_e.pdf

Public Health Agency of Canada. (2006b). *Sexually transmitted infection in Canadian street youth: Findings from enhanced surveillance of Canadian street youth, 1999–2003.* Ottawa, ON: Author. Retrieved from http://www.phac-aspc.gc.ca/std-mts/reports_06/pdf/sti-street_youth_e.pdf

Public Health Agency of Canada. (2008). *Canadian guidelines for sexual health education.* Ottawa, ON: Author. Retrieved from http://www.phac-aspc.gc.ca/publicat/cgshe-ldnemss/index-eng.php

Public Health Agency of Canada. (2009). *Transfusion transmitted injuries section: Transfusion transmitted diseases/infections.* Ottawa, ON: Author.

Public Health Agency of Canada. (2010). *Population-specific HIV/AIDS report: Aboriginal peoples.* Ottawa, ON: Author. Retrieved from http://www.phac-aspc.gc.ca/aids-sida/publication/ps-pd/aboriginal-autochtones/chapter-chapitre-3-eng.php

Public Health Agency of Canada. (2011). *Report on sexually transmitted infections in Canada: 2009.* Ottawa, ON: Author. Retrieved from http://www.catie.ca/sites/default/files/2009%20Report%20on%20STI%20in%20Canada_EN.pdf

Public Health Agency of Canada. (2012a). *HIV and AIDS in Canada: Surveillance report to December 31, 2011.* Ottawa, ON: Author. Retrieved from http://www.catie.ca/sites/default/files/PHAC_HIV-AIDS_2011%20Report_Eng-Fr.pdf

Public Health Agency of Canada. (2012b). *Hepatitis C in Canada: 2005–2010 Surveillance report.* Ottawa, ON: Author. Retrieved from http://www.phac-aspc.gc.ca/sti-its-surv-epi/hepc/surv-eng.php

Public Health Agency of Canada. (2012c). *Fact sheet: People in prison.* Ottawa, ON: Author. Retrieved from http://www.phac-aspc.gc.ca/aids-sida/pr/sec4-eng.php#ab

Public Health Agency of Canada. (2013–2014). *Canadian guidelines on sexually transmitted infections.* Ottawa, ON: Author. Retrieved from http://www.phac-aspc.gc.ca/std-mts/sti-its/cgsti-ldcits/index-eng.php#toc

Public Health Agency of Canada. (2013a). *Sexual health and sexually transmitted infections.* Ottawa, ON: Author. Retrieved from http://www.phac-aspc.gc.ca/std-mts

Public Health Agency of Canada. (2013b). *Human Immunodeficiency Virus: HIV screen and testing guide.* Ottawa, ON: Author. Retrieved from http://www.phac-aspc.gc.ca/aids-sida/guide/hivstg-vihgdd-eng.php

Public Health Agency of Canada. (2013c). *At a glance—HIV and AIDS in Canada: Surveillance report to December 31, 2012.* Ottawa, ON: Author. Retrieved from http://www.phac-aspc.gc.ca/aids-sida/publication/survreport/2012/dec/index-eng.php

Public Health Agency of Canada. (2013d). *Canadian immunization guide: Evergreen edition.* Ottawa, ON: Author. Retrieved from http://www.phac-aspc.gc.ca/publicat/cig-gci/index-eng.php#toc

Public Health Agency of Canada. (2013e). *The chief public health officer's report on the state of public health in Canada, 2013: Infectious disease—The never ending threat.* Ottawa, ON: Author. Retrieved from http://www.phac-aspc.gc.ca/cphor-sphc-respcacsp/2013/index-eng.php

Public Health Agency of Canada. (2014a). *Notifiable diseases on-line.* Ottawa, ON: Author. Retrieved from http://dsol-smed.phac-aspc.gc.ca/dsol-smed/ndis/index-eng.php

Public Health Agency of Canada. (2014b) *Your immunization schedule.* Ottawa, ON: Author. Retrieved from http://www.phac-aspc.gc.ca/im/iyc-vve/schedule-calendrier-eng.php

Rekart, M. L. (2005). Sex work harm reduction. *The Lancet, 366*, 2123–2134.

Rowniak, S. (2009). Safe sex fatigue, treatment optimism, and serosorting: New challenges to HIV prevention among men who have sex with men. *Journal of the Association of Nurses in AIDS Care, 20*(1), 31–38.

Shier, M., & Bryson, P. (2007). Vaccines. *Journal of Obstetrics and Gynaecology Canada, 29*(8), S51–S54.

Shriver, S. P., Byer, C. O., Shainberg, L. W., & Galliano, G. (2002). *Dimensions of human sexuality* (6th ed.). Boston, MA: McGraw-Hill.

Shoveller, J., Knight, R., Davis, W., Gilbert, M., & Ogilvie, G. (2012). Online sexual health services: Examining youth's perspectives. *Canadian Journal of Public Health, 103*(1), 14–18.

Small, W., Shoveller, J., Moore, D., Tyndall, M., Wood, E., & Kerr, T. (2011). Injection drug users' access to a supervised injection facility in Vancouver, Canada: The influence of operating policies and local drug culture. *Qualitative Health Research, 21*(6), 743–756.

Society of Obstetricians and Gynaecologists of Canada. (2012). *Contraception: Contraception methods.* Ottawa ON: Author.

Society of Obstetricians and Gynaecologists of Canada. (n.d.). *Prevention.* Retrieved from http://hpvinfo.ca/prevention

Statistics Canada. (2011). *Aboriginal peoples in Canada: First Nations People, Metis and Inuit.* Retrieved from http://www12.statcan.gc.ca/nhs-enm/2011/as-sa/99-011-x/99-011-x2011001-eng.cfm

White, M., & Dorman, S. M. (2001). Receiving social support online: Implications for health education. *Health Education Research: Theory and Practice, 16*(6), 693–707.

Werb, D., Kerr, T., Buxton, J., Shoveller, J., Richardson, C., Montaner, J., & Wood, E. (2013). Patterns of injection drug use cessation during an expansion of syringe exchange services in a Canadian setting. *Drug and Alcohol Dependence, 132,* 535–540.

Wood, E., Kerr, T., Montaner, J. S., Strathdee, S. A., Wodak, A., Hankins, C. A., . . . Tyndall, M. W. (2004a). Rationale for evaluating North America's first medically supervised safer-injecting facility. *The Lancet Infectious Diseases, 4*(5), 301–306.

Wood, E., Kerr, T., Small, W., Li, K., Marsh, D. C., Montaner, J. S. G., & Tyndall, M. W. (2004b). Changes in public order after the opening of a medically supervised safer injecting facility for illicit injection drug users. *Canadian Medical Association Journal, 171*(7), 731–734.

## ABOUT THE AUTHORS

**Wendi Lokanc-Diluzio**, RN, BN (University of Calgary), MN (University of Calgary), PhD (University of Calgary), has worked in public health since 1997. Since 2002, Wendi has worked as a Sexual and Reproductive Health Specialist for Alberta Health Services, where she provides leadership in the area of child and youth sexual health promotion, service provider education and training, and program evaluation.

**Tammy Troute-Wood**, RN, BScN (British Columbia Institute of Technology), MN (Athabasca University), has worked in the area of reproductive health since 1994. Tammy has worked at Alberta Health Services, Sexual and Reproductive Health, as a clinic nurse, as a sexual and reproductive health specialist, and with the education and health promotion teams. Tammy has also worked as a labour and delivery nurse and at the Regional Fertility Program in Calgary.

Acknowledgements: We would like to thank Janet Wayne, Janet Hettler, and Alison Nelson for their contributions to previous editions.

# CHAPTER 32

## Emergency Preparedness and Disaster Nursing

*Betty Schepens and Lucia Yiu*

### LEARNING OUTCOMES

**After studying this chapter, you should be able to:**

1. Define the various types of disasters and their consequences.

2. Describe some of the key activities involved in public safety and emergency preparedness in Canada.

3. Explain the roles and responsibilities of the Public Health Agency of Canada in emergency preparedness.

4. Identify the key functions of community health nurses before, during, and following a disaster.

5. Articulate the use of the Jennings Disaster Nursing Management Model in responding effectively to emergencies or disasters.

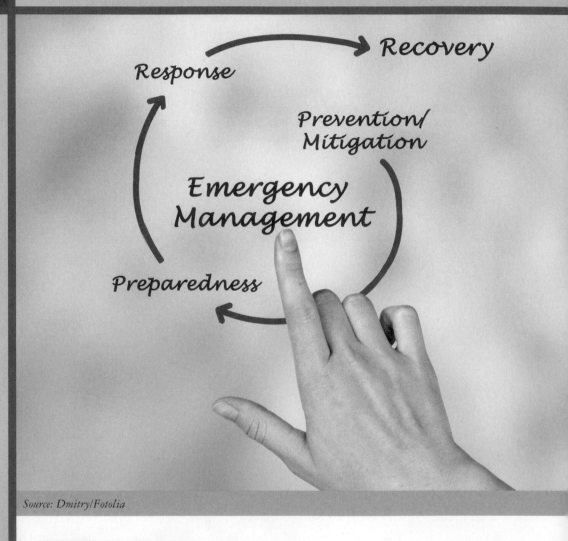

*Source: Dmitry/Fotolia*

## INTRODUCTION

In the last decade, over 2.6 billion people in more than 45 countries worldwide experienced health threats as a result of natural disasters or social and economic crises; enormous efforts were required to save lives and reduce illness and suffering (World Health Organization, 2007, 2014). Different types of disasters vary in severity, and each with its own degree of death, mass injury, illness, and loss. How a disaster will impact a community depends upon the individual community's social, cultural, economic, and health makeup. In order to respond effectively in a disaster situation across different communities, special expertise in emergency management is required.

Emergency preparedness and disaster nursing is an emerging specialty. Since Florence Nightingale demonstrated to the world that nurses have a critical role in health and illness, nursing has continued to expand its scope of practice. The Canadian Nurses Association (CNA) (2014) states that registered nurses must be well prepared to respond and provide essential services to people affected by disasters with a goal to preserve health and safety in these communities. This chapter highlights different types of disasters, and how the Incident Management System (IMS) is used to manage major incidents. It provides an overview of the role of community health nurses (CHNs) in community emergency preparedness planning and in disaster situations. The Jennings Disaster Nursing Management Model will be introduced to guide CHNs in understanding disaster nursing.

## DISASTERS IN CANADA

According to the Canadian Disaster Database (Public Safety Canada, 2013a), chemical and fuel spills, floods, snowstorms, and forest fires were the most common disasters in Canada in the last decade (see Table 32.1). Emergencies and disasters never fail to impact and alter the lives of people and their environment.

## WHAT IS A DISASTER?

**Disasters** typically occur suddenly and can be caused by nature, human error, biological hazards, or infectious diseases. They include earthquakes, floods, fires, hurricanes, cyclones, major storms, volcanic eruptions, spills, air crashes, droughts, epidemics, food shortages, and civil strife (Landesman, 2012). Disasters often are perceived as random killers. They affect public safety and leave communities with long-term adverse socioeconomic, health, and environmental effects. Individuals at greatest risk include vulnerable or priority groups such as women, children, the elderly, the poor, and people with mental and physical disabilities (Burkle, 2006). Life-threatening conditions brought on by disasters and the adverse health effects borne of these conditions often result in increased mortality and morbidity.

## Types of Disasters

**Natural Disasters**  **Natural disasters** are unpredictable; they can happen very quickly or slowly. However, with advance warning, such as weather reports, the impacts can sometimes be mitigated. Some examples of natural disasters include

| Table 32.1 | **Selected Canadian Disasters** | |
|---|---|---|
| **Date and Location** | **Disaster** | **Human Consequences (Number of People)** |
| 1900 Ottawa and Hull | Fire | 15 000 evacuated, 7 dead |
| 1918 to 1925 Canada | Spanish flu | 2 million people ill, over 50 000 died |
| 1936 Canada | Heat wave (2-week) | 1180 died |
| 2000 Ontario (Walkerton) | Drinking water contamination | 7 died, 2300 injured |
| 2003 Canada (Toronto) | SARS epidemic | 44 died (of 438 cases) |
| 2003 southeastern B.C. and southwestern Alberta | Forest fires | ~50 000 evacuated |
| 2005 Alberta (16 communities) | Floods | 2 dead<br>7028 evacuated, ~40 000 homes damaged |
| 2009 across Canada | Biological epidemic | 425 fatalities, 8582 injured/infected |
| 2009 British Columbia | Wildfire | 20 000 evacuated |
| 2010 Newfoundland[1] | Hurricane | 7000+ affected |
| 2011 Alberta | Wildfire | 12 055 evacuated |
| 2011 Goderich, Ontario | Tornado | 1 died, 37 injured |
| 2013 Alberta | Flood | 100 000+ evacuated |
| 2013 Lac-Mégantic, Quebec | Runaway train derailed and exploded | 42 died, 5 missing |
| 2013 Toronto, Ontario[2] | Ice storm | 230 000 affected (without power) |
| 2015 Northern Alberta[3] | Wildfires | ~5000 people evacuated<br>Shut down oil sands production |

Source: Adapted from Public Safety Canada. (2013a). Canadian Disaster Database. Ottawa, ON: Government of Canada. Retrieved from http://cdd.publicsafety.gc.ca/rslts-eng.aspx?cultureCode=en-Ca&boundingBox=&provinces=1,2,3,4,5,6,7,8,9,10,11,12,13&eventTypes=&eventStartDate=%2719000101%27,%2720131231%27&injured=&evacuated=&totalCost=&dead=&normalizedCostYear=1

Sources: [1]CBC News. (2010, September 22). *Hurricane Igor attacks Newfoundland.* Retrieved from http://www.cbc.ca/news/canada/newfoundland-labrador/hurricane-igor-attacks-newfoundland-1.935880

[2]CBC News (2013, December 23). *Toronto ice storm leaves 230,000 without power.* Retrieved from http://www.cbc.ca/news/canada/toronto/toronto-ice-storm-leaves-230-000-without-power-1.2473543

[3]Huffpost Alberta. (2015, August 13). *Wildfires in Northern Alberta close highway, cover skies in smoke.* Retrieved from http://www.huffingtonpost.ca/2015/06/29/wildfires-alberta_n_7690662.html

droughts, heat waves, ice storms, cold waves, heavy snow-falls, earthquakes, cyclones, tornadoes, flood or thunder-storms, tsunamis, volcanoes, wildfires, train derailments, and plane crashes. Recent incidents of natural disasters are the December 24, 2004, earthquake, which triggered a massive tsunami that hit Southeast Asia, leaving 280 931 dead; the earthquake in Haiti on January 12, 2010 that left approxi-mately 150 000 dead; and the March 11, 2011, earthquake that triggered a tsunami followed by nuclear explosion in Japan left 15 883 dead, 9500 missing, 26 992 injured, and 185 000 displaced, and with effects of radioactivity that may last for 30 years in these communities (CNN, 2013). (See also Photo 32.1.)

**Man-Made Disasters** Man-made disasters often result in mass numbers of civilian injuries and deaths. Bioterrorism, bombings, and technical disasters, such as nuclear disasters and oil spills, are all examples of man-made disasters.

The September 11, 2001, terrorist attacks on the World Trade Center in New York and the Pentagon in Washington in the United States are among the most recent and well-watched examples of a man-made disaster. Twenty-five Canadians were among the 2977 killed when terrorists flew commercial airliners into the World Trade Center towers (Weinreb, 2007).

**Bioterrorism** is the intentional use of a micro-organism to cause infection or death. The release of smallpox or anthrax with the intent to infect humans is an example of a bioterror-ist attack. Ideologically or politically inspired bombings, civil and political disorder as seen in countries at war, and riots resulting in social instability are also examples of man-made disasters.

Technological malfunctions can occur in industrial sites and can be triggered by a natural disaster. Contamination of the water or food supply; the unintentional release of deadly airborne substances such as anthrax; fires; explosions; oil spills;

and exposure to hazardous materials are all conduits for technological disasters. Building or bridge collapses, transpor-tation crashes, dam or levee failures, nuclear reactor accidents, and breaks in water, gas, deep sea oil drilling, and sewer lines may also result in a disaster of this type (CBC, 2010; Landesman, 2012). Both man-made and natural disasters leave people injured, put emergency responders at risk, and have a lasting financial, environmental, or health impact on the communities they affect.

**Epidemics** An **epidemic** can occur when an infectious disease spreads rapidly, affecting a large number of individuals within a population, community, or region. This can quickly lead to an emergency situation if the right conditions exist. Conditions such as a densely populated area, lack/loss of proper sanitation and hygiene practices, lack of equipment and supplies, lack of experienced professional personnel to manage the epidemic, and lack of or disrupted public health services may provide a breeding ground for an epidemic. Epidemics with high levels of morbidity and mortality often lead to economic and social disruptions.

Epidemics become **pandemics** when the infection becomes widespread in different parts of the globe and affects a significantly higher proportion of the population than nor-mal. The emergence of a swine-origin influenza A (H1N1) virus in humans in Mexico in early 2009 that spread around the world is an example of how an infectious disease response can escalate to the declaration of a global influenza pandemic within months, as reported by the Public Health Agency of Canada (PHAC) (2010).

## PUBLIC SAFETY AND EMERGENCY PREPAREDNESS IN CANADA

Disaster preparedness and response at a national and provin-cial or territorial level ensures support for public health authorities and other officials who are responsible for man-aging the health of their community before, during, and after a disaster occurs. Public health officials attend to pre-vention of infectious disease and injury. They routinely con-duct surveillance for infectious disease and they work in collaboration with other agencies within the health sector. They have governmental jurisdiction to oversee the public's health, and they use triage skills in disaster situations (PHAC, 2012).

Emergency management and preparedness responses in Canada begin at the local level. Local municipalities have the first responsibility in managing an emergency, and if their capacity is exceeded they call on their respective province, which in turn can call on the federal government for assis-tance. Therefore, local emergency preparedness plans are key to the success in managing emergencies. Some countries have an opposite response chain of command in place: all responses to large-scale emergencies and disasters are initiated at the federal level.

## Government Authority and Legislative Framework

Federal legislation with respect to emergencies and emergency preparedness is found in three complementary acts: the Emergencies Act, the Emergency Preparedness Act, and the Emergency Management Act. The first two legislations were enacted in 1988, at which time the Emergencies Act replaced the War Measures Act as the source of the federal government's authority to act in the event of a national emergency. The Emergency Management Act replaces parts of the Emergency Preparedness Act.

**The Emergencies Act** The **Emergencies Act** (Ministry of Justice, 2014a) allows the federal government to grant the use of special powers to ensure the safety and security of Canadians during a national emergency. The Emergencies Act defines a **national emergency** as "an urgent and critical situation of a temporary nature that seriously endangers the lives, health or safety of Canadians and is of such proportions or nature as to exceed the capacity or authority of a province to deal with it, or seriously threatens the ability of the Government of Canada to preserve the sovereignty, security and territorial integrity of Canada, and cannot be effectively dealt with under any other law of Canada" (p. 8).

The federal government intervention is restricted to only the most serious emergency situations, while respecting the authority of the provinces and territories to govern accordingly within their own geographical jurisdictions.

There are four categories of national emergency:

1. *public welfare emergencies*, such as a major natural disaster or accident, which are beyond the authority of the province or territory in which the disaster occurs to address;
2. *public order emergencies*, wherein there is a serious security threat to the nation;
3. *international emergencies* arising from acts of coercion or intimidation or the serious use of force or violence, which threaten the sovereignty, security, or territorial integrity of Canada or its allies; and
4. *a state of war*, either active or imminent, involving Canada or its allies.

It is important to note that the extraordinary powers extended by the federal government must be tailored to the specific disaster event, and may not exceed what is necessary to deal with the particulars of the situation at hand. The Emergencies Act is not designed to justify the arbitrary or excessive use of power on the part of the federal government.

**The Emergency Preparedness Act** The **Emergency Preparedness Act** (Ministry of Justice, 2014b) functions as companion legislation to the Emergencies Act. While the Emergencies Act provides the authority for government action, the Emergency Preparedness Act provides a basis for the planning and programming necessary to address disasters of all kinds. Specifically, the Emergency Preparedness Act addresses the need for co-operation between the provinces and territories at the federal level to establish responsibilities and the need for public awareness, and provides a structure for training and education.

**The Emergency Management Act** The **Emergency Management Act** (Ministry of Justice, 2014c) replaces parts of the Emergency Preparedness Act to strengthen the government's readiness to respond to major emergencies by defining the roles and responsibilities for all federal ministers. It also enhances information sharing between various levels of government and the private sector. It provides direction for critical infrastructure protection as this is one of the emerging challenges of modern emergency management (Public Safety Canada, 2013b). Critical infrastructure consists of physical and information technology facilities, networks, services, and assets that are vital to the health, safety, security, or economic well-being of Canadians and for the effective functioning of governments in Canada. Public Safety Canada developed the Federal Emergency Response Plan, which is the Government of Canada's "all-hazards" response plan. This plan applies to domestic emergencies and to international emergencies with a domestic impact.

## Emergency Management

**Emergency management** is an essential discipline involving a diverse group of skilled professionals, with the ultimate responsibility resting with the government to assess and deal with risk in an effort to protect the health and safety of the public. A "crisis" or "emergency" is a threatening condition that requires urgent action. Effective emergency management action can avoid the escalation of an event into a disaster. Emergency management involves plans and institutional arrangements to engage and guide the efforts of government, non-government, voluntary, and private agencies in comprehensive and coordinated ways to respond to the entire spectrum of emergency needs (Haddow, Bullock, & Coppola, 2011).

The four areas of emergency management in the life-cycle process of a disaster include:

1. mitigating or preventing the effects of an emergency;
2. preparing for emergencies or disasters;
3. responding to an emergency or disaster to reduce the impact on public loss; and
4. recovering from an emergency or disaster by assisting communities to return to normal (Veenema, 2013).

## Hazard Identification Risk Assessment

Emergency response plans generally use an all-hazards approach where activities will be applicable to any type of emergency. Communication and media plans, business continuity plans, employee health and safety plans, and procurement of supplies and purchasing plans are examples of strategies generic to all response plans. By completing a Hazard Identification Risk Assessment (HIRA), organizations can prioritize specific threats based on risk of probability and consequence or impact. **Probability** is the likelihood of an event occurring within a given time period. **Impact** assesses the level or degree to which the hazard will affect three critical dimensions: human, physical infrastructure, and business impacts. (See MyNursingLab for an example of an assessment tool.)

All levels of government as well as public health agencies and hospitals use this process. Community-level response organizations, such as public health units and hospitals, need to incorporate the individual response plans into a local coordinated community response plan. For example, a fire services agency is the lead for responding to a hazardous materials spill in the community, whereas the public health unit and the hospital would have supporting roles. In comparison, public health would be the lead in responding to a community infectious disease outbreak, or a pandemic, and the local first responder agencies would have supporting roles.

Effective hazard identification risk assessment strategies combined with interagency coordination can and will prepare an agency for response, mitigate the effects of the emergency, and assist in recovery and evaluation activities.

## Organizational Structure and Chain of Command: National Incident Management System

An international system known as the **National Incident Management System (NIMS)** was developed by the Department of Homeland Security in the United States and released in March 2004. The NIMS was adopted by the Government of Canada as the IMS, which now provides the framework for all levels of government in Canada to develop emergency response plans regardless of the nature of the incident or its level of complexity.

## Incident Management System

The **Incident Management System (IMS)** is a standardized, function-driven model used by agencies throughout North America to manage and respond to emergencies. A similar version, the **Incident Command System (ICS)**, is used at on-site emergency scenes by first responders using a formal command approach. Public health authorities use the IMS as an operational framework for emergency preparedness and response planning. The benefits of the IMS are to enhance capacity, streamline resources, improve communication, and facilitate the co-operation of activities and interoperability among organizations.

The basic IMS structure consists of five components: command, operations, planning, logistics, and finance and administration (see Table 32.2). The pertinent functional components are established only when necessary, depending on the magnitude of the emergency. The IMS framework allows the staff to communicate directly with other healthcare jurisdictions and other emergency response organizations to coordinate the distribution of medical supplies from federal and provincial stockpiles to the front line by using the logistics section personnel at federal, provincial, and local health unit levels. An example can be seen in Alberta's pandemic influenza plan (available from www.health.alberta.ca/documents/APIP-Pandemic-Plan-2014.pdf).

---

| Table 32.2 | The IMS Structure |
|---|---|

The IMS Structure consists of the following five components:

**COMMAND** includes these five key positions:

- Executive Lead – authorizes all activities pertaining to the investigation and/or intervention
- Incident Manager – manages all the required day-to-day activities while conducting public health investigation and/or intervention
- Liaison Officer – represents the Incident Manager to outside organizations
- Communication Officer – responsible for all internal and external messaging
- Safety Officer – responsible to ensure the protection of the health and safety of staff

**PLANNING** assesses the situation and prepares an Incident Action Plan that prioritizes objectives, identified required resources, and assigned activities for a specified time period.

**OPERATION** implements all activities in the Incident Action Plan such as mass immunization clinics and the operation of telephone hotlines.

**LOGISTICS** is responsible for the procurement and maintenance of required supplies, physical space, and technological support.

**FINANCE AND ADMINISTRATION** coordinates and manages human resources and volunteers, all purchases and expenditures, and maintains a record of all activities during the emergency. (See Canadian Research Box 32.1.)

Source: Ontario Agency for Health Protection and Promotion (Public Health Ontario). (2015). *Public health emergency preparedness: An IMS-based workshop. Base scenario. Facilitator's guide.* Toronto, ON: Queen's Printer for Ontario. Reprinted (or adapted) with the permission of Public Health Ontario.

**CANADIAN RESEARCH BOX 32.1**

**What supports are most effective for disaster-relief volunteers?**

Fahim, C., O'Sullivan, T., & Lane, D. (2014). Supports for health and social service providers from Canada responding to the disaster in Haiti. *PLoS Curr, 13*(6). doi:10.1371/currents. dis.8821e785b58ec43043c7e46c82885409

After the earthquake that shook Port-au-Prince in Haiti on January 12, 2010, that county relied on international humanitarian aids to recover from this natural disaster. This qualitative study explored the effectiveness of various supports made available to health and social service providers who were deployed to Haiti in response to the disasters during or after the 2010 earthquake. A single, semi-structured interview was conducted with 21 Canadian health professionals from a variety of organizations between December 2011 and February 2012. The researchers used Strauss and Corbin's structured approach to grounded theory to explore the participants' perceptions with what might enhance the success in their relief work. Themes and relationships were extracted from the interviews. The participants (71%) indicated that they need to improve training supports, such as pre-deployment training and de-briefing at departure and on their return. Also, psychological and emotional supports—in particular, integration of mental health workers in the response team, communication, and leadership—are crucial to improve the experience and effectiveness of their work. Organizations also need to be self-sufficient to lead various logistics, including flights, transportation, passports, vaccinations, food and water, equipment repair, and emergency medical support.

**Discussion Questions**

1. Based on the perceptions of the Canadian health workers deployed to Haiti, which functional components have they validated that should be in place in any basic IMS?

2. As organizations carry out disaster-relief efforts, what are the critical elements that will ensure success in their relief work?

## CRISES IN PUBLIC HEALTH

The face of emergency preparedness in Canada has been shaped by recent events that highlighted the gaps and weaknesses in the Canadian public health system and infection control capacity.

## The Walkerton E-Coli Experience

In 2000, improper execution of safe water practices in Walkerton, Ontario, led to the contamination of the town's water supply by E-coli O157:H7 and *Campylobacter jejuni* bacteria. One year later, the same strain of E-coli contaminated the drinking water in North Battleford, Saskatchewan. The Walkerton Commission of Inquiry Reports (O'Connor, 2002) highlighted the need for safe drinking water and ways to reduce the risk of infection and death.

## Sudden Acute Respiratory Syndrome

In 2003, Canadians again faced the need for emergency response following the outbreak of sudden acute respiratory syndrome (SARS). SARS emerged from China in 2002 and spread quickly across the globe to Toronto (Naylor, 2003). Following these events, there were calls for a renewal in the national public health system. All stressed the need for the federal government to provide funding support and to take a stronger leadership role to strengthen the public health infrastructure and health-promotion efforts in Canada (Kirby, 2003; Kirby & LeBreton, 2002).

"Learning from SARS: Renewal of Public Health in Canada: A Report of the National Advisory Committee on SARS and Public Health," known as the Naylor Report (2003), addressed a lack of capacity in the clinical and public health systems and epidemiological investigation of the outbreak, dysfunctional relationships between various orders of governments, absence of protocols for data or information sharing among different government levels, and inadequate business processes between and across jurisdictions for outbreak management and emergency response. The report recommends a Canadian Agency for Public Health with a chief public health officer of Canada heading the agency and reporting to the Minister of Health, development of a national health strategy with specific health targets and benchmarks, public health partnership programs to build capacity in public health at the local or municipal level, and a national strategy to renew and sustain public health human resources (including public health nurses, public health physicians, infection control practitioners, and microbiologists). The report also draws attention to the role of CHNs in emergency preparedness, and notes that the contributions by public health nurses during the SARS outbreak had received little public attention.

## Listeriosis

The listeriosis outbreak in 2008 linked to deli meats produced at a Maple Leaf plant in Ontario was a significant public health event. The collective efforts of local and regional health authorities, provincial and territorial governments, and federal officials detected and contained the outbreak following three weeks of higher-than-expected case reports of listeriosis in Ontario. Eventually, seven provinces were implicated in the outbreak. Of the 56 confirmed cases (75% in Ontario) and two probable cases, there were 20 deaths across five provinces (PHAC, 2008). Consequently, recommendations were made to improve the management of food-borne outbreaks, from clarifying the roles, responsibilities, and relationships of personnel involved to providing PHAC's staff with training and practice in outbreak and emergency response.

## Pandemic H1N1 Flu Virus

Influenza, or the flu, is a common viral respiratory infection that accounts for approximately 12 200 hospitalizations and 3500 deaths annually. In the spring of 2009, H1N1 was a new strain of the influenza virus with outbreaks that started in Mexico and spread to Canada within weeks. The first Canadian cases of H1N1 were confirmed on April 26, 2009. As the H1N1 flu virus spread around the world, the World Health Organization (WHO) declared it a pandemic influenza virus (PHAC, 2014).

Influenza pandemics are difficult to predict. At the very outset of the pandemic, the PHAC called on the National Microbiology Laboratory for laboratory assistance, and five Public Health Agency scientists helped with testing in Mexico over the course of six weeks. The PHAC was the first to characterize the entire genomic sequence of the pandemic H1N1 influenza virus; it was instrumental in making a significant contribution to international scientific understanding of this novel strain.

Canada experienced two waves of H1N1 in 2009: the first between April 12 and August 29 and the second in early November. Canada's second wave of H1N1 resulted in four to five times more hospitalizations and deaths compared with the first wave. Because H1N1 was a new strain of influenza, a large number of populations had little to no natural immunity to the virus. Those with higher rates of hospitalization and mortality were the Aboriginal people, pregnant women, and individuals with at least one underlying medical condition. Over 400 people in Canada died due to pandemic H1N1.

## Roles and Responsibilities for Public Health

As public health faced these recent crises, such as SARS, contaminated water, food poisoning, and H1N1, various commission reports recommended that even though many emergency response organizations were using some form of the IMS there should be one common emergency response system "to bring an orderly, consistent, and flexible chain of command and control within an emergency response" (Campbell, 2005, p. 322). Further, it was pointed out that the healthcare system needs to be properly funded in order to plan and deliver public health programs and emergency medical services. This would help build a cohesive public health model, establish infection control networks and standards, improve emergency preparedness, develop a communications infrastructure in the event of an emergency, enhance surveillance, and increase enrolment in key public health professions.

## THE PUBLIC HEALTH AGENCY OF CANADA

Following the terrorist attacks of September 11, 2001, and the outbreak of SARS, Emergency Preparedness Canada was created and renamed Public Safety Canada (PS) in 2003. This was to ensure that federal departments and agencies responsible for national security and the safety of Canadians could work more closely together.

On September 24, 2004, the Government of Canada established the Public Health Agency of Canada (PHAC) and appointed the first chief public health officer (CPHO) of Canada. The agency provides leadership in promoting health, investigating and controlling disease outbreaks, supporting public health infrastructure, and fostering collaboration across and between governments. PHAC and PS work with the provincial and territorial governments to coordinate a unified response to any national public health emergency (PHAC, 2006). The 2006 Public Health Agency of Canada Act (Government of Canada, 2014) recognized the agency with enabling legislation and by establishing the dual role of the CPHO as head of the PHAC and lead public health professional in Canada.

## PUBLIC HEALTH RESPONSE IN A DISASTER

Public health preparedness for all types of disasters, especially infectious disease emergencies, has become essential in today's world. CHNs must learn from past disasters that include infection prevention and control in mass casualty incidents, public education, internal and external communication, and building partnerships with outside agencies (Rebmann, Carrico, & English, 2008). As the largest group of healthcare professionals in any given jurisdiction, CHNs must play pivotal advocacy and leadership roles to facilitate agency-specific and community-wide preparations for health-related emergencies and disasters. (See Canadian Research Box 32.2.)

---

### CANADIAN RESEARCH BOX 32.2

**What is our understanding of mass casualty incidents?**

Turris, S. A., Lund, A., & Bowles, R. R. (2014). An analysis of mass casualty incidents in the setting of mass gatherings and special events. *Disaster Med Public Health Prep, 16,* pp. 1–7. Retrieved from http://www.researchgate.net/publication/261741235_An_Analysis_of_Mass_Casualty_Incidents_in_the_Setting_of_Mass_Gatherings_and_Special_Events (PMID: 24735776)

This collaborative research among the School of Nursing, the Department of Emergency Medicine, and the Centre for Applied Research at the University of British Columbia analyzed the literature for mass casualty incidents (MCIs) and mass gatherings (MGs) from 1982 to 2012 to guide emergency preparedness services. Their findings revealed that of the 290 MCIs, the most frequent MCIs involved people under crowded conditions (55.9%), hazards, e.g., airplane crashes, pyrotechnic displays, car crashes, boat collisions (19.6%), structural failures, e.g., building code violations, balcony collapses (13.1%), deliberate events (9%), and toxic exposures (2.4%). These MCIs took place in North America (27%), Asia (24%), Europe (24%), Africa (17%), South America (9%), the Middle East (9%), and Australasia (1%). The researchers recommended that a centralized database be created to guide prevention efforts and minimize the effects of MCIs during MGs.

#### Discussion Questions

1. Give examples of at least three types of MGs.
2. Give at least three examples of categories of mass casualties or incidents.
3. What are the possible actions and implications to prevent MCIs?

## Phases of Disaster Response

Federal, provincial or territorial, and local public health professionals are responsible for the health of their communities in both preparing for a disaster and responding once a disaster has occurred. The seven phases of a disaster response for public health activities in preparing and responding to a disaster are as follows (Landesman, 2012):

1. *Planning phase* is guided by the basic public health concepts to disaster management;
2. *Prevention phase* involves activities to control or prevent outbreaks, organize services and treatment, manage injuries, and provide long-term counselling and mental health interventions;
3. *Assessment phase* is where the incidence of disease and causal factors will be determined when a disaster occurs;
4. *Response phase* follows the assessment phase to communicate the disaster management plans and community needs;
5. *Surveillance phase* is used to establish syndromic information about the disaster in the community;
6. *Recovery phase* is where resources will be mobilized to meet the community needs; and
7. *Evaluation phase* is carried out to determine whether emergency plans and disaster response are effective and efficient.

Each phase is linked to specific responsibilities and skill sets possessed by a network of public health professionals for disaster planning and relief.

## Stages of Emergency Management

In some provinces in Canada, such as in Ontario, emergency management programming is organized into five stages: prevention, mitigation, preparedness, response, and recovery, as outlined by the Ontario Ministry of Health and Long-Term Care [OMOHLTC] (2008).

1. *Prevention* involves activities taken to prevent or avoid an emergency or disaster. The eradication of smallpox is an example of a prevention strategy.
2. *Mitigation* involves actions that can reduce the impact of an emergency or disaster. Influenza vaccination and infection prevention and control measures are health-specific examples of mitigation.
3. *Preparedness* involves measures that are in place before an emergency occurs and that will enhance the effectiveness of response and recovery activities, such as developing plans, tools, and protocols; establishing communication systems; conducting training; and testing response plans.
4. *Response* involves the coordinated actions that would be undertaken to respond to an emergency or disaster. This could include the mobilization of providers, the coordination of healthcare services, and the acquisition of necessary equipment and supplies.
5. *Recovery* involves activities that help communities recover from an emergency or disaster and return to a state of normalcy.

This includes activities to restore services, rebuild infrastructure, and carry out the ongoing treatment and care for the sick or injured. It may also include prevention or mitigation measures designed to avert a future emergency (e.g., vaccination to prevent a future outbreak).

## Integrated Community Emergency Preparedness

While provincial and federal emergency preparedness and response-planning parameters can provide local community emergency planners with a variety of tools, templates, and structure, local community emergency response mechanisms are often led by first-responder agencies, such as police, fire, and emergency medical services, to manage incidents related to health or non-health types of emergencies. As infectious disease–related emergencies begin to appear more often, local planners must engage all healthcare professionals and agencies in planning for a health-related emergency. In this instance, the healthcare sector becomes the lead or command agency with emergency-response agencies having a supporting role. There needs to be consensus and collaboration as to agency and professional roles in advance of any emergency. Public health agencies may facilitate these discussions and challenge key community stakeholders to develop, implement, and maintain a comprehensive preparation, response, and recovery plan for health emergencies. CHNs need to become familiar with local agency emergency plans and key agency personnel, and utilize their community mobilization skills to assist in identifying and developing the required health infrastructure to ensure emergency response readiness, surge capacity, and sustainability.

Public health units or departments in provinces across Canada have mandated requirements for fundamental public health programs and services (see Figure 32.1). In Ontario, a review of the 1997 Mandatory Program and Services Guidelines identified a need to add new standards and protocols. In 2008, the Emergency Preparedness Program Standard was added to the revised and newly named Ontario Public Health Standards (OPHS) (OMOHLTC, 2008).

The goal of the Public Health Emergency Preparedness Program is to enable and ensure a consistent and effective response to public health emergencies and emergencies with public health impacts. The Emergency Preparedness Standards and Protocol (OMOHLTC, 2009) identifies the minimum expectations for programs and services by providing direction on how health units must operationalize specific requirements. Key components of the Emergency Preparedness Standard and Protocol include the following:

- identifying and assessing the relevant hazards and risks to public health;
- developing a continuity of operations plan;
- developing an emergency response plan utilizing the IMS;
- developing and implementing 24/7 notification protocols for communications with staff, community partners, and government bodies;

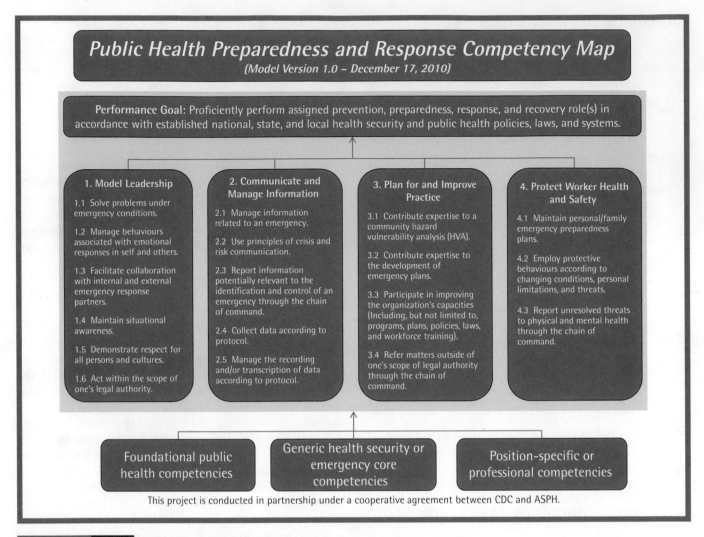

## Public Health Preparedness and Response Competency Map
### (Model Version 1.0 – December 17, 2010)

**Performance Goal:** Proficiently perform assigned prevention, preparedness, response, and recovery role(s) in accordance with established national, state, and local health security and public health policies, laws, and systems.

**1. Model Leadership**

1.1 Solve problems under emergency conditions.

1.2 Manage behaviours associated with emotional responses in self and others.

1.3 Facilitate collaboration with internal and external emergency response partners.

1.4 Maintain situational awareness.

1.5 Demonstrate respect for all persons and cultures.

1.6 Act within the scope of one's legal authority.

**2. Communicate and Manage Information**

2.1 Manage information related to an emergency.

2.2 Use principles of crisis and risk communication.

2.3 Report information potentially relevant to the identification and control of an emergency through the chain of command.

2.4 Collect data according to protocol.

2.5 Manage the recording and/or transcription of data according to protocol.

**3. Plan for and Improve Practice**

3.1 Contribute expertise to a community hazard vulnerability analysis (HVA).

3.2 Contribute expertise to the development of emergency plans.

3.3 Participate in improving the organization's capacities (Including, but not limited to, programs, plans, policies, laws, and workforce training).

3.4 Refer matters outside of one's scope of legal authority through the chain of command.

**4. Protect Worker Health and Safety**

4.1 Maintain personal/family emergency preparedness plans.

4.2 Employ protective behaviours according to changing conditions, personal limitations, and threats.

4.3 Report unresolved threats to physical and mental health through the chain of command.

| Foundational public health competencies | Generic health security or emergency core competencies | Position-specific or professional competencies |
|---|---|---|

This project is conducted in partnership under a cooperative agreement between CDC and ASPH.

**FIGURE 32.1** Public Health Preparedness and Response Competency Map

*Source:* Association of Schools and Programs of Public Health. (2010, December 17). *Public health preparedness and response core competency model* (p. 2). Retrieved from http://www.cdc.gov/phpr/documents/perlcPDFS/PreparednessCompetencyModelWorkforce-Version1_0.pdf

- increasing public awareness regarding emergency preparedness activities;
- delivering emergency preparedness and response education and training for board of health staff and officials; and
- exercising or testing the continuity of the operations plan, the emergency response plan, and the 24/7 notification protocols.

## ROLE OF COMMUNITY HEALTH NURSING ORGANIZATIONS IN DISASTERS

### Canadian Nurses Association

The Canadian Nurses Association (CNA) provides information related to global nursing issues, including disasters. The CNA has partnered with PHAC's Centre for Emergency Preparedness and Response to provide expertise and consultation

in developing the role of nurses in a national emergency plan. The CNA (2012) articulates the integral role that the nursing profession plays in all aspects of emergencies, including prevention, mitigation, preparedness, response, and recovery. In order for an effective, coordinated community emergency response to take place, effective inter-professional collaboration and shared responsibilities among professionals in non-governmental organizations, such as the health, social services, safety, transportation, meteorology, and voluntary sectors, must be developed and nurtured before emergencies occur. (See Table 32.3.)

## THE JENNINGS DISASTER NURSING MANAGEMENT MODEL

The literature has a limited number of disaster planning models to guide nurses in responding to a disaster. Jennings-Sanders (2004) described **disaster nursing** as the "systematic and flexible utilization of knowledge and skills specific to disaster-related nursing, and the promotion of a wide range of activities to minimize the health hazards and life-threatening damage caused by disasters in collaboration with other specialized fields" (p. 69). The Jennings Disaster Nursing Management Model, originally introduced to teach disaster nursing to nursing students, is an effective framework to assist CHNs in planning for and managing disasters. Nursing process is used in the four phases of the Jennings Disaster Nursing Management Model to assess, plan, implement, and evaluate provision of care in a community's response to disasters.

## Phases of a Disaster

**Phase I (Pre-Disaster)** This phase involves assessing resources and risks and planning to achieve primary prevention, such as providing information to help the public at large prepare for a disaster. During this phase, the nurse must be able to respond effectively by identifying and allocating human resources and material resources such as shelters, planning co-operative agreements with other community agencies, defining the roles of everyone involved, assisting special-needs groups to develop plans, and developing or activating the disaster plan.

**Phase II (Disaster Occurs)** In this phase the nurse assumes multiple roles: providing care, education, and case management to disaster victims using a holistic approach that considers emotional, physical, psychosocial, and cultural aspects of care to improve the overall health of disaster victims. The impact of a disaster varies in time and severity. Children, older adults, and people with mental illness are among the highest-risk groups for serious mental health morbidity and mortality. CHNs must recognize symptoms of serious mental illness and depression, and must make every effort to reduce devastating outcomes (Landesman, 2012). Their own family safety, pet care, and personal safety at work, as well as food, water, sleep, shelter, and rest periods while at work, are also of concern to nurses responding in the event of an emergency (Jennings-Sanders, 2004).

CHNs may find themselves working in different roles, such as operating a walk-in clinic, working in a shelter or evacuation centre, and triaging people at mass clinics while providing prophylactic medication or administering vaccine. They act as a case manager to liaise between the victim and a community agency or clinic. Nurses must recognize problems through diagnosis and, through secondary prevention, provide immediate treatment, including making referrals to an emergency room or community site where a clinic has been organized.

**Phase III (Post-Disaster)** During this phase, the nurse performs tertiary prevention through assessment, planning, and implementation. Nurses ensure that victims in the disaster are receiving treatment, and they decrease disabilities through tertiary preventive interventions such as rehabilitation. Nurses will also assess the emergency disaster plan and evaluate the severity of the disaster on the community. They will coordinate recovery operations to help local residents of the community reduce their exposure to risk and disease. They will apply epidemiological principles to ensure that the community does not become infected with disease, and they will implement infection-control measures.

**Phase IV (Positive Client/Population Outcomes)** In this phase, nurses measure the overall impact of the disaster to organize the coordination of community services to help residents in their recovery, reduce mortality rates, and reduce healthcare costs while improving the health status of the client and the population. Positive outcomes include increased community relations, improved knowledge of disasters, improved disaster nursing plans, and decreased costs related to the disaster.

## The Nursing Process

Community mobilization skills and collaboration competencies are crucial to these first two phases. Table 32.3 illustrates how the phases of a disaster are linked to the nursing process.

Nurses play a critical role during all phases of a disaster emergency response system. They need to be knowledgeable of current emergency preparedness frameworks, structures, and responses within their own professional practice and place of employment. To effectively contribute during a disaster, CHNs must apply nursing process and be competent to respond in an emergency in areas such as leadership, communication and managing information, planning for and improving practice, and protecting worker health and safety, as outlined in Table 32.3. CHNs are accountable for having a basic understanding and knowledge of competencies related to emergency preparedness, management, and response activities.

**Public Health Nurses in Public Health Surge Events** Public health nursing skills and competencies are critical to bioterrorism preparedness and a public health nurse response (Berkowitz, 2002; Patillo, 2003). **Surge capacity** is defined as the "healthcare system's ability to expand quickly beyond normal services to meet an increased demand for medical care in the event of bioterrorism or other large-scale public health emergencies" (Agency for Healthcare Research and Quality, 2004). Surge capacity typically addresses acute care facility issues such as equipment, supplies, and personnel. It does not, however, address public health's role in population-based care.

**Public health surge interventions** are those that "improve access and availability of limited health resources for the entire population" (Burkle, 2006). Mass immunization clinics during a pandemic are an example of a public health surge event. The operations of mass immunization clinics during a pandemic would overwhelm public health agencies but would have a minimal effect on hospital systems. **Medical triage** differs from public health triage in that medical triage sorts individuals to maximize the number of lives saved, and **public health triage** is the sorting or identifying of populations for priority interventions (Polivka et al., 2008). The population-based model of care used in public health practice during non-surge events needs to continue during surge events associated with public health triage.

Based on Jakeway, C., Larosa, G., Cary, A., & Schoenfisch, S. (2008). The Role of Public Health Nurses in Emergency Preparedness and Response: A Position Paper of the Association of State and Territorial Directors of Nursing. Public Health Nursing, 25(4), 353–361.

**Table 32.3  Phases of Disaster Linked to the Nursing Process**

**Examples of Each Disaster Phase Aligned with the Nursing Process**

Preparedness, response, and recovery focuses on the public health infrastructure needed to monitor the environment, assess population needs, and allocate resources in times of disaster.

| Disaster Cycle | Definition* | Assessment | Planning | Implementation | Evaluation |
|---|---|---|---|---|---|
| Preparedness | Preparedness includes prevention, protection, and mitigation.  It comprises "the capabilities necessary to avoid and/or prevent a disaster, as well as to reduce the loss of life and property by lessening the impact of disasters."  Elimination of threats before a disaster strikes. | Assess the region for populations at risk for access and functional needs during times of disaster.  Conduct a hazard vulnerability assessment for threats and hazards that pose the greatest risk. | Develop a care plan to address access and functional needs of populations during times of disaster.  Complete this assurance function in collaboration with stakeholders to address needs such as sheltering in place, evacuation, and mass casualty surge capabilities. | Conduct training, drills, and exercises related to the care of individuals, families, and communities during disasters, focusing on populations with access and functional needs in an identified region. | Evaluate the training, drills, and exercises related to the care of populations with access and functional needs in disasters, identifying gaps and remaining needs.  Evaluate operational plans for preparedness, response, and recovery for populations with access and functional needs. |
| Response | | | Collaborate with response partners to develop plans for triage algorithms that determine appropriate care and sustenance logistics for populations, based on their symptoms and co-morbid conditions (e.g., chronic disease). | Identify and place public health nurses and other support personnel to provide care according to the developed algorithms.  Ensure that logistics are in place to support community care during the crisis period.  Conduct ongoing rapid needs assessments during the response phase in order to meet population needs. | Participate in ongoing response planning during the incident (e.g., the IMS and its Planning "P").  Participate in service planning and provide real-time adjustment on the basis of real-time public health response evaluation.  Ensure needed and necessary public health nursing care. |

| Table 32.3 | Continued | | | |
|---|---|---|---|---|
| Recovery | | Work with community stakeholders to plan for any long-term health concerns following an incident, getting ahead of the curve by identifying key resources and critical care logistics. | Participate in the reconstitution of critical services and the sustainment of the health and social infrastructure.<br><br>Assist the community to find its "new normal" post-disaster. | Conduct evaluation of the long-term impact of disaster consequences on the whole community, promoting public health essential services through public health nursing. |

\*Definitions retrieved from http://www.fema.gov/mission-areas

Source: Association of Public Health Nurses. (2013). *The role of public health nurses in emergency and disaster preparedness, response, and recovery: A position paper.* (pp. 7–8). Copyright © 2014 by Association of Public Health Nurses (APHN). Used with permission of APHN. Retrieved from http://www.apha.org/NR/rdonlyres/5B42E252-FA95-4AED-AD0C-2C878633A842/0/APHN_RoleofPHNinDisasterPRR_FINALJan14.pdf

# SAFETY OF VULNERABLE/PRIORITY POPULATIONS

Nursing organizations and home health nurses (HHNs) must know the types of disasters and biological agents that could occur or be released in their community to be able to provide medical management for their clients while ensuring their own personal protection when responding to an emergency. Management must provide education and training of HHNs to understand the agency emergency preparedness plan, document skill sets of each staff member, know how to answer questions, and establish a clear communication plan in an emergency response (Sawyer, 2003).

Clients receiving home care may be ventilator dependent, so their life is threatened if an electrical failure should occur. Many clients may be hearing impaired, be unable to access a telephone due to physical limitations, and have no close support from their family members who may live out of town. The Hazard Vulnerability Analysis assessment tool can be used by HHNs to determine the level of risk to their caseload of clients by focusing on "preparation" and "prevention" (Rodriguez & Long, 2006). In the event of an emergency, HHNs are in an excellent position to provide increased surveillance of those patients who make up their caseload. After assessing the client's home environment, family, social support networks, and community partners, the HHN can develop a plan to ensure communication, protect the client from death, and reduce the impact of a disaster on those most susceptible. As participants in a community emergency, HHNs can also report any suspected evidence of a biological agent, monitor and support those individuals who are quarantined in their homes, and offer skills in health screening and administer vaccines at community sites.

In order to ensure that vulnerable and priority populations are protected in the event of an emergency or disaster, long-term care facilities and community-based support services must be integrated into local and regional disaster planning to provide for clear communication and appropriate response plans. Knowledge of the current and evolving health status of vulnerable and priority populations within a community will assist in the response and recovery outcomes for those affected by an emergency or disaster.

To date, there has been limited guidance on preparedness activities addressing at-risk populations. However, efforts are being made to provide emergency-preparedness information to at-risk populations and many innovative practices to better serve at-risk communities are being developed. The need for information exchange is significant in all phases of emergency management and particularly important in the case of vulnerable populations. Nurses play a critical role in facilitating this exchange of knowledge and information and are often the advocacy voice for at-risk and vulnerable populations. Health and social service agencies are starting to incorporate emergency-preparedness activities into their high-risk client's care plans. Information and education on the contents of a 72-hour personal or family emergency-preparedness kit is provided by nurses as part of home visiting care plans.

## CASE STUDY

In February 2007, the WHO notified that a pandemic influenza emergency had been declared in the world. The WHO confirmed that the avian influenza (H5N1) virus had killed 1 million people in Asia as a result of human-to-human transmission. The virus was spreading across Europe. It was estimated that in three months the strain would arrive in North America from Asia and Europe. The PHAC informed provincial and territorial governments that they needed to implement their pandemic plans at the provincial or territorial and community levels. Local public health units then took the lead in each community to implement pandemic plans.

### Discussion Questions

1. Determine the type of disaster in an avian influenza pandemic.

2. Describe the steps you would take to prepare for this pandemic situation.

## CONCLUSION

This chapter has outlined the types of disasters and challenges to which the nursing profession must learn to competently respond during a community disaster. It describes how the federal government works collaboratively with the provinces, territories, and individual communities from prevention to recovery of a disaster. Disaster mitigation efforts involve leadership from the PHAC; the chief public health officer; and established emergency procedures, legislation, regulations, and processes to build the current framework and legislation essential to healthcare delivery during any emergency.

Canadian nurses must develop an agenda that strengthens education in disaster nursing. An understanding of disaster training, combined with community health and public health nursing experience, and technological knowledge strengthen the role of public health nurses in emergency preparedness and response. New knowledge can be translated to action when nursing research is applied to emergency response practice, education, and health policy. CHNs play a vital role in emergency preparedness. They are key facilitators in the community mobilization process. Nurses contribute to the capacity to conduct surveillance; they educate health professionals, volunteers, and the public; they assess needs and allocate resources; they provide healthcare services; they evaluate response measures; and they make decisions about resource allocation where resources are limited (CNA, 2014).

Nurses comprise the largest group of health professionals in any given jurisdiction. A strong, effective public health workforce of CHNs must be established to meet the challenges of unpredictable threats from disaster on the community. By becoming knowledgeable and competent in emergency preparedness and disaster nursing concepts, principles, and skills, nurses can participate in healthcare policy development processes at the local community, provincial, and federal levels and within the nursing profession.

## KEY TERMS

bioterrorism    p. 580
disaster    p. 579
disaster nursing    p. 586
Emergencies Act    p. 581
emergency management    p. 581
Emergency Management Act    p. 581
Emergency Preparedness Act    p. 581
epidemic    p. 580
impact    p. 582
Incident Command System (ICS)    p. 582
Incident Management System (IMS)    p. 582
man-made disasters    p. 580
medical triage    p. 587
national emergency    p. 581
National Incident Management System (NIMS)    p. 582
natural disasters    p. 579
pandemics    p. 580
probability    p. 582
public health surge interventions    p. 587
public health triage    p. 587
surge capacity    p. 587

## STUDY QUESTIONS

1. Describe the types of disasters and their consequences.

2. What are the essential elements to respond effectively in a disaster situation?

3. Distinguish among the Emergencies Act, the Emergency Preparedness Act, and the Emergency Management Act.

4. Explain the four areas of emergency management in the life-cycle process of a disaster.

5. What expertise should nurses possess in order to respond effectively in a disaster situation?

6. List the core competencies and skills and public health services required for pandemic planning.

7. Distinguish medical triage from public health triage.

After working through these questions, go to the MyNursingLab at www.pearsoned.ca/mynursinglab to check your answers.

## INDIVIDUAL CRITICAL-THINKING EXERCISES

1. What competencies do beginning nurses require to be able to respond to mass casualty incidents?

2. What technical skills do nurses require to respond during an emergency?

3. What must CHNs do in the event of a disaster?

4. Discuss what CHNs must consider following a disaster.

5. How does the PHAC play a key role in emergency preparedness?

## GROUP CRITICAL-THINKING EXERCISES

1. A tornado has left many families without homes. Local politicians and emergency response planners have declared a disaster in the area and ordered citizens to evacuate to a shelter.

   a) Discuss what essential public health services are needed in this situation.

   b) How would nursing students assist in this emergency response?

2. What special considerations need to be given when a disaster takes place in developing countries or communities?

3. Discuss what lessons were learned from disasters such as the SARS crisis for emergency preparedness planning.

## REFERENCES

Agency for Healthcare Research and Quality. (2004). *Bioterrorism and health system preparedness: Emerging tools, methods, and strategies.* Retrieved from http://archive. ahrq.gov/news/ulp/bioteleconf

Berkowitz, B. (2002). Public health nursing practice: Aftermath of September 11, 2001. *Online Journal of Issues in Nursing, 7*(3), Manuscript 4. Retrieved from www .nursingworld.org/MainMenuCategories/ANAMarketplace/ ANAPeriodicals/OJIN/TableofContents/Volume72002/ No3Sept2002/September11PublicHealthNursing.aspx

Burkle, F. M. (2006). Population-based triage management in response to surge-capacity requirements during a large-scale bioevent disaster. *Academic Emergency Medicine: Official Journal of the Society for Academic Emergency Medicine, 13*(11), 1118–1129.

Campbell, A. (2005). *The SARS Commission second interim report: SARS and public health legislation.* Retrieved from http:// www.health.gov.on.ca/en/common/ministry/publications/ reports/campbell05/campbell05.pdf

Canadian Nurses Association. (2012). Emergency preparedness and response (Position Statement). Ottawa, ON: Author. Retrieved from https://www.cna-aiic.ca/~/media/cna/page-content/pdf-en/ ps119_emergency_preparedness_2012_e.pdf?la=en

Canadian Nurses Association. (2014). *Emergency and pandemic preparedness.* Retrieved from http://www.cna-aiic.ca/en/on-the-issues/better-health/infectious-diseases/emergency-and-pandemic-preparedness

CNN. (2013, September 20). *Japan earthquake–Tsunami fast facts.* Retrieved from http://www.cnn.com/2013/07/17/ world/asia/japan-earthquake—tsunami-fast-facts

Government of Canada. (2014). *Public Health Agency of Canada Act, S.S. 2006, c.5.* Retrieved from http://lois-laws.justice. gc.ca/PDF/P-29.5.pdf

Haddow, G. D., Bullock, J. A., & Coppola, D. (2011). *Introduction to emergency management* (4th ed.). Burlington, MA: Elsevier Inc.

Jennings-Sanders, A. (2004). Teaching disaster nursing by utilizing the Jennings Disaster Nursing Management Model. *Nurse Education in Practice, 4,* 69–76.

Kirby, M., & LeBreton, M. (2002, October). *The health of Canadians: The federal role, final report.* Vol. 6: Recommendations for Reform. The Standing Senate Committee on Social Affairs, Science and Technology. Retrieved from http:// www.parl.gc.ca/37/2/parlbus/commbus/senate/com-e/soci-e/ rep-e/repoct02vol6-e.htm

Kirby, M. (2003, November). *Reforming health protection and promotion in Canada: Time to act.* The Standing Senate Committee on Social Affairs, Science and Technology. Retrieved from http://www.parl.gc.ca/Content/SEN/Committee/372/ soci/rep/repfinnov03-e.htm

Landesman, L. Y. (2012). *Public health management of disasters: The practice guide* (3rd ed.). Washington, DC: American Public Health Association.

Ministry of Justice. (2014a). *Emergency Act. R.S.C. 1985, c. 22* (4th Supp.). Retrieved from http://laws-lois.justice.gc.ca/ PDF/E-4.5.pdf

Ministry of Justice. (2014b). *Emergency Preparedness Act,* Repealed, 2007, c15, s.13. Retrieved from http://laws. justice.gc.ca/en/showtdm/cs/E-4.6

Ministry of Justice. (2014c). *Emergency Management Act,* S.C., 2007, c.15. Retrieved from http://laws-lois.justice.gc.ca/ PDF/E-4.56.pdf

Naylor, D. (2003). *Learning from SARS: Renewal of public health in Canada: A report of the National Advisory Committee on SARS and Public Health.* Ottawa, ON: Public Health Agency of Canada. Retrieved from http://www.phac-aspc. gc.ca/publicat/sars-sras/naylor

O'Connor, D. R. (2002). *Walkerton Commission of Inquiry reports: A strategy for safe drinking water.* Toronto, ON: Ontario Ministry of the Attorney General. Retrieved from http://www. attorneygeneral.jus.gov.on.ca/english/about/pubs/walkerton/ part1/WI_Summary

Ontario Ministry of Health and Long-Term Care. (2008, revised 2014). *Ontario public health standards 2008.* Toronto, ON: Queen's Printer for Ontario. Retrieved from http:// www.health.gov.on.ca/en/pro/programs/publichealth/ oph_standards/docs/ophs_2008.pdf

Ontario Ministry of Health and Long-Term Care. (2009). *Emergency preparedness protocol.* Toronto, ON: Queen's Printer for Ontario. Retrieved from http://www.health.gov.on.ca/ english/providers/program/pubhealth/oph_standards/ophs/ progstds/protocols/ep_protocol_09.pdf

Patillo, M. M. (2003). Mass casualty disaster nursing course. *Nurse Educator, 28*(6), 271–275.

Polivka, B. J., Stanley, S. A. R., Gordon, D., Taulbee, K., Kieffer, G., & McCorkle, S. M. (2008). Public health nursing competencies for public health surge events. *Public Health Nursing, 25*(2), 159–165.

Public Health Agency of Canada. (2006). *Highlights from the Canadian pandemic influenza plan for the health sector.* Retrieved from http://www.icid.com/files/Marg_Pop_ Influenza/1_Canadian_Pandemic_Influenza_Plan_for_the_ Health_Sector.pdf

Public Health Agency of Canada. (2008). *Lessons learned: Public Health Agency of Canada's response to the 2008 listeriosis outbreak.* Retrieved from http://www.phac-aspc.gc.ca/fs-sa/ listeria/2008-lessons-lecons-eng.php

Public Health Agency of Canada. (2010). *Lessons learned review: Public Health Agency of Canada and Health Canada response to the 2009 H1N1 pandemic.* Retrieved from http://www. phac-aspc.gc.ca/about_apropos/evaluation/reports-rapports/2010-2011/h1n1/f-c-operation-eng.php

Public Health Agency of Canada. (2012). *Emergency preparedness and response.* Retrieved from http://www.phac-aspc.gc.ca/ ep-mu/index-eng.php

Public Health Agency of Canada. (2014). *Influenza.* Retrieved from http://www.phac-aspc.gc.ca/influenza/index-eng.php

Public Safety Canada. (2013a). *Canadian Disaster Database.* Ottawa, ON: Government of Canada. Retrieved from http:// cdd.publicsafety.gc.ca/rslts-eng.aspx?cultureCode=en-Ca&bou ndingBox=&provinces=1,2,3,4,5,6,7,8,9,10,11,12,13&event Types=&eventStartDate=%2719000101%27,%2720131231 %27&injured=&evacuated=&totalCost=&dead=&normalized CostYear=1

Public Safety Canada. (2013b). *Emergency management.* Retrieved from http://www.publicsafety.gc.ca/cnt/mrgnc-mngmnt/index-eng.aspx

Rebmann, T., Carrico, R., & English, J. F. (2008). Lessons public health professionals learned from past disasters. *Public Health Nursing, 25*(4), 344–352.

Rodriguez, D., & Long, C. O. (2006). Preparedness for the home healthcare nurse. *Home Healthcare Nurse, 24*(1), 21–27.

Sawyer, P. P. (2003). Bioterrorism: Are we prepared? *Home Healthcare Nurse, 21*(4), 220–223.

Veenema, T. G. (Ed.). (2013). *Disaster nursing and emergency preparedness for chemical, biological, and radiological terrorism and other hazards* (3rd ed.). New York, NY: Springer.

Weinreb, A. (2007, January 24). Defence Minister acknowledges 9/11 deaths of Canadians. *Canadian Free Press.* Retrieved from http://www.canadafreepress.com/2007/weinreb012407.htm

World Health Organization. (2007). *Working for health: An introduction to the World Health Organization.* Geneva, Switzerland: Author. Retrieved from http://www.who.int/about/brochure_en.pdf?ua=1

World Health Organization. (2014). *Emergency and essential surgical care.* Retrieved from http://www.who.int/surgery/en

## ABOUT THE AUTHORS

**Betty Schepens**, RN (St. Clair College), BScN (University of Windsor), DPA (University of Western Ontario), is the Manager of Infectious Diseases and Emergency Preparedness Programs at the Chatham-Kent Public Health Unit (Chatham, Ontario). She has experience as a classroom and clinical nursing instructor with St. Clair College. She served as the municipal representative on the Essex Kent and Lambton District Health Council. Betty is a member of the Registered Nurses' Association of Ontario (RNAO), the Ontario Association of Emergency Managers (OAEM), and the Community and Hospital Infection Control Association (CHICA). She was recognized by the Ministry of Health and Long-Term Care when asked to present best practices on community partnerships in emergency preparedness programming during the launch of the revised public health standards and protocols in 2008.

**Lucia Yiu**, RN, BScN, BA (University of Windsor), BSc (University of Toronto), MScN (University of Western Ontario), is an Associate Professor in the Faculty of Nursing at the University of Windsor, and an educational and training consultant in community nursing. She has worked overseas and served on various community and social services committees involving local and district health planning. Her practice and research include multicultural health, international health, experiential learning, community development, breast health, and program planning and evaluation. Lucia is the recipient of the 2014 Community Health Nurses of Canada Award of Merit.

## Global Health

*Aliyah Dosani and Judith Gleeson*

# CHAPTER
# 33

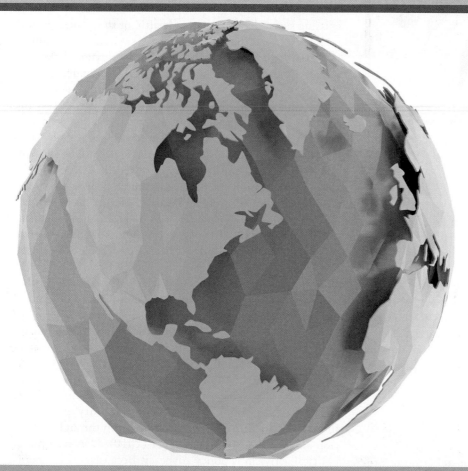

*Source: Ivan Kireiev/Shutterstock*

> *"Public health/community health nurses know that caring is a principle of social justice as well as an essential and global human need which is expressed in different ways across cultures and practice domains."*
>
> (Canadian Public Health Association, 2010)

## LEARNING OUTCOMES

**After studying this chapter, you should be able to:**

1. Describe and discuss the evolution of strategies to decrease inequities in health status globally.

2. Recognize the difference between global health, international health, and public health.

3. Critically appraise the political, cultural, and economic impacts on global health.

4. Evaluate the consequences of globalization on nursing issues, including nurse migration and global citizenship.

5. Incorporate a social justice perspective in understanding and responding to global health inequities.

6. Integrate ethical considerations when working in global health.

## INTRODUCTION

Working in an increasingly dynamic, diverse, and borderless world requires community health nurses (CHNs) to understand and address issues that may be vastly complex when working with individuals, families, groups, communities, and populations. Canada's multicultural society (see Photo 33.1) necessitates that CHNs appreciate and value various cultural and global contexts in order to work effectively and efficiently with diverse groups of people. In this chapter, we will provide an overview of

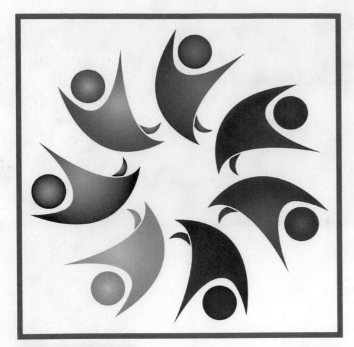

**PHOTO 33.1** In Canada, diversity is viewed as a strength

*Source: Glopphy/Fotolia*

globalization and global health from economic, political, and cultural perspectives. We will then consider some consequences of globalization for the nursing profession, specifically the role of the CHN. We will take a social justice lens when considering these issues, with a key focus on addressing health inequities. We will end this chapter by reflecting on global health ethics for CHNs who choose to work in this exciting and developing area of practice. Using the notion of global citizenship to conceptualize nursing practice, community health nursing roles and practices, local and global, will be critically examined.

# GLOBALIZATION

**Globalization** has been defined as "a constellation of processes by which nations, businesses, and people are becoming more connected and interdependent via increased economic integration, communication exchange, and cultural diffusion" (Labonte & Togerson, 2005, p. 158). These interdependent processes have far-reaching effects, and taken together, the globalization process generates unbalanced outcomes for populations both between and within countries. While there is nothing inherently good or bad about the flow of capital, labour, and knowledge around the world, questions may arise in regard to who governs this flow and who benefits from it (Navarro, 1999). Thus far, the evidence indicates that while globalization has promoted advances in technology, science, communication, and cross-national interdependencies, it has also increased wide disparities in access to the societal resources and the

opportunities they afford (Leuning, 2001; Taylor, 2009). Disparities in access have given rise to much discussion and debate regarding the implications of globalization for health and health for all.

There is strong evidence indicating that most of the **global burden of disease** and, more specifically, health inequalities are caused by social determinants of health (Labonte & Torgerson, 2005). The Bangkok Charter of the World Health Organization [WHO] (2005) identifies the global factors affecting health as (a) increasing inequalities within and between countries, (b) new patterns of consumption and communication, (c) commercialization, (d) global environmental change, and (e) urbanization. These factors compound the negative effects of the already existing social determinants of health, or those social factors influencing health such as income, shelter, peace, education, and food access. Globalization can be viewed through various lenses including social, political, economic, and cultural (Steger, 2013). This is significant because one of the core competencies for public health nurses is to assess the impact of the broad social, cultural, political, and economic determinants of health (Community Health Nurses of Canada, 2009). More specifically, CHNs need to be aware of power in relationships, giving voice to vulnerable populations, in this case working with resource-poor populations, within the context of global health. Refer to Table 33.1 for an overview of key characteristics of global health education. Villeneuve (2008) appealed to nurses globally to give priority to eliminating disparities. For Villeneuve (2008), this is the core goal of nursing for the 21st century. In addition, the Canadian Nurses Association (CNA) believes that reducing health inequities globally is a nursing obligation (2012). One of the ways this can be achieved is through nurses' involvement in **political activism** (Falk-Rafael, 2006). Clearly, one of the roles of CHNs in Canada is activism. The Canadian Public Health Association (CPHA) delineates advocacy in terms of activities of CHNs, including using collaborative approaches, advocating for change, and showing a strong commitment to **equity** and **social justice** by speaking out for equity in health through legislation and policy-making activities (2010). One example of political activism is policy advocacy. Because health inequities ultimately result from the attitudes, beliefs, and actions of those who are not experiencing inequities (yet have the power to change conditions), it is important for nurses to engage with the public and advocate in order for their perspective to be heard when setting the policy agenda (Reutter & Kushner, 2010).

# GLOBAL HEALTH—WHAT IS IT?

As we increasingly witness events of global concern, including emerging infectious diseases, pandemics, bioterrorism, and migration of health professionals, the role of various healthcare professionals must be revisited. The traditionally national focus of the health sector urgently needs to make

| Table 33.1 | Key Characteristics of Global Health Education | | |
|---|---|---|---|
| **Category** | **Characteristics** */**/† | **Implication** | **Rationale** |
| **Object** | Focuses on social, economic, political, and cultural forces which influence health across the world* | Learning opportunities in "global health" focus on the underlying structural determinants of health | To ensure that educational interventions cover the social, economic, political and cultural aetiology of ill health, and not merely its disease-oriented symptoms on a global level |
| | Concerned with the needs of developing countries; with health issues that transcend national boundaries; and with the impact of globalisation* | Learning opportunities in "global health" link territorial up to supraterritorial dimensions of underlying structural determinants of health | To ensure that educational interventions clarify the links between territorial health situations (either domestic ones and/or situations in other countries) and their underlying transborder and global determinants |
| **Orientation** | Toward "health for all"**/† | Learning opportunities in "global health" should adopt and impart the ethical and practical aspects of achieving "health for all" | To ensure that educational interventions are relevant to people's needs on community, local, national, international, and global levels. |
| | Toward health equity**/† | Learning opportunities in "global health" should emphasise issues of health equity (or health inequity) within and across countries | To ensure that educational interventions orientate on the challenge of achieving health equity worldwide |
| **Outcome** | Identification of actions | Learning opportunities in "global health" facilitate the identification of actions (by the student) undertaken to resolve problems either top-down or—more importantly—bottom-up | To ensure that educational interventions foster critical thinking and present options for professional engagement on different dimensions towards "health for all" and health equity |
| **Methodology** | Cross-disciplinarity* | Learning opportunities in "global health" involve educators and/or students from various disciplines and professions | To ensure that educational interventions lead to an understanding of influences on health beyond the bio-medical paradigm and respect the importance of sectors other than the health sector in improving health |
| | Bottom-up learning and problem-orientation | Learning-opportunities in "global health" require unconventional methods for teaching and learning | To ensure that educational interventions clarify the relevance for the health workforce to deal with transborder and/or global determinants of health |

Deduced from: *Rowson et al (2007) cited in [29]; **Koplan et al (2009) [35]; †WHO (1984, 1995, 2005) [38-40]

Source: Bozorgmehr, K., Saint, V. A., & Tinnemann, P. (2011). The "global health" education framework: A conceptual guide for monitoring, evaluation and practice. *Globalization and Health, 7,* 8.

greater shifts in order to provide health services across borders and to remote regions within countries in equitable ways. While many definitions of global health exist, Koplan et al. (2009) provide a comprehensive explanation of the differences between global health, international health, and public health. Koplan et al. (2009) characterize **global health** as an area for study, research, and practice that places a priority on improving health and achieving equity for all people worldwide (see Table 33.2). Areas of healthcare that are often identified as explicitly associated with understanding and addressing the effects of globalization on health are public health, international health, and global health. While distinctions are made between these terms (which has implications for understanding the unique

| Table 33.2 | Comparison of Global Health, International Health, and Public Health | | |
|---|---|---|---|
| | **Global Health** | **International Health** | **Public Health** |
| Geographical reach | Focuses on issues that directly affect health but that can transcend national boundaries | Focuses on health issues of countries other than one's own, especially those of low income and middle income | Focuses on issues that affect the health of the population of a particular community or country |
| Level of co-operation | Development and implementation of solutions often requires global co-operation | Development and implementation of solutions usually requires bi-national co-operation | Development and implementation of solutions do not usually require global co-operation |
| Individuals or populations | Embraces both prevention in populations and clinical care of individuals | Embraces both prevention in populations and clinical care of individuals | Mainly focused on prevention programs for populations |
| Access to health | Health equity among nations and for all people is a major objective | Seeks to help people of other nations | Health equity within a nation or community is a major objective |
| Range of discipline | Highly interdisciplinary and multidisciplinary within and beyond health sciences | Embraces a few disciplines but has not emphasized multidisciplinary | Encourages multidisciplinary approaches, particularly within health sciences and social sciences |

Source: Koplan, J. P., Bond, T. C., Merson, M. H., Reddy, K. S., Rodriguez, M. H., Sewankambo, N. K., & Wasserheit, J. N. (2009). Towards a common definition of global health. *The Lancet, 373,* 1993–1995. Used by permission of Elsevier Inc. – Health Sciences Division.

primary objectives of each), public, international, and global health share a common concern for preventing disease and promoting health for communities and whole populations. The distinctions exist in terms of geographical considerations and how people and organizations work together. The WHO Commission on Social Determinants of Health (CSDH) brought together a global evidence base indicating that obvious health inequities exist between continents, between countries, and within countries (WHO, 2008) (see Canadian Research Box 33.1). Reducing these inequities in health requires attention to the social determinants of health (Friel & Marmot, 2011).

### CANADIAN RESEARCH BOX 33.1

**Is it easier to learn about community health nursing if you are placed in a different country?**

Mawji, A., Lind, C., Loewen, S., Underwood, M., & Thompson-Isherwood, R. (2014). "Slapped in the face with it": Internalizing community health concepts from an international practice setting. *International Journal of Applied Science and Technology, 4*(2), 29–36.

In 2011, a group of eight nursing students from the University of Calgary, Canada, travelled to the Dominican Republic (DR) to complete their practice component in community health nursing. Students spent 12 days immersed in a local culture learning to integrate and apply community health concepts in partnership with a community. The authors carried out an exploratory study using a descriptive, qualitative approach in order to answer the broad research question, "What is nursing students' personal and professional learning when engaged in community health community health practice in a resource-poor country?"

The results were grouped into four themes: social justice, relationships, asset-based community development, and personal transformation. In the social-justice domain, the main issues identified by the students were extreme poverty, racial discrimination, and gender inequality. In the area of relationships, students identified the relational culture they witnessed in the DR as a huge strength for the community. Their experience also helped the students to develop a real understanding of the value of asset-based community development. One student said, "I learned that addressing health issues within a community starts with the people themselves . . . we were there to provide guidance, help where needed, but mainly it is the community itself [that creates the change]" (p. 32). For many of the students, the chance to experience a community health placement in a global context was personally and professionally transformative. Furthermore, the students who completed their community health placement in the DR gained a comprehensive understanding of a number of foundational concepts of community health and showed subsequent transferability of their knowledge to other practice settings.

### Discussion Questions

1. Can you think of the context you were brought up in (Canadian or otherwise) where you witnessed similar community-based social injustice?

2. Based on your answer to question 1 above, and knowing what you do now about community health nursing, are there ways in which a community health nurse could have intervened?

3. When you read about the community health learning that took place in DR, think about whether or not you would have been willing to be placed in a different country context.

# THE EVOLUTION OF GLOBAL HEALTH EQUITY POLICY

## Health for All Movement

As discussed in Chapter 8, in 1978, WHO member states convened for an international conference on primary health care in Alma-Ata, USSR (now Almaty, Kazakhstan). The outcome was the **Declaration of Alma-Ata**, which expressed "the need for urgent action by all governments, all health and development workers, and the world community to protect and promote the health of all the people of the world" (WHO, 1978, p. 1). The declaration led to the formation of the Health for All movement, which pledged that health could be achieved for all by the year 2000. While the original goal is yet to be achieved, the Health for All strategy set an important direction for health equity policy and health programming.

## Millennium Development Goals

In September 2000, after a series of United Nations conferences and summits, world leaders convened at United Nations Headquarters in New York to accept the United Nations Millennium Declaration. This led to global partnership to address the **Millennium Development Goals (MDGs)** and identify specific health-related targets to be achieved by 2015. The eight goals are as follows:

1. eradicate extreme hunger and poverty;
2. achieve universal primary education;
3. promote gender equality and empower women;
4. reduce child mortality;
5. improve maternal health;
6. combat HIV/AIDS, malaria, and other diseases;
7. ensure environmental sustainability; and
8. develop a global partnership for development (United Nations, 2000).

The MDGs provide a framework of time-bound goals and targets through which progress can be measured, using a baseline of 1990 (United Nations, 2000). Table 33.3 presents an evaluation of progress toward meeting selected targets from information available as of June 2013. The latest available data for most indicators refer to 2011 to 2013. While many targets have been met, or are expected to have been met by 2015, others demonstrate that progress is insufficient to reach the target if prevailing trends persist, or that there has been no progress or even, in some cases, a deterioration. In a few countries, there has been insufficient data available to evaluate progress made to date.

In 2010 a United Nations summit on the MDGs took place in New York from September 20 to 22. This summit concluded with the adoption of a global action plan to achieve the eight anti-poverty goals by their 2015 target date. However, various challenges were apparent, including persistent inequalities; food and nutrition insecurity; knowledge challenges; growing environmental footprints; conflict, violence, and insecurity;

governance deficits at all levels; and shifting demographics (e.g., migration, urbanization, and aging). This pointed to a critical need to find new approaches to promote global health equity. This new approach led to the initiation of the Sustainable Development Goals (United Nations System Task Team on the Post- 2015 UN Development Agenda, 2012).

## Sustainable Development Goals

The outcome document of the 2010 MDG Summit (United Nations Secretary-General, 2010) requested the Secretary-General to initiate thinking on the global development agenda beyond 2015. This ultimately led to discussions at the 2012 Rio+20 Conference to devise a roadmap to move forward with the MDG agenda. The outcome document of the 2012 Rio+20 Conference on Sustainable Development instigated an inclusive process to develop a set of **Sustainable Development Goals**. The process of arriving at this new framework is member state–led, with broad participation from external stakeholders, such as civil society organizations, the private sector and businesses, and academia and scientists (United Nations Sustainable Development Solutions Network, 2013). The Sustainable Development Solutions Network (SDSN) has established 12 thematic groups that are *solution oriented* rather than research oriented. The goal is to stimulate governments, UN agencies, and the public toward discovery of practical solutions to the greatest challenges of sustainable development. The 12 thematic areas are:

1. macroeconomics, population dynamics, and planetary boundaries;
2. reducing poverty and building peace in fragile regions;
3. challenges of social inclusion: gender, inequalities, and human rights;
4. early childhood development, education, and transition to work;
5. health for all;
6. low-carbon energy and sustainable industry;
7. sustainable agriculture and food systems;
8. forests, oceans, biodiversity, and ecosystem services;
9. sustainable cities: inclusive, resilient, and connected;
10. good governance of extractive and land resources;
11. global governance and norms for sustainable development; and
12. redefining the role of business for sustainable development (United Nations Sustainable Development Solutions Network, 2013).

Seventeen Sustainable Development Goals have been developed from these 12 thematic areas and are listed below. Martens, Akin, Maud, and Mohsin (2012) recognize the importance of these diverse impacts of globalization on health. Furthermore, it is important to note that global health is inextricably linked to globalization, suggesting a focus on both global interdependence in health and how economic, environmental, political, and social processes—on a worldwide scale—affect people's health (Rowson et al., 2012).

**Table 33.3**  Evaluation of Progress toward Millennium Development Goals

| Goals and Targets | Africa | | Asia | | | | Oceania | Latin America & the Caribbean | Caucasus & Central Asia |
|---|---|---|---|---|---|---|---|---|---|
| | Northern | Sub-Saharan | Eastern | South-Eastern | Southern | Western | | | |
| **GOAL 1 | Eradicate extreme poverty and hunger** | | | | | | | | | |
| Reduce extreme poverty by half | low poverty | very high poverty | moderate poverty* | moderate poverty | very high poverty | low poverty | very high poverty | low poverty | low poverty |
| Productive and decent employment | large deficit in decent work | very large deficit in decent work | large deficit in decent work | large deficit in decent work | very large deficit in decent work | large deficit in decent work | very large deficit in decent work | moderate deficit in decent work | moderate deficit in decent work |
| Reduce hunger by half | low hunger | very high hunger | moderate hunger | moderate hunger | high hunger | moderate hunger | moderate hunger | moderate hunger | moderate hunger |
| **GOAL 2 | Achieve universal primary education** | | | | | | | | | |
| Universal primary schooling | high enrolment | moderate enrolment | high enrolment | high enrolment | high enrolment | high enrolment | — | high enrolment | high enrolment |
| **GOAL 3 | Promote gender equality and empower women** | | | | | | | | | |
| Equal girls' enrolment in primary school | close to parity | close to parity | close to parity | parity | parity | close to parity | close to parity | parity | parity |
| Women's share of paid employment | low share | medium share | high share | medium share | low share | low share | medium share | high share | high share |
| Women's equal representation in national parliaments | low representation | moderate representation | moderate representation | low representation | low representation | low representation | very low representation | moderate representation | low representation |
| **GOAL 4 | Reduce child mortality** | | | | | | | | | |
| Reduce mortality of under-five-year-olds by two-thirds | low mortality | high mortality | low mortality | low mortality | moderate mortality | low mortality | moderate mortality | low mortality | moderate mortality |

## Table 33.3　Continued

| Goals and Targets | Africa | | Asia | | | | Oceania | Latin America & the Caribbean | Caucasus & Central Asia |
| --- | --- | --- | --- | --- | --- | --- | --- | --- | --- |
| | Northern | Sub-Saharan | Eastern | South-Eastern | Southern | Western | | | |
| **GOAL 5 | Improve maternal health** | | | | | | | | | |
| Reduce maternal mortality by three-quarters | low mortality | very high mortality | low mortality | moderate mortality | high mortality | low mortality | high mortality | low mortality | low mortality |
| Access to reproductive health | moderate access | low access | high access | moderate access | moderate access | moderate access | low access | high access | moderate access |
| **GOAL 6 | Combat HIV/AIDS, malaria, and other diseases** | | | | | | | | | |
| Halt and begin to reverse the spread of HIV/AIDS | low incidence | high incidence | low incidence | low incidence | low incidence | low incidence | low incidence | low incidence | intermediate incidence |
| Halt and reverse the spread of tuberculosis | low mortality | moderate mortality | low mortality | moderate mortality | moderate mortality | low mortality | high mortality | low mortality | moderate mortality |
| **GOAL 7 | Ensure environmental sustainability** | | | | | | | | | |
| Halve proportion of population without improved drinking water | high coverage | low coverage | high coverage | moderate coverage | high coverage | high coverage | low coverage | high coverage | moderate coverage |
| Halve proportion of population without sanitation | high coverage | very low coverage | low coverage | low coverage | very low coverage | moderate coverage | very low coverage | moderate coverage | high coverage |
| Improve the lives of slum-dwellers | moderate proportion of slum-dwellers | very high proportion of slum-dwellers | moderate proportion of slum-dwellers | high proportion of slum-dwellers | high proportion of slum-dwellers | moderate proportion of slum-dwellers | moderate proportion of slum-dwellers | moderate proportion of slum-dwellers | — |
| **GOAL 8 | Develop a global partnership for development** | | | | | | | | | |
| Internet users | high usage | moderate usage | high usage | high usage | moderate usage | high usage | low usage | high usage | high usage |

Source: United Nations, based on data and estimates provided by: Food and Agriculture Organization of the United Nations; Inter-Parliamentary Union; International Telecommunication Union; UNAIDS; UNESCO; UN-Habitat; UNICEF; UN Population Division; World Bank; World Health Organization – based on statistics available as of June 2013. Compiled by Statistics Division, Department of Economic and Social Affairs, United Nations. Used with permission of United Nations. http://www.un.org/millenniumgoals/pdf/report-2013/2013_progress_english.pdf

**17 Sustainable Development Goals**

- Goal 1. End poverty in all its forms everywhere.
- Goal 2. End hunger, achieve food security and improved nutrition, and promote sustainable agriculture.
- Goal 3. Ensure healthy lives and promote well-being for all, at all ages.
- Goal 4. Ensure inclusive and equitable quality education and promote lifelong learning opportunities for all.
- Goal 5. Achieve gender equality and empower all women and girls.
- Goal 6. Ensure availability and sustainable management of water and sanitation for all.
- Goal 7. Ensure access to affordable, reliable, sustainable, and modern energy for all.
- Goal 8. Promote sustained, inclusive, and sustainable economic growth; full and productive employment; and decent work for all.
- Goal 9. Build resilient infrastructure, promote inclusive and sustainable industrialization, and foster innovation.
- Goal 10. Reduce inequality within and among countries.
- Goal 11. Make cities and human settlements inclusive, safe, resilient, and sustainable.
- Goal 12. Ensure sustainable consumption and production patterns.
- Goal 13. Take urgent action to combat climate change and its impacts (acknowledging that the United Nations Framework Convention on Climate Change is the primary international, intergovernmental forum for negotiating the global response to climate change).
- Goal 14. Conserve and sustainably use the oceans, seas, and marine resources for sustainable development.
- Goal 15. Protect, restore, and promote sustainable use of terrestrial ecosystems; sustainably manage forests; combat desertification; and halt and reverse land degradation, and halt biodiversity loss.
- Goal 16. Promote peaceful and inclusive societies for sustainable development; provide access to justice for all; and build effective, accountable, and inclusive institutions at all levels.
- Goal 17. Strengthen the means of implementation and revitalize the global partnership for sustainable development (United Nations, 2014).

# GLOBALIZATION, GLOBAL HEALTH, AND ECONOMICS

In the economic and social domains, nurses need to develop an understanding of the global economy, including the effects of the spread of neo-liberal economic policies on equity and health (see Photo 33.2). Neo-liberalism is a political and economic ideology that privileges the free market economy and promotes the "rolling back" of the state. This results in less government intervention, increased privatization of services, limited universal social protection programs, and a promotion of individual rather than collective responsibility for health (Raphael, Curry-Stevens, & Bryant, 2008). As a result of globalization, the link between trade and health must be addressed on a global scale (see Photo 33.3). This is because as we become more integrated as a world, it becomes more important to consider different policy areas together. The **World Health Organization (WHO)** and the **World Trade Organization (WTO)** came together to evaluate the implications of global trade agreements on health. Five key trade agreements were identified to have relevance for health:

1. the General Agreements on Tariffs and Trade (GATT);
2. the Agreement on the Application of Sanitary and Phytosanitary Measures (SPS);
3. the Trade Agreement on Technical Barriers to Trade (TBT);
4. Trade-Related Aspects of Intellectual Property Rights (TRIPS); and
5. the General Agreement on Trade in Services (GATS).

These trade agreements were found to have an impact on the following global health issues: infectious disease control, food safety, tobacco control, environment, access to drugs, access and provision of health services, and food security (WTO & WHO, 2002). Additional issues, such as biotechnology, information technology, and traditional knowledge were also considered. One example under the GATS impacts health services in the form of nurse migration.

## Nurse Migration

Globalization has had far-reaching effects in terms of the nursing workforce as evidenced by the migration of nurses from majority world countries to minority world countries (Dwyer, 2007; Kingma, 2006; McElmurry et al., 2006). This movement of nurses from already resource-constrained countries is contrary to primary health care equity and inconsistent with the "Health for All" principles. Health worker migration and international recruitment have a very particular significance to **primary health care (PHC)**. The World Health Report in 2006 estimated that the world lacks about 4 million health workers if a minimum level of health outcomes is to be achieved, significantly hindering the attainment of the health-related MDGs (Painter, 2000).

For the past several decades, international recruiting has been a strategy to relieve nurse shortages in recipient countries. This takes nurses away from where they are needed the most (from their source countries) and may mask problems in recipient countries (Bach, 2003; Tejada de Rivero, 2003). McElmurry et al. (2006) argue that in order to satisfy the philosophical approaches to PHC (see Chapter 8), nurse migration needs to (1) leave majority world countries enhanced rather than depleted, (2) contribute to country health outcomes consistent with essential care for all people, (3) be based on community participation, (4) address common nursing labour issues, and (5) involve equitable and clear financial arrangements. Managing nurse migration will facilitate the achievement of health equity in primary health care.

The nursing labour force is a commodity operating within a capitalist world economy (Herdman, 2004), with the

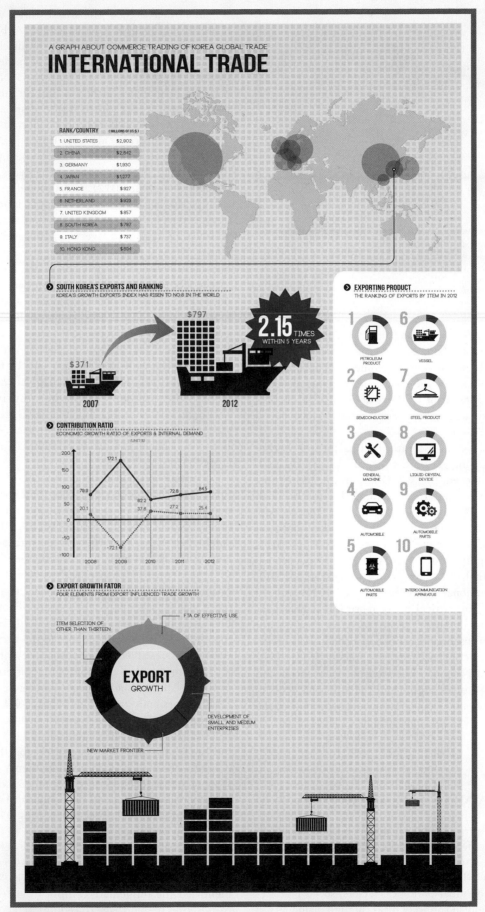

A GRAPH ABOUT COMMERCE TRADING OF KOREA GLOBAL TRADE

# INTERNATIONAL TRADE

| RANK/COUNTRY | (MILLIONS OF US $) |
|---|---|
| 1. UNITED STATES | $2,902 |
| 2. CHINA | $2,842 |
| 3. GERMANY | $1,930 |
| 4. JAPAN | $1,277 |
| 5. FRANCE | $927 |
| 6. NETHERLAND | $923 |
| 7. UNITED KINGDOM | $857 |
| 8. SOUTH KOREA | $797 |
| 9. ITALY | $737 |
| 10. HONG KONG | $694 |

**SOUTH KOREA'S EXPORTS AND RANKING**
KOREA'S GROWTH EXPORTS INDEX HAS RISEN TO NO.8 IN THE WORLD

$371 — 2007

$797 — 2012

**2.15 TIMES WITHIN 5 YEARS**

**EXPORTING PRODUCT**
THE RANKING OF EXPORTS BY ITEM IN 2012

1 PETROLEUM PRODUCT
2 SEMICONDUCTOR
3 GENERAL MACHINE
4 AUTOMOBILE
5 AUTOMOBILE PARTS
6 VESSEL
7 STEEL PRODUCT
8 LIQUID CRYSTAL DEVICE
9 AUTOMOBILE PARTS
10 INTERCOMMUNICATION APPARATUS

**CONTRIBUTION RATIO**
ECONOMIC GROWTH RATIO OF EXPORTS & INTERNAL DEMAND
(UNIT:%)

79.9 — 172.1 — 62.2 — 72.8 — 84.5
20.1 — -72.1 — 37.8 — 27.2 — 25.4

2008 2009 2010 2011 2012

**EXPORT GROWTH FATOR**
FOUR ELEMENTS FROM EXPORT INFLUENCED TRADE GROWTH

ITEM SELECTION OF OTHER THAN THIRTEEN

FTA OF EFFECTIVE USE

**EXPORT GROWTH**

DEVELOPMENT OF SMALL AND MEDIUM ENTERPRISES

NEW MARKET FRONTIER

PHOTO 33.2 Economics has a direct impact on health

*Source: Getfile/Shutterstock*

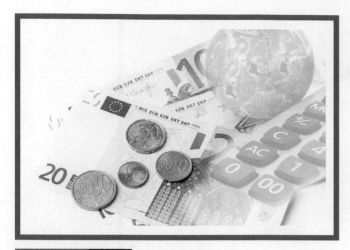

**PHOTO 33.3** Nurses need to understand the link between health and trade on a global scale

*Source: Pimpic/Shutterstock*

potential to become exploited and oppressed in an environment in which the focus has been on economic factors rather than on the social and cultural outcomes of globalization. Hence, any examination of the social determinants of health requires critical appraisal of issues related to social justice, human rights, and sustainability on local and global levels (Allen & Ogilvie, 2004).

Since the debates about international health worker recruitment and its impact on the health system have been increasingly pronounced, the WHO has been working on a Code of Practice on the International Recruitment of Health Personnel. Workforce migration is a complex and multi-dimensional global health challenge and a number of issues, including international recruitment practices, mutuality of employment benefits, and national health workforce sustainability, are being discussed (WHO, 2010). The International Council of Nurses (ICN) issued a position statement on ethical nurse recruitment that condemns recruitment of nurses from countries that do not have sound human resource planning and denounces unethical recruitment practices that exploit nurses (ICN, 2007; ICN, 2008). The ICN's position statement on retention and migration respects nurses' rights and the potential benefits of migration but identifies migration as a symptom of the problem of dysfunctional health systems.

# GLOBALIZATION, GLOBAL HEALTH, AND CULTURE

**Culture** is "the learned, shared, and transmitted values, beliefs, norms, and life ways of a particular culture that guides thinking, decisions, and actions in patterned ways and often intergenerationally" (Leininger 2006, p. 13). Aspects of culture (including individual biological factors, social practices and rules, and the global spread of ideas through dialogue) can affect health.

In an increasingly globalized world, we need to understand other cultures. This is reinforced by one of the core competencies for community health nurses, which indicates that nurses should demonstrate skill in dealing with diversity and high levels of ambiguity (CHNC, 2009). When working in global health, two important concepts for the nurse to consider are **cultural pluralism** and **cultural relativism** (Johnson, 2007). Cultural pluralism involves valuing and honouring all cultures equally. Taking this perspective encourages CHNs to be open-minded and respect others' beliefs, values, behaviours, and ways of life (Racher & Annis, 2012). Cultural relativism is a related concept that also encourages an appreciation of cultural differences but, furthermore, "rejects assumptions of superiority of one's culture and averts ethnocentrism" (Racher & Annis, 2012, p. 159). Cultural relativism involves respecting culture and honouring diversity and it supports the idea of a "cultural mosaic" as seen in Canada. CHNs practising in global health contexts may encounter various cultural practices that have implications for health. For example, skin lightening is practised in various countries including the Middle East, Asia, and Latin America (Peregrino, Moreno, Miranda, Rubio, & Leal, 2011), female infanticide in India (Mittal, Khanna, Khanagwal, & Paliwal, 2013), widow shunning and widow burning in India (Mastey, 2009), and child brides in Ethiopia (Gage, 2013). Another example of a cultural practice that has health implications is that of female genital mutilation (FGM), which is discussed next.

**Female genital mutilation (FGM)** encompasses all procedures that involve partial or total removal of the external female genitalia or other injury to the female genital organs for non-medical reasons (WHO, 2013a). It is usually conducted on young girls between infancy and 15 years of age. While this is widely practised around the world, it has no health benefits for girls and women. In Africa alone, an estimated 101 million girls have had this procedure done, often against their will. As a result, FGM is considered a human rights violation by many (WHO, 2013a). Approximately 140 million females around the world are living with the health consequences of FGM at present.

Due to increased globalization, registered nurses working in the global health arena may find themselves working with communities and populations where FGM is prevalent. One way in which registered nurses can unpack this complex cultural practice and its consequences for health is to use the public health nursing discipline-specific competencies (CHNC, 2009). For example, competency 2.7 involves supporting individuals, families, groups, and communities to identify risks to health and make informed choices about protective and preventive health measures. This can be accomplished by communicating such risks to health. (For more details on risk communication, please refer to Chapter 8.) These can be communicated by discussing both immediate and long-term consequences of FGM. The WHO (2013a) has identified the immediate complications to include "severe pain, shock, haemorrhage (bleeding), tetanus or sepsis (bacterial infection), urine retention, open sores in the genital region, and injury to nearby genital tissue." Long-term consequences may include recurrent bladder and urinary tract infections, infertility, increased risk of childbirth complication and newborn deaths, and the possibility of later corrective surgeries (WHO, 2013a). Once risks have been identified and discussed, the nurse may facilitate a discussion on the role of power dynamics in relationships and help women to find a voice to resist others' imposing this practice on them (competency 2.7—"describe the role of power in relationships by giving voice to the vulnerable").

Since FGM has been recognized as a human rights issue (WHO, 2013a), this presents registered nurses with an opportunity to "recognize opportunities to promote social justice" (competency 2.9, CHNC, 2009). While helping girls and women find a voice to resist this practice can be viewed as a way to promote social justice, registered nurses also need to be cognizant of possible negative outcomes of women speaking out. For example, women who have spoken out have been stigmatized in many ways. First, they may be stigmatized by healthcare professionals simply for being from a non-Western culture. Second, they may be stigmatized because Western discourse has identified FGM as harmful. And finally, by speaking out they may be viewed as betraying their own culture (Khaja, Lay, & Boys, 2010). Despite the fact that the practice of FGM is distasteful to Western cultures, registered nurses need to be mindful that FGM is a valued and accepted societal norm in many cultures around the world (Goldenstein, 2013). This implies the need to incorporate concepts related to cultural safety and cultural relativism, and to discuss issues relating to FGM with sensitivity. This is significant in order to establish and maintain good working relationships and to promote a culture of reciprocity and learning from each other without judgment.

# GLOBALIZATION, GLOBAL HEALTH, AND POLITICS

In order to influence the policy agenda, nurses need to develop their understanding of how power structures influence the policy process, identify key stakeholders in the policy process, build credibility with the stakeholders, and understand that policy development can be a lengthy process (CNA, 2009). Specific skills that nurses need to develop in order to engage politically include lobbying, working with the media, and writing policy briefs. Increasingly, nurse educators are arguing for the development of curricula that address skill development in such areas (Carnegie & Kiger, 2009; Reutter & Kushner, 2010). Please refer to Figure 33.1 for an illustrative depiction of this process. Using FGM as an example, nurses can enact competency 3A.8, to "advocate for the reduction of inequities in health through legislative and policy-making activities" (CHNC, 2009). The first step in meeting this competency is to be aware of current political developments on this particular issue. This has included a statement in 2008 by the WHO and UN organizations pledging to eliminate FGM, a 2010 WHO global strategy to

stop healthcare providers from engaging in any act of FGM, and a United Nations resolution in 2012 to eliminate FGM worldwide (WHO, 2013a). Specific to Canada, registered nurses need to be aware of article 268 of the Canadian Criminal Code, which states that a parent who performs FGM on their child may be charged with aggravated assault. In the instance that the parent agrees to have FGM performed by another party, the parent can still be convicted as a party to the offence. Furthermore, under section 273.3, it is a crime to remove a child under the age of 18 from Canada in order to perform FGM (Government of Canada, 2013).

The second step is for registered nurses to engage in the issue through advocacy, policy making, and awareness-building activities. For example, registered nurses may engage in the WHO (2013a) efforts to eliminate FGM in multiple ways. First, registered nurses can engage in building evidence so that the knowledge generated can help build effective policy around FGM. This can include evidence about how to effectively eliminate FGM and how to care for those who have experienced FGM. This is in line with the CNA code of ethics in terms of promoting justice, promoting health and well-being, and preserving dignity (2008). Second, registered nurses can play a role in strengthening the health sector response by being aware of agency guidelines and policies when working with women who have undergone FGM. This includes preparing oneself through education to provide safe, compassionate, competent, and ethical care (CNA, 2008). Finally, registered nurses can increase their role in advocacy by contributing to the development of publications and advocacy tools for local, regional, and global efforts to end FGM (WHO, 2013a). This often entails working across sectors and disciplines including health, education, finance, justice, and women's affairs (WHO, 2013a). Engaging in this type of work will assist in decreasing the inequity between the health status of men and women in countries where FGM is being practised as well as decreasing the inequities in health status that are observed between Western and non-Western countries.

As a result of globalization, we need to be aware of any potential cultural consequences. Holton (2000) offers three perspectives concerning globalization's impact on culture. First, the concept of **homogenization** suggests that global culture is becoming standardized around a Western or American pattern. This is sometimes called the "McDonaldization" of culture. Second, the **polarization** perspective proposes that global cultures are becoming increasingly dichotomized around Western and non-Western ways of life. Sometimes Western cultures are described as individualistic, or cold, and non-Western cultures are viewed as community-centred, or warm (Lanier, 2000). The third view point is that of **hybridization**, where intercultural exchange occurs. This exchange offers opportunities for cultural elements from a variety of sources to merge and form an amalgamated culture. Nurses working in global health need to be aware of the ways in which globalization has affected and continues to affect culture. This understanding will enhance culturally safe care and promote equity in health among diverse cultural groups.

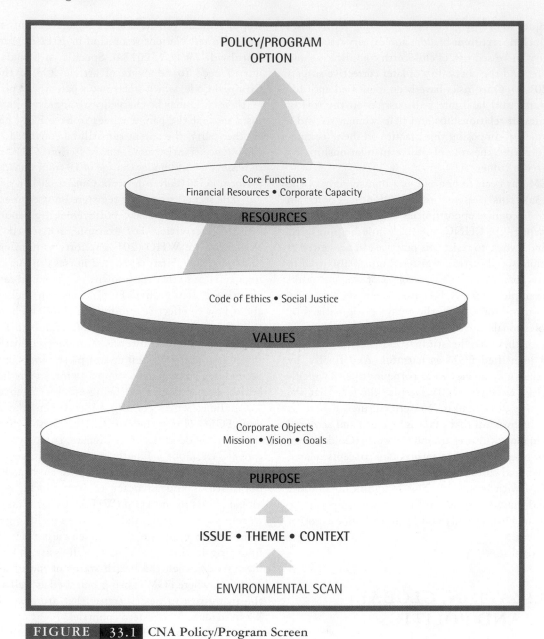

**POLICY/PROGRAM OPTION**

Core Functions
Financial Resources • Corporate Capacity

**RESOURCES**

Code of Ethics • Social Justice

**VALUES**

Corporate Objects
Mission • Vision • Goals

**PURPOSE**

**ISSUE • THEME • CONTEXT**

**ENVIRONMENTAL SCAN**

**FIGURE 33.1** CNA Policy/Program Screen

*Source:* Canadian Nurses Association. (2010). *Social justice: A means to an end . . . an end in itself* (2nd ed.). Ottawa: Author. Reprinted with permission. Further reproduction prohibited.

# GLOBALIZATION OF NURSING AND GLOBAL CITIZENSHIP

Due to increased globalization, nurses need to be educated as global citizens who have a moral responsibility and professional competency to care and promote health beyond their local communities and national institutions (Chavez, Peter, & Gastaldo, 2008). The new global interdependence calls for all people across the globe to extend their thinking about moral responsibility and health beyond their local communities and national citizenship to become citizens of the world (Crigger, Branningan, & Barid, 2006). Nussbaum (1997) describes three necessary capacities for the cultivation of global citizenship. The first is the capacity to examine ourselves and our traditions critically, which is known as **reflexivity**, and it involves scrutinizing our beliefs, traditions, and habits to ensure that they are consistent and justifiable. Specific to nursing, Crigger et al. (2006) suggest that **global citizenship** begins in nursing training when nursing students become sensitized to their own culturally established perspectives on healthcare. These nursing students become capable of identifying and challenging underlying values and assumptions of their nursing education and practice, as well as of the healthcare system. The work highlighted in Canadian Research Box 33.2 is a good example of global citizenship.

**CANADIAN RESEARCH BOX 33.2**

**What is the contribution of maternal perinatal distress on preterm birth and infant survival and mother–infant interaction?**

Premji, S., on behalf of MiGHT—Maternal Infant Global Health Team (Global Collaborators in Research) (in alphabetical order): Ms. Dorcas Akoya Amunga, Ms. Dorcus Asmai, Dr. Susan Dahinten, Dr. Farooq Ghani, Dr. Saleem Iqbal, Dr. Imtiaz Jehan, Dr. Zeenatkhanu Kanji, Mr. Adam King, Dr. Nicole Letourneau, Dr. Aliyah Mawji, Dr. Alliya Mohamed, Dr. Joseph Wangira Musana, Dr. Haider Ali Naqvi, Dr. Christopher T. Naugler, Ms. Christine Omukani Okoko, Dr. M. Sarah Rose, Dr. Pauline Samia, Ms. Kiran Shaikh, Ms. Rozina Shazad, Ms. Salima Sulaiman, Ms. Rose Swai, Mr. Josephat Wambua, Dr. Saba Wasim. (2014). Allostatic load as a framework to examine the effect of perinatal distress on preterm birth and infant health with emphasis on low- and middle-income countries. *Maternal and Child Health Journal, 18*(4), 15. doi:10.1007/s10995-014-1479-y

The authors of this article undertook an interpretive review of the literature in order to determine the impact that perinatal distress has on preterm birth in pregnant women in low- and middle-income countries (LMIC). A conceptual framework to identify any potential casual links from perinatal distress to preterm birth and infant health (i.e., infant survival and mother–infant interaction) was then developed. The main finding was that perinatal distress (stress, anxiety, or depression) was significantly higher in LMIC as compared to high-income countries. Factors related to the determinants of health as well as social, cultural, and political contexts in the LMIC were found to negatively influence women's maternal health. Furthermore, it was found that women in these countries may be more vulnerable to poorer pregnancy outcomes. An important recommendation of the authors of this study was to build research capacity by forming collaborations between researchers in high-income countries and those in LMIC in order to build new knowledge.

### Discussion Questions

1. Discuss some of the social, cultural, and political factors that might adversely affect the mental health of women in LMIC.
2. How can community nurses (in partnership with others) support women in the perinatal period?
3. How could the community nurse integrate culturally safe care into her practice with this population?

Nussbaum's (1997) second capacity for global citizenship entails **moral cosmopolitanism**, which means adopting the fundamental view of all people as fellow citizens who have equal moral worth and deserve equal moral consideration (Friedman, 2000). Global citizenship, however, does not mean that we need to give up our unique local preferences and familial, ethnic, or religious responsibilities. Instead, as fellow citizens of the world, all people are part of our community of respect and concern, which at times means that concerns may constrain our local interests.

The third capacity is **narrative imagination**, which requires the ability to imagine what it might be like to be a person different from yourself, and to allow such imaginings to inform an understanding of others' experiences, emotions, desires, and life stories (Nussbaum, 1997). Being exposed to other cultures and people is one aspect of developing this kind of narrative imagination as part of cultivating global citizenship. It also requires a politicized understanding of how we are all situated in relation to one another across the globe. Global citizenship, then, comes partly through critical-thinking skills expressly focused on challenging oppressive power relations, along with a commitment to social change, social justice, and reflexivity (Painter, 2000).

One way of challenging oppressive power relationships in the hopes of achieving social justice is global health diplomacy. Within a **global health diplomacy** framework, state and non-state actors work together to increase the prominence of health issues in foreign policy decision making (Labonte & Gagnon, 2010). Usually key actors in global health diplomacy include those working in public health, international affairs, management, law, and economics (WHO, 2013b). The alliance between health, foreign policy, and trade is at the "cutting edge of global health diplomacy" (WHO, 2013b). The WHO has a large role to play in global health diplomacy. In this area, its goals are as follows:

- to support the development of a more systematic and proactive approach to identify and understand key current and future changes impacting global public health; and
- to build capacity among member states to support the necessary collective action to take advantage of opportunities and mitigate the risks for health (WHO, 2013b).

The significance of including global health issues in the foreign policy agenda is that health affects the global dimensions of security, economics, and social justice (Kickbusch, 2011). With respect to security, global health diplomacy focuses on preventing the spread of pathogens across borders and responds to humanitarian conflicts, natural disasters, and emergencies. In the economic domain, global health diplomacy is concerned with improving the socioeconomic status of countries in efforts to improve health. One example of this is supporting fair trade in global goods and services. Lastly, social justice is emphasized, reinforcing that health is a human right, supporting the United Nation's MDGs (discussed earlier in this chapter), advocating access to medicines and primary health care, and calling for investment in various global health initiatives (Kickbusch, 2011). While the focus of global health diplomacy has largely been on infectious diseases such as influenza and SARS, there has been a call to also consider various chronic diseases, such as obesity prevention within the global health diplomacy agenda (Blouin & Dube, 2010). Engaging in global health diplomacy presents both opportunities and challenges for health. In the past, nation states have focused on health and policy within their own national boundaries. However, the

**A Village—Developed by Sylvia Loewen and Aliyah Dosani**

Avillage has decided it needs a hospital. The government will not pay for a hospital, so the village leaders put in a request to a local non-governmental organization (NGO) working in their country. You now work for the NGO and are part of a delegation sent to work with the community. You learn the village has 100 000 people, and 50% of them are under 18 years of age. Severe vomiting and diarrhea accounts for much of the illness and 5–10% of infant deaths. The estimate is that 10% of the children have tuberculosis (a respiratory disease). Two years ago, five children died due to measles, and on average they lose at least one child to tetanus each year. It is a six-hour bus ride to the nearest centre with health services. The bus arrives in the evening and the villagers usually sleep on the sidewalk outside the public health office until it opens. The health centre vaccinates children on a first-come, first-served basis.

The community gathers together often to provide support to its members in whatever way they can. This may include sharing food, shelter, clothing, and any other basic necessities of life. A group of community women often come together to share resources as they sew clothing for their children. At times, sharing of staple food such as cornmeal may occur.

Children can attend the government school if their parents can afford a uniform, supplies, and the books. One teacher offers Saturday morning basic reading and arithmetic classes free of charge to children who cannot afford school. He accepts 30 children for each term for his free classes.

About half the population lives in make-shift housing. They use back alleys to urinate, but for bowel movements they usually go up the hill to where there are trees that offer privacy. The same teacher that offers free classes on Saturdays taught the villagers to dig small holes to use as latrines to keep the area cleaner. The village gets its water from a stream that runs down from the hill and through the town. In spring time the water flows rapidly but in late summer it is sluggish.

### Discussion Questions

1. Which of the Sustainable Development Goals outlined above relate to this case study?

2. How would you as a community health nurse work with the community to identify three priority areas for action on health?

3. Suppose the priority areas identified with the stakeholders are education, sanitation, and immunization. Suggest some short-term and long-term goals in relation to these three areas.

determinants of health often are influenced by global forces and need to be addressed through global strategies. The challenge is to capitalize on the benefits and diminish the harm of globalization, while keeping our eye on human rights and equity (Owen & Roberts, 2005).

## Postcolonial Feminism

**Postcolonialism** may be described as a theory and political movement that challenges Western authority and its ethnocentric ideas that naturalize the current global economic and political order rather than problematize them as the consequence of centuries of colonialism (Loomba, 2005). Postcolonialism seeks to explain people's lives in places and times other than "the West," celebrate pluralism, and strongly critique any assumptions about universal knowledge. Given that nations and communities are social constructs supported by particular notions of gender, race, and class, **postcolonial feminism (PCF)** offers a theoretical lens through which to address the intersections of such social "locations" and to explore their corresponding forms of oppression that are inherently part of everyday experiences (Anderson et al., 2003; Loomba, 2005).

The usefulness of this perspective for cultivating global citizenship is that it sheds light on inequities in any global context and facilitates examination of the complex nature of health issues. It explicitly calls on nurses to critique current global (including Canadian) disparities in health and health-care arising from such phenomena as sexism, racism, or the imposition of Eurocentric colonialist views over Aboriginal Canadian knowledge and other indigenous ways of understanding health and healing (Chavez et al., 2008).

PCF represents an opportunity for nurses to acknowledge their multiple social and cultural locations as individuals and healthcare professionals. It challenges deeply held certainties about the "right way" to provide care and considers all knowledge as being situated with a given place and within the power relations therein. Using this perspective enables us to consider multiple perspectives on meanings of health and illness (Anderson & McCann, 2002), as well as the complex issues associated with the global locations of nursing practice and caregiving. For instance, as an international profession, nursing faces invisibility in the healthcare decision-making processes, and nurses' working conditions are difficult (Lunardi, Peter, & Gastaldo, 2002). In addition, nurses are subjected to much lower wages and appalling working conditions in certain nations and there is considerable variation in such conditions among institutions within the same country.

Through its focus on gender, PCF is also a useful framework to examine the common unpaid and low-prestige nature of caregiving, despite being an essential activity for the well-being and health of nations (Bover & Gastaldo, 2005). For example, the inclusion of women in the paid labour market in high-income countries has not been accompanied by increased caregiving roles for men but was rather followed by the migration of women from middle- and low-income countries, such as Filipina nannies coming to Canada and Latin American caregivers for the elderly going to Spain.

## Internationalization of Nursing Research

Nursing research worldwide is highly influenced by, among other things, the availability of professionals to engage in research work, access to research training and graduate programs, and working conditions for academics and practitioners. Some nursing research is situated within the domain of biomedical research, which has been criticized for its lack of commitment toward the disease treatment and prevention for the pathologies and conditions that affect the majority of the world's population. This phenomenon is known as the **90/10 divide**, which refers to the fact that only 10% of all international funding for biomedical research is dedicated to studying problems associated with 90% of the world's global burden of disease (Resnik, 2004).

Another element to be considered is that high-income countries' researchers are the majority of the world's nursing scientists, who are educated and funded to study local and national issues. In addition, studies are frequently published in English, which is called now the 21st-century language of science (Gennaro, 2009), constituting a barrier for nurses from low- and medium-income countries. In this context, English-speaking scientists become producers of knowledge, while researchers and practitioners in other countries are reduced to being the consumers or are altogether disconnected from new findings or knowledge exchange (Mancia & Gastaldo, 2004). In order to address these issues, nurse researchers need to work on building networks that employ PCF lenses, or other equitable frameworks, to guide their collaborations and set research agendas that tackle health promotion and healthcare needs of diverse populations, including the issues faced by communities and professionals in resource-constrained settings.

# GLOBAL HEALTH ETHICS

Community health nursing necessarily involves making ethical decisions in daily practice (see Chapter 6). Ethical theory helps to guide such decisions and has been expressed in codes of ethics and standards of practice (Community Health Nurses of Canada, 2011, revised). **Global health ethics** is a particular avenue of ethical theory that closely aligns with public health ethics, moves beyond traditional bioethical principles, draws from the philosophy of health as a human right, and acknowledges work in this area as largely involving vulnerable populations (Pinto & Upshur, 2009). Benatar, Daar, and Singer (2003) argue that it is imperative to move beyond individually focused biomedical ethical principles to a more comprehensive approach that focuses on improving health globally: a shift in mindset that requires "a realization that health, human rights, economic opportunities, good governance, peace and development are all intimately linked within a complex interdependent world" (p. 108).

Global health ethics can guide moral decision making in settings other than one's home community, from the perspective of the nurse as global citizen. Situations involving moral dilemmas for researchers and practitioners alike in international settings are innumerable. Some examples include using the already scant resources of host agencies to become culturally familiar with primary health care practices; working through translators, which places a burden on locals who are already overworked and may impede natural flow of care, and balancing learned local standards of care with what is drawn from one's own ethnocentric knowledge so that interventions are culturally appropriate without being problematic. Pinto and Upshur (2009) suggest four principles for global health research ethics that also apply to primary health care nursing work: humility, introspection, solidarity, and social justice. **Humility** refers to "recognizing one's limitations and being open to learning from all sources" (p. 7). **Introspection**, or reflection, is a "rigorous examination of one's motives and being aware of one's own privilege" (p. 8). **Solidarity** refers to "working to ensure that goals and values are aligned with those of the community and seeing indigenous views of health and healthcare as an opportunity to understand a problem from the perspective of those receiving care" (p. 8). Finally, social justice addresses the "need to diminish the gross inequities observed, to understand power relationships and networks at interpersonal, organizational, and international levels, to explicitly consider equity in examining health systems, and to always familiarize oneself with the political and human rights conditions of the places visited" (p. 9).

## CONCLUSION

CHNs as global citizens look past the dominant emphasis on individual care (commonly disconnected from social, economic, political, and cultural contexts); engage critically and reflexively with social, historical, and political issues; and develop their capacity in identifying tensions between personal professional interests and global interests. A nurse who can exercise her or his global citizenship professionally works from the premise that people's experiences of health and illness are culturally and geographically located. In addition, it is important to recognize that the majority of the people in the world live under severe social and economic inequities and suffer from preventable or curable diseases. Unfortunately, the majority of people in this world experience an enormous amount of unnecessary human suffering. Nurses working in the global health arena should have the ability to address the health concerns of the majority of the world's population. Projects related to "Health for All" are those that engage in the construction of sustainable, publicly run sanitation and safe water programs; develop affordable, healthy food and housing initiatives; and build national healthcare systems (Chavez et al., 2008). Nurses, the largest group of health professionals in the world, are strategically located and needed to leverage this position to advocate for global health in this globalized world.

## KEY TERMS

90/10 divide    p. 607
cultural pluralism    p. 602
cultural relativism    p. 602
culture    p. 602
equity    p. 594
Declaration of Alma-Ata    p. 597
female genital mutilation (FGM)    p. 602

## STUDY QUESTIONS

1. Differentiate among public health, international health, and global health.

2. Discuss efforts made to decrease inequity in health status among people around the world.

3. Why is it important for CHNs in Canada to learn about globalization and global health?

4. What are the key characteristics of global health education?

5. What are the five key trade agreements that have relevance for health?

6. Identify the three capacities needed to develop global citizenship.

7. How can the notion of global citizenship guide your nursing practice?

> After working through these questions, go to the MyNursingLab at www.pearsoned.ca/mynursinglab to check your answers.

## INDIVIDUAL CRITICAL-THINKING EXERCISES

1. Define global citizenship in your own words and describe it using examples from your own life story or that of those close to you.

2. Imagine you are working in a First Nations community in Canada.

   a. In what ways might you see the effects of globalization on the community?

   b. How might the Sustainable Development Goals apply to First Nations Canadian communities?

3. As you have come to understand the role of CHNs throughout the whole text, how do you now understand this role specific to a global health perspective?

4. Write a brief rebuttal to the following statement: "Public health, international health, and global health are really all the same anyway, so making distinctions in language is not meaningful or useful."

## GROUP CRITICAL-THINKING EXERCISES

1. "When spider webs unite, they can tie up an elephant."
   —Ethiopian proverb

   Imagine forming a web of connections among global health topics raised in this chapter that brings together the health issues, the sociopolitical global context, and corresponding concerns for nursing. Take a few minutes to individually draw a "global health and nursing" web representing what you have imagined, labelling/identifying its various strands. Share your drawing with the group, explaining the following:

   ■ Your identification of the central strands that give strength to the whole web (i.e., foundational ideas) and those strands that may be further out in the web (i.e., those that are important but not central).

   ■ Your understanding of the points where the strands connect as points where nurses may take action (i.e., how issues, context, and nursing concerns come together to direct care in global health).

2. Chen is waiting to be seen in the outpatient clinic with her granddaughter, who looks to be about 10 years old. It is about 6:30 p.m. when a primary health care nurse invites them into her office for assessment and discovers that Mrs. Chen has only recently arrived in Canada and speaks no English. The nurse does not like to use family members as interpreters but the hospital interpreters and the Cantonese-speaking receptionist have left for the day. Not knowing what else to do, the nurse begins the interview with the help of the granddaughter acting as interpreter. In carrying out some open-ended questions, the nurse realizes that Mrs. Chen may be seriously depressed. She wants to ask more focused questions to assess the risk of suicide, but feels uncomfortable about posing these questions through Mrs. Chen's granddaughter. As a group, discuss the following:

   a. What global health issues arise in this situation?

   b. What are the implications for nursing practice that would reflect global citizenship?

3. Imagine that you are in a remote, resource-constrained area of a majority world country, working in a health clinic staffed only by one nurse and two lay health workers. Write a letter home describing your imagined experience. Tell the person to whom you are writing about (a) situations in which your taken-for-granted assumptions have been challenged, (b) where you felt discomfort in taking action or

felt great confidence, and (c) when you felt marginalized in some way. Read your letters to one another in the group and discuss how these experiences can be understood through postcolonial feminism.

## REFERENCES

Allen, M., & Ogilvie, L. (2004). Internationalization of higher education: Potential and pitfalls for nursing education. *International Nursing Review*, 73–80.

Anderson, J. M., & McCann, E. K. (2002). Toward a post-colonial feminist methodology in nursing research: Exploring the convergence of post-colonial and black feminist scholarship. *Nurse Researcher, 9*(3), 7–27.

Anderson, J., Perry, J., Blue, C., Brown, A., Henderson, A., Khan, K. B., . . . Smye, V. (2003). Rewriting cultural safety within the postcolonial and postnational feminist project: Toward new epistemologies of healing. *Advances in Nursing Science, 26*(3), 196–214.

Bach, S. (2003). *International migration of health workers: Labour and social issues*. Geneva, Switzerland: International Labour Office.

Benatar, S. R., Daar, A. S., & Singer, P. A. (2003). Global health ethics. The rationale for mutual caring. *International Affairs, 79*(1), 107–138.

Blouin, C., & Dube, L. (2010). Global health diplomacy for obesity prevention: Lessons from tobacco control. *Journal of Public Health Policy, 31*(2), 244–255. doi:10.1057/jphp.2010.4

Bover, A., & Gastaldo, D. (2005). La centralidad de la familiacomorecurso en el cuidado domiciliario: Perspectivas de género y generación [The centrality of the family as a resource in home care: Gender and generational perspectives]. *Revista Brasileira de Enfermagem, 58*(1), 9–16.

Carnegie, E., & Kiger, A. (2009). Being and doing politics: An outdated model or 21st century reality? *Journal of Advanced Nursing, 65*(9), 1976–1984.

Canadian Nurses Association. (2008). *Code of ethics for registered nurses*. Ottawa, ON: Author. Retrieved from http://www.cna-aiic.ca/~/media/cna/files/en/codeofethics.pdf

Canadian Nurses Association. (2009). *CNAs influencing public policy: Capacity building strategies and tactics*. (3rd ed.). Ottawa ON: Author.

Canadian Nurses Association. (2012). *Global health partnerships retrospective*. Ottawa, ON: Author. Retrieved from http://www.cna-aiic.ca/~/media/cna/page-content/pdf-fr/global_health_partnership_program_2012_e.pdf?la=en

Canadian Public Health Association. (2010). *Public health – Community health nursing practice in Canada: Roles and activities* (4th ed.). Ottawa, ON: Author. Retrieved from http://www.cpha.ca/uploads/pubs/3-1bk04214.pdf

Chavez, F. S., Peter, E., & Gastaldo, D. (2008). Nurses as global citizens: A global health curriculum at the University of Toronto, Canada. In V. Tschudin & A. J. Davis (Eds.), *The globalization of nursing* (pp. 175–186). Oxford, UK: Radcliffe.

Community Health Nurses of Canada. (2009). *Public health nursing discipline specific competencies version 1.0*. St. John's, NL: Author. Retrieved from http://chnc.ca/documents/PHNCompetenciesFinalReportMarch312009.pdf

Community Health Nurses of Canada. (2011, revised). *Canadian community health nursing: Professional practice model & standards of practice*. St. John's, NL: Author. Retrieved from https://www.chnc.ca/documents/CHNC-ProfessionalPracticeModel-EN/index.html

Crigger, N., Brannigan, M., & Baird, M. (2006). Compassionate nursing professionals as good citizens of the world. *Advances in Nursing Science, 29*(4), 15–26.

Dwyer, J. (2007). What's wrong with the global migration of health care professionals? Individual rights and international justice. *Hastings Center Report, 37*(5), 36–43.

Falk-Rafael, A. (2006). Globalization and global health: Towards nursing praxis in the global community. *Advances in Nursing Science, 29*(1), 2–14.

Friel, S., & Marmot, M. G. (2011). Action on the social determinants of health and health in equities goes global. *Annual Review of Public Health, 32*, 225–236. doi:10.1146/annurev-publhealth-031210-101220

Friedman, M. (2000). Educating for world citizenship. *Ethics, 110*(3), 586–601.

Gage, A. J. (2013). Association of child marriage with suicidal thoughts and attempts among adolescent girls in Ethiopia. *Journal of Adolescent Health, 52*, 654–656. http://dx.doi.org/10.1016/j.jadohealth.2012.12.007

Gennaro, S. (2009). Searching for knowledge. *Journal of Nursing Scholarship, 41*(1), 1–2.

Goldenstein, R. A. (2013). Female genital cutting: Nursing implications. *Journal of Transcultural Nursing, published online*, 1–7. doi:10.1177/1043659613493441

Government of Canada. (2013). Criminal Code. Ottawa, ON: Minister of Justice. Retrieved from http://laws-lois.justice.gc.ca/PDF/C-46.pdf

Herdman, E. (2004). Globalization, internationalism and nursing. *Nursing and Health Sciences, 6*, 237–238.

Holton, R. (2000). Globalization's cultural consequences. *The ANNALS of the American Academy of Political and Social Science, 520*, 140–152. doi:10.1177/000271620057000111

International Council of Nurses. (2007). *Ethical nurse recruitment: Position statement*. Geneva, Switzerland: Author. Retrieved from http://www.icn.ch/images/stories/documents/publications/position_statements/C03_Ethical_Nurse_Recruitment.pdf

International Council of Nurses. (2008). *Nurse retention and migration: Position statement*. Geneva, Switzerland: Author. Retrieved from http://www.icn.ch/images/stories/documents/publications/position_statements/C06_Nurse_Retention_Migration.pdf

Johnson, T. H. (2007). Cultural relativism: Interpretations of a concept. *Anthropological Quarterly, 80*(3), 791–802.

Khaja, K., Lay, K., & Boys, S. (2010). Female circumcision: Toward an inclusive practice of care. *Health Care for Women International, 31*(8), 686–699. doi:10.1080/07399332.2010.490313

Kickbusch, I. (2011). Global health diplomacy: How foreign policy can influence health. *British Medical Journal, 342* (d3154). doi:10.1136/bmj.d3154

Kingma, M. (2006). *Nurses on the move: Migration and the global health care economy*. Ithaca, NY: Cornell University Press.

Koplan, J. P., Bond, T. C., Merson, M. H., Reddy, K. S., Rodriguez, M. H., Sewankambo, N. K., & Wasserheit, J. N. (2009). Towards a common definition of global health. *The Lancet, 373,* 1993–1995.

Labonte, R., & Torgerson, R. (2005). Interrogating globalization, health and development: Towards a comprehensive framework for research, policy, and political action. *Critical Public Health, 15*(2), 157–179.

Labonte, R., & Gagnon, M. L. (2010). Framing health and foreign policy: Lessons for global health diplomacy. *Globalization and Health, 6,* 14. Retrieved from http://www.globalizationandhealth.com/content/6/1/14

Lanier, S. A. (2000). *Foreign to familiar.* Hagerstown, MD: McDougal.

Leuning, C. J. (2001). Advancing a global perspective: The world as classroom. *Nursing Science Quarterly, 14,* 298–303.

Leininger, M. (2006). Culture care diversity and universality theory and evolution of the ethnonursing method. In M. Leininger & M. R. McFarland (Eds.), *Culture care diversity and universality: A worldwide nursing theory* (2nd ed., pp. 1–41). Boston, MA: Jones and Bartlett.

Loomba, A. (2005). *Colonialism/Postcolonialism* (2nd ed.). New York, NY: Routledge.

Lunardi, V., Peter, E., & Gastaldo, D. (2002). Are submissive nurses ethical? Reflecting on power anorexia. *Revista-Brasileira de Enfermagem, 55*(2), 183–188.

Mancia, J. R., & Gastaldo, D. (2004). Production and consumption of science in a global context. *Nursing Inquiry, 11*(2), 65–66.

Martens, P., Akin, S., Maud, H., & Mohsin, R. (2012). Is globalization healthy: A statistical indicator analysis of the impacts of globalization on health. *Globalization and Health, 6*(16), 1–14. Retrieved from http://www.globalizationandhealth.com/content/pdf/1744-8603-6-16.pdf

Mastey, N. (2009). Examining empowerment among Indian widows: A qualitative study of the narratives of Hindu widows in North Indian ashrams. *Journal of International Women's Studies, 11*(2), 191–198.

McElmurry, B. J., Solheim, K., Kishi, R., Coffia, M. A., Woith, W., & Janepanish, P. (2006). Ethical concerns in nurse migration. *Journal of Professional Nursing, 22*(4), 226–235.

Mittal, P., Khanna, K., Khanagwal, V. P., & Paliwal, P. K. (2013). Female infanticide: The innocence murdered again. *Journal of Indian Academic Forensic Medicine, 35*(2), 181–183.

Navarro, V. (1999). Health and equity in the world in the era of "globalization." *International Journal of Health Services, 29*(2), 215–226.

Nussbaum, M. C. (1997). *Cultivating humanity: A classical defense of reform in liberal education.* Cambridge, MA: Harvard University Press.

Owen, J. W., & Roberts, O. (2005). Globalization, health and foreign policy: Emerging linkages and interests. *Globalization and Health, 1*(12). Retrieved from http://www.globalizationandhealth.com/content/pdf/1744-8603-1-12.pdf. doi:10.1186/1744-8603-1-12

Painter, J. (2000). Critical human geography. In R. J. Johnston, D. Gregory, G. Pratt, & M. Watts (Eds.), *The dictionary of human geography* (4th ed., pp. 126–128). Oxford, UK: Blackwell.

Peregrino, C. P., Moreno, M. V., Miranda, S. V., Rubio, A. D., & Leal, L. O. (2011). Mercury levels in locally manufactured Mexican skin-lightening creams. *International Journal of Environmental Research and Public Health, 8*(6), 2516–2523. doi:10.3390/ijerph8062516

Pinto, A. D., & Upshur, R. E. (2009). Global health ethics for students. *Developing World Bioethics, 9*(1), 1–10.

Racher, F. E., & Annis, R. C. (2012). Honouring culture and diversity in community practice. In R. Vollman, E. T. Anderson, & J. McFarlane (Eds.), *Canadian community as partner: Theory and multidisciplinary practice* (3rd ed., pp. 154–176). Philadelphia, PA: Lippincott, Williams & Wilkins.

Raphael, D., Curry-Stevens, A., & Bryant, T. (2008). Barriers to addressing the social determinants of health: Insights from the Canadian experience. *Health Policy, 88*(2–3), 222–235.

Resnik, D. B. (2004). The distribution of biomedical research resources and international justice. *Developing World Bioethics, 4*(1), 42–57.

Reutter, L., & Kushner, K. E. (2010). Health equity through action on the social determinants of health: Taking up the challenge in nursing. *Nursing Inquiry, 17*(3), 269–280.

Rowson, M., Willot, C., Hughes, R., Maini, A., Martin, S., Miranda, J. J., . . .Yudkin, J. S. (2012). Conceptualising global health: Theoretical issues and their relevance for teaching. *Globalization and Health, 8*(36), 1–8. Retrieved from http://www.globalizationandhealth.com/content/pdf/1744-8603-8-36.pdf

Steger, M. B. (2013). *Globalization: A very short introduction.* Oxford, U.K.: Oxford University Press.

Taylor, S. (2009). Wealth, health and equity: Convergence to divergence in late 20th century globalisation. *British Medical Bulletin, 91*(1), 29–48.

Tejada de Rivero, D. A. (2003). Alma-Alta revisited. *Perspectives in Health, 8,* 3–7.

United Nations. (2000). *Millennium summit (6-8 September 2000).* Used with permission of United Nations. Retrieved from http://www.un.org/en/events/pastevents/millennium_summit.shtml

United Nations. (2014). General Assembly August 12, 2014: Report of the open working group of the General Assembly on Sustainable Development Goals. Retrieved from http://www.un.org/ga/search/view_doc.asp?symbol=A/68/970&Lang=E

United Nations Secretary-General. (2010). *Keeping the promise: A forward-looking review to promote an agreed action agenda to achieve the Millennium Development Goals by 2015.* Retrieved from http://www.un.org/en/mdg/summit2010

United Nations Sustainable Development Solutions Network. (2013). *Membership.* Retrieved from http://unsdsn.org/membership/about-our-network

United Nations System Task Team on the Post-2015 UN Development Agenda. (2012). *Realizing the future we want for all: Report to the Secretary-General.* Retrieved from http://www.un.org/en/development/desa/policy/untaskteam_undf/untt_report.pdf

Villeneuve, M. (2008). Yes we can! Eliminating health disparities as part of the core business of nursing on a global level. *Policy, Politics and Nursing Practice, 9*(4), 334–341.

World Health Organization. (1978). Declaration of Alma Alta: International conference on primary health care, Alma-Ata, USSR, 6–12. Europe: Reprinted with permission from World Health Organization. Author. Retrieved from http://www.who.int/publications/almaata_declaration_en.pdf

World Health Organization. (2005). Bangkok Charter of Health Promotion. From the 6th Global Conference on Health Promotion, Bangkok, Thailand, August 11, 2005. Retrieved from http://www.who.int/healthpromotion/conferences/6gchp/hpr_050829_%20BCHP.pdf

World Health Organization. (2008). *Closing the gap in a generation: Health equity through action on the social determinants of health.* Geneva, Switzerland: World Health Organization. Retrieved from http://www.who.int/social_determinants/thecommission/finalreport/en/index.html

World Health Organization. (2010). *A World Health Organization code of practice on the international recruitment of health personnel: Background paper.* Geneva, Switzerland: Author.

World Health Organization. (2013a). *Female genital mutilation.* Fact Sheet 241. Retrieved from http://www.who.int/mediacentre/factsheets/fs241/en

World Health Organization. (2013b). Trade, foreign policy, diplomacy and health: Global health diplomacy. Reprinted with permission from World Health Organization. Retrieved from http://www.who.int/trade/diplomacy/en

World Trade Organization & World Health Organization. (2002). *WTO agreements and public health: A joint study by the WHO and WTO secretariat*: Geneva, Switzerland: Authors.

## ABOUT THE AUTHORS

**Aliyah Dosani**, RN, BN, MPH, PhD, is an Associate Professor in the School of Nursing and Midwifery, Faculty of Health, Community and Education at Mount Royal University in Calgary Alberta. She holds a PhD from the University of Calgary with a specialization in population/public health. Her nursing practice includes instructing students in the Bachelor of Nursing Program, population/public health, community health nursing, and legal issues in nursing. Her work generally focuses on maternal, newborn, and child health. Her research interests include working with vulnerable populations through community-based programs and interventions. She also shares a passion for global health issues.

**Judith Gleeson**, RN, PhD, is an Associate Professor in the School of Nursing and Midwifery, Faculty of Health, Community and Education at Mount Royal University, Calgary. She teaches courses in community health, health equity, and global health. Her research program is focused on health policy, social justice, and community service learning.

# CHAPTER 34

# Challenges and Future Directions

*Aliyah Dosani and Lucia Yiu*

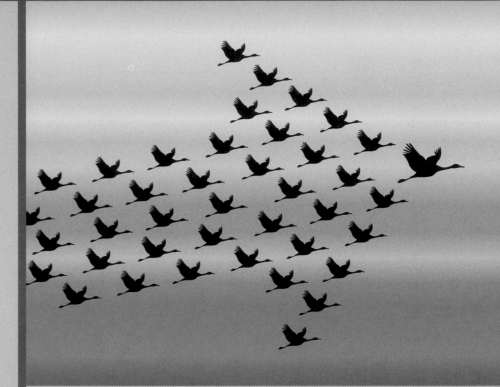

Source: Harish Marnad/Shutterstock

## INTRODUCTION

Community health nurses (CHNs) work in a variety of settings where people live, work, play, worship, and learn. They attend to the diverse social determinants of health that influence the opportunity for optimal health across the lifespan, and they use collaborative actions to promote, protect, and restore the health of the population (Canadian Public Health Association, 2010; Community Health Nurses of Canada, 2011, revised). In 1978, the World Health Organization called on the nations to implement the primary health care strategy to achieve "Health for All" by the year 2000 (see Chapter 8). The Canadian Nurses Association (CNA) also has been a strong advocate for primary health care (PHC) for the past 35 years. Today, the CNA asks nurses to play an even greater role in leading PHC initiatives and to examine the challenges and/or barriers that hinder us from advancing our health systems (CNA, 2015).

While studying certain chapters of this textbook, you have come to understand how the various social determinants of health could and do influence health at different levels—from individual, family, group, aggregate, community, system, and society or population to the global scale. Social issues such as poverty, homelessness, violence, and food insecurity contribute to both physiological and psychological stress that pose health risks to individuals across the lifespan (Garg, Sandel, Dworkin, Kahn, & Zuckerman, 2012). The opportunities for CHNs to influence change are limitless. However, CHNs must be well prepared to address the challenges in practice, education, research, and leadership.

## EVOLVING PRACTICE

In the 2006 discussion paper "Toward 2020: Visions for Nursing," Rosemary Goodyear (as cited in Villeneuve & MacDonald, 2006) described the dramatic change in the role of nurses and the care they will provide in the near future. It was noted that "communities are moving away from doctors as primary care providers and are more open to alternative providers like NPs and RNs" (p. 94). The 2012 Ontario Health Action Plan also emphasized the need for an accountable and responsive health system where there will be improved access, better value, and superior quality services to meet the health needs of the communities (Ontario Ministry of Health and Long-Term Care, 2012). On our horizon there will be more opportunity for nurses and other healthcare providers to work together to provide community-based care. We will also use evidence-based practice more effectively to shape our nursing practice. As we see rising rates of various illnesses such as cancers, lung diseases, and obesity, it is imperative that we develop expert knowledge and skills in health promotion, illness prevention, and disease management for our population.

As described in the "Toward 2020" discussion paper (Villeneuve & MacDonald, 2006), self-care is the "largest contributor to the creation and maintenance of health" (p. 95), and it takes place "in the socio-environmental–political-cultural context of the individual and is influenced by resources available" (p. 95). The second-largest contributor is identified as "all the community health and social resources in place to support health and keep people well" (p. 95). This further reinforces the need for CHNs to provide a supportive environment for people to attain good health in their own communities—where they live, work, learn, worship, and play. CHNs will be working with various healthcare providers to care for their clients in a shared-care model.

According to the Canadian Institute of Health Information [CIHI] (2013), 61.6% of nurses worked in hospital settings and 15.4% worked in community settings in 2012. By 2020, these percentages will be reversed, with two-thirds working in community-based care. In the near future, nurses will have a much stronger and more visible presence as they develop and implement health-promotion and illness-prevention programs in schools, workplaces, and various community settings.

How are we preparing for such changes? First, let's look at changes in nursing practice, specifically community health nursing practice. The demographics of the Canadian population are changing, as seen in the age stratifications, the cultural mix, and the increase in Aboriginal populations. The "one size" approach will no longer fit all. Strategies to improve population health will need to be targeted to specific groups. As the Canadian population becomes increasingly diverse, nurses must know who their populations are and what their health needs are. CHNs must be mindful to move beyond cultural sensitization and awareness, and direct their care to promoting cultural safety, cultural harmony, and fostering individual and community cultural differences.

We all are witnessing the grave concerns of increasing healthcare costs over the last few decades and we anticipate that this trend will continue in the future. We see merging or elimination of services, labour disputes, and long wait lists to name a few of the challenges in the healthcare arena. With longer life expectancy, we encounter various chronic illnesses such as cancer, diabetes, heart conditions, debilitating arthritis, and Alzheimer's disease during our life course. Instead of viewing the aging population as a burden to the healthcare system, it is even more important for CHNs to continue to find ways to provide the best quality essential care in the most cost-effective and efficient ways. We must acquire proficient skills when assessing community needs and engaging the community and stakeholders from various sectors to find solutions to issues that are surfacing at the community level of practice. In doing so, we must take an asset-based focus to leverage the strengths of various population groups and communities. To achieve optimal health for their community, CHNs must work collaboratively with multidisciplinary teams to achieve a well-integrated system that reduces service duplication and fragmentation while improving access and enhancing the quality of life for their clients across the lifespan.

As we live in our fast-paced and ever-evolving technological world, we already have seen innovations in telemedicine, computers, robots, mobile applications, and various other devices that allow our clients to easily access health information and to communicate their health needs and progress with their healthcare providers. To be proactive, CHNs can participate in developing technological innovations to enhance client care. They may be involved in technological advances in terms of refining existing information and data-based management systems, and by creating various applications that may be used on various devices to monitor diabetic clients or clients living with various heart conditions. CHNs may also be involved in creating various ideas pertaining to community resources, including breastfeeding assistance for new mothers or monitoring the safety of frail and dependent clients.

Over the last few years we have seen an explosion in the numbers of devices that are used to monitor our physical activity. CHNs may also explore their role in this important primary prevention initiative. In the pursuit of social justice and equity to achieve health for all, CHNs face new health challenges in helping individuals and populations through chronic disease management, reducing dependence on hospital services, and supporting people in their various community settings. Also, the need for emergency preparedness will not diminish but will always be present, albeit with a variety of concerns, ranging from infectious diseases such as measles outbreaks, HIV/AIDS, and H1N1 to natural and man-made disasters. As healthcare providers speak of the need to strengthen the primary care model to ensure that people will have a range of health services when they enter the health system, we must never forget to work from the philosophy of primary health care—that health promotion and illness prevention will be key to reducing healthcare costs and to ensuring our communities are in the healthiest state possible. Furthermore, CHNs must envision what role they can play as leaders and change agents as they plan and implement appropriate care for their community clients.

## RESPONSIVE EDUCATION

Community health nursing has always been part of baccalaureate nursing curricula, with a broad-based approach and the individual, family, group, aggregate, community, system, and society or population identified as clients. Within community health nursing practice, public health nursing primarily focuses on population health and primary health care (CHNC, 2009), while home health and other forms of community nursing focus more on direct care or primary care (CHNC, 2010).

In a 2008 pan-Canada survey conducted by the Faculty of Nursing at McMaster University, public health nurses identified the following key learning needs that were important to support their practice: (a) understanding of theoretical and application of concepts in health promotion and epidemiology; (b) methods to conduct program planning and evaluation; (c) using informatics, research findings, and harm reduction strategies; (d) engaging in collaborative intersectoral partnerships; (e) providing culturally relevant care; and (f) advocating for healthy public policies (Schofield et al., 2009). These findings ignited the urgency for nurse educators to rethink and to strengthen teaching methods in order to prepare competent nurses to practise in community settings.

The Canadian Association of Schools of Nursing (CASN) created a sub-committee to address public health education. Members of the sub-committee work with nurse educators, employers, and other stakeholders to examine the competencies and that might change basic nursing curricula. CASN (2010) created guidelines for universities to select quality community clinical placements for students. Additionally, expected qualifications for faculty advisors and preceptors were also outlined in this document. The CASN (2014) further assembled an expert task force made up of both educators and practitioners, and developed entry-level competencies in public health nursing practice for undergraduate nursing students. Prodigious efforts were made to ensure that competencies exist to define how public health nurses (PHNs) should apply knowledge and skills to address the determinants of health and to build relationships with communities in order to achieve population

health. Creating an online resource of teaching strategies in public health nursing to increase the capacity of nurse educators to teach these competencies is also in the CASN's plan. Once again, leadership demonstrated by nurse educators is contributing to redefining and strengthening public health competencies of CHNs. This is one way to achieve health for all. While it is important to recognize what the entry-level competencies for PHNs need to be, we must never lose sight of other competencies that can be categorized as generalist community health nursing skills required of graduates. Because of the anticipated shift to community-based nursing, we must be mindful of new and emerging community health nursing roles.

Graduate opportunities are also increasing in number, scope, and variety. Specific to community health nursing, the Canadian Nurse Practitioner Initiative (CNPI) of the CNA worked with provincial organizations and schools of nursing to create curricula for primary health care nurse practitioner programs. Also, graduate nursing students have opportunities to tailor Master of Nursing degrees to a community health specialty or to consider one of the new interdisciplinary Master of Public Health programs that are springing up across the country. Furthermore, schools of public health exist in several universities—representing additional opportunities for advanced interdisciplinary work and research in community health with a strong nursing contribution. Research in community health nursing is also increasing.

While the CASN has taken on a leadership role nationally to promote and strengthen nursing education, the responsibility for us to excel in the practice of community health lies with committed and well-prepared nurse educators (CHNC, 2014; Matuk & Horsburgh, 1992). It is imperative for nurse educators to share such responsibility as they are in the position to prepare our future generations in nursing. They must address and reinforce the entry to practice competencies in all areas in nursing, including community health nursing, throughout their curricula. In addition, safe and effective clinical placements will need to continue to be provided, where students will work with diverse populations (CHNC, 2014). More importantly, as we continue to move toward the shared-care practice model, nurse educators will also need to create opportunities for their students to engage in interprofessional education for collaborative, client-centred practice.

## ADVANCING RESEARCH

Throughout this book, we included selected Canadian nursing research studies to address various aspects of community health nursing practice. The ultimate goal of any type of health research is to improve the quality of life for individuals, families, communities, systems, and populations. Over the last decade, we have seen an increase in the literature around methods of engaging in research at the community and population levels, including participatory action research (PAR) and population health intervention research (PHIR). While PAR is not new, it has come to the forefront again as more emphasis is being placed on working *with* communities (Gillis & Jackson, 2002). The ultimate goal of PAR is to build capacity among community members and associated stakeholders in order to empower them to engage in some form of social change (Macdonald, 2012). We have learned that community-based participatory research is the preferred model of engaging in research that is community based (Blumenthal, Diclemente, Braithwaite, & Smith, 2013). The use of PAR is particularly important in resource-poor countries where much health-promotion work takes place at the grassroots level. CHNs must find a way to engage communities in this important research work.

It will be increasingly important for CHNs to be familiar with and use PHIR to inform their nursing practice. The goal of PHIR is to "produce knowledge about policy, programs, and events that have the potential to impact health at the population level" (Hawe, Di Ruggiero, & Cohen, 2012, p. e468). Such research is useful in framing primary prevention initiatives, including interventions to alter the underlying sociocultural and environmental risks that will ultimately decrease health inequities (Benach, Malmusi, Yasui, Marinez, & Muntaner, 2011; Hawe et al., 2012; Rose, 1992). Hence, PHIR identifies the decisions that people make, including the choice and power that individuals in decision-making positions have, that ultimately result in some people being rich and others poor (Hawe et al., 2012).

Looking to the future, CHNs will need to be a part of generating sound evidence for practice. In addition, CHNs will need to strategically place themselves at various levels of decision making within health systems and governments if we are to see significant improvements in health equity. As we begin to see the shift to community-based care, it is crucial for CHNs to focus on broader and societal-level factors that impact the health of populations and to become increasingly involved in higher-level initiatives that address the root causes of such inequities in health status among various communities and among population groups. In order for research to be more applicable to community health settings, we must seek rigour in external validity and generalizability to maximize the public health significance of the research (Hohmann & Shear, 2002). This means that CHNs will need to excel in the research process, from conceiving research ideas within teams, to data collection and analysis, and finally to disseminating the results. We know that women, visible minority populations, the elderly, people living in rural areas, and marginalized populations are often underrepresented in research (Cottler et al., 2013). CHNs must find a way to use their rapport-building skills to engage various communities and population groups in the research process and as research participants. At the same time, care must be taken to avoid further marginalization of various populations that are under threat. Furthermore, in keeping in line with the principles of primary health care, it is important for CHNs to keep public participation at the forefront of their research initiatives, regardless of the country that they may be working in.

To be responsive to the needs of the communities and society, educational institutions, healthcare employers, professional nursing associations, and individual CHNs need to follow developments in research. Nurse educators must be aware of the current research that is being undertaken at the community and population levels so that graduating nurses are prepared to engage in community health nursing practice in a meaningful way—either by being involved in the research process or utilizing the results of these types of research to inform their nursing practice. They can act as role models and help develop a culture of nursing research and cultivate curiosity when working with their students early on in the profession. Employers must be able to influence working conditions so that CHNs may have various opportunities to either engage in research activities or have sufficient resources at their disposal to make informed practice decisions based on evidence.

CHNs must continue to contribute to the national picture and research efforts through knowledge about, and data from, our local communities. One example of this is the Community Health Research Unit at the University of Ottawa (http://aix1.uottawa.ca/~nedwards/chru) that brings CHNs from all sections to share ideas as they examine current issues in community nursing practice. When national, provincial, and local community health nursing associations, as well as individual CHNs, incorporate such evidence into their practice, we see community health nursing practice move forward.

## VISIONARY LEADERSHIP

To create dynamic synergy, it is essential for CHNs to build leadership capacity by working with multidisciplinary teams on common health issues, with a goal to achieve health outcomes that would align with community needs (Careau et al., 2014). Humphreys et al. (2015) describe the importance of understanding how various models of leadership affect health disparities, conflict resolution and negotiation, and community organizing. CHNs are in an ideal position to act as leaders while working in the community setting. While working collaboratively with other professionals as well as community members, the team members focus on "developing leaders that are able to build a shared vision within a group/organization/community and who facilitate the distribution of leadership processes according to the group's expertise, as well as act as a catalyst for shared decision-making processes and collective actions" (Careau et al., 2014, p. 43). Ultimately, the goal is to develop leadership capacity, building within community members themselves such that community empowerment can be achieved.

We must never forget what community health is and how we, as practitioners, evolved from the past to where we are today. We must also be able to anticipate what our future goals might be, both locally and nationally. To this end, CHNs must be well informed of how socioeconomic and political trends and environmental changes, such as global warming, may impact the health of various communities. The CHNC (2015) has developed leadership competencies to guide CHNs. Leadership competency statements have been developed for the following areas: system transformation, leading self, engaging others, and developing coalitions. It will be up to us to make a concerted effort to ensure that our voices are heard and that we stand together to protect the health of Canadians. We must, at the same time, position ourselves and partner with nurses in other countries to influence and support healthcare on a global scale. The challenges of preparing practitioners in community health nursing and producing the evidence on which our practice is based will continue to arise. We must stress the importance of using frameworks such as the determinants of health to assist CHNs in proactively planning for the future and positioning ourselves as co-creators of change in practice. And at the heart of it all will be our nurse–client relationships, with a focus to promote and protect the health of the community.

So, what of the future? While it is difficult to know for sure what the future holds for us, we can anticipate a few things. One is that nurses, including CHNs, have the skills and knowledge to be a political force for the health of Canadians, if we so choose. It is important for CHNs to demonstrate a united front. By supporting our professional organizations locally, nationally, and globally; by being proactive in the political process; and by using our knowledge to affect and effect healthy public policy, we can contribute significantly to influencing the movement and direction of healthcare in Canada. In doing so, we will be promoting equity and social justice in various communities nationwide and around the world.

The future of our profession and how well it will advance relies on the synergy of our new nurse graduates. We are certain that our new nurse graduates will help advance community health nursing! What an exciting future to behold!

## REFERENCES

Benach, J., Malmusi, D., Yasui, Y., Marinez, J. M., & Muntaner, C. (2011). Beyond Rose's strategies: A typology of scenarios of policy impact on health and health inequalities. *International Journal of Health Services, 41*(10), 1–9.

Blumenthal, D. S., Diclemente, R. J., Braithwaite, R., & Smith, S. A. (Eds.). (2013). *Community based participatory research: Issues, methods, and translation to practice* (2nd ed.). New York, NY: Springer Publishing Company, LLC.

Canadian Association of Schools of Nursing. (2010). *Guidelines for quality community health nursing clinical placements for baccalaureate nursing student.* Retrieved from http://casn.ca/vm/newvisual/attachments/856/Media/CPGuidelinesFinal March.pdf

Canadian Association of Schools of Nursing. (2014). *Entry-to-practice public health nursing competencies for undergraduate nursing education.* Ottawa, ON: Author.

Canadian Institute for Health Information. (2013). *Regulated nurses, 2012: Summary report.* Retrieved from https://secure.cihi.ca/free_products/RegulatedNurses2012Summary_EN.pdf

Canadian Nurses Association. (2015). *RNs leading in PHC.* Retrieved from http://www.cna-aiic.ca/en/on-the-issues/better-health/primary-health-care/rns-leading-in-primary-health-care

Canadian Public Health Association. (2010). *Public health–community health in Canada: Roles and activities* (4th ed.). Ottawa, ON: Author. Retrieved from http://www.chnc.ca/documents/PublicHealth-CommunityHealthNursinginCana daRolesandActivities2010.pdf

Community Health Nurses of Canada. (2009). *Public health nurses discipline specific competencies.* St. John's, NL: Author. Retrieved

from http://www.chnc.ca/documents/competencies_june_2009_english.pdf

Community Health Nurses of Canada. (2010). *Home health nursing competencies.* St. John's, NL: Author. Retrieved from http://www.chnc.ca/documents/HomeHealthNursingCompetenciesVersion 1March2010.pdf

Community Health Nurses of Canada. (2011, revised). *Canadian community health nursing: Professional practice model & standards of practice.* St. John's, NL: Author. Retrieved from https://www.chnc.ca/documents/CHNC-ProfessionalPracticeModel-EN/index.html

Community Health Nurses of Canada. (2014). *CHNC position statement: Community Health Nursing Education.* St. John's, NL: Author. Retrieved from https://www.chnc.ca/documents/PositionStatementCHNEducationFINAL2015March1.pdf

Community Health Nurses of Canada. (2015). *Leadership for competencies for public health practice in Canada.* St. John's, NL: Author. Retrieved from http://chnc.ca/documents/LCPHPC-EN

Careau, E., Biba, G., Brander, R., van Dijk, J. P., Verma, S., Paterson, M., & Tassone, M. (2014). Health leadership education programs, best practices, and impacts on learners' knowledge, skills, attitudes, and behaviors and system change: A literature review. *Journal of Healthcare Leadership, 6,* 39–50. doi:http://dx.doi.org/10.2147/JHL.S61127

Cottler, L. B., McCloskey, D. J., Aguilar-Gaxiola, S., Bennett, N. M., Strelnick, H., Dwyer-White, M., . . . Evanoff, B. (2013). Community needs, concerns, and perceptions about health research: Findings from the clinical and translational science award sentinel network. *American Journal of Public Health, 103*(9), 1685–1692. doi:10.2105/AJPH.2012.300941

Garg, A., Sandel, M., Dworkin, P. H., Kahn, R. S., & Zuckerman, B. (2012). From medical home to health neighborhood: Transforming the medical into a community-based health neighborhood. *The Journal of Pediatrics, 160*(4), 535–536.e1. doi:10.1016/j.jpeds.2012.01.001

Gillis, A., & Jackson, W. (2002). *Research methods for nurses: Methods and interpretation.* Philadelphia, PA: F. A. Davis Company.

Hawe, P., Di Ruggiero, E., & Cohen, E. (2012). Frequently asked questions about population health intervention research. *Canadian Journal of Public Health, 103*(6), e468–e471.

Hohmann, A. A., & Shear, M. K. (2002). Community-based intervention research: Coping with the "noise" of real life in study design. *American Journal of Psychiatry, 159*(2), 201–207. doi:http://doi.org/10.1176/appi.ajp.159.2.201

Humphreys, B. P., Couse, L. J., Sonnenmeier, R. M., Kurtz, A., Russell, S. M., & Antal, P. (2015). Transforming LEND leadership training curriculum through the maternal and child health leadership competencies. *Maternal and Child Health Journal, 19,* 300–307. doi:10.1007/s10995-014-1587-8

MacDonald, C. (2012). Understanding participatory action research: A qualitative research methodology option. *Canadian Journal of Action Research, 13*(2), 34–50.

Matuk, L., & Horsburgh, M. (1992). Toward redefining public health nursing in Canada: Challenges for education. *Public Health Nursing, 9*(3), 149–154.

Ontario Ministry of Health and Long-Term Care. (2012). *Ontario action plan for health care.* Toronto, ON: Queen's Printer for Ontario. Retrieved from http://health.gov.on.ca/en/ms/ecfa/healthy_change/docs/rep_healthychange.pdf

Rose, G. (1992). *The strategy of preventive medicine.* Oxford, UK: Oxford University Press.

Schofield, R., Valaitus, R., Akhtar-Danesh, N., Baumann, A., Martin-Misner, R., & Underwood, J. (2009). *Phase 2:* *Strengthening the quality of community health nursing practice: A pan-Canadian survey of community health nurses' continuing education needs study.* Hamilton, ON: McMaster University. Retrieved from http://www.chnc.ca/documents/Phase2 StrengtheningtheQualityofCommunityHealthNursing Practice.pdf

Villeneuve, M., & MacDonald, J. (2006). *Toward 2020: Visions for nursing.* Ottawa, ON: Canadian Nurses Association.

## ABOUT THE AUTHORS

**Aliyah Dosani**, RN, BN, MPH, PhD, is an Associate Professor in the School of Nursing and Midwifery, Faculty of Health, Community and Education at Mount Royal University in Calgary Alberta. She holds a PhD from the University of Calgary with a specialization in population/public health. Her nursing practice includes instructing students in the Bachelor of Nursing Program, population/public health, community health nursing, and legal issues in nursing. Her work generally focuses on maternal, newborn, and child health. Her research interests include working with vulnerable populations through community-based programs and interventions. She also shares a passion for global health issues.

**Lucia Yiu**, RN, BScN, BA (University of Windsor), BSc (University of Toronto), MScN (University of Western Ontario), is an Associate Professor in the Faculty of Nursing at the University of Windsor, and an Educational and Training Consultant in community nursing. She has worked overseas and served on various community and social services committees involving local and district health planning. Her practice and research include multicultural health, international health, experiential learning, community development, breast health, and program planning and evaluation. Lucia is the recipient of the 2014 Community Health Nurses of Canada Award of Merit.

# Appendix A: The Canadian Community Health Nursing Standards of Practice

## INTRODUCTION

The Canadian Community Health Nursing Standards of Practice (the Standards) represent a vision for excellence in community health nursing. The Standards define the practice of a registered nurse in the specialty area of community health nursing. They build on the generic practice expectations of registered nurses and identify the practice principles and variations specific to community health nursing in Canada. The Standards apply to community health nurses who work in the areas of practice, education, administration and research.

## PURPOSE OF STANDARDS OF PRACTICE

- Define the scope and depth of community nursing practice
- Establish criteria and expectations for acceptable nursing practice and safe, ethical care
- Provide criteria for measuring actual performance
- Support ongoing development of community health nursing
- Promote community health nursing as a specialty and provide the foundation for certification of community health nursing by the Canadian Nurses Association
- Inspire excellence in and commitment to community nursing practice
- Set a benchmark for new community health nurses.

## USING THE STANDARDS OF PRACTICE

- Nurses in clinical practice use the standards to guide and evaluate their practice.
- Nursing educators include the standards in course curricula to prepare new graduates for practice in community settings.
- Nurse administrators use the standards to direct policy and guide performance expectations.
- Nurse researchers use the standards to guide the development of knowledge specific to community health nursing.

## COMMUNITY HEALTH NURSING PRACTICE

*Community health nurses value caring, principles of primary health care, multiple ways of knowing, individual and community partnerships, empowerment, and social justice.*[xviii]

Community health nursing acknowledges its roots and traditions, embraces advances, and recognizes the importance of the need to continually evolve as a dynamic nursing specialty[i]. (see Figure 2. History of Community Health Nursing)

A new nurse entering community health practice will likely need at least two years to achieve the practice expectations of these specialty Standards. Strong mentorship, leadership and peer support, as well as self directed and guided learning all contribute to the achievement of the expertise required.

Community health nurses practice in a variety of specialty care services and work in a variety of settings (See Appendix F - *Community Health Nursing by Area of Practice*). Home health nursing and public health nursing are linked historically through common beliefs, values, traditions, skills and above all their unique focus on promoting and protecting community health.

Evolving from centuries of community care by laywomen and members of religious orders, community health nursing started to gain recognition as a nursing specialty in the mid-1800s. Florence Nightingale and Lillian Wald as well as organizations such as the Victorian Order of Nurses, the Henry Street Settlement and the Canadian Red Cross Society have permanently shaped community health nursing. During the 20th century, public health and home health nursing emerged from common roots to represent the ideals of community health nursing. Community health nursing is situated on a foundation of ethical practice and caring.[i]

**FIGURE  2**  History of Community Health Nursing

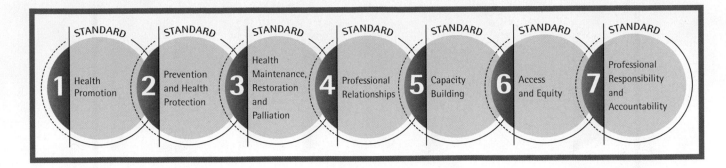

Home health nursing and public health nursing differ in their client and program emphasis. Both Public Health Nurses[vi] and Home Health Nurses[vii] have discipline specific competencies that define the integrated knowledge, skills, and attributes required to achieve the standards. (See Appendix G for a diagram depicting the *Relationship Between Standards and Competencies.*

Community health nurses view health as a dynamic process of physical, mental, spiritual and social well-being. Health includes self-determination, realization of hopes and needs, and a sense of connection to the community.[i] Community health nurses consider health as a resource for everyday life that is influenced by circumstances, beliefs and the determinants of health. The determinants of health are factors and conditions that affect health status and include social, cultural, political, economic, physical and environmental health determinants. Additional determinants of health specific to aboriginal populations have also been identified. (See also Appendix C – *Determinants of Health*)

A *Glossary of Terms,* which further describes relevant concepts and terms related to community health nursing practice can be found at http://chnc.ca/nursing-publications.cfm

## STANDARDS OF PRACTICE FOR COMMUNITY HEALTH NURSES

STANDARD 1: HEALTH PROMOTION
STANDARD 2: PREVENTION AND HEALTH PROTECTION
STANDARD 3: HEALTH MAINTENANCE, RESTORATION AND PALLIATION
STANDARD 4: PROFESSIONAL RELATIONSHIPS
STANDARD 5: CAPACITY BUILDING
STANDARD 6: ACCESS AND EQUITY
STANDARD 7: PROFESSIONAL RESPONSIBILITY AND ACCOUNTABILITY

## Standard 1: Health Promotion

Community health nurses integrate health promotion into their practice. *"Health promotion is the process of enabling people to increase control over, and to improve, their health"*[xiii]

### The Community Health Nurse. . .

a. Collaborates with individuals, families, groups, communities, populations or systems to do a comprehensive assessment of assets and needs, acknowledging that differences exist in assets and needs of different members of the population.

b. Uses a variety of information sources including community wisdom to access high quality data and research findings related to health at the international, national, provincial, territorial, regional and local levels to plan programs and services.

c. Seeks to identify the root causes of illness, disease and inequities in health.

d. Considers socio-political issues that may underlie individual, family, group, community, population or system problems. (See Appendix C- *Determinants of Health*)

e. Recognizes the impact of specific issues such as political climate, will, values and culture, historical context, client readiness, and social and systemic structures on health.

f. Facilitates planned change with the individual, family, group, community, population or system (See Figure 3. Population Health Promotion Model) See Appendix H – *Health Promotion)*

g. Demonstrates knowledge of determinants of health and effectively implements multiple health promotion strategies. (See Appendix H – *Health Promotion*)

h. Identifies strategies for change that will make it easier for people to make healthier choices.

i. Collaborates, along with other sectors, with the individual, family, group, community or population, to support them to overcome health inequities and take responsibility for maintaining or improving their health by

- Identifies the level of intervention necessary to promote health.
- Identifies which determinants of health require action or change to promote health.
- Uses a comprehensive range of strategies to address health-related issues.

**FIGURE 3** Population Health Promotion Model

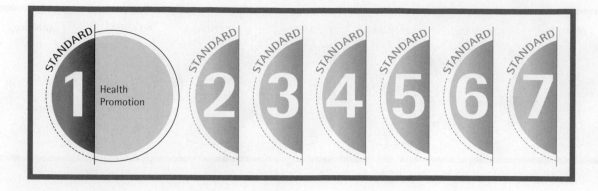

increasing their knowledge, influence and control over the determinants of health.

j. Understands and uses social marketing, media and advocacy strategies, in collaboration with others, to raise awareness of health issues and place issues of social justice and health equity on the public agenda.

k. Applies relevant theories and concepts (e.g. Stages of Change Theory,[xix]; Self-Efficacy Theory,[xx] Assets and Strengths [xxi], Community Mobilization[xxii]) to shift social norms and change behaviours in partnership with others while working on enabling factors to overcome barriers in the social and physical environment.

l. Uses a client centered approach to help the individual, family, group, community and population to identify strengths and available resources to access health and take action to address their needs

m. Evaluates and modifies population health promotion programs as needed in partnership with the individual, family, group, community, population or system in partnership with individuals, employers and policy makers.

## Standard 2: Prevention and Health Protection

Community health nurses integrate prevention and health protection activites into practice. These activities are often mandated by government programs to minimize the occurrence of diseases or injuries and their consequences.

### The Community Health Nurse. . .

a. Participates in surveillance activities; analyzes and utilizes this data to identify and address health issues within a population or community.

b. Recognizes patterns and trends in epidemiological data and service delivery and initiates strategies to improve health.

c. Recognizes the differences between the levels of prevention (primary, secondary, tertiary) and selects the appropriate level of intervention.

d. Facilitates informed decision making for protective and preventive health measures.

e. Helps individuals, families, groups, communities, populations or systems identify potential risks to health including contributing to emergency and/or disaster planning, being knowledgeable about specific emergency / disaster plans and promoting awareness of the plan(s) amongst individuals, families, groups and communities.

f. Uses harm reduction principles grounded in the concepts of health equity and social justice, to identify and reduce or remove risk factors in a variety of environments and settings including homes, neighbourhoods, workplaces, schools and street.

g. Provides prevention and protection services for the individual, family, group or community to address issues such as communicable disease, injury, chronic disease, physical environment (e.g. clean air, water, land) and community emergencies or disasters.

h. Applies epidemiological principles for planning strategies such as screening, surveillance, immunization,

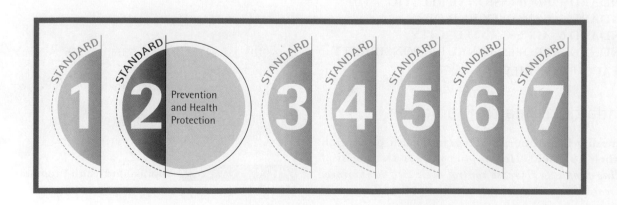

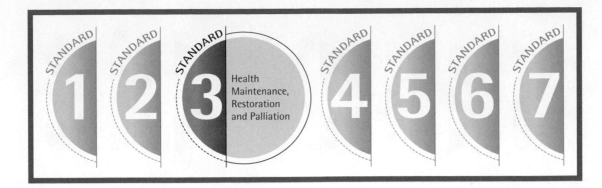

communicable disease response and outbreak management, and education.

i. Engages in collaborative, interdisciplinary and intersectoral partnerships to address health risks of the individual, family, group, community, population or system recognizing that some individuals and groups are disproportionately affected.

j. Collaborates to develop and use follow-up systems to facilitate continuity of care.

k. Practices in accordance with legislation and regulation relevant to community health practice (e.g. public health legislation, child protection legislation and provincial/territorial/federal regulatory frameworks). In addition, when relevant, practices in accordance with complementary sub specialty standards e.g. occupational health nursing; parish nursing.

l. Evaluates practice (personal, team, intersectoral and interprofessional collaborative practice) in achieving outcomes such as reduced communicable disease, injury, chronic disease or impacts of a disease process.

## Standard 3: Health Maintenance, Restoration and Palliation

Community health nurses integrate health maintenance, restoration and palliation into their practice. These are systematic and planned methods to maintain maximum function, improve health and support life transitions including acute, chronic or terminal illness and end of life care.

### The Community Health Nurse. . .

a. Assesses the health status and functional competence of the individual, family, group, community, population or system within the context of their environmental and social supports.

b. Develops mutually agreed upon plans and priorities for care with the individual, family, group, community, population or system.

c. Identifies a range of strategies including health promotion, health teaching, disease prevention and direct clinical care strategies along with short and long-term goals and outcomes.

d. Maximizes the ability of an individual, family, group, community, population or system to take responsibility for and manage their health needs according to resources and personal skills available.

e. Supports informed decision making; acknowledges diversity, unique characteristics and abilities; and respects the individual, family, group, community or population's specific requests.

f. Adapts community health nursing techniques, approaches and procedures to health challenges and the challenges related to equity in health in a particular community situation or setting.

g. Uses knowledge of the community to link with and refer to community resources or develop appropriate community resources as needed.

h. Facilitates maintenance of health and the healing process for the individual, family, group, community, population or system in response to significant health emergencies or other community situations that negatively impact health.

i. Evaluates outcomes systematically and continuously in collaboration with the individual, family, group, community, population or system including other health practitioners and inter-sectoral partners.

## Standard 4: Professional Relationships

Community health nurses connect with others to establish, build and nurture professional relationships. These relationships promote maximum participation and self determination of the individual, family, group, community or population.

### The Community Health Nurse. . .

a. Builds a network of relationships and partnerships with a wide variety of individuals, families, groups, communities, organizations and systems (e.g. community and volunteer service organizations, businesses, faith communities and with health professionals and other sectors) to address health-related issues and support health equity.

b. Uses a holistic and comprehensive mix of community and population based strategies such as coalition building, inter-sectoral collaboration, partnerships and networking to overcome health inequities.

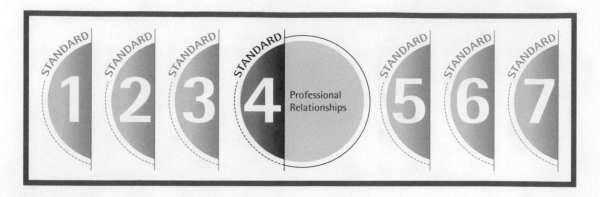

c. Assesses individual, family, groups, community and system beliefs, attitudes, feelings and values about health and health inequities and their potential effect on the relationship and intervention.

d. Recognizes her or his personal beliefs, attitudes, assumptions, feelings and values about health and their potential effect on interventions/strategies.

e. Is aware of and uses culturally relevant communication strategies when building relationships. Communication may be verbal or non-verbal, written or graphic. It may involve face-to-face, telephone, group, print or electronic methods.

f. Respects, trusts and supports or facilitates the ability of the individual, family, group, community, population or system to identify, solve and improve their own health issues.

g. Involves the individual, family, group, community, population or system as an active partner, applying community development principles, to identify relevant needs, perspectives and expectations.

h. Recognizes and promotes the development of health enhancing social support networks as an important determinant of health.

i. Maintains awareness of community resources, values and characteristics.

j. Promotes and supports linkages with appropriate community resources when the individual, family, group, community, population or system is ready to receive them (e.g., hospice or palliative care, parenting groups).

k. Maintains professional boundaries in long-term relationships in the home or other community settings where professional and social relationships may become blurred.

l. Negotiates an end to the relationship, in a professional manner, when appropriate (i.e., when the client demonstrates readiness and assumes self-care, when the goals for the relationship have been achieved, or based on the direction of the organization/employer).

m. Evaluates the nurse/client relationship as part of regular practice assessment.

## Standard 5: Capacity Building

Community health nurses build individual and community capacity by actively involving and collaborating with individuals, families, groups, organizations, populations communities and systems. The focus is to build on strengths and increase skills, knowledge and willingness to take action in the present and in the future.

### The Community Health Nurse. . .

a. Works collaboratively with the individual, family, group, community, population or system (including other health care providers) to identify needs, strength, available resources and strategies for action.

b. Uses community development principles and facilitates action to support the priorities of the *Jakarta Declaration* (See Figure 4)

c. Engages the individual, family, group, community, population or system in a consultative process from a foundation of equity and social justice.

d. Recognizes and builds on the readiness of the individual, family, group, community or system to participate and act.

e. Uses empowering strategies such as mutual goal setting, visioning and facilitation.

f. Understands group dynamics and effectively uses facilitation skills to support group development.

g. Helps the individual, family, group, community or system to participate in issue resolution to address their determinants of health.

h. Helps groups and communities to gather available resources that support taking action to address their health issues.

i. Actively shares knowledge with other professionals and community partners and appreciates the importance of collaborative team work.

The Jakarta Declaration identified the following priorities;
1. Promote social responsibility for health
2. Increase investments for health development
3. Consolidate and expand partnerships for health
4. Increase community capacity and empower the individual
5. Secure an infrastructure for health promotion.

**FIGURE    4    The Jakarta Declaration**[xv]

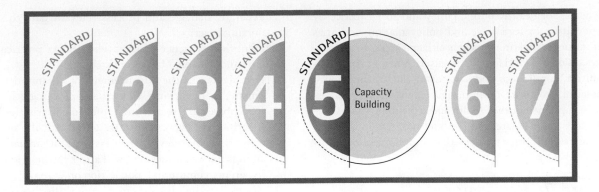

j. Supports the individual, family, group, community, and population to advocate for themselves.

k. Encourages lifestyle choices that support health.

l. Applies principles of social justice and advocates for those who are not yet able to take action for themselves.

m. Uses a comprehensive mix of strategies to address unique needs and to build individual, family, group, community, population or system capacity.

n. Supports community action to influence policy change in support of health.

o. Actively works with community partners including health professionals to build capacity for health promotion.

p. Evaluates the impact of change on the health outcomes of the individual, family, group, community, population or system.

## Standard 6: Access and Equity

**Community health nurses facilitate access and equity by working to make sure that resources and services are equitably distributed throughout the population and reach the people who most need them.**

### The Community Health Nurse...

a. Assesses and understands the capacity of the individual, family, group, community, population or system.

b. Assesses, in collaboration with partners, the norms, values, beliefs, knowledge, resources and power structures of the client (individual, family, group, community, population or system).

c. Identifies and facilitates universal and equitable access to available services.

d. Collaborates with colleagues and with other members of the health care team and community partners to promote effective working relationships that contribute to comprehensive client care and optimal client care outcomes.

e. Collaborates with individuals, families, groups, communities, populations or systems to identify and provide programs and methods of delivery that are acceptable to them and responsive to their needs across the life span.

f. Provides culturally sensitive care in diverse communities and settings.

g. Supports the individual, family, group, community and population's right to choose alternate health care options.

h. Advocates for equitable access to health and other services and equitable resource allocation.

i. Mobilizes resources to support health by coordinating and planning care, services, programs and policies.

j. Refers, coordinates or facilitates access to services in the health sector and other sectors.

k. Adapts practice in response to the changing health needs of the individual, family, group, community, population or system.

l. Uses strategies such as home visits, outreach and case finding to overcome inequities and facilitate access to services and health-supporting conditions for potentially vulnerable populations (e.g., persons who are ill, elderly, young, poor, immigrants, isolated or have communication barriers).

m. Analyzes and addresses the impact of the determinants of health on the opportunities for health for individuals, families, groups, communities, populations and systems.

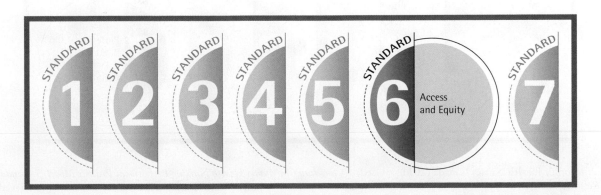

n. Advocates for healthy public policy and social justice by participating in legislative and policy-making activities that influence determinants of health and access to services.

o. Takes action with and for individuals, families, groups, communities, populations and systems at the organizational, municipal, provincial, territorial and federal levels to address service gaps, inequities in health and accessibility issues.

p. Monitors and evaluates changes and progress in access to relevant community services that support the determinants of health.

## Standard 7: Professional Responsibility and Accountability

**Community health nurses demonstrate responsibility and accountability as a fundamental component of their professional and autonomous practice.**

### The Community Health Nurse...

a. Assesses and identifies risk management issues and takes preventive or corrective action individually or in partnership to protect individuals, families, groups, communities, **populations, and organizations from unsafe,** unethical, illegal or socially unacceptable circumstances.

b. Identifies ethical dilemmas about whether responsibility for issues lie with the individual, family, group, community, population, or system or with the nurse or the nurse's employer.

c. Makes decisions using ethical standards and principles, taking into consideration one individual's rights over the rights of another, individual or societal good, allocation of scarce resources, and quantity versus quality of life.

d. Seeks help with problem solving, as needed, to determine the best course of action when responding to ethical dilemmas, risks to human rights and freedoms, new situations and new knowledge.

e. Provides leadership by creating change within communities and systems.

f. Advocates for societal change to support health for all based on the concepts of health equity and social justice.

g. Uses current evidence and informatics (including information and communication technology) to identify, generate, manage and process relevant data to support nursing practice.

h. Identifies and acts on factors which affect practice autonomy and delivery of quality care.

i. Participates in the advancement of community health nursing by mentoring students and new practitioners.

j. Participates in research and professional activities.

k. Identifies and works proactively (individually or by participating in relevant professional organizations) to address nursing issues that will affect the individual, family, group, community, population or system.

l. Appreciates and develops teamwork skills that contribute proactively to the quality of the work environment by identifying needs, issues and solutions, using conflict resolution skills and collaborative decision making.

m. Provides constructive feedback to peers as needed to enhance community health nursing practice.

n. Documents community health nursing activities in a timely and thorough manner (includes telephone advice and work with individuals, families, groups, communities, populations and systems).

o. Advocates for effective and efficient use of community health nursing resources.

p. Uses reflective practice to continually assess and improve personal community health nursing practice.

q. Seeks professional development experiences that are consistent with: current community health nursing practice; new and emerging issues; the changing needs of the population; the evolving knowledge of the impact of inequities or social injustices; determinants of health; and emerging research.

r. Acts on legal obligations (applicable provincial / territorial / federal legislation) to report to relevant authorities any situations involving unsafe or unethical care. This care may be provided by family, friends or other individuals and involve or be directed toward children or vulnerable adults.

s. Identifies desired outcomes and related indicators in collaboration with individuals, families, groups, communities, populations, systems or the workplace.

t. Uses available resources to systematically evaluate the achievement of desired outcomes including the availability, acceptability, efficiency, and effectiveness for quality improvement in community health nursing practice and the work environment.

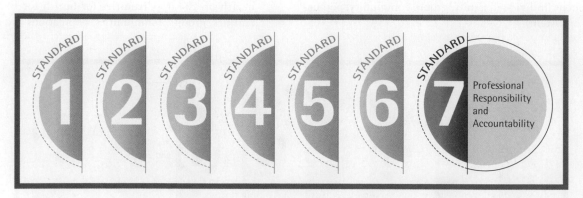

*Source:* Community Health Nurses Canada (2011, revised) – *Canadian Community Health Nursing Professional Practice Model & Standards of Practice Revised March* 2011 (pp. 7–23; 33–35). Used by permission of Community Health Nurses Association of Canada. Retrieved from https://www.chnc.ca/documents/CHNC-ProfessionalPracticeModel-EN/index.html#/1/

# Appendix B: Public Health Nursing Discipline Specific Competencies

Public Health Nursing Competencies are the integrated knowledge, skills, judgement and attributes required of a public health nurse to practice safely and ethically. Attributes include, but are not limited to attitudes, values and beliefs. (Canadian Nurses Association Code of Ethics, 2008)

## 1. PUBLIC HEALTH AND NURSING SCIENCES

This category includes key knowledge and critical thinking skills related to: the public health sciences (behavioural and social sciences, biostatistics, epidemiology, environmental public health, demography, workplace health, prevention of chronic diseases, infectious diseases, psychosocial problems and injuries) as well as nursing theory, change theory, economics, politics, public health administration, community assessment, management theory, program planning and evaluation, population health principles, community development theory, and the history of public health. Competency in this category requires the ability to apply knowledge in practice.

*A public health nurse is able to . . .*
1.1 Apply knowledge about the following concepts: the health status of populations; inequities in health; the determinants of health and illness; social justice; principles of primary health care; strategies for health promotion; disease and injury prevention; health protection, as well as the factors that influence the delivery and use of health services.
1.2 Apply knowledge about the history, structure and interaction of public health and health care services at local, provincial/territorial, national, and international levels.
1.3 Apply public health and nursing sciences to practice and synthesize knowledge from a broad range of theories, models and frameworks.
1.4 Critically appraise knowledge gathered from a variety of sources.
1.5 Use evidence and research to inform health policies, programs and practice:
  ■ contribute to the development and generation of evidence-based nursing
  ■ use available resources to systematically plan and evaluate public health nursing practice
1.6 Pursue lifelong learning opportunities in the field of public health that are consistent with: current public health nursing practice; new and emerging issues; the changing

needs of individuals, families, groups and communities; emerging research and evolving information about the impact of the determinants of health.
1.7 Integrate multiple ways of knowing into practice.

## 2. ASSESSMENT AND ANALYSIS

This category describes the core competencies needed to collect, assess, analyze and apply information (including data, facts, concepts and theories). These competencies are required to make evidence-based decisions, prepare budgets and reports, conduct investigations and make recommendations for policy and program development. Community members are involved in identifying and reinforcing those aspects of everyday life, culture and political activity that are conducive to health.

*A public health nurse is able to . . .*
2.1 Recognize that a health concern or issue exists:
  ■ apply principles of epidemiology
  ■ conduct comprehensive community assessments with individuals, families, groups and communities using quantitative and qualitative strategies
  ■ recognize patterns and trends in epidemiological data and service delivery
  ■ assess the impact of the broad social, cultural, political and economic determinants of health.
2.2 Identify relevant and appropriate sources of information, including community assets, resources and values in collaboration with individuals, families, groups, communities and stakeholders.
2.3 Collect, store, retrieve and use accurate and appropriate information on public health issues.
2.4 Analyze information to determine appropriate implications, uses, gaps and limitations.
2.5 Assess impact of specific issues on health such as political climate and will; values and culture; social and systemic structures; settings; as well as the individual, family, group, and community's readiness and capacity.
2.6 Assess the health status and functional competence of individuals, families, groups, communities or populations within the context of their environmental and social supports.
2.7 Determine the meaning of information, considering the ethical, political, scientific, socio-cultural and economic contexts:
  ■ identify attitudes, beliefs, feelings and values about health and their effect on relationships and interventions

- support individuals, families, groups and communities to identify risks to health and make informed choices about protective and preventive health measures
- describe the role of power in relationships by giving voice to the vulnerable
- demonstrate skill in dealing with diversity and high levels of ambiguity.

2.8 Recommend specific actions based on the analysis of information:

- identify a range of appropriate interventions including health promotion; health protection; disease and injury prevention and clinical care using a multi strategy and multi target approach
- identify short and long term goals
- identify outcome indicators
- identify research questions.

2.9 Recognize opportunities to promote social justice.

# 3. POLICY AND PROGRAM PLANNING, IMPLEMENTATION, AND EVALUATION

This category describes the core competencies needed to effectively choose options, and to plan, implement and evaluate policies and/or programs in public health. This includes the management of incidents such as outbreaks and emergencies.

## 3(A). Policy Development

*A public health nurse is able to . . .*

3A.1 Describe selected policy options to address a specific public health issue.

3A.2 Describe the implications of each policy option, especially as they apply to the determinants of health and recommend or decide on a course of action.

3A.3 Develop a plan to implement a course of action taking into account relevant evidence, legislation, emergency planning procedures, regulations and policies.

3A.4 Implement a policy.

3A.5 Support community action to influence policy change.

3A.6 Build community capacity to improve health and address health inequities.

3A.7 Advocate for healthy public policy and services that promote and protect the health and well-being of individuals, families, groups and communities.

3A.8 Advocate for the reduction of inequities in health through legislative and policy making activities.

## 3(B). Program Planning

*A public health nurse is able to . . .*

3B.1 Describe selected program options to address a specific public health issue.

3B.2 Describe the implications of each option, especially as they apply to the determinants of health and recommend or decide on a course of action.

3B.3 Develop a plan in collaboration with individuals, families, groups and communities to implement a course of action that is responsive to needs taking into account relevant evidence, legislation, emergency planning procedures, regulations and policies.

## 3(C). Implementation and Intervention

*A public health nurse is able to . . .*

3C.1 Take action, across multiple levels, to address specific public health issues by using a comprehensive mix of public health strategies to address unique needs and to build individual, family, group and community capacity.

3C.2 Facilitate planned change with individuals, families, groups, communities, systems or population(s) by applying the Population Health Promotion Model, primary health care principles and appropriate change theory.

3C.3 Demonstrate the ability to integrate relevant research and implement evidence informed practice.

3C.4 Participate in collaborative, interdisciplinary and intersectoral partnerships to enhance the health of individuals, families, groups, communities and populations.

3C.5 Maximize the capacity of the individual, family, group or community to take responsibility for and to manage their health needs according to resources available and personal skills.

3C.6 Set and follow priorities and maximize outcomes based on available resources.

3C.7 Fulfill functional roles in response to a public health emergency.

3C.8 Facilitate access to services in the health sector and other sectors.

3C.9 Adapt practice in response to the changing health needs of the individual, family, group and community and in response to the unique characteristics of the setting.

3C.10 Take action to protect individuals, families, groups and communities from unsafe or unethical circumstances.

3C.11 Advocate in collaboration with, and on behalf of, and with individuals, families, groups and communities on social justice related issues.

## 3(D). Evaluation

*A public health nurse is able to . . .*

3D.1 Evaluate an action, policy or program in a systematic and continuous manner by measuring its effect on individuals, families, groups or communities.

3D.2 Evaluate programs in relation to determinants of health and health outcomes.

3D.3 Evaluate programs in partnership with individuals, families, groups, communities and other stakeholders.

# 4. PARTNERSHIPS, COLLABORATION, AND ADVOCACY

This category captures the competencies required to influence and work with others to improve the health and well-being of the public through the pursuit of a common goal. This includes the concepts of: social justice, which is the fair distribution of society's benefits and responsibilities and their consequences (Canadian Nurses Association, Code of Ethics, 2008); partnership and collaboration, which is to optimize performance through shared resources and responsibilities; advocacy, which is to speak, write or act in favour of a particular cause, policy or group of people and aims to reduce inequities in health status or access to health services.

*A public health nurse is able to . . .*

4.1 Advocate for societal change in support of health for all:
  - collaborate with partners to address public health issues and service gaps in order to achieve improved health outcomes
  - build coalitions, intersectoral partnerships and networks
  - facilitate the change process to impact the determinants of health and improve health outcomes.
4.2 Use skills such as team building, negotiation, conflict management and group facilitation to build partnerships and to support group development.
4.3 Mediate between differing interests in the pursuit of health and well-being, and advocate for appropriate resource allocation and equitable access to resources.
4.4 Advocate for healthy public policies and services that promote and protect the health and well-being of individuals and communities.
4.5 Involve individuals, families, groups and communities as active partners to identify assets, strengths and available resources and to take action to address health inequities, needs, deficits and gaps.

# 5. DIVERSITY AND INCLUSIVENESS

This category identifies the competencies required to interact effectively with diverse individuals, families, groups and communities in relation to others in society as well to recognize the root causes of disparities and what can be done to eliminate them (Canadian Nurses Association, Code of Ethics, 2008). It is the embodiment of attitudes and actions that result in inclusive behaviours, practices, programs and policies.

*A public health nurse is able to . . .*

5.1 Recognize how the determinants of health (biological, social, cultural, economic and physical) influence the health and well-being of specific population groups.
5.2 Address population diversity when planning, implementing, adapting and evaluating public health programs and policies.

5.3 Apply culturally-relevant and appropriate approaches with people from diverse cultural, socioeconomic and educational backgrounds, and persons of all ages, genders, health status, sexual orientations and abilities.

# 6. COMMUNICATION

Communication involves an interchange of ideas, opinions and information. This category addresses numerous dimensions of communication including internal and external exchanges; written, verbal, non-verbal and listening skills; computer literacy; providing appropriate information to different audiences; working with the media and social marketing techniques.

*A public health nurse is able to . . .*

6.1 Communicate effectively with individuals, families, groups, communities and colleagues:
  - use verbal, non-verbal and written or graphic communication skills
  - speak and write in plain language
  - use multi-sensory forms of communication to address unique communication styles
  - use culturally relevant communication when building relationships.
6.2 Interpret information for professional, nonprofessional and community audiences.
6.3 Mobilize individuals, families, groups and communities by using appropriate media, community resources and social marketing techniques.
6.4 Use current technology to communicate effectively.

# 7. LEADERSHIP

This category focuses on leadership competencies that build capacity, improve performance and enhance the quality of the working environment. They also enable organizations and communities to create, communicate and apply shared visions, missions and values.

*A public health nurse is able to . . .*

7.1 Describe the mission and priorities of the public health organization where one works, and apply them in practice.
7.2 Contribute to developing key values and a shared vision to assess, plan and implement public health programs and policies in the community by actively working with health professionals and in partnership with community partners to build capacity.
7.3 Use public health and nursing ethics to manage self, others, information and resources and practice in accordance with all relevant legislation, regulating body standards and codes (e.g., provincial health legislation, child welfare legislation, privacy legislation, Canadian Nurses Association Code of Ethics for registered nurses).
7.4 Contribute to team and organizational learning in order to advance public health goals.

7.5 Contribute to the maintenance of organizational performance standards.

7.6 Demonstrate an ability to build capacity by sharing knowledge, tools, expertise and experience:
  - participate in professional development and practice development activities
  - mentor students and orient new staff
  - participate in research and quality assurance initiatives.

# 8. PROFESSIONAL RESPONSIBILITY AND ACCOUNTABILITY

This category addresses a number of dimensions including the recognition that nurses are accountable for their actions and are responsible for making sure they have the required knowledge and skills needed to ensure the delivery of safe, compassionate, competent and ethical care. It includes the competencies required to maintain quality work environments and relationships needed in a professional practice. Public Health nurses are responsible for initiating strategies that will address the determinants of health and generate a positive impact on people and systems. They are accountable to a variety of authorities and stakeholders as well as to the individual and community they serve. This range of accountabilities places them in a variety of situations with unique ethical dilemmas.

*A public health nurse is able to . . .*

8.1 Demonstrate professionalism in independent practice in multiple settings with multiple stakeholders.

8.2 Apply ethical standards and principles taking into consideration appropriate public health and nursing ethics.

8.3 Consult as needed to determine the best course of action in response to: ethical dilemmas, safety issues, risks to human rights and freedoms, new situations and new knowledge.

8.4 Use reflective practice to continually assess and improve practice:
  - examine practice in relation to personal and individual, family, group or community attributes, existing knowledge and context
  - adapt public health nursing techniques, approaches and procedures to the challenges in a particular community situation or setting.

8.5 Advocate for effective, efficient and responsible use of resources.

8.6 Act upon legal and professional obligations, and practices in accordance with relevant legislation.

8.7 Contribute to the quality of public health nursing work environments by identifying needs, issues, solutions and mobilizing colleagues by actively participating in team and organizational structures and mechanisms.

*Source:* Community Health Nurses of Canada (2009). *Public Health Nursing Discipline Specific Competencies Version 1.0* (pp. 2–10). Reproduced by permission of Community Health Nurses Association of Canada. Retrieved from http://www.chnc.ca/members/documents/PHNCompetenciesPrintReadyFinalEnglish.pdf

# Appendix C: Home Health Nursing Competencies

## 1. ELEMENTS OF HOME HEALTH NURSING

These elements and associated competencies focus on the nursing activities, functions, goals and outcomes that are central to home health nursing practice.

## a. Assessment, Monitoring and Clinical Decision Making

*The home health nurse is able to . . .*

  i. conduct comprehensive autonomous and/or collaborative health assessments to determine the health status, functional and psychosocial needs and competence of clients and their families within the context of their environment and social supports
 ii. apply critical thinking skills and creative problem-solving analysis when making clinical decisions
iii. analyze information to determine appropriate nursing actions, implications, applications, gaps and limitations
 iv. collaborate with health care team members and others who are involved with the client, to determine appropriateness and availability of required services
  v. incorporate a combination of basic and advanced knowledge of health and nursing across the lifespan and the health-illness continuum
 vi. keep knowledge current and use evidence to inform practice to ensure optimal case management
vii. assess the safety of the home environment with the goal of optimizing client safety and taking actions to support a safe work environment for all members of the home health care team

## b. Care Planning and Care Coordination

*The home health nurse is able to . . .*

  i. plan and prioritize visits to meet the health and scheduling needs of clients
 ii. use the nursing process to collaboratively develop, coordinate and implement mutually agreed upon care plans, negotiating priorities in care with clear treatment and outcome goals and supporting client navigation and transition through the continuum of care
iii. support clients and families to build on their strengths to attain or maintain a desired health status within available resources

 iv. anticipate the need for alternative ways of providing services and use creative problem solving skills to overcome obstacles in delivery of client care, i.e., weather, lack of resources, etc.
  v. ensure discharge planning is integrated within the care plan and occurs in collaboration with the client, family, health care team and community
 vi. promote an integrated assessment and develop a unified care and treatment plan that is collaboratively carried out by team members to maximize continuity of care within a client-centered approach
vii. appreciate and understand the roles and responsibilities and the contributions of other regulated and unregulated health workers involved in the client care plan
viii. facilitate and coordinate access to other members of the multidisciplinary team such as primary care providers, specialist physician, community pharmacist, nurses, and other allied health professionals to address a specific health issue
 ix. collaboratively evaluate care plan interventions through reassessment and ongoing evaluation of results and adapt them to the changing conditions of the client and the client's family

## c. Health Maintenance, Restoration and Palliation

*The home health nurse is able to . . .*

  i. assist clients and families to maintain and/or restore health by using a comprehensive mix of strategies to address their health needs across the life span and illness continuum
 ii. understand and/or educate clients, their families/caregivers and colleagues in the safe and appropriate use and maintenance of various types of equipment, technology and treatments to maintain health and assist clients and families to integrate them into their everyday life/routine
iii. communicate effectively with clients and families while supporting them through the decision making process about end of life issues
 iv. use basic and advanced nursing skills to perform and adapt complex procedures in the home health setting
  v. recognize when specialized counselling beyond the scope of nursing is required and facilitate an appropriate referral
 vi. respond to the ever-changing and evolving health care needs of the client and family by strategically revising interventions and therapies
vii. self-identify the need for assistance when not familiar with care requirements and seek support to assure continued excellence in care

## d. Teaching and Education

*The home health nurse is able to . . .*

i. assess the knowledge, attitudes, level of motivation, values, beliefs, behaviours, practices, stage of change, and skills of the client/family

ii. consider and integrate into educational planning the factors that may impact the client/family's ability to learn. For example: environment, readiness, willingness, literacy level, educational background, socioeconomic situation, health status, etc.

iii. interpret and explain complex information for clients and families

iv. apply appropriate learning principles, teaching methods and educational theories to educational activities

v. include family, volunteers and caregivers in teaching and education

vi. evaluate the effectiveness of health education interventions

## e. Communication

*The home health nurse is able to . . .*

i. use effective listening, verbal and non-verbal communication skills to understand the client's perspective and be understood by the client, family and other caregivers involved in the care

ii. use effective interviewing skills and strategies to engage in constructive dialogue with clients and their families

iii. use effective communication skills to engage, connect, appreciate, respond, empathize and support the empowerment of others

iv. identify and use strategies to overcome language and communication barriers

v. maintain a focused approach amidst multiple distractions within the home environment

vi. employ negotiation and conflict management skills

vii. use techniques that are client-centered, client-driven, and strength-based when counselling clients

viii. use documentation as an effective communication tool

ix. use technology to effectively communicate and manage client care in a confidential manner

## f. Relationships

*The home health nurse is able to . . .*

i. optimize the health of the client and caregiver(s) by establishing and maintaining a therapeutic nurse–client relationship based on mutual trust, respect, caring, and listening within the context of being "a guest in the house"

ii. acknowledge the contribution that the family/caregiver provides to client health in a way that makes them feel valued and respected and support them to maintain relationships that support effective care

iii. work effectively and non-judgementally in a wide range of environments with varying conditions of cleanliness

iv. use skills such as team building, negotiation, conflict management and group facilitation to build and sustain partnerships

v. involve clients and families as active partners to identify assets, strengths and available resources

## g. Access and Equity

*The home health nurse is able to . . .*

i. advocate for healthy public policies and accessible, inclusive and integrated services that promote and protect the health and well-being of all individuals and communities

ii. apply culturally-relevant and appropriate approaches with people of diverse cultural, socioeconomic and educational backgrounds, and persons of all ages, genders, health status, sexual orientations and abilities

iii. recognize opportunities to promote social justice and advocate in collaboration with, and on behalf of clients and families on related issues to give voice to the vulnerable

iv. optimize allocation of human, financial, and infrastructure resources in order to provide a safe and accessible health delivery system

v. advocate for the reduction of inequities in health by participating in legislative and policy making activities

## h. Building Capacity

*The home health nurse is able to . . .*

i. mobilize clients, families and others to take action to address health needs, deficits and gaps accessing and using available resources

ii. assist the client and their family to recognize their capacity for managing their own health needs according to available resources

iii. assist colleagues, partners and/or clients to support and build on the capacities that are inherent in the individual, families and the communities to influence policy change

iv. demonstrate cultural competency when addressing client care issues and when working in an environment where there may be levels of ambiguity

v. adapt and be flexible and responsive to the changing health needs of the client and family

## 2. FOUNDATIONS OF HOME HEALTH NURSING

These competencies focus on the core knowledge and primary health care philosophy that is central to home health nursing practice.

## a. Health Promotion

*The home health nurse is able to . . .*

i. facilitate planned change with clients and families by applying and incorporating health promotion theory, primary health care principles and change theory into practice

ii. recognize how the determinants of health influence the health and well-being of clients and families

iii. assess the impact specific issues may have on the client's health such as political climate; priorities, values and culture; social and systemic structures and settings

iv. assess the readiness and capacity of the client and family to make changes to promote their health

## b. Illness Prevention and Health Protection

*The home health nurse is able to . . .*

i. apply nursing sciences to practice and evaluate, synthesize and apply knowledge from a broad range of theories, models, frameworks and practice

ii. use critical thinking to consider the ethical, political, scientific, socio-cultural and economic contexts to determine the meaning of information related to client health care needs

iii. support clients and families to identify risks to health and make informed choices about protective and preventive health measures

iv. take action to protect clients, families and groups from unsafe or unethical circumstances

v. participate in collaborative, interdisciplinary and intersectoral partnerships to enhance the health of clients and families

## 3. QUALITY AND PROFESSIONAL RESPONSIBILITY

These competencies focus on practice activities and/or strategies by which the home health nurse promotes quality of care and demonstrates professional responsibility.

## a. Quality Care

*The home health nurse is able to . . .*

i. initiate, lead and participate in risk management and quality improvement activities to measure effectiveness of services, cost implications and processes

ii. initiate and participate in critical incident reviews

iii. evaluate nursing interventions in a systematic and continuous manner by measuring their effect on clients and families

iv. evaluate programs in relation to determinants of health and health outcomes

v. contribute to the quality of work environments by identifying needs, issues, solutions and actively participating in team and organizational quality improvement processes

vi. understand the financial aspects of care and be accountable for effective, efficient and responsible use of time and resources when delivering care to clients and families

## b. Professional Responsibility

*The home health nurse is able to . . .*

i. demonstrate professionalism, leadership, judgement and accountability in independent practice in multiple settings with multiple stakeholders

ii. practice independently and autonomously providing client centered services in a wide variety of settings where nursing care and services are needed

iii. use reflective practice to continually assess and improve practice

iv. integrate multiple ways of knowing into practice

v. contribute to the development and generation of evidence-informed nursing practice

vi. pursue lifelong learning opportunities to support professional practice

vii. use nursing ethics, ethical standards and principles and self-awareness to manage self and practice in accordance with all relevant legislation, regulatory body standards, codes and organizational policies

viii. describe the mission, values and priorities of the health organization where one works

ix. participate in the advancement of home health nursing by mentoring students and new practitioners

x. recognize and understand that one's attitudes, beliefs, feelings and values about health can have an effect on relationships and interventions

*Source:* Community Health Nurses of Canada (2010). *Home Health Nursing Competencies Version 1.0 March 2010.* (pp. 3–9). Reproduced by permission of Community Health Nurses Association of Canada. Retrieved from https://chnc.ca/documents/ HHNursingCompetenciesFINALEnglish.pdf

# Index

Note: Page numbers followed by *f* or *t* represent figures or tables respectively.